Mosby's COMPREHENSIVE REVIEW OF
Practical Nursing
For NCLEX-PN

Mosby's COMPREHENSIVE REVIEW OF Practical Nursing

For NCLEX-PN

Editor

Mary O. Eyles, PhD, RN

Director, Education
Kessler Medical Rehabilitation Research and
Education Corporation (KMRREC)
West Orange, New Jersey

Associate, Department of Physical Medicine
and Rehabilitation
University of Medicine and Dentistry of New Jersey
New Jersey Medical School
Newark, New Jersey

(formerly) Director of Continuing Education
National Association for Practical Nurse
Education and Service, Inc. (NAPNES)

13th EDITION

with 88 illustrations

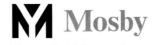 Mosby

A Harcourt Health Sciences Company
St. Louis   London   Philadelphia   Sydney   Toronto

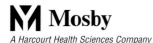

A Harcourt Health Sciences Company

Vice President, Nursing Editorial Director: Sally Schrefer
Senior Editor: Loren Wilson
Developmental Editor: Nancy L. O'Brien
Project Manager: Deborah L. Vogel
Project Specialist: Ann E. Rogers
Book Design Manager: Bill Drone
Cover Designer: Teresa Breckwoldt

THIRTEENTH EDITION

NCLEX-PN is a registered trademark of the National Council of State Boards of Nursing, Inc.

Mosby, Inc.
A Harcourt Health Sciences Company
11830 Westline Industrial Drive
St. Louis, Missouri 63146

Printed in the United States of America.

Library of Congress Cataloging in Publication Data
Mosby's comprehensive review of practical nursing—13th ed./editor, Mary O. Eyles.
    p.; cm.
  Includes bibliographical references and index.
  ISBN 0-323-01166-7
  1. Practical nursing—Outlines, syllabi, etc.   2. Practical nursing—Examinations,
  questions, etc.   I. Title: Comprehensive review of practical nursing.   II. Eyles, Mary O.
  [DNLM: 1. Nursing, Practical—Examination Questions.   2. Nursing,
  Practical—Outlines. WY 18.2M8938 2000]
  RT62.M62 2000
  610.73'076—dc21

                                                                00-055398

01 02 03 04 CL/KPT 9 8 7 6 5 4 3 2

This text is dedicated to all individuals and organizations involved in the profession of practical/vocational nursing for their knowledge, skills, and abilities in promoting and providing excellence in patient care within the United States and Canada.

CONTRIBUTING AUTHORS

Sandra G. Brewer, BA, RN
Coordinator/Professor–Nursing
Georgian College of Applied Arts and Technology
Owen Sound, Ontario, Canada
Canadian Content for Chapter 1 and Chapter 2

Kathy K. Clark, MSN, RN, CPN
Director of Quality Improvement and Education
CareMed Chicago Home Health Agency
Chicago, Illinois
Chapter 8, Pediatric Nursing

Mary O. Eyles, PhD, RN
Director, Education
Kessler Medical Rehabilitation Research and Education
    Corporation (KMRREC)
West Orange, New Jersey
*Chapter 1, Introduction for Students Preparing for the Licensure
    Examination*

Patricia M. Jacobson, MSN, BSN, RN
Nursing Instructor
Bullard Havens RVTS
Bridgeport, Connecticut
Chapter 3, Pharmacology
Chapter 7, Maternity Nursing

Sharon Laney, MSN, RN
Coordinator, School of Practical Nursing
Indiana County Technology Center
Indiana, Pennsylvania
Chapter 2, Review of the Basics
Chapter 4, Nutrition
Chapter 5, Medical-Surgical Nursing
Chapter 9, Nursing Care of the Aging Adult

Kim Inman Smith, MSN, MA, BSN, RN
Instructor, Practical Nursing Program
Shelton State Community College
Tuscaloosa, Alabama
Chapter 6, Mental Health Nursing

Russlyn St. John, MSN, RN
Practical Nursing Coordinator
St. Charles County Community College
St. Peters, Missouri
Chapter 10, Emergency Nursing

Rose Wilcox, MEd, BSN, RN
(formerly) Teacher Coordinator
School of Practical Nursing
Columbus Public Schools
Columbus, Ohio
Chapter 5, Medical-Surgical Nursing

CONTRIBUTING ITEM WRITERS

Karen Danielson, BSN, RN
Assistant Professor
North Central State College
Mansfield, Ohio

Lajuana B. Jordan, MSN, BSN, RN
Assistant Professor/Program Director
Danville Community College
Danville, Virginia

Joyce Martin, MS, BSN, RN
Vocational Nursing Instructor
Tyler Junior College
Tyler, Texas

Dale R. Miller, BSN, RN, CCRN
Practical Nursing Instructor
Coosa Valley Technical Institute
Rome, Georgia

Deborah Toth, MSN, BSN, RN
Director of Allied Health
EHOVE Career Center
Milan, Ohio

Vera Webster, MS, BSN, RN
Practical Nursing Instructor
Kaw Area Technical School
Topeka, Kansas

REVIEWERS

Sally Flesch, PhD, EdS, MA, BSN, RN
Professor and Department Chair
Black Hawk College
Moline, Illinois

Barbara Jorenby, MA, BSN, RN
Nursing Instructor
Dakota County Technical College
Rosemount, Minnesota

Linda L. Kerby, MA, BSN, BA, RN
Educational Consultant
Leawood, Kansas

Carla Lehman, BSN, RN
Nursing Instructor
Hutchinson Community College
McPherson, Kansas

Nola Ormrod, MSN, RN
Nursing Director and Associate Professor
Centralia College
Centralia, Washington

Joann E. Potts Peuterbaugh, MSN, RN
LPN Coordinator
Alton School District
Alton, Illinois

Shirley Stamford, BSN, RN
Nursing Instructor
Hillsborough County School of Practical Nursing
Tampa, Florida

Carol A. Storm, MSN, BSN, BA, RN, CS
Director, B.M. Spurr School of Practical Nursing
Reynolds Memorial Hospital
Glen Dale, West Virginia

Yvonne VanDyke, MSN, BSN, RN
Program Coordinator
Austin Community College
Austin, Texas

Kathleen N. Young, BSN, RN
Practical Nursing Instructor
Greater Altoona Career Technology Center
Altoona, Pennsylvania

Mosby's Comprehensive Review of Practical Nursing for NCLEX-PN has been developed to provide individuals preparing for entry or reentry into nursing at the practical/vocational nurse level with a dependable source of information as they prepare to become valued members of today's health care team. The most current, up-to-date developments in health care and in the field of practical/vocational nursing are incorporated in the text as each contributor has recently been or is currently active in practical/vocational nursing education.

In this thirteenth edition of *Mosby's Comprehensive Review of Practical Nursing for NCLEX-PN,* the basic practical/vocational nursing curriculum is addressed, from concepts basic to all levels of nursing to the complexities of specialty areas, while incorporating the nursing process throughout. This text also refers to the 1999-2000 approved listing of NANDA nursing diagnoses (see Appendix A for a complete listing). Although the LP/VN is not solely responsible for the formulation of a nursing diagnosis, the practical nurse does assist the registered professional nurse by collecting data essential to formulating a nursing diagnosis.

The text contains ten chapters: Chapter 1 is an introduction to the use of the text and its contents, while offering ways in which one can improve test-taking skills; Chapter 2 covers basic skills, fundamental nursing concepts of the practical/vocational nurse curriculum, and today's trends in nursing and health care in the United States and Canada; Chapters 3 and 4 cover Pharmacology and Nutrition for complete coverage of content found in the NCLEX-PN exam. Chapters 5 through 10 cover the more complex nursing concepts encountered in the various specialty areas of nursing, such as medical-surgical nursing, obstetrics, pediatrics, mental health, gerontology, and emergency nursing.

The thirteenth edition has been thoroughly revised and updated to reflect current nursing practice. Each chapter's content is organized in a concise outline format to enhance study, and is followed by review questions to help you determine how much you have learned in that particular subject area before you advance to the next chapter. Answers and rationales for correct and incorrect answer options follow the review questions.

Two comprehensive exams are included at the end of the text, each containing 250 questions following the style of those on the National Council Licensure Examination for Practical Nurses (NCLEX-PN). The correct answer and rationales for both correct and incorrect answer options are also provided following each exam.

The thirteenth edition of *Mosby's Comprehensive Review of Practical Nursing for NCLEX-PN* has doubled the total number of practice questions available with this text. Along with the chapter review questions and the two comprehensive examinations, a CD-ROM containing 1,200 additional test items is packaged with this book. The questions on this CD-ROM are *not* repeated in the text. The CD-ROM provides both review and test modes of content-specific or comprehensive exams. To reinforce study and build confidence, it is suggested that students practice answering questions on a computer to simulate the NCLEX-PN computer adaptive test.

For the sake of clarity and consistency, the word *nurse* is used to indicate a practical/vocational nurse. The recipient of care is termed the *patient* to provide consistency as well, although we acknowledge that the term *client* may be preferred and has been used in some cases within this text.

The editor and contributors of this text have the utmost respect for and recognize the LP/VN as a valued member of today's health care team providing quality nursing care to patients nationwide. It is because of this respect and recognition that this text has been developed, with the hope that individuals preparing for entry or reentry into nursing at the practical/vocational nurse level will find a dependable source with which to prepare to become that valued member of today's health care team.

As coordinating editor, I would like to thank all of those individuals who have worked so diligently in the preparation of this text, that is, all the contributors and item writers, as well as all those at Mosby, especially Nancy O'Brien, without whom this text would not have been possible. I would also like to extend a special note of thanks to my husband, Robert, for being so supportive of our efforts during the revision of this text.

To those who will use this text, we wish the very best as you enter into a service that will offer you the greatest satisfaction of all: the satisfaction of extending caring and a helping hand, your hand, to those in need.

Welcome to the caring profession: *welcome to nursing.*

Mary O. Eyles, PhD, RN

CONTENTS

4 NUTRITION, 149

5 MEDICAL-SURGICAL NURSING, 181

6 MENTAL HEALTH NURSING, 353

7 MATERNITY NURSING, 389

8 PEDIATRIC NURSING, 449

COMPREHENSIVE EXAMINATIONS

ANSWERS AND RATIONALES FOR COMPREHENSIVE EXAMINATIONS

Mosby's COMPREHENSIVE REVIEW OF
Practical Nursing
For NCLEX-PN

CHAPTER 1

Introduction for Students Preparing for the Licensure Examination

The practice of nursing is regulated by law in each state, the District of Columbia, Guam, Puerto Rico, and the Virgin Islands for the express purpose of public protection. The state board of nursing in each of the above is charged with upholding the regulation of such law. To do so each state board requires that qualified individuals take a licensing examination prepared by the National Council of State Boards of Nursing (The National Council). Puerto Rico has developed its own licensing examination and does not use the one prepared by The National Council. However, content covered in its examination closely parallels that in the National Council Licensure Examination for Practical Nurses (NCLEX-PN). This book provides a valuable review tool regardless of the licensure examination taken. A special note appears at the end of the chapter for Canadian readers.

The NCLEX-PN covers all areas of the practical/vocational nursing curriculum and has been designed to test your nursing knowledge, including your ability to apply the principles of the knowledge to given clinical situations in a safe and effective manner. Periodic revision of the NCLEX-PN test plan can be expected because of the continually changing face of nursing. Nevertheless, such changes do not compromise your use of this text as you prepare for the licensing examination.

WHY REVIEW?

The purpose of this text is threefold: (1) to assist you in determining the extent of your nursing knowledge relative to your areas of specific strengths and weaknesses, (2) to increase your understanding of nursing knowledge through additional study, and (3) to increase your familiarity with and ability to respond to written test questions and corresponding clinical situations similar to those presented in the NCLEX-PN licensing examination.

The National Council's test plan for the NCLEX-PN consists of one essential content dimension, "client need." This serves to provide a structure that is universal in defining the skills and competencies necessary to provide safe and effective nursing care. The dimension of "client need" is therefore critical to ensure the final intent of the examination: to protect the public through safe practitioners. A more detailed description of the test plan, including the percentage of questions allocated to each category and subcategory of the client need dimension are provided in Box 1-1.

EFFECTIVE STUDY AND THE USE OF THIS TEXT

The key to effective study and the use of this text can be determined only by you. The review is presented in a manner that is easily adaptable to various forms of study habits, in addition to familiarizing you with timed tests/examinations.

Each chapter outlines a specific content area within the practical/vocational nurse curriculum, followed by a set of questions relative to that particular content area. The correct answers and the rationales for both the correct and the incorrect responses are found at the end of the chapter. Rationales are provided for all four answer choices for each question. The rationale for the correct answer is listed first, followed by the other rationales.

All questions have been classified by *cognitive level, nursing process, client need,* and *level of difficulty.* These classifications follow the question number in the Answers and Rationales portion of the chapter:

First classification or word = the *cognitive level* of the question

Knowledge, comprehension, application, or *analysis*

Second classification or word = the *phase of the nursing process*

Assessment, planning, implementation, or *evaluation*

Third classification or word(s) = one of the 10 *client need* subcategories

Coordinated care; safety and infection control; growth and development; prevention and early detection of disease; coping and adaptation; psychosocial adaptation; basic care and comfort; pharmacological therapies; reduction of risk potential; or *physiological adaptation*

(See Box 1-1 for a more detailed outline of *client need* categories and subcategories.)

Box 1-1 Test Plan for the National Council Licensure Examination for Practical/Vocational Nurses: Percentage of Items Relative to Each *Client Need* Subcategory in NCLEX-PN

Safe, Effective Care Environment
Coordinated Care (6%-12%)
Includes all collaborative efforts with other members of the health care team necessary to facilitate delivery of effective patient care

Safety and Infection Control (7%-13%)
Includes all means taken to protect patients and health care personnel from environmental hazards

Health Promotion and Maintenance
Growth and Development Through the Life Span (4%-10%)
Includes all efforts taken to assist the patient and their significant others in the normal expected stages of growth and development from conception through advanced old age

Prevention and Early Detection of Disease (4%-10%)
Includes efforts taken to provide patient care relative to prevention and early detection of health problems

Psychosocial Integrity
Coping and Adaptation (6%-12%)
Includes efforts taken to promote the patient's ability to cope, adapt, and/or problem solve situations related to illnesses or stressful events

Psychosocial Adaptation (4%-10%)
Includes all participatory efforts in providing care for patients with acute or chronic mental illness

Physiological Integrity
Basic Care and Comfort (10%-16%)
Includes all means to provide comfort and assistance in the performance of activities of daily living

Pharmacological Therapies (5%-11%)
Includes all means by which to provide care relative to the administration of medication and monitoring of patients receiving parental therapies

Reduction of Risk Potential (11%-17%)
Includes all measures taken to reduce the patient's potential for development of complications or health problems relative to treatments, procedures, or existing conditions

Physiological Adaptation (13%-19%)
Includes all participatory efforts taken to provide care to patients with acute, chronic, or life-threatening physical health conditions

Additional Considerations
Integrated throughout the test plan are additional concepts and processes that are essential to the safe and effective practice of entry-level practitioners. These are the *nursing process, care, communication, cultural awareness, documentation, self-care,* and *teaching/learning.* Entry-level scope of practice, relative to these integrated concepts and processes, is determined by the laws and statutes of each jurisdiction/state.

Modified from NCLEX-PN Test Plan for National Council Licensure Examination for Practical Nurses, 1998. Adapted with permission of the National Council of State Boards of Nursing, Chicago, Illinois.

Letters in parenthesis = the *difficulty of the question*

The letter (a) signifies that more than 75% of students should answer the question correctly.

The letter (b) signifies that between 50% and 75% of students should answer correctly.

The letter (c) signifies that between 25% and 50% of students should answer correctly.

You may want to start with the questions to determine areas in which you need more study and then return to review the outline of that particular chapter. Concentrate study efforts on those areas in which you scored low (i.e., less than 80% to 85% of the questions answered correctly). Should you need more in-depth study, you may refer to texts from the bibliography found at the end of each chapter, your own nursing texts, or current nursing journals.

Once you have completed the review and corresponding questions of all chapters, you are ready to take the two comprehensive examinations. Each comprehensive examination contains 125 questions and should take 2 hours to complete. Time yourself with your alarm clock or have someone else monitor your time.

In April 1994 the National Council began administering the NCLEX-PN examination via computerized adaptive testing (CAT), a change from the traditional paper-and-pencil method of testing. To use this text effectively in preparation for CAT, we suggest that you darken your answer choice on the chapter review questions and the comprehensive examination questions. Marking your answers in this manner permits you to focus all your concentration on answering the questions.

Computerized adaptive testing (CAT) allows candidates to take the examination at their own pace. There is no set minimum amount of time for the examination; however, there is a maximum time of 5 hours. In addition to the questions at the end of each chapter, this review book contains two examinations, each having two parts, simulating the NCLEX-PN examination content. Each part of the examinations contains 125 questions, which should be completed in 2 hours. Even though time may no longer be a major concern, becoming more proficient in time-management skills will be to your advantage during the actual examination. Proper use of this text not only increases your nursing knowledge but also increases your self-confidence in your test-taking abilities.

Remember, intelligence plays a vital role in your ability to learn. However, being "smart" involves more than just intelligence. Being practical and applying common sense are also part of the learning experience.

Regardless of how you choose to study, following simple study guides may be helpful:

1. Establish priorities and the goals by which to achieve those priorities.
2. Enhance organizational skills by developing a checklist and creating ways to improve your ability to retain information (e.g., index cards, which are easy to carry and review whenever you have a spare moment).
3. Enhance time-management abilities by designing a study schedule that best suits your needs, considering the following:
   - Amount of time needed
   - Amount of time available
   - "Best" time to study
   - Allowance for emergencies/free time
4. Prepare for study by considering the following:
   - An environment that will be conducive to learning
   - The appropriate study material
   - Planned study sessions alone or with friend/group
   - A formal review course

A note of warning: do not expect to achieve the maximum benefits of this text by cramming a few days before the examination. It doesn't work. Instead, organize planned study sessions, by yourself or with others, over a reasonable period of time, in an environment that you find relaxing, stress free, and supportive of the learning process.

TEST-TAKING SKILLS

By now you more than likely have been exposed to a variety of testing in both objective and subjective forms. The licensing examination, however, deals only with the objective type and more precisely with the objective multiple choice form of testing. Although this form of testing may be familiar to you, let's take a look at how you can avoid some common test-taking errors:

1. Answer the question that is asked. To do so you need to read, not scan, the situation and the question carefully, looking for key words or phrases. Do not read anything into the question or apply what you did in a similar situation during one of your clinical experiences. Think of each question as pertaining to an ideal situation. No one is trying to trick you. Each question contains a stem (the main intent of the question), followed by four plausible answers or alternatives that either complete a statement or answer the question presented. Only one of the alternatives is the best answer; the remaining three alternatives are known as distractors, so named because they are written in such a way that they could be the correct answer and so distract you to a certain degree. However, your nursing knowledge will lead you to the correct answer.

   For example:

   Which of the following hormones is secreted only during early pregnancy?
   - Estrogen
   - Progesterone
   - Follicle-stimulating hormone (FSH)
   - Human chorionic gonadotropin (HCG)

   The correct answer is HCG. The alternatives are female hormones and are intended to distract you; however, the key phrase, "only during early pregnancy," is the clue to the correct answer.

2. Listen to the examiner and follow directions carefully. All candidates will be given a short training session, which includes a keyboard tutorial complete with a practice session. No prior computer experience is necessary. Should you have any question regarding the directions, ask the examiner for clarification.

3. Have confidence in your initial response to a question, because it probably is the correct answer. If you are unable to answer immediately, eliminate the alternatives you know are incorrect and proceed from there. Remember, although a time factor is not involved, don't spend an excessive amount of time on any one question. One minute is the recommended time allotted to any question. Not all questions consume a full minute; some may take only 20 or 30 seconds to read and answer. With CAT, skipping questions or going back to review and/or change responses is not possible. In fact, you must answer the question because you will not be able to continue with the examination until you do so.

4. Avoid taking a wild guess at an answer; however, should you feel insecure about a question, eliminate the alternatives you believe are definitely incorrect. This approach increases your chances of randomly selecting the correct answer. Although there is no penalty for guessing on the NCLEX-PN examination, the subsequent question will be based, to an extent, on the response to a given question; that is, if you answer a question incorrectly, the computer will adapt the next question accordingly based on your knowledge/skill performance on the examination to that point.

5. Above all, begin with a positive attitude about yourself, your nursing knowledge, and your test-taking abilities. A positive attitude is achieved through self-confidence gained by studying effectively. Stated simply, this means (a) answering questions (assessment), (b) organizing study time (planning), (c) reading and further study (implementation), and (d) again answering questions (evaluation).

Being emotionally prepared for an examination is also a key factor in your success; however, proper use of this text over an extended period of time (5 to 6 months before the actual examination) ensures your understanding of the mechanics of the examination as well as increases your confidence about your nursing knowledge. Practicing a few relaxation techniques may also prove helpful, especially on the day of the examination. Relaxation techniques such as deep breathing, imagery, head rolling, shoulder shrugging, rotating and stretching of the neck, leg lifts and heel lifts with feet flat on the floor can effectively reduce tension while causing little or no distraction to those around you. It is recommended that you do one or two of the techniques intermittently to avoid becoming too tense. The more tense you are, the longer it will take you to relax.

Some additional advice before you begin your review sessions or take the licensing examination:

- Many times the correct answer is the longest alternative given; however, don't count on it. Individuals who prepare the examination are also aware of this fact and attempt to avoid offering you any such "helpful hints."
- Avoid looking for an answer pattern or code. Many times four or five consecutive questions have the same letter or number for the correct answer.
- Key words or phrases in the stem of the question, such as *first, primary, early,* or *best,* are also important. Likewise, words such as *only, always, never,* and *all* in the alternatives are frequently evidence of a wrong response; as in life, there are no real absolutes in nursing. Of course, there are exceptions to every rule, so answer with care.
- Be alert for grammatical inconsistencies. If the response is intended to complete the stem (an incomplete sentence) but makes no grammatical sense to you, it could be a distractor rather than the correct answer. However, test developers try to eliminate such inconsistencies.
- Look for options that are similar in nature; if all are correct, you should know that it is either a poor question or that all are incorrect, the latter of which is most likely. For example, if the answer you are seeking is directed to a specific treatment and all but one option deals with signs and symptoms, then you would be correct in choosing the treatment specific option, because it totally excludes the other three options.
- Identify option components as correct or incorrect; being alert for correct/incorrect option components (parts) could help you eliminate a wrong answer. For example, if you were

being asked to identify a specific diet, your knowledge about that condition would help you to choose the correct response, even though you can't recall the exact diet (cholecystectomy = low fat, high protein, low calorie).
- Look for specific determiners; be alert for words in the stem of the item that are the same or similar in nature to those in one or two of the options. For example, if the item relates to and identifies stroke rehabilitation as its focus and only one of the options contains the word *stroke* in relation to *rehabilitation,* you are safe in identifying this as the correct response.
- Be aware that information from previously asked questions may help you respond to other examination questions.
- Be alert for details. Specific details given in the stem of the item, such as "behavioral and/or clinical changes within a certain time period" can give you a clue regarding the most appropriate response.
- You have at least a 25% chance of selecting the correct answer. Should you feel uncertain about a question, eliminate those choices you think are wrong and then call on your knowledge, skills, and abilities to choose from the remaining responses.
- The night before the examination you may wish to review some material, but then relax and get a good night's sleep. Remember to set your alarm or to have someone wake you. In the morning allow yourself plenty of time to dress comfortably, have breakfast, and arrive at the testing site a few minutes early. Be sure you know where to park and where the test will be given. Also, remember to take eyeglasses (if needed), your admission card, and second proof of identity. Being prepared will reduce your stress/tension level. Remember that positive attitude.

NCLEX-PN

The number of questions will vary in CAT and will be based on the candidate's performance, which measures knowledge, skills, and abilities. All successful candidates will answer no fewer than 75 questions or a maximum of approximately 195 questions within the 5-hour time frame. Rest periods (one mandatory after the first 2 hours of testing and one optional following the next 90 minutes of testing) and the computer tutorial are included as part of the 5-hour testing session. Tests are scored to determine the number of correct answers (raw score). The raw score is then equated to a standard score, which simply indicates where a candidate stands relative to the minimum passing score set by his or her particular state board of nursing. Scores reflect the "pass" or "fail" status of the candidate, with the majority of the boards using the same pass/fail score as determined via a statistical analysis by the National Council.

A candidate who fails will receive a diagnostic profile, which will assist him/her to focus further study efforts for retaking the examination.

The examination has been developed with the basic knowledge necessary for the practice of practical/vocational nursing. It contains test items reflecting the cognitive levels of knowledge, comprehension, application, and analysis.

Although the test plan focuses on one major dimension, that of client need, keep in mind that the elements of accountability, nutrition, anatomy and physiology, growth and development, documentation, communication, fundamentals, and patient education are included throughout the examination (see Box 1-1).

Please note that the NCLEX-PN examination may contain test items (questions) that are being validated for future NCLEX-PN examinations, which are not identifiable to the test taker. Whether you answer these questions correctly or incorrectly, you do not gain or lose points. As already stated, these test items are being validated (tested) for use in future NCLEX-PN examinations.

In all likelihood, no two candidates will be given the same questions to answer, because the examination is individualized according to the candidate's knowledge and skills while meeting test plan requirements.

A SPECIAL NOTE FOR CANADIAN CANDIDATES

Nursing is regulated in each province in Canada. A designated body of nurses in each province has the responsibility for setting minimum standards of safe practice for Practical Nurses (PNs), thus ensuring the client and the public a consistent standard of nursing care in any setting. To be allowed to practice as a PN, qualified individuals are required to take a registration/licensure examination before receiving a certificate of competence. All provinces except Quebec use the Canadian Practical Nurse Registration Examination (CPNRE). The CPNRE is prepared by Assessment Strategies Incorporated (ASI), previously known as the Canadian Nurses Association Testing division (CNAT). Examinations are available in both English and French. The Quebec government regulates the licensure of practical nurses in the province of Quebec.

The Canadian Practical Nurse Registration Examination (CPNRE) is offered three times a year—every January, May, and September. The examination consists of a core component and two supplementary components. The core component is presented in two parts and is administered on 1 day. The core part of the examination is competency-based, containing 190 to 210 questions total. The two supplementary components to the examination test the areas of medication administration and intravenous/infusion therapy and are administered only in those jurisdictions in which the competencies are applicable. The CPNRE is a multiple-choice examination. All questions require a single-choice answer, as do the questions in this book.

The CPNRE tests fundamental core competencies an entry-level practical nurse is required to have to practice safely and effectively. These competencies represent outcomes of combined knowledge, abilities, skills, attitudes, and judgment that practical nurses possess. The total examination is planned to test knowledge of safe and effective practice, covering all areas of practical nursing across the life span in a variety of areas of practice. Your knowledge of biological, psychological, and social sciences is tested, as well as your knowledge of nursing and your ability to apply principles of professionalism and ethical judgment. All participating provinces and territories have had opportunity for input into the preparation of the examination; thus, the examination reflects common health problems encountered across the life span that are representative of practical nurse educational curricula across the country.

The CNA Blueprint for the Practical Nurse/Nursing Assistant Registration/Licensure Examination (1996) identifies major concepts and content areas covered in the examination and outlines the competencies on which the examination is based. Currently these competencies are under review, and it is expected that the new competencies, as well as a new examination

format, will be implemented by September 2001. The following 1996 CNA Blueprint used for the PN/NA Registration/Licensure Examination is adapted with permission from Assessment Strategies, Inc., Ottawa, Canada. This blueprint is subject to change with the 2001 administration of the Canadian Practical Nurse Registration Examination (CPNRE).

Framework for the Development of the Examination

Competency Categories

Client care*	83%
Communication	10%
Personal and professional responsibilities	7%

*Nursing Process is tested throughout the client care section.

Taxonomy of Questions

Cognitive Domain

Knowledge/comprehension	20%-30%
Application	55%-65%
Critical thinking	5%-10%

Affective Domain

Attitudes and judgment	5%-10%

Contextual Variables
1. Client age and gender

Age group	Target Percentage of Items on the Core Component of the Examination	Target Percentage (males)	Target Percentage (females)
Child and adolescent (18 years)	24%-30%	12%-15%	12%-15%
Adult (19-64 years)	29%-47%	14%-23%	15%-24%
Older adult (65+ years)	29%-41%	12%-18%	17%-23%

2. Client culture: The examination is designed to include items representing the variety of cultural backgrounds found in Canada.
3. Client health situation: In the examination the clients are viewed holistically, including their biophysical, psychosocial, and spiritual dimensions.
4. Health care environment: Because the PN/NA works in a variety of settings and contexts where competencies are equally applicable, the examination specifies health care environment only where it is required to provide guidance to the candidate.

In your review, study all areas to be tested, and budget your time appropriately. This text has three main purposes: (1) to assist you in determining the extent of your nursing knowledge relative to your specific areas of strength and weakness, (2) to increase the understanding of your nursing knowledge through additional study, and (3) to increase your familiarity with and ability to respond to written test questions and corresponding clinical situations. Although the questions in this text are geared to the American NCLEX-PN examination and therefore include questions on medication administration and intravenous infusion that are not applicable throughout Canada, the majority of the questions are directly applicable to all Canadian PNs. Using this text with your notes and other textbooks will focus your attention on the material applicable to your program, which is the bulk of this text. This book should not be used for last-minute cramming, but rather should be used as an adjunct to planned study, and for practicing examination questions with instant feedback. Refer to sections on effective study and test-taking skills earlier in this chapter.

CONCLUSION

You started preparation for the licensing examination the first day you began your nursing program. Every lecture, quiz, examination, term paper, and clinical experience had definite purpose and meaning. This thirteenth edition of *Mosby's Comprehensive Review of Practical Nursing for NCLEX-PN* has been developed as a culmination of this preparation process. It is now in your hands, for only your initiative and dedication to achieving a long-awaited goal will be rewarded with success.

Before you move on to the next chapter, answer the test questions on the following page to see just how sharp your test-taking skills are.

HOW SHARP ARE YOUR TEST-TAKING SKILLS?
Take the Following Examination and Find Out!

The following is a hypothetical examination in which, if you are aware of the pitfalls of test construction, you could possibly achieve a score of 100%. We hope you have some fun with this short quiz, which tests only test wiseness skills, not content knowledge.

1. The purpose of the cluss in furmpalling is to revove:
① Cluss-Prags
② Tremalls
③ Cloughs
④ Plumots

2. Trassing is true when:
① Lusp trasses the vom
② The viskal flane, if the viskal is donwil or zortil
③ The belgo frulla
④ Dissels liks easily

3. The sigla frequently overfesks the trelsum because:
① All siglas are mellious
② Siglas are always votial
③ The trelsum is usually tarious
④ No trelsa are feskable

4. The fribbled breg will minter best with an:
① Derst
② Morst
③ Sortar
④ Ignu

5. The reasons for tristal doss are:
① The sabs foped and the doths tinsed
② The kredges roted with the orts
③ Few rakobs were accepted in sluth
④ Most of the polits were thonced

6. Which of the following is/are always present when trossels are being gruven?
① Rint and vost
② Vost
③ Shum and vost
④ Vost and plone

7. The mintering function of the ignu is most effectively carried out in connection with:
① A razma tol
② The groshing stantol
③ The fribbled breg
④ A frally sush

8. ①
②
③
④

Reprinted with permission of the test creator Sorush Batmangelich, Assistant Professor, Department of Physical Medicine and Rehabilitation, Rush Medical College, Chicago, Ill; Medical Education Consultant and President, BATM.

ANSWERS AND RATIONALES

Because of the nature of the test questions in Chapter 1, only the correct response and the rationale for the correct response will be given.

1. ① Cluss appears in the stem and this response; this response is also the longest alternative.

2. ② This response is the longest alternative.

3. ③ All, always, and *no* in answer #1, #2, and #4 eliminate them as possible correct answers; nothing is ever that definite; also #3 is the longest alternative.

4. ④ Although the sentence makes no sense, the fourth alternative appears to be more grammatically correct than the other three.

5. ① The stem asks for more than one reason; this response is the only one of the four that offers more than one reason.

6. ② Proper reading of the stem and a close look at the possible answers reveal that the second response appears in the other responses as well, making it the only possible correct answer.

7. ③ Some of the terms used in this question may seem familiar to you, and well they should, as they also appeared in a previous question (#4)—a definite clue to the correct answer.

8. ④ Yes, there is a correct answer even though there is no stem or actual responses; if you haven't already figured it out, there was a definite "answer pattern" created (#1, #2, #3, #4, #1, #2, #3, #4).

CHAPTER 2

Review of the Basics: Trends in the United States and Canada, Nursing Concepts, and the Nursing Process

Nursing is an ongoing relationship with patients in various stages of development and at different points of the health-illness continuum. Basic to nursing are knowledge of the patient as a person, factors contributing to health and illness, the ability to problem solve, and the ability to perform nursing skills. Nurses also appreciate the history of their profession and respect the ethical and legal aspects of rendering nursing care. This chapter reviews the history of practical/vocational nursing and the functions of its professional organizations; discusses the basic concepts of effective nursing care, while focusing on professional obligations and patient rights; and outlines changes in the health care delivery system and how these changes relate to the practice of LP/LVN.

HEALTH–ILLNESS
Health Defined

A. According to the World Health Organization (WHO), health is "a state of complete physical, mental, and social well-being and not merely an absence of disease or infirmity"
B. According to Abraham H. Maslow, health exists when all human needs are satisfied
C. According to Hans Selye, health exists when an individual is in a relative state of adaptation to his or her environment
D. In 1990 *Healthy People 2000 National Health Promotion and Disease Prevention Objectives* were published in an effort to reduce preventable diseases, disabilities, and deaths. The three goals of *Healthy People 2000* include increasing span of healthy life; reducing health disparities; and achieving access to preventative services

Illness Defined

A. No one definition exists
B. Illness exists when disease is present, when an individual believes he or she is ill (subjective symptoms), or when (objective) signs of illness are detected by the individual or the professional
C. Illness exists when all basic human needs are not satisfied
D. Illness is a state of disturbance in the body's homeostasis, either of body structure and function or emotional or sociological functioning

Health–Illness Continuum

A. An individual is rarely either totally healthy or totally ill
B. The individual's position is constantly changing in the balance between health and illness
C. The individual's position on the continuum is determined by need satisfaction, the stage of disease progression, and his or her perception of relative health or illness

VARIABLES INFLUENCING HEALTH BELIEFS AND PRACTICES

A. Many variables influence a person's perception of health and illness
B. Internal variables include the patient's developmental stage, knowledge level, perception of functioning, emotional factors, and religious/spiritual views
C. External variables include the patient's family practices, socioeconomic status, and cultural practices

TRENDS IN NURSING
Practical/Vocational Nursing in the United States
HISTORY

A. Practical/vocational nursing evolved to provide better use of nursing personnel and to ease the shortage of nurses
B. The first school to train practical/vocational nurses was the Ballard School in New York City, founded in 1893. This 3-month program taught care of chronic invalids, elderly persons, and children
C. In 1907 the Thompson School was founded in Brattleboro, Vermont. The Household Nursing Association School of Attendant Nursing was founded in Boston in 1918.
D. In the 1940s there were about 50 approved programs; during the 1950s the number of schools of practical/vocational nursing grew. Most programs were extended to 12 months, placing emphasis on integrating class instruction with clinical experience
E. In 1956 Public Law 911 appropriated millions of dollars for the improvement and expansion of practical/vocational nurse training. The United States Office of Education established a practical nurse education service
F. Today more than 1000 practical/vocational nursing schools are located in hospitals, colleges, and vocational-technical schools providing instruction to more than 50,000 students each year
G. There are approximately 500,000 practical/vocational nurses licensed in the United States and three U.S. territories (Guam, Puerto Rico, and the Virgin Islands)

EDUCATION

A. Practical/vocational nursing programs must meet requirements and be approved by the state board of nursing
B. Practical/vocational nursing schools of high standards may voluntarily apply for national accreditation by the National League for Nursing Accrediting Commission (NLNAC)
C. Admission requirements to practical/vocational nursing programs vary, but generally applicants must
   1. Be at least 17 years of age
   2. Have a high school diploma or equivalent
   3. Have good physical and mental health
   4. Be of good moral character
D. The curriculum incorporates content and concepts from the biological and physical sciences, behavioral sciences, and principles and practices of nursing
E. The curriculum includes nursing theory and clinical practice, which provide the students with learning opportunities to meet physical and psychosocial needs of mothers and infants, children, medical-surgical patients, the elderly, and patients with long-term illnesses
F. Graduates receive a diploma or certificate and are eligible to take the practical/vocational nurse licensing examination
G. Practical/vocational nursing is the entry level into the practice of nursing

ROLE RESPONSIBILITIES

A. The licensed practical/vocational nurse (LP/VN) has a vital and effective role as a member of the health care team
B. The LP/VN provides direct nursing care to patients whose conditions are stable under the supervision and direction of a registered nurse or physician
C. The LP/VN assists the registered nurse with the care of patients whose conditions are unstable and complex
D. The LP/VN, adhering to the nursing process, observes, assesses, records, reports, and performs basic therapeutic, preventive, and rehabilitative procedures
E. LP/VNs work in acute and long-term care hospitals, nursing homes, physician's offices, ambulatory care facilities, home health agencies, community agencies, schools, and industries
F. To identify the abilities of the beginning practitioner in practical/vocational nursing, see Box 2-1

CONTINUING EDUCATION

A. Each LP/VN is responsible for maintaining competency and increasing level of knowledge
B. The rapid growth of nursing and medical knowledge and advances in technology require nurses to keep up to date

---

Box 2-1   National Association for Practical Nurse Education and Service: Statement of Practical/Vocational Nurse Entry-Level Competencies

Assessment

Uses basic communication skills in a structured care setting

Obtains specific information from patients through goal-directed interviews

Participates in the identification of physical, emotional, spiritual, cultural, and overt learning needs of patients by collecting appropriate data

Analyzes data collected in relation to patients' pathophysiology

Planning

Determines priorities and plans nursing care accordingly

Formulates and/or collaborates in developing written nursing care plans

Participates in developing preventive or long-term health plans for patients and/or families

Implementation

Protects the rights and dignity of patients and families

Uses basic communication skills in a structured care setting

Safely performs therapeutic and preventive nursing procedures, incorporating fundamental biologic and physiologic principles in giving individualized care

Observes patients and communicates significant findings to the health care team

Conducts incidental teaching and supports and reinforces the teaching plan for a specific patient and/or family

Evaluation

Evaluates, with guidance if necessary, the care given and makes necessary adjustments

Records evaluations of the results of nursing actions

Identifies own strengths and weaknesses and seeks assistance for improvement of performance

Professional Responsibilities

Recognizes the LP/VN's role in the health care delivery system and articulates that role with those of other health care team members

Maintains accountability for own nursing practice within ethical and legal framework

Serves as a patient advocate

Accepts role in maintaining and developing standards of practice in providing patient care

Participates in nursing organizations

Seeks further growth through educational opportunities

C. The LP/VN must take advantage of learning opportunities through in-service programs where employed; attending seminars and workshops available through institutions, school, official, or voluntary organizations; and reading professional journals

D. Membership in nursing organizations provides continuing education opportunities, usually at a lower cost to members

HEALTH CARE TEAM

A. Members of the health care team vary depending on the patient's needs and goals

B. Constant team members are
   1. Physicians: diagnose and prescribe
   2. Nurses: plan and carry out nursing care
   3. Patient and family: participate in planning care

C. Other team members include certified nursing assistants, unlicensed assistive personnel, physical therapists, social workers, occupational therapists, respiratory therapists, dieticians, clergy, and others

D. Successful nursing care depends on the interaction and cooperation of all members of the team

E. The LP/VN collaborates with team members

The LP/VN Role in Leadership

A. Dossett (1992) defines leadership as the use of one's skills to influence others to perform to the best of their ability

B. The number of LP/VN positions in extended-care facilities is increasing. LP/VNs are being placed in the role of charge nurse, responsible for assigning unlicensed assistive personnel job tasks

C. Assigning is within the scope of practice of the LP/VN and involves allotting tasks that are in the job description of unlicensed assistive personnel

---

Box 2-2   Examples of Tasks Assigned to Unlicensed Assistive Personnel

Bathing
Vital signs
Feeding
Maintaining safety
Grooming
Weights
Transferring/ambulating
Intake and output

D. The LP/VN must know agency policy and job descriptions of unlicensed assistive personnel before assigning tasks

E. Tasks assigned may include assistance with activities of daily living and uncomplicated tasks. See Box 2-2 for examples of tasks that may be assigned

F. Provide clear, concise descriptions of what tasks are to be accomplished. Provide time frame and give feedback and praise for staff members' efforts

G. The LP/VN is legally liable for improper assigning of tasks

DELEGATION

A. Many states are debating the issue of delegation as it pertains to the LP/VN scope of practice

B. Bernard and Walsh (1995) define delegation as the process of assigning part of one person's responsibility to another qualified person, with their consent. Delegation is a transfer of responsibility and authority while maintaining accountability

C. LP/VNs must ensure that the Nurse Practice Act of their state permits delegation. The Nurse Practice Act should authorize specific tasks to be delegated

D. The LP/VN must ensure that the delegatee has demonstrated the appropriate level of competency to perform the delegated task

CONFLICT RESOLUTION

A. Conflict results when one person's expectations or rights cross with those of another person's

B. LP/VNs in leadership roles need to become accustomed to resolving conflicts

C. The steps in conflict resolution include recognition, clarification, negotiation (compromise), and decision making

D. In addition to conflict resolution, LP/VNs must address common individual problems. See Box 2-3 for examples of individual problem areas

E. LP/VNs have an ethical and legal responsibility to report substance abuse among peers. See Box 2-4 for signs of substance abuse

F. Drug addiction among nurses is 30 to 100 times greater than among the general population

G. Most states have impaired professional programs

Legislation Related to Practice of LP/VN
NURSE PRACTICE ACT

A. Nursing is subject to laws passed by the state's legislature

B. Laws pertaining to nursing are in the state's nurse practice act

C. The nurse practice act varies from state to state. Some states define the practice of nursing, whereas others describe what a nurse may or may not do in the practice of nursing

D. The nurse practice act also provides for some type of nursing board to regulate nursing practice and procedures for:
   1. Approval of nursing schools and curriculum requirements
   2. Licensure and renewal
   3. Grounds for suspension and revocation of licensure

E. The LP/VN must practice nursing within the legally defined scope of his or her state's nurse practice act

STATE BOARDS OF NURSING

A. Administer the state nurse practice act

B. Membership on the board varies from state to state, usually consists of RNs, LP/VNs, and consumers appointed by the governor

C. In most states, both professional and practical/vocational nursing practice are under the same board; some states have two boards, one for each

D. Functions
   1. Enforces established educational requirements of schools of nursing
      a. Surveys program to determine if preestablished standards are being met
      b. Approves new programs that meet standards
      c. Withholds or withdraws approval from programs that do not meet standards
   2. Controls licensure
      a. Administers the NCLEX-PN licensure examination
      b. Grants license to authorized applicants

Box 2-3   Employee Problem Areas

Excessive tardiness/absence
Excessive use of phone for personal phone calls
Negative attitudes/not being a team player
Poor quality of work
Substance abuse

Box 2-4   Recognition of Substance Abuse

Personality changes
Frequent sick calls
Glassy eyes, slurred speech
Changes in attitude toward others

---

   c. Renews license
   d. Denies, suspends, or revokes license for cause
   3. Conducts investigations and hearings relating to charges of unsafe nursing practice
   4. Interprets the nurse practice act based on past practice, standard of care, and information from other states

LICENSURE

A. Protects the public from unqualified practitioners

B. A license is mandatory to practice nursing

C. Permits use of title LPN or LVN

D. Qualifications vary from state to state but most require the following for licensure
   1. Graduation from an approved program in practical/vocational nursing
   2. Proof of moral character
   3. Minimum score on the nationally administered examination

E. License must be renewed for a small fee at regular intervals

F. Many states require LP/VN to submit proof of continuing education before license will be renewed

G. License may be revoked or suspended for acts of misconduct or incompetence such as drug addiction or conviction of a felony

H. Licensure by endorsement occurs when a state board of nursing reviews the credentials of a nurse licensed in another state and determines that the nurse meets the qualifications of their state

EXAMINATION

A. As of 1994, all states administer the National Council of State Boards of Nursing (NCSBN) examination as a computer adaptive test (CAT). This test, the National Council Licensure Examination for Practical Nurses (NCLEX-PN), is used to determine if the LP/VN candidate is prepared to practice nursing safely. It tests knowledge of nursing care and ability to apply that knowledge in a clinical situation

B. Testing occurs in more than 1200 computer testing sites throughout the nation. Candidates schedule a testing date following graduation. Testing occurs throughout the year, 6 days per week, 15 hours per day. Each examinee sits at an individual computer terminal and answers questions on the screen. The candidate's answer to each question determines the next question to be presented. No two persons receive the same test

C. The test stops when the candidate's ability level has been estimated at a predetermined degree of accuracy. There is a minimum number of questions that must be answered, and a maximum time allotment for the test (5 hours). Some candidates will complete the test in less than 5 hours

Ethical Principles: Code of Ethics

A. Principles established by professional group as a means of self-regulation
B. Each LP/VN is responsible for upholding the professional standards of conduct and ethics

Legal Implications for the LP/VN

RESPONSIBILITIES

A. Function within the scope of state nurse practice act
B. Maintain standards of care (Box 2-5)
C. Function according to employer or agency policy
D. Apply the skills and knowledge that a prudent LP/VN with comparable training would apply in a similar situation
E. Maintain complete and accurate patient records
F. Maintain confidentiality

DELIVERY OF NURSING CARE

A. Functional method: each nursing team member is assigned specific tasks (e.g., obtaining and recording all vital signs, administering all medications)
B. Team nursing: a group of patients are cared for by a team consisting of professional nurses, practical/vocational nurses, nurses' aides, and student nurses
C. Primary nursing
  1. One nurse assigned to patient from admission to discharge, usually registered nurse
  2. Total responsibility for care on all shifts
  3. Coordinates care with other health workers, for example, LP/VN, aide

ILLEGAL ACTIONS

A. Torts—civil law
  1. An act or wrong committed by one person against another that results in injury or damage
  2. Can be either the commission or omission of an act
  3. Acts of negligence include
    a. Professional misconduct
    b. Performing care incorrectly
    c. Illegal or immoral conduct
    d. Examples include
      (1) Administration of wrong medication
      (2) Administration of medication or treatment to wrong patient
      (3) Failure to ensure safety through use of side rails or restraints as ordered by the physician
      (4) Failure to prevent injury while applying heat
      (5) Gross negligence: patient's life is endangered or lost—often results in criminal action
B. Intentional torts
  1. Legal liability exists even if no damage occurs to the other person
  2. May not be covered by malpractice insurance

Box 2-5   Standards of Practice for the LP/VN

The LP/VN provides individual and family-centered nursing care

Follow principles of nursing process in meeting specific needs of patients of all ages in the areas of safety, hygiene, nutrition, medication, elimination, psychosocial, cultural, and respiratory needs
Apply appropriate knowledge, skills, and abilities in providing safe, competent care
Apply principles of crisis intervention in maintaining safety and making appropriate referral when necessary
Use effective communication skills
- Communicate effectively with patients, family, significant others, and members of the health care team
- Maintain appropriate written documentation
Provide appropriate health teaching to patients and significant others in the areas of
- Maintenance of wellness
- Rehabilitation
- Use of community resources
Serve as a patient advocate
- Protect patients' rights
- Consult with appropriate others when necessary

The LP/VN fulfills the professional responsibilities of the practical/vocational nurse

Know and apply the ethical principles underlying the profession
Know and follow the appropriate professional and legal requirements
Follow the policies and procedures of the employing institution
Cooperate and collaborate with all members of the health care team to meet the needs of family-centered nursing care
Demonstrate accountability for own nursing actions
Maintain current knowledge and skills in the area of employment

Modified from Standards of Practice for LP/VN.
Adopted in 1985 by the National Association for Practical Nurse Education and Service, Silver Spring, Md.

---

  3. Assault and battery
    a. Assault
      (1) Definition: threat or attempt to make bodily contact with another person without that person's consent with intent to injure
      (2) Example: threatening to restrain or physically punish patient if he or she does not cooperate
    b. Battery
      (1) Definition: act of making unauthorized contact with another
      (2) Example: nurse actually restrains patient
  4. False imprisonment
    a. Definition: unwarranted restriction of another person by force or threat of force
    b. Examples: detaining patient in hospital against his or her will; unwarranted use of restraints

c. Patient who wishes to leave hospital against advice of physician may be asked to sign a release; cannot detain patient if he or she refuses to sign

5. Invasion of privacy
   a. Definition: unauthorized disclosures about a patient even if information is true
   b. Examples
      (1) Release of patient's medical information
      (2) Exposure of patient during procedures or transportation

6. Defamation
   a. Definition: attack on the name, business, or professional reputation of another through false and malicious statements to a third person
   b. Types
      (1) Slander: oral statement
      (2) Libel: written statement

OTHER LEGAL ASPECTS

A. Good Samaritan laws
   1. Laws that give certain persons legal protection when giving aid at the scene of an accident; not all states cover nurses
   2. Purpose: to encourage people to give assistance at the scene of an emergency
   3. These laws do not make it legally necessary for a nurse to assist
   4. When nurses do assist, they are expected to use good judgment in deciding whether an emergency exists
   5. The LP/VN is expected to give a standard of care that a reasonable LP/VN with comparable training would give in similar circumstances

B. Child abuse
   1. All states have laws that require reporting known or suspected cases of child abuse
   2. The laws grant immunity from civil suits to those who are required to report child abuse

C. Narcotics
   1. The Federal Controlled Substances Act of 1970 is a federal law that regulates the manufacture, sale, prescription, and dispensing of narcotics and other harmful drugs
   2. Violation of the law by a nurse is a felony and will result in revocation of the LP/VN license

D. Wills
   1. A legal declaration of how a person (testator) wishes to dispose of his or her property after death
   2. For a will to be valid, the testator must be of sound mind and acting without force
   3. No legal reason for the nurse not to witness a will; the witness is only witnessing the person's signature, not the contents of the will
   4. A beneficiary of the will must not witness it

E. Malpractice insurance
   1. Professional liability policies cover liability arising out of the rendering of or failure to render professional service
   2. Policy is safeguard against suits for damages; can be expensive to prove innocence
   3. Can be purchased from nursing organizations, bargaining organizations, and private insurance companies
   4. Provides monetary award of damages within specified limits of the policy, also legal fees, court costs, and payment of bond

5. Employer's insurance protects employee only while on duty

Patient's Rights
BILL OF RIGHTS

A. Patients have the right to courteous, individual care given without discrimination as to race, color, religion, sex, marital status, national origin, or ability to pay
B. A patient's bill of rights is a statement of what the patient can expect from the institution
C. The following is paraphrased from the Patient's Bill of Rights adopted by the American Hospital Association. The patient should:
   1. Be given considerate and respectful care
   2. Obtain from the physician complete current information concerning diagnosis, treatment, and prognosis in terms he or she can be reasonably expected to understand
   3. Receive from the physician information necessary to give informed consent prior to the start of any procedure or treatment
   4. Be allowed to refuse treatment to the extent permitted by law and be informed of the medical consequences of that action
   5. Be given every consideration of privacy concerning his or her own medical care program
   6. Expect that all communications and records pertaining to his or her care be treated as confidential
   7. Expect that within its capacity a hospital must make reasonable response to the request of a patient for services
   8. Obtain information as to any relationships of the patient's hospital to other health care and educational institutions insofar as his or her care is concerned
   9. Be advised if the hospital proposes to engage in or perform human experimentation affecting the patient's care or treatment
   10. Expect reasonable continuity of care
   11. Examine and receive an explanation of the bill regardless of the source of payment
   12. Know what hospital rules and regulations apply to the patient's conduct

STANDARD OF CARE

A. Patients are entitled to a safe, competent standard of nursing care no matter who administers it (RN, LP/VN, student)
B. The LP/VN is accountable for his or her own actions and must ensure that the patient receives qualified care
C. If the LP/VN thinks that the patient assignment is beyond his or her ability, the LP/VN must discuss the matter with the registered nurse before carrying it out
D. Standard of care is established by:
   1. State nurse practice act
   2. Institution's job description
   3. Hospital policies and procedures
   4. Patient's nursing care plan

PATIENT ADVOCATE

A. An advocate acts on behalf of another person and stands up or speaks up on behalf of that person
B. Patient has the right to information needed to make informed decisions freely and without pressure

C. The responsibility of the LP/VN is to:
1. Maintain standard of care
2. Support patients in the decisions they make
3. Inform physician when the patient apparently does not understand what is going to happen to him or her
4. Observe and speak out regarding instances of incompetent, unethical, or illegal practice by any member of the health care team
5. Know hospital policy regarding procedure to follow when patients' rights are being violated
D. Many hospitals employ a patient representative who serves as a liaison between patient and institution and who has the power to act to resolve patients' problems

CONSENT FORMS

A. Before any invasive procedure can be performed, the patient must give written consent, except in extreme emergency, when failure to treat may be considered negligence
B. Patient must be fully informed of the extent of the proposed procedure, risks and benefits, alternatives, and their consequences
C. Consent must be obtained by the physician, whose duty it is to advise the patient
D. Consent may be withdrawn by the patient prior to the procedure

PATIENT'S MEDICAL RECORDS: THE CHART

A. The chart is a legal document
B. Provides a written account of the patient's hospitalization
C. May be used as evidence in courts of law; records only information related to patient's health problem
D. Information contained in records must be held in confidence
E. Only authorized persons should have access to patient's records
F. Most states consider medical records the property of the hospital, and the contents the property of the patient

Nursing Organizations

A. Membership
1. LP/VN has the responsibility to join a professional organization and support practical/vocational nursing by becoming an active member
2. Membership provides:
   a. Fellowship and interaction with other LP/VNs
   b. Opportunity to enhance and strengthen role of LP/VNs
   c. Means to keep current on issues relating to practical/vocational nursing
   d. A voice in planning policies of the association
   e. Continuing education opportunities
B. National Association for Practical Nurse Education and Service (NAPNES)*
1. NAPNES was organized in 1941 to promote the development of sound practical/vocational nursing education and to promote advancement and recognition of the LP/VN as a member of the health team
2. Membership includes:
   a. Regular members: LP/VNs, practical nursing educators, other registered nurses, general educators,

physicians, hospital and nursing home administrators, practical nursing students, and interested lay persons
   b. Student members: students in state-approved schools of practical/vocational nursing
   c. Agency members: hospitals, nursing homes, schools of practical nursing, alumni groups, civic organizations, and other institutions or groups in harmony with NAPNES objectives
3. Functions and activities listed by NAPNES:
   a. Serves as clearinghouse for information about practical/vocational nursing, including information about functions and roles of LP/VNs
   b. Publishes *Journal of Practical Nursing,* a monthly magazine
   c. Prepares publications useful to faculties in schools of practical/vocational nursing
   d. Sponsors workshops and seminars for LP/VNs and practical nursing educators in conjunction with state LP/VN associations, universities, and national organizations
   e. Engages in activities aimed at protecting and strengthening position of LP/VNs and cooperates with state LP/VN associations in activities of this kind
   f. Provides consultation to state LP/VN constituencies on matters relating to their organization and programs
   g. Sponsors "national certification" in pharmacology and long-term care for LP/VNs
C. National Federation of Licensed Practical Nurses (NFLPN)*
1. NFLPN was organized in 1949 to foster high standards in practical nursing and to promote practical nursing
2. Membership limited to LP/VNs and student practical/vocational nurses
3. Affiliate membership is available to individuals who are not LP/VNs or students but are interested in the work of NFLPN
4. There are many state associations
5. Functions of the NFLPN:
   a. Provides leadership for LP/VNs employed in the United States
   b. Fosters high standards of practical/vocational nursing education and practice
   c. Encourages every LP/VN to make continuing education a priority
   d. Achieves recognition for LP/VNs and advocates the effectiveness of LP/VNs in every type of health care facility
   e. Interprets the role and function of the LP/VN for the public
   f. Represents practical/vocational nursing through relationships with other national nursing, medical, and allied health organizations, legislators, government officials, health agencies, educators, and other professional groups
   g. Serves as the central source of information on the new and changing aspects of practical/vocational nursing education and practice

---

Box 2-6   National League for Nursing Statement Supporting Practical/Vocational Nursing and Practical/Vocational Nursing Education*

The Executive Committee of the Council of Practical Nursing Programs of the National League for Nursing believes that practical/vocational nursing is a vital component of the occupation of nursing and supports those who elect practical/vocational nursing as a permanent career choice. The minimal educational credential for entry into practical/vocational nursing is a diploma or certificate.

Nursing is an occupation that exists on a continuum, and education for nursing can be developed at different levels of knowledge and skills required to fulfill identified yet different nursing roles. The nursing profession has an obligation to society to develop sound and efficient patterns for nursing education that meet the varied nursing needs of society and permit educational options for those who wish them.

Practical/vocational nurses are involved in the nursing process. Practical/vocational nurses, with the supervision and direction of a registered nurse or physician, utilize the nursing process to give direct care to patients whose conditions are considered to be stable. This care encompasses observation, assessment, recording, reporting to appropriate persons, and performing basic therapeutic, preventive, and rehabilitative procedures. When patients' conditions are unstable and complex, the practical/vocational nurse assists and collaborates with the registered nurse in the provision of care.

The practical/vocational nurse is prepared for employment in health care settings in which the policies and protocols for providing patient care are well defined and in which supervision and direction by a registered nurse or physician are present. These settings may be acute or long-term care hospitals, nursing homes, home health agencies, and ambulatory care facilities.

Practical/vocational nurses function within the definition and framework of the regulations set forth by the nurse practice act of the state in which they are employed. The practice of practical/vocational nursing requires licensure, which is the responsibility of the board of nursing in each state, in order to protect the public and safeguard nursing practice.

Education of the practical/vocational nurse is characterized by its consistent emphasis on the clinical practice experience necessary to meet common nursing problems. The curriculum—based on concepts from the physical and biologic sciences that underlie nursing measures and the behavioral science concepts necessary to individualize care—is a planned sequence of correlated theory and clinical experience.

On completion of the program of study in practical/vocational nursing, the graduate demonstrates the specific competencies related to assessment, planning, implementation, and evaluation of nursing care as identified by the Council of Practical Nursing Programs.

The licensed practical/vocational nurse is responsible for maintaining and updating her or his competencies. Adequate orientation and continuing inservice education are responsibilities of the employing agency. However, the practical/vocational nurse must take advantage of other opportunities for continuing self-improvement and, if desired, career advancement.

Opportunities for career mobility without undue penalty must exist in the system of nursing education to provide for changing career goals.

*Issued in 1982, reaffirmed in 1987.

D. National League for Nursing (NLN)*
   1. The NLN was organized in 1952 by combining the National League for Nursing Education and six other national nursing organizations
   2. Membership includes:
      a. Individual membership; anyone interested in nursing; registered nurses, LP/VNs, student nurses, consumers
      b. Agency membership: hospitals, nursing homes, public health agencies, schools of nursing
   3. Functions are:
      a. Defining and furthering good standards for all nursing service
      b. Defining and promoting good standards for institutions giving nursing education on all levels
      c. Helping to extend facilities to meet these services when necessary
      d. Helping in proper distribution of nursing education and nursing service
      e. Working to improve organized nursing services in hospitals, public health agencies, nursing homes, and other agencies; accrediting community public health nursing services; developing criteria and other self-evaluation tools
      f. Working to improve nursing education programs; the National League for Nursing Accrediting Commission (NLNAC), acts as an accrediting agency for all levels of nursing education
      g. Constructing, processing, and providing preadmission, achievement, and qualifying tests
      h. Gathering and publishing information about trends in nursing, personnel needs, community nursing services, and schools of nursing
   4. Official journal is *Nursing and Health Care*
   5. In 1984 the NLN Council of Practical Nursing Programs adopted a resolution that recognized the NFLPN as the official organization for LP/VNs. See Box 2-6
E. National Council of State Boards of Nursing (NCSBN)*
   1. Established in 1978 to strengthen and coordinate the credentialing of nurses nationally

---

* www.nln.org

* www.ncsbn.org

2. Membership open to any state board of nursing; presently composed of 53 state boards
3. Maintains a liaison with national organizations that represent nursing
4. Controls the NCLEX, which prepares the LP/VN and RN licensure examinations
F. American Nurses Association (ANA)*
    1. National organization for registered nurses formed in 1896 as the Nurses Association Alumnae; renamed ANA in 1911
    2. Concerned with standard of nursing practice and promoting general welfare of the professional nurse
    3. Membership limited to registered nurses
    4. Publishes *American Journal of Nursing (AJN),* a monthly magazine
G. Alumni associations
    1. Organization of graduates from the LP/VN's respective school
    2. Membership provides a means of:
        a. Keeping informed of school's progress
        b. Offering suggestions to improve programs
        c. Providing continuing education
        d. Facilitating social activities with classmates and other graduates
        e. Offering scholarships to future students

Practical Nursing in Canada
HISTORY
A. There has always been a person working as an assistant to the professional nurse
B. During and following World War II there was a shortage of nurses; to meet this need, hospitals began a variety of short courses on the job
C. In response to these many and varied short courses, the Canadian Nurses Association developed a syllabus for a course to be used as a guide by provincial nursing associations with the aim of standardizing courses
D. The title for graduates suggested by the CNA was "nursing assistant"
E. In 1940 Ontario was the first province to pass legislation protecting the title "certified nursing assistant"
F. In 1941 the Registered Nurses Association of Ontario opened a demonstration school in London, Ontario, to determine the feasibility of training an auxiliary group; the course lasted 6 months and had a grade 8 admission requirement
G. Following the war, arrangements were made through the Department of Veterans Affairs, the national and provincial nursing associations, and the departments of health and education in each province to organize courses to meet the needs of people released from the armed services
H. Standardized courses, developed across the country, were offered to the public in such places as hospitals, secondary schools, and technical/vocational schools, as well as independent schools
I. Each province assumed responsibility for supervising the course of instruction, evaluating the programs, and registering/licensing the graduates, plus designating their title: this accounts for the variation in title, program lengths,

and responsibilities of the nursing assistant across the country
J. In 1971 the Ontario Association for Nursing Assistants began discussions with the other provinces to form a national organization
K. In 1975 the Canadian Association of Practical Nursing Assistants (CAPNA) was incorporated; all provinces are affiliated except Quebec
L. There are currently approximately 84,000 practical nursing/nursing assistants in Canada

EDUCATION
A. Practical nursing/nursing assistant (PN/NA) programs must meet requirements of the registering/licensing body in each province/territory
B. There is no national accreditation body for nursing in Canada
C. Admission requirements vary from province to province and the territories; a high school diploma or its equivalent is usually required
D. The curriculum incorporates content and concepts from the biologic and psychosocial sciences, as well as principles and practice of nursing
E. The curriculum includes nursing theory and clinical practice, which provide the students with learning opportunities to meet physical, psychosocial, and spiritual needs of patients across the life span
F. Graduates receive a diploma or certificate and are eligible to take the certification/licensing examination in their jurisdiction

RESPONSIBILITIES OF THE CANADIAN PRACTICAL NURSE/NURSING ASSISTANT
A. The PN/NA has a vital and effective role as a member of the health care team
B. The PN/NA provides direct nursing care to patients whose conditions are stable. Depending on the provincial standards and the setting, care may be provided independently, or with varied amounts of supervision and direction from a registered nurse, a registered psychiatric nurse (in certain provinces), or a physician
C. In certain provinces the PN/NA may be responsible for direct supervision/direction of unregulated care providers in stable settings
D. The PN/NA aids the registered nurse with the care of patients whose conditions are unstable and complex
E. The PN/NA using the nursing process observes, assesses, records, reports, and performs basic therapeutic, preventive, and rehabilitative procedures
F. The PN/NA works in acute and long-term care hospitals, nursing homes, physicians' offices, ambulatory care facilities, home health agencies, public health agencies, community agencies, and industry
G. The PN/NA uses the nursing process, that is, assessment, planning, implementation, and evaluation in delivering nursing care in all settings
H. The PN/NA practices within the legal and ethical boundaries for the province/territory

CONTINUING EDUCATION
A. Each PN/NA has the responsibility to maintain competency and increase level of knowledge

B. The rapid growth of medical knowledge and advances in technology make it necessary that PN/NAs keep up to date
C. The PN/NA must take advantage of learning opportunities through in-service programs where employed; attending seminars and workshops available through institutions and schools, official, or voluntary organizations; and reading professional journals
D. Membership in nursing organizations provides continuing education opportunities, usually at a lower cost to their members

LEGISLATION RELATED TO THE PRACTICE OF PRACTICAL NURSING IN CANADA

A. Legislation
1. Nursing is subject to legislation passed by each province/territory
2. Laws pertaining to nursing are specific to each province/territory
3. The regulating body is designated through legislation in each province/territory
4. Each province/territory designates a body to approve and review nursing schools
B. Regulatory body: each province/territory has either an independent body such as a council or a college or a professional association responsible for the practice of its members
C. Registration/licensure
1. Each province/territory determines the title held by the PN/NA in that jurisdiction
2. Registration/licensure ensures the public of a minimum standard of safe nursing care
3. Registration protects the title of the registrant only; licensure also protects the practice of nursing
4. Licenses are usually renewed annually
5. Licenses may be revoked or suspended for acts of misconduct, negligence, or incompetence as outlined in legislation
D. Examination
1. All provinces and territories except Quebec purchase the Canadian Nurse Association examinations
2. The CNA examination for PN/NAs is held three times a year, in January, May, and September
3. All provinces and territories administer the examination on the same day
4. Passing scores are determined by each province or territory; 350 is generally required
5. Quebec administers its own examinations

CANADIAN NURSING ORGANIZATIONS

A. Membership
1. The PN/NA has the responsibility to join a professional organization and support PN/NAs by becoming an active member
2. Membership provides
   a. Fellowship and interaction with other PN/NAs
   b. Opportunity to enhance and strengthen role of PN/NAs
   c. Means to keep current on issues relating to the PN/NA
   d. A voice in planning policies of the association
   e. Continuing education opportunities
   f. Malpractice insurance (most provinces)

B. Canadian Association of Practical Nursing/Nursing Assistants (CAPNNA)
1. CAPNNA (formerly CAPNA) was formed in 1971 and incorporated in 1975. CAPNNA is a voluntary association currently representing members of associations from all provinces and the territories with the exception of Quebec. It can be accessed through each organization
2. Membership includes
   a. Association member: a member of any provincial or territorial association of PNs/NAs that belongs to CAPNNA
   b. Affiliate member: individual PNs/NAs from province or territories that do not belong to CAPNNA are entitled to membership upon payment of the prescribed annual fee
3. CAPNNA objectives are
   a. To promote the concept of health
   b. To promote the high standards and uniformity of nursing education to achieve reciprocity
   c. To interpret and promote the Practical Nurse/Nursing Assistant role on the health team
   d. To safeguard the interest, professional identity, and practice of the Practical Nurse/Nursing Assistant
   e. To promote and encourage an attitude of mutual understanding and unity among all provincial and/or territorial associations
   f. To safeguard and promote the autonomy and self-governance of the Practical Nurse/Nursing Assistant
   g. To promote nursing research that facilitates the provision of quality nursing care for the people of Canada
   h. To participate in the provision and development of an effective, efficient, patient-centered interdisciplinary approach to the delivery of health care services

TRENDS IN DELIVERY OF HEALTH CARE

A. Traditionally the health care focus was on diagnosis and treatment of disease
B. Trends
1. Emphasis on prevention of illness and maintenance of health
2. Decrease in length of hospital stay
3. Rise in home health care
C. Reason for changes in delivery of health care
1. Technological advances: scientific knowledge has provided early diagnosis and effective treatment of diseases
2. Consumer movement: the public has exerted pressure for the right to health at an affordable price through legislative action
3. Population change: life expectancy has significantly increased with an increase in the number of elderly and a declining birth rate
4. Nature of disease pattern is changing: decrease in acute diseases with an increase in chronic and degenerative diseases
5. Continuing scrutiny of health care costs
D. Related health problems
1. Growing technology and use of complex scientific equipment has caused
   a. Increase in cost of health care; even a short hospitalization can be financially crippling

b. Fragmentation of care caused by increased number of health workers required by technology
2. Increased population has caused health problems related to air, noise, and water pollution with overcrowding and unsanitary living conditions
3. Aging population: more likely for elderly persons to become ill and to develop chronic and degenerative diseases
4. Uneven distribution of health care facilities and resources available to
   a. Elderly, poor, and minorities
   b. Rural areas and inner cities
5. Cost capitation: managed care strategy that provides a fixed payment for all members (patients) for each pay period (usually a year); profit attained by keeping patients out of expensive care setting; focuses on health promotion for cost containment; risk for patient related to denied payment for expensive, high-tech treatments

Disease Prevention and Maintenance of Health

LEVELS OF HEALTH CARE

A. Primary
   1. Promotion of health and prevention of disease including
      a. Immunization against infectious diseases
      b. Health education such as nutrition counseling
      c. Physical fitness program
      d. Research to find cause of disease
   2. Primary care takes place in prenatal centers, well-baby centers, schools, and health maintenance organizations
B. Secondary
   1. Early diagnosis and treatment to stop progress of disease
   2. Prevention of complications
   3. The largest and most expensive segment of the health care delivery system
   4. Secondary care usually takes place in hospitals, but also occurs in clinics and physicians' offices
C. Tertiary
   1. Rehabilitation after illness to return the patient to a level of maximum functioning
   2. Involves assessing patient's strengths and weaknesses, assisting the patient to increase strengths and cope with limitations, assisting with rehabilitation measures, and encouraging self-care
   3. Agencies providing tertiary care are rehabilitation hospitals, skilled nursing homes, and hospices
   4. Other groups involved with rehabilitation are special interest groups such as Alcoholics Anonymous and Reach to Recovery

BARRIERS TO PREVENTIVE HEALTH CARE

A. High cost
   1. Preventive measures not always covered under insurance plan
   2. Lower socioeconomic groups unable to finance cost
B. Inconvenience
   1. Clinics usually open during day
   2. Difficult to get appointment with physician
C. Unpleasantness of diagnostic or treatment measures accompanied by fear of pain
D. Fear of findings causes many to seek care only after symptoms are acute

ROLE OF LP/VN

A. To act as a role model by promoting personal health
   1. Assess own health status through regular physical and dental examinations
   2. Observe basic principles of personal hygiene and avoid products known to be harmful to health such as tobacco and drugs
   3. Provide for adequate rest, sleep, and nutrition
   4. Participate in primary care programs
   5. Obtain treatment of any infection or injury
B. LP/VN functions within the health care system
   1. Promote health: patient teaching
   2. Prevention of disease: provide safe environment for patients; encourage and participate in screening programs
   3. Discovery and treatment of disease by assisting physician with patient's physical examination, making observations, collecting specimens and data, and performing procedures as ordered
   4. Rehabilitation: assist patients with rehabilitation procedures

HEALTH CARE AGENCIES

A. The LP/VN should know what resources are available, what services they provide, and how to make use of the services
B. International agency
   1. The World Health Organization (WHO) is an agency of the United Nations established in 1948
   2. WHO assists nations to strengthen and improve their health services by providing advisory service in disease control
C. Official agencies in the United States—federal, state, and local—are supported by tax dollars and are accountable to the public
   1. Department of Health and Human Services (DHHS)
      a. Administration of federal programs relating to health is under the jurisdiction of the DHHS
      b. The DHHS has five divisions
         (1) Social Security Administration (SSA): administers the national system of health, old age, survivor, and disability insurance
         (2) Health Care Financing Administration (HCFA) created in 1977 to oversee the Medicare and Medicaid programs
         (3) Office of Human Development Services: administers programs on aging, children, youth and families, and native Americans
         (4) Public Health Service (PHS): involved with improving and protecting the health and environment of the United States; the major components of the PHS include
            (a) Centers for Disease Control and Prevention (CDC)
            (b) Food and Drug Administration (FDA)
            (c) Health Resources and Services Administration (HRA)
            (d) National Institutes of Health (NIH)
            (e) Alcohol, Drug Abuse, and Mental Health Administration
         (5) Family Support Administration
   2. State health departments
      a. Supported by tax funds from the state

b. Functions vary among the states; usually responsible for licensing of hospitals, nursing homes, and undertakers; health education materials; vital statistics; and communicable disease control
3. Local health department functions also vary; the general functions include
  a. Keeping vital statistics
  b. Reporting communicable disease
  c. Maternal and child health services
  d. Environmental sanitation; inspecting food establishments
D. Voluntary agencies
1. Depend on voluntary contributions for funds
2. Concerned with prevention and solution of specific health problem
3. Provide funds for research and educational projects
4. National organizations function through state or local chapters; examples of voluntary agencies are
  a. The American Cancer Society
  b. The American Diabetes Association
  c. The American Heart Association
  d. The American Red Cross
  e. The National Society for the Prevention of Blindness
E. Health service providers: presently a realignment of services is shifting care from acute hospital settings to ambulatory and home care
1. Hospitals
  a. Short-term facilities provide acute care for patients undergoing treatment for health problems
  b. Long-term facilities provide service over an extended period for patients with chronic or long-term health problems; rehabilitation as well as recreational and occupational therapy are stressed
2. Nursing homes, also called long-term or extended-care facilities; the federal government has established two categories of nursing homes
  a. Skilled nursing facility (SNF), which provides 24-hour nursing service for the recuperating resident who no longer needs intensive nursing but still requires skilled nursing
  b. Intermediate care facility (ICF), which provides regular nursing care, but not around the clock, for residents not capable of living by themselves
3. Hospices
  a. Care provided to assist the terminally ill patient to achieve the highest possible quality of life
  b. The goal is to maintain the patient in his or her own environment
  c. Care is provided in the home by home care nurses
4. Home care
  a. Provides continuity and comprehensive health service for individuals who do not need to be hospitalized but who require more than ambulatory care
  b. Services provided vary from homemaker services to skilled nursing care
  c. Estimated skilled nursing care may be provided at one third of the cost of hospitalization
5. Ambulatory care: care provided on outpatient basis
6. Geriatric day-care centers: patients are cared for during the day at the center and returned home during the evening

F. Financing health care
1. Health maintenance organizations (HMOs)
  a. Provide comprehensive health services to participants on a prepaid basis
  b. Emphasize primary care to prevent costly illness and hospitalization
  c. Do not cover illness outside service area
2. Related health insurance plans/organizations
  a. Preferred provider organization (PPO): network of health care agencies that offer insurance plan enrollees services at reduced rates; cost is higher for medical service from outside providers
  b. Exclusive provider organization (EPO): PPO insurance plan that does not reimburse for services of providers outside the network
  c. Point of service (POS): plan that uses a primary care physician to refer patients to additional services within the plan; unauthorized use of services costs more
3. Medicare and Medicaid are government-supported health insurance programs created in 1965 by an amendment to the Social Security Act
  a. Medicare, title XVIII, provides medical care to older adults receiving Social Security benefits regardless of their need, to people with permanent disabilities, and to those with end stages of renal disease
  b. Medicaid, title XIX, was designed to defray expenses that Medicare did not provide for older adults in need; it also provides services for the poor; program is jointly sponsored with matching funds from federal and state governments; today the states contribute a larger share than the federal government
4. Diagnosis-related groups (DRGs)/managed care
  a. DRGs established to determine Medicare reimbursement, averages costs of care based on diagnosis. Being phased out because of managed care systems
  b. Managed care: various methods for financing and organizing the delivery of health care in which costs are lowered by controlling the provision of services
  c. Both DRGs and managed care have caused early discharges, decreased acute care census, and reevaluation of need for in-hospital care for many diagnoses

FACTORS INFLUENCING HEALTH-ILLNESS
Growth and Development of the Adult
A. Growth is change in physical size and functioning
B. Development is change in psychosocial functioning
C. Growth and development progress from the simple to the complex and in orderly sequences
D. Individuals grow and develop at different rates
E. Most growth has occurred by adulthood
F. Certain tasks must be accomplished in each stage of development
G. Stages cannot be skipped; each must be accomplished before the next
H. Stages and tasks of adult development
1. Young adulthood (18 to 40 years)
  a. Characteristics
    (1) The "prime" of biological life
    (2) Reproductive capacity is at its height
    (3) A generally healthy period of life

b. Tasks
   (1) Developing a set of personal moral values
   (2) Establishing a personal identity and lifestyle
   (3) Establishing intimate relationships outside the family
   (4) Establishing own family/support unit
   (5) Establishing a career: a field of work
   (6) Achieving independence

2. Middle adulthood (40 to 65 years)
  a. Characteristics
   (1) Physical changes develop gradually: diminishing strength, energy, and endurance, wrinkles, graying and loss of hair, changes in vision, menopause, and weight increases
   (2) Beginning of chronic illnesses: cancer and heart disease
   (3) Decreased demands of parenthood, with children achieving independence
   (4) Increased demands of aged parents
   (5) Expected period of work and financial success
   (6) A period sometimes involving crisis: the "empty nest," realization that lifelong dreams are yet unmet
  b. Tasks
   (1) Adjusting to changes: physical, family, and social
   (2) Recognizing own mortality
   (3) Developing concern beyond the family: future generations and society in general

3. Older adulthood (over 65 years)
  a. Characteristics
   (1) Much variation in levels of functioning and health
   (2) Retirement often brings fixed income
   (3) Most are undergoing the normal physical changes of the aging process
   (4) Most maintain active lifestyles
  b. Tasks
   (1) Adjusting to loss of friends and family members
   (2) Adapting to the physical changes of the aging process
   (3) Adapting to psychosocial changes: relationships with children, retirement, housing
   (4) Review life and prepare for death

4. Development of the family
  a. Understanding the patient's role in the family, the influence of the family on the patient, and the developmental stage of the family helps to better understand the patient and his or her feelings and needs
  b. Characteristics
   (1) Traditional: wife, husband, and perhaps children
   (2) Nontraditional but common
    (a) Single parent (usually the mother) as a result of death, divorce, or never having been married
    (b) Communal: unrelated adults with or without children in a group setting
  c. Stages and tasks
   (1) Marriage
    (a) Establishing a home
    (b) Establishing individual responsibilities

    (c) Establishing a gratifying sexual relationship
    (d) Establishing good communication
   (2) Child-rearing stage
    (a) Taking on new responsibilities: financial and maintaining an optimal atmosphere for growth and development
    (b) Continuing efforts to maintain communication among all family members
    (c) Adapting to changes that occur as children become independent
   (3) Postparental stage
    (a) A crisis period caused by lifestyle changes, or
    (b) A relaxed period with fewer parental demands
    (c) More time available for hobbies and personal pleasures

Environmental (External) Factors

A. Physical agents
  1. Heat: may lead to heat exhaustion or heat stroke
  2. Ultraviolet rays of the sun: produce sunburn
  3. Cold: may cause hypothermia, frostbite, or even death, especially in the very young or very old
  4. Electric current: may cause shock, burns, or death

B. Chemical agents
  1. Taken accidentally or intentionally
  2. Taken by ingestion, such as medicine overdose
  3. Inhaled, such as gases, insecticidal sprays, and factory emissions

C. Cultural background: the beliefs and practices common to a group of people and passed down from generation to generation
  1. Cultural practices influence food habits, reactions to illness, family interactions, and health practices
  2. The nurse needs to be aware of patient's cultural practices and beliefs to meet needs in a way most beneficial to the patient

D. Religious background
  1. Religious practices may affect health practices
  2. Complying with a patient's religious practices may help reduce anxiety during illness
  3. Must be aware of the patient: may follow all, some, or none of the religion's practices; may turn to or completely away from them while ill
  4. The nurse must know the practices of the major religions and learn about others when the occasion arises to best meet the patient's needs (Table 2-1)

E. Socioeconomic level
  1. Economic level may influence accessibility of health care
  2. Lack of social and economic resources may contribute to disturbed mental health
  3. Substandard living accommodations and sanitation may predispose to diseases such as tuberculosis

F. Infectious agents
  1. Microorganisms: small living organisms that can only be seen with a microscope
   a. Pathogens: disease-producing organisms
   b. Nonpathogens: organisms that do not usually cause disease

TABLE 2-1 Common Religious Practices

Religion	Clergy	Sabbath	Practices
Judaism Reform Conservative Orthodox	Rabbi	Sundown Friday to sundown Saturday	Observation of Kosher laws Meat and dairy products not served at the same meal No pork products Only fish with scales and fins may be eaten Circumcision of male child Are excused from dietary practices when ill
Protestantism Episcopal Methodist Presbyterian Baptist Others	Priest Minister	Sunday	Sacraments of baptism and communion
Catholicism Roman Others	Priest	Sunday	Sacraments of baptism, confession, communion, confirmation, marriage, holy orders, anointing of the sick (last rites) Critically ill infants may be baptized by the nurse Abstention from meat on Ash Wednesday and on Fridays during Lent (40 days from Ash Wednesday to Easter) Some still abstain from meat on all Fridays Many feel they must attend mass each week—can be performed at the bedside
Jehovah's Witnesses	Every member is a minister	Sunday	Do not accept blood products
Seventh Day Adventists	Elder	Sundown Friday to sundown Saturday	Abstain from pork and pork products
Islam	Imam	Friday	Alcohol and pork products are forbidden
The Church of Jesus of Latter-Day Saints (Mormons)	Elder	Sunday	Abstain from tobacco, coffee, tea, colas, alcohol

   c. Normal flora: microorganisms that normally live on or in an individual's body
2. Types of microorganisms
   a. Bacteria
   b. Viruses
   c. Fungi
   d. Protozoa
   e. Rickettsia

Internal Factors

A. Congenital factors
   1. Defined as being present at birth
   2. Defects may be hereditary, caused by malformation during intrauterine life, or a result of birth injuries
   3. Maternal infections, such as German measles, during the first trimester of pregnancy often result in congenital defects
   4. Certain drugs, including alcohol, are implicated in congenital defects
B. Hereditary factors
   1. Defined as being transmitted via the genes from parents to offspring
   2. Can produce conditions such as phenylketonuria (PKU), hemophilia, or sickle cell disease
C. Body defense mechanisms
   1. Methods used by the body to protect itself from invasion by disease-producing substances
   2. First barriers are unbroken skin and mucous membranes
   3. Tears wash foreign particles including some microorganisms from the eyes
   4. The normally acid secretions of the vagina usually destroy pathogens
   5. Cilia (hairlike projections) in the nose, trachea, and bronchi sweep pathogens out of the respiratory tract
   6. Reflexes such as coughing and sneezing rid the body of pathogens
   7. Inflammatory reaction
     a. A local reaction that occurs when tissue is injured by physical agents, chemical agents, or microorganisms
     b. Signs: redness, heat, pain, swelling, and limited movement
     c. After an injury the inflammatory process begins: there is increased blood flow to the area; leukocytes move out of capillaries to the area; phagocytes begin

TABLE 2-2   Principal Electrolytes

Principal Electrolytes	Normal Serum Value	Problems Associated With Excess	Problems Associated With Deficit
Na^+ (sodium)	134-145 mEq/L	Dry mucous membranes, thirst, restlessness	Confusion, weakness, coma (hyponatremia)
K^+ (potassium)	3.6-5 mEq/L	Nausea, vomiting, diarrhea, irritability, cardiac standstill (hyperkalemia)	Weakness, cardiac arrhythmias (hypokalemia)
Ca^{++} (calcium)	9-11 mg/dl	Nausea, vomiting, muscle weakness (hypercalcemia)	Muscle cramps, tetany, convulsions (hypocalcemia)

to engulf and digest bacteria; pus forms from dead pathogens and dead tissue; healing begins

    d. Conditions caused by inflammation commonly end with the suffix itis, (e.g., vaginitis and cystitis)

8. Immune response
    a. The body's response to the invasion of foreign protein substances: bacteria, viruses, foods, chemicals, and tissue
    b. Antigen: any invading substance that can trigger the immune response
    c. Antibody: proteins (gamma globulins) produced by the body to defend against the invading antigen

D. Immunity
1. The state of being resistant to a particular pathogen
2. Active immunity: occurs when the individual produces his or her own antibodies
    a. Results naturally after having had a specific disease such as chickenpox, or
    b. Acquired after the administration of
      (1) Vaccines made up of living or killed organisms such as the measles vaccine
      (2) Toxoids made of neutralized toxins (poisons) produced by bacteria such as tetanus
3. Passive immunity: results from receiving antibodies developed by another source (animal or human)
    a. Received naturally by fetus from mother: lasts only about 6 months
    b. Acquired from the administration of
      (1) Immune serum, usually from animals: provides short-term immunity to a specific organism such as that causing rabies
      (2) Gamma globulin, usually from humans: also provides short-term immunity to a specific organism such as hepatitis
4. Autoimmunity
    a. Antibodies are produced by the body against its own tissues
    b. Thought to be a factor in diseases such as rheumatoid arthritis and rheumatic fever

E. Fluid and electrolyte balance
1. 50% to 60% of adult body weight is body fluid
2. 75% to 80% of a young child's weight is body fluid
3. Body fluids consist mostly of water
4. Electrolytes are substances that when dissolved in water become electrically charged ions (Table 2-2)

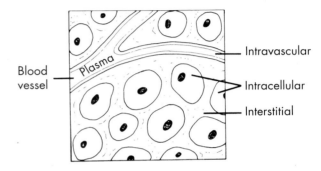

Figure 2-1.   Body fluid compartments. Intracellular, inside the cells; extracellular, outside the cells. Extracellular compartments may be either interstitial, between the cells, or intravascular, in the vessels.

5. Amounts of fluid and electrolytes must be normal at all times for the body to be in homeostasis (a state of equilibrium)
6. Fluids and electrolytes are present in "compartments" but constantly flow between the compartments to maintain balance (Figure 2-1)

F. Tissue and wound healing
1. Healing is affected by a person's general condition, age, nutritional status, the blood supply to the area, and extent of the injury
2. Many injured tissues are repaired by cell regeneration: cells replaced by identical or similar cells
    a. Tissues of the skin, digestive and respiratory tracts, and bone regenerate well
    b. Nervous, muscle, and elastic tissues have little ability to regenerate
3. When regeneration cannot take place, granulation tissue is formed, which eventually becomes a scar
4. Formation of scar tissue often leaves disfigurement, such as after burns, or diminished function, such as in heart tissue after myocardial infarction
5. Types of wounds
    a. Incision: clean wound made by sharp instrument
    b. Contusion: closed wound; bruise; made with blunt force; underlying tissue is damaged
    c. Abrasion: rubbed or scraped off skin or mucous membrane

TABLE 2-3   Wound Healing

Type of Healing	Type of Wound	How Healing Occurs
First intention	Minimal tissue damage Simple incision	Without infection No separation of wound edges Results in minimal scar
Second intention	Decubitus ulcer Severe burn	Wound edges do not join Spaces between wound edges fill with granulation tissue Results in scar
Third intention	Dehisced suture line	Wound edges come together at first, then reopen Results in scar and possibly contraction of surrounding tissue

    d. Puncture: small opening or hole made by a pointed instrument
    e. Laceration: tear or rip leaving jagged edges
  6. Wound healing is classified by first, second, or third intention (Table 2-3)

CONCEPTS BASIC TO NURSING
Reducing the Spread of Microorganisms
A. Infectious disease chain
  1. Presence of pathogenic organisms
  2. A susceptible host: susceptibility affected by
    a. Nutritional status
    b. Age
    c. Personal health habits
    d. Medical treatments in progress (radiation therapy and bone marrow–depressing drugs)
    e. Trauma
    f. Chronic illness
    g. Stress
    h. Fatigue
  3. Portal of entry to the body: break in skin or mucous membrane, vaginal opening, or blood
  4. Reservoir: Microorganisms multiply and increase in number in the bladder, lungs, or throat
  5. Modes of transmission (movement/spread) of microorganisms
    a. By contact (excreta or used tissues)
    b. By air, on droplets (sneezing and coughing)
    c. On fomites (books and stethoscopes)
    d. In food or water
    e. By vectors (animals and insects)
  6. Portal of exit from the body: mouth, nose, rectum, skin, blood, or reproductive tract
B. Measures to reduce the spread by breaking the chain (interrupting the process)
  1. Hand washing: most important measure
  2. Medical asepsis: practices that limit the numbers, growth, and spread of microorganisms (clean technique)
    a. Linens: no shaking or holding against uniform
    b. Use of antiseptics and disinfectants
    c. Anything touching the floor is not to be used
  3. Surgical asepsis: practices that eliminate microorganisms and their spores from sterile items or areas (sterile technique)
    a. Used in operative procedures, delivery room, and caring for patients with breaks in skin and for proce-

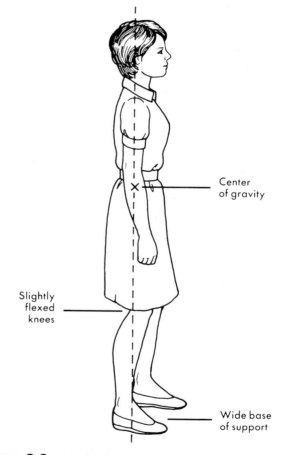

Figure 2-2.   Body alignment. Lateral view of adult with alignment of head, neck, spine, slightly flexed knees, and wide base of support. (Adapted from Sorrentino SA: *Textbook for nursing assistants,* ed 5, St Louis, 2000, Mosby.)

Center of gravity
Slightly flexed knees
Wide base of support

dures that enter sterile body cavities (e.g., bladder, lung, and vein)
    b. General principles
      (1) Sterile items become nonsterile (contaminated) when touched by anything that is not sterile
      (2) Sterile field that becomes wet is considered nonsterile
      (3) Sterile items out of eyesight or below waist level are considered nonsterile

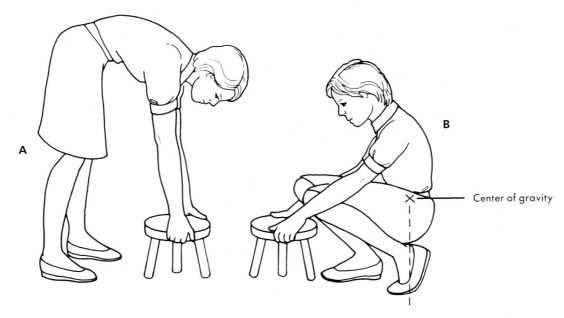

Figure 2-3. **A,** Lifting with poor body mechanics: using back muscles. **B,** Lifting with good body mechanics: using leg muscles with object close to body. (Adapted from Sorrentino SA: *Textbook for nursing assistants,* ed 5, St Louis, 2000, Mosby.)

(4) Nurses need to develop a sterile conscience (self-judgment of whether aseptic practices have been broken) and act accordingly
  c. Means of sterilization
    (1) Steam under pressure: autoclave
    (2) Boiling
    (3) Liquid chemicals
    (4) Gas
4. Isolation and barrier techniques (protective asepsis): practices that limit the transfer of microorganisms either from the infected person or to a highly susceptible person
  a. Category-specific isolation
    (1) Enteric: to reduce spread of pathogens via feces (e.g., hepatitis A)
    (2) Respiratory: to reduce spread of pathogens through the air (e.g., pneumonia)
    (3) TB isolation: to reduce exposure in health care settings; gown and particulate respirator mask, patient in negative air pressure isolation room
    (4) Strict: to reduce spread of pathogens by air or contact (e.g., chickenpox)
    (5) Drainage/secretion: to reduce spread of pathogens by contact with the infected person or contaminated articles (linens) (e.g., draining wounds)
    (6) Universal blood and body fluid (universal precautions): used by everyone to prevent transmission by direct or indirect contact with blood or body fluids (e.g., AIDS)
    (7) Care of severely compromised patients: to protect a highly susceptible person (with lowered resistance) from becoming infected (e.g., leukemia)

  b. Disease-specific isolation: each disease receives its specific protective measures—historically used for tuberculosis, not used much anymore
  c. Standard precautions: guidelines recommended by the CDC to control and reduce the risk of transmission of blood-borne and other pathogens; a combination of Universal (Blood and Body Fluid) Precautions and Body Substance Isolation; applies features to all patients receiving care regardless of diagnosis or presumed infection status; applies to blood, all body fluids, nonintact skin, and mucous membranes
C. Types of infections
  1. Nosocomial: acquired as a result of hospitalization
  2. Local: confined to a relatively small, specific area (e.g., a wound)
  3. Systemic: infection spreads throughout body

Body Mechanics

A. Defined as efficient use of the body's structure and muscles
B. Applies to patients as well as nurses
C. Use of good body mechanics helps to prevent injuries, conserve energy, and prevent fatigue
D. Principles of good body mechanics
  1. Maintain proper alignment (posture): head, neck, and spine should be in a straight line with feet 10 to 12 inches (25 to 31 cm) apart and pointed straight ahead and knees slightly flexed (Figure 2-2)
  2. Maintain a wide base of support: keep feet separated to provide balance (see Figure 2-2)
  3. Keep center of gravity directly above the base of support (see Figure 2-2)
E. Points to remember
  1. Use largest and strongest muscles (legs, arms, and shoulders) when moving or lifting heavy objects (Figure 2-3)

2. Do not let your back do the work
3. Roll, slide, push, or pull an object rather than lift it
4. Keep objects close to your body when lifting or moving; avoid reaching, twisting or bending unnecessarily
5. Point feet in the direction of movement
6. Use devices whenever possible: patient lifters, trapeze, turning sheets, and rolling carts
7. Get assistance when necessary
8. Have the patient help as much as possible when being moved or lifted

Communication

A. Definition: exchange of messages between two or more people, including information, thoughts, and feelings
B. Purposes in nursing
   1. To establish a meaningful, helping relationship between nurse and patient
   2. To transmit information between health care workers
C. Means
   1. Verbal
   2. Written
   3. Nonverbal
D. Guidelines
   1. Verbal communication
      a. Introduce self, stating name and title
      b. Be sincerely interested in the patient
      c. Be an attentive, active listener
      d. Stand or sit close to the patient
      e. Allow the patient to express thoughts and feelings freely without fear of being judged
      f. Clarify what has been said to ensure understanding
      g. Ask open-ended questions rather than questions resulting in yes or no answers, "What has happened to change your mind?"
      h. Use incomplete sentences: "you are afraid that . . ."
      i. Report information accurately and thoroughly
      j. Report abnormal findings immediately
      k. Maintain confidentiality
   2. Written communication
      a. Record information clearly, concisely, and accurately
      b. Nurses' notes are part of a legal document
         (1) Use pen
         (2) Use only standard abbreviations
         (3) Do not erase or obliterate errors (Figure 2-4)
         (4) Leave no blank spaces
         (5) Sign the note at the time it is written
         (6) Date and time each entry
      c. Formats for nurses' notes
         (1) Narrative: in paragraph form (Figure 2-5, B)
         (2) SOAP: Subjective data, Objective data, Assessment, Plan (Figure 2-5, A)
         (3) PIE: Problem, Intervention, Evaluation
         (4) Focus charting: Data (assessment); Action (planning/implementation); Response (evaluation) (Figure 2-5, C)

      (5) Charting by exception: used with flow sheets, pertinent data charted at beginning shift, only changes in treatments or patient condition noted after that; must include details on patient status for accurate monitoring
   3. Nonverbal communication
      a. Exchanging messages by body posture, movements, gestures, and touch
      b. Often a more accurate expression of what is being thought or felt than verbal expression

Basic Human Needs

A. Definition: described by the psychologist Abraham Maslow as those needs that must be met for humans to function at their highest possible level
B. Used by many nurses as a systematic guide for assessment
C. Premises
   1. There is a hierarchy of needs; lower level needs must be met before higher level ones can be addressed
   2. People will usually be able to meet their own needs
   3. When people are unable to meet their own needs, intervention is required
   4. In caring for the whole person, the nurse is involved in helping to meet the basic needs as well as in dealing with signs and symptoms of disease
   5. Chronological age is not a variable in ascending the hierarchy of needs
D. Hierarchy of needs (Figure 2-6)
   1. Physiological: oxygen, water, food, elimination, rest and sleep, activity, sexuality, and relief of pain
   2. Safety and security: protection from injury, maintenance of body defenses, structure and order in both the environment and relationships, and freedom from anxiety
   3. Love and belonging: not just romantic love but a feeling of affection (the need for caring relationships)
   4. Esteem: a feeling of worth and value to both self and others
   5. Self-actualization: reaching one's fullest potential

THE NURSING PROCESS

A. Definition: a set of predetermined steps used by nurses to identify and to help solve patient problems
B. Purposes
   1. To provide planned, coordinated, and individualized patient care
   2. To communicate problems and approaches among all those providing patient care

4/18/92	PROBLEM #6 – Drainage on Cast, ⓛ
4PM	lateral aspect of knee
	S – "I have no pain or numbness."
	O – Toes pink, warm, mobile. VS stable
	A – Normal postoperative drainage
	P – Mark area of drainage. Reassess
	patient and cast q ½ hr.
	Elaine Stevens, L.P.N.

A

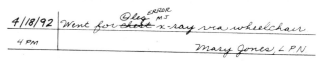

| 4/18/92 | Went for ~~chest~~ leg x-ray via wheelchair |
| 4 PM | *Mary Jones, L.P.N.* |

Figure 2-4.   Correcting an error in a nurse's note.

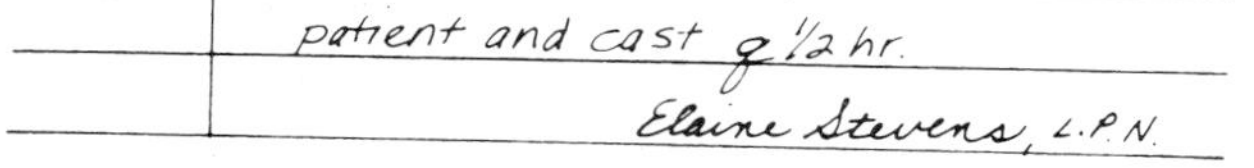

Figure 2-5.   **A,** Nurse's note in SOAP format.

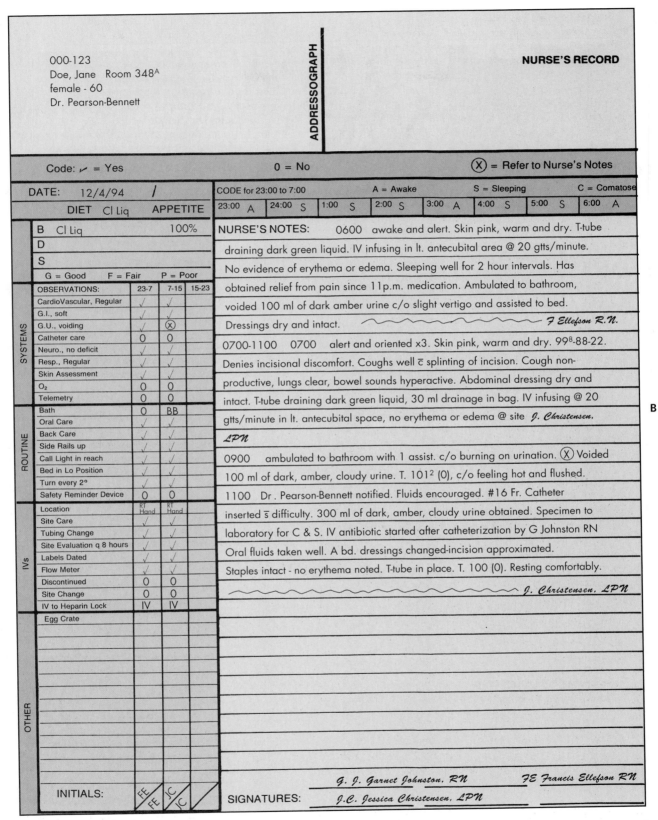

ADDRESSOGRAPH	NURSE'S RECORD
000-123 Doe, Jane Room 348ᴬ female - 60 Dr. Pearson-Bennett	

Code: ✓ = Yes	0 = No	Ⓧ = Refer to Nurse's Notes

DATE: 12/4/94 /	CODE for 23:00 to 7:00	A = Awake	S = Sleeping	C = Comatose

DIET Cl Liq APPETITE	23:00 A	24:00 S	1:00 S	2:00 S	3:00 A	4:00 S	5:00 S	6:00 A

NURSE'S NOTES: 0600   awake and alert. Skin pink, warm and dry. T-tube draining dark green liquid. IV infusing in lt. antecubital area @ 20 gtts/minute. No evidence of erythema or edema. Sleeping well for 2 hour intervals. Has obtained relief from pain since 11p.m. medication. Ambulated to bathroom, voided 100 ml of dark amber urine c/o slight vertigo and assisted to bed. Dressings dry and intact. ～～～～～～～～～ *F Ellefson R.N.*

0700-1100   0700   alert and oriented x3. Skin pink, warm and dry. 99^8-88-22. Denies incisional discomfort. Coughs well c̄ splinting of incision. Cough non-productive, lungs clear, bowel sounds hyperactive. Abdominal dressing dry and intact. T-tube draining dark green liquid, 30 ml drainage in bag. IV infusing @ 20 gtts/minute in lt. antecubital space, no erythema or edema @ site *J. Christensen.*

LPN

0900   ambulated to bathroom with 1 assist. c/o burning on urination. Ⓧ Voided 100 ml of dark, amber, cloudy urine. T. 101^2 (0), c/o feeling hot and flushed.

1100   Dr. Pearson-Bennett notified. Fluids encouraged. #16 Fr. Catheter inserted s̄ difficulty. 300 ml of dark, amber, cloudy urine obtained. Specimen to laboratory for C & S. IV antibiotic started after catheterization by G Johnston RN Oral fluids taken well. A bd. dressings changed-incision approximated. Staples intact - no erythema noted. T-tube in place. T. 100 (0). Resting comfortably.

～～～～～～～～～ *J. Christensen. LPN*

B Cl Liq		100%
D		
S		
G = Good	F = Fair	P = Poor

	OBSERVATIONS:	23-7	7-15	15-23
SYSTEMS	CardioVascular, Regular	√	√	
	G.I., soft	√	√	
	G.U., voiding	√	Ⓧ	
	Catheter care	0	0	
	Neuro., no deficit	√	√	
	Resp., Regular	√	√	
	Skin Assessment	√	√	
	O₂	0	0	
	Telemetry	0	0	
ROUTINE	Bath	0	BB	
	Oral Care	√	√	
	Back Care	√	√	
	Side Rails up	√	√	
	Call Light in reach	√	√	
	Bed in Lo Position	√	√	
	Turn every 2°	√	√	
	Safety Reminder Device	0	0	
IVs	Location	RT Hand	RT Hand	
	Site Care	√	√	
	Tubing Change	√	√	
	Site Evaluation q 8 hours	√	√	
	Labels Dated	√	√	
	Flow Meter	√	√	
	Discontinued	0	0	
	Site Change	0	0	
	IV to Heparin Lock	IV	IV	
OTHER	Egg Crate			

INITIALS:	FE / FE	JC / JC	

SIGNATURES: *G. J. Garnet Johnston. RN*   *FE Francis Ellefson RN*
J.C. Jessica Christensen. LPN

Figure 2-5—cont'd.   **B,** Narrative charting.   *Continued*

DATE	12/7	
TIME	FOCUS	NURSES NOTES
1400	post-op pain	Ambulating in hall c̄ moderate assist. I.V. infusing
		@ 20 gtts/min. Still feels warm, main concern is
		incisional pain, splinting is helpful. Positioned in
		bed c̄ pillows for support. Medicated for pain.
		Practiced relaxation breathing exercises. *J. Christensen LPN*
1400	pain/fever	States, "I am more comfortable and relaxed now." Skin warm
		and dry. T. 99⁶ (O). c/o some burning on urination,
		less than in a.m. Taking fluids well. Urine light
		yellow and less cloudy ⟿ *J. Christensen LPN*

Figure 2-5—cont'd.   **C,** Focus charting nurse's notes.

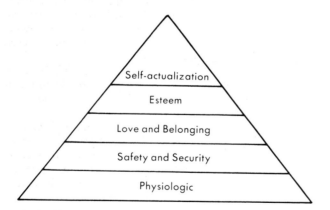

Figure 2-6.   Hierarchy of basic human needs as described by Maslow.

C. The process: names of steps differ slightly according to various sources but include the following
  1. Assessment: gathering and organizing of data; statement of patient problems (unmet needs); the nursing diagnosis
  2. Planning: setting goals to be accomplished and constructing a plan of action to accomplish the goals
  3. Implementation: carrying out the nursing actions to accomplish the goals and solve the problem (meet the need)
  4. Evaluation: determining whether the goal was accomplished and the problem solved

Assessment: A Continuous Process

A. Sources of data
  1. Patient
  2. Family or significant others
  3. Patient's chart
    a. Physician's order sheet
    b. Nurses' notes
    c. Laboratory reports
      (1) Blood chemistry
        (a) Electrolytes: see fluid and electrolyte balance
        (b) Creatinine: assesses kidney function
      (2) Complete blood count (CBC): assesses adequacy of the various blood cells: red, white, and platelets
      (3) Blood sugar (BS) or glucose: fasting (FBS) or postprandial (after meals)
    d. X-ray reports
      (1) Chest x-ray examination: assesses condition of lungs and size of heart
      (2) Upper gastrointestinal (UGI) series: assesses condition of esophagus, stomach, and duodenum with barium sulfate used as the contrast medium
      (3) Barium enema (BaE): assesses condition of colon with barium sulfate used as the contrast medium
      (4) Gallbladder series (GBS): assesses condition of the gallbladder with radiopaque dye

e. Electrocardiogram (ECG) reports: assesses the electrical activity of the heart
f. Biopsy reports: assesses a tissue specimen for cell changes
g. Progress notes of other health care workers
   (1) Physician
   (2) Social worker
   (3) Dietician
   (4) Physical therapist
   (5) Occupational therapist
   (6) Respiratory therapist
4. Nursing report
B. Subjective versus objective data
  1. Subjective data
    a. Information reported by the patient
    b. Information that is not observable by another person
      (1) Pain
      (2) Nausea
      (3) Anxiety
      (4) Dizziness
      (5) Ringing in the ears (tinnitus)
      (6) Numbness
  2. Objective data
    a. Information gathered through the senses: sight, hearing, smell, and feel
    b. Information gathered with a measuring instrument: thermometer, sphygmomanometer, and scale
      (1) Vital signs
      (2) Weight, height
      (3) Hematuria
      (4) Wheezing
      (5) Edema
      (6) Cyanosis
C. Methods of gathering data
  1. Formal interviewing (communication with patient or family or significant others): usually on patient's admission to the hospital
    a. Gather data on age, occupation, reason for hospitalization, medications, allergies, previous hospitalizations, previous illnesses, prostheses, valuables, and special diet
    b. Gather data on difficulty with activities of daily living (ADLs), sleep, elimination, activity, eating, and any special needs
  2. Listening
  3. Observation of the patient and attached equipment
    a. Use an orderly approach
      (1) Head-to-toe
      (2) System-by-system
      (3) Basic human needs
    b. Look for signs and symptoms of disease or change in disease
  4. Physical examination
    a. Methods
      (1) Inspection
      (2) Palpation
      (3) Percussion
      (4) Auscultation
    b. Assisting with the physical examination
      (1) Be sure that the patient understands the examination and why it is being done
      (2) Gather equipment

      (3) Position patient appropriately (Figure 2-7)
      (4) Drape covers to provide for privacy
      (5) Collect patient data using:
        (a) Interviewing
        (b) Auscultation
        (c) Inspection
        (d) Palpation
        (e) Examination
      (6) After the examination make the patient comfortable and safe, following orders, if any
      (7) Chart the procedure and patient's reactions; note specimens obtained
  c. The practical nurse's role in assisting with diagnostic examinations
    (1) Explain procedure to the patient
    (2) Explain and carry out specific requirements
      (a) Nothing by mouth (NPO) or special meals
      (b) Clothing
      (c) Positioning
      (d) Medications
    (3) Chest x-ray examinations: no metal objects in view of x-ray (zippers, bra fastenings, necklaces, and pins)
    (4) Blood studies: see agency's procedure manual for requirements of various studies
    (5) UGI series: nothing by mouth after midnight (NPO p- MN), medication or enema to eliminate barium after the x-ray examination
    (6) BaE: low-residue meal evening before, NPO p- MN, medications or enema to clear colon before and after x-ray examination
    (7) Excretory urogram or intravenous pyelogram (IVP): NPO p- MN, medications to clear colon before x-ray examination; uses iodine-based dye; notify physician if patient is allergic to iodine or shellfish
    (8) GBS: fat-free meal evening before, NPO p- MN, oral ingestion of dye tablets; dye is iodine based; check patient for iodine or shellfish allergy
    (9) Lumbar puncture: signed consent form is required; empty bladder and bowel before procedure; patient lies curled on side with head almost touching knees; nurse faces patient holding shoulders and knees; patient remains flat in bed after procedure
    (10) Arteriogram-visualization of an artery after injection of a radiopaque dye. Patient stays still for a period of time because of chance for bleeding at injection site
    (11) Bronchoscopy-visualization of the bronchi using a scope. Patient's throat is sometimes anesthetized. Check for a gag reflex after procedure before fluids are given
5. Measurement of vital signs: to assess functioning of cardiovascular and respiratory systems
  a. Temperature
    (1) Normal ranges
      (a) Axillary: 96° F to 98° F
      (b) Oral: 97° F to 99° F
      (c) Rectal: 98° F to 100° F
      (d) Tympanic: 97° F to 99° F

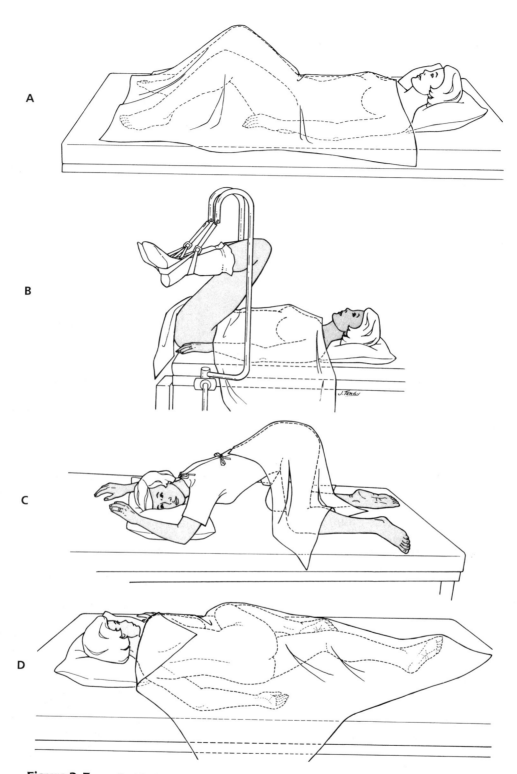

Figure 2-7. Positioning and draping for the physical examination. **A,** Dorsal recumbent position. **B,** Lithotomy position. **C,** Knee-chest position. **D,** Sims' position. (Adapted from Sorrentino SA: *Textbook for nursing assistants,* ed 5, St Louis, 2000, Mosby.)

(2) Oral temperature
- (a) Mercury thermometer left in place 2 to 4 minutes or according to agency policy
- (b) Electronic thermometer left in place until final reading is indicated
- (c) Wait 10 minutes if the patient has been eating, smoking, drinking a hot or cold beverage, or chewing gum
- (d) Contraindications
  - Patient is receiving oxygen
  - Patient is irrational or unconscious
  - Patient is under 5 years of age
  - Patient is breathing through the mouth
  - Patient is prone to seizures
  - Patient recently had oral surgery or mouth trauma
  - Patient is on suicide precautions

(3) Rectal temperature
- (a) Mercury thermometer held in place 3 to 4 minutes or according to agency policy
- (b) Electronic thermometer held in place until final reading is indicated
- (c) Lubricate before inserting; insert 1 to 1½ inches (3.75 cm)
- (d) Contraindications
  - Rectal or perineal surgery
  - Diseases of the rectum
  - Diarrhea
  - Use with caution in patients with cardiovascular disease
  - Use with caution in restless or combative patients

(4) Axillary temperature
- (a) Mercury thermometer held in place 10 minutes
- (b) Electronic thermometer held in place until final reading is indicated
- (c) Pat dry the axilla before inserting; hold arm close to side

(5) Tympanic temperature
- (a) Press "On" button and apply disposable cover on probe tip
- (b) Seal ear opening with probe; seal outer ear opening in infants
- (c) Press "Scan" button and read temperature after beeper sounds
- (d) Discard probe cover and replace thermometer in recharger
- (e) Contraindications
  - Recent exposure to cold air
  - Inflammatory ear condition
  - Excessive cerumen accumulation

b. Pulse: the beat of the heart heard at the apex or felt at specific sites as a wave of blood flows through an artery
(1) Observe rate, rhythm, and strength
(2) Normal adult range: 60 to 80 beats/min varies greatly among individuals; rate is more rapid for children
(3) If rate or rhythm is irregular, take pulse apically and count for 1 full minute

(4) Variations
- (a) Bradycardia: slow heart rate—under 60 beats/min
- (b) Tachycardia: fast heart beat—over 100 beats/min
- (c) Irregular: intervals between beats are uneven
- (d) Thready: weak pulse—easily obliterated
- (e) Bounding: very strong pulse—difficult to obliterate

(5) Sites: felt with fingertips at places where an artery crosses over muscle or bone close to the skin and at the apex of the heart
- (a) Temporal
- (b) Carotid
- (c) Brachial
- (d) Radial
- (e) Femoral
- (f) Popliteal
- (g) Pedal
- (h) Apical: heard with stethoscope

(6) Apical-radial pulse: to detect a difference between rates at the two sites (the pulse deficit)
- (a) Requires two people: one taking the radial pulse and one taking the apical pulse
- (b) Must be counted simultaneously for 1 full minute
- (c) Apical rate can never be lower than the radial rate

c. Respiration: the process of inhaling and exhaling air into and out of the lungs; one inhalation plus one exhalation equals one respiration
(1) Observe rate, rhythm, and depth; normal adult range is 14 to 20 respirations per minute; varies greatly with activity level; rate is higher for children
(2) Patient must not be aware that respirations are being observed
(3) Variations
- (a) Apnea: absence of breathing
- (b) Tachypnea: rapid breathing
- (c) Stertorous: noisy breathing; snoring
- (d) Cheyne-Stokes: rhythmic repeated cycles of slow shallow respirations increasing in depth rate, then gradually becoming slower and more shallow, followed by a period of apnea; often precedes death
- (e) Dyspnea: difficulty breathing
- (f) Orthopnea: breathing is possible only while in an upright position
- (g) Kussmaul's: paroxysms of dyspnea often preceding diabetic coma

(4) Count respirations for 1 full minute if rate is abnormal or rhythm is irregular

d. Blood pressure (BP): force exerted by the blood against the walls of the arteries (measured in millimeters [mm] of mercury [Hg])
(1) Normal adult range is 60 to 80 mm Hg diastolic, 90 to 120 mm Hg systolic, varies among individuals and with activity
(2) Can be measured at brachial artery or popliteal artery

(3) Be sure cuff is proper size for the individual
(4) Terminology
   (a) Systolic: pressure in the arteries during contraction of the heart
   (b) Diastolic: pressure in the arteries during relaxation of the heart
   (c) Hypotension: lower than normal blood pressure—under 100/60
   (d) Hypertension: higher than normal blood pressure—140/90
   (e) Pulse pressure: difference between systolic and diastolic pressures
   (f) Pulse oximetry: Noninvasive continuous monitor of blood oxygen saturation
      ■ Normal adult range: 95% to 100%
      ■ Report readings under 90%, indicate hypoxia. SaO$_2$ under 70% is life-threatening
      ■ Clip-on or adhesive probe attaches to finger, toe, earlobe, or bridge of nose
      ■ Uses light for reading; do not block light on probe. Area being assessed should be clean, dry, and without nail polish
      ■ Rotate clip q4h, adhesive-check for proper clip position with alarms
      ■ Check abnormal readings with arterial blood gases

6. Measurement of weight and height
   a. Weight
      (1) Should be done before breakfast
      (2) Should be done in same amount of clothing each day; shoes should be off
      (3) Can use results in establishing medication dosages, gain or loss of body fluid, and nutritional status
      (4) Can use standing, chair, or stretcher scale; be sure scale is balanced
   b. Height
      (1) Have patient be in bare feet, standing on a paper towel
      (2) Have patient stand tall
      (3) Can use in determining some medication dosages and anesthesia requirements

7. Collection of specimens
   a. General guidelines
      (1) Follow your agency's procedure for collection, container, labels, requisitions, and recording
      (2) Label all specimen containers correctly and send with a laboratory requisition
      (3) Send specimens to the laboratory promptly
      (4) Wear protective gloves
      (5) Wash hands thoroughly after handling specimen
   b. Urine specimens
      (1) Urinalysis: routine examination of urine
         (a) Patient and container need only be clean
         (b) Often collected as part of admission procedure
      (2) Culture and sensitivity
         (a) Clean-catch, midstream: genitalia and meatus are cleansed; specimen is taken after stream has started but before voiding is completed
         (b) Catheterized specimen: by using sterile technique and equipment
      (3) 24-hour specimens: first voiding is discarded and time is noted; all urine for the next 24 hours is collected; see agency policy for type of container and storage methods
      (4) Sugar and acetone testing
         (a) Urine should be obtained 30 to 60 minutes before meal or at designated time
         (b) Double-voided specimen gives more accurate results
            ■ Have patient empty bladder
            ■ Collect specimen as soon as patient can void again
            ■ May need additional fluids to produce specimen
         (c) Test specimen with Tes-tape, Clinitest, Clinistix, or Keto-diastix; follow manufacturer's directions precisely for accurate results
         (d) Report results immediately to medication nurse
         (e) Record results in proper place
      (5) Specimens from indwelling catheter
         (a) Closed drainage system must be maintained
         (b) Specimens must be obtained from specimen "port" with needle and syringe by sterile technique
   c. Stool specimens
      (1) Collect in clean bedpan
      (2) Use tongue depressor or wooden spatula to transfer stool to specimen container
      (3) Types of testing
         (a) For blood: occult (guaiac, Hematest); patient must be on a red meat–free diet 3 days before test
         (b) For culture and sensitivity: use sterile container
         (c) For ova and parasites: stool must still be warm when it reaches the laboratory
   d. Sputum specimens
      (1) Best collected in the morning before breakfast
      (2) Patient first rinses mouth with water
      (3) Instruct patient to take deep breath, cough deeply, and expectorate into container
      (4) Specimen must be from the lung, not just mouth saliva
   e. Blood specimen: capillary puncture, e.g., blood glucose testing. May be finger stick for child/adult, heel stick for infant. May require agency certification
      (1) Explain procedure to patient; warn that it does hurt
      (2) Assemble equipment: gloves, alcohol swab, lancet, collector, gauze or cotton ball, and adhesive bandage
      (3) Wash hands; don gloves
      (4) Enhance blood supply by applying warmth; do not milk site

(5) Puncture side of nondominant finger or side of heel

(6) Puncture with lancet; wipe away first drop of blood; collect sample

(7) Apply pressure to site; apply bandage

f. Blood specimen: venipuncture; requires puncture of vein for collection of several ml of blood for variety of laboratory tests; agency certification usually required

   (1) Explain procedure to patient; procedure hurts

   (2) Assemble equipment: gloves, tourniquet, alcohol swabs, sterile gauze pads, tape, a sharps container, appropriate vacuum tubes, vacuum adaptor, and double-ended needle

   (3) Wash hands, don gloves

   (4) Hyperextend arm for ease of access to antecubital vein; apply tourniquet; have patient make fist

   (5) Clean site with alcohol; pull skin taut from below site; insert needle (bevel up) at 5-degree angle

   (6) Once needle "pops" into vein, slide vacuum tube onto needle; remove and replace tubes as each fills

   (7) Remove final tube; loosen tourniquet; lay gauze over puncture site, remove needle and apply pressure to site

   (8) Immediately discard needle into sharps container; label tubes before leaving patient's side

g. Other specimens

   (1) Vomitus: may be tested for blood

   (2) Gastric analysis: examination of stomach contents; obtained by aspirating from nasogastric tube

   (3) Wound drainage: if infection is suspected

D. Statement of patient problems requiring nursing intervention

1. Identifying unmet basic human needs resulting in a problem for the patient

2. Identifying problems arising from the patient's signs and symptoms

3. Actual problems: those that the patient is currently having

4. Potential problems: those that may develop and should be prevented from occurring (Box 2-7)

E. Nursing diagnosis: the practical nurse assists the registered nurse in formulating nursing diagnosis

---

Box 2-7   Actual and Potential Unmet Basic Needs and Problems

Situation: At 7 AM, Mrs. Clayton tells the nurse that she has a productive cough. She states that it began about 3 AM and continues.

Actual problem: productive cough
Actual unmet need: rest and sleep
Potential unmet need: oxygen
Potential problem: decreased oxygen

Planning Patient Care

A. Definition: process of setting priorities, determining patient-centered goals, and deciding on nursing actions to achieve the goals; ends with writing of the nursing care plan

B. Setting priorities

1. Problems that are life threatening are of highest priority

2. When no single problem seems more important than the others, the patient may help determine priorities

C. Determining goals/expected outcomes

1. Stated in terms of patient behavior so that achievement can easily be evaluated

2. Whenever possible patients should be involved in setting goals

3. Long-term goals are those hoped for in the future, usually set by the registered nurse

4. Short-term goals are those sought immediately or in the near future

D. Decisions about which nursing measures to use are based on sound knowledge of current nursing practice, principles, rationales, and judgment

E. Written nursing care plan provides continuity of patient care

Implementation of Nursing Measures

A. Principles

1. Preparation

a. Nurse: must know how, when, and why measure is to be performed, checking for a physician's order when necessary

b. Patient/family/significant others

   (1) To reduce anxiety, patients need to know what measure is to be performed and why, as well as what is expected of them

   (2) May need special preparation for the specific measure: positioning, medications, attire

c. Have all necessary equipment ready and in working order

2. Performance

a. Nurse must have knowledge of and ability to perform measure and to seek help when necessary

b. Medical asepsis is always followed: surgical asepsis and standard precautions are followed as required

c. Work must be organized to conserve nurse's and patient's energy and to meet patient's need for security

d. Assessment of patient's response to the measure is ongoing

3. Aftercare

a. Patient made safe and comfortable

b. Equipment cleaned and returned to proper place or disposed of

c. Evaluation of results of the measure and whether it helped achieve the goal

4. Reporting and recording

a. Significant observations immediately

b. When the measure was performed and the results

Evaluation of Plan of Care

A. Criteria for evaluation

1. Has the need been met?

2. Is the problem solved or being solved?

3. Has the goal/expected outcome been achieved?

B. Revision of the nursing care plan
   1. Based on evaluation of effectiveness
   2. Practical nurse collaborates with the registered nurse in revising problem list, goals, and nursing measures

MEASURES TO MEET OXYGEN NEEDS

A. Assessment: color, level of consciousness, vital signs, presence of cough (productive or nonproductive), nature of sputum (amount, consistency, and color), and energy level
B. General measures
   1. Encourage exercise and activity to help expand lungs, providing better oxygenation
   2. Bedridden patients must be turned and positioned every 2 hours (q2h) to prevent pooling of secretions in the lungs and capillary congestion that may lead to decubitus ulcer formation because of tissue hypoxia
   3. Encourage coughing and deep breathing at least q2h for inactive or bedridden patients to help with oxygenation and bringing up secretions
   4. Ensure adequate fluid intake to keep secretions thin, thus easier to expectorate
C. Use of nebulizer (aerosol)
   1. Method of delivering medications directly to the respiratory tract
   2. Nebulizer breaks liquids into a mist of droplets, which are inhaled
D. Incentive spirometer: to improve inspiratory volume
   1. With lips sealed around a mouthpiece, the patient takes a deep breath, holds it for 3 seconds, and slowly exhales

   2. The spirometer indicates with a light or small plastic balls reaching an indicated level whether the patient has inhaled the desired volume
E. Intermittent positive pressure breathing (IPPB) therapy
   1. Forces the patient to inhale more deeply, allowing better oxygenation and loosening of secretions
   2. May be attached to oxygen or compressed air
   3. Humidity is provided, usually by normal saline solution
   4. Medications may be added
   5. Patient should be sitting up during treatment and encouraged to cough up secretions after treatment
F. Chest physical therapy
   1. Postural drainage: use of various positions so that gravity can assist in removal of secretions (Figure 2-8)
   2. Percussion is a manual technique of striking the chest wall over the affected area with cupped hands in a rhythmic motion
   3. Vibration is a manual compression and tremor-like motion with hands or mechanical device against chest wall of affected area done during exhalation
   4. Nurse positions patient so affected areas are vertical and gravity can assist in drainage
   5. Position also depends on diagnosis and condition
   6. Schedule before or at least 2 hours after meals. Provide emesis basin and tissues; oral hygiene after treatment
   7. This therapy is contraindicated in patients with lung abscess or tumors, pneumothorax, and diseases of the chest wall

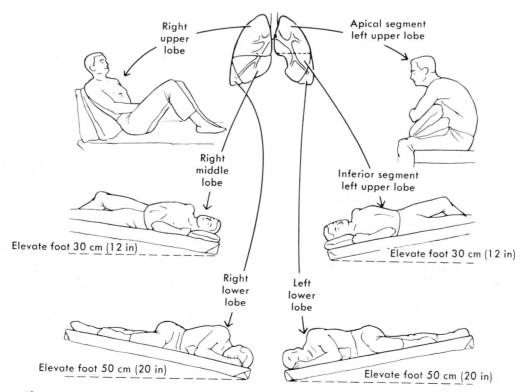

Figure 2-8.   Positions for postural drainage. (From Phipps WJ, Sands JK, Marek JF, editors: *Medical-surgical nursing: concepts and clinical practice,* ed 6, St Louis, 1999, Mosby.)

G. Suctioning: oral, nasopharyngeal, or tracheal
   1. To remove accumulated secretions blocking airway or to obtain sputum specimen
   2. Usually a sterile procedure
   3. Introduce catheter gently; do not apply suction while introducing catheter
   4. Suction intermittently for no more than 10 seconds
   5. Slowly withdraw catheter by rotating motion while suctioning continues
   6. Unless there are copious amounts of secretions, wait 30 seconds between suctionings
   7. Repeat procedure until all excess secretions are removed
   8. Administer oxygen before and between suctionings if needed
H. Administration of oxygen
   1. Safety precautions
      a. Caution patients and visitors that smoking is prohibited
      b. Post warning sign on door or bed: NO SMOKING—OXYGEN IN USE
      c. Do not use heating pads, electric blankets, or electric razors
      d. Do not use woolen blankets
      e. Secure oxygen tanks so they do not tip over
   2. Physician's order is required for method of administration, rate of oxygen flow, or concentration
   3. Oxygen must always be humidified
   4. Nasal cannula: prongs fit into nares
      a. Turn oxygen on and check flow through prongs before positioning on patient
      b. Adjust strap after placing cannula on patient
      c. Periodically check that there is sufficient water in humidity source
      d. Periodically check patient's nares and behind ears for pressure
      e. Periodically assess patient for changes in condition

5. Oxygen by mask: simple; Venturi (delivers oxygen in precise concentrations)
   a. Proceed as with nasal cannula
   b. Fit mask snugly to face and adjust strap
   c. Periodically assess patient and equipment as with nasal cannula
   d. If condition warrants, may obtain order to change mask to nasal cannula for meal-time
I. Care of patient with a tracheostomy
   1. Tracheotomy: opening into the trachea
   2. Tracheostomy: tracheal opening, which normally has a tracheal tube
   3. Tube is either metal or plastic, which is usually cuffed (Figures 2-9 and 2-10)
   4. Tube is held securely in place with cotton ties around the neck (Figure 2-11)
   5. Ties are changed with extreme caution to prevent patient from coughing out tube
   6. A gauze dressing is placed under the tube to absorb secretions; dressing must be changed every shift
   7. Inner cannula is removed, cleaned with peroxide and pipe cleaners, and rinsed with normal saline at least once a shift by sterile technique; commercially prepared kits are available
   8. Skin around stoma is cleansed with peroxide, rinsed with saline, and assessed at least once a shift
   9. Tube must be suctioned frequently. Patient is often apprehensive and needs frequent reassurance
   10. Patient may take oral feedings if ordered, cuff must be inflated at all times
J. Medication classifications: refer to Chapter 3 for more detailed information on drugs that affect the respiratory system
   1. Respiratory stimulants
   2. Respiratory depressants
   3. Those acting on mucous membranes: administered orally or as spray or vapor
      a. Mucolytics
      b. Expectorants
   4. Bronchodilators

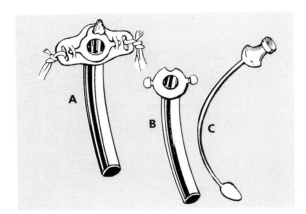

Figure 2-9.   Metal tracheostomy tube. **A,** Outer cannula. **B,** Inner cannula. **C,** Obturator. (From Harkness GA, Dincher JR: *Medical-surgical nursing: total patient care,* ed 10, St Louis, 2000, Mosby.)

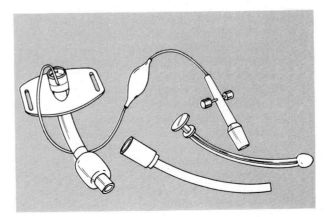

Figure 2-10.   Cuffed tracheostomy tube. (From Harkness GA, Dincher JR: *Medical-surgical nursing: total patient care,* ed 10, St Louis, 2000, Mosby.)

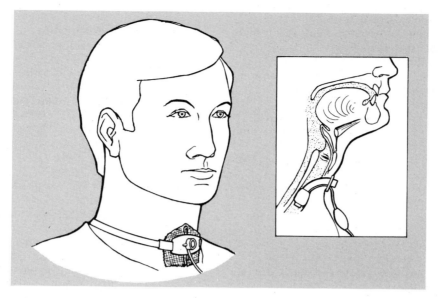

Figure 2-11.   Tracheostomy tube in place. (From Harkness GA, Dincher JR: *Medical-surgical nursing: total patient care,* ed 10, St Louis, 2000, Mosby.)

MEASURES TO MEET FLUID NEEDS

A. Assessment: daily weights, comparison of intake and output, appearance of urine, presence of edema, fluid preferences, and skin turgor
B. Fluid excess (edema)
 1. Associated with heart and kidney disease: body unable to rid itself of excess fluid
 2. Can result from excessive intravenous (IV) fluids
 3. Observed as edema as well as weight gain and reduced urine output
 4. Sites of edema: eyes, fingers, ankles, and sacral area
C. Fluid deficit (dehydration)
 1. Associated with inadequate fluid intake, diarrhea, excessive perspiration, vomiting, bleeding, and increased urine output
 2. Observed as dry skin and mucous membranes, thick mucus, poor skin turgor, behavioral changes, or changes in vital signs
D. Measuring intake and output
 1. Measure all fluids taken in: IV, tube feedings, and obvious fluids such as water, milk, ice cream, gelatin, custard, and soup
 2. Measure all fluids leaving the body: urine, vomitus, diarrhea, gastric secretions, and blood
 3. Know capacity of agency's fluid containers
 4. Set measuring containers on level surface to read measurements accurately
 5. Record and total amounts in appropriate places
E. Administering IV fluids
 1. Assess site of needle insertion
  a. Infiltration: fluid entering subcutaneous tissues instead of vein; area is pale, cool, and swollen
  b. Phlebitis: inflammation of vein; area is red, warm, and swollen
 2. Assess tubing: no kinks; no leakage along entire length of tubing; tubing should be labeled and changed every 48 to 72 hours or per agency policy
 3. Assess rate of flow

 4. Assess container
  a. It must match physician's order
  b. Check that the amount absorbed is on schedule
F. Medication classifications—diuretics: refer to Chapter 3 for more detailed information

MEASURES TO MEET NUTRITIONAL NEEDS

A. Assessment: weight/height ratio, weight changes, skin and mucous membranes, food preferences, meal patterns, ability to eat, and appetite
B. Preparing for meals
 1. Environment
  a. Control odors, noise, and unpleasant sights; remove soiled equipment and linens
  b. Avoid stressful situations before and during mealtime
 2. Patient
  a. Provide oral hygiene and opportunity for elimination and hand washing
  b. Position comfortably, preferably in sitting position
 3. Meal tray
  a. Ensure correct tray for correct patient
  b. Arrange tray to be accessible to patient
  c. Assist in opening containers, removing covers, and cutting and preparing food
  d. Serve trays first to patients able to feed themselves
C. Assisting the patient to eat
 1. Place napkin across chest
 2. Explain what foods and liquids are on the tray
 3. Prepare foods and feed in order of patient's preference
 4. Encourage the patient to assist as much as possible
 5. Do not rush: allow time to chew and swallow
 6. Talk with the patient during meal
 7. Provide opportunity for hand washing and oral care
D. Gastric gavage (tube feeding)
 1. Used when patient is unable to eat, swallow, or take in adequate quantities of food

2. Blended foods and fluids (commercially or agency prepared) are passed to the stomach through a nasogastric tube either intermittently or by slow continuous drip
3. Check amount, frequency, and type ordered by physician
4. Feeding must be at room temperature before administering
5. Placement of tube must be checked before feeding begins
   a. Nasogastric or nasoduodenal tubes
      (1) By aspirating stomach contents with a syringe
      (2) Inject 10 cc of air into large bore feeding tube while simultaneously listening with a stethoscope over the stomach to hear a whooshing sound
      (3) Small-bore feeding tube must have radiographic confirmation prior to beginning of feeding
   b. Gastrostomy or jejunostomy tubes
      (1) Aspirate stomach contents with a syringe
      (2) Measure, record, and return aspirated contents
6. Place patient in sitting position
7. Aspirate tube for stomach contents. Hold feeding if greater than 100 cc of residual is obtained
8. Administer feeding slowly: 200 ml during 30- to 45-minute period
9. Feeding should be followed by ordered amount of water
10. Clamp tube after completion of feeding to prevent air entering stomach
11. If nausea, vomiting, diarrhea, or cramps occur, rate may be too fast or patient may be intolerant of feeding or volume or the feeding may be too concentrated
12. Tube may be left in place between feedings or removed after each feeding as ordered by physician
13. Have patient remain in sitting position for 45 minutes to help prevent aspiration

E. Medication classifications: refer to Chapter 3 for more detailed information
   1. Vitamin supplements
   2. Mineral supplements

MEASURES TO MEET URINARY ELIMINATION NEEDS

A. Assessment: intake/output ratio, color, odor, amount, and consistency of urine, frequency of urination, and continence
B. Common problems of urination
   1. Incontinence: inability to control voiding
      a. Requires frequent skin care and linen change
      b. May be reduced with scheduled toileting
      c. May be secondary to medications (diuretics)
   2. Retention: inability to void
      a. If adequate amounts of fluid have been taken in, no more than 8 hours should pass between voidings, except during sleeping hours
      b. Palpation of bladder can determine distention of full bladder
   3. Anuria: no urine being produced by the kidneys
   4. Dysuria: difficult or painful urination ("burning")
C. Assisting with urination
   1. Offer bedpan or urinal at regularly scheduled times
   2. Keep bedpan or urinal and toilet tissue within easy reach for patients who can assist themselves

3. Keep call signal within easy reach
4. Provide privacy
5. Hearing the sound of running water or having warm water poured over the perineum may induce voiding
6. Provide opportunity for hand washing after urination

D. Care of patient with retention catheter
   1. Presence of indwelling catheter greatly predisposes patient to urinary tract infection
   2. Opening a closed urinary system is to be avoided
   3. Drainage container must be kept below level of the bladder but must not touch the floor
   4. Drainage tubing must be free of kinks; catheter taped to patient's leg allowing slack
   5. Drainage container is emptied at end of shift or if container becomes nearly full; urine is measured, assessed, and amount recorded
   6. Catheter care is given at least once per shift and after every bowel movement
      a. Meatus and catheter are cleansed with soap and water; from meatus down catheter and away from body
      b. Removal of crusts and secretions from meatus and catheter may require use of hydrogen peroxide
      c. A bacteriostatic ointment is often ordered to be applied to the meatus
   7. Unless contraindicated, fluid intake should reach 2000 to 3000 ml/24 hr

E. Catheterization
   1. "Straight": catheter removed at end of procedure (intermittent catheterization) often ordered to relieve urine retention, obtain a sterile urine specimen, or to measure residual urine after voiding
   2. Indwelling, retention or Foley: catheter is left in place in bladder
   3. Assemble equipment: sterile catheterization tray or disposable kit containing catheter, basin, container with lid (for specimen, if ordered), cotton balls, antiseptic solution, lubricant, sterile gloves, and drape
   4. For indwelling catheterization, add Foley catheter, syringe, solution for inflating balloon, drainage bag with tubing, and tape for securing catheter
   5. After explaining procedure to patient and ensuring privacy, place female in dorsal recumbent position and male in supine position
   6. Place equipment on an over-the-bed table or between patient's legs; using sterile technique open package, don gloves, and place drape
   7. For female patient, while holding labia apart, cleanse vulva and meatus well going from front to back toward vagina; use cotton ball for one stoke only before discarding
   8. For male patient, cleanse around penis from meatus toward base using each cotton ball once around
   9. Insert catheter into meatus (3 to 4 inches [7.5 to 10 cm] in female and 6 to 8 inches [15 to 20 cm] in male) until urine flows; advance catheter one more inch, drain urine (no more than 750 ml at one time to prevent hypovolemic shock); remove catheter ("straight") or inflate balloon and connect drainage tubing (indwelling)

F. Intermittent bladder irrigation (hand bladder irrigation)
   1. To rid bladder and catheter of clots or mucus; to instill antibiotic or other solutions

2. Open technique
   a. Assemble equipment: sterile solution (type and amount as ordered), sterile container for solution, bulb syringe, and basin for return flow
   b. Disconnect catheter from drainage tube over empty basin; protect ends from contamination
   c. Allow solution to flow in by gravity or gentle pressure; drain by gravity or gentle solution; repeat until returns are clear or ordered amount of solution has been used
   d. Subtract amount of solution used from amount of returns; record output
3. Closed technique
   a. Assemble equipment: 20- to 30-ml syringe with needle, alcohol swabs, solution ordered, and clamp
   b. Draw solution into syringe by sterile technique
   c. Clamp tubing distal to needle entry point
   d. Cleanse resealable rubber entry port on drainage tubing with alcohol swab
   e. Insert needle into port
   f. Inject fluid into catheter
   g. Remove needle
   h. Release clamp and allow fluid to drain into drainage bag
   i. Observe fluid return
   j. Repeat until ordered amount of solution has been used
   k. Empty drainage bag, subtracting amount of irrigant from total; record urine output
G. Continuous bladder irrigation (through and through or three-way irrigation)
   1. To prevent clot formation; to reduce obstruction of catheter; to circulate antibiotic or other solutions continuously in bladder
   2. Equipment: patient has three-way catheter or needs sterile Y tube connector attached to regular two-way catheter's drainage channel; large bottle or bag of solution, with tubing attached, hanging from IV pole
   3. With three-way catheter: using sterile technique
      a. Remove plug from irrigating channel; protect plug and tubing from contamination
      b. Insert solution tubing into irrigating channel
   4. With two-way catheter: using sterile technique
      a. Attach single end of sterile Y tube connector to catheter
      b. Attach drainage tubing to one end of Y
      c. Attach solution tubing to other end of Y
   5. Start solution flow at rate ordered by physician
   6. Observe fluid return through drainage tubing
   7. Replace solution bottle or bag as it becomes nearly empty
   8. Empty drainage container as it becomes nearly full and when solution container is replaced
   9. Subtract amount of irrigant solution from total amount of drainage to record actual urine output
H. Removal of indwelling catheter
   1. Assemble equipment: syringe without needle, underpad, basin, urinal or bedpan, toilet tissue, and protective gloves
   2. After explaining procedure and ensuring privacy, place pad under patient
   3. Remove tape from catheter and patient's leg
   4. Put on protective gloves
   5. Place basin under patient's meatus
   6. Insert syringe into balloon channel; fluid will return on its own
   7. After all fluid has returned, gently pull on catheter to remove it
   8. If resistance is met, stop and obtain assistance
   9. Assist patient to wash perineum
   10. Teaching
      a. Patient should continue to drink fluids
      b. Burning on urination may occur during first few voidings
      c. Complete continence and normal voiding pattern may take awhile to return
      d. Instruct patient to void into bedpan or urinal so that the color, consistency, and amount of urine can be assessed
   11. Encourage relaxation: anxiety may inhibit ability to void
   12. Continue to assess bladder distention, intake/output ratio, and patient complaints until normal patterns of elimination are achieved
I. Medication classifications
   1. Cholinergics: to induce bladder contraction (bethanechol [Urecholine] and neostigmine [Prostigmin])
   2. Anticholinergics: to reduce bladder spasms and urinary frequency (methantheline [Banthine] and flavoxate hydrochloride [Urispas])

MEASURES TO MEET BOWEL ELIMINATION NEEDS

A. Assessment: the patient's pattern of elimination; amount, color, consistency, odor, and shape of stool; patient's activity level; amount and type of food and fluid intake; passage of flatus; abdominal distention
B. Common problems of elimination
   1. Constipation: passage of dry, hard feces
   2. Diarrhea: frequent passage of liquid or unformed stools
   3. Impaction: formation of a hardened mass of stool in the lower bowel forming an obstruction to the passage of normal stool; often characterized by the frequent seepage of small amount of liquid stool
   4. Abdominal distention: swollen abdomen caused by retention of flatus in the intestines
C. General nursing measures
   1. Encourage intake of roughage in the diet: fresh fruits and vegetables and whole grain breads and cereals
   2. Encourage intake of adequate amounts of fluids unless contraindicated: 2000 to 3000 ml/day
   3. Encourage maximum amount of physical activity
   4. Encourage patient to respond to the urge to defecate
   5. Position patient comfortably and provide adequate time and privacy for elimination
   6. Provide access to call signal and toilet tissue
   7. Provide opportunity for hand washing after elimination
D. Rectal tube
   1. To assist in expelling flatus
   2. Assemble equipment: rectal tube with flatus bag or waterproof pad, lubricant, glove, and tape
   3. After explaining procedure and providing privacy, position patient in left lateral (Sims') position

4. With gloved hand insert lubricated tube 2 to 4 inches (5 to 10 cm) into rectum
5. Tape tube to patient's buttock and leave in place no longer than 20 to 30 minutes
6. Note passage of flatus or stool; report and record findings

E. Rectal suppository
1. To stimulate peristalsis and aid stool elimination; to soothe painful rectum or anus, to administer medications
2. Assemble equipment: suppository as ordered, glove, bedpan, and toilet tissue
3. Suppository begins to melt at room temperature, providing its own lubrication
4. Separate buttocks and with gloved index finger insert pointed end of suppository into anus
5. Gently insert 3 to 4 inches (7.5 to 10 cm) into rectum
6. Hold buttocks together until initial urge to defecate has passed
7. Best results occur within 30 minutes

F. Commercially prepared pre-filled enema
1. To promote bowel or flatus movement
2. Assemble equipment: enema (usually 120 ml), underpad, bedpan, toilet paper, and gloves
3. After explaining procedure and providing privacy, place patient in left lateral (Sims') position
4. With gloved hand insert prelubricated tip of enema to the hub and squeeze container until most of solution is instilled
5. Encourage patient to retain solution until urge to defecate is felt
6. Place call signal, bedpan, and toilet tissue within easy reach
7. If patient uses toilet, instruct not to flush so that results can be assessed

G. Oil-retention enema
1. To soften and lubricate stool, promoting easier passage
2. Often followed by cleansing enema
3. Equipment and administration are the same as for commercially prepared enema above
4. Encourage patient to retain oil 30 to 60 minutes

H. Cleansing enemas
1. To relieve constipation or flatus or to cleanse the bowel before diagnostic procedures, surgery, or childbirth
2. Solutions used as ordered by physician
   a. Tap water: can cause fluid and electrolyte imbalance
   b. Soap solution: 5 ml of liquid soap to 1000 ml of water; can irritate mucous membranes of bowel
   c. Saline solution: can cause fluid and electrolyte imbalance
3. Assemble equipment: disposable enema kit containing enema bag, tubing with clamp, liquid soap, and lubricant; waterproof underpad; solution at a temperature no greater than 105° F; bedpan and toilet tissue; IV pole; protective gloves
4. After explaining procedure and providing privacy, place patient in left lateral (Sims') position
5. Put on protective gloves
6. Insert lubricated tubing about 3 to 5 inches (7.5 to 12.5 cm) into rectum

7. With bottom of enema bag hanging 12 inches (30 cm) above anus or 18 inches (45 cm) above mattress, slowly administer 500 to 1000 ml of solution
8. If patient complains of cramping or has difficulty retaining solution
   a. Slow administration rate, or
   b. Temporarily stop flow
   c. Encourage slow, deep breathing through the mouth
9. After fluid has been administered, assist patient to bathroom or onto bedpan or commode; instruct patient not to flush toilet so that results can be assessed
10. If enemas are ordered "until clear," repeat procedure until returns are clear of stool (or of barium after barium enema)
11. Observe patient during procedure for signs of weakness or fatigue, which would necessitate stopping the procedure to allow rest

I. Digital removal of fecal impaction
1. Breaking up the hard fecal mass and removing it
2. Assemble equipment: gloves, waterproof underpad, lubricant, and bedpan
3. Liberally lubricate gloved index finger
4. With patient in left lateral (Sims') position, gently insert finger into hardened mass of stool
5. Gently break off small pieces of the stool, bringing them out and placing them in the bedpan
6. Assess patient for signs of weakness and fatigue; this is an uncomfortable, tiring procedure and may need to be intermittently stopped
7. Assist patient to bedpan: disimpaction may induce defecation

J. Colostomy irrigation
1. To regulate the discharge and drainage of fecal contents and flatus
2. Time of irrigation depends on physician's order and patient's own established routine; when colostomy has become regulated, irrigation may be only done every other day; some patients never irrigate their colostomy
3. Assemble equipment
   a. Irrigating appliance (types vary)
   b. Irrigating container (enema bag)
   c. Tubing and catheter (may be part of enema kit)
   d. Irrigating solution: usually 500 to 1000 ml of tap water or physiologic saline solution at 100° F
   e. Lubricant
   f. Drainage bag (may be part of irrigating appliance) and bedpan if not using on toilet
   g. Waterproof underpad if being performed in bed
   h. Fresh colostomy appliance, dressing, or stoma pad
   i. IV pole
   j. Protective gloves
4. After explaining procedure and ensuring privacy, place patient on toilet (most convenient) or in bed in left lateral (Sims') position
5. Put on protective gloves
6. Raise irrigation container 18 inches (45 cm) above stoma, clear catheter of air, lubricate catheter, introduce catheter through irrigating appliance, and insert catheter into stoma 2 to 6 inches (5 to 15 cm); do not advance if resistance is met
7. Allow solution to flow slowly and remove catheter; return is usually completed within 45 to 60 minutes

8. When return is completed, remove irrigating appliance, wash and dry abdomen, and apply fresh colostomy appliance, dressing, or stoma pad as indicated
9. Record character and amount of returns, patient's tolerance, and degree of assistance provided by patient
K. Medication classifications: refer to Chapter 3 for more detailed information on drugs that affect the gastrointestinal (GI) system
    1. Stool softeners
    2. Laxatives/cathartics
    3. Antidiarrhetics

MEASURES TO MEET REST AND SLEEP NEEDS

Rest and sleep are necessary for restoring physical and mental well-being, reducing stress and anxiety, and maintaining the ability to attend to and concentrate on activities of life.
A. Assessment: normal number of hours of sleep, usual bedtime, usual bedtime habits or practices, sleep difficulties, daytime fatigue, usual methods of obtaining rest, and sleep medications being used
B. Physician's orders for rest must be clarified: is bed rest ordered to provide rest for a damaged heart, the entire body, or an injured part such as a foot?
C. Providing for rest and sleep
    1. Promote relaxation: provide diversions, pain relief, clean, wrinkle-free bed, a noise-free and odor-free room, and easy access to bedside equipment and call signal; give a relaxing back rub
    2. Reduce patient's anxiety level by allowing time for the patient to talk about stressful or fear-producing situations
    3. If possible, position patient in usual sleeping position with amount of covers desired
    4. Plan and organize care to allow the patient uninterrupted rest and sleep periods
    5. Give sleeping medication if ordered and if required by the patient
D. Medication classifications: refer to Chapter 3 for more detailed information
    1. Sedatives: to reduce anxiety
    2. Hypnotics: to induce sleep

MEASURES TO MEET ACTIVITY AND EXERCISE NEEDS

Physical activity is necessary for proper functioning of all body systems as well as for promotion of emotional well-being; immobility can lead to physical as well as emotional disability
A. Assessment: posture, ability to walk, ability to turn and move in bed, usual activity level, and skin condition
B. Patient's activity and exercise level is ordered by the physician
    1. Bed rest (BR): patient is confined to bed
    2. Bathroom privileges (BRP): although confined to bed, patient may perform urinary and bowel elimination in the bathroom
    3. May dangle: although confined to bed, patient may sit on edge of bed with legs and feet hanging down over side of bed and supported by footstool
        a. Often accompanied by orders for frequency and duration of dangling time (e.g., dangle every shift for 10 minutes)
        b. Provide footstool
        c. Assess vital signs
        d. Stay with patient to assess tolerance and assist back to bed
    4. Allow to chair: although patient may sit in chair, he or she is not permitted to ambulate any farther
    5. Out of bed (OOB) ad lib: can and should perform as much activity out of bed as desired
    6. Encourage patients to perform as much activity as orders permit
C. Dangers of immobility
    1. Atelectasis: collapse of lung caused by reduced depth and rate of respirations or obstruction of lungs by excessive secretions
    2. Hypostatic pneumonia: caused by pooling of lung secretions and the resulting congestion
    3. Thrombus formation: caused by reduced rate of blood flow through the veins and prolonged coagulation time
    4. Constipation: caused by slowed peristaltic action
    5. Contractures: permanent shortening of muscles leading to joint immobility
    6. Skin breakdown and decubitus ulcer formation caused by prolonged pressure and reduced circulation to an area
    7. Development of urinary tract infections and kidney stones caused by stasis of urine and demineralization of bones
D. Measures to prevent dangers of immobility
    1. Coughing and deep breathing
        a. Performed q2h
        b. Patient should be in semi-Fowler's position and take 10 deep breaths followed by deep cough to raise secretions
    2. Turning and repositioning q2h
    3. Range-of-motion (ROM) exercises: to maintain full range and flexibility of joint movement
        a. Performed 8 to 10 times on each joint at least qd
        b. Passive range-of-motion (PROM): performed for the patient
        c. Active range-of-motion (AROM): performed by the patient
        d. Each joint is put through all its possible movements (Figure 2-12)
    4. Maintain adequate fluid intake (2000 to 3000 ml/day)
    5. Provide for adequate nutritional intake
    6. Frequent skin care, keeping skin clean, dry, and lubricated
E. Devices used to help prevent dangers of immobility
    1. Footboard: to prevent plantar flexion (footdrop)
        a. Soles of patient's feet are flat against board and in good alignment
        b. Board should be padded
    2. Bed cradle: to keep weight of bed covers off a body part
    3. Alternating pressure mattress: changes pressure on body parts in contact with the mattress
        a. Only one layer of loosely pulled linen should be between mattress and patient
        b. Keep pins and other pointed objects away from this mattress
    4. Sheepskin: provides a soft surface, reducing skin abrasion

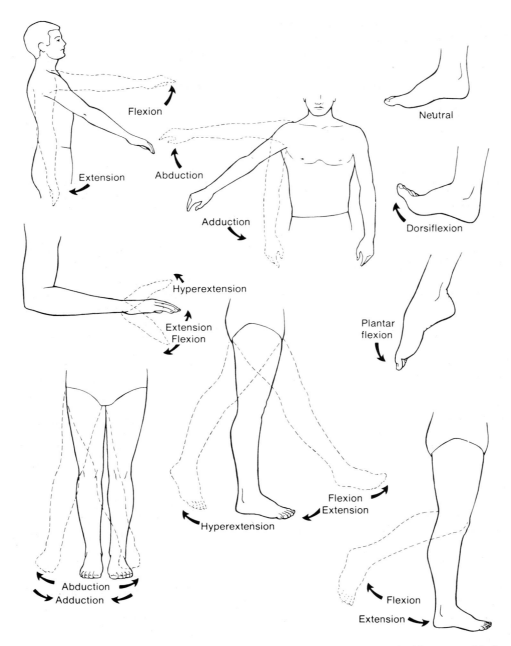

Figure 2-12.   Range of joint motions. (From Beare PG, Myers JL: *Adult health nursing,* ed 3, St Louis, 1998, Mosby.)

5. Special beds such as the CircOlectric allow patient's position to be changed more readily
6. Venodixie boots: prevent thrombophlebitis
7. Antiembolism stockings

MEASURES TO MEET PAIN RELIEF NEEDS

Individuals (including nurses) vary in their perception of and response to pain. Pain is often intensified in the presence of anxiety and fatigue and the absence of distraction.

A. Assessment: intensity, onset, duration, quality, and location of pain, patient's nonverbal responses to pain: behavior, change in vital signs, and nausea; factors associated with the pain: activity and visitors; pain relief measures

B. Therapeutic relationship may help reduce anxiety, thus reducing pain level
C. Altering contributing factors: relieving constipation and nausea; eliminating environmental disturbances such as bright lights, odors, and noise
D. Providing diversional activities: television, radio, and visitors
E. Repositioning, back rub, and tightening linens
F. Application of heat or cold if ordered
G. Relaxation
  1. To reduce muscle tension
  2. First need
    a. A comfortable position
    b. A quiet environment

c. Focus on something outside the body, such as a word to repeat, an object to look at, or something to imagine
3. Techniques
   a. Exercises in which various muscle groups are alternately tensed and relaxed
   b. Exercises in which various muscle groups are alternately stretched and relaxed
   c. Breathing techniques similar to those used in the Lamaze method of childbirth (controlled and focused)
   d. Biofeedback: learning to control normally autonomic body functions
      (1) Muscle tension is monitored
      (2) Subject receives feedback as to the success of attempts to control functions
H. TENS: Transcutaneous electrical nerve stimulation; small, battery-operated device that provides continuous mild electric current to skin
   1. Clean skin with alcohol before applying electrodes on or around pain site
   2. No tingling indicates controls are too low; pain or muscle spasm indicates controls are too high
I. Medication classifications: refer to Chapter 3 for more detailed information
   1. Placebo: inactive substance administered to satisfy the patient's need for a drug
      a. Pain relief after administration is probably a result of anxiety reduction
      b. Relief felt after a placebo does not mean there was no pain
   2. Analgesics
      a. Narcotics
      b. Nonnarcotics

MEASURES TO MEET SAFETY AND HYGIENE NEEDS

Individuals are usually capable of meeting these needs themselves, but in strange environments and in times of stress and illness, help is often needed. Individuals need protection from injury, maintenance of intact skin and mucous membranes and of body alignment, and structure and order in their environment

A. Assessment
   1. Protection from injury: level of consciousness, ability to move, and knowledge of environment, equipment, and patient's medications
   2. Maintenance of intact skin and mucous membranes and alignment: personal hygiene, condition of skin, mucous membranes, joints, and posture
   3. Structure and order in the environment: arrangement of personal belongings, cleanliness of patient's unit, environmental conditions, and potential hazards
B. Measures to protect from injury
   1. Bed side rails: use whenever bed is above its lowest level; use for patients who are unconscious, disoriented, or confused or for children
   2. Call signal: should always be within patient's reach; patient should know how to use it
   3. Restraints (patient protectors/patient protective devices)
      a. Require physician's order to place and remove unless there is an emergency and patient is in immediate need of protection

b. Used to restrict movement of the individual or of one or more extremities
c. Explain to patient and family why restraint is being used
d. Remain quiet and calm while applying restraint to reduce patient's fear and stress
e. Apply restraint securely enough to provide protection but loosely enough to permit circulation and lung expansion
f. Periodically check pulses and skin integrity distal to the restrained extremity (radial, pedal pulses)
g. Continue to provide patient with all necessary nursing care including turning, fluids, hygiene, and opportunity for elimination
h. Secure restraint to bed frame rather than to bed rail
i. Types of restraints
   (1) Sheet around waist to secure patient in chair
   (2) Jacket or vest, mitts, ankle and wrist restraints
   (3) Safety belts
j. Measures to avoid restraints
   (1) Reorientation measures
   (2) Alarms and monitors
   (3) Specialized chairs
4. Reduce environmental hazards
   a. Proper care of hospital equipment
      (1) Equipment should be stored properly
      (2) All apparatus, equipment, and furnishings should be kept in good repair
      (3) All apparatus, equipment, and furnishings should be used correctly
   b. Prevention of fire
      (1) Proper care and use of electrical equipment
      (2) Prohibition of smoking in bed
      (3) Observance of oxygen safety measures
   c. Prevention of accidents
      (1) Keep floor dry, clean, and free of litter
      (2) Place rubber tips on crutches, canes, and walkers
      (3) Dispose of dressings and needles properly
      (4) Have frequent fire drills
      (5) Lock wheels on beds, wheelchairs, and stretchers
      (6) Maintain good lighting
   d. Protect from microorganisms and pests
      (1) Hand washing and maintenance of medical asepsis
      (2) Proper disinfection and sterilization
      (3) Minimize food storage in patient unit
5. Transferring patient from bed
   a. Protect from falling by using transfer belt and having patient wear sturdy shoes rather than slippers
   b. Two or three people may be required to transfer helpless or heavy patients
   c. Be sure bed and stretcher wheels and wheelchairs are in locked position
   d. Make use of lifting devices such as Hoyer lift
   e. Use good body mechanics
C. Measures to promote and maintain intact skin and mucous membranes
   1. Bed making: dry, tight, wrinkle-free bed helps maintain skin integrity as well as provide for comfort
      a. Assemble equipment: sheets, spread, blanket, pillow, and pillow covering

b. Care of soiled linens
   (1) Always place on a surface above floor or in individual laundry bags
   (2) Deposit in linen hamper (disposable "linens" are available and are used especially for patients with communicable diseases)
c. Types of bed making
   (1) Closed bed is made in preparation for new patient
   (2) Open bed is occupied but patient is out of bed
   (3) Occupied bed is made with patient in it
   (4) Fracture or orthopedic bed is made from head to foot
   (5) Postanesthetic or recovery bed is made to receive patient easily from stretcher (Figure 2-13)
d. Bed positions
   (1) Low Fowler's: head is raised (gatched) 18 to 20 inches (45 to 50 cm) above flat bed level
   (2) Semi-Fowler's: head is raised 45 degrees and knee is gatched 15 degrees
   (3) High Fowler's: head of bed is raised to a 90-degree angle
   (4) Trendelenburg's: head is lower than the level of the feet (no gatch)

2. Daily bath
   a. Clean, dry, intact, and healthy skin and mucous membranes are first line of defense against microorganisms
   b. Bath time is also important for establishing relationship with patient and for assessment
   c. Some patients do not desire, need, or require complete bath each day
   d. Bed bath: given to patient who is restricted to bed or helpless in bathing self
   e. Assisted bath: patient bathes as much of self as possible; may need assistance with back, feet, legs, and perineum
   f. Tub bath or shower: for patient who is capable of doing so; must have physician's order
   g. Commercial sponge bath packets: contain moisturizing cleansing agent; warm in microwave; decreases heat loss, skin drying, exposure, and task time
3. Skin care
   a. Use soap sparingly; rinse well with warm water; pat skin dry
   b. Lotions prevent dry skin
   c. Gently massage bony prominences with lotion to promote circulation

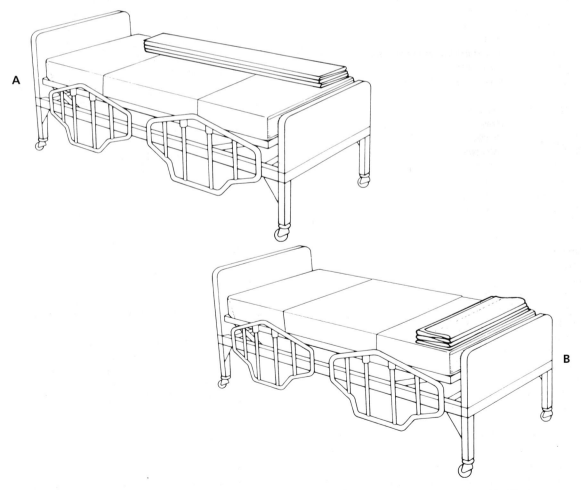

Figure 2-13. Postanesthetic beds. **A,** With top linens fan folded lengthwise to the side of bed. **B,** With top linens fan folded from the head of the bed to the foot. (Adapted from Sorrentino SA, Gorek B: *Textbook for long-term care assistants,* ed 3, St Louis, 2000, Mosby.)

d. Use deodorant or antiperspirant as necessary

e. Avoid heavy use of powder, which can cake, causing skin irritation

4. Mouth care

   a. Routine mouth care: use of toothbrush, mouthwash, or substitutes

   b. Special mouth care: more frequent routine care plus the judicious use of glycerin and lemon swabs or hydrogen peroxide if ordered

   c. Care of dentures

      (1) Clean dentures over towel-lined basin of water to reduce chance of breakage if dropped

      (2) Hold dentures with gauze or cloth to prevent dropping

      (3) Clean with tepid water; hot water may change shape

      (4) Store dentures in clearly marked denture cup with tepid water in drawer of bedside stand when not in patient's mouth

5. Hair care

   a. Comb or brush daily; groom as desired

   b. If tangled

      (1) Use 95% alcohol for oily hair

      (2) Use mineral oil for dry hair

      (3) Start at ends working toward scalp

      (4) Hold hair close to head to prevent pulling

   c. Braid long hair if not objectionable to patient

   d. Shampoo as often as necessary and as patient's condition permits

   e. Give pediculosis (lice) treatment as ordered by physician

      (1) Commercial preparations are available

      (2) Use fine-toothed comb to remove nits (eggs)

      (3) Patient may be isolated to avoid spread

6. Nail care: daily and as indicated; must have physician's order to cut nails; extreme care must be used with patients with diabetes or circulatory problems

   a. Scrub under nails as necessary

   b. Cut nails even with tips of fingers and toes

   c. Round fingernails to curve with fingertips

   d. Cut toenails straight across

7. Decubitus (pressure) ulcer care: assess areas over all bony prominences, such as sacrum, heels, elbows, hips and shoulder blades, and along edges of casts and braces

   a. Contributing factors

      (1) Crumbs or food particles in the bed

      (2) Exposure to moisture such as urine

      (3) Wrinkles in sheets

      (4) Unrelieved pressure for longer than 2 hours

      (5) Conditions that restrict movement

      (6) Poor nutritional or fluid balance states

   b. Treatment

      (1) "An ounce of prevention is worth a pound of cure"—turn and reposition q2h

      (2) Identify high-risk patients

      (3) Report and initiate care for beginning signs of redness, whiteness, or breaks in skin

      (4) Use devices such as sheepskin, egg-crate mattress, alternating-pressure mattress, water mattress, or Clinitron bed

      (5) Avoid use of waterproof underpads

      (6) Use special cleansing agents and dressings as ordered by physician or as indicated by agency policy

8. Use turning sheet to move and turn patient with minimum of friction, which may cause abrasions

D. Measures to maintain body alignment

1. Encourage good posture while sitting, standing, and lying

2. Bed-lying positions

   a. Supine: lying on back

   b. Prone: lying on abdomen with head turned to the side

   c. Side-lying (Sims'): lying on side with upper hip and knee sharply flexed

3. Reposition patient at least q2h

4. Guidelines for proper positioning

   a. Normal body curves must be supported by small pillows or pads: use "bridging" techniques

   b. Joints that are normally flexed need support

   c. Bony prominences need to be protected from pressure

   d. Use devices such as sandbags or rolls to keep joints and body parts positioned

   e. Periodically check patient for discomfort or difficulties

   f. Ensure that patient can reach call signal

E. Measures to promote structure and order in the patient's environment

1. Physical factors

   a. Lighting

      (1) Lighting should be indirect except for reading or for procedures

      (2) General lighting should be diffused

      (3) Sunlight promotes healing and feeling of well-being

   b. Waste disposal: trash, human excretions, and soiled dressings and linens should be discarded according to agency's procedures

2. Esthetic factors

   a. Sound

      (1) Music therapy promotes rest and relaxation

      (2) Noise causes fatigue and anxiety

   b. Decor

      (1) Pastel colors (yellow or pink) are soothing and relaxing

      (2) Harsh colors (red or black) overstimulate senses

      (3) Flowers and pictures enhance environment

   c. Odors

      (1) Foul or strong odors should be eliminated by means of room deodorizer or removal of causative agent

      (2) Mild, fragrant odors reduce antiseptic smell and patient embarrassment

   d. Privacy: curtains, screens, and proper draping should be used as indicated to reduce embarrassment and protect patient dignity

3. Care of the environment: varies according to agency policy

   a. Responsibilities of housekeeping and ancillary services (central supply and maintenance)

      (1) Daily damp dusting and floor cleaning

(2) Scrubbing, disinfecting, sterilizing, and storing of equipment after patient transfer, discharge, or death

(3) Repairing or replacing defective equipment or furnishings

b. Responsibilities of the nursing personnel

(1) Place bedside table, call signal, phone, and personal articles within patient's reach

(2) Straighten and damp dust bedside unit (includes care of flowers)

(3) Care for patient belongings (clothing, valuables, glasses, dentures, and prostheses)

(4) Prevent cross-infection between patients

OTHER THERAPEUTIC NURSING MEASURES
Wound Care

A. Cleaning the wound: if a wound culture is ordered, always obtain the specimen prior to cleansing

1. Commonly used antiseptics
   a. 70% alcohol
   b. Povidone-iodine (Betadine)
2. Hydrogen peroxide to remove dry and crusted secretions
3. Always clean from innermost to outermost aspect of wound

B. Wound irrigation

1. To remove secretions or excessive discharge from surfaces or body cavities or to apply moist heat
2. May use clean or sterile technique depending on area to be irrigated
3. Assemble equipment: may vary according to area to be irrigated (disposable kits are available)
   a. Container to hold irrigating solution
   b. Container for return flow of solution
   c. Irrigating solution
   d. Irrigator: usually bulb syringe or large plunger-type syringe
   e. Protection for patient and linens
   f. Gloves; masks and goggles if needed
   g. Replacement dressing if indicated

C. Dressing changes

1. Dressing: material placed on a wound or incision to protect, absorb drainage, or promote healing
2. Dressings are classified by method of application
   a. Clean
   b. Sterile
   c. Moist or dry
3. Disposable kits or hospital-assembled kits
4. Types of dressing material
   a. Gauze
   b. Petrolatum gauze
   c. Telfa
5. Material for securing dressings
   a. Tape: in various widths
      (1) Adhesive
      (2) Paper
      (3) Nonallergic
   b. Montgomery straps
   c. Bandages and binders
6. Nurse may be responsible for changing dressing or assisting physician in changing dressing

7. Initial change of postoperative dressing is done by physician unless an order specifies otherwise
8. Dressings that are not to be changed should be reinforced with additional material if drainage seeps through

D. Care of patient with wound infection

1. Infection may be local (confined to wound) or systemic (generalized throughout body), often depending on the causative organism
2. Signs of local infection result from increased circulation and accumulation of waste in the area
   a. Redness, heat, pain, and swelling
   b. Purulent drainage
   c. Loss of function
   d. Changes in vital signs
3. Signs of systemic infection
   a. Increase in temperature, pulse, and respirations (TPR); possible decrease in blood pressure
   b. Nausea and vomiting
   c. General malaise
   d. Loss of appetite
4. Basic principles of treatment
   a. Physical and mental rest
   b. Elevation and rest of infected part
   c. Application of heat or cold
5. Special treatment may include
   a. Pharmacological (sulfonamides and antibiotics)
   b. Incision and drainage of wound
   c. Debridement: removal of foreign, infected, or necrotic tissue
6. Infection control committee investigates and follows up infections occurring in an agency

Bandages

A. Applied to give support, immobilize a part, apply pressure, or hold dressings
B. Types of bandages
   1. Strips or rolls of gauze, cotton flannel, or elastic material
   2. Many widths, depending on purpose and part to be bandaged
C. Types of basic turns in bandaging
   1. Circular
   2. Spiral
   3. Spiral reverse
   4. Recurrent
   5. Figure-of-eight
D. Safety factors
   1. Apply in direction from distal to proximal
   2. Apply tight enough to serve purpose but loose enough to permit circulation (presence of pulse)
   3. Do not fasten over bony prominence, area of pressure, or a wound
   4. Part being bandaged should remain in functional position

Binders

A. Purposes
   1. Support: abdomen or chest
   2. Hold dressings in place
   3. Apply pressure
B. Types
   1. Straight
   2. Tailed: T-binder, four-tailed, or scultetus (many-tailed)

Antiembolism Stockings

A. Purposes
   1. To help maintain circulation
   2. To prevent thrombi or phlebitis formation
B. Application and maintenance
   1. Exact size is obtained by measuring calf or leg length and circumference
   2. Be sure legs are clean and dry before applying
   3. Apply with patient lying down; stockings should fit evenly and smoothly; no wrinkles
   4. Periodically check foot and leg for redness, irritation, swelling, and presence of pulse
   5. Stockings should be removed daily for bathing and skin inspection purposes. Occasional laundering is necessary

Application of Heat and Cold

A. Physiological principles
   1. Cold applications (by constricting blood vessels) prevent or reduce swelling, stop bleeding, decrease suppuration, and reduce pain
   2. Heat applications (by dilating blood vessels) increase supply of oxygen and nutrients to body cells and increase amount of toxins and excess fluids carried away
B. Types of cold applications
   1. Dry: ice bag, ice cap, ice collar, and hypothermic devices
   2. Moist: cold packs and compresses
C. Nursing observations
   1. White, mottled skin
   2. Frostbite
   3. Numbness
   4. Lowered body temperature

D. Guidelines
   1. Caps and bags are two-thirds filled and air is removed
   2. Containers are closed securely
   3. Caps and bags are always covered
   4. Application is removed every half hour for 1 hour
   5. Ice is replaced frequently
   6. These treatments are contraindicated or used only with great care in patients with poor circulation or impaired sensation
   7. Physician's order is always required
E. Types of heat applications
   1. Dry: hot water bottle, sunlight, heating pad, and incandescent, ultraviolet, and infrared lights
   2. Moist: warm compresses, hot soaks, hot packs, and K pad units
F. Nursing observations
   1. Redness
   2. Swelling
   3. Pain
   4. Change in vital signs
   5. Loss of function in part
G. Guidelines
   1. Always requires physician's order
   2. Carefully observe body parts that are very sensitive and burn easily (eyes, neck, and inner aspect of arm)
   3. Bottles and pads are always covered
   4. Never allow patient to lie on heating device
   5. Check for faulty electrical wiring
   6. Never use safety pins with electric devices
   7. Check body temperature frequently
   8. Check distance of heating bulbs from body area; should be at least 18 inches (45 cm) away

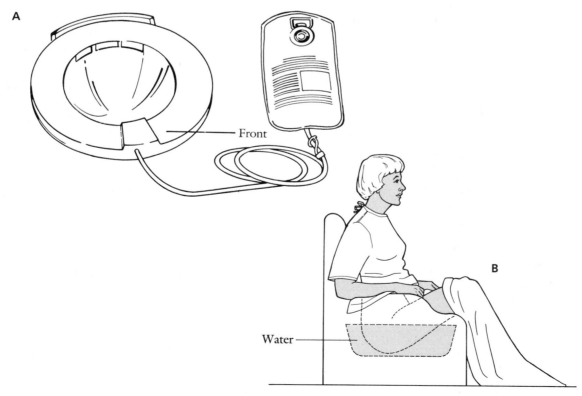

Figure 2-14. Sitz baths. **A,** Disposable. **B,** Built-in. (Adapted from Sorrentino SA: *Textbook for nursing assistants,* ed 5, St Louis, 2000, Mosby.)

9. Wring out compresses well to prevent burn; if area is infected, use compresses only once and discard
10. Agency policy may require application of a thin layer of petrolatum to area receiving heat

H. Special baths
   1. Hot (sitz) or cold (Figure 2-14)
   2. Medicated

MEASURES FOR EYE, EAR, AND THROAT DISORDERS
Eye Treatments

A. Hot compresses
   1. Assemble equipment: sterile basin of solution as ordered, gauze pad, heating device, paper bag, and protective gloves
   2. Put on protective gloves
   3. Apply thin layer of petrolatum over lid
   4. Wring out gauze pad with hands (if clean technique) or with two pairs of forceps (if sterile technique) and allow pad to stop steaming; apply compress slowly until patient is accustomed to heat, or allow patient to apply compress if able
   5. Try to keep compress on eyelid only; if lid is inflamed, compress may be placed on lid and cheek; if eyeball is inflamed, compress may be placed on lid and brow
   6. Change compresses every 30 to 60 seconds for 15 to 20 minutes as ordered
   7. If discharge is present, use clean pad each time compress is applied
   8. Use two sets of equipment if both eyes are involved

B. Irrigation
   1. Assemble equipment: basin of sterile solution as ordered at 95° F to 100° F, medicine dropper or ear syringe, basin for return flow, cotton balls to protect uninvolved eye and to dry treated eye, and face towel to protect bed; separate irrigating tip is needed for each eye

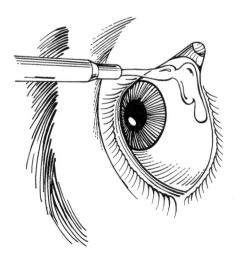

Figure 2-15.   Irrigation of the eye. The nurse turns the patient's head toward the eye that is to be irrigated. Solution flows from the inner canthus to the outer canthus of the eye. The irrigator is held less than 4 inches (10 cm) away from the eye. The patient may assist by retracting the lower eyelid and collecting irrigating solution with absorbent material. (From Elkin MK, Perry AG, Potter PA: *Nursing interventions and clinical skills*, ed 2, St Louis, 2000, Mosby.)

   2. Direct flow of solution into conjunctival sac from inner angle to outer angle of eye; position patient toward affected side (Figure 2-15)

Ear Treatment: Irrigation

A. Assemble equipment: sterile ear syringe, solution as ordered at 105° F to 108° F, basin for return flow, and towel to protect bed
B. Position patient: patient may lie down, but sitting position is preferred, with head tilted slightly so that affected ear is downward; patient may hold basin for return flow, if able
C. Retract pinna, in direction according to age, to expose orifice of external canal; direct flow gently against side of canal; interrupt irrigation if pain or dizziness occurs and notify physician

Throat Treatments

A. Throat swab
   1. Assemble equipment: sterile applicators, tongue blade, medication as ordered, tissue wipes, flashlight, and paper bag
   2. When swabbing throat, avoid stimulating gag reflex by not touching uvula
B. Throat culture
   1. Assemble equipment: sterile culture tube, applicator, and tissue wipes
   2. After touching sides and back of throat with applicator, put applicator in culture tube without contaminating inside of tube by breaking off top of applicator that was touched by fingers
C. Throat irrigation
   1. Assemble equipment: irrigating container, solution as ordered at 110° F, tubing with rubber tip on end, tissue wipes, basin for return flow, towel to protect patient; protective gloves
   2. Put on protective gloves
   3. Have patient tilt head forward over basin and breathe through nose; discourage deep breathing
   4. Have patient do treatment if able
   5. Hold container slightly above patient's mouth; direct flow toward affected area
      a. Irrigation may be interrupted for patient's comfort
      b. Flow should not be directed toward uvula or base of tongue
   6. Tilt patient's head to one side and then the other to facilitate results

MEASURES FOR GASTROINTESTINAL DISORDERS
Gastric Intubation

A. Purposes
   1. To administer gavage feedings
   2. To obtain specimens (gastric analysis and cytology)
   3. To irrigate or cleanse (lavage)
   4. For decompression (suction)
B. Tube locations
   1. Nose to stomach: nasogastric
   2. Mouth to stomach: orogastric
   3. Artificial opening into stomach: gastrostomy
C. Insertion of tube
   1. Is not always the responsibility of a licensed practical/vocational nurse (LP/VN): refer to your agency's policy

2. Assemble equipment: flashlight, tongue blade, stethoscope, cup of water, irrigating syringe, water-soluble lubricant, 12- to 18-gauge French tube, gloves, and towel to protect patient's clothing
3. If rubber tube is used, it should be chilled first
4. Place patient in semi-Fowler's position with towel protecting clothing
5. Approximate distance of tube insertion is the length from tip of nose to ear lobe to xiphoid process
6. Apply water-soluble lubricant to tip of tube; if intubation is for cytology study, tube is lubricated with water or saline solution
7. With gloved hands hold tube 3 inches (7.5 cm) from tip, place into nostril or mouth, and advance
8. Have patient flex neck and take repeated shallow breaths when tube passes into pharynx (about 3 inches [7.5 cm])
9. Have patient swallow while advancing tube

D. Checking placement of tube
   1. Check back of throat with tongue blade and flashlight to see if coiling has occurred
   2. Aspirate stomach contents; may need to advance tube if no stomach contents are obtained
   3. While injecting 5 ml of air, use stethoscope to listen for air entering stomach
   4. Observe patient's respirations and note ability to speak; respirations may be labored or patient will be unable to speak if tube is in trachea or lungs

E. Securing tube (Figure 2-16)
   1. Anchor with strip of tape; secure to nose and cheek if nasogastric; avoid resting tube on side of nares to avoid irritation or necrosis
   2. Tube may be looped through a rubber band and attached to patient gown with safety pin for added security

F. Removal of tube
   1. Clamp tube
   2. Remove anchoring tape
   3. Put on protective gloves
   4. Draw tube through towel so that it is wiped of secretions
   5. Have patient inhale and exhale slowly
   6. Pull tube with one continuous, rapid motion
   7. Have basin ready if patient vomits

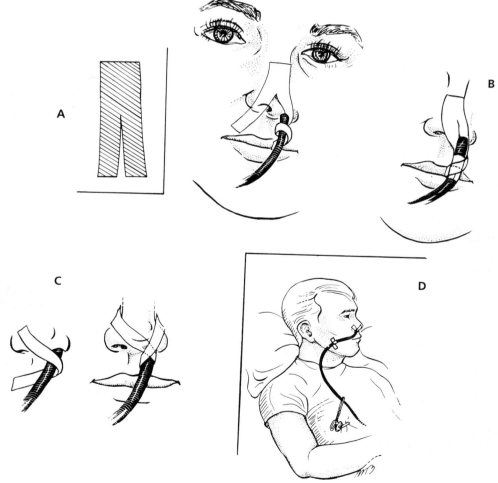

Figure 2-16. Securing the nasogastric tube. **A,** A length of adhesive tape is split for use in anchoring the tube to the nostril. **B,** The unsplit portion is affixed to the nose: one of the split portions is wrapped around the tube, and then the other portion is wrapped around the tube. **C,** A narrow strip of tape may be used to secure the tube. **D,** The tube is taped to the nostril and cheek and clamped or connected to suction. (From Dison N: *Clinical nursing techniques,* ed 4, St Louis, 1975, Mosby.)

Suction and Irrigation

A. Nasogastric or GI tubes (Levin, Cantor, Miller-Abbott, or Salem sump) may be connected to mechanical suction apparatus
B. Suction
   1. Rate is ordered by physician or according to agency policy
   2. May be intermittent or continuous
   3. Collection container is emptied and rinsed; amount of drainage is measured and recorded at end of shift and when container becomes nearly filled
   4. Turn off or clamp off suction when assessing for bowel sounds. Suction may mimic the sounds of peristalsis
C. Irrigation
   1. Check orders for frequency, solution type, amount, and method of aspiration (force or gravity)
   2. Assemble equipment: solution as ordered, container for solution, basin for return flow, irrigating syringe (bulb or plunger type), and protective pad
   3. Fill syringe and free it of air
   4. Instill solution into tube slowly and gently
   5. Allow solution to return by aspirating or by gravity
   6. Remove syringe and reconnect to suction if ordered
D. Patients with indwelling tubes should be given frequent mouth and nose care
E. Accurate measurement of intake and output (subtracting irrigating solution) is essential

MEASURES FOR VAGINAL CARE
Perineal Care

A. Assemble equipment: solution as ordered, cotton balls (or washcloth) for cleansing and drying, gloves, perineal pad with belt, and bedpan
B. With gloved hands put patient on bedpan; pour solution over vulva, clean with cotton balls or washcloth; dry vulva; make patient comfortable
C. If using bottle method, fill bottle with warm water and squeeze solution over vulva; dry, wiping from urinary meatus toward anus and wiping only once with each cotton ball

Vaginal Irrigation (Douche)

A. Assemble equipment: irrigating container with solution as ordered, tubing with douche tip, clamp, cotton balls for drying, gloves, perineal pad with belt, bedpan, and bed protection
B. Have patient void; place on bedpan, or patient may administer to self in bathroom if able
C. Insert tip down and back into vagina
D. Give irrigation under low pressure; have solution flowing before inserting douche tip; rotate douche tip until prescribed amount is used
E. If patient is on bedpan, raise head of bed slightly to allow fluid to drain into bedpan

MEASURES FOR PATIENTS UNDERGOING SURGERY
Preoperative Preparation

A. Psychosocial aspects
   1. Nurse assesses patient's knowledge and expected results of surgery
   2. Anxiety may interfere with preoperative teaching
   3. Extremely frightened patients may respond poorly to surgery
   4. Planned, individualized, simple explanations will enhance patient cooperation and reduce anxiety
   5. Nurse assesses and responds to patient's religious needs
   6. Common preoperative fears
      a. Fear of mutilation
      b. Fear of death
      c. Fear of change in family role
      d. Fear of pain
   7. Family or significant others must understand measures taken to prepare patient
   8. Family or significant others should participate in explanations and encouragement
B. Physical preparation
   1. Explain preoperative tests (CBC, ECG, urinalysis, x-ray examinations)
   2. Explain, demonstrate, and have patient practice any special postoperative exercises that will need to be done (turning, deep breathing, and pumping feet)
   3. Follow preoperative orders as prescribed by physician (enema, diet, and medications)
   4. Prepare appropriate skin area (see agency procedure manual)
   5. Care for valuables
   6. Follow and complete preoperative checklist
      a. Informed consents for surgery and anesthesia signed and witnessed
      b. Nail polish, prostheses, jewelry, and makeup removed
      c. Patient dressed in hospital gown only
      d. Hygienic measures performed (bath with mouth care and voiding or catheterization)
      e. Vital signs collected and recorded and abnormalities reported
      f. Identification and allergy bracelets in place
C. Observations and procedures recorded
D. After patient leaves for operative procedure, prepare postoperative bed and unit

Postoperative Care

A. Immediate care
   1. Ensure and maintain patent airway
   2. Maintain adequate circulation
   3. Observe for complications at operative site and in general (hemorrhage, shock, swelling, and severe pain). Carefully observe dependent areas of the body for concealed hemorrhage
   4. Assess and secure dressing, drainage, and IV tubing
   5. Assess mental status (orientation)
   6. Position patient properly; keep patient warm
   7. Assess vital signs as often as ordered or more frequently, as condition warrants
   8. Follow physician's orders
   9. Report signs of restlessness, excessive drainage, or abnormal reactions
   10. Support patient and family by briefly answering questions and offering explanations
B. Routine care
   1. Follow physician's orders
   2. Assess and record vital signs frequently during first 24 hours; report changes immediately
   3. Assess dressing or surgical site frequently
   4. Give oral hygiene as needed

5. Have patient turn, deep breathe, and, unless contraindicated, cough and exercise legs at least q2h
6. Assess and record intake and output (patient may need order for catheterization if he or she does not void within 6 to 8 hours after surgery)
7. Assist patient with passive or active exercises unless contraindicated
8. Encourage and assist patient to ambulate as much as orders permit
9. Perform daily assessment
   a. Lungs: breath sounds and cough
   b. Circulation: color, temperature, capillary refill of extremities; pain in legs or chest and IV site
   c. GI tract: nausea, vomiting, distention, bowel sounds, and passage of flatus
   d. Urine: amount, color, odor, and frequency
   e. Mental status: withdrawal, confusion, anxiety, or restlessness
10. Offer pain medication

MEASURES RELATED TO RADIATION THERAPY

A. Radiation
   1. Radiate: to send out rays (light, heat, or roentgen)
   2. Radiation is used in diagnosis and therapeutic treatment of various conditions (especially for malignancies)
   3. Types of radiation
      a. Alpha rays: harmless; do not travel far
      b. Beta rays: more penetrating; stop at person's body surface
      c. Gamma rays: very penetrating
B. Types of therapy
   1. Infrared lamp
   2. Ultraviolet
   3. Diatherapy
   4. Roentgen ray (x-ray: low voltage, external)
   5. Betatron, cobalt, cesium (high voltage, external)
   6. Internal radiation
      a. Implants (skin surface, intratumor, intracavitary)
      b. Liquid forms of radioisotopes
      c. Injection (intracavitary, systemic)
C. Radiation therapy and the nurse
   1. Internal implant
      a. Explain procedure and precautions to patient and family or significant others
         (1) Patient needs to know that he or she will be in isolation and how many days isolation is likely to last
         (2) Patient should know that nursing personnel and visitors will be spending a minimal amount of time at the bedside and yet will be available when needed
      b. Ensure good fluid intake unless contraindicated
      c. Have patient move about as little as possible
      d. Assess for signs of radiation reactions (nausea, vomiting, or skin irritation)
      e. Communicate frequently with patient from doorway without entering room
      f. Use precautions at all times
   2. Radiation precautions with implant
      a. "RADIATION IN USE" sign with directions posted on patient's door

b. No staff member or visitor spends more than 1 hour per day with patient; care must be well organized
c. Pregnant women and children should not enter the patient's room
d. Check placement of implant q4h
e. Wear gown and gloves while handling excreta, secretions, and utensils. Excreta may need to be double flushed in toilet, know agency policy
f. Wash contaminated gloves with soap and water before removing
g. Wash hands with soap and water
h. If implant becomes dislodged, call radiologist immediately—do not touch implant

   3. Nursing care for specific situations
      a. Therapy involving mouth
         (1) Oral hygiene with brushing teeth (or dentures) should be done 3 times a day (tid)
         (2) Smoking should be discouraged
         (3) Teeth should be assessed for change in condition; if changes observed, notify physician
         (4) Male patient should not shave if jaw is being treated
      b. Uterine therapy
         (1) Bed rest is maintained to prevent displacement of implant
         (2) Bedpan is inspected for loss of implant before contents are discarded
         (3) Foley catheter with continuous irrigation may be ordered to reduce bladder irritation
         (4) Vaginal irrigation may be ordered after removal of implant
      c. Radioactive gold administered intraperitoneally
         (1) Leakage on dressings appears bright red and may be confused with blood
         (2) Dressings should be wrapped in newspaper and disposed of in special container
   4. External radiotherapy
      a. Explain procedure to patient and family or significant others
      b. Never remove skin markings
      c. Avoid washing the marked area
      d. Do not apply ointments, creams, or powders to marked area
      e. Encourage good fluid intake and nutrition
      f. Observe for radiation reactions

MEASURES CONCERNING PATIENT'S DEPARTURE

A. Transferring patient
   1. Patient may be transferred from one service to another, from one floor to another, or from one agency to another
   2. Physician's order is required
   3. Transfer patient ambulatory, by wheelchair, or on stretcher; follow agency's policy
   4. Explain transfer to patient; be sure all personal belongings are transferred with patient
   5. Avoid transferring during mealtime or change of shift to reduce confusion
   6. Make proper charting notations; notify significant others

B. Discharging patient
1. Written order by physician is required
2. Nurse's responsibilities
   a. Gather and check all personal belongings with patient
   b. Make sure patient understands all instructions regarding diet, medications, treatments, and follow-up appointments
   c. Notify family as necessary
   d. Accompany patient to exit
   e. Make proper charting notations
3. Discharge planning
   a. Begins after initial nursing assessment and is included on care plan
   b. Nursing interventions are directed toward eventual discharge of patient
   c. Planning consists of teaching patient and family or significant other
      (1) Cause of illness
      (2) Drugs, treatments, and diet
      (3) Health care follow-up
      (4) Functions within limitations

CARING FOR THE DYING

A. Signs of approaching death
1. Patient is pale with pinched expression of anxiety
2. Eyes are glazed and dull; pupils do not react to light
3. Mouth remains partially open unless patient attempts to speak; speech is mumbled and often confused
4. Muscle tone becomes flaccid
5. Skin is cool and clammy and may be mottled; this is caused by diminished circulation; body temperature is often elevated
6. Respirations are rapid and shallow, often progressing to Cheyne-Stokes
7. Pulse becomes weak and thready
8. Patient may be diaphoretic, thirsty, and incontinent of urine and feces
B. Five stages in the process of reaction to a terminal illness or to dying: refer to Chapter 6 for more detailed information relative to death and dying
1. Denial
2. Anger
3. Bargaining
4. Grief/depression
5. Acceptance
C. Nursing care of dying patient
1. Give symptomatic nursing care
2. Give good personal hygiene
3. Turn patient frequently
4. Give treatments and medications as long as possible or until discontinued
5. Carry out desires of patient, family, or significant others as far as possible
6. Be available to provide emotional support and privacy to patient, family, or significant other
7. Remember that hearing may be the last sense to fail

D. Spiritual needs of patient
1. Fulfill needs as requested by patient, family, or significant other
2. Continue to adhere to patient's individual religious beliefs
E. Care of body after death (postmortem care): physicians pronounce death in most cases. Registered nurses may pronounce death (in some states) under special circumstances (hospice patients)
1. Lower head of bed
2. Leave one pillow under head to prevent congestion of blood in vessels of face
3. Close eyes
4. Place dentures in mouth immediately and close mouth
5. Clean body; follow agency's policy for removal of drains, IV needle and tubing, dressings, and tubes
6. Straighten body and place in natural position
7. Allow viewing of body by family or significant other if they desire
8. Wrap in shroud and label with tags according to agency policy
9. Gather, pack, label, and care for patient's personal belongings
10. Record observations, procedures, disposition of valuables, and time of death; complete records

SUGGESTED READINGS

Becker BG, Fendler DT: *Vocational and personal adjustments in practical nursing,* ed 7, St Louis, 1994, Mosby.

Bernhard LA, Walsh M: *Leadership: the key to the professionalization of nursing,* ed 3, St Louis, 1995, Mosby.

Blair L: *Passport to practical and vocational nursing,* St Louis, 1998, Mosby.

Christensen BL, Kockrow EO: *Foundations of nursing,* ed 3, St Louis, 1999, Mosby.

Cole G: *Fundamental nursing concepts and skills,* ed 2, St Louis, 1996, Mosby.

DuGas BW, Esson L, Ronaldson SE: *Nursing foundations: a Canadian perspective,* ed 2, Scarborough, Ontario, 1999, Prentice Hall.

Dunham-Taylor J, Penny Marquette R, Pinczuk JZ: Surviving capitation, *AJN* 96:26, 1996.

Elkin MK, Perry AG, Potter PA: *Nursing interventions and clinical skills,* St Louis, 2000, Mosby.

Ellis JR, Nowlis EA, Bentz PM: *Modules for basic nursing skills, modules I and II,* ed 6, 1996, Lippincott-Raven.

Grossman D: Cultural dimensions in home health nursing, *AJN* 96:33, 1996.

Kerr JR, Sirotnik MK: *Potter and Perry Canadian fundamentals of nursing,* St Louis, 1997, Mosby.

McDevitt MJ: A(TENS)tion!, *Nursing* 25:46, 1995.

Potter PA, Perry AG: *Basic nursing, a critical thinking approach,* ed 4, St Louis, 1999, Mosby.

Stolley JM: Freeing your patients from restraints, *AJN* 95:26, 1995.

Sullivan EJ, Decker PJ: *Effective leadership and nursing management in nursing,* ed 4, Upper Saddle River, 1997, Prentice Hall Health.

Wheeler SR: Helping families cope with death and dying, *Nursing* 26:25, 1996.

REVIEW QUESTIONS

1. A 59-year-old female patient arrives at the physician's office complaining of severe back pain. Which of the following questions would be most important to ask when gathering information for the physician?
   ① "Are you allergic to any drugs?"
   ② "Can you point to where the pain is?"
   ③ "How have you treated the pain at home?"
   ④ "Are you experiencing any other symptoms?"

2. A patient is being prepared for sealed internal radiation therapy for cervical cancer. The nurse can help reduce the patient's anxiety by emphasizing that:
   ① Pain medication will be offered regularly
   ② Visitors will be limited during this treatment
   ③ The nurse will be available whenever needed
   ④ The patient will not be radioactive during this treatment

3. A patient begins to leave a physician's office after receiving instructions concerning a scheduled cholecystectomy. Which of the following is the correct rationale for reviewing the preoperative instructions prior to the patient's leaving?
   ① Repetition increases learning
   ② Physicians use very technical terms
   ③ Patient anxiety may have interfered with understanding
   ④ Preoperative documentation requires teaching reinforcement by the nurse

4. When performing a throat culture, the nurse swabs the sides of the throat before the back in order to:
   ① Delay stimulating the gag reflex
   ② Stimulate production of secretions
   ③ Avoid contamination of the culture site
   ④ Obtain adequate specimens for culture

5. One hour after the nurse applies an elastic bandage to a patient's sprained ankle, the patient complains of tingling and burning in the toes. The nurse should:
   ① Palpate for pedal pulses
   ② Reapply the bandage less snugly
   ③ Instruct her to elevate the affected foot
   ④ Encourage her to wiggle her toes every 2 hours

6. During a surgical dressing change, the nurse notes that there is copious purulent drainage along the reddened incision site. These symptoms most likely indicate:
   ① Local infection
   ② Systemic infection
   ③ Necrosis of the wound
   ④ Nosocomial wound contamination

7. When performing wound irrigations, the nurse can best be protected by:
   ① Raising the bed to a workable height
   ② Explaining the procedure to the patient
   ③ Hand washing before and after the procedure
   ④ Donning appropriate personal protective equipment

8. Which of the following patients is most at risk for decubitus formation?
   ① A 20-year-old with an L4 injury confined to a wheelchair
   ② A 6-year-old in skeletal traction for a fractured right femur
   ③ An ambulatory 90-year-old patient with Alzheimer's disease
   ④ A 75-year-old male on bed rest following total knee replacement

9. A patient is 1 day postoperative gastric resection. The patient has a nasogastric tube attached to low-intermittent suction and complains of severe thirst. The nurse's next course of action is:
   ① Call the physician for an order allowing ice chips
   ② Instill approximately 100 ml of normal saline into his tube
   ③ Explain that he must remain NPO until the tube is removed
   ④ Assist the patient in brushing his teeth and rinsing his mouth

10. A nurse assigns an unlicensed assistive personnel (UAP) to medicate a patient complaining of a headache. In assigning this task the nurse is:
    ① Prioritizing patient care
    ② Responsive to patient complaints
    ③ Enhancing the UAP's sense of self-worth
    ④ Delegating an inappropriate task to ancillary personnel

11. In a managed care environment, the nurse has an ethical responsibility to the patient to:
    ① Provide only allowable services
    ② Assume the role of patient advocate
    ③ Interpret insurance coverage for the patient
    ④ Determine level of care based upon insurance benefits

12. A patient, newly admitted to a nursing home, complains of difficulty in sleeping. The patient states that he routinely takes sleeping pills in order for him to fall asleep. Which of the following is the nurse's best response to the patient's statement?
    ① "We really don't like our residents to use sleeping pills."
    ② "It's not unusual to have difficulty sleeping in a new setting."
    ③ "Let me try to make you comfortable first before giving you a sleeping pill."
    ④ "I'm certain your doctor will reorder the medication for you when I tell him tomorrow."

13. When performing an intermittent bladder irrigation, the nurse discontinues instilling fluid if the:
    ① Irrigant returns are clear
    ② Irrigant returns are bloody
    ③ Returns equal the fluid instilled
    ④ The patient complains of bladder spasm

14. A patient has returned to the unit following a transurethral resection of the prostate (TURP). The nurse notes that the bedside drainage unit is filled with red urine and numerous large clots. The abdomen is distended, and the bladder can be palpated above the symphysis pubis. Which of the following is the nurse's first course of action?
    ① Change the patient's position
    ② Notify the surgeon of your findings
    ③ Check the chart for bladder irrigation orders
    ④ Document your observations on the flow sheet

15. A male patient has just been admitted in acute respiratory distress. The physician has prescribed nasal oxygen

at 3 L/min and has ordered that a Foley catheter be inserted. In light of this patient's condition, the most appropriate position for this procedure is:
① Supine
② Dorsal recumbent
❸ High Fowler's with knees flat
④ High Fowler's with knees gatched

16. Bacterial contamination of indwelling catheters in home care patients can often be avoided by:
① Scheduling weekly catheter changes
② Administration of prophylactic antibiotics
❸ Daily cleansing of meatus and catheter with soap and water
④ Thorough cleansing of the meatus with appropriate antiseptic solution

17. A patient who is 1 day postop abdominal hysterectomy has a urinary catheter, a Penrose drain, and an IV of dextrose 5% in Ringer's lactate infusing at 100 ml/hour. The patient is complaining of a sense of urinary urgency and lower abdominal pressure and requests an injection of Demerol. Which of the following is the nurse's <u>first</u> course of action?
① Check when this patient was last medicated for pain
② Request that the physician change the IV flow rate order
❸ Determine that urine is draining into the bedside drainage unit
④ Assure the patient that catheters often cause this type of discomfort

18. A patient is recovering in the same-day surgery unit, after undergoing cataract repair to the left eye. How should the nurse best assist the patient in regards to delivering the lunch tray?
① Offer to feed the patient
② Remove all hot fluids from the tray
❸ Describe the tray in clock fashion to the patient
❹ Place the tray so that the patient does not have to strain to reach it

19. A patient of African-American descent is admitted with status asthmaticus and presents as very dyspneic and uncomfortable. Due to the dark complexion, how should the nurse assess for the symptom of cyanosis?
❶ By examining his oral mucosa
② Monitoring vital signs hourly
③ Observing lips and nail beds
❹ Applying a pulse oximeter probe

20. A patient with insulin controlled diabetes mellitus, residing in a long-term care facility, calls the nurse to her room because she has been vomiting during the night and is now feeling weak and lightheaded. Which of the following nursing interventions would take priority?
① Taking her blood pressure
❷ Performing a glucometer test
③ Instructing her to remain in bed today
④ Having her maintain a clear fluid diet for the day

21. The physician has ordered a patient's IV to infuse at 100 ml per hour. The IV was started at 7:00 PM. When the nurse rounds at 11:00 PM, 200 ml fluid has infused into the patient. The nurse's initial course of action is to:
① Notify the physician that the IV has infiltrated

② Note the amount on the patient's intake and output record
❸ Check the tubing and infusion site for possible obstructions
④ Change the rate of flow until the correct amount has infused

22. The volume of a patient's Foley catheter bedside drainage unit is most accurately measured by:
① Holding the drainage bag up at eye level
② Approximating output from the markings on the drainage unit
③ Emptying the urine into a bedpan and noting what level it reaches
❹ Pouring the urine into a measuring container on a flat eye-level surface

23. Which of the following nursing measures would best address the comfort needs of a patient with a newly inserted tracheostomy tube?
❶ Providing a pad and pencil within reach
② Having tissues easily available to the patient
❸ Reassuring the patient that nurses are always nearby
④ Arranging to have telephone service discontinued temporarily

24. An elderly patient is receiving nasal oxygen at 2 L/min and has been placed on bed rest. During the evening, the patient complains that her feet are cold. The nurse's best response is to:
❶ Offer the patient cotton socks
② Bring the patient a woolen blanket
③ Place a hot water bottle under the patient's feet
④ Assure the patient that this is a common complaint for her diagnosis

25. The nurse has been assigned to perform colostomy care for a patient who has had a recent hemicolectomy. The nurse can best determine how the patient tolerated the procedure by:
❶ Noting all objective signs and symptoms during the procedure
② Asking the patient if anything is bothering him during the procedure
③ Questioning the patient regarding his well-being at the end of the treatment
❹ Observing the patient's verbal and nonverbal actions throughout the procedure

26. The chief reason that the nurse explains procedure steps and purpose to the patient prior to performing a treatment is:
① It diminishes the likelihood of malpractice suits
❷ Patient anxiety is decreased with understanding
③ It allows the patient the opportunity to refuse the treatment
④ It provides the nurse with an opportunity to mentally review the procedure

27. Which instruction is most appropriate for a patient with copious bronchial secretions?
① "Decrease fluid intake to solidify bronchial secretions."
❷ "Tracheal suctioning is the best method for removing heavy secretions."
❸ "Try to drink several glasses of juice or water daily to loosen secretions."

④ "You'll find it easier to breathe if you sit up straight during postural drainage treatments."

28. When contributing to the nursing care plan, the nurse knows that an example of a short-term goal is:
    ① Assist patient in range-of-motion exercises
    ❷ Patient will transfer from bed to chair this week
    ③ Patient will return to previous level of functioning
    ④ Physical activity will improve muscle tone and function

29. The measure of blood glucose control in a patient with diabetes mellitus is best determined by:
    ① Regular evaluation of glucose tolerance tests
    ❷ Home blood glucose monitoring several times daily
    ③ Daily monitoring of sugar and acetone content in the urine
    ④ Measurement of sugar and acetone in double-voided specimens

30. When instructing a patient in the procedure for collecting stools for occult blood, the nurse explains to the patient that:
    ① Diarrhea stools are unacceptable sources for this examination
    ② The specimen should be kept warm until delivery to the laboratory
    ❸ Small samples should be taken from two separate areas of the stool
    ④ The specimen should only be obtained from stool areas containing blood

31. A patient with heart failure is beginning a treatment regimen that includes diuretic medications. Which of the following instructions regarding obtaining weights should the nurse reinforce to the patient?
    ❶ Weigh each morning upon arising
    ② Weigh 1 hour after taking medication
    ③ Weigh each time a medication is omitted
    ④ Weigh only when shortness of breath develops

32. When preparing a patient for X-ray examination, the nurse takes care to instruct the patient to:
    ① Remove all undergarments for better visualization
    ② Fast from food and fluids 12 hours prior to the exam
    ③ Layer clothing to avoid chilling during the examination
    ❹ Remove all pins and jewelry in the path of the X-ray exam

33. While documenting the care of a home care patient, the nurse realizes that significant information was mistakenly omitted from yesterday's notes. The nurse should:
    ① Rewrite the notes after discarding the original
    ② Include yesterday's observations in today's note
    ❸ Document the observations in a dated addendum
    ④ Write "error" and initial it after drawing a line through the notes

34. The nurse is providing hospice care for a patient with terminal bone cancer. Tonight the patient is weeping and states "I can't take any more of this, I wish you would just give me something to end it all." The nurse's best response would be:
    ❶ "You can't take any more of this?"
    ❷ "I'll get you something for the pain"
    ③ "It would be unethical for me to do something like that."

④ "I'm sure you'll feel much better after you've had some sleep."

35. An elderly patient required a Foley catheter following hip surgery. Lab tests now indicate that the patient has developed a *Pseudomonas aeruginosa* urinary tract infection. In light of this patient's medical history, the nurse would suspect that this is a (an):
    ① Superinfection
    ❷ Nosocomial infection
    ③ Autoimmune response
    ④ Antibiotic resistance response

36. A mother has brought her child to see the pediatrician because the child, who has chickenpox, has developed a high fever and ear pain. As the office nurse, you would:
    ❶ Immediately bring the child into a closed examination room
    ② Suggest that the child see the physician in the emergency room
    ③ Have the child wear a face mask if he must be near any other patients
    ④ Tell the mother to avoid letting the child touch any toys in the waiting room

37. When moving heavy physical therapy equipment onto a patient's bed, nurses know that they can best avoid personal injury by:
    ❶ Carrying the equipment close to the body
    ② Sliding equipment from the floor to the bed
    ③ Using the back muscles to do the major lifting
    ④ Holding the equipment at arm's length from the body

38. Which of the following breakfasts would be appropriate to serve to a postpartum mother observing Kosher diet rules?
    ❶ Oatmeal, poached egg, whole wheat toast with jelly, grapefruit, tea
    ② Blueberry pancakes with syrup, pork sausage, fresh orange, coffee
    ③ Creamed chipped beef on toast, corn flakes, yogurt, sliced melon, milk
    ④ Scrambled eggs and bacon, bagel and cream cheese, orange juice, tea

39. When collecting a patient's psychosocial history, the nurse questions religious affiliation because:
    ❶ Religion may affect health practices
    ② It determines whether the patient should receive last rites
    ③ Certain religious denominations offer social supports to ill members
    ④ The patient may wish to have specific clergy notified of hospitalization

40. During the past decade health care trends have caused nursing care to be:
    ① Greatly diminished in scope
    ② More focused on treatment of illness
    ❸ Less concentrated in the acute care setting
    ❹ Based on technology rather than treatment

41. As a professional, the nurse is ethically bound to:
    ① Regularly file for relicensure
    ② Maintain active membership in professional nursing organizations

④ Keep abreast of changing trends and technologies within the field

④ Campaign for political programs that guarantee nursing employment

42. Nurses completing incident reports following medication errors should be sure to:
    ① Correct the error as quickly as possible
    ② Notify the patient and his family of the error
    ③ Document completion of the incident report on the patient's chart
    ● Note the medication administered as well as notification of the physician

43. Licensing laws regulate the practice of nursing to:
    ● Protect the public from injury
    ● Guarantee the best possible nursing care
    ③ Ensure that every nurse has good moral character
    ④ Support nurse employment by limiting the competition

44. A nurse has been assigned to help teach a patient regarding the use of a new blood glucose monitor. The nurse is unfamiliar with the equipment. The nurse's best course of action would be to:
    ① Refuse the assignment, since he/she is unprepared
    ● Have the charge nurse explain the equipment to him/her
    ③ Use a different, more familiar monitor for teaching the patient
    ④ Have the patient demonstrate what he knows concerning the monitor

45. A patient is preparing for discharge after incision and drainage of an infected hand wound. The nurse has been assigned to review the instructions concerning home care of the wound. The nurse, finding the patient sitting and watching TV, should approach the patient by saying:
    ① "This should only take us a few minutes if you listen carefully."
    ● "Would you mind if I turn off your TV while we discuss your wound care?"
    ③ "I can see that you're busy right now, so I'll come back later if I have time."
    ④ "Wound care can be very complicated, so we may be practicing this for a while."

46. To ensure optimum evacuation, patients receiving sodium phosphate (Fleet) enemas should be encouraged to:
    ① Expel the enema immediately following instillation
    ● Retain the enema solution for at least 5 minutes
    ③ Receive the enema while seated on the commode
    ④ Rest quietly in bed immediately following enema instillation

47. During the bed bath procedure, the nurse reduces the chance of infection by:
    ① Thoroughly rinsing and drying all skin folds
    ● Applying clean gloves before beginning the bath
    ● Using separate wash cloth sections for each eye
    ④ Changing the bath water after bathing each extremity

48. The rules and regulations governing the practice of nursing in the United States are made by:
    ● Each state's legislative body
    ● Each state's board of nursing
    ③ The National Council of State Boards of Nursing

④ The Joint Commission of Accreditation of Health Care Organizations

49. When first ambulating a patient, the nurse encourages the patient to dangle at the bedside to:
    ① Increase joint flexibility
    ② Assess the patient's ability to move unassisted
    ● Prevent the complication of orthostatic hypotension
    ④ Align the patient's extremities for optimum ambulation

50. A patient has spent several weeks in traction for a leg fracture. During the morning bath he confides in you that he keeps hearing voices in the room, although he knows he is alone. The nurse's best response would be:
    ● "Tell me more about these voices."
    ● "Have you ever had this happen before?"
    ③ "Ignore them. You've been alone in this room too long."
    ④ "That's interesting, but tell me more about how your leg is feeling."

51. An elderly patient has arrived at the physician's office complaining of ear pain, vertigo, and impaired hearing. The physician has ordered a normal saline ear irrigation to loosen embedded ear wax. Following this procedure, the nurse would take care to:
    ① Retract the pinna of the ear
    ● Determine the patient's tolerance of movement
    ③ Encourage the patient to remain supine for several hours
    ④ Thoroughly dry the ear canal with cotton-tipped applicators

52. A female patient has been admitted to the hospital unit with a fever of unknown origin. The physician has ordered urine and blood specimens for culture as well as a broad-spectrum antibiotic. The nurse should:
    ● Obtain the specimens before beginning antibiotic therapy
    ② Ask the physician to clarify which procedure should be performed first
    ③ Begin the antibiotic therapy immediately before obtaining the specimens
    ④ Obtain the blood, start the medication, and tell the patient to call when she is able to void

53. When applying sterile gloves, the nurse is careful to:
    ① Handle only the outside of each glove
    ● Pick the first glove up by the inside of the cuff
    ③ Keep the gloves on the sterile field throughout the procedure
    ④ Insert his/her fingers under the outside cuff to apply the first glove

54. Which of the following observations would indicate that the nurse should withhold a tube feeding?
    ● Oozing at the gastrostomy site
    ② Absence of an adequate gag reflex
    ● Presence of more than 100 ml of residual feeding
    ④ Absence of residual feeding when the gastrostomy tube is suctioned

55. Patients receiving gastrostomy tube feedings may experience gastric bloating and diarrhea if:
    ● The feeding formula is changed
    ② The feeding is delivered by electronic pump infusion

③ The patient does not remain upright for 1 hour after infusion

④ The gastrostomy tube is not adequately flushed following each feeding

56. If a patient complains of the urge to defecate after the nurse begins to administer a tap water enema, the nurse should:
① Adjust the tube location while maintaining fluid flow
② Lower the enema bag while instructing the patient to breathe deeply
③ Reassure the patient that the discomfort should pass in a few minutes
④ Immediately discontinue the procedure to allow patient bowel evacuation

57. The nurse knows that a patient undergoing nasogastric (NG) suction may soon have the tube removed when:
① The patient no longer complains of nausea
② Bowel sounds are heard in all four quadrants
③ Scant drainage is present on the surgical dressing
④ There is no gastric drainage into the suction container

58. An elderly patient who underwent emergency resection of the colon 2 days ago is receiving intravenous fluids and has a nasogastric tube attached to low continuous suction. The nurse notes that the patient is hiccoughing and complaining of nausea. The nurse's first course of action is to:
① Irrigate the tube to assess for blockage
② Call the physician for medication orders
③ Retape the tube to decrease throat irritation
④ Position the patient to diminish the risk of emesis aspiration

59. During a sterile dressing change, the nurse should dispose of soiled dressings:
① In the dirty utility room
② In the patient's bedside trash
③ On the sterile waterproof barrier
④ In a waterproof container away from the sterile field

60. When cleansing an open wound, the nurse should:
① Apply constant pressure
② Forcefully irrigate all wound areas
③ Scrub encrusted areas thoroughly
④ Work from cleanest to dirtiest areas

61. Which of the following should the nurse carefully document following surgical dressing changes?
① The specific location of the wound
② The characteristics of the suture line
③ The type of antibiotic cleansing solution
④ The patient's emotional response to the surgical procedure

62. When the nurse performs a skin puncture blood collection on a newborn infant, special care is taken to:
① Pierce only the center of the fingertip
② Limit punctures to the soles of the feet
③ Avoid piercing the center of the infant's heel
④ Avoid puncturing fingers on the dominant hand

63. During venipuncture, the tourniquet should be released:
① As soon as an appropriate vein is palpated
② Before withdrawing the needle from the patient's vein
③ After application of a bandage to the venipuncture site
④ As soon as blood begins flowing into the specimen tube

64. Placing the patient's arm in a downward position during venipuncture helps to:
① Dilate blood vessels for better access
② Diminish patient discomfort during the procedure
③ Prevent backflow of any chemical additives in the blood tubes
④ Prevent any unnecessary arm movement during the procedure

65. Blood specimen tubes should be labeled with the patient's name and date:
① Before the venipuncture procedure
② Upon receipt of the physician's order
③ Before leaving the venipuncture patient's side
④ Before delivery of the specimen tubes to the laboratory

66. Which of the following lab studies should be included in the plan of care for patients receiving total parenteral nutrition (TPN) infusions?
① Blood glucose
② Complete blood count
③ Hemoglobin and hematocrit
④ Erythrocyte sedimentation rate

67. When changing the dressing of a new PEG (gastric) tube insertion site, the nurse always cleanses the exit site:
① With a vigorous back-and-forth, sweeping motion
② Circularly, from the center of the exit site outward
③ Downward, from the side farthest away to the side closest
④ Upward, through the center of the site, then down each side

68. The nurse is evaluating the effectiveness of a patient's intravenous therapy. Which of the following symptoms would lead the nurse to suspect the patient may have circulatory overload?
① Bounding pulse, dyspnea, and cough
② Pain, edema, and erythema at the infusion site
③ Pain, edema, and a palpable venous cord at the infusion site
④ Fever, chills, and purulent discharge from the IV insertion site

69. A patient, receiving the first dose of IV ampicillin, begins complaining of itching upon infusion of the drug. The nurse notes that her back and abdomen are covered by red wheals. The nurse's next course of action is to:
① Discontinue the IV immediately and notify the physician
② Discontinue the IV, and set up for a restart in opposite arm
③ Discontinue the piggyback, restart original fluid, and notify the physician
④ Reassure her regarding this normal reaction and apply ointment to the rash

70. A patient has undergone complicated abdominal surgery and is now receiving TPN via a central venous catheter. During the morning bath, the patient suddenly becomes dyspneic, anxious, and cyanotic. The nurse finds that the TPN is disconnected from the central line. The nurse should first:
① Initiate the hospital's protocol for respiratory emergency
② Reconnect the TPN ports after swabbing them with alcohol

③ Place the patient on his left side with his head below chest level

④ Place the patient in high Fowler's position to assist his respiratory efforts

71. When a patient has died, the nurse should schedule postmortem care:
   ① Before family viewing of the body
   ② Following transport of the body to the morgue
   ③ As quickly as possible to decrease tension on the unit
   ④ After allowing the family the opportunity to view the body

72. A patient has just undergone a lumbar puncture and questions why he must remain flat in bed for several hours. The nurse's best response is:
   ① "You are less likely to fall if you remain quiet today."
   ② "It is easier for the nurses to check for any complications this way."
   ③ "This position prevents any increased blood loss from the spine area."
   ④ "This position allows your body to readjust pressure around your brain."

73. A patient wants to know why wet-to-dry dressings are being used to treat his stasis leg ulcer. The nurse's best response would be that this treatment:
   ① Increases circulation to the wound
   ② Cleans the wound by removing dead tissue and debris
   ③ Promotes the absorption of drainage by capillary action
   ④ Decreases pain by lowering edema along wound edges

74. When preparing a feeding pump for a patient's tube feeding, the nurse knows that the pump should be filled with:
   ① The full day's supply of formula
   ② One full can of formula each time
   ③ Eight hours' worth of feeding each time
   ④ No more than a 2-hour supply each time

75. Which of the following is a critical nursing measure when caring for patients undergoing nasogastric (NG) suctioning?
   ① Mouth care every 2 hours
   ② Thorough skin care to the nares
   ③ Turn and position every 2 hours
   ④ Maintain accurate intake and output record

76. A 16-year-old female has just returned to the unit following a tonsillectomy. Which of the following routes would be most appropriate for measuring her body temperature?
   ① Oral
   ② Rectal
   ③ Axillary
   ④ Tympanic

77. While assisting an elderly nursing home resident with a bath, you observe that the skin is dry and that the resident has been scratching. A priority in planning this resident's care is to:
   ① Avoid bathing her
   ② Call the physician
   ③ Avoid the use of soap
   ④ Apply a medicated lotion

78. Before beginning a new tube feeding via a nasogastric tube, the nurse must first:
   ① Measure and replace any residual feeding
   ② Warm the feeding to approximately 105° F

③ Check for correct tube placement in the stomach
④ Dislodge encrusted formula with a warm water flush

79. The nurse has requested an unlicensed assistive personnel (UAP) to assist in moving a paralyzed patient up in bed. Which of the following is an appropriate instruction to the UAP for this procedure?
   ① Stand one step back from the bed while lifting
   ② Keep your back straight and your knees flexed
   ③ Keep your knees straight and your back flexed
   ④ Keep your feet close together for balance

80. When monitoring a patient receiving IV therapy, which of the following observations may indicate infiltration?
   ① Poor skin turgor
   ② Redness at insertion site
   ③ Warmth at insertion site
   ④ Swollen area above catheter

81. When considering the need for application of restraints on an elderly confused patient, the nurse knows that restraints:
   ① Provide patients with a sense of security
   ② Should be applied only after receiving a physician's order
   ③ Are applied loosely on elderly patients to prevent skin abrasion
   ④ Must be tied to side rails to allow faster removal in an emergency

82. When preparing to administer oxygen via nasal cannula, the nurse attaches the oxygen flowmeter to a container of sterile distilled water to:
   ① Decrease the danger of oxygen combustion
   ② Increase the patient's level of oxygen absorption
   ③ Remove any particle contaminants from the tubing
   ④ Prevent drying the patient's nasooropharyngeal mucosa

83. A patient refuses morning care and states that he does not like to bathe in the morning; he prefers an evening shower. Which of the following is the nurse's best response?
   ① "The staff is too busy to provide for an evening shower."
   ② "The staff will do its best to provide for an evening shower."
   ③ "Bathing in the morning makes one feel more refreshed."
   ④ "Hospital routine requires nurses to provide for bathing in the morning."

84. When working in a long-term care facility, which one of the following actions would be considered unethical?
   ① Reporting UAPs for sneaking food out of the kitchen on break
   ② Going to the dementia unit and looking at your (resident) neighbor's chart
   ③ Calling a resident's husband to come sit with her because she asked you to
   ④ Asking the business office to lock up $400 that you found under a resident's pillow

85. Which of the following is the correct sequence of events to follow should a fire occur in a facility?
   ① Notify the switchboard, extinguish flames, close doors, and remove persons
   ② Call for help, remove persons, confine the fire, and extinguish any flames present

● Rescue persons, activate the alarm, confine the fire, and extinguish any flames present

④ Activate the alarm, confine the fire, remove any persons present, and use fire extinguisher

86. The nurse is caring for a patient whose left arm is restrained. Which of the following assessment data would indicate circulatory impairment of the restrained extremity?
   ① Fingers are pink and warm
   ❷ Bluish discoloration of nail beds
   ③ Ability to freely move fingers on both hands
   ④ Capillary refill times are less than 3 seconds

87. The nurse is caring for a patient who has been placed in protective isolation. When planning care for the patient, the nurse is aware that the primary goal in caring for a patient in protective isolation is:
   ① To protect the health care workers caring for the patient
   ② Limit the psychological impact of being isolated on the patient
   ❸ Reduce the number of organisms that may come in contact with the patient
   ④ Prevent the infectious process from spreading to other patients on the patient unit

88. Which of the following actions is the appropriate way for a nurse to correct a mistaken entry made in charting?
   ① Use an eraser to remove the entry
   ❷ Line out the entry, date, and initial it
   ③ Recopy the entry and destroy the original sheet
   ④ Paint over the entry using white correction fluid

89. The nurse has applied a warm, moist soak to a patient's leg. After what length of time would the nurse return to remove the soak?
   ① 2-3 minutes
   ❷ 15-30 minutes
   ③ 2-3 hours
   ④ 4-6 hours

90. A patient has a nasogastric tube inserted to decompress the stomach prior to surgery. The patient asks what the purpose of the tube is. Which of the following responses by the nurse is correct?
   ① "The tube is meant to assist your bowels to move."
   ❷ "Fluids and gas will be removed from your GI tract."
   ③ "The tube will stop gastric juice from being secreted."
   ④ "The tube will speed your healing time after the surgery."

91. Which of the following is the best method for the nurse to use to check that a large bore nasogastric tube is in the stomach?
   ① Obtain a chest radiograph
   ② Attach the tube to wall suction
   ③ Irrigate with 30 cc of sterile saline
   ❹ Instill 20 cc of air and listen for a "whoosh" over the stomach

92. A nurse is inserting a retention catheter in a female patient. The nurse suspects that the tip of the catheter may have been contaminated before it could be inserted into the meatus. The nurse's next course of action is to:
   ❶ Request a coworker to bring another sterile catheter
   ② Use betadine to decontaminate the tip of the catheter
   ③ Discontinue the procedure, discard the entire sterile tray

④ Go ahead with the procedure, the tip is probably not contaminated

93. The nurse is instructing an unlicensed assistive personnel (UAP) to place an ostomy pouch on a patient, ensuring that the pouch fits snugly. The UAP inquires as to why the ostomy pouch must be so tight. The nurse's best response is:
   ① "The pouch must stay on a long time because they are expensive."
   ② "The pouch has to stay on when the patient takes a bath or shower."
   ❸ "The pouch may leak if it's loose, causing the skin to become excoriated."
   ④ "If the pouch stays on well, the smell of the drainage can be better contained."

94. A patient is scheduled for abdominal surgery. The nurse is planning the patient's care and is aware that the reason for a "nothing by mouth" order before an operation is because:
   ① Anesthesia stops the digestive process
   ② Energy from food is not needed during surgery
   ③ There is normally vomiting in the recovery phase
   ❹ An empty stomach reduces the chance for aspiration of stomach contents

95. A nurse is suctioning secretions from a patient's nasal artificial airway. The nurse applies suction for no longer than"
   ① 3 seconds
   ❷ 10 seconds
   ③ 30 seconds
   ④ 1 minute

96. Which of the following arrhythmias is the most dangerous and life threatening?
   ① A sinus arrhythmia
   ② An atrial arrhythmia
   ③ An AV nodal arrhythmia
   ❹ A ventricular arrhythmia

97. The simplest method for a nurse to use to open a patient's airway is to:
   ① Perform a mouth sweep
   ② Turn the head to one side
   ❸ Tilt the head back and lift the chin
   ④ Perform a modified jaw thrust maneuver

98. An older adult is being evaluated for placement in a long-term care facility. The patient's family questions why some individuals the same age as their family member are in much better health. Which of the following is the nurse's best response?
   ① "Disease strikes different individuals at different times."
   ② "All the elderly will eventually fall victim to some chronic problem."
   ❸ "There is much variation among the elderly in regards to health and functioning."
   ④ "Most elderly patients will eventually become incapacitated and need a nursing home."

99. A coworker approaches a nurse with concerns that a small bore feeding tube may not be properly placed. The coworker reports that she did not hear the characteristic "whoosh" when she instilled air in the tube. Which of the following methods should the nurse advise his/her coworker to use to establish placement of the tube?
   ❶ Obtain a chest radiograph

② Attach the tube to suction
③ Irrigate the tube with 30 cc of sterile saline
④ Place the end of the tube in a glass of water and watch for bubbles

100. In planning for the medical supply needs of an elderly home health care patient, the nurse should be aware that the older adult's income level:
① Gradually increases with retirement
② Remains virtually unchanged through the years
❸ Becomes predominantly "fixed" upon retirement
④ Gradually decreases throughout life and retirement

101. The nurse is interviewing a 52 year-old patient who presents to a physician's office complaining of feelings of hopelessness and depression. Which of the following statements made by the patient would reflect life changes common to this age group?
① "I can't imagine starting my life over again."
② "My lifestyle will change so much after my retirement."
❸ "My kids have all left home and I feel so depressed now."
④ "The prospect of all this time on my hands is driving me crazy."

102. The nurse is planning an exercise program for a group of elderly individuals who have a history of cardiopulmonary disease. Which of the following activities would best meet the exercise needs of the individuals?
① Jogging
❷ Walking
③ Ski machines
④ Rowing machines

103. A patient of the Jehovah's Witness faith is scheduled for surgical repair of a hip fracture. Which of the following preoperative orders may conflict with this patient's religious practices?
① Incentive spirometry q4 hours while awake
② Coughing, deep breathing, and leg exercises q2h
❸ Type and cross for 2 units packed red blood cell (PRBCs)
④ Magnetic resonance imaging (MRI) of the right hip region

104. A nurse is caring for a patient who has a hearing impairment. Which of the following measures should the nurse do first?
① Call the hospital's American Sign Language practitioner
❷ Ask significant others how patient communicates at home
③ Arrange for a family member to stay with the patient continually
④ Arrange for a social worker to visit with patient and family members

105. A patient complains to the nurse that he is having difficulty sleeping at night. Which of the following should be the nurse's first course of action?
① Administer the patient's pain medication
② Call the physician to obtain an order for a sedative/hypnotic
③ Assure patient that no one will awaken him during the night
❹ Ask the patient what normal bedtime rituals are at his home

106. A patient asks the nurse why his eyes water and his nose runs during episodes of hay fever. Which of the following responses best describes the reason?
❶ The body is attempting to flush out the irritant
② The hay fever response is an autoimmune reaction
③ These are normal reflexes that the body uses in times of stress
④ The hay fever is actually an allergic response to grasses and trees

107. A patient presents to the emergency room following an auto accident. Which of the following problems would the nurse consider the most emergent?
① The blood glucose level is high at 396 mg/dl
② The patient has a 3 cm laceration of his left eye
❸ The patient is complaining of shortness of breath
④ A distraught family member is crying in the hallway

108. A patient with a healing stage III decubitus ulcer asks the nurse if the ulcer will leave a scar once it heals. Which of the following is the most correct response by the nurse?
① "Sometimes there is a scar and sometimes there isn't."
② "I don't think you should worry about that right now."
❸ "Usually there is a scar present with this type of healing."
④ "I think you should ask your doctor about that tomorrow."

109. A patient has an indwelling urinary retention catheter. The nurse is to obtain a sterile urine specimen from the patient. To do this the nurse should:
① Remove the patient's catheter and have him/her void
② Remove the urine from the balloon port with a syringe
❸ Collect the specimen from the sampling port on the drainage tube with a syringe
④ Disconnect the catheter from the drainage tubing and let urine drain into the specimen container

110. A patient complains of extreme pain when the nurse begins to inflate the balloon of a newly inserted urinary retention catheter. The most probable cause of the patient's pain is:
① The balloon has ruptured
② The balloon is being inflated too rapidly
❸ The balloon is not in the bladder but in the urethra
④ The patient is complaining due to the nature of the procedure

111. While transporting a patient to the radiology department in a wheelchair, the nurse should place the urinary drainage bag from her retention catheter:
① On the patient's lap
② Clipped to patient's front robe pocket
③ On the IV pole that is attached to the wheelchair
❹ Hung from the side- or backrail of the wheelchair that is below hip level

112. A nurse is assisting a physician in inserting a chest tube to resolve a pneumothorax. To drain the air from the patient's lung, the nurse assists the physician to place the chest tube:
① Laterally, near the apex of the lung
❷ Anteriorly, near the base of the lung
③ Posteriorly, near the base of the lung
❹ Anteriorly, near the apex of the lung

113. The nurse is planning to place a patient into isolation. The patient has a white blood cell count of 2000 /mm³ and has been receiving chemotherapy and radiation for 3 weeks. Which of the following types of isolation would the nurse place the patient?
    ① Strict
    ② Enteric
    ❸ Protective/reverse
    ④ Blood and body fluid precautions

114. The nurse is "prepping" a patient's skin prior to surgery. The purpose of clipping a patient's hair from the surgical site prior to surgery is to:
    ① Allow for less discomfort from the surgery
    ② Facilitate suturing of the incision after the surgery
    ❸ Reduce the incidence of infection at the surgical incision
    ④ Allow for better visualization of the site during the surgery

115. Which of the following methods would be the best way for the nurse to determine the effectiveness of preoperative teaching?
    ① Have the patient verbalize what has been taught
    ② Have the patient take a written, comprehensive quiz
    ③ Ask the patient to teach another patient how to do the skill
    ❹ Ask the patient to perform the skill for you, describing each step

116. Which of the following immediate postoperative orders would a nurse question for a patient who has received spinal anesthesia?
    ① Encourage fluids
    ② Bathroom privileges in AM
    ③ Clear liquids, advance diet as tolerated
    ❹ Keep head of bed elevated at 45 degrees

117. A nurse is applying a bandage to a patient's foot, ankle, lower leg, and knee. Where should the nurse begin bandaging the extremity?
    ❶ At the foot
    ② At the knee
    ③ At the ankle
    ④ At the middle of the leg

118. When the nurse places a patient's arm in a sling, the wrist should be:
    ❶ Level with the elbow
    ② Slightly lower than the elbow
    ❸ Slightly higher than the elbow
    ④ At least 6 inches lower than the elbow

119. In an emergency situation, which of the following is the first priority of patient care?
    ① Obtaining the victim's past medical history
    ② Controlling bleeding from a compound fracture
    ❸ Maintaining an open airway for adequate oxygenation
    ④ Performing a survey at the scene of the victim's accident

120. A victim has been rescued from near-freezing water after being submerged for nearly 1 hour. The nurse's assessment reveals he is breathless, pulseless, and hypothermic. What is the rationale for the nurse beginning CPR?
    ① The patient must be "warmed up" before death can be pronounced

    ② The near-drowning victim needs to have water removed from the lung
    ③ The cold water may have raised metabolism and revival may be possible
    ❹ Cold water temperatures slow the rate of cellular death, and revival may be possible

121. The nurse is caring for a patient who has had an arteriogram. Post-test care specific to this diagnostic test includes:
    ① Giving enemas until clear
    ② Maintaining the patient on NPO status
    ③ Ambulating the patient every 1 to 2 hours
    ❹ Checking pulses distal to the catheter insertion site

122. Blood urea nitrogen and creatinine levels are useful in determining if damage has occurred in the:
    ① Liver
    ❷ Kidneys
    ③ Muscles
    ④ Intestines

123. Of the following procedures, which one necessitates performance of a post-test gag reflex?
    ① Angiogram
    ② Arteriogram
    ③ Mammogram
    ❹ Bronchoscopy

124. A nurse needs to obtain a sputum specimen from a patient. At which time of day would it be easier for the nurse to obtain the specimen?
    ① After a meal
    ② Between meals
    ❸ In the morning
    ④ In the evening

125. When teaching a patient concerning respiratory care, which of the following measures would the nurse recommend to prevent respiratory secretions from becoming thick and difficult to expectorate?
    ① Adequate sleep
    ② Regular exercise
    ③ A nourishing diet
    ❹ A generous fluid intake

126. Which of the following would indicate to the nurse that a patient may need sputum suctioned from his respiratory tract?
    ① A respiratory rate of 22/min
    ② A heart rate that is tachycardic
    ❸ A gurgling noise in his airway
    ④ Expectorates a large amount of green mucus

127. A terminally ill adult refuses further therapy. In such situations, it is generally agreed that:
    ❶ The patient has the right to make such a decision
    ② Only the patient's physician has the authority to make such a decision
    ③ The patient and family as a group should come to this decision together
    ④ Health care workers should make every effort to dissuade patients from refusing therapy

128. The nurse is speaking with a family concerning hospice care for an elderly relative. The nurse advises the family that one of the basic assumptions of hospice care is that the:
    ① Terminally ill patient is encouraged to work through his feelings alone

② Bond between the terminally ill person and his family members is maintained

③ Majority of personal care of the person is performed around the clock by RNs

④ Hospice workers place primary emphasis on assisting family members through the grieving process

129. The nurse learns that a patient has an advanced directive. This document ensures that:
① Only lifesaving heroic measures will be utilized
② The patient's right to make decisions about his death will be honored
③ Physician will not attempt to dissuade the patient from any treatment plans
④ The family's rights to make final decisions concerning the care of the terminally ill patient will be honored

130. When should the nurse begin preparing for a patient's discharge?
① When the patient is admitted to the hospital
② After the discharge instructions are written by the physician
③ During the patient's last 2 or 3 days of hospitalization
④ After procedures take place that may necessitate a convalescent period

131. Which of the following nursing actions is performed on patients with known or suspected renal calculi?
① Flank massage
② Urine reductions
③ Straining all urine
④ Restricting fluid intake

132. While collecting a 24-hour urine specimen, the nurse should:
① Discard every other void
② Save all urine that the patient voids
③ Insert a retention catheter for the 24-hour period
④ Send each void to the lab in a separate specimen cup

133. A postoperative patient is complaining of "gas pains." Which of the following nursing interventions would aid in relieving the patient's discomfort?
① Maintain the patient on bed rest
② Contact the physician for medication
③ Insert a rectal tube for 30 minutes
④ Encourage the use of straws for drinking liquids

134. When the nurse collects a specimen for ova and parasites, the nurse should ensure that:
① The specimen is refrigerated
② A sterile specimen cup is used for collection
③ The specimen is placed in a preservative solution for transport
④ The specimen should be sent to the lab immediately after obtaining it

135. An 8-month-old child is admitted to pediatrics with a diagnosis of hyperemesis and dehydration. Which of the following signs and symptoms of dehydration might the nurse observe in the child?
① Weight gain and hypotension
② Weight loss and hypertension
③ Oliguria and poor skin turgor
④ Moist, pink mucous membranes

136. A patient has had a cast applied to his right leg. He begins to complain of pain in the ankle area and asks for pain medication. The nurse's assessment finds that the toes are warm to touch, he can move them, and he has good capillary refill. The nurse concludes that:
① The patient is reacting to having the cast applied
② The cast is most likely on too tight, causing pressure
③ From the assessment data, the patient has circulatory impairment
④ The pain is probably due to the fracture itself and may require pain medication

137. A nurse observes a patient trying to scratch the inside of his cast with a fork. Which of the following is the primary reason why this action could cause difficulty?
① Infections may occur if the skin is broken
② He may poke a hole in the cast or damage it
③ It is unsanitary to use a food utensil to scratch down his cast
④ The patient would not be able to feel if he would injure himself

138. When the integrity of the skin has been damaged or broken as in an abrasion or decubitus ulcer, the body loses some of its ability to:
① Resist infections
② Produce antibodies
③ Eliminate waste products
④ Maintain correct body alignment

139. A patient asks the nurse to clip her fingernails. If the nurse is permitted to clip the nails, which of the following techniques should be utilized?
① Clip nails straight across
② Clip nails with rounded edges
③ Clip nails with square corners
④ Clip nails as short as possible

140. A nurse has been asked to shave a male patient. Which of the following patient disorders may prevent the nurse from performing the shave?
① A bleeding disorder
② An emotional disorder
③ A respiratory disorder
④ A neurological disorder

141. The nurse is performing mouth care on an unconscious patient. In which of the following positions should the nurse place the patient?
① Prone, with head turned to one side
② Supine, with suction equipment nearby
③ In semi-Fowler's position, with a towel under the chin
④ In a side-lying position, with head turned to the side

142. During a preoperative assessment on a patient, the nurse finds that the patient experiences sleep apnea. The nurse recognizes sleep apnea as a:
① Problem caused by snoring or overeating
② Problem that is increased if the patient is overly nervous or upset
③ Syndrome that is transitory in nature and not considered dangerous
④ Syndrome that can cause symptoms of daytime tiredness and fatigue

143. Which of the following is the best way for the nurse to assess the intensity of a patient's pain?
① Ask the patient how long he/she has been experiencing the pain
② Ask the patient to point to the location of the pain they are feeling

❸ Ask the patient to rate their pain on a scale of 1 (mild) to 10 (severe)

④ Ask the patient to gauge their pain using words such as "bad" or "severe"

144. A patient is learning to walk with crutches. After traveling down the hallway, the patient complains of numbness in his axilla and tingling of his fingers. The nurse should:
① Switch the patient to a walker
② Notify the physician of possible nerve damage to the arm
❸ Adjust the crutch length and review appropriate crutch technique with the patient
④ Provide padding to the patient's axilla and assist the patient in doing range-of-motion exercises

145. A patient has right-sided weakness from the effects of a cerebrovascular accident. The patient begins to use a cane. The nurse instructs the patient to use the cane in the left hand and to move the cane simultaneously with:
① Both arms
② Both feet
③ The left leg
❹ The right leg

146. A nurse observes that a terminally ill patient's respirations appear to have periods of apnea interspersed with increasing and decreasing respiratory depth and rate. The nurse recognizes that this pattern of breathing may indicate approaching death and is termed:
① Dyspnea
② Tachypnea
③ Kussmaul's
❹ Cheyne Stokes

147. A nurse is assessing an individual on bed rest for possible edema. Where might the nurse find edema in a patient who is confined to bed?
① Feet
② Hands
③ Calves
❹ Sacrum

148. A nurse is instructing an unlicensed assistive personnel (UAP) to administer a nonmedicated vaginal douche to an elderly patient. Which of the following statements made by the UAP signifies understanding of the procedure?
① "The patient should wait to void until after the douche is given."
② "The tip should be inserted and then instillation of fluid can begin."
❸ "The fluid should be already flowing when I place the douche into the vagina."
④ "The fluid should be instilled using lots of pressure to make sure the vagina gets clean."

149. A patient who is scheduled to undergo a mastectomy in the morning states to the nurse, "I am afraid my husband will no longer love me after the surgery." Which of the following is the nurse's best response to this statement?
① "You shouldn't feel that way. Everything will be fine."
② "I think the anxiety of your surgery is causing you undue worry."
❸ "You are afraid that your husband might no longer find you attractive?"
④ " I think you should sleep on it, you'll feel better about it in the morning."

150. Which of the following vital signs collected by the nurse from adult patients should be considered abnormal and needs to be reported?
① Oral temperature 99° F, Pulse 68, Respirations 20, BP 122/80
❷ Rectal temperature 102° F, Pulse 100, Respirations 22, BP 118/50
③ Axillary temperature 97.8° F, Pulse 88, Respirations 20, BP 138/70
④ Tympanic temperature 98.5° F, Pulse 74, Respirations 16, BP 120/84

151. A patient who is on a 1000 cc/day fluid restriction because of renal insufficiency is observed to be consuming a large amount of water from the water faucet in her room. The nurse approximates that she may have consumed over 3000 cc in a short period. The nurse should expect that the patient's weight will:
❶ Increase
② Decrease
③ Remain the same, as the patient will just rid herself of excess fluid
④ Remain the same, as the patient needed the water due to her dehydrated state

152. A nurse is caring for a patient who has a diagnosis of dysphagia. Which of the following should be included in this patient's plan of care?
① Facial exercises
❷ Special feeding precautions
③ Allow extra time for formation of words
④ Referral to an occupational therapist for assessment

153. A patient is recovering from a hemorrhoidectomy and is receiving oxygen via face mask. Which of the following methods for obtaining temperature should the nurse use?
① Oral
② Rectal
③ Axillary
❹ Tympanic

154. A patient is being monitored by pulse oximetry utilizing a clip-on probe. The machine alarms and the oxygen saturation reads 60%. The patient is sitting up in bed and talking with his family. What is the nurse's first course of action?
① Call the physician immediately
② Begin oxygen therapy at 3 L/min nasal cannula
❸ Adjust the clip-on probe on the finger or move it to another finger
④ Remove family members from the room to better deal with this emergency

155. A patient recovering from a respiratory ailment is confined to bed rest. Which of the following positions should the nurse place the patient in to facilitate the best respiratory effort?
① Sims'
② Supine
③ Low Fowler's
❹ High Fowler's

156. A nurse obtains a positive hemoccult test on a patient's stool. Which of the following statements made by the patient would lead the nurse to question the validity of the test results?
① "I love my coffee. I drink 4 or 5 cups a day."
② "I wish they would stop giving me that blue gelatin, I am sick of it!"

③ "I really enjoyed the steaks I've had on my tray the past two evenings."

④ "The hospital must have its own garden, judging by the amount of vegetables they feed you."

157. A patient who performs home glucose testing tells the nurse that she can never seem to get enough blood from her finger to do the test. Which of the following methods should the nurse advise the patient to do to increase blood flow to the fingertips?

① "Milk the finger down towards the fingertips."

② "Hold your fingers in the air for a few minutes before the test."

❸ "Apply a warm, moist compress over the fingers a few minutes before the test."

④ "Collect blood from more than one finger in order to get enough blood for the test."

158. A nurse is packing a surgical incision with a 2×2 gauze pad soaked in saline solution. The nurse drops the wet gauze pad on the edge of the sterile field. What should the nurse do next?

① Pick up the gauze pad and put it in the wound

❷ Leave the gauze where it fell and prepare a new one

③ Pick up the gauze and rinse it out in the saline solution before using

❹ Begin anew, with a new sterile tray, dressings, and gloves

159. A patient is scheduled to begin IPPB treatments. The patient asks the nurse the purpose of these treatments. The nurse's best response is that the treatments:

❶ Are useful in dislodging secretions

② Give the patient incentives to increase inhalation

③ Allow gravity to assist in the removal of secretions

❹ Forces the person to inhale more deeply, increasing oxygenation

160. A patient is receiving 75% humidified oxygen via a tracheostomy collar. The patient requires suctioning. Which of the following actions should the nurse perform that will be safe for the patient?

① Restrain the patient

❷ Administer supplemental oxygen to the patient

③ Apply suction while carefully advancing the catheter

④ Use a rotating motion while carefully advancing the catheter

161. Which of the following techniques should be utilized by the nurse when obtaining a patient's blood pressure?

① Place the arm above the level of the heart

② Have the patient extend the arm with palm downward

③ Place the cuff 1 inch above the position of the radial artery

❹ "Match up" the arrow on the cuff to the area where the brachial artery was palpated

162. The nurse is assessing a patient's circulatory status by checking all peripheral pulses. When the nurse assesses pulses she is using the technique of:

❶ Palpation

② Percussion

③ Inspection

④ Auscultation

163. Which of the following fluids should be measured and factored in a patient's fluid output?

❶ Vomitus

② IV fluids

③ Perspiration

④ Tube feedings

164. A nurse is assessing a patient's IV site and administration set. Which of the following requires corrective action by the nurse?

① The IV site is clean and dry

② There is fluid in the IV container

❸ The tubing was changed 5 days ago

④ There is no swelling or redness at the site

165. Which of the following actions would assist in reducing the incidence of aspiration in a patient receiving a tube feeding?

① Clamp tube after feeding has infused

② Flush tube with water after each feeding

③ Dilute the feedings to half-strength solutions

❹ Remain in an upright position for 45 minutes after feeding

166. A patient had an indwelling urinary catheter removed 6 hours ago. The patient relates to the nurse that burning was experienced after the first post-catheter void. Which of the following is the nurse's best response?

① "I think you may have a urinary tract infection."

② "I will need to contact the physician about that."

❸ "Sometimes that happens after a catheter is removed."

④ "Let me collect a sterile urine specimen from you now."

167. The nurse is inserting a nasogastric tube into a patient. Which of the following would indicate that the tube is in the patient's trachea?

❶ The patient is unable to speak

② The nurse can't see the tube in the back of the throat

③ The patient blows the nose and blood is present on the tissue

④ The nurse notes that the tube has a return of light green drainage

168. A hospitalized patient is ordered both an oil retention enema and a cleansing enema. Which of the following statements correctly explains the rationale for administering these enemas?

① The enemas work together to stimulate peristalsis

❷ The oil retention enema softens the stool and the cleansing enema stimulates peristalsis

③ If the oil retention enema does not work to evacuate the bowel, then the cleansing enema can be given

④ The cleansing enema is generally given to soften the stool 30 minutes prior to the oil retention enema

169. A patient has a "straight cath, prn" order. Which of the following may indicate that the patient may need to have the straight catheter inserted?

❶ The patient has not voided in 4 hours

② The patient has consumed 2000 cc of fluid in 6 hours

③ The patient had an incontinent episode 30 minutes ago

❹ The patient voids 5 to 10 cc of amber-colored urine every hour

170. A patient presents to a physician's office with complaints of constipation for 6 days. Which of the following statements made by the patient during the health history may be contributing to the constipation?

① "I exercise almost every day."

② "I eat plenty of raw vegetables."

❸ "I am not a big water drinker."

④ "I go to the bathroom when I feel the need."

171. Which of the following postprocedure orders should the nurse expect after a patient receives a barium enema?
    ① NPO × 3 days
    ② Straight cath, prn
    ③ Remain flat in bed until AM
    ④ Cleansing enemas until clear

172. An unlicensed assistive personnel (UAP) inquires as to why a patient's arm is contracted into a flexion position. Which of the following statements by the nurse answers the UAP's question?
    ① "A physical therapy consult is needed to help this patient."
    ② "The muscles of the arm must have been damaged in some way."
    ③ "The muscles are permanently shortened due to the effects of immobility."
    ④ "The arm is just temporarily frozen, range-of-motion exercises should restore it."

173. A nurse is providing care to a patient with a tracheostomy. Which of the following actions poses the most risk to the patient?
    ① Suctioning
    ② Cleansing the stoma
    ③ Changing the trach ties
    ④ Cleansing the inner cannula

174. An elderly postoperative patient has an order to be ambulated a few hours after surgery. The patient becomes upset with the nurse and wants to know why he should ambulate so soon after surgery. Which of the following is the best response by the nurse?
    ① "You know what they say, if you don't use it you might lose it."
    ② "Please get out of bed now. You can ask your doctor in the morning."
    ③ "Your doctor always orders his patients out of bed right after surgery."
    ④ "Walking will keep the fluids in your lungs moving, so bacteria will not grow."

175. A nurse is applying antiembolic stockings on a patient prior to surgery. The patient inquires why the stockings need to be so snug. The nurse responds that snugness is needed because:
    ① "They do not do their job if they are too loose."
    ② "The stockings pool blood in your legs during surgery."
    ③ "They are meant to exercise the muscles of the legs while you are in surgery."
    ④ "They help to prevent blood clots from developing by pushing blood toward the heart"

176. Which of the following would be an appropriate short-term nursing goal for a patient with an ankle fracture who is just learning to walk with crutches?
    ① Patient will have decreased need for pain medication
    ② Patient will be able to use crutches appropriately within 3 weeks
    ③ Patient will walk length of hallway with crutches, three times per day
    ④ Patient will walk without crutches or supportive devices within 3 months

177. The nurse is visiting a home health care patient and his family. The family reports that the patient is easily agitated, especially when he is in the dining room, which is a noisy room, decorated with red walls and carpeting. Which of the following should the nurse recommend to the family?
    ① "Try to keep the patient as active as possible."
    ② "Taking him to the mall or store should help."
    ③ "Spending time in a quiet, light-colored room could help."
    ④ "Spending time watching TV or listening to the radio may calm him."

178. The nurse is attempting to remove some dry and crusted secretions from a patient's Foley catheter. Which of the following solutions should the nurse use if soap and water are ineffective?
    ① Alcohol
    ② Betadine
    ③ Sterile saline
    ④ Hydrogen peroxide

179. A patient returns from surgery with a large, abdominal dressing in place. As the evening progresses, the nurse notes that some drainage has seeped through the dressing. Which of the following is the nurse's best course of action?
    ① Change the dressing
    ② Reinforce the dressing with additional gauze
    ③ Remove the dressing and leave the wound open to air
    ④ Remove the dressing and send it to the lab for culture

180. A nurse is using wet-moist saline dressings to debride a patient's stage III decubitus ulcer. The patient asks the purpose of using this type of dressing. Which of the following is the nurse's best response?
    ① "The wet dressing soothes the damaged tissue."
    ② "The wet dressing keeps the wound from getting infected."
    ③ "The saline is eventually absorbed into the body, promoting healing."
    ④ "The drying of the dressing helps to remove any drainage or dead skin."

181. A nurse is applying heat to the leg of a patient with cellulitis of the leg. Which of the following facts in the patient's medical history necessitates the need for the nurse to take special precautions?
    ① Blindness
    ② Paraplegia
    ③ Hypertension
    ④ Diabetes mellitus

182. Which of the following substances should the nurse apply to the eyelid of a patient who is to receive a warm compress to the eye?
    ① Saline
    ② Betadine
    ③ Petrolatum
    ④ Antibiotic ointment

183. When irrigating a patient's NG tube, special care is taken by the nurse to add the irrigating fluid to the patient's:
    ① Intake
    ② Output
    ③ IV fluids
    ④ Oral fluids

184. A nurse is assessing a patient's incision line. Which of the following data may indicate infection?
    ① Area surrounding the sutures is red and swollen
    ② Some of the sutures have fallen out of the incision line

③ No drainage around the sutures, surrounding skin is pink

④ Sutures are all intact, small amount of serosanguinous drainage present

185. The nurse is preparing to irrigate a patient's infected left eye. The nurse should position the patient:
① On his back
② On his left side
③ On his right side
④ In Semi-Fowler's position

186. A patient being admitted to a long-term care facility inquires why he must undergo a routine TB test. The nurse should respond by advising the patient that:
① It is a rule that all patients admitted have to have one
② He will need to take the issue up with his primary physician
③ He needs to take the screening exam whether he likes it or not
④ This is a routine screening exam that is used to safeguard the resident's health

187. A 50-year-old female visits the physician's office for a routine physical. During the health history it is determined that the patient has never had a mammogram. The nurse is aware that mammograms:
① Are done when breast cancer is suspected
② Should be done every 1 to 2 years as a routine screening exam
③ Are not necessary if the woman does not have a history of breast cancer in the family
④ Are difficult for the woman to undergo and therefore are only recommended every 5 to 10 years

188. A nurse is assisting an unlicensed assistive personnel (UAP) to set up a footboard on a patient's bed. The UAP asks the nurse why a footboard would be used. The nurse's best response is:
① "A footboard will assist in maintaining good abduction."
② "It will prevent the patient from developing thrombophlebitis."
③ "The footboard will keep the foot from developing plantar flexion."
④ "The patient will be able to use the board to help push herself up in bed."

189. A nurse is making the decision to purchase liability insurance. The nurse should keep in mind that professional liability coverage:
① Costs the same in all health care settings
② Protects the nurse from prosecution for criminal acts
③ Does not cover acts outside the scope of nursing practice
④ Provides coverage to the nurse for his/her entire professional career

190. A practical nurse is working at a home health care agency. Under what form of supervision is the nurse practicing?
① None, the nurse is self-employed
② The directives of the state board of nursing
③ The owner of the home health care agency
④ The direction of a physician or registered nurse

191. A nurse overhears a terminally ill cancer patient state to his family members, "If I get over this cancer thing, I will travel with the church's missionary to South Africa next spring." Which stage of the dying process is this patient exhibiting?
① Anger
② Denial
③ Bargaining
④ Depression

192. A nurse is caring for a patient with hypostatic pneumonia. Which of the following assessment data is most important for this patient?
① Lung sounds
② Bowel sounds
③ Peripheral pulses
④ Neurological exam

193. An elderly patient has had a urinary catheter for 1 month. During a routine urinalysis it is found that the patient has an infection caused by *E. coli*. Given the patient's history the nurse suspects that the infection is a(an):
① Secondary infection
② Nosocomial infection
③ Autoimmune reaction
④ Antibiotic resistant strain

194. In planning care for a patient who is paralyzed, the nurse should plan to reposition the patient at least:
① Once a shift
② Every 2 hours
③ Every 4 hours
④ Every 30 minutes

195. Which of the following is the responsibility of the Canadian provincial regulatory bodies?
① Setting and administering examinations
② Reporting acts of criminal negligence to the police
③ Passing laws pertaining to the practice of nursing
④ Establishing minimum levels of safe nursing practice

196. Which of the following descriptions best reflects the role of the Canadian practical nurse/nursing assistant?
① Able to work independently in all settings
② Works under the direct supervision of an RN
③ Works as an integral part of the health care team
④ Cares for only those patients whose conditions are stabilized

197. Which of the following is registration intended to protect?
① The public
② The individual registrant
③ The title of the registrant
④ The level of nursing practice

198. Which of the following regulates Canadian registration?
① Federal legislation
② Provincial legislation
③ Municipal legislation
④ Professional associations

199. Which of the following is registration/licensure designed to protect?
① The public
② The practice of nursing
③ Level of the practitioner
④ Individual registrants

200. Which of the following organizations is responsible for admission requirements to practical nursing/nursing assistant programs?
① Individual educational institutions
② Provincial professional associations

③ Provincial licensing bodies
④ The Canadian Association of Practical Nursing/Nursing Assistants (CAPNNA)

201. Which of the following organizations offers malpractice insurance to practical nurses/nursing assistants?
① CAPNNA
② Provincial licensing bodies
③ Provincial professional associations
④ Private insurance companies

202. Which of the following statements best describes membership in CAPNNA?
① It is voluntary and optional for PNs/NAs
② It is mandatory in each province/territory
③ It is included with membership in affiliated organizations
④ It is automatic with registration/licensure

203. The PN/NA maintains competence by:
① Writing a yearly examination
② Taking advantage of learning opportunities
③ Demonstrating skill level to his/her employer
④ Completing designated seminars and workshops

204. Laws pertaining to nursing in Canada are:
① Set by nursing regulatory bodies
② The same as in the United States
③ Specific to each province/territory
④ Specific to the nursing practice setting

ANSWERS AND RATIONALES

1. Application, assessment, basic care and comfort (b)
   ❷ Assessing the exact location of the pain assists in determining cause and treatment.
   ① Establishing existence of drug allergies does not address the diagnosis of pain.
   ③ This may help determine treatment but will not aid in diagnosis.
   ④ This does not address the characteristics of the pain.

2. Application, implementation, coping and adaptation (b)
   ❸ This statement reduces fear of abandonment and alleviates fear of needs not being met.
   ① Pain medication is not commonly needed during this procedure.
   ② Limiting visitors increases anxiety and causes feelings of isolation.
   ④ The patient and his/her secretions are radioactive during treatment.

3. Application, assessment, reduction of risk potential (b)
   ❸ Anxiety often interferes with the patient's ability to listen to or comprehend instructions.
   ① The patient needs to understand the instructions, not memorize them.
   ② The terms used by the physician are not known.
   ④ The rationale for nursing actions should not be to solely satisfy documentation requirements.

4. Comprehension, implementation, reduction of risk potential (b)
   ❶ Stimulating the gag reflex may result in vomiting.
   ② Secretions do not originate in the throat area.
   ③ Contamination of the culture site is not of primary consideration.
   ④ The size of the specimen is not a concern with a throat culture.

5. Application, assessment, reduction of risk potential (b)
   ❶ This intervention gathers more information before determining course of action.
   ② This may not be the course of action, more data is needed.
   ③ Elevating the foot will reduce edema, but does not address the numbness and tingling.
   ④ Wiggling her toes will not alleviate the numbness and tingling.

6. Application, assessment, physiological adaptation (b)
   ❶ Symptoms of a local infection include edema, erythema, and purulent drainage.
   ② Symptoms of systemic infection include general symptoms of GI upset, malaise, fever, increased pulse, and respirations.
   ③ Necrotic wounds contain blackened, not red tissue.
   ④ Not enough information is given to come to this conclusion.

7. Comprehension, implementation, safety and infection control (a)
   ❹ This action best protects the nurse against the specific dangers of wound irrigation, such as splashing or spraying of blood and body fluids.
   ① Common knowledge states that the bed should be at a workable height for all procedures.
   ② Explaining the procedure alleviates patient anxiety; it does not protect the nurse.
   ③ Handwashing is indicated before and after all patient procedures.

8. Comprehension, planning, reduction of risk potential (c)
   ❶ Individuals with spinal cord injuries suffer from immobility complicated by impaired sensory function.
   ② Patients in skeletal traction retain skin sensation and can assist with relieving pressure.
   ③ Ambulatory patients are at low risk for decubitus formation.
   ④ Immobility is short-term and skin sensation is not limited.

9. Application, implementation, basic care and comfort (b)
   ❹ Mouth care relieves the discomfort related to the mouth dryness caused by mouth breathing.
   ① This is unwarranted; this situation does not warrant immediate medical attention.
   ② This causes a potential for electrolyte imbalance.
   ③ The response does not address patient discomfort.

10. Comprehension, planning, coordinated care (b)
    ❹ Assigning ancillary personnel to give out medications is most likely not under the person's scope of practice and may result in injury to the patient and a lawsuit for the nurse.
    ① Not enough information is given about the nurse's other tasks for this to be correct; the issue is still inappropriate delegating of tasks.
    ② There is no guarantee that the UAP will respond quickly to patient complaints.
    ③ Safeguarding patients takes priority over increasing self-esteem.

11. Application, implementation, coordinated care (b)
    ❷ The nurse protects the patient's best interests in all care situations.
    ① Allowable services may not always meet the patient's needs.
    ③ The nurse is not the representative of the insuring agency.
    ④ Level of care is based upon patient needs, not allowable benefits.

12. Application, assessment, basic care and comfort (c)
    ❸ The resident may fall asleep if he is made comfortable, medication can be given at a later time if he is unable to sleep; try the most basic comfort measures first.
    ① This closes communication without addressing the problem.
    ② This is true and reassuring but doesn't address the problem.
    ④ Nurse is not engaging in the conversation and blocks communication.

13. Application, implementation, basic care and comfort (c)
    ❹ Bladder pain may indicate a complication, such as a blockage, and requires further assessment.
    ① This is an expected outcome of the procedure.
    ② This may be the reason that the irrigation was ordered.
    ③ Returns may be lower than amount instilled because of patient's position.

14. Application, planning, basic care and comfort (c)
    ❸ This assessment data signifies a catheter blockage that may be alleviated with bladder irrigation.

① Position changes will not relieve an obstructed catheter.

② The assessment data can be expected, nurse can proceed within scope of practice without notifying physician.

④ The nurse should act on these observations, not document them.

15. Application, assessment, physiological adaptation (b)
❸ This addresses the patient's respiratory status while allowing for efficient completion of the procedure.
① This would further compromise the patient's respiratory distress.
② This would further compromise the patient's respiratory distress and does not allow visualization for the procedure.
④ The gatched knees would interfere with the performance of the procedure.

16. Application, implementation, reduction of risk potential (b)
❸ This reduces bacterial counts at the entry point to the bladder.
① Multiple invasive procedures predispose the patient to infection
② Unnecessary antibiotic medication encourages the development of resistant organisms.
④ Antiseptic solutions are irritating to mucosa.

17. Application, assessment, physiological adaptation (c)
❸ Urinary urgency and lower abdominal pressure are symptoms of a full bladder; the catheter may be malfunctioning or blocked.
① The cause of the pain must first be determined.
② This is not related to the patient's physical discomfort.
④ This response fails to address the patient's discomfort.

18. Application, implementation, physiological adaptation (b)
❸ This allows the patient to be independent and feed herself.
① This denies the patient's independence.
② This denies the patient their full nourishment and is unnecessary if precautions are taken.
④ This does not address the patient's impaired vision.

19. Application, assessment, basic care and comfort (a)
❶ Cyanosis is a blue tinge to the skin or oral mucosa that indicates poor oxygenation.
② Vital signs indicate cardiopulmonary status and not cyanosis.
③ Cyanosis is difficult to assess in the lips or nails of individuals with dark complexions.
④ Pulse oximetry measures the amount of oxygen in capillary blood, not cyanosis.

20. Application, implementation, reduction of risk potential (c)
❷ Blood glucose levels are a significant assessment for individuals with diabetes, especially during illness.
① Although helpful, this is not a priority for this patient, at this time.
③ This may not be indicated for this particular patient, and the glucometer takes precedence.
④ This may not be indicated; further assessment data is needed.

21. Application, evaluation, basic care and comfort, (c)
❸ A delayed infusion of IV solution is often caused by obstruction of the rate of flow; the action allows for further assessment of the problem.
① Not enough data has been collected to make this assumption.
② These data indicate further action on the nurse's part.
④ Changing the rate of flow places the patient at risk for injury.

22. Knowledge, implementation, basic care and comfort (a)
❹ The most accurate measurement of fluid level is at eye level, in a firm container on a level surface.
① The flexibility of the drainage bag interferes with accurate measurement.
② Approximation is not an accurate measure.
③ Bedpan markings are approximations.

23. Application, implementation, coping and adaptation (b)
❶ This enables the patient to communicate his/her needs.
② This is a secondary comfort measure; communication of needs would be a primary patient concern.
③ The presence of the nurse is more important than reassurances.
④ This does not address the patient's comfort.

24. Comprehension, implementation, safety and infection control (b)
❶ This provides a warm, absorbent covering for the feet without combustion danger.
② Wool can create sparks, which is dangerous in an oxygen-rich environment.
③ Poor circulation and sensation in the elderly place them at high risk for injury with heat application.
④ This does not address the patient's overall discomfort.

25. Comprehension, evaluation, basic care and comfort (b)
❶ A full assessment includes both subjective and objective data.
② Objective signs do not address cues that the patient himself can provide when evaluating progress.
③ Limiting data collection to subjective information ignores the observable, measurable symptom not offered by the patient.
④ Data must be gathered throughout the procedure to fully determine their effect upon the patient.

26. Comprehension, planning, reduction of risk potential (b)
❷ Knowledge of the procedure diminishes patient fear, which improves patient cooperation and promotes the expected outcome of the procedure
① Competent nursing practice reduces the likelihood of malpractice suits.
③ Procedures are not explained to avoid them, although this may be a secondary aspect of patient teaching.
④ The nurse must review the procedure before explaining it to the patient to provide complete information.

27. Application, implementation, physiological adaptation (b)
❸ Increased fluid intake decreases the tenacity of respiratory secretions, making sputum removal easier.
① Low hydration makes respiratory secretion thicker and more difficult to expel.
② Tracheal suctioning is invasive and should only be employed if the patient is unable to expel secretions independently.

④ Postural drainage relies on gravity to assist with expulsion of secretions; affected lung areas vary and must be vertical for this to occur.

28. Application, planning, coordinated care (b)
❷ This is an expected outcome of the nursing action that should occur within a short period of time.
① This is a nursing intervention. It outlines the actual nursing activity.
③ This is a long-term goal, outlining the overall purpose of the nursing actions.
④ This is a rationale; it explains why the action is being implemented.

29. Comprehension, assessment, reduction of risk potential (c)
❷ Frequent and regular home blood glucose monitoring best determines the stability of the patient's blood sugar.
① The glucose tolerance test is a diagnostic procedure for diabetes; it does not measure how well the diabetic is controlling the disease.
③ Sugar and acetone urine testing is not as accurate a blood glucose measure because of the delay of processing blood glucose through the kidneys and bladder.
④ Double voiding provides a more accurate urine test but is still less accurate than blood glucose monitoring.

30. Knowledge, implementation, reduction of risk potential (a)
❸ This procedure increases the likelihood of detecting occult blood in the stool.
① Diarrhea stools are acceptable sources provided they are not contaminated with urine.
② Stools for ova and parasites must be kept warm and delivered to the lab immediately.
④ Occult blood is hidden or unseen blood.

31. Application, implementation, reduction of risk potential (b)
❶ Weight should be measured at the same time each day, in the same clothing.
② The patient should weigh one time each day; the patient may be taking medication several times a day at different intervals.
③ Medication should never be omitted; a more accurate measurement is weighing each morning.
④ This is a symptom of advanced heart failure; daily weights will indicate early symptoms.

32. Comprehension, implementation, reduction of risk potential (b)
❹ Metal objects will interfere with X-ray visualization.
① There is not enough information to assume that undergarments are contraindicated.
② There is not enough information provided to assume that this is a fasting exam.
③ Clothing may interfere with some types of X-ray examinations.

33. Application, implementation, coordinated care (b)
❸ A dated addendum can be added to the chart if appropriately noted.
① No part of the legal chart may be discarded or altered.
② Addendums to the chart must be dated for clarity of information.

④ Omission of information is not an error; an addendum should be made for the omitted information.

34. Application, implementation, coping and adaptation (c)
❶ A reflective statement that encourages further communication.
② This does not respond to the patient's statement and impairs communication.
③ This response diminishes the patient's individuality and does not address the patient's concerns.
④ This response is false reassurance and blocks communications.

35. Comprehension, evaluation, safety and infection control (b)
❷ A nosocomial infection is an infection acquired during the course of a hospital stay or as a result of a medical treatment (urinary catheter).
① A superinfection is an illness produced by growth of a resistant organism during antimicrobial therapy.
③ An autoimmune response is the immune reaction of the body against its own tissues.
④ Antibiotic resistance is the continued growth of pathogenic organisms during antibiotic therapy.

36. Application, implementation, safety and infection control (b)
❶ This measure limits any patient contact with others, as chickenpox is spread by both droplet and direct contact.
② This places emergency room patients at risk.
③ The mask addresses only one mode of infection.
④ This measure addresses only one mode of infection.

37. Knowledge, planning, safety and infection control (a)
❶ Carrying the equipment close to the body places it over the base of support, diminishing the strain on back muscles.
② Sliding the equipment from the floor to the bed is unwieldy and disrupts the bedding.
③ Leg muscles, which are stronger, should be involved in the lift effort to limit the danger of injury.
④ Holding the equipment at arm's length places it out of the base of support and strains arm and back muscles.

38. Application, implementation, coping and adaptation (b)
❶ This provides a well-balanced meal while observing kosher dietary practices.
② A kosher diet forbids pork and pork products.
③ A kosher diet does not allow mixing of meat with dairy products.
④ Kosher diets forbid the mixing of meat with dairy products; bacon is a pork product.

39. Knowledge, assessment, coping and adaptation (b)
❶ Religious beliefs influence the patient's choice of treatment, as well as the patient's belief about the cause of illness.
② Last rites is a religious practice limited to the Roman Catholic religion.
③ This is not the primary reason for gathering this information; the nurse needs to understand the patient's health practice beliefs to plan care.
④ The nurse collects data concerning religion in order to plan the patient's plan of care.

40. Comprehension, evaluation, coordinated care (a)
- ❸ The movement toward cost reduction has shifted health care delivery out of hospitals and into long-term care, home care, and skilled nursing facilities.
- ① The scope of nursing practice has increased with technological advances in health care.
- ② The focus of all health care delivery has moved to wellness promotion rather than illness treatment.
- ④ Nursing remains patient centered. Treatment is more technology-based but still involves direct contact with the patient by the nurse.

41. Application, planning, safety, and infection control (b)
- ❸ Maintaining skill levels guarantees safe, effective, nursing practice.
- ① Regular relicensure is a legal requirement for nursing practice.
- ② Maintenance of membership in a professional organization helps the nurse to keep abreast of changes in the field.
- ④ This action promotes professionalism but is not an ethical issue.

42. Application, implementation, coordinated care (b)
- ❹ This clarifies the error and the corrective measure.
- ① An incident report is completed after the error is corrected.
- ② The family is not notified unless they have power of attorney.
- ③ An incident report is an internal record and is never documented on the patient's chart.

43. Comprehension, implementation, coordinated care (b)
- ❶ Licensing laws are public safety measures.
- ② Licensing laws establish minimum standards.
- ③ Moral character is a subjective measure that can only be minimally established by licensing law.
- ④ Licensing laws do not limit the numbers of applicants to nursing practice.

44. Application, planning, coordinated care (c)
- ❷ Collaborating with fellow nurses is an important measure for guaranteeing quality care.
- ① The nurse has a responsibility to update skills and knowledge necessary for patient care.
- ③ This action fails to meet the patient's need to understand the equipment he/she will use.
- ④ The nurse will have no point of reference for determining if the patient's knowledge is correct.

45. Application, implementation, coping and adaptation (c)
- ❷ Instruction should take place in a distraction-free environment; asking permission to turn off the TV recognizes the individuality of the patient and makes him/her more receptive to instruction.
- ① This is a belittling approach toward the patient and fails to establish a teaching environment.
- ③ Self-care teaching is an important aspect of this patient's care.
- ④ This does not establish a teaching environment and prejudices the patient.

46. Application, planning, basic care and comfort (b)
- ❷ Retention of the enema increases its effectiveness.
- ① The enema may be expelled before it has been fully effective.
- ③ This position does not allow for adequate visualization of the procedure and risks injury to the rectum.
- ④ This ignores the patient's need to evacuate the enema.

47. Knowledge, implementation, basic care and comfort (b)
- ❸ Using separate wash cloth sections for each eye prevents spread of organisms from one eye to the other.
- ① Rinsing and drying skin folds reduces skin irritation.
- ② Clean gloves are a useless protective mechanisms if hands are immersed in bath water.
- ④ Changing bath water after bathing each extremity maintains the warmth of bath water.

48. Knowledge, implementation, coordinated care (b)
- ❶ Each state passes nurse practice acts that define and determine the scope of nursing within that state.
- ② The state's board of nursing administers the nurse practice acts.
- ③ The National Council of State Boards of Nursing is a professional association composed of the state boards of nursing and administers the licensing examination for nurses.
- ④ JCAHO is a professional association organized to promote standards for health care.

49. Comprehension, implementation, reduction of risk potential (b)
- ❸ Bed rest often causes pooling of blood in the lower extremities, resulting in poor blood flow to the brain when a patient arises quickly.
- ① Range of motion exercises improve joint flexibility.
- ② Assessment of the patient's ability is ongoing throughout the ambulation procedure.
- ④ Although this can take place during dangling, the chief purpose is to balance one's blood pressure.

50. Application, assessment, coping and adaptation (b)
- ❶ Further assessment of the patient's complaint is necessary before determining action.
- ② This encourages a yes or no answer. Answer #1 allows for more information.
- ③ This discourages communication by diminishing the importance of the patient's complaint, and it fails to allay the patient's fears.
- ④ This discourages communication by changing the topic, and it fails to allay the patient's fears.

51. Application, implementation, reduction of risk potential (c)
- ❷ Vertigo is a common side effect of this treatment.
- ① The pinna of the ear is retracted during the procedure.
- ③ Most patients can resume activity shortly after treatment.
- ④ Use of cotton-tipped applicators in the ears can lead to injury.

52. Application, implementation, reduction of risk potential (b)
- ❶ Culture specimens can be inaccurate if obtained while the patient is receiving antibiotics.
- ② There is no need for clarification; this is a standard nursing function.
- ③ Antibiotics will interfere with microbial growth on the specimen cultures.
- ④ Antibiotics will interfere with microbial growth on the urine culture.

53. Comprehension, implementation, safety and infection control (b)
- ❷ Handling the glove on the inside guarantees that the nurse's bare, nonsterile hand will not contaminate the sterile exterior of the glove.

① Contamination occurs if the nurse's nonsterile hand touches the sterile exterior of the glove.

③ Keeping the gloves on the sterile field throughout the gloving procedure risks contamination of the field.

④ Contamination occurs if the nonsterile hand touches the outside of the glove.

54. Application, assessment, basic care and comfort (c)

❸ This may indicate delayed gastric emptying; further feedings could induce vomiting.

① Gastrostomy site oozing is a common occurrence that requires skin integrity measures, but it does not indicate a need to withhold feedings.

② An absence of the gag reflex is actually an indicator for tube feedings.

④ No residual feeding return usually indicates full absorption of the feeding.

55. Comprehension, evaluation, basic care and comfort (b)

❶ The most common cause of GI discomfort in a patient receiving tube feedings is formula intolerance.

② Electronic pump infusion is a common, nonirritating delivery route for tube feedings.

③ Remaining upright for 1 hour after feeding reduces the likelihood of reflux and vomiting.

④ Failing to correctly flush the tube after each feeding eventually leads to tube blockage.

56. Application, implementation, basic care and comfort (b)

❷ This measure should relax the patient, allow the colon to adjust to the fluid flow, and allow the patient to retain more of the enema fluid for better results.

① Maintaining fluid flow will increase the urge to defecate.

③ This is a false reassurance.

④ Allowing the patient to defecate too soon will decrease the effectiveness of the procedure.

57. Application, planning, reduction of risk potential (b)

❷ Bowel sounds indicate the return of GI function; the NG tube is in place to empty stomach contents until the GI tract can resume active peristalsis.

① The patient should not be nauseated if the NG tube is operating effectively, and does not mean that the patient no longer needs GI suction.

③ Drainage indicates wound healing progress, not GI function.

④ Absence of gastric drainage may indicate a problem with the NG suction rather than a return of GI function.

58. Application, assessment, basic care and comfort (c)

❶ Hiccoughing and nausea are indications of accumulated gastric secretions; the most likely cause for this would be something interfering with gastric suction.

② Full assessment of the patient's condition must be made before contacting the physician.

③ Throat irritation is not the most likely cause of the GI symptoms.

④ Clearing any blockage to the GI suction will most likely diminish nausea, making measures for possible emesis unnecessary.

59. Application, implementation, safety and infection control (a)

❹ This prevents contamination of the environment with wound drainage.

① The nurse cannot leave the patient's bedside during a sterile procedure.

② Leaving soiled dressing materials in the bedside trash creates odor problems and the potential for spread of pathogens.

③ This contaminates the sterile field.

60. Comprehension, implementation, basic care and comfort (b)

❹ This prevents bacterial spread into the wound.

① Pressure on a wound diminishes bleeding; it would interfere with wound cleansing.

② Forceful wound irrigation disrupts healing tissue.

③ Scrubbing disrupts healing tissue.

61. Application, evaluation, coordinated care (b)

❷ Healing, as well as complications, is best determined by inspection of the actual wound.

① This is unnecessary unless there is more than one wound present.

③ An antibiotic cleanser cannot be used without a physician's order.

④ Although this is important, it is not directly relevant to the dressing change procedure.

62. Knowledge, implementation, reduction of risk potential (b)

❸ Bony structures of the heel are just below this site, which places the child at risk for osteomyelitis.

① The newborn fingertip is too small, with inadequate blood vessels.

② There is inadequate skin depth at this site.

④ Newborn fingers are too small to use for blood collection.

63. Knowledge, implementation, basic care and comfort (b)

❹ Once blood begins to enter the specimen tube, the tourniquet is released to allow unrestricted blood flow.

① Releasing the tourniquet causes the veins to recede, hindering access.

② Keeping the tourniquet on during the blood draw lengthens the procedure and promotes venispasm.

③ This would promote bruising at the venipuncture site.

64. Comprehension, implementation, basic care and comfort (c)

❸ Chemical additives have a greater potential for backflow into the patient's vein if they rest against the tube stopper.

① Tourniquet application dilates the blood vessels for access.

② The nurse's personal approach and skill level prevent patient discomfort.

④ Preventing unnecessary arm movement decreases vein injury and patient discomfort.

65. Knowledge, planning, reduction of risk potential (b)

❸ The specimen tubes should be labeled as soon as the blood has been obtained.

① Labeling tubes before the procedure may be wasteful if the venipuncture is unsuccessful.

② Loose labeled specimen containers create a potential for donor error.

④ Unlabeled specimen tubes may be mislabeled with the wrong patient's name.

66. Application, planning, pharmacological therapies (c)

❶ Blood glucose measurements often determine the adequacy of the TPN solution concentration and flow rate.

② Complete blood cell count is a blood test measuring the various cell components of the blood; it is not a priority assessment in TPN therapy.

③ Hemoglobin and hematocrit tests measure blood volume and oxygen-carrying capacity; TPN is a nutritional IV therapy.

④ Erythrocyte sedimentation rate is a blood test that indicates inflammatory conditions such as rheumatic fever or endocarditis; there is no link to TPN therapy.

67. Application, implementation, basic care and comfort (b)

❷ Surgical tube sites are cleansed concentrically, from the cleanest area outward, to minimize contamination of the wound.

① Scrubbing the site disrupts wound healing and can contaminate the wound.

③ This brings distal organisms into the surgical site.

④ This is not an effective measure for cleaning ostomy sites; there is a potential for missing areas under the ostomy tube.

68. Comprehension, evaluation, reduction of risk potential (c)

❶ Bounding pulse, dyspnea, and cough are symptoms of heart failure, caused by the inability of the heart to pump excessive IV fluid volume.

② These are symptoms of IV infiltration.

③ These are symptoms of phlebitis.

④ These are symptoms of a systemic infection.

69. Application, implementation, pharmacological therapies (c)

❸ These are symptoms of an allergic reaction; this action removes the allergen while preserving the IV line.

① This causes the patient pain and undue risk if the IV must be restarted.

② This causes the patient undue risk and pain; it will not correct the problem and if the allergic reaction worsens, an IV line may be needed quickly.

④ This is not a normal reaction, and the nurse cannot apply medication without an order.

70. Application, assessment, pharmacological therapies (c)

❸ The symptoms indicate air embolism; placing the patient in this position prevents the embolism from moving from the right atrium.

① Despite the respiratory symptoms, this is a circulatory emergency, and the patient needs to be positioned to prevent further injury.

② TPN ports should be reconnected after the patient is positioned.

④ Placing the patient in high Fowler's position allows embolism dispersal to vital organs and will not diminish the patient's distress.

71. Knowledge, planning, coping and adaptation (a)

❶ Cleansing and preparing the body before family viewing decreases the stress of the situation.

② Postmortem care is always completed before the body is moved.

③ Family and patient needs are the priority of unit function.

④ The family will be less stressed if the patient's body is clean and has a more normal appearance.

72. Comprehension, implementation, reduction of risk potential (b)

❹ It takes approximately 4 to 6 hours for spinal fluid pressure to stabilize following lumbar puncture; fewer neurological side effects occur if bed rest is maintained during this period.

① Falling may occur because of vertigo, but this explanation is not as inclusive as answer #4.

② The nursing staff's convenience is not a reason for remaining flat.

③ Although the position may limit spinal fluid leakage, there should be scant or no blood loss from the procedure.

73. Comprehension, planning, basic care and comfort (b)

❷ The drying and subsequent removal of wet-to-dry dressings creates mechanical debridement of wounds.

① This is not the chief effect of this wound treatment; application of moist heat or increased patient activity would increase circulation.

③ Wet-to-damp dressing promote absorption of wound secretions.

④ Wet-to-dry dressings have no effect on wound edema.

74. Knowledge, implementation, safety and infection control (a)

❸ Formula hang time should not exceed 8 hours, because bacteria will multiply in the feeding once it is opened and kept at room temperature.

① One day's supply of formula may require 16 to 20 hours of infusion time, providing an environment for bacterial growth.

② More than one can of formula can be hung for efficiency, as long as the solution is not open at room temperature for more than 8 hours.

④ A 2-hour time frame is inefficient and unnecessary.

75. Application, implementation, basic care and comfort (b)

❹ An accurate intake and output record is necessary for correct calculation of the patient's fluid replacement needs.

① Mouth care is an important comfort measure for the patient undergoing GI suction, but it is not as critical as I & O.

② Thorough skin care of the nares is important for skin integrity, but fluid balance is more critical.

③ Turning and positioning the patient may promote better GI drainage and will prevent decubitus formation, but fluid balance measures are more critical.

76. Application, implementation, physiological adaptation (b)

❹ Tympanic thermometers measure core body temperature noninvasively.

① Throat surgery forces oral breathing, causing an inaccurate oral reading.

② Rectal thermometer reading is uncomfortable and embarrassing to the patient.

③ Axillary readings are too reliant upon placement and environmental factors for accuracy.

77. Application, planning, growth and development (b)

❸ Soap has a drying effect on the skin of the elderly.

① The resident must be clean.

② There is no indication that this is a medical issue.

④ This requires a physician's order; nursing interventions should be tried first.

78. Comprehension, implementation, basic care and comfort (b)
    ❸ Because of the danger of aspiration, fluids should not be introduced into a nasogastric tube until correct placement has been verified.
    ① Although this is a part of the procedure, the primary step is verification of tube location.
    ② The feeding need only be room temperature.
    ④ Fluid should never be introduced into a nasogastric tube until placement in the stomach is verified.

79. Knowledge, implementation, coordinated care (b)
    ❷ This position will relieve strain on back muscles and uses the strongest muscles for lifting.
    ① To prevent injury, personnel must stand close to the object being lifted.
    ③ This puts undue strain on the back muscles.
    ④ This causes a narrow base of support; a wide base of support is needed for stability.

80. Application, evaluation, pharmacological therapies (b)
    ❹ Edema found above the catheter is indicative of infiltration.
    ① Poor skin turgor is a symptom of dehydration.
    ② Redness at the site is a symptom of infection or phlebitis.
    ③ Warmth at the insertion site is indicative of infection or phlebitis.

81. Knowledge, implementation, safety and infection control (a)
    ❷ Legal constraints make restraints a medically ordered procedure.
    ① Restraints often increase patient restlessness and powerlessness.
    ③ Too loose application increases patient injury risk.
    ④ Side rails cannot be lowered in an emergency if restraints are tied to them.

82. Knowledge, implementation, physiological adaptation (b)
    ❹ Oxygen has a drying effect on mucous membranes.
    ① Ventilating oxygen through water will not reduce its combustibility.
    ② The patient's level of oxygen absorption is related to liter flow, not humidity.
    ③ Particle contamination is not a factor in oxygen therapy.

83. Application, implementation, coping and adaptation (b)
    ❷ This response recognizes the patient's need for self-determination.
    ① This response fails to value the patient's needs.
    ③ This response imposes the nurse's values on the patient.
    ④ An inflexible response that fails to recognize patient individuality.

84. Comprehension, evaluation, coordinated care (b)
    ❷ The resident's chart is private and the nurse should not view the chart unless involved in direct patient care.
    ① This is inappropriate behavior and must be reported.
    ③ This is an appropriate intervention based upon the patient's wishes.
    ④ This is a most appropriate action; the incident requires further investigation.

85. Application, planning, safety and infection control (a)
    ❸ Taking people out of harm's way is always the first step in the event of fire.
    ① This sequence of events does not put the patient's safety first.
    ② This sequence does not place the patient's safety first.
    ④ Preserving the safety of the patient is always the first step in the event of a fire.

86. Application, assessment, reduction of risk potential (b)
    ❷ Cyanotic nail beds are indicative of diminished circulation.
    ① Warm, pink fingers are signs of good circulation.
    ③ This assessment finding is important and indicates good perfusion.
    ④ Circulatory impairment is indicated if capillary refill times are greater than 3 seconds.

87. Application, planning, safety and infection control (b)
    ❸ The primary goal in caring for a patient in protective isolation is to limit the amount of contact the patient has with organisms that may be brought into the room on the hands and body of individuals.
    ① The risk present is to the patient, not health care workers (who should be following blood and body fluid measures).
    ② Although it is important to minimize the impact of being isolated on patients in any type of isolation, the goal of therapy is to minimize the risk to the patient.
    ④ This is not the primary goal for protective isolation and it has not been established that the patient has an infectious process.

88. Application, implementation, coordinated care (b)
    ❷ By lining out the entry, others may still read the original entry; dating and initialing it is the proper procedure that signifies accountability.
    ① This is improper and does not allow for others to see the original mistake.
    ③ This would be destroying property belonging to the hospital; it is considered falsifying records.
    ④ Using correction fluid does not allow others to see the original message.

89. Application, evaluation, basic care and comfort (b)
    ❷ Most soaks are left on for this period of time, which allows for maximum vasodilation.
    ① This period of time is not sufficient to allow for vasodilation.
    ③ The compress would have become cold, causing vasoconstriction.
    ④ This period of time is too long; the compress would cause vasoconstriction instead of vasodilation.

90. Application, implementation, basic care and comfort (b)
    ❷ A tube that is being inserted to decompress the stomach will result in fluids and gas being removed.
    ① Increasing peristalsis is not the action that the NG tube is performing.
    ③ An NG tube will not inhibit the secretion of gastric secretions.
    ④ This response does not answer the patient's question concerning the purpose of the tube.

91. Application, implementation, basic care and comfort (c)
    ❹ This is the acceptable method for checking the placement of a large bore nasogastric tube.

① Although this would confirm placement of the tube, there are easier, less-expensive methods for obtaining this information.

② If the tube is in the patient's respiratory tract, the suction could cause damage to mucous membranes.

③ This could be potentially dangerous and may cause aspiration if the tube is in the patient's respiratory tract.

92. Application, implementation, safety and infection control (b)

❶ This response preserves the sterile catheter tray, while ensuring that a sterile catheter is used.

② Betadine will merely disinfect, not sterilize, the tip of the catheter; this is not an acceptable procedure.

③ There is no reason to discontinue the procedure or discard the sterile tray, when maintaining sterility can be achieved by obtaining a new catheter.

④ The nurse must maintain a sterile conscious, if instinct says the tip is contaminated, the nurse should obtain a new catheter.

93. Application, implementation, basic care and comfort (b)

❸ The major reason for ostomy pouches to fit snugly is so that the drainage will not excoriate the surrounding skin.

① Although this is a true statement, this is not the major reason for a snug fitting appliance.

② Normally, pouches can be removed when the patient takes a bath; this is not the major reason for a snug-fitting appliance.

④ Although this is true, it is not the major reason for a snug-fitting appliance.

94. Comprehension, planning, reduction of risk potential (b)

❹ An NPO order ensures that the stomach will be empty, therefore decreasing the chance for aspiration if the patient vomits after surgery.

① Anesthesia does slow down the digestive process, but it does not stop it.

② The energy needs of a surgical patient increase, not decrease.

③ Vomiting does not normally occur, and if the stomach is empty, aspiration is less likely to occur.

95. Application, implementation, physiological adaptation (b)

❷ This period of time allows the nurse to effectively remove secretions and not interrupt the patient's normal breathing pattern for too long a time.

① This is not an adequate period of time to remove secretions.

③ Thirty seconds is too long to keep a patient from their normal breathing patterns.

④ The patient is not able to breathe during the suctioning, and this period of time is too long an interruption of normal breathing patterns.

96. Comprehension, evaluation, reduction of risk potential (b)

❹ In general, ventricular arrhythmias are the most dangerous and potentially life threatening.

① A sinus arrhythmia may cause difficulty, but is generally not life threatening.

② An atrial arrhythmia is not as dangerous as a ventricular arrhythmia.

③ An AV nodal arrhythmia can cause serious consequences but is not as dangerous as a ventricular arrhythmia.

97. Application, implementation, physiological adaptation (b)

❸ This is the acceptable method for opening an airway of a patient who is not suspected of having a spinal cord injury; it is also the simplest method.

① Performing a mouth sweep is done to remove foreign objects from the mouth, potentially opening an airway; however, the head and chin must still be maneuvered after this procedure is done.

② Turning the head to one side will not open an airway.

④ This maneuver is difficult to perform and is done on patients with a suspected spinal cord injury.

98. Application, assessment, growth and development (c)

❸ This statement recognizes the individuality of older people, where chronological age is not a good indicator of functional ability.

① Disease may not occur in all individuals.

② This is untrue; many elderly do not develop chronic health problems.

④ Only 5% of elderly individuals actually live in a nursing home.

99. Application, evaluation, basic care and comfort (c)

❶ The proper method for establishing the patency of a small-bore feeding tube is to obtain a chest radiograph.

② If the tube is in the patient's respiratory tract, the suction may cause damage to the mucosa.

③ This could cause aspiration if the tube is in the respiratory tract.

④ This method may not work; given the small bore of the feeding tube, a chest radiograph is a more exact way of establishing patency.

100. Knowledge, planning, growth and development (b)

❸ The older adult routinely faces a "fixed" amount of income after retirement.

① The older adult does not typically have an increase in their income with retirement.

② As with everyone, income levels change depending on life's circumstances.

④ Income levels may change, but does not typically decrease throughout life.

101. Comprehension, assessment, growth and development (a)

❸ This statement reflects some of the developmental changes that occur in middle-age patients (empty nest syndrome).

① Although this is a personal statement, it could be made by a variety of age groups.

② Most individuals retire in their 60s, and this patient would not typically have this concern yet.

④ This is an ambiguous statement that requires further investigation.

102. Application, planning, prevention and early detection of disease (a)

❷ Walking is a nonstressful, pleasant activity especially beneficial for those individuals who have chronic health problems; it also preserves the joints of elderly individuals.

① Jogging may be too stressful for the elderly, especially to those with cardiopulmonary disease.

③ Ski machines may be too vigorous activity and place undue strain on joints.

④ Rowing machines may also be too vigorous, especially to those with cardiopulmonary disease.

103. Application, evaluation, coping and adaptation (b)

❸ Individuals of the Jehovah's Witness faith do not accept blood or blood products and may question why a type and cross would be done.

① This is normal preoperative teaching that does not conflict with this particular religion's beliefs.

② Coughing, deep breathing, and leg exercises should not conflict with this particular religion's beliefs.

④ This noninvasive procedure does not conflict with Jehovah's Witness beliefs.

104. Application, assessment, coping and adaptation (b)

❷ Collecting data concerning normal home practices allows the nurse to plan care effectively for the patient and is a priority.

① It has not been ascertained that this is necessary.

③ This may not be possible and the nurse must communicate effectively with the patient.

④ This is appropriate; however, the nurse must first establish communication with the patient.

105. Application, planning, basic care and comfort (b)

❹ The nurse may be able to provide the patient with some comfort measures that he engages in at home, or otherwise meet the patient's needs.

① The patient is not complaining of pain.

② It has not been determined that the patient needs a sedative, more information from the patient is needed.

③ This is an unrealistic reassurance and does not address the patient's complaint.

106. Application, implementation, reduction of risk potential (c)

❶ This response best describes the reason for the runny nose and watery eyes, which is the question the patient posed.

② This is not clearly established and it does not answer the patient's question.

③ This may be a normal reflex; however, the patient is asking why it happens during hay fever season.

④ This is true but does not describe the reason for the watery eyes and runny nose.

107. Application, planning, physiological adaptation (b)

❸ This complaint could be life threatening and is of priority.

① This blood glucose level does need to be corrected; however, respiratory status takes priority.

② This small laceration will need to be attended to after the shortness of breath is addressed.

④ The family member does need to be attended to at some time; however, the shortness of breath is of primary importance.

108. Application, implementation, basic care and comfort (b)

❸ The ulcer will fill in from the inside and upward, which leaves a scar.

① This is a flip response that demeans the individual.

② This response does not recognize the needs of the patient.

④ The physician may be consulted, but the question is asked of the nurse who has the ability to answer it.

109. Comprehension, implementation, reduction of risk potential (a)

❸ By using a syringe and withdrawing the urine using the provided sampling port, the nurse can obtain a sterile specimen without breaking the continuity of the system.

① This action would not produce a sterile specimen and would necessitate putting the catheter back in the patient.

② Water should come out of the balloon port on the catheter, not urine; this action would deflate the catheter balloon, causing dislodgement.

④ Urine is no longer sterile after it has been sitting in the bottom of the drainage bag; a sterile urine specimen is needed.

110. Application, evaluation, basic care and comfort (b)

❸ The pain is most likely due to inflating the balloon while it is in the urethra; the nurse should make sure that the catheter is advanced into the bladder before inflating the balloon.

① If the balloon ruptures, it should not cause pain and the result would be that the catheter could not be considered indwelling.

② Although not a wise practice, this action should not cause pain if the catheter is in the bladder.

④ The patient complained during balloon inflation, and therefore the pain must be connected to this action.

111. Application, implementation, reduction of risk potential (b)

❹ This placement ensures that the tubing will be below the urinary bladder; therefore the urine will not travel back up the drainage tube, an action that could result in a urinary tract infection.

① This position may result in urine traveling back up the drainage tubing, potentially causing a urinary tract infection.

② This position may result in urine traveling back up the drainage tubing back to the bladder.

③ This position is also too high, resulting in urine traveling back up the drainage tubing.

112. Application, implementation, physiological adaptation (c)

❹ Air, being a gas, would be floating in the uppermost portion of the lung, and to drain that air, the chest tube would have to be positioned near the front of the lung, at the apex.

① This position may not facilitate the removal of the air in the patient's lung.

② Drainage and blood collects in the bottom, or base of the lung; air floats toward the anterior, upper surface.

③ This position facilitates removal of drainage and blood, but not air.

113. Application, planning, safety and infection control (b)

❸ The patient's low WBC count makes him susceptible to infection and a protective isolation would limit the number of organisms with which he came into contact.

① This method of isolation is normally used for patients who have an infectious, communicable disease.

② Enteric precautions are designed for those individuals who have an infection that spreads via the fecal route.

④ These precautions are used by all health care personnel for all patients.

114. Comprehension, implementation, reduction of risk potential (b)
    ❸ Clipping hair from the potential surgical site and surrounding area reduces the number of microorganisms present on the hair and skin, reducing the incidence of infection.
    ① Removal of hair does not lessen discomfort from the surgical procedure.
    ② If the incision is sutured, the amount of hair at the site will not affect that practice.
    ④ Although this may be true, this is not the primary purpose for clipping hair before surgery.

115. Comprehension, evaluation, coordinated care (c)
    ❹ A return demonstration of the skill coupled with verbalization of the steps is considered the best way of evaluating the knowledge base of the individual.
    ① The patient may be able to tell you what he/she has learned but not be able to perform it.
    ② Taking a quiz is anxiety producing for patients and will evaluate only the knowledge base of the individual, not the skill base.
    ③ Although this would be an excellent way to determine the effectiveness of the teaching, it is generally anxiety producing and inappropriate for the nurse to ask a patient to teach another patient.

116. Comprehension, evaluation, physiological adaptation (b)
    ❹ Normally, individuals who have had spinal anesthesia are to remain flat for specified length of time after surgery (4 to 6 hours) to prevent headache.
    ① This is an appropriate order.
    ② Generally, surgical patients can get out of bed after 4 to 6 hours of lying flat.
    ③ This order allows the patient to advance their diet as they tolerate fluids.

117. Application, implementation, basic care and comfort (b)
    ❶ The nurse bandages the extremity from the foot upwards, facilitating venous return, and reducing the incidence of swelling due to the bandaging.
    ② If the nurse bandages from the knee down to the foot, venous return is compromised and swelling of the foot may occur.
    ③ If the nurse begins bandaging at the ankle, swelling of the foot may occur and this technique does not facilitate venous return to the heart.
    ④ Bandaging from the middle of the leg, either upward or downward, will not facilitate venous return and may cause swelling above and below the bandage.

118. Application, implementation, basic care and comfort (b)
    ❸ This position allows for venous return, decreasing the incidence of swelling of the arm and hand.
    ① This position may not allow for adequate venous drainage and may cause swelling.
    ② If the arm and hand are in a dependent position from the elbow, swelling will occur.
    ④ This position is not only uncomfortable, but swelling will occur in the arm and hand.

119. Comprehension, planning, physiological adaptation (b)
    ❸ Adequate oxygenation is always the first priority in any emergency situation.
    ① Although important, this cannot be accomplished unless a patent airway is established.

② A victim's airway must be established before controlling bleeding.
④ This is not a priority nursing action and may be performed by ancillary personnel.

120. Application, implementation, physiological adaptation (c)
    ❹ Cold water lowers metabolism, slowing cellular death. A patient may be revived because of this effect after hours of being submerged.
    ① The reason for doing CPR is not to warm the patient up, but to try to revive him.
    ② Performing CPR may result in removing water from the lung, however this is not the reason for performing CPR.
    ③ Cold water lowers metabolism, allowing for a possible revival.

121. Application, implementation, reduction of risk potential (b)
    ❹ It is important to assess the neurovascular status of extremities that are distal to the catheter insertion site; checking pulses is a common method for assessing neurovascular status.
    ① This is not indicated for patients that have had an arteriogram.
    ② It is not necessary to maintain the patient on NPO status.
    ③ Ambulation immediately following the procedure can cause bleeding from the catheter insertion site.

122. Knowledge, implementation, reduction of risk potential (b)
    ❷ Elevated BUN and creatinine levels indicate damage to the kidneys.
    ① These levels are not indicators of liver function.
    ③ Damaged muscles do not result in elevated BUN and creatinine levels.
    ④ These levels cannot determine damage to the intestines.

123. Comprehension, planning, reduction of risk potential (a)
    ❹ A bronchoscopy utilizes passage of a scope into the respiratory tract; it is important to check for a gag reflex prior to giving the patient fluids.
    ① An angiogram does not necessitate checking a gag reflex.
    ② Arteriograms are not performed near the respiratory tract and do not require performance of a gag reflex.
    ③ Mammograms are performed on breast tissue and do not require performance of a gag reflex posttest.

124. Application, planning, reduction of risk potential (b)
    ❸ It is generally easier to obtain a sputum specimen in the morning because of stasis of secretions during the night; as the individual awakens and moves about, a specimen can sometimes be obtained.
    ① This is not a good time to obtain a specimen; the patient may have difficulty producing one.
    ② This may be a good time to obtain a specimen, but early morning is still the best time.
    ④ Specimens are normally harder to obtain in the evening, because the patient has been active during the day.

125. Application, implementation, physiological adaptation (b)
    ❹ A generous fluid intake liquefies secretions, allowing them to be more easily expectorated.

① Adequate sleep is important in any treatment plan, however, it does not keep secretions from becoming thick.

② Although important, regular exercise does not directly liquefy secretions.

③ A nourishing diet is important in the treatment plan, but does not directly liquefy secretions.

126. Application, assessment, physiological adaptation (b)
❸ The gurgling noise signifies that the patient is unable to control his secretions and should be assisted by suctioning.

① Although rapid, many individuals with a respiratory ailment are tachypneic, which does not indicate that suctioning is needed.

② When patients need suctioning, their heart rate normally does increase; however, it is not itself an indicator for suctioning.

④ If the patient is able to expectorate his mucus, he does not need to be suctioned.

127. Comprehension, implementation, coordinated care (a)
❶ The adult patient has the right to refuse any or all therapy and must be given the opportunity to formulate a living will.

② The patient may consult with the physician, but the patient has the right to make the decision independently.

③ The decision is the patient's, however he/she may consult with a variety of individuals.

④ As a rule, nurses assist in curing patients; when cure is not possible, health care workers should uphold the patient's wishes.

128. Comprehension, implementation, coordinated care (b)
❷ Hospice encourages the patient and his family members to work through the dying process together.

① Although the patient may be introspective at times, hospice encourages communication between the patient and the family.

③ Registered nurses check on the patient frequently, but the majority of care does fall on the family.

④ Hospice workers do assist family members through the grieving process; however, the patient and family are encouraged to work through these feelings together.

129. Comprehension, planning, coordinated care (b)
❷ An advance directive ensures that the patient or designee can make decisions concerning treatment before death.

① The patient or patient advocate will dictate which measures will be utilized as death approaches.

③ The physician must uphold the patient's wishes; however, the physician has the right to advise the patient concerning a treatment plan.

④ The patient designates a patient advocate to make end-of-life decisions; these decisions are based on the patient's wishes, not the family's.

130. Comprehension, planning, coordinated care (b)
❶ Planning for discharge should begin on the day of admission to the hospital.

② This does not give adequate time to organize community resources if the patient needs them.

③ It is difficult to predict when a patient will be discharged; planning should begin well before discharge.

④ The plan of care for the patient should be evaluated each day, making changes based on the procedures or treatments that the patient has.

131. Comprehension, implementation, reduction of risk potential (b)
❸ Urine is strained on patients with known or suspected calculi to collect stones for evaluation.

① Flank massage is not indicated for patients with renal calculi.

② Urine reductions are indicated for patients with diabetes mellitus.

④ Fluids are generally encouraged in patients who have suspected renal calculi.

132. Comprehension, implementation, reduction of risk potential (b)
❷ In order for the proper laboratory tests to be completed, all voided urine must be collected.

① In a 24-hour urine specimen, all urine is collected that the patient voids in a 24-hour period.

③ There is no discernible reason to insert a retention catheter, unless the patient is incontinent.

④ All urine is sent to the lab in one large, dark container.

133. Comprehension, implementation, physiological adaptation (b)
❸ Inserting a rectal tube will stimulate peristalsis and relieve the abdominal pain and pressure.

① Normally, activity if possible will help to relieve the pain of flatus.

② Nonpharmaceutical interventions can usually alleviate this type of discomfort.

④ This action will decrease the amount of additional gas buildup but will not relieve the immediate discomfort.

134. Comprehension, implementation, reduction of risk potential (b)
❹ The presence of ova and parasites can only be detected when the specimen is still warm.

① This action will not allow lab personnel to find ova and parasites; the specimen must be warm.

② It is not necessary to use a sterile specimen cup. The GI tract is not sterile.

③ Nothing should be added to the specimen prior to transport to the lab.

135. Application, assessment, basic care and comfort (b)
❸ Symptoms of dehydration include decreased urine output and poor skin turgor.

① Weight gain is indicative of hypervolemia.

② Hypertension is indicative of hypervolemia.

④ Moist, pink, mucous membranes are a symptom of balanced fluid status.

136. Application, evaluation, physiological adaptation (b)
❹ All assessment data indicate that the circulatory status of the extremity is intact and that the pain is from the fracture itself.

① This response disregards the patient's complaints.

② The assessment data do not indicate that the cast is too tight.

③ The assessment data do not indicate that the patient has any circulatory impairment.

137. Application, implementation, physiological adaptation (b)
❶ The patient may cause a break in his skin, introducing bacteria from the cast, skin, and fork into the wound.

② Although this is a concern, causing an infection is the primary reason for dissuading this practice.

③ No sharp object should be used to scratch down and inside a cast.

④ Unless the patient has decreased sensation as a result of another malady, he should feel if he injures himself; this is not the primary reason for discouraging this practice.

138. Knowledge, planning, basic care and comfort (b)

❶ The skin is the body's first line of defense, and a break in this defense reduces the body's ability to resist infections.

② A break in the skin does not necessarily decrease the body's ability to produce antibodies.

③ Although the skin does assist in eliminating perspiration, a break in the skin does not reduce this substantially.

④ The ability to maintain correct body alignment should not be affected by a break in the skin.

139. Comprehension, implementation, basic care and comfort (b)

❷ Fingernails should be clipped with slightly rounded edges; toenails should be clipped straight across.

① Toenails should be clipped straight across.

③ Clipping the fingernails in this manner may cause injury from scratching, and it is unattractive.

④ This may cause infection and injury if the nails are too short.

140. Comprehension, implementation, basic care and comfort (b)

❶ A patient with a bleeding disorder may preclude the nurse from completing the shave; further investigation is necessary before proceeding.

② A patient with an emotional disorder would most likely not stop the nurse from shaving the patient.

③ Patients with respiratory disorders may need frequent rest periods, but shaving with a manual razor should not pose a problem for the patient.

④ A patient with a neurological disorder should not preclude the nurse from completing the task.

141. Application, implementation, basic care and comfort (b)

❹ If possible, the patient should be placed on the side with head turned to the side; this facilitates removal of secretions and decreases the chance of aspiration.

① This is too difficult a position to place an unconscious patient in, although it would facilitate secretion drainage.

② The patient should be placed so that secretions naturally fall from the mouth, suction is an appropriate device that should be near.

③ The patient needs to be flat and side lying; this position does not facilitate secretion drainage.

142. Comprehension, planning, basic care and comfort (b)

❹ Sleep apnea is a disorder that results in frequent waking during the night, causing daytime fatigue.

① This disorder is not normally caused by snoring or overeating.

② Sleep apnea is not increased if the patient is nervous or upset.

③ Individuals with sleep apnea can have the disorder for a long period of time.

143. Comprehension, assessment, basic care and comfort (b)

❸ This allows the patient to easily describe the intensity of the pain to the nurse, and allows for evaluation of treatment options.

① This will not assess the intensity of the pain, only the duration.

② This response allows the patient to locate the pain but does not describe intensity.

④ These words are too subjective; the word *bad* may have different meanings to the nurse and patient.

144. Application, implementation, basic care and comfort (b)

❸ The crutch length is too long, causing compression of the nerves in the axilla; adjusting the crutches and teaching the patient to place weight on his hands will alleviate the problem.

① There is no indication that the patient needs a walker instead of a crutch.

② The pain and tingling is most likely caused by compression of a nerve, not nerve damage.

④ This does not correct the problem, which is improper crutch length and technique.

145. Comprehension, implementation, basic care and comfort (b)

❹ The patient should use the cane to take weight off of her weak extremity, the right side.

① This will not assist the patient in walking.

② This may confuse the patient and will not effectively limit weight bearing on the right side.

③ Holding the cane in the left hand and moving it with the left leg will not limit weight bearing on the right side.

146. Application, assessment, basic care and comfort (b)

❹ Cheyne Stokes respirations are characterized by rhythmic breathing with a varying depth and rate of respirations, with periods of apnea; it is commonly seen in patients who are approaching death.

① Dyspnea is difficulty breathing, and although this patient is having difficulty breathing, the question asks for the specific breathing pattern that is being observed.

② Tachypnea is fast breathing, or increased rate; the patient does not exhibit tachypnea.

③ Kussmaul's is a type of breathing seen in individuals who have diabetes mellitus; it is characterized by paroxysms of dyspnea.

147. Application, assessment, basic care and comfort (b)

❹ Patients on bedrest normally have their feet and head elevated; therefore excessive tissue fluid would fall into the sacral area.

① Individuals who are ambulatory are most likely to notice edema of the feet.

② Individuals who are bedfast may eventually develop edema of the hands; however, initially it is normally found in the sacral area.

③ As the edema progresses, calves may become edematous; however, calf edema is more common in the ambulatory individual.

148. Application, implementation, coordinated care (b)

❸ This response signifies a correct step in the procedure for administering a vaginal douche.

① The patient should be encouraged to void before the douche is instilled.

② The fluid should already be flowing as the enema enters the vagina.

④ Low pressure is used when instilling the fluid to decrease tissue trauma.

149. Application, implementation, coping and adaptation (b)

❸ By paraphrasing the statement and restating it in the form of a question, the nurse is able to illicit more information about the patient's feelings.

① This belittles the patient's concern and gives false reassurance.

② Anxiety may be heightening this patient's worries, but this response belittles the patient's fears.

④ This response neither validates the patient's concerns nor encourages expression of feelings.

150. Comprehension, evaluation, physiological adaptation (b)

❷ These vital signs are abnormal, signify a fever, and should be reported.

① All vital signs are normal for adult patients.

③ Axillary temperatures may be unreliable; however, all these vital signs are within normal limits.

④ All vital signs are within normal limits.

151. Comprehension, evaluation, basic care and comfort (b)

❶ Due to the patient's inability to excrete fluids, the patient's weight will likely increase because of the excess fluid.

② The patient's weight will not decrease, because the excess fluid will not be able to be eliminated.

③ Because of the patient's diagnosis, she will not be able to rid herself of the fluid.

④ The patient is most likely hypervolemic and not dehydrated.

152. Comprehension, planning, basic care and comfort (b)

❷ The patient has difficulty swallowing and will need special feeding precautions taken.

① Facial exercises will not assist in helping the patient to swallow.

③ The patient may or may not have difficulty forming words; however, if dysphagia is present, then special feeding precautions must be instituted.

④ This may be necessary and needs to be determined, but the plan of care needs to address the swallowing difficulty.

153. Application, planning, physiological adaptation (b)

❹ A tympanic temperature will give an accurate reading and should be used as the oral and rectal routes are not indicated for this patient.

① The oral route should not be used because the patient is receiving oxygen.

② The rectal surgery precludes using this route.

③ The axillary method is the most unreliable of the methods listed; the tympanic temperature is the best choice for this patient.

154. Comprehension, assessment, physiological adaptation (b)

❸ If the patient's oxygen saturation was truly 60%, the patient would be in distress; the more likely cause for the alarm is that the probe has become dislodged.

① The need for this action has not been established.

② The nurse would need to report to the physician and receive orders to complete this task.

④ There is no need for this action at this time.

155. Application, planning, physiological adaptation (b)

❹ The patient in high Fowler's position is virtually sitting upright, which facilitates the greatest chest expansion.

① This side-lying position will not allow the patient to achieve full chest expansion.

② This flat position will not maximize the patient's chest expansion.

③ Low Fowler's position is not high enough to maximize chest expansion.

156. Comprehension, evaluation, reduction of risk potential (b)

❸ The presence of meat in this patient's system will cause the hemoccult test to be positive, whether or not there is actually blood in his stool; the patient should be free of red meat for 2 to 3 days for the test to be considered accurate.

① Ingestion of coffee should have no bearing on the test results.

② The gelatin should not cause the developer slide to turn blue (indicating the presence of blood).

④ Lots of fiber should not have any bearing on the test results.

157. Application, implementation, reduction of risk potential (c)

❸ Application of heat should dilate the blood vessels of the fingers and increase blood flow to the area.

① Milking the finger may cause an inaccurate reading on the machine.

② This will prevent blood from reaching the fingertips; fingers could be held downward to facilitate filling.

④ This practice is not only painful but also may affect the accuracy of the reading.

158. Application, implementation, safety and infection control (b)

❷ This choice allows the nurse to maintain sterility and reduce cost to the patient.

① This would be unsanitary; the gauze was wet and was not entirely on the sterile field, which may not be waterproof.

③ The gauze pad became contaminated during the time it was on the sterile field's edge, and rinsing it in saline solution will not resterilize it.

④ There is no need to begin again; the situation can be resolved without the additional expense to the patient of beginning again.

159. Comprehension, implementation, reduction in risk potential (b)

❹ An IPPB treatment works by forcing the person to inhale deeply, which will increase airflow, increase oxygenation, and assist in loosening secretions.

① Manual or mechanical chest physiotherapy is better able to dislodge secretions.

② Incentive spirometry is useful in increasing tidal volume of inhalations.

③ This statement describes how postural drainage assists patients.

160. Application, implementation, physiological adaptation (b)
    ❷ The patient needs to have oxygen supplemented; the patient is accustomed to oxygen and must have it supplied in increased amounts before the suctioning procedure; failure to do so may cause hypoxia.
    ① There is no indication that restraints are needed.
    ③ Suction is never applied when advancing the catheter.
    ④ The patient needs to have oxygen prior to advancing the suction catheter.

161. Application, implementation, reduction in risk potential (b)
    ④ To obtain an accurate measurement, the arrow on the cuff should be positioned where the brachial artery was palpated, which will result in appropriate cuff pressure of the artery.
    ① This may result in an inaccurate, low reading.
    ② The patient's arm should be extended with palm up.
    ③ The cuff is positioned 1 inch above the brachial artery.

162. Application, assessment, physiological adaptation (b)
    ❶ The nurse palpates the peripheral pulse.
    ② The technique of percussion is used when evaluating the status of fluid, drainage, or air in a cavity.
    ③ Inspection requires observation of the patient, without touching the patient.
    ④ Auscultation is listening for sounds; the apical pulse is evaluated in this manner.

163. Knowledge, implementation, basic care and comfort (a)
    ❶ A patient's emesis should be measured and added to the output for that period of time.
    ② IV fluids are considered as part of a patient's intake.
    ③ The water loss that results from perspiration is insensible and can not be measured.
    ④ The volume of tube feedings is added to a patient's intake.

164. Application, assessment, pharmacological therapies (b)
    ❸ This is too long for IV tubing to hang without being changed; normally IV tubing is changed every 2 to 3 days; the nurse needs to hang a new IV bag and tubing to decrease the incidence of infection.
    ① The IV site is not infected, no action is required.
    ② Fluid in the IV container signifies that there is enough to infuse into the patient, depending on the flow rate; if the tubing does not need changing, the bag would not need to be changed.
    ④ Normal IV site, no action is needed.

165. Comprehension, implementation, reduction of risk potential (b)
    ❹ By remaining in an upright position, the tube feeding is less likely to travel back up the esophagus and be aspirated by the patient.
    ① This is a common practice; however, it does not assist in reducing the risk of aspiration.
    ② This is a very appropriate action but does not reduce the risk for aspiration.
    ③ This may cause the patient to lose calories and should not be done unless physician ordered; it has no bearing on aspiration.

166. Application, assessment, basic care and comfort (b)
    ❸ Burning on urination is to be expected after a catheter is removed and needs to be acted upon only if it persists.

① There is no evidence of this yet; however, if other symptoms develop and the burning does not decrease, action may need to be taken.
② It has not been established that the physician need be called.
④ The nurse needs a physician's order to obtain a urine specimen; if the burning continues, the physician may need to be called.

167. Application, implementation, basic care and comfort (b)
    ❶ If the tube is in the patient's trachea, air will not flow to vibrate the vocal cords, and the patient will be unable to speak.
    ② This signifies that the tube is still in the nasal cavity.
    ③ A small amount of blood is indicative of tissue trauma from inserting the tube.
    ④ This would signify that the tube was in the stomach.

168. Comprehension, planning, basic care and comfort (b)
    ❷ This statement correctly explains the actions of each enema.
    ① Although both enemas may stimulate peristalsis somewhat, the cleansing enema is designed for this purpose.
    ③ The oil retention enema is given to soften stool, not given specifically to evacuate the bowel.
    ④ The oil retention enema is the enema given to soften the stool and is normally given before the cleansing enema.

169. Comprehension, assessment, basic care and comfort (b)
    ❹ The patient may be unable to fully expel all urine from the bladder; further assessment is indicated to assess the fullness of the urinary bladder, but this response is the best indicator that the patient may need the catheter.
    ① Without further data, this would not indicate that the patient needs the catheter.
    ② The urinary bladder should be palpated to assess fullness; the consumption of large amounts of fluids is not an indication that the catheterization is needed.
    ③ The patient's bladder is most likely empty if the incontinent episode occurred; further assessment is needed.

170. Comprehension, assessment, basic care and comfort (b)
    ❸ The patient may not be drinking enough fluids, and this may contribute to the problem.
    ① Exercise assists in establishing normal bowel function.
    ② Vegetables supply fiber, which should assist in establishing normal bowel patterns.
    ④ It is important to defecate as soon as the need is felt.

171. Comprehension, planning, reduction of risk potential (b)
    ❹ Because of the barium in the bowel, cleansing enemas will be ordered to decrease the chance of fecal impaction from the barium.
    ① Unless further procedures are ordered, the patient should not have to be NPO for any length of time.
    ② This is not an order that is normally associated with a barium enema.
    ③ There should be no reason for a patient that has had a routine barium enema to remain flat in bed.

172. Comprehension, implementation, coordinated care (b)
    ❸ This response is the definition of a contracture; the muscle is permanently shortened because of the effects of immobility.
    ① This does not address the UAP's question.

② An injury may have precipitated the decreased mobility, but the contracture is directly due to the effects of immobility.
④ Once contracted, the arm will remain this way permanently and ROM exercises will not restore it.

173. Comprehension, implementation, physiological adaptation (b)
❸ Changing the trach ties poses the most risk, as the patient could cough out the trach tube, thereby losing the patency of the airway.
① Suctioning should pose limited risk if performed in a safe manner.
② Limited risk, cleansing the stoma does not directly effect the airway.
④ As long as trach ties are in place, cleansing the inner cannula should not pose a risk.

174. Comprehension, implementation, reduction of risk potential (b)
❹ This is the most correct, appropriate response by the nurse because it addresses the patient's question.
① Although humorous, this answer is demeaning and does not answer the question.
② This response belittles the patient and shifts responsibility for explanation to another person.
③ The patient wants to know why he needs to get out of bed; this response does not answer that question.

175. Application, implementation, basic care and comfort (a)
❹ This is the most logical response to the question and describes the action of the stockings.
① This does not tell the patient why the stockings are needed or why they should be snug.
② This is not the purpose for the stockings.
③ Although the muscles of the legs are compressed by the stockings, the reason they need to be snug is so that blood is pushed back toward the heart.

176. Comprehension, planning, coordinated care (b)
❸ This is a short-term, easily measurable goal for this patient.
① The emphasis of this plan of care is how well the patient will walk with crutches, not how long he/she can go without pain medication.
② This goal may be long term, and most patients do not need 3 weeks to learn to walk with crutches.
④ This is an example of a long-term goal.

177. Comprehension, implementation, basic care and comfort (b)
❸ Patients are generally calmer when they are in a quiet, stress-free environment; pastel shades of carpeting and wall decorations are also calming.
① Although exercise is important, a lot of physical activity may overstimulate the patient.
② This may cause the patient to become overstimulated.
④ These activities may overly stimulate the patient.

178. Knowledge, implementation, basic care and comfort (b)
❹ Hydrogen peroxide's oxidizing capabilities make it a good choice for removing hardened secretions.
① Alcohol should not be used on the rubber Foley catheter, because it will cause drying and cracking.
② Betadine is an antiseptic and should not be used to remove secretions.
③ If soap and water were ineffective, sterile saline will not remove the secretions.

179. Application, implementation, basic care and comfort (b)
❷ The first surgical dressing should be changed by the surgeon; therefore, the dressing should be reinforced until further orders can be obtained.
① The nurse is unsure of what is under the dressing; changing a fresh postoperative dressing requires a physician's order.
③ Removing the dressing would require a physician's order.
④ Dressings are not routinely sent to the laboratory, and there is no order to change the dressing.

180. Application, implementation, reduction of risk potential (b)
❹ The term *debride* means to cleanse a wound, and this is the purpose of this type of dressing.
① The dressing may soothe the tissue, but this is not the purpose of the dressing.
② Unless impregnated with an antibiotic solution, the dressing has no antiinfective qualities.
③ The saline evaporates from the dressing, and as it dries the gauze adheres to the tissue that needs to be removed.

181. Application, implementation, reduction of risk potential (b)
❷ The patient that has decreased sensation to extremities is at increased risk for injury as a result of the application of heat.
① As long as the nurse explains the entire procedure to the patient, special precautions do not need to be taken for patients who are blind.
③ Patients with hypertension are not at increased risk from the effects of the heat application.
④ Although patients with diabetes mellitus may have neuropathy, which would place them at risk, the paraplegic individual remains the person at most risk from the heat application.

182. Knowledge, planning, reduction of risk potential (b)
❸ A thin layer of petrolatum (petroleum jelly) should be place between the compress and the patient's eyelid to reduce damage to the eye area.
① Saline will not protect the eye from the heat.
② Betadine is an antiseptic solution and should not be applied anywhere near the eye area.
④ Unless ordered, the antibiotic ointment is not placed on the lid.

183. Application, implementation, basic care and comfort (b)
❶ The irrigating fluid is added to the patient's intake in a special column of the I & O record; the resulting drainage back of the fluid is added to the patient's output.
② The drainage of the irrigant is added to the patient's output.
③ The NG irrigating fluid is not added to the IV fluids column.
④ The NG irrigant is not given orally and should not be added into the oral intake.

184. Application, assessment, physiological adaptation (b)
❶ The presence of redness and swelling indicate that infection may be present in the incision line.
② This does not directly indicate infection.
③ This is normal assessment data and indicates adequate healing.

④ At times a small amount of bloody drainage may be observed in a new incision line; this does not indicate infection.

185. Application, implementation, basic care and comfort (b)
   ❷ The patient should be placed on his left side so that the infected drainage will flow away from the other eye.
   ① Drainage may flow into the right eye, causing infection.
   ③ If the patient is on his right side, drainage will flow from the left to the right eye.
   ④ The drainage will not be able to flow away from the patient's face.

186. Comprehension, implementation, prevention and early detection of disease (b)
   ❹ Most long-term care facilities routinely test for tuberculosis upon admission; this is a routine screening done to protect the patients in the facility.
   ① This does not validate the patient's concern nor explain the rationale for the test.
   ② This response appears to be antagonistic and does not help the patient.
   ③ Once again, this response will only antagonize the patient, not explain the rationale for the test.

187. Comprehension, implementation, prevention and early detection of disease (b)
   ❷ Most physicians recommend that women over the age of 40 undergo mammograms every 1 to 2 years.
   ① Mammograms are screening exams and are done on women over the age of 40 whether or not cancer is suspected.
   ③ All women should receive mammograms, women with strong family histories may be screened as often as every 6 months.
   ④ Mammograms are not difficult for women, although they may be embarrassing to some women; mammograms are recommended every 1 to 2 years after the age of 40.

188. Application, implementation, basic care and comfort (b)
   ❸ The footboard is used to keep the feet in proper alignment and decrease the incidence of plantar flexion.
   ① An abductor pillow assists in maintaining an abducted state of the legs.
   ② Antiembolic stockings are better able to keep the patient from developing thrombophlebitis, although a footboard can be used to do pedal pushes, thereby exercising the calf muscles.
   ④ This may be true, but is not the purpose of the board.

189. Comprehension, planning, coordinated care (b)
   ❸ Liability insurance only covers the nurse while performing professional duties.
   ① Malpractice insurance costs vary from agency to agency.
   ② Malpractice insurance protects the nurse from financial damages.
   ④ Malpractice insurance must be renewed periodically.

190. Knowledge, implementation, coordinated care (b)
   ❹ The LP/VN functions in home care settings under the direction of a physician or registered nurse.
   ① LP/VNs cannot be self-employed, they must always work under the supervision of a physician or registered nurse.

② The state board of nursing does not directly supervise nurses.
   ③ The LP/VN can only function under the supervision of a physician or registered nurse.

191. Comprehension, assessment, coping and adaptation (b)
   ❸ The patient is bargaining with God for his life.
   ① There is no evidence of anger in his statement.
   ② The patient accepts his diagnosis; he just wishes to change it.
   ④ The patient does not appear depressed at this time.

192. Comprehension, assessment, physiological adaptation (b)
   ❶ Given the patient's diagnosis, lung sounds are the most important assessment criteria.
   ② Although important, bowel sounds are not the most important assessment data for this patient.
   ③ The patient's lung sounds are of paramount importance.
   ④ There is no indication that a neurological exam is warranted for this patient; lung sounds remain the top priority.

193. Comprehension, evaluation, safety and infection control (b)
   ❷ The catheter most likely was the reservoir for the infection.
   ① There is no indication that a primary infection is present.
   ③ Urinary tract infections are not normally due to an autoimmune response.
   ④ There is no evidence that the patient received antibiotics.

194. Knowledge, planning, basic care and comfort (b)
   ❷ Generally, most individuals need to be repositioned at least every 2 hours to prevent ulcer formation.
   ① This is not a frequent enough turning schedule.
   ③ The nurse should reposition the patient at least every 2 hours.
   ④ Although pressure ulcers would not develop on this turning schedule, the patient would be excessively disturbed.

195. Knowledge, legal/professional, coordinated care (a)
   ❹ Provision of safe care is the responsibility of each province.
   ① Other than in Alberta and Quebec, certification/registration/licensing examinations are set by CNAT.
   ② Laws are passed by the provincial legislature.
   ③ Regulatory bodies decide whether there is negligence in the individual practice of nursing and are completely autonomous from the court system.

196. Comprehension, legal/professional, coordinated care (a)
   ❸ All members of the health care team work together.
   ① The PN/NA may be under the direction of an RN in some settings. In others the PN/NA works independently or may direct others (e.g., UCPs).
   ② The RN is responsible for the direction, not the supervision, of the PN/NA.
   ④ The PN/NA cares for a variety of patients with different degrees of responsibility, depending on the complexity of care required.

197. Knowledge, legal/professional, coordinated care (a)
   ❸ The purpose of registration is to prohibit those not registered from using the title.

① The standards of care set by the regulatory bodies protect the public.

② Each registrant is responsible for his/her own practice.

④ Licensure protects the actual acts within the practice of nursing.

198. Knowledge, legal/professional, coordinated care (a)

❷ Health care delivery is the responsibility of the provinces.

① Federal legislation applies to matters of national or international nature (e.g., testing new drugs).

③ Regulatory bodies are provincial, not local or municipal.

④ Professional associations are provincial, not local, and have a lobbying function only with regard to legislation.

199. Comprehension, legal/professional, coordinated care (a)

❷ Licensure protects the practice of nursing through legislation, which provides mechanisms for charging those practicing without a license.

① It is the role of the licensing body to protect the public by setting and ensuring implementation of minimum standards of safe practice.

③ Licensure indicates the level of the practitioner.

④ The individual registrant is protected while providing safe care within the minimum standards of practice of the licensing body.

200. Knowledge, legal/professional, coordinated care (a)

❸ Provincial licensing bodies are responsible for setting admission requirements for their own jurisdiction.

① Educational institutions may only set admission requirements for general interest courses.

② Provincial professional associations may make recommendations regarding, but do not set, admission requirements.

④ CAPNNA is a voluntary professional association representing provincial professional associations and as such has nothing to do with admission requirements.

201. Knowledge, legal/professional, coordinated care (a)

❸ Malpractice insurance is not mandatory in Canada, and is offered as a reason to join voluntary professional associations.

① CAPNNA is the professional voice for PNs/NAs in Canada and has nothing to do with the practice of individual members.

② The role of the licensing bodies is to protect the public; therefore it would be seen as conflict of interest to provide malpractice insurance.

④ Private insurance companies do not provide malpractice insurance for PNs/NAs; it is handled through the provincial associations.

202. Knowledge, legal/professional, coordinated care (a)

❸ Every member of each affiliated provincial/territorial association is a member of CAPNNA upon payment of association fees.

① Membership is voluntary and optional to individuals in provinces not affiliated with CAPNNA or in provinces where the professional association and licensing body are not the same.

② Membership is not mandatory in any province/territory.

④ Membership in CAPNNA is only automatic with membership in affiliated provincial/territorial associations.

203. Knowledge, legal/professional, coordinated care (a)

❷ Each PN/NA has the responsibility to maintain competency and increase level of knowledge.

① Examinations are written only for initial registration/licensing.

③ Maintaining skill level, as well as other competencies, is the responsibility of the individual PN/NA.

④ The PN/NA may choose to attend a variety of educational programs to maintain and increase competence; these would vary among registrants, depending upon individual needs.

204. Knowledge, legal/professional, coordinated care (a)

❸ In Canada the provinces/territories are given responsibility for developing legislation related to nursing.

① The regulatory body in each province/territory is designated by legislation; it does not develop the legislation.

② The legal systems in Canada and in the United States are different in most aspects, including how nursing is regulated.

④ The legislation gives the regulatory body the authority to set standards for nursing in a variety of settings; specific directions are not outlined in the legislation.

CHAPTER 3

Pharmacology

This chapter covers two major areas: (1) administration of medications and (2) pharmacological aspects of nursing care. The nursing process as it applies to drugs and drug administration is explained and integrated throughout the text.

Calculation of dosage and intravenous infusion rate, principles of medication administration, procedures and sites for medication administration, blood transfusion administration, and pediatric drug administration are reviewed.

The major classifications of drugs are presented as to their action, adverse effects, and nursing process application. Commonly used clinical drugs are listed with generic name and brand name.

The role of the licensed practical/vocational nurse (LP/VN) in the administration of medications is determined by the state nurse practice acts and agency policy. However, knowledge of drugs has a significant impact on the quality of nursing care provided each patient by the LP/VN.

PHARMACOLOGY AND THE NURSING PROCESS

A. Assessment: a systematic collection of subjective and objective data on the patient, drug, and environment
B. Planning: prioritize the nursing diagnosis, specify the goals and outcome criteria, and the time when these should be achieved
C. Implementation: consists of initiation and completion of the nursing care plan as defined by the nursing diagnosis and outcome criteria
D. Evaluation: an ongoing monitoring of the patient's response to drug therapy

Assessment

A. Assessing the patient
   1. Variables
      a. Growth and development related to age
      b. Body build
      c. Past and present history
      d. Nutritional practices
      e. Allergies
      f. Sociocultural beliefs
      g. Knowledge of disease and drugs
      h. Cognitive function
      i. Physical challenges
      j. Physical assessment: vital signs, height, weight, laboratory results, and results of diagnostic tests
   2. Medication history
      a. Over-the-counter (OTC) medications
      b. Prescription medications
      c. Street drugs
      d. Smoking, alcohol, or caffeine-related products
      e. Problems with drug therapy in the past (i.e., allergies or adverse effects)
      f. Cultural beliefs
B. Assessing the drug
   1. Medication order
      a. From a physician or other licensed individual
      b. Contains patient's name, date order was written, name of medication, dosage (size, frequency, and number of doses), route, signature of prescriber
      c. Accurate, legible, need for clarification
   2. Types of medication orders
      a. Routine or standard
      b. Prn order: given on a "when necessary" basis
      c. Single order: to be given only once
      d. Stat order: to be given only once and immediately
      e. Standing order: established for all patients with a specific condition
C. Institutional level management: drug distribution systems
   1. Floor stock
   2. Individual patient medication system: a supply of medication is dispensed and labeled for a particular patient
   3. Unit dose: individual doses of each medication ordered

Planning

A. Establish priorities: weighing the importance of one problem against another
B. Goal setting: objective, measurable, and realistic with an established time period for achievement of the outcome; should reflect expected changes through nursing care
C. Outcome criteria: provide a standard of measure that can be used to move toward the goal

Implementation

A. Requires constant communication with patient and health care team
B. Proper administration of medication
   1. Approach to patient
      a. "Therapeutic use of self" attitude of nurse
      b. Consistency of approach
      c. Informed consent for patients
      d. Compliance and right to refuse
   2. Utilizes the five rights:
      a. Right drug
      b. Right dose
      c. Right time
      d. Right route
      e. Right patient
   3. Measures to support the therapeutic or desired effect: nursing actions can complement drug therapy or minimize unpleasant adverse reactions
   4. Observation for desired therapeutic effect
      a. Establish baseline
      b. Establish observational parameters—vital signs, laboratory data—to evaluate effectiveness of medications
C. Teaching patients
   1. Explain drug, dose, side effects, food-drug interactions, time schedule, etc.
   2. Identify need for teaching
   3. Establish realistic teaching goals
   4. Select teaching methods
   5. Implement teaching
   6. Evaluate effectiveness
D. Accurate documentation (form is set by agency policy): some institutions consider this the sixth right
   1. Information must be complete and accurate
   2. Documentation must be done immediately after administration
   3. Legal implications: if drug administration is not documented, it is assumed not to have been administered
   4. Data should include
      a. Observations relevant to therapeutic effects
      b. Actions taken to prevent or treat adverse reactions
      c. Time when a drug is discontinued
      d. Reason(s) for discontinuation of drug
      e. Reasons for refusal/noncompliance of patient
E. Dosage form and route
   1. Factors influencing route of administration
      a. Specific chemical and physical properties of the drug
      b. Pathological condition of the patient
      c. Adequacy of medication compliance
   2. Dose: amount of drug to be given at one time
   3. Dosage: regulation of the frequency, size, and number of doses
   4. Dosage form: final product administered to the patient
      a. Preparations for oral use
         (1) Liquids
            (a) Aqueous solutions: substances dissolved in water and syrups
            (b) Aqueous suspensions: solid particles suspended in liquid
            (c) Syrup: medication dissolved in a concentrated solution of a sugar to which flavors may have been added
            (d) Emulsions: fats or oils suspended in liquid with an emulsifier

(e) Spirits: alcohol solution

(f) Elixirs: aromatic sweetened alcoholic and water solution

(g) Tinctures: alcoholic extract of plant or water solution

(h) Fluid extract: concentrated alcoholic extract of plant or vegetables

(i) Extract: syrup or dried form of pharmacologically active drug

(2) Solids

(a) Capsules: soluble case (usually gelatin) that contains liquid, dry, or beaded particles; capsules may be timed release or sustained action (slow, continuous dissolution for an extended period of time)

(b) Tablets: compressed powdered drug(s) in small discs

▪ Enteric-coated tablets: coated with a second layer of material to prevent dissolution in stomach; disintegrates in small intestine to prevent stomach irritation

▪ Press-coated or layered tablet: contain a second layer of material pressed on or around it, which allows incompatible ingredients to be separated and dissolve at different rates

▪ Caplets: a coated tablet in the shape of a capsule

▪ Troches/lozenges: medicated tablets that dissolve slowly in the mouth

(c) Powders/granules: loose or molded drug substances for drug administration with or without liquids

b. Preparations for parenteral use

(1) Ampules: sealed glass containers for liquid injectable medications

(2) Vials: glass containers with a rubber stopper, usually for multiple doses; contains liquid or powdered medications

(3) Cartridge/tubex: single-dose unit of parenteral medication to be used with a specific injecting device

(4) Intravenous solutions: must be sterile and particle free

(a) Continuous infusion may be used for fluid replacement with or without medication

(b) Intermittent runs as a secondary administration set (piggy-back) hung separately from the primary set via a secondary tubing

(c) Heparin lock or angiocath: a port site for direct administration or intermittent IV medications without the need for a primary IV solution

c. Preparations for topical use

(1) Liniments: liquid suspension for lubrication that are applied by rubbing

(2) Lotions: liquid suspensions that can be protective, emollient, cooling, astringent, antipruritic, cleansing, etc.

(3) Ointment: semi-solid medicine in a base for local, protective, soothing, astringent, or transdermal application for systemic effects (such as nitroglycerine, scopolamine, and estrogen)

(4) Paste: thick ointment used primarily for skin protection

(5) Plasters: solid preparations that are adhesive, protective, or soothing

(6) Creams: emulsions that contain an aqueous and an oily base

(7) Aerosols: fine powders or solutions in volatile liquids that contain a propellent

(8) Transdermal patches: patches containing medication that is absorbed continuously through the skin and acts systemically

(9) Powder: a finely ground drug or combination of drugs

d. Preparations for use on mucous membranes

(1) Drops are aqueous solutions with or without gelling agent (to increase retention time in the eye); drops can be used for eyes, ears, or nose

(2) Topical installation of an aqueous solution of medications usually for topical action but occasionally used for systemic effects, including enemas, douches, mouthwashes, throat sprays, and gargles

(3) Aerosol sprays, nebulizers, and inhalers deliver aqueous solutions of medication in droplet form to the target membrane, such as bronchial tree (bronchodilators)

(4) Foams are powders or solutions of medication in volatile liquids with a propellant, such as vaginal foams for contraception

(5) Suppositories usually contain medicinal substances mixed in a firm but malleable base to facilitate insertion into a body cavity (i.e., rectal or vaginal)

e. Miscellaneous drug delivery systems

(1) Intradermal implants are pellets containing a small deposit of medication that are inserted in a dermal pocket. Usually used to administer hormones such as testosterone or estradiol

(2) Micropump system is a small, external pump, attached by belt or implanted, that delivers medication via a needle in a continuous, steady dose. Examples include insulin, anticancer chemotherapy, and opioids

F. Dosage route: means of access to the site of action or systemic circulation. Divided into three classifications

1. Enteral: administered directly into gastrointestinal tract

a. Oral: drug is ingested and absorbed from stomach or small intestine; convenient and economical; can irritate stomach; may be destroyed by digestive juices

b. Rectal: drug inserted into rectum and absorbed through mucous membrane; may be used in unconscious or vomiting patient

2. Parenteral: in practice, parenteral means administration by the use of a needle; drugs must be sterile and aseptic technique must be utilized

a. Intradermal: drug injected directly under the skin; amount of drug is small and absorption is slow; examples of use include allergy testing, TB testing, and small amounts of anesthesia

b. Subcutaneous: drug injected under the skin into subcutaneous fascia; ideally solutions are limited to no more than 1 cc of solution; examples of use include insulin, heparin, and morphine

c. Intramuscular: injected into muscle mass; relatively rapid absorption result of good blood supply; larger volumes up to 5 cc can be given

d. Intravenous: drug injected into the vein for immediate effect; permits direct control of blood drug concentrations; used when an immediate effect is desired; can be given by injection or infusion; useful in emergency situations; precautions must be taken to avoid infiltration

e. Epidural (this route is performed by a physician; however, the nurse is responsible for assisting and monitoring sites and effects): a catheter implanted beneath the skin with its tip in the epidural space; the drug diffuses into the central spinal fluid, bypassing the blood brain barrier; frequently used in the management of acute and chronic pain

f. Intraarterial (this route is performed by a physician; however, the nurse is responsible for assisting and monitoring sites and effects): drug injected directly into an artery

g. Intraarticular (this route is performed by a physician; however, the nurse is responsible for assisting and monitoring sites and effects): drug injected directly into a joint

h. Intraspinal (this route is performed by a physician; however, the nurse is responsible for assisting and monitoring sites and effects): drug injected directly into spinal canal

3. Percutaneous: application of medications to the skin or mucous membranes; may be used for local or systemic effects

a. Sublingual: drug dissolved under tongue and absorbed through mucous membrane of mouth; can irritate oral mucosa; number of drugs given this way is limited—nitroglycerine is primary example

b. Buccal: drug dissolved between cheek and gum and absorbed through mucous membrane of the mouth

c. Lungs: drug inhaled as a gas or aerosol; useful for drugs intended to act directly on the lungs

d. Vaginal: drug inserted into the vagina and absorbed through the mucous membrane

e. Ophthalmic: drug applied to the eye in form of drops or ointments; must be sterile

f. Otic or aural: drugs applied in the ear

g. Nasal: drugs applied to the nasal cavity by dropper or atomizer

h. Transdermal: patch applied to skin that provides controlled release of medication

Evaluation

A. Therapeutic goals: evaluate therapeutic effectiveness of drugs

B. Diagnostic goals: observe for potential adverse reactions

C. Teaching goals: verify patient's knowledge of drug or ability to perform a skill necessary for administration of the drug

D. Patient compliance: evaluate adherence by the patient to a prescribed plan of treatment

SOURCES OF DRUGS

A. Animals
B. Plants

C. Microorganisms
D. Synthetic chemical substances
E. Food substances

DRUG NAMES

A. Generic: the official, established nonproprietary name assigned to a drug; a drug is licensed under its generic name; often less expensive than brand names

B. Brand (trademark): a name assigned to a drug by its manufacturer; the copyright restricts the use of this name to the specific manufacturer

C. Chemical: the exact designation of the chemical structure as determined by the rules of accepted systems of chemical nomenclature

D. A drug may be considered a prescription drug, which means it requires a legal prescription to be dispensed, or it may be a nonprescription or over-the-counter (OTC), which may be purchased without a prescription

DRUG LEGISLATION

A. Food, Drug, and Cosmetic Act: 1938 (amended 1952, 1962)
  1. Contains detailed regulations to ensure that drugs meet standards of safety and effectiveness
  2. Requires physician's prescription for legal drug purchase
B. Controlled Substances Act: 1970
  1. Defines drug dependency and drug addiction
  2. Classifies drugs according to potential abuse and medical usefulness
  3. Establishes methods for regulating manufacture, distribution, and sale of controlled substances
  4. Establishes education and treatment programs for drug abuse
C. Controlled substances schedule

Schedule I:	Drugs that have a high potential for abuse and are not approved for medical use in the United States (e.g., cocaine)
Schedule II:	Drugs that have a high potential for abuse but have a currently accepted medical use in the United States; abuse may lead to severe psychological or physical dependence (e.g., morphine sulfate)
Schedule III:	Drugs that have a lower potential for abuse than those in schedules I and II; abuse may lead to high psychological or low-to-moderate physical dependence (e.g., aspirin [Empirin] with codeine)
Schedule IV:	Drugs that have some potential for abuse; abuse may lead to limited psychological or physical dependence (e.g., diazepam [Valium])
Schedule V:	Drugs that have the lowest potential for abuse; products that contain moderate amounts of controlled substances that may be dispensed by the pharmacist without a physician's prescription but with some restrictions such as amount, record keeping, and other safeguards (e.g., Robitussin A-C)

PRINCIPLES OF DRUG ACTION

A. The physiological means by which a drug exerts its desired effects
B. Examples include increasing or decreasing the rate at which a cell or tissue functions or replacing something that is needed by the body

PHARMACOKINETICS

A. The study of what actually happens to a drug from the time it enters the body until it leaves the body
B. Includes onset, peak, and duration of the drug

Mechanisms of Drug Therapy

A. Dissolution: disintegration of dosage form; dissolution of an active substance
B. Absorption: the process that occurs between the time a substance enters the body and the time it enters the bloodstream
C. Distribution: the transport of drug molecules within the body to receptor sites
D. Metabolism: biotransformation; the way in which drugs are inactivated by the body
E. Excretion: elimination of a drug from the body

Variables that Affect Drug Action

A. Dosage
B. Route of administration
C. Drug-diet interactions: food slows absorption of drugs; some foods containing certain substances react with certain drugs
D. Drug-drug interactions
   1. Additive effect: occurs when two drugs with similar actions are taken together
   2. Synergism (potentiation): a total effect of two similar drugs that is greater than the sum of the effects if each is taken separately
   3. Interference: occurs when one drug interferes with the metabolism or elimination of a second drug, resulting in intensification of the second drug
   4. Displacement: occurs when one drug is displaced from a plasma protein-binding site by a second, causing an increased effect of the displaced drug
   5. Antagonism: a decrease in the effects of drugs caused by the action of one on the other
E. Age
   1. Fetus: metabolism and elimination mechanisms immature
   2. Newborn: organ systems not fully developed
   3. Children: depends on age and developmental stage
   4. Elderly adults: physiological changes may alter a drug's actions in the body
F. Body weight: affects drug action mainly in relation to dosage
G. Pregnancy: influence on drug interactions can be pronounced
H. Pathological condition: disease processes are capable of altering drug mechanisms (e.g., patients with kidney disease have increased risk of drug toxicity)
I. Psychological considerations: attitudes and expectations influence patient response (e.g., anxiety can decrease effect of analgesics)

Adverse Reactions to Drugs

A. Idiosyncratic reaction: unusual, unexpected reaction usually the first time a drug is taken
B. Allergic reactions: stimulate antibody reactions from the immune system of body
   1. Urticaria (hives)
   2. Anaphylaxis: severe allergic reaction involving cardiovascular and respiratory systems; may be life threatening
C. Gastrointestinal effects
   1. Anorexia
   2. Nausea, vomiting
   3. Constipation
   4. Diarrhea
   5. Abdominal distention
D. Hematological effects
   1. Blood dyscrasia
   2. Bone marrow depression
   3. Blood coagulation disorders
E. Hepatotoxicity
   1. Hepatitis
   2. Biliary tract obstruction or spasms
F. Nephrotoxicity: renal insufficiency or failure; kidney stones
G. Drug dependence
   1. Physiological: physical need to relieve shaking; pain
   2. Psychological: need to relieve feeling of anxiety; stress
H. Teratogenicity: ability of a drug to cause abnormal fetal development

Tolerance and Cross Tolerance

A. Tolerance: acclimation of the body to a drug over a period of time so that larger doses must be given to achieve the same effect
B. Cross tolerance: tolerance to pharmacologically related drugs

Sources of Drug Information

A. Resource people
   1. Pharmacists
   2. Physicians
   3. Registered nurses
B. Poison control centers
C. Published sources of information
   1. *United States Pharmacopeia (USP)* and *National Formulary (NF)*
      a. Official reference books
      b. Establish legally binding standards to which drugs must conform
      c. Revised every 5 years with periodic supplements
   2. Package insert: Food and Drug Administration (FDA)—approved label for drug products in the United States
   3. *Physicians' Desk Reference (PDR)*
      a. Published annually with interim supplements
      b. Contains information supplied by manufacturers
      c. Is most useful for finding drugs according to brand name
   4. American Hospital Formulary Service
      a. Contains data on almost every drug available in the United States
      b. Kept current by periodic supplements
   5. Pharmacology textbooks; drug reference books/cards
   6. Nursing journals

Nursing Process

A. Assessment: Obtain data on patient regarding problems related to
1. Route of administration
2. Elimination or metabolism (pay particular attention to persons with renal or hepatic disease)
3. Baseline laboratory values
4. Patient teaching needs

B. Planning
1. Proper timing of dosage
2. Ways to improve the effectiveness of the drug
3. Instruction of patient concerning the drug

C. Implementation
1. Proper method of administration
2. Proper timing of dosage
3. Instruction of patient concerning the drug

D. Evaluation
1. Effectiveness of drug:
   a. Subjective: questioning the patient for expected response of the drug (i.e., pain relief or reduction in symptoms)
   b. Objective: monitoring physical response by the nurse (i.e., decreased blood pressure, or increased cardiac regularity)
2. Presence of side effects, adverse reactions
3. Effectiveness of patient teaching
4. If therapy is ineffective, examine possible causes such as drug interactions

ADMINISTERING MEDICATIONS
Calculation of Dosage

A. Practical nurse responsibility
1. Abide by the guidelines of the health care agency
2. Check for accuracy in dosage calculation before preparing and administering drug
3. Check calculations with another knowledgeable person
4. Measure doses exactly as prescribed by physician

B. Systems of measurement
1. Household system: measurements commonly used in the home; not as accurate as other systems; following are examples:
   a. 1 teaspoon (tsp or t) = 60 drops (gtt)
   b. 3 or 4 tsp = 1 tablespoon (tbsp or T)
2. Apothecary system: an older system but one that continues to be used in dosage calculations
   a. Common units of measurements
      (1) Weight: grain (gr)
      (2) Volume
         (a) 60 minims (♏) = 1 dram (dr or ℨ)
         (b) 8 dr = 1 ounce (oz or ℥)
   b. Notations in this system use lowercase Roman numerals; quantities less than 1 are expressed as common factors: exception: one half is written as $\overline{ss}$
3. Metric system: international decimal system
   a. Common units of measurement
      (1) Weight: unit is expressed in terms of the gram (g)
         (a) Prefix *kilo* indicates 1000
         (b) Prefix *milli* indicates ⅟₁₀₀₀
         (c) 1 g = 1000 milligrams (mg)
      (2) Volume: unit is expressed in terms of the liter (L)
         (a) Prefix milli indicates ⅟₁₀₀₀
         (b) 1 L = 1000 milliliters (ml)

   b. Notations in this system use Arabic numbers; fractions are expressed as decimals
4. Equivalents between systems: a given quantity considered to be of equal value to a quantity expressed in a different system; some common approximate equivalents are
   a. 1 kilograms (kg) = 2.2 pounds (lb)
   b. 1 g = 15 gr
   c. 60 mg = 1 gr
   d. 1 cubic centimeter (cc) = 1 ml
   e. 1000 ml = 1 quart (qt)
   f. 30 ml = 1 oz
   g. 1 ml = 15 or 16 ♏
   h. 1 tsp = 4 or 5 ml
   i. 1 ml = 15 or 16 gtt

C. Mathematics of conversion within and between systems; ratio and proportion method:
1. Household

   EXAMPLE: 3 tsp = _____ gtt
   teaspoons : drops :: teaspoons : drops
   1 : 60 :: 3 : *x*
   x = 180
   Answer: 3 tsp = 180 gtt

2. Apothecary system

   EXAMPLE: 3 oz = _____ dr
   ounces : drams :: ounces : drams
   1 : 8 :: 3 : *x*
   x = 24
   Answer: 3 oz = 24 dr

3. Metric system

   EXAMPLE: 250 mg = _____ g
   milligram : gram :: milligram : gram
   1000 : 1 :: 250 : *x*
   1000 *x* = 250
   x = 0.25
   Answer: 250 mg = <u>0.25</u> g

4. Conversion between systems

   EXAMPLE: gr ⅙ = _____ mg
   grains : milligrams :: grains : milligrams
   1 : 60 :: ⅙ : *x*
   1*x* = 60 × ⅙
   x = 10
   Answer: gr ⅙ = <u>10</u> mg

D. Dosage calculations: The dose for oral tablets, capsules, and liquids or solutions for injections can be calculated by using the following formula:

$$\frac{\text{Desired dose (D)}}{\text{Dose on hand (H)}} \times \text{Quantity (Q)} = \text{Amount to be given}$$

EXAMPLE: Give 500 mg of tetracycline (Achromycin) using capsules containing 250 mg

$$\frac{D}{H} \times Q = \frac{500 \text{ mg}}{250 \text{ mg}} \times 1 \text{ capsule} =$$

Answer: 2 capsules

EXAMPLE: Physician orders digoxin 0.125 mg to be given orally; stock bottle is labeled "Digoxin 0.25 mg" scored tablets

$$\frac{D}{H} \times Q = \frac{0.125 \text{ mg}}{0.25 \text{ mg}} \times 1 \text{ tablet} =$$

Answer: 0.5 tablet or ½ tablet

EXAMPLE: Erythromycin suspension 750 mg is ordered orally. The bottle is labeled 250 mg/5 ml

$$\frac{D}{H} \times Q = \frac{750 \text{ mg}}{250 \text{ mg}} \times 5 \text{ ml} =$$

Answer: 15 ml

EXAMPLE: Morphine sulfate gr ¼ is to be given by subcutaneous injection; the vial is labeled "Morphine Sulfate gr ½/ml"

$$\frac{D}{H} \times Q = \frac{\text{gr } ¼}{\text{gr } ½} \times 1 \text{ ml} =$$

Answer: 0.5 ml

EXAMPLE: Penicillin 600,000 units is to be given by intramuscular injection; the vial is labeled "Penicillin 300,000 units per ml"

$$\frac{D}{H} = Q = \frac{600,000 \text{ units}}{300,000 \text{ units}} \times 1 \text{ ml} =$$

Answer: 2 ml

NOTE: This formula can be used with any system of measurement. When two systems are involved, it is necessary to convert to the system of measurement of the dose on hand.

EXAMPLE: Codeine sulfate gr $\overline{ss}$ is ordered by mouth; on hand are codeine sulfate tablets labeled 30 mg

STEP 1: conversion between systems
grain : milligram :: grain : milligram
1 : 60 :: ½ : x
$x = 60 \times ½$
$x = 30$
Answer: codeine gr $\overline{ss}$ = 30 mg

STEP 2: Formula

$$\frac{D}{H} \times Q = \frac{30 \text{ mg}}{30 \text{ mg}} \times 1 \text{ ml} =$$

Answer: 1 tablet

Calculation of Drip Rate for Intravenous Infusion

A. Information that must be known
1. Volume of solution to be infused
2. Length of time over which this volume is to be infused
3. Number of drops per milliliter delivered by the administration set being used
B. The drip rate may be calculated as follows:
1. Find the volume of fluid to be administered per hour

$$\frac{\text{Milliliters of fluid to be infused}}{\text{Number of hours for infusion}} = \text{Milliliters of fluid per hour}$$

2. Find the volume of fluid to be administered per minute

$$\frac{\text{Milliliters of fluid per hour}}{60 \text{ min/hr}} = \text{Milliliters to run per minute}$$

3. Multiply the milliliters of fluid to run per minute by the number of drops per milliliter delivered by the infusion set; this gives the number of drops that should fall in the drip chamber per minute

Milliliters per minute × Drops per milliliter = Drops per minute

EXAMPLE: Administer 1000 ml of dextrose 5% in water (D5W) over 8 hours using an infusion set that delivers 10 gtt per minute

$$\frac{1000 \text{ ml}}{8 \text{ hr}} = 125 \text{ ml/hr}$$

$$\frac{125 \text{ ml/hr}}{60 \text{ min/hr}} = 2.1 \text{ ml/min}$$

2.1 ml/min × 10 gtt/ml =
Answer: 21 gtt/min

EXAMPLE: Administer 250 ml of dextrose 5% in water over 8 hours using a microdrip infusion set that delivers 60 gtt per minute

$$\frac{250 \text{ ml}}{8 \text{ hr}} = 31.25 \text{ ml/hr}$$

$$\frac{31.25 \text{ ml/hr}}{60 \text{ min/hr}} = 0.52 \text{ ml/min}$$

0.52 ml/min × 60 gtt/ml = 31.2 gtt/min
Answer: 31 gtt/min

C. If the administration rate has been ordered as milliliters per hour, step 1 above is omitted
D. Alternate formula to calculate drip rate:

$$\frac{\text{Milliliters to administer} \times \text{Drops per milliliter}}{\text{Hours to run} \times = 60 \text{ min/hr}}$$
= Drops per minute

EXAMPLE: Administer 1000 ml of D5W over 8 hours using an infusion set that delivers 10 gtt/min

$$\frac{1000 \text{ ml} \times 10 \text{ gtt/ml}}{8 \text{ hr} \times 60 \text{ min/hr}} =$$

Answer: 21 gtt/min

E. Adjust the flow rate to the number of drops per minute as calculated; assess the fluid volume at hourly intervals to see that the fluid is being administered at the desired rate; the calculated drip rate is an approximation of the actual flow rate; the type of solution, additives, position of the patient or infusion tubing, height of the reservoir, and volume of fluid in the container can influence the actual drip rate; the practical nurse should verify computations with another knowledgeable person before readjusting the drip rate to ensure volume delivery for the prescribed time

Methods of Administering Medications

A. Nurse's responsibilities
1. Knowledge of drug
   a. Its actions
   b. Ranges of dosage
   c. Methods of administration
   d. Common use
   e. Adverse reactions
   f. Contraindications
   g. Patient education
2. Assess patient regarding history of allergies or sensitivities to drugs
3. Be aware of and follow agency's policy regarding procedure by which the medication order is checked
4. Know agency's system of medication distribution
   a. Cards
   b. Kardex/Medex
   c. Computer printout sheet
5. Know occasions when drugs may be withheld
   a. Fasting for diagnostic tests or surgery; illness
   b. Required laboratory blood work before medication administration
   c. Specific guidelines for certain drugs, for example, apical pulse rate before cardiotonics or blood pressure (BP) readings before antihypertensive agents

6. Position the patient to properly administer medications; assist as needed
7. Observe the "5 rights" of medication administration
   a. *Right patient*
   b. *Right drug*
   c. *Right dose*
   d. *Right route*
   e. *Right time*
8. Inform patient of any anticipated change in normal body functions such as drowsiness, nausea, or change in color of urine
9. Report patient noncompliance or adverse reactions to other responsible person, that is, registered nurse or physician
10. Be aware of and follow procedure for controlled substances
11. Remain with patient until medication is taken
12. Never leave medications at patient's bedside unless specifically ordered
13. Ensure accuracy in drug calculation; when in doubt, verify with other responsible person, that is, registered nurse or pharmacist
14. Check expiration date on all medication labels and orders
15. Accurately document medications given and, if omitted or refused, document reason
16. Document effectiveness of medication
17. Be aware of and follow agency procedure in event of medication error
18. Acknowledge and respect patient's request to refuse medication

B. Safety measures in preparing medications
   1. Environment
      a. Quiet
      b. Free from distractions
      c. Good lighting
   2. Do not leave prepared medications unattended; keep in a locked area
   3. Read each label three times
      a. When reaching for the container
      b. Immediately before pouring the medication
      c. When replacing or discarding the container
   4. Transport drugs for administration by using trays or carts that allow the identifying information and the medication container to be kept together safely
   5. Do not allow tray or cart to be left out of sight during administration
   6. Make positive identification of patient before administering the medication, preferably by checking the patient's identification bracelet; having patient state his or her name; having second person identify patient
   7. Remain with the patient until patient takes the medication
   8. Document necessary supplemental information according to agency policy, for example, pulse rate, blood pressure, site of application or injection
   9. Guidelines for drug safety at home
      a. Keep each drug in original, labeled container
      b. Be sure labels are legible
      c. Discard any outdated medications
      d. Always finish a prescribed drug unless otherwise instructed

      e. Dispose of drug in sink or toilet
      f. Do not give one family member a drug prescribed for another family member
      g. Refrigerate medications if required
      h. Read labels carefully and follow all instructions

C. Oral administration of medications
   1. General information
      a. Simplest and most convenient route
      b. Liquid preparations
         (1) Pour into a container placed on a flat surface
         (2) Read at eye level
         (3) Measure amount by using the bottom of meniscus
      c. Irritating drugs should be dissolved or diluted and given with food or immediately after a meal
      d. Distasteful oral medications can be disguised, for example, by having patient suck on a piece of ice for a few minutes to numb taste buds, by storing oily medications in a refrigerator, by having patient use a straw, or by mixing medication with a small amount of fruit juice, milk, applesauce, or gelatin; always inform patient that a food vehicle contains the medication
      e. For patients who have difficulty swallowing tablets, some tablets may be crushed to facilitate swallowing; be aware of contraindications for crushing of certain medications, for example, enteric coated tablets, or of opening capsules containing timed-release medications
      f. Liquid medications that are harmful to teeth, for example, liquid iron preparations, should be administered with a straw placed at the back of the tongue
   2. Specific procedure is described in Table 3-1

D. Parenteral administration of medications: administration by a route other than through the enteral or gastrointestinal (GI) tract, such as intradermal, subcutaneous, intramuscular, or intravenous routes
   1. General information: maintain surgical aseptic technique in preparation and administration; it is preferable to use prepackaged, disposable sterile needles and syringes
   2. Selection of syringe and needle: thick or oily solutions require a large lumen; short needles are used for children and adults with little adipose tissue; obese individuals may require longer needles to ensure delivery of medications to proper tissue level (Table 3-2)
   3. Putting the drugs into the syringe
      a. Manufacturer prefilled syringes or cartridges: contain the name and dose of the drug and the intended parenteral route; should not be given by any route other than the one specified
      b. Rubber-capped vials: single or multidose container; solution or powder form; dry form of drug dissolved according to label instructions; to remove the drug
         (1) Remove the soft metal cover on top of the vial
         (2) Using friction; wipe the rubber cap with a pledget soaked with antiseptic solution
         (3) Fill syringe with air equal to amount of solution to be withdrawn to increase pressure within the vial and to facilitate withdrawal of solution

TABLE 3-1   Administration of Oral Medications

Suggested Action	Rationale
Wash hands before and practice medical asepsis while preparing and administering medication	Careful hand washing and separate medication cups prevent cross-contamination between nurse and patients
Check the order and read the label three times while preparing the drug	Frequent checking prevents errors and ensures accuracy
Pour tablets and capsules into the cap of a stock container and then transfer proper amount into medication cup	Pouring medications into the nurse's hand contaminates the tablet or capsule
Pour liquids from the side of the bottle opposite the label	Liquid that may spill onto the label makes reading the label difficult
Transport medications to patient's bedside carefully	Prevents accidental or deliberate disarrangement of medications
Keep medications in sight at all times	For safety reasons
Identify patient carefully	Illness and different environment can often cause confusion
Assist patient to an upright position as necessary	Proper positioning facilitates swallowing
Offer sufficient water or other permitted fluids	Liquids allow for ease in swallowing and help to dissolve solid drugs
Remain with patient until each medication is swallowed	Patient may discard unwanted medications or may accumulate them with intent to harm himself or herself
Document each medication administered, promptly and according to agency's policy; report/document medications not taken	The patient's chart is a legal record; prompt documentation avoids the possibility of repeating administration of the same drug
If patient's intake is being measured, record the amount of fluid taken with the medication	All fluids taken are to be recorded for determining total intake

TABLE 3-2   Selection of Syringe and Needle

Type of Injection	Syringe Size	Needle Size
Intradermal	1 ml calibrated in tenths or hundreths of a milliliter or in minims	26 or 27 gauge, ½ or ¾ inch
Subcutaneous	2, 2½, or 3 ml calibrated in 0.1 ml	25 gauge, ½ or ⅝ inch
Intramuscular	2-5 ml calibrated in 0.2 ml	10 or 22 gauge, 1½ inch
Insulin (subcutaneous)	Insulin syringe 1-2 ml calibrated in units	25, 26, or 27 gauge, ½ or ⅝ inch

(4) Insert needle into the rubber cap while holding the needle in a slightly lateral position to prevent a piece of the stopper from entering the vial

(5) Inject the air and remove prescribed amount of solution while holding the syringe in a vertical position

c. Glass ampules: prescored or unscored tops; constricted neck ampules require that solution be in base of ampule

(1) Quickly snap finger on the stem to move the solution into the base of the ampule

(2) Hold the ampule in one hand

(3) Protecting the fingers of the other hand with a sterile, dry gauze pledget, break off the stem of the ampule; check solution for fragments of glass

(4) Insert needle into the opened ampule, avoiding needle contamination by not touching the rim of the ampule with the needle

(5) Keep needle under solution and withdraw the prescribed amount of the solution

4. Skin preparation

a. Heavily soiled skin in area of intended injection site should be washed with soap and water

b. Antiseptic-soaked gauze or pledget is then used to disinfect injection site and thus prevent injection of harmful organism into body tissue

(1) Wipe in a circular motion, starting at point of injection and moving outward to carry debris away from injection site

(2) Use firm pressure and friction when wiping to help remove soil

5. Reduce discomfort

a. Use sharp needle

b. Use appropriate gauge

c. Select site free of irritation or nodules from previous injections

d. Numb skin receptors: cold compresses or ice cube over injection site

e. Hold tissue taut or compress tissue to form a pad, depending on type of injection

f. Be sure there is no solution on the needle

g. Help patient to relax

TABLE 3-3   Administration of Subcutaneous Injection

Suggested Action	Rationale
Verify physician's order and read medication three times; check expiration date	Ensures accuracy and prevents errors
Obtain and assemble equipment maintaining sterile technique	Prevents contamination
Draw the drug into syringe and protect needle with sterile needle cover	Exposure to air or contact with moist surface contaminates needle
Identify patient by identification bracelet and by having patient state name, if possible	Prevents potential medication error
Select appropriate injection site and cleanse area with antiseptic pledget, using firm, circular motion moving outward from injection site	Friction helps to clean skin and decreases possibility of introducing bacteria into body
Grasp the tissue surrounding the injection site and hold it to form a cushion pad	Ensures placement of medication into subcutaneous tissue and helps prevent deposition of medication into muscle tissue
Inject the needle quickly at an angle of 45 to 90 degrees, depending on the quality and amount of tissue and length of needle	Ensures placement of medication into subcutaneous tissue
After needle is in proper tissue level, release grasp of the tissue	Reduces discomfort of injection
Aspirate to determine whether needle is in a blood vessel	Prevents discomfort and possible serious reaction if medication is injected into vein
If there is no blood return, inject solution slowly	Reduces discomfort by reducing pressure in subcutaneous tissue
Withdraw needle quickly	Reduces discomfort
Massage area gently, unless contraindicated with certain medications	Helps to distribute the solution and hasten absorption of the medication

    h. Insert needle without hesitation
    i. Aspirate when appropriate
    j. Inject solution slowly
    k. Remove needle quickly
    l. Massage area after injection unless contraindicated with certain medications or certain routes (i.e.: intradermal; z-track)
6. Care of equipment after injections: use needle disposal unit; follow agency policy
7. Injection sites
    a. Intradermal injection: solutions injected directly under the epidermis into the dermis (10- to 15-degree angle)
      (1) Absorption occurs slowly through the capillaries
      (2) Common site: inner aspect of the forearm
    b. Subcutaneous injection: solutions injected into the subcutaneous layer of the skin (45- to 90-degree angle)
      (1) Common sites
        (a) Outer aspect of upper arm
        (b) Thigh
        (c) Lower abdomen
        (d) Upper back
      (2) Suggested procedure for subcutaneous injection is described in Table 3-3
    c. Intramuscular injection: solutions injected into the muscular layer of tissue (90-degree angle)
      (1) Common sites
        (a) Dorsogluteal site
        (b) Ventrogluteal site
        (c) Vastus lateralis muscle
        (d) Deltoid muscle
        (e) Posterior triceps muscle
        (f) Rectus femoris muscle
      (2) Suggested procedure for intramuscular injection is described in Table 3-4
    d. Z-track injection: technique used to prevent damage to and staining of the skin and subcutaneous tissues; common site is the upper outer quadrant of the gluteal region
    e. Intravenous infusion: administration of a large amount of fluid into a vein
      (1) Purposes
        (a) To restore or maintain electrolyte balance
        (b) To supply drugs for immediate effect
        (c) To replace nutrients and vitamins
        (d) To replace blood loss
      (2) Nurse practice acts and agency policy dictate who may administer intravenous infusions
      (3) Nurse's responsibilities for intravenous infusion
        (a) Verifying physician's order
        (b) Calculating rate of flow
        (c) Monitoring rate of flow
        (d) Assessing patient for adverse reactions
          ■ Infiltration
          ■ Circulatory overload
          ■ Thrombophlebitis
    f. Hyperalimentation: total parenteral nutrition (TPN), that is, an intravenous infusion containing

TABLE 3-4   Administration of Intramuscular Injection

Suggested Action	Rationale
Verify physician's order and read medication label three times; check expiration date	Ensures accuracy and prevents errors
Obtain and assemble equipment, maintaining sterile technique	Prevents contamination
Draw the drug into syringe; create small air bubble in the syringe; protect needle with sterile needle cover	Air bubble forces medication out of needle shaft when injected; exposure to air or contact with most surfaces contaminates needle
Identify patient by identification bracelet and by having patient state name, if possible	Prevents potential medication error
Have the patient assume appropriate position according to site selected	Helps to relax muscles and eases discomfort
Select appropriate injection site and cleanse area with antiseptic pledget, using firm, circular motion moving outward from injection site	Friction helps to clean the skin, thus decreasing possibility of introducing bacteria into body tissue
Press down and hold tissue taut over the injection site	Ensures needle reaches muscle layer
Hold syringe at 90-degree angle and quickly thrust needle into the tissue	Minimizes discomfort
Aspirate to determine whether needle is in a blood vessel	Prevents discomfort and possible serious reaction if medication injected into vein
If there is no blood return, inject medication slowly, followed by the air bubble	Reduces discomfort and allows medication to disperse into the tissue; air bubble clears medication from needle
Withdraw needle quickly	Reduces discomfort
Massage area gently, unless contraindicated with certain medications	Helps to distribute the solution and hasten absorption of the medication

sufficient nutrients to sustain life; provides amino acids, glucose, vitamins, and electrolytes for those patients unable to ingest nutrients normally for extended periods and for whom standard infusions are inadequate

g. Blood transfusion: infusion of whole blood from a healthy person into a recipient's vein
   (1) Blood is typed and cross matched before administration to determine compatibility
   (2) Nurse's responsibility for blood transfusion
      (a) Check and double-check
         ▪ The labels
         ▪ The numbers
         ▪ The Rh factor
         ▪ Compatibility
      (b) Stay with patient for at least the first 5 minutes after transfusion is started
      (c) Monitor rate of transfusion
      (d) Assess patient for signs of adverse reactions
         ▪ Hemolytic reaction: stop transfusion immediately, keep vein open with slow drip normal saline solution, and notify physician; indications include
            □ Headache
            □ Sensations of tingling
            □ Difficulty in breathing
            □ Pain in lumbar region or legs
         ▪ Allergic reactions: stop transfusion immediately and notify physician; indications include
            □ Pruritus
            □ Hives (urticaria)
            □ Difficulty in breathing
         ▪ Febrile reactions resulting from contaminant in the blood: usually occurs late in the transfusion or after it is completed; indications include
            □ Flushed skin
            □ Elevated temperature
            □ Chills, muscular spasms
            □ General malaise
            □ Signs of systemic infection
         ▪ Circulatory overload can lead to pulmonary edema; indications include
            □ Increased pulse rate
            □ Dyspnea
            □ Respiratory distress
            □ Moist coughing
            □ Expectoration of blood-tinged mucus
         ▪ Anticoagulant reaction: indications include
            □ Tingling in the fingers
            □ Muscular cramping
            □ Convulsions

h. Blood extracts: specific components of whole blood that meet specific needs of the patient
   (1) Packed red blood cells (RBCs)
   (2) Plasma
   (3) Human albumin
   (4) Fibrinogen
   (5) Gamma globulin

PEDIATRIC DRUG ADMINISTRATION
General Rules

A. Pediatric drug therapy should be guided by the child's age, weight, and level of growth and development
B. The nurse's approach to the child should convey the impression that he or she expects the child to take the medication
C. Explanation regarding the medication should be based on the child's level of understanding
D. The nurse must be honest with the child regarding the procedure
E. It may be necessary to mix distasteful medication or crushed tablets with a small amount of honey, applesauce, or gelatin
F. Never threaten a child with an injection if he or she refuses an oral medication
G. All medications should be kept out of the reach of children, and medications should never be referred to as candy

Calculating the Pediatric Dose

Safe dosage ranges of drugs are less well defined for children than for adults. Not all drug dosage ranges for children are listed in the literature. It is not the nurse's responsibility to determine the dose of a drug for the infant or child, but at times it may be necessary to verify or calculate a dose as a fraction of the adult dose. The following methods may be used:

A. Body surface area: considered most accurate; requires a nomogram—a device for rapid estimation of body surface area

$$\text{Child's dose} = \frac{\text{Body surface area (in square meters)}}{1.73 \text{ m}^2} \times \text{Adult dose}$$

B. Clark's rule: based on weight and used for children at least 2 years old

$$\text{Child's dose} = \frac{\text{Weight (in pounds)}}{150} \times \text{Adult dose}$$

C. Young's rule: based on age and used for children at least 2 years old

$$\text{Child's dose} = \frac{\text{Age (in years)}}{\text{Age (in years)} + 12} \times \text{Adult dose}$$

D. Fried's rule: used for children less than 2 years old

$$\text{Child's dose} = \frac{\text{Age (in months)}}{150} \times \text{Adult dose}$$

Identifying the Patient

A. Check the child's identification bracelet
B. Ask the older child his or her name

Oral Medication

Verify, calculate, and document all medications
A. Infants
1. Draw up liquid medication in a dropper or a syringe without the needle
2. Elevate infant's head and shoulders; hold infant in a feeding position
3. Depress the chin with the thumb to open infant's mouth
4. Using the dropper or syringe, direct the medication toward the inner aspect of the infant's cheek and release the flow of medication slowly

5. Release the thumb and allow the infant to swallow
6. Liquid medication can also be measured into a nipple and the infant allowed to suck the medication through the nipple
7. Crushed tablets can be mixed with a small amount of honey or applesauce and fed slowly with a teaspoon
B. Toddlers
1. Draw up medication in a syringe or measure into a medication cup
2. Elevate the child's head and shoulders
3. Place the syringe in the child's mouth and slowly release the medication, directing it toward the inner aspect of the cheek, or allow the child to hold the medicine cup and drink it at own pace; offer praise
C. School-age children
1. When the child is old enough to take medicine in tablet or capsule form, direct him or her to place the medicine near the back of the tongue and to immediately swallow fluid such as water or juice
2. Offer the child praise after he or she has taken medication

Intramuscular Injection

A. Infants
1. Common site: largest muscle group is the quadriceps femoris, located in the anterolateral thigh; largest muscle of this group is the vastus lateralis, situated on the anterior surface of the midlateral thigh
   a. Place infant in supine position
   b. Compress muscle tissue at upper aspect of thigh, pointing the nurse's fingers toward the infant's feet
   c. Needle is inserted at a 90-degree angle; maximum length of needle for an infant is 1 inch (2.5 cm)
2. Alternate site: rectus femoris muscle, located on the anterolateral surface of the upper thigh; needle is inserted at a 45-degree angle and is directed toward the knee
B. Toddlers and school-age children: common sites are
1. Dorsogluteal muscle; upper outer quadrant; gluteal muscle does not develop until child begins to walk; should be used for injections only after the child has been walking for a year or more
2. Ventrogluteal muscle: a dense muscle mass; the disadvantage is that the site is visible to the child
3. Deltoid muscle may be used for older, larger children
4. Lateral and anterior aspect of thigh: upper outer quadrant of thigh

Administration of Injections

A. Infants
1. Place infant in a secure position to avoid movement of the extremity
2. Usually, have a second person to secure the infant
3. Hold, cuddle, and comfort the infant after the injection
B. Toddlers and school-age children
1. Have syringe and needle completely prepared before contact with the child
2. Keep needle outside of child's visual field
3. Explain, according to the child's developmental age, the reason for an injection and where it will be given; do not say "it won't hurt"
4. Inspect injection site before injection for tenderness or undue firmness

5. Have a second person available to help secure the child and offer comfort during the procedure
6. Allow the child to express fears
7. Perform the procedure quickly and gently
8. Praise the child for his or her behavior after the injection

CENTRAL NERVOUS SYSTEM
Depressants
A. Characteristics of drug-induced central nervous system (CNS) depression
   1. Mild: disinterest in surroundings, inability to focus on a topic or to initiate talking or movement, slowed pulse and respirations
   2. Moderate or progressive: drowsiness or sleep, decreased muscle tone and ability to move, diminished acuity of all sensations—touch, vision, hearing, heat, cold, or pain
   3. Severe: unconsciousness or coma, loss of reflexes, respiratory failure, death
B. Barriers to effective pain management
   1. Fear of developing tolerance
      a. Tolerance is rarely seen in clients with severe acute or chronic pain
      b. Usually an increase in pain is due to progression of disease or complications
   2. Fear of addiction
      a. Risk of addiction in hospitalized patients is minimal
      b. Psychological dependence is rare in hospitalized patients
      c. Patients with cancer pain may be titrated to large amounts of opioids to control pain without producing the adverse effects of respiratory depression or excessive sedation
   3. Fear of respiratory depression
      a. Tolerance develops to the respiratory depression effect but not to the analgesia effect
      b. Significant respiratory depression is rarely seen because medication has been titrated to meet an individual's requirement
   4. Children are often untreated or inadequately treated for pain
   5. Elderly patients need careful assessment
      a. Close monitoring to reduce the chances of over- or undertreatment
      b. Greater chance for adverse affects
      c. May have diminished circulatory processes affecting the absorption of medications
C. Analgesics: drugs that relieve pain
   1. Opioid analgesics: act on the central nervous system; alter the patient's perception of pain; more often used for severe pain
      a. Examples include the following: morphine is prototype; natural or synthetic agents that have a morphine-like effect; additional examples found in Table 3-5
      b. Adverse reactions and contraindications
         (1) Depresses respiratory and cough centers in the medulla
         (2) Use cautiously in patients with impaired respiratory function and with patients with head injury, because it will obscure CNS evaluation

         (3) Inhibits gastric, biliary, and pancreatic secretions; depresses gastrointestinal tract; can cause nausea, vomiting, and constipation
         (4) Stimulates release of antidiuretic hormone, resulting in decreased urine volume; can cause urinary retention
         (5) Induces hypotension
         (6) Decreases heart rate
         (7) Causes pupillary constriction
         (8) Pruritus
   2. Nonopioid/antiinflammatory analgesics: act at the site of the pain; do not alter the patient's perception; used more frequently for mild to moderate pain; act by sensitizing peripheral pain receptors; are often combined with opioid analgesics to enhance pain control in severe pain; NSAIDs are indicated for conditions when an antiinflammatory effect is desired.
      a. Examples can be found in Table 3-6
      b. Agents
         (1) Acetylsalicylic acid (aspirin): effective in management of low-intensity pain
            (a) Adverse reactions
               ▪ Gastric irritation
               ▪ Ulceration and gastric bleeding
               ▪ Intoxication (salicylism): tinnitus, reversible hearing loss, hyperventilation, fever, metabolic acidosis, vomiting, hypokalemia, convulsions, coma, and death
            (b) Drug interactions with aspirin
               ▪ Anticoagulants: increase likelihood of bleeding
               ▪ Alcohol: increases likelihood of gastrointestinal irritation and bleeding
         (2) Acetaminophen (Datril, Tylenol): effective in management of low-intensity pain; does not produce gastric irritation or alter platelet function and bleeding times as does aspirin; does not interact with oral anticoagulants; prolonged use or frequent high doses can cause liver and kidney damage
         (3) Nonsteroidal antiinflammatory drugs (NSAIDs): effective in treatment of osteoarthritis, degenerative joint disease, rheumatic diseases
            (a) Adverse reactions
               ▪ Heartburn/indigestion
               ▪ Nausea/vomiting
               ▪ Constipation or diarrhea
               ▪ Fluid retention
               ▪ Hypertension
               ▪ Dizziness
               ▪ Blurred vision
               ▪ Skin rash
            (b) Drug interactions vary because of the chemical makeup of the various NSAIDs
               ▪ Used with caution in elderly patients who are prone to upper GI, hepatic, or renal effects
               ▪ Given with anticoagulants may increase risk of GI ulcers or hemorrhage
               ▪ Given concurrently may reduce the effectiveness of hypertensive agent

TABLE 3-5   Selected Opioid Dosage Forms: Pharmacokinetic Overview

Drug/Dosage Form	Onset of Action (min)	Peak Effect (min)	Duration of Action (hr)
codeine			
oral	30–45	60–120	4
IM	10–30	30–60	4
SC	10–30		4
hydrocodone (Hycodan)			
oral	10–30	30–60	4–6
hydromorphone (Dilaudid)			
oral	30	90–120	4
IM	15	30–60	4–5
IV	10–15	15–30	2–3
SC	15	30–90	4
rectal	Not available	Not available	6–8
levorphanol (Levo-Dromoran)			
oral	10–60	90–120	4–5
IM	Not available	60	4–5
IV	Not available	Within 20	4–5
SC	Not available	60–90	4–5
meperidine (Demerol)			
oral	15	60–90	2–4 (usually 3)
IM	10–15	30–50	2–4 (usually 3)
IV	1	5–7	2–4 (usually 3)
SC	10–15	30–50	2–4 (usually 3)
methadone			
oral	30–60	90–120	4–6*
IM	10–20	60–120	4–5*
IV		15–30	3–4
morphine			
oral			
solution,† syrup,‡ tablets	10–30	60–120	4–5
extended-release tablets§	—	—	8–12
IM	10–30	30–60	4–5
IV		20	4–5
SC	10–30	50–90	4–5
epidural‖	15–60	—	Up to 24
intrathecal‖	15–60	—	Up to 24
rectal**	20–60	—	4–5
oxycodone			
oral	Not available	60	3–4
controlled release	Not available	3–4	12
oxymorphone (Numorphan)			
IM	10–15	30–90	3–6
IV	5–10	15–30	3–4
SC	10–20	Not available	3–6
rectal	15–30	120	3–6
propoxyphene (Darvon)			
oral	15–60	120	4–6

From McKenry LM, Salerno E: *Pharmacology in nursing,* ed 20, St Louis, 1998, Mosby.
*With active metabolites and continuous dosing, half-life and duration of action may increase to 22 to 48 hours.
†Roxanol, M.O.S., MSIR.
‡Morphite, Morphitex-1, Morphitec-5 (not commercially available in United States).
§MS Contin, Roxanol SR.
‖Duramorph (preservative-free).
**RMS suppositories.

TABLE 3-6   Nonsteroidal Antiinflammatory Drugs: Pharmacokinetics, Dosing, and Comments

NSAID	Onset of Action (hr)	Half-life (hr)	Usual Adult Dosage (mg/day)	Comments*
Acetic Acids				
diclofenac (Voltaren)	0.5	1.2–2	50 mg tid or qid	Has less effect on platelet aggregation than most other NSAIDs. Used to treat arthritis, pain, primary dysmenorrhea, and acute gout attacks.
etodolac (Lodine)	0.5	6–7	200, 300, or 400 mg tid or qid	Also has uricosuric effects. Gastrointestinal distress and ulceration reported less often.
indomethacin (Indocin)	0.5	4–6	25 or 50 mg bid to qid	Higher risk for GI effects and renal function impairment than other agents. Use cautiously in persons with epilepsy, depression, and Parkinson's disease because it may aggravate these conditions.
ketorolac (Toradol)	IM-10 min (dose dependent)	PO-4 IM-6	30 mg IM/IV q6h, then 10 mg PO q4-6h	Should not be given by any route for longer than 5 days. Risk of GI bleeding and other severe effects increases with duration of treatment. Do not give preoperatively or intraoperatively if bleeding control is necessary. Severe allergic reactions or anaphylaxis may occur with first dose.
nabumetone (Relafen)	—	22	500, 750, or 1000 mg daily (hs) or in two divided doses	Pro-drug (inactive), converted to active metabolite (6-MNA) in liver. Absorption increased by food and milk. Has lower reports of GI ulceration and bleeding than other NSAIDs.
sulindac (Clinoril)	—	8	150–200 mg bid	Renal calculi and biliary obstruction containing sulindac metabolites reported although it is less likely than most NSAIDs to cause renal toxicity.
tolmetin (Tolectin)	—	5	400 mg tid	High evidence of anaphylactic reactions and may also cause serum sickness or flu-like syndrome.
Fenamates				
meclofenamate (Meclomen)	1	2–3	50 mg tid or qid	Less effect on platelet aggregation than most other NSAIDs. Use cautiously in persons on sodium-restricted diet.
mefenamic acid (Ponstel)	—	2	250 mg q6h	Less effect on platelet aggregation but can prolong prothrombin time. Used for short-term treatment of pain and dysmenorrhea; also for acute gouty attacks and vascular headaches.
Oxicams				
paroxicam (Feldene)	2–4	24	20 mg daily or 10 mg bid	Contraindicated in renal impairment. May cause flu-like syndrome. May accumulate in elderly women.

From McKenry LM, Salerno E: *Pharmacology in nursing,* ed 20, St Louis, 1998, Mosby.
CAP, Capsule; *ERC,* extended-release capsules; *ERT,* extended-release tablets.
*All oral NSAIDs should be taken with 8 oz of water with person remaining upright for at least 15 to 30 minutes afterward.

Continued

TABLE 3-6   Nonsteroidal Antiinflammatory Drugs: Pharmacokinetics, Dosing, and Comments—cont'd

NSAID	Onset of Action (hr)	Half-life (hr)	Usual Adult Dosage (mg/day)	Comments*
Propionic Acids				
fenoprofen (Nalfon)	—	3	300 to 600 mg tid or qid	Contraindicated in persons with renal impairment. Food decreases absorption and peak serum levels; therefore administer 30 minutes before or 2 hr after meals unless GI distress occurs, then administer with milk.
flurbiprofen (Ansaid)	—	5.7	100 mg daily bid or tid	Similar to other agents in this category. Currently under study in transdermal patch to treat soft tissue lesions.
ibuprofen (Motrin, Advil)	0.5	2	300 to 800 mg tid or qid	Available in tablets, liquid, and OTC. May decrease blood glucose levels. Incidence of GI side effects less than with aspirin.
ketoprofen (Orudis)		CAP– 1.6 ERC– 5.4 ERT–3- 4	25 to 75 mg tid or qid	Can cause fluid retention and increase in creatinine levels, especially in persons receiving diuretics and the elderly. Monitor renal function closely.
naproxen (Naprosyn)	1	13	250, 375, or 500 mg bid	Available in liquid, tablet, and extended-release tablets. Use tablets and liquid with caution in persons on sodium-restricted diet.
oxaprozin (Daypro)		21–25	600 mg daily or bid	Has a long half-life that accumulates with chronic dosing. Half-life may be 40 to 60 hr or more, which increases with age. Discontinue oxaprozin at least 1 to 2 weeks before elective surgery because it has greater tendency to cause perisurgical bleeding.
Salicylates				
diflunisal (Dolobid)	1	8–12	250–500 mg bid	Higher risk of causing renal impairment but less apt to cause antiplatelet effect than other NSAIDs. Does not have any antipyretic effects.

From McKenry LM, Salerno E: *Pharmacology in nursing*, ed 20, St Louis, 1998, Mosby.
CAP, Capsule; *ERC,* extended-release capsules; *ERT,* extended-release tablets.
*All oral NSAIDs should be taken with 8 oz of water with person remaining upright for at least 15 to 30 minutes afterward.

- Alcoholic beverages produce a synergistic effect with NSAIDs in causing GI bleeding
3. Nursing assessment: determine character, location, onset, contributing factors, duration of pain, time of last-dose: presence of head injury; hepatic or renal failure
4. Nursing management
   a. Determine the most effective way to manage the pain: drug versus nondrug measure (i.e., positioning, turning)
   b. Obtain vital signs
      (1) Be alert to hypotension/hypertension
      (2) Analyze rate and character of respiration
      (3) Withhold drug and notify physician in presence of respiratory depression: respiratory rate of 10 or less respirations per minute or a decrease of 8 or more respirations per minute from baseline data
   c. Caution patient to remain quiet after drug administration to decrease possible nausea and vomiting
   d. Implement safety measures: use side rails and advise patient to remain in bed if there are changes in mental status, alterations in judgment, or unsteadiness
   e. Initiate intake and output records to determine effectiveness of bladder function
   f. Determine efficacy of bowel activity
   g. Patient instruction concerning
      (1) How to take drug
      (2) Safe storage in the home
      (3) Avoidance of driving
      (4) Danger of simultaneous administration of alcohol or other CNS depressant with narcotics

5. Nursing evaluation
   a. Have patient rate pain before and after administration on a scale of 1 to 10 and document
   b. Observe for decreased restlessness and anxiety and ability of the patient to function
   c. Instruct patient to request pain medication before pain becomes severe
D. Narcotic antagonists
   1. Action: reverses CNS and respiratory depression caused by overdose of narcotics
   2. Agents

Examples	Comment
Levallorphan tartrate (Lorfan)	If effects of the narcotic persist, repeat doses may be necessary
Naloxone hydrochloride (Narcan)	
Naltrexone hydrochloride (Trexan)	

   3. Adverse reactions and contraindications
      a. Arrhythmias
      b. Hypertension
      c. Hypotension
      d. Nausea/vomiting
      e. Return of severe pain
   4. Failure to improve indicates need to investigate other causes of CNS and respiratory depression
E. Dependency: the total psychophysical state of one addicted to drugs or alcohol who must receive an increasing amount of the substance to prevent the onset of abstinence symptoms
   1. Rarely seen in hospitalized patients who are taking medication for pain relief, not euphoric effects
   2. Symptoms include runny nose, gooseflesh, tearing, yawning, muscle twitching, abdominal cramping, insomnia, nausea and vomiting, diarrhea
   3. Methadone hydrochloride is used for detoxification and maintenance
   4. With acute toxicity, the usual cause of death is respiratory depression; treated with support to respiration and with a narcotic antagonist
F. Anesthetics: provide a pain-free experience during an operative procedure along with a relaxed state of mind and sense of security
   1. General anesthetics: provide loss of pain sensation, loss of consciousness, loss of memory, and loss of voluntary and some involuntary muscle activity
      a. Inhalation agents: the following are examples

Cyclopropane	Methoxyflurane (Penthrane)
Ether	Nitrous oxide
Halothane	

      b. Intravenous agents: the following are examples

Droperidol (Inapsine)	Methohexital sodium (Brevital)
Droperidol-Fentanyl citrate (Innovar)	Thiamylal sodium (Surital)
Ketamine hydrochloride	Thiopental sodium (Pentothal)

   2. Regional anesthetics: provide loss of sensation and motor activity in localized areas of the body
      a. Types
         (1) Topical
         (2) Infiltration
         (3) Peripheral nerve blocks
         (4) Spinal
         (5) Epidural
         (6) Caudal
      b. Agents: the following are examples

Carbocaine	Pontocaine
Novocain	Xylocaine
Nupercaine	

   3. Nursing assessment
      a. Preoperative: obtain health history including allergies, psychological status, physiological baseline data: inform patient about surgical procedure
      b. Intraoperative: implement safety measures in presence of explosive or flammable agents
      c. Postoperative: determine vital signs and respiratory function
   4. Nursing management
      a. Preoperative: prepare patient physically and psychologically; initiate measures to prevent complications: deep breathing and bed exercises; administer preoperative medications; initiate safety measures and provide quiet environment
      b. Intraoperative: maintain quiet during stage 2 anesthesia; position patient properly and pad pressure points adequately; transfer patient from operating table in a smooth, coordinated manner to avoid severe hypotension
      c. Postoperative: preserve quiet atmosphere; maintain airway, assess pain carefully and have patient rate on a scale of 1 to 10 and document; prevent complications by encouraging deep breathing and coughing, etc.
   5. Nursing evaluation
      a. Preoperative: effects of preoperative medication
      b. Intraoperative: ongoing evaluation of patient's status, usually the responsibility of the anesthesiologist
      c. Postoperative: concerned with pulmonary complications, thrombophlebitis, infection, or other complications, postanesthesia nausea, vomiting, hypotension, tachycardia
G. Anticonvulsants: drugs used to control seizures
   1. Action: not completely understood; thought to depress neuron excitability and to modify the ability of brain tissue to respond to stimuli that initiate seizure activity
   2. Agents

Examples	Adverse Reactions
a. Long-acting barbiturates Mephobarbital (Mebaral) Phenobarbital (Luminal) Primidone (Mysoline)	Sedation, drowsiness, tolerance, nystagmus, ataxia, anemia, congenital malformations in fetus; sudden withdrawal can induce convulsions

b. Hydantoins
Ethotoin (Peganone)
Mephenytoin (Mesantoin)
Phenytoin (Dilantin)

Nystagmus, ataxia, slurred speech, tremors, nervousness, drowsiness, fatigue, overgrowth of the gums (gingival hyperplasia), occasional folic acid or vitamin D deficiency; congenital malformations in fetus

c. Succinimides
Ethosuximide (Zarontin)
Methsuximide (Celontin)
Phensuximide (Milontin)

Gastrointestinal irritation, dizziness, drowsiness, headache, fatigue

d. Oxazolidinediones
Trimethadione (Tridione)

Serious allergic dermatitis, kidney and liver damage, vertigo, photophobia, spontaneous abortion, congenital malformations

e. Benzodiazepines
Clonazepam (Clonopin)
Diazepam (Valium)

Drowsiness, ataxia, personality changes

f. Miscellaneous
Acetazolamide (Diamox)
Carbamazepine (Tegretol)

Loss of appetite, drowsiness, confusion
Drowsiness, dizziness, ataxia, double vision, gastrointestinal upset

Lidocaine hydrochloride (Xylocaine)

Depressed heart action

Paraldehyde

Bronchopulmonary irritation, thrombophlebitis at intravenous injection site

Valproic acid (Depakene)

Gastrointestinal distress, sedation

3. Nursing assessment: observe course of the seizure; assist in case finding; assess baseline data with concentration on areas known to be affected by the drug, e.g., phenytoin (Dilantin): assess mouth, teeth, and gums for development of gingival hyperplasia
4. Nursing management: instruct patient concerning
   a. Drug characteristics
   b. Importance of taking medication even when patient is seizure free; awareness that reaching a therapeutic level may take time
   c. Impairment of absorption of the anticonvulsant when taken with milk or antacids
   d. Wearing or carrying identification indicating seizure activity and drugs and dosages being taken
   e. Reducing gastric irritation by taking drug with meals
   f. Good gum massage and oral care after each meal
5. Nursing evaluation: continued medical follow-up; blood level tests
H. Skeletal muscle relaxants: drugs used to treat muscle spasticity
   1. Action: Inhibits nerve impulse transmission by blocking polysynaptic pathways in the spinal cord

2. Agents

Examples	Adverse Reactions
a. Drugs to treat spasticity Baclofen (Lioresal)	Drowsiness incoordination, gastrointestinal upset
Dantrolene sodium (Dantrium)	Liver damage
Diazepam (Valium)	Drowsiness, incoordination
b. Drugs to treat muscle spasm Carisoprodol (Rela, Soma)	Drowsiness, dizziness
Chlorphenesin carbamate (Maolate)	
Chlorzoxazone (Paraflex)	
Cyclobenzaprine hydrochloride (Flexeril)	
Dantrolene (Dantrium)	
Diazepam (Valium)	
Methocarbamol (Delaxin, Robaxin)	
Meprobamate (Miltown, Equanil)	
Orphenadrine citrate (Flexon, Norflex)	

3. Nursing assessment: obtain baseline data, focusing on spasticity, including degree, aggravating factors, associated pain, and interference with activities of daily living (ADLs); observe baseline liver function studies
4. Nursing management: monitor for drug effectiveness and side effects; institute safety measures if drowsiness occurs; teach patient to avoid alcohol and CNS depressants
5. Nursing evaluation: at regular intervals, assess the continuing degree of spasticity
I. Antiparkinsonian drugs: drugs used in the management of Parkinson's disease
   1. Action: restores action of the neurotransmitter dopamine to the basal ganglia of the brain or blocks the effects of excessive action of acetylcholine
   2. Agents

Examples	Adverse Reactions
a. Anticholinergics Benztropine mesylate (Cogentin)	Dry mouth, constipation, urinary retention, blurred vision; impairment of recent memory, confusion, insomnia, and restlessness
Biperiden (Akineton)	
Cycrimine hydrochloride (Pagitane hydrochloride)	
Ethopropazine hydrochloride (Parsidol)	
Procyclidine hydrochloride (Kemadrin)	
Trihexyphenidyl hydrochloride (Artane, Pipanol, Tremin)	

b. Antihistamines — Sedation
   Chlorphenoxamine
      hydrochloride
      (Phenoxene)
   Diphenhydramine
      hydrochloride
      (Benadryl)
   Orphenadrine citrate
      (Disipal)
c. Other drugs
   Amantadine — Dry mouth, constipa-
      hydrochloride   tion, urinary reten-
      (Symmetrel)   tion, blurred vision
   Levodopa (Dopar, — Nausea, vomiting,
      Larodopa)   anorexia, ortho-
                         static hypotension,
                         GI bleeding, cough,
                         hoarseness, dys-
                         pnea, blurred vision,
                         increased sex drive
   Carbidopa-levodopa — Same as Levodopa
      (Sinemet)

J. Sedatives, hypnotics, antianxiety drugs
   1. Sedatives: small dose to calm an anxious patient
   2. Hypnotics: larger dose to induce sleep
   3. Antianxiety drugs (minor tranquilizers): drugs used to treat anxiety
   4. Barbiturates: classified according to duration of action: ultra short acting, short acting, intermediate acting, and long acting
      a. Action: produce CNS depression ranging from sedation to anesthesia
      b. Adverse reactions
         (1) Mild withdrawal symptoms: rebound REM sleep, nightmares, daytime agitation, and a "shaky" feeling—dosage must be decreased gradually
         (2) Acute overdose: depression of medullary centers regulating respiration and cardiovascular system—tachycardia, hypotension, loss of reflexes, marked depression of respiration
      c. Agents: the following are examples

Amobarbital (Amytal, Tuinal)	Pentobarbital (Nembutal)
Butabarbital sodium (Butalan, Butisol Sodium)	Phenobarbital (Luminal)
	Secobarbital (Seconal)

   5. Benzodiazepines
      a. Action: produce CNS depression
      b. Adverse reactions: daytime sedation, motor incoordination, dizziness, headaches; schedule IV substances
      c. Agents: the following are examples

Chlordiazepoxide hydrochloride (Librium)	Flurazepam hydrochloride (Dalmane)
Clorazepate dipotassium (Tranxene)	Lorazepam (Ativan)
	Oxazepam (Serax)
Diazepam (Valium)	Prazepam (Verstran, Centrax)

6. Miscellaneous
   a. Action: produce CNS depression; generally short acting
   b. Agents

Examples	Adverse Reactions
Chloral betaine (Beta-Chlor)	Gastric irritation; schedule IV substance
Chloral hydrate (Noctec)	Gastric irritation; schedule IV substance
Ethchlorvynol (Placidyl)	Muscular weakness; schedule IV substance
Glutethimide (Doriden)	Dilated pupils, dry mouth; schedule III substance
Hydroxyzine hydrochloride (Vistaril)	Dry mouth, hypotension, blurred vision, urinary retention
Meprobamate (Equanil, Miltown)	Schedule IV substance
Methaqualone (Quaalude, Sopor, Parest)	Paresthesia, peripheral neuropathy; schedule II substance
Methyprylon (Noludar)	Schedule II substance

7. Nursing assessment: give special attention to vital signs, level of consciousness, sleep patterns
8. Nursing management: observe for signs of CNS depression; identify nondrug solutions to sleep problems; monitor safety aspects of patient care
9. Nursing evaluation: review purpose for which drug is given and observe effectiveness; instruct patient concerning self-medication, medical follow-up, and drug-dependence potential

K. Alcohol
   1. Action: produces CNS depression: sedation, disinhibition, sleep, anesthesia; vasodilation; gastric irritation
   2. Effects of an acute overdose: death, accidents, hangover, upset stomach, thirst, fatigue, headache, depression, anxiety; chronic toxicity can lead to liver, esophagastrointestinal and cardiovascular disorders
   3. Withdrawal symptoms after chronic use: tremors, anxiety, tachycardia, increased blood pressure, diaphoresis, anorexia, nausea, vomiting, insomnia, hallucinations, seizures, delirium tremens
   4. Withdrawal therapy: one of the benzodiazepines; restoration of normal metabolic functions, and vitamin B_1, B_{12}, and folic acid
   5. Aversion therapy: disulfiram (Antabuse) given to detoxified patient who wishes to avoid drinking again; produces unpleasant reaction in presence of alcohol: flushing, throbbing in head and neck, respiratory difficulty, nausea, copious vomiting, diaphoresis, fainting, dizziness, blurred vision, confusion

Psychotherapeutic Agents

A. Antidepressants: Characteristic of drug-induced prevention or relief of depression
   1. Tricyclic antidepressants
      a. Action: primarily used to relieve symptoms of endogenous depression; also used to treat mild exogenous depression

b. Agents: the following are examples

Amitriptyline hydro- chloride (Elavil)	Imipramine hydrochloride (Tofranil)
Clomipramine hydrochloride (Anafranil)	Nortriptyline hydrochloride (Aventyl hydrochloride, Pamelor)
Doxepin hydrochloride (Adapin, Sinequan)	

2. Monoamine oxidase (MAO) inhibitors
   a. Action: relieve symptoms of severe reactive or endogenous depression that has not responded to tricyclic antidepressant therapy, electroconvulsive therapy, or other modes of psychotherapy
   b. Agents: the following are examples
      Isocarboxazid (Marplan)
      Phenelzine sulfate (Nardil)
      Tranylcypromine sulfate (Parnate)
3. Heterocyclic antidepressants
   a. Action: second generation antidepressant; inhibits the reuptake of norepinephrine; fewer long-term side effects; individual agents have to be considered for advantages and disadvantages
   b. Agents: the following are examples
      amoxapine (Asendin)
      bupropion (Wellbutrin)
      maprotiline (Ludiomil)
      trazodone (Desyril)
4. Selective serotonin reuptake inhibitors (SSRIs)
   a. Action: used to treat depression
   b. Agents: the following are examples
      fluoxetine (Prozac)
      paroxetine (Paxil)
      sertraline (Zoloft)
5. Nursing assessment
   a. Obtain complete health history
   b. History of insomnia, fatigue, or loss of motivation
   c. Observe motor movements, facial expression, and posture
   d. Assess for any feelings of suicide; potential for suicide is inherent in any severely depressed patient until a significant remission occurs
   e. Administer with caution to patients with increased intraocular pressure, prostatic hypertrophy, history of urinary retention, or history of glaucoma, because tricyclic antidepressants possess significant anticholinergic properties
   f. Check medication history carefully for extensive drug interactions
   g. Use extreme caution with patients with cardiovascular disease because of potential for conduction defects
   h. Initial dose in adolescent and debilitated patients should be lower and increased gradually
6. Nursing management: administer medication with food to avoid gastric distress
7. Nursing evaluation: observe for adverse effects, such as drowsiness
8. Patient teaching
   a. Stress compliance of taking medication as ordered
   b. Instruct patient to avoid using alcohol with sleeping pills and hay fever or cold medications, because doing so increases the effects of these medications

c. Teach patient to report anticholinergic side effects (blurred vision, altered thought processes, constipation, urinary retention, and eye pain, which may be indicative of glaucoma)
   d. Food containing tyramine should not be ingested for at least 2 to 3 weeks after discontinuation of therapy; educate patient and family on dietary restrictions
   e. Teach patient that therapeutic effects take 2 to 3 weeks
   f. Instruct patient not to discontinue medication quickly after long-term use; may cause nausea, headache, malaise
B. Antipsychotic drugs
   1. Phenothiazines/thioxanthenes
      a. Action: primarily to reduce or relieve symptoms of acute and chronic psychoses, including schizophrenia, schizoaffective disorders, and involutional psychoses
      b. Agents: the following are examples

Chlorpromazine (Thorazine)	Trifluoperazine hydrochloride (Stelazine)
Promazine hydrochloride (Sparine)	Triflupromazine hydrochloride (Vesprin)
Thioridazine hydrochloride (Mellaril)	

   2. Nursing assessment: obtain complete health history, current use of medications, and possibility of pregnancy; obtain history of emotional unrest, agitation, paranoid ideation, delusions, and inability to cope with reality
   3. Nursing management: administer medication with food or milk to avoid or reduce gastric distress
   4. Nursing evaluation: observe for adverse effects such as urinary retention, change in vision, sore throat with fever, muscle spasms, trembling or shaking of hands, skin rash, yellow tinge to skin or eyes, uncontrollable movements of the tongue
C. Antimanic drugs: used to treat manic-depressive psychoses in the acute manic phase; also used to prevent recurrent episodes of mania in the manic-depressive patient
   1. Agent: Lithium carbonate (Lithane, Carbolith)
   2. Nursing assessment: obtain complete health history, possibility of pregnancy, and medications currently being taken; observe for restlessness, hyperactivity, aggressiveness
   3. Nursing management: ensure adequate fluid and electrolyte balance
   4. Nursing evaluation: monitor serum lithium levels to avoid drug toxicity and reduce side effects
   5. Patient teaching: stress compliance of taking medication as ordered; instruct patient to wear medical identification tag

Stimulants

Stimulants are medically accepted only for treatment of narcolepsy, hyperkinetic behavior in children, and obesity. Occasionally they are used for depression in the elderly and to reverse respiratory depression from CNS depressants.
A. Amphetamines
   1. Action: increase the release and effectiveness of catecholamine neurotransmitters in the brain and peripheral nerves and create increased alertness and sensitivity to stimuli

2. Adverse reactions
   a. Gastrointestinal system: vomiting, diarrhea, abdominal cramps, dry mouth, anorexia
   b. Central nervous system: restless behavior, tremor, irritability, talkativeness, insomnia, mood changes, excessive aggressiveness, confusion, panic, increased libido
   c. Autonomic nervous system: headache, chilliness, palpitation, pallor or facial flushing
   d. Children: growth retardation
3. Agents: the following are examples

Amphetamine sulfate
Dextroamphetamine sulfate (Dexedrine, Ferndex)
Methamphetamine hydrochloride (Desoxyn)

Methylphenidate (Ritalin)
Pemoline (Cylert)

4. Nursing assessment: obtain thorough history of patient's presenting problem; obtain vital signs, weight, and height in children
5. Nursing management: monitor height, weight, and vital signs; inquire about relief of subjective symptoms such as insomnia, agitation, headache, and irritability; begin preparation of patient and family for long-term management; teach patient that last daily dose should be taken at least 6 hours before retiring
6. Nursing evaluation: success of goals of therapy evaluated
   a. Hyperkinesis: less hyperactivity and a more normal attention span
   b. Narcolepsy: ability to remain awake and alert during specified appropriate time periods
B. Appetite suppressants: used to help control obesity
   1. Action: exert an anorectic effect on the appetite-control center in the brain
   2. Agents

Examples	**Adverse Reactions/ Comments**
Amphetamine sulfate (Benzedrine)	See Amphetamines
Benzphetamine (Didrex)	See Amphetamines
Caffeine	Nervousness, jitteriness, gastrointestinal bleeding, nausea, vomiting, excessive CNS stimulation, and convulsions
Caffeine sodium benzoate injection	Same as Caffeine
Dextroamphetamine sulfate (Dexedrine)	See Amphetamines
Diethylpropion hydrochloride (Propion, Tenuate)	Dry mouth, constipation; schedule IV drug
Doxapram hydrochloride (Dopram)	Dizziness, apprehension, disorientation
Fenfluramine hydrochloride (Pondimin)	Sedation and depression; schedule IV drug
Mazindol (Sanorex)	Insomnia, dizziness, agitation; schedule III drug

Methamphetamine hydrochloride (Desoxyn, Obedrin-LA)	See Amphetamines
Nikethamide (Coramine)	Hypertension, tachycardia, tremors, flushing, increased body temperature, convulsion
Phendimetrazine tartrate (Bacarate)	Gastrointestinal distress; schedule III drug
Phenmetrazine hydrochloride (Preludin)	Schedule II drug; see Amphetamines
Phentermine hydrochloride (Adipex-P, Fastin, Tora)	Insomnia; schedule IV drug
Phenylpropanolamine hydrochloride (Acutrim, Control, Diadax, Dexatrim)	Blood pressure increases
Theophylline	Increased heart rate, nervousness, jitteriness, nausea, vomiting, excessive CNS stimulation, and convulsions

3. Nursing assessment: obtain vital signs and weight; discuss usual eating habits and establish reasonable goals for losing weight
4. Nursing management: promote weight reduction; monitor for adverse reactions; offer support
5. Nursing evaluation: instruct patient concerning medication and its potential for drug abuse; assess achievement of goal—weight loss
C. Respiratory stimulants (analeptics): used to stimulate respiration when it has been depressed by drugs, asphyxiation, or electric shock
   1. Action: stimulates central nervous system medullary centers controlling respiration, vasomotor tone, and vagal tone
   2. Agents: see Amphetamines
   3. Nursing assessments: check respiratory rate and depth of respirations; may measure vital capacity and arterial blood gas levels
   4. Nursing management: monitor vital signs with focus on respirations; keep suction machine at bedside
   5. Nursing evaluation: observe whether patient is breathing at a rate and depth nearing normal and whether short-term hospitalization is necessary

AUTONOMIC NERVOUS SYSTEM
Cholinesterase Inhibitors (Cholinergic Agents)
A. Description: drugs that produce a physiologic response similar to that of acetylcholine released on nerve stimulation
B. Action
   1. Direct-acting cholinergic stimulants: mimic the action of acetylcholine
   2. Indirect-acting cholinergic stimulants: inhibit the enzyme cholinesterase, which acts to limit acetylcholine action
C. Effects
   1. Vasodilation
   2. Lowered blood pressure

3. Slowing of heart rate
4. Salivation
5. Perspiring
6. Increased tone and movement in the gastrointestinal and genitourinary systems
7. Increased tone and contractility in striated muscles
D. Adverse reactions: heart block, arrhythmias, hypotension, hypertension, nausea, vomiting, cramps, diarrhea, heartburn, muscle weakness, increase in intraocular pressure, urinary retention (bethanechol)
E. Agents: the following are examples

Ambenonium chloride (Mytelase Chloride, Mysuran)
Demecarium bromide (Humorsol)
Echothiophate iodide (Phospholine iodide)
Bethanechol (Urecholine)
Edrophonium chloride (Tensilon)
Isoflurophate (Floropryl)
Neostigmine bromide (Prostigmin)
Pyridostigmine bromide (Mestinon)

F. Nursing assessment: history of lung disease, hyperthyroidism, prostate enlargement; patients with obstruction of the intestine or renal disease should not use these products
G. Nursing management: monitor vital signs; insert rectal tube to relieve flatus; inform patient that drug is not a cure; it only relieves symptoms (myasthenia gravis)
H. Nursing evaluation: observe for adverse reactions, bowel activity, intake and output records; therapeutic response in the treatment of myasthenia gravis—increased muscle strength, hand grasp, improved muscle gait, absence of labored breathing (if severe)

Parasympathetic Blocking Agents (Parasympatholytic or Cholinergic Blocking Agents)

A. Action: prevent acetylcholine released by nerve stimulation from exerting its effects
B. Effects:
1. Gastrointestinal: slows peristalsis
2. Heart: increases rate
3. Secretions: depresses all body secretions including perspiration and respiratory, salivary, pancreatic, and gastric secretions
4. Eye: dilates pupils (mydriasis); paralyzes ciliary muscles; increases intraocular pressure
C. Adverse reactions: dry skin, delirium, tachycardia, convulsions, mydriasis, hypertension, dry mouth, urinary retention
D. Agents

Examples	Clinical Uses
Atropine sulfate	Adjunct to anesthesia, antispasmodic, cardiac stimulant
Cyclopentolate hydrochloride (Cyclogyl)	Mydriatic, cycloplegic
Homatropine hydrobromide	Mydriatic, cycloplegic
Scopolamine hydrobromide (Hyoscine)	Sedative-hypnotic, adjunct to anesthesia, antiemetic, mydriatic, cycloplegic
Isopropamide iodide (Darbid)	Antispasmodic
Methantheline bromide (Banthine)	Antispasmodic
Propantheline bromide (Pro-Banthine)	Antispasmodic
Benztropine mesylate (Cogentin)	Antiparkinsonian agent
Procyclidine hydrochloride (Kemadrin)	Antiparkinsonian agent
Trihexyphenidyl hydrochloride (Artane)	Antiparkinsonian agent

E. Nursing assessment: monitor vital signs; tachycardia; bowel functions; stimulation or depression of central nervous system; elevation in temperature; respiratory status; history of urinary difficulty, familial history of glaucoma
F. Nursing management: maintain oral hygiene for dry mouth; initiate methods to prevent abdominal distention and constipation; initiate safety measures in presence of blurred vision
G. Nursing evaluation: establish intake and output records when these drugs are given to elderly males; observe for effectiveness of drug

Neuromuscular Blocking Agents

A. Action: act at the striated neuromuscular junction to produce paralysis of the voluntary muscles
B. Effects
1. Produce muscular relaxation for insertion of endotracheal tubes during surgical interventions
2. Protect against violent thrashing that occurs with electroconvulsive therapy
3. Alleviate spasms that accompany tetanus
C. Adverse reactions: paralysis of respiration, which may be reversed with neostigmine or Tensilon
D. Agents: the following are examples

Decamethonium bromide (Syncurine)
Pancuronium bromide (Pavulon)
Succinylcholine chloride (Anectine)
Tubocurarine chloride (Tubarine)

E. Nursing assessment: elicit medical history: asthma, myasthenia gravis remission; potassium blood levels
F. Nursing management: cardiopulmonary resuscitation skills—have resuscitative equipment available; monitor vital signs
G. Nursing evaluation: observe for early signs of flaccid paralysis in muscles of face, neck, eyes
H. Know that patient may appear to be asleep but can still hear

Sympathomimetic Drugs: Adrenergic Stimulants

A. Actions
1. Act directly on adrenergic receptors to produce either excitation or inhibition of a particular effector organ
2. Act indirectly by releasing the stored catecholamines norepinephrine and epinephrine
B. Major effects
1. Excitation of the heart, both its rate and force of contraction

2. Excitation and constriction of smooth muscles in peripheral blood vessels
3. Inhibition and relaxation of smooth muscles in bronchi, gastrointestinal tract, and skeletal muscle blood vessels
4. Metabolism: release of fatty acids from adipose tissue and increased gluconeogenesis in muscle and liver
5. Excitation of functions controlled by central nervous system, for example, respiration
6. Suppression of appetite
7. Lessening of fatigue

C. Adverse reactions: anxiety, apprehension, headache, arrhythmias, cerebral hemorrhage, heart failure, pulmonary edema

D. Agents

Examples	Clinical Indications
Dopamine hydrochloride (Intropin)	Hypotension
Ephedrine hydrochloride (Bronkotabs)	Bronchospasms, nasal decongestion, allergy
Epinephrine bitartrate (Medihaler-Epi)	Acute or chronic bronchial asthma, allergic disorders, acute hypersensitivity to drugs
Epinephrine hydrochloride (Adrenalin Chloride)	Cardiac arrest, heart block, acute asthma, adjunct to local anesthesia, acute hypersensitivity to drugs
	Ophthalmic use: control hemorrhage, decrease intraocular pressure
Isoproterenol hydrochloride (Isuprel)	Bronchodilation, cardiac stimulant
Isoproterenol sulfate (Medihaler-Iso)	Bronchodilation
Mephentermine sulfate (Wyamine)	Maintain blood pressure during anesthesia
Metaraminol bitartrate (Aramine)	Hypotension
Naphazoline hydrochloride (Privine)	Nasal decongestion
Norepinephrine bitartrate (Levophed, Noradrenalin)	Shock, cardiac arrest
Nylidrin hydrochloride (Arlidin)	Peripheral vascular disease

E. Nursing assessment: obtain history of hyperthyroidism, diabetes, hypertension, emotional lability, heart disease

F. Nursing management: monitor vital signs; check infusion rate often; observe for infusion infiltration; record bowel and urinary activity; teach patient to keep fluid intake to at least 2000 ml/day to reduce viscosity of secretions.

G. Nursing evaluation: monitor effect on blood pressure, pulse rate, and regularity of heart rate; observe for therapeutic and adverse effects

Adrenergic Receptor Blockers and Neuron Blockers

A. Action: interfere with peripheral adrenergic activity by blocking alpha and beta receptors, by depleting peripheral neural stores of norepinephrine, and by inhibiting peripheral sympathetic activity through an action on the central nervous system

B. Adverse reactions: postural hypotension, miosis, inhibition of ejaculation, headache, intense vasoconstriction, diarrhea, nausea, disturbances of vision, insomnia, depression

C. Agents

Examples	Clinical Indications
Clonidine (Catapres-TTS)	Chronic hypertension
Ergoloid mesylate (Hydergine)	Mental and emotional complaints of the elderly
Guanethidine monosulfate (Ismelin)	Hypertension
Methyldopa (Aldomet)	Hypertension
Metoprolol tartrate (Lopressor)	Chronic hypertension, angina prophylaxis
Nadolol (Corgard)	Chronic hypertension, angina prophylaxis
Phenoxybenzamine hydrochloride (Dibenzyline)	Peripheral vascular disease
Phentolamine mesylate (Regitine)	Hypertension secondary to pheochromocytoma, adrenal tumor surgery
Prazosin hydrochloride (Minipress)	Chronic hypertension
Propranolol hydrochloride (Inderal)	Chronic hypertension, angina prophylaxis, cardiac dysrhythmias, migraine headaches
Reserpine (Serpasil)	Chronic hypertension
Timolol maleate (Timoptic)	Glaucoma
Tolazoline hydrochloride (Priscoline)	Peripheral vascular disease

D. Nursing assessment: ascertain if patient has history of ulcer disease, diabetes, ulcerative colitis, emotional depression, renal problems, coronary heart disease, predisposition to asthma, or congestive heart failure

E. Nursing management: aim instruction toward patient compliance; administer medications with meals or milk; maintain safety measures in presence of postural hypotension; monitor vital signs

F. Nursing evaluation: observe for therapeutic and adverse reactions; observe for changes in sleep patterns and appetite and depression or suicidal tendencies; observe for interactions with other arrhythmias or channel blockers; may cause additive effect; interaction with insulin or hypoglycemic agents could alter insulin requirements and mask signs of hypoglycemia

Ganglionic Agents

A. Action: reduces sympathetic tone, particularly in the cardiovascular system

B. Adverse reactions: postural hypotension, pupillary dilation, blurring vision, dry mouth, constipation

C. Agents

Examples	Clinical Indications
Mecamylamine hydrochloride (Inversine)	Hypertensive crisis, chronic hypertension
Trimethaphan camsylate (Arfonad)	Hypertensive crisis

D. Nursing assessment: obtain baseline vital signs; assess factors contributing to hypertension such as diet, weight, exercise, and lifestyle
E. Nursing management: instruction aimed at patient compliance
F. Nursing evaluation: observe for therapeutic effects and adverse reactions

RESPIRATORY SYSTEM
Antihistamines
A. Action: blocks histamine effects at the receptor site
B. Adverse reactions: sedation, drowsiness, dry mouth, blurred vision, urinary retention, constipation; can also stimulate the nervous system, especially in children, causing insomnia, irritability, and nervousness
C. Agents

Examples	Clinical Indications
Brompheniramine maleate (Dimetane)	Colds, allergies
Carbinoxamine maleate (Clistin)	Colds, allergies
Chlorpheniramine maleate (Chlor-Trimeton, Teldrin, Chlortab)	Colds, allergies
Clemastine fumarate (Tavist)	Allergies
Cyproheptadine hydrochloride (Periactin)	Pruritus
Dexchlorpheniramine maleate (Polaramine)	Colds, allergies
Dimethindene maleate (Forhistal)	Colds, allergies
Diphenhydramine hydrochloride (Benadryl)	Allergic reactions, motion sickness, mild parkinsonism
Fexofenadine hydrochloride (Allegra)	Allergies
Loratidine (Claritin)	Allergies
Meclizine hydrochloride (Bonine)	Motion sickness
Methdilazine hydrochloride (Tacaryl)	Pruritus
Promethazine hydrochloride (Phenergan, Promine, Remsed, Zipan)	Sedation, pruritus, motion sickness, nausea, vomiting
Trimeprazine tartrate (Temaril)	Pruritus
Tripelennamine hydrochloride (Pyribenzamine)	Colds, allergies

D. Nursing assessment: obtain vital signs; assess respiratory and cardiovascular status; ascertain if patient has history of allergy and extent and type of rash if present
E. Nursing management: monitor respiratory response, vital signs, urinary and bowel function
F. Nursing evaluation: observe for therapeutic effects and adverse reaction; instruct patient on dangers of operating machinery and to wear medical identification tag in presence of allergies; therapeutic response: includes absence of allergy symptoms, itching

Prophylactic Asthmatic Drugs
A. Action: indicated for prevention of bronchospasms and bronchial asthma attacks; inhibits the release of histamines from mast cells
B. Adverse reactions: cough, hoarseness, dry mouth or throat, nasal congestion, sneezing and bad taste in mouth
C. Agent: cromolyn sodium (Intal)
D. Nursing assessment: helps prevent but does not relieve asthma attacks; client should be advised that it may be as long as 4 weeks before the drug is fully beneficial
E. Nursing evaluation: therapeutic effect would be a reduction in the number of attacks, reduced cough, decreased sputum production, and/or a decreased need for other asthma drugs

Nasal Decongestants
A. Action: sympathomimetic agents (see the Autonomic Nervous System) when applied to nasal mucosa or taken orally constrict the smooth muscle of arterioles in the nasal mucosa and thus reduce blood flow and edema
B. Adverse reactions: rebound nasal congestion if used too frequently; nervousness, irritability
C. Agents: the following are a few examples of the numerous preparations available

Afrin	Neo-Synephrine
Allerest	Privine
Contac	Sine-Off
Coricidin	Sinutab
Dristan	Sudafed

D. Nursing assessment: obtain history of irritants or environmental conditions contributing to symptoms and such objective data as respiratory rate and vital signs
E. Nursing management: instruct patient regarding medication use
F. Nursing evaluation: monitor for therapeutic effects and adverse reactions

Expectorants, Antitussives, Mucolytic Drugs
A. Definitions
  1. Expectorant: increases output of respiratory tract fluid that coats the bronchi and trachea
  2. Antitussive: suppresses cough
  3. Mucolytic: breaks up viscous mucus to allow for ease in expectoration of drainage
B. Adverse reactions
  1. Expectorants: nausea, drowsiness; iodide base drugs: skin rash, metallic taste, fever, skin eruptions, mucous membrane ulcerations, salivary gland swelling
  2. Antitussives: nausea, dizziness, constipation
  3. Mucolytics: gastrointestinal upset
C. Agents: the following are examples
  1. Expectorants: Robitussin, iodinated glycerol (Organidin), potassium iodide
  2. Antitussives: codeine, hydrocodone bitartrate, dextromethorphan hydrobromide (Romilar), Benylin, benzonatate (Tessalon)
  3. Mucolytics: acetylcysteine (Mucomyst), Alevaire
D. Nursing assessment: obtain history relevant to cough, vital signs, and such objective data as character and quantity of secretions

E. Nursing management: monitor symptoms, vital signs, and amount of secretions with mucolytics
F. Nursing evaluation: instruct patient regarding drugs, how/when to take them and when they should be discontinued; encourage patients with persistent coughs to seek follow-up treatment

Bronchodilators
A. Action: act on bronchial cells to dilate the bronchioles
B. Adverse reactions: CNS stimulation, increased heart rate, muscle tremors, headache, nausea, epigastric pain, bronchospasms
C. Agents: the following are examples

Aminophylline
Dyphylline (Dilin, Protophylline)
Ephedrine sulfate (Slo-Fedrin)
Epinephrine (Sus-Phrine)
Epinephrine bitartrate (AsthmaHaler, Medihaler-Epi, Primatene Mist)
Epinephrine hydrochloride (Adrenalin Chloride)
Isoetharine hydrochloride (Bronkosol)

Isoetharine mesylate (Bronkometer)
Isoproterenol hydrochloride (Iprenol, Isuprel hydrochloride)
Metaproterenol sulfate (Alupent, Metaprel)
Oxtriphylline (Choledyl)
Terbutaline sulfate (Brethine, Bricanyl)
Theophylline (many preparations)

D. Nursing assessment: obtain relevant history and vital signs; note amount and characteristics of secretions
E. Nursing management: monitor vital signs and lung sounds, closely monitor intravenous drugs; teach patient to increase fluid intake to 2000-3000 ml/day
F. Nursing evaluation: observe for therapeutic effects; instruct patient regarding drug knowledge and usage

CARDIOVASCULAR SYSTEM
Drugs to Improve Circulation
A. Action: vasoconstriction (direct- and indirect-acting sympathomimetic amines cause release of norepinephrine, which stimulates alpha receptors and thus produces vasoconstriction)
B. Adverse reactions: headache, anxiety, palpitation, nausea, vomiting, insomnia, tremors
C. Agents: the following are examples

Dobutamine hydrochloride (Dobutrex)
Dopamine hydrochloride (Intropin)
Epinephrine hydrochloride (Adrenalin Chloride)
Isoproterenol hydrochloride (Isuprel hydrochloride)
Mephentermine sulfate (Wyamine)

Metaraminol bitartrate (Aramine)
Methoxamine hydrochloride (Vasoxyl)
Norepinephrine bitartrate (Levarterenol bitartrate; Levophed)
Phenylephrine hydrochloride (Neo-Synephrine hydrochloride, Isophrin)

D. Principal clinical use: treatment of cardiogenic and anaphylactic shock; to maintain blood pressure in life-threatening situations and during anesthesia

E. Nursing assessment: obtain pulse, respirations, and blood pressure; note level of consciousness
F. Nursing management: use infusion-control device to monitor intravenous administration; monitor vital signs frequently
G. Nursing evaluation: observe for therapeutic effects

Vasodilator Drugs (Antianginal Drugs)
A. Action: dilate arterioles and veins to lower blood pressure, which reduces workload on the heart and decreases the heart's oxygen demand; increases circulation to cardiac muscle
B. Adverse reactions: flushing, headache, dizziness
C. Agents: the following are examples

Amyl nitrite (Vaporole)
Erythrityl tetranitrate (Cardilate)
Isosorbide dinitrate (Iso-Bid, Isordil, Sorbide, Sorbitrate)
Mannitol hexanitrate (Nitranitol)

Nitroglycerin (Nitro-Bid)
Nitroglycerin lingual aerosol (Nitrolingual Spray)
Nitroglycerin ointment, 2% (Nitrol)
Pentaerythritol tetranitrate (Peritrate)
Trolnitrate phosphate (Metamine)

D. Nursing assessment: obtain vital signs and history relevant to onset and duration of pain
E. Nursing management: observe and monitor for additional angina attacks; instruct patient about prescribed drugs
F. Nursing evaluation: observe for therapeutic effects

Vasodilator Drugs for Peripheral Vascular Disease
A. Action: work directly on vascular smooth muscle to cause relaxation or stimulate beta receptors in blood vessels to produce vasodilation
B. Adverse reactions: gastrointestinal upset, flushing, hypotension, dizziness, increased heart rate, headache
C. Agents: the following are examples

Cyclandelate (Cyclospasmol)
Ergoloid mesylates (dihydrogenated ergot alkaloids; Hydergine)
Isoxsuprine hydrochloride (Vasodilan)

Nylidrin hydrochloride (Arlidin, Rolidrin)
Papaverine hydrochloride (many trade names)
Tolazoline hydrochloride (Priscoline)

D. Nursing assessment: obtain history of onset and course of vascular disease; assess blood pressure, pulses, including peripheral pulses, mental status, and color and temperature of affected extremities
E. Nursing evaluation: observe for therapeutic and adverse effects
F. Nursing management: monitor presenting signs and symptoms; instruct patient regarding medications

Antihypertensives
Several subgroups of drugs can lower blood pressure
A. Action
  1. Adrenergic drugs
    a. Beta-1 adrenergic receptor antagonists (beta-

blockers): reduce cardiac output; reduce renin release from kidney (blocks response to sympathetic impulses)

   b. Alpha-1 adrenergic receptor antagonists: prevent norepinephrine from constricting blood vessels to increase resistance to blood flow

2. Centrally acting antihypertensive drugs that inhibit the activity of the sympathetic nervous system: decrease sympathetic tone and activate alpha receptors in the medulla that decrease heart rate and cardiac output
3. Vasodilators: relax arteriolar smooth muscle
4. Vasodilators in hypertensive emergencies: rapidly relax smooth muscle

B. Adverse reactions: bradycardia, hypotension, nasal congestion, reflex tachycardia, dry mouth, fluid retention, arthralgia, depression, drowsiness
C. Agents: the following are examples

1. Beta adrenergic receptor antagonists
   Metoprolol tartrate (Lopressor)
   Nadolol (Corgard)
   Propranolol hydrochloride (Inderal)
2. Alpha adrenergic receptor antagonists
   Phenoxybenzamine hydrochloride (Dibenzyline)
   Phentolamine mesylate (Regitine)
   Prazosin hydrochloride (Minipress)
3. Drugs interfering with norepinephrine
   Deserpidine (Harmonyl)
   Guanethidine monosulfate (Ismelin)
   Rauwolfia serpentina (Raudixin)
   Reserpine (Serpasil, Sandril)
4. Centrally acting antihypertensive drugs
   Clonidine hydrochloride (Catapres)
   Methyldopa (Aldomet)
5. Vasodilators
   Hydralazine hydrochloride (Apresoline)
   Minoxidil (Loniten)
6. Vasodilators: hypertensive emergencies
   Diazoxide (Hyperstat)
   Sodium nitroprusside (Nipride)
   Trimethaphan camsylate (Arfonad)

D. Nursing assessment: obtain vital signs and additional baseline data, such as weight, diet, and serum electrolyte levels for electrolyte imbalances
E. Nursing management: monitor vital signs, intake and output, weight, blood studies; instruct patient regarding drugs
F. Nursing evaluation: observe for therapeutic effects and adverse reactions
G. Patient teaching: stress the importance of knowing acceptable ranges of blood pressure and pulse; taking medication as ordered; preventing orthostatic hypotension; and reporting asthmalike signs and symptoms
1. Patients who suspect pregnancy should not use ace inhibitors, the "pril" drugs (i.e., Captopril)
2. Beta blockers, the "olol" drugs (i.e., Metroprolol), should not be used by patients with COPD, because these drugs can cause bronchospasm and wheezing
3. Beta blockers and thiazide diuretics cause the most severe sexual dysfunction

Diuretics

A. Action: increase the excretion of sodium ion and thus increase urine flow
B. Agents

Examples	Adverse Reactions
1. Ethacrynic acid (Edecrin)	Dehydration, thrombosis, emboli, electrolyte imbalance
Furosemide (Lasix)	Acute dehydration, sodium and potassium depletion, calcium loss, dermatitis, blood dyscrasias
2. Thiazide diuretics Bendroflumethiazide (Naturetin) Benzthiazide (Aquatag, Urazide) Chlorothiazide (Diuril) Chlorthalidone (Hygroton) Cyclothiazide (Anhydron) Hydrochlorothiazide (Esidrix, HydroDiuril) Hydroflumethiazide (Saluron) Methyclothiazide (Enduron) Metolazone (Zaroxolyn) Polythiazide (Renese) Trichlormethiazide (Diurese, Naqua)	Fluid and electrolyte imbalance, increased calcium serum levels, gastrointestinal irritation, dizziness, headache, paresthesias, blood dyscrasias, allergy, hypotension

3. Carbonic anhydrase inhibitors

Examples
Acetazolamide (Diamox) Ethoxzolamide (Cardrase, Ethamide)

4. Potassium-sparing diuretics

Examples	Adverse Reactions
Spironolactone (Aldactone)	Hyperkalemia, fatal cardiac dysrhythmias, endocrine alterations, blood dyscrasias
Triamterene (Dyrenium)	

C. Nursing assessment: perform total patient assessment with emphasis on presenting signs and symptoms, vital signs, and laboratory blood studies
D. Nursing management: to foster drug therapy such as by restriction of fluid and diet; monitor weight, intake and output, and vital signs
E. Nursing evaluation: observe for therapeutic effects and adverse reactions; instruct patient regarding drugs and diet, prevention of orthostatic hypotension

Cardiotonic Drugs (Cardiac Glycosides)

A. Action: act directly on myocardial cells to increase contractility and thus cardiac output; slows heart rate
B. Adverse reactions: anorexia, nausea, vomiting, bradycardia, weakness, fatigue, visual dimming, double vision, altered color vision, mood alterations, hallucinations, dysrhythmias
C. Toxic reactions, contusion, heart block, PVCs
D. Agents: the following are examples

Digitoxin (Crystodigin)
Digoxin (Lanoxin)

E. Nursing assessment: obtain baseline data, weight, vital signs, electrocardiogram (ECG) results
F. Nursing management: monitor vital signs, weight, fluid intake and output, serum electrolyte level, especially potassium; instruct patient regarding drugs, eating foods high in potassium
G. Nursing evaluation: observation for therapeutic effects and adverse reactions

Drugs to Control Dysrhythmias

A. Action: slow conduction through atrioventricular (AV) node; block effects of vagal nerve stimulation; block beta adrenergic stimulation; suppress automaticity; increase electrical threshold for stimulation
B. Agents

Examples	Adverse Reactions
Atropine	Dry mouth, cycloplegia, mydriasis, fever, urinary retention
Bretylium tosylate (Bretylol)	Anginal attacks, bradycardia, hypotension
Deslanoside (Cedilanid-D)	Bradycardia, premature ventricular beats, atrioventricular tachycardia, anorexia, nausea, vomiting
Digitoxin (Crystodigin, Purodigin)	
Digoxin (Lanoxin)	
Disopyramide phosphate (Norpace)	Dry mouth, constipation, urinary retention, blurred vision
Lidocaine (Xylocaine without epinephrine)	Muscle twitching, respiratory depression, convulsions, coma
Phenytoin (Dilantin)	Bradycardia, cardiac arrest, nausea, dizziness, drowsiness
Procainamide hydrochloride (Pronestyl)	Hypotension, decreased cardiac output, gastrointestinal distress
Propranolol hydrochloride (Inderal)	Bradycardia, lowered cardiac output, bronchospasm
Quinidine sulfate (Cin-Quin, Quinora)	Peripheral vasodilation, hypotension, gastrointestinal distress
Quinidine gluconate (Duraquin)	
Quinidine polygalacturonate (Cardioquin)	

C. Nursing assessment: obtain baseline data, history of subjective and objective symptoms, vital signs
D. Nursing management: monitor vital signs; instruct patient regarding drugs; maintain therapeutic blood levels by administering around the clock
E. Nursing evaluation: observe for therapeutic effects and adverse reactions

Anticoagulants

A. Action: inhibit the aggregation of platelets; interfere with any of the steps leading to the formation of fibrin
B. Adverse reactions: hemorrhage, hematuria, melena, rashes, depression of bone marrow
C. Agents: the following are examples

1. Antiplatelet drugs
   Aspirin
   Dipyridamole (Persantine)
2. Heparin sodium (Liquaemin Sodium, Panheprin, Lipo-Hepin)
3. Coumarins
   Dicumarol
   Phenprocoumon (Liquamar)
   Warfarin sodium (Coumadin, Panwarfin)
4. Indanediones
   Anisindione (Miradon)
   Enoxaparin (Lovenox)

D. Nursing assessment: obtain baseline data relevant to general condition of the patient, history of problems with clots, and blood coagulation studies: prothrombin time (PT), partial thromboplastin time (PTT), platelet count, and clotting times
E. Nursing management: monitor blood coagulation studies carefully; use infusion monitoring device for constant infusions of heparin; have drug antidotes readily available
F. Nursing evaluation: observe for therapeutic effects and adverse reactions
G. Patient teaching: stress home safety factors to prevent tissue trauma and bleeding; advise to avoid foods high in vitamin K; avoid aspirin, dextran, dipyridamole, and nonsteroidal antiinflammatory drugs that increase risk of bleeding; instruct patient to observe excreta for signs of bleeding
H. Drug interactions
   1. Drugs potentiating response: clofibrate (Atromid S), disulfiram (Antabuse), neomycin sulfate, phenylbutazone (Butazolidin), salicylates, sulfisoxazole (Gantrisin)
   2. Drugs diminishing response: barbiturates, cholestyramine (Questran), ethchlorvynol (Placidyl), glutethimide (Doriden), griseofulvin (Grifulvin-V)
I. Antidotes
   1. Heparin: protamine sulfate
   2. Coumarins: vitamin K

Thrombolytic Drugs

A. Action: promote the digestion of fibrin to dissolve the clot
B. Agents: enzymes urokinase and streptokinase
C. Adverse reaction: hemorrhage
D. Special considerations: reserved for use in acute pulmonary embolism, deep vein thrombosis, or peripheral arterial occlusion; posttreatment: treated with heparin
E. Nursing assessment: obtain baseline data relevant to size, location, and symptoms of clot; vital signs and peripheral pulses for adequate circulation to extremities

F. Nursing management: used only in acute care setting; monitor laboratory blood studies and for signs of clot dissolution
G. Nursing evaluation: observe for therapeutic effects and adverse reactions

Hemostatic Agents

A. Action: inhibit the dissolution of blood clots
B. Adverse reactions: nausea, cramps, dizziness, tinnitus, thrombophlebitis, flushing, vascular collapse
C. Agents

Examples	Clinical Indications
1. Systemic agents	Used in special surgical situations
Aminocaproic acid (Amicar)	
Menadiol sodium diphosphate (Synkayvite)	Correction of secondary hypoprothrombinemia, correction of severe vitamin K deficiency
Menadione sodium bisulfite (Hykinone)	
Phytonadione; vitamin K (AquaMEPHYTON, Konakion, Mephyton)	Oral anticoagulant overdose emergency
2. Local hemostatic agents Absorbable gelatin sponge (Gelfoam)	Control bleeding in wound or at operative site

D. Nursing assessment: obtain baseline data relevant to type, location, and amount of bleeding, appropriate laboratory blood studies, and general condition of patient
E. Nursing management: monitor appropriate laboratory blood studies
F. Nursing evaluation: observe for therapeutic effects and adverse reactions

Drugs That Lower Blood Lipid Levels

A. Action: in general these drugs lower blood lipid concentrations
NOTE: no present proof that lowering blood lipid concentrations will reverse or halt atherosclerosis
B. Adverse reactions: bloating, nausea, constipation, muscle cramps, impotence, flushing, weight loss, insomnia, water retention
C. Agents: the following are examples

Cholestyramine resin (Questran)   Lovastatin (Mevacor)
Colestipol hydrochloride (Colestid)   Niacin; nicotinic acid (Nicobid, Niac, Nicolar)

D. Nursing assessment: obtain baseline data relevant to weight, serum cholesterol and triglyceride levels, blood pressure, and dietary history
E. Nursing management: observe for any new symptoms; instruct patient regarding drugs; restrict intake of fats, cholesterol, and alcohol; stop smoking; follow recommended exercise program

F. Nursing evaluation: observe for adverse effects; monitor blood levels for therapeutic effects

Drugs That Treat Nutritional Anemias

A. Action: supplement or replace essential vitamins and minerals
B. Agents

Examples	Adverse Reactions
1. Iron salts Ferrous sulfate (Feosol, Fer-In-Sol, Fero-Gradumet, Mol-Iron)	Acute toxicity: acute nausea and vomiting, metabolic acidosis, extensive liver and kidney damage
Ferrous gluconate (Fergon, Ferralet Plus, Entron)	Chronic toxicity: bronze coloration of skin, development of diabetes mellitus, heart failure
Ferrocholinate (Chel-Iron, Kelex) Ferrous fumarate (Ferranol, Feostat) Iron dextran injection (Imferon)	
2. Antidote for iron toxicity Deferoxamine mesylate (Desferal)	
3. Vitamin B_{12} Cyanocobalamin (Betalin 12 Crystalline, Redisol, Rubramin PC, Sytobex) Hydroxocobalamin (alphaRedisol)	Virtually free of adverse reactions
4. Folic acid for anemia Folic acid (Folvite) Leucovorin calcium	Nontoxic

C. Nursing assessment: obtain baseline data for vital signs, weight, dietary history, blood studies, and presence of neurological symptoms
D. Nursing management: monitor blood studies, vital signs
E. Nursing evaluation: observe for therapeutic effects and adverse reactions; instruct patient regarding medications; use z-track techniques when injecting iron to avoid staining of skin
F. Patient teaching: expect dark or black stools and the possibility of gastrointestinal distress; nutritionally balanced diet
G. Folic acid has been shown to prevent neural tube defects

GASTROINTESTINAL SYSTEM
Drugs That Increase Tone and Motility

A. Action: cholinomimetic action to stimulate or restore intestinal tone or urinary bladder tone
B. Adverse reactions: salivation, skin flushing, sweating, diarrhea, abdominal cramps
C. Agents: bethanechol chloride (Urecholine); neostigmine methylsulfate (Prostigmin)
D. Nursing assessment: obtain baseline data regarding vital signs, bowel sounds, fluid intake and output, bowel activity

E. Nursing management: stay with patient at least 15 minutes after administration to observe for adverse reactions; monitor vital signs, fluid intake and output, bowel activity
F. Nursing evaluation: observe for therapeutic effects and adverse reactions

Drugs That Decrease Tone and Motility (Anticholinergics)

A. Action: inhibit gastric secretion and depress gastrointestinal motility
B. Adverse reactions: dry mouth, mydriasis, blurred vision, tachycardia, constipation, and acute urinary retention
C. Agents: the following are examples

Atropine sulfate	Homatropine methylbromide (Homapin)
Belladonna extract	Oxyphencyclimine hydrochloride (Daricon)
Belladonna tincture	
Dicyclomine hydrochloride (Bentyl, Di-Spaz)	Propantheline bromide (Pro-Banthine)
Diphemanil methylsulfate (Prantal)	Thiphenamil hydrochloride (Trocinate)
Glycopyrrolate (Robinul)	Tridihexethyl chloride (Pathilon)

D. Nursing assessment: obtain baseline data for vital signs; frequency and character of stools and presence of occult blood in stools; ability to empty bladder
E. Nursing management: monitor vital signs
F. Nursing evaluation: observe for therapeutic effects and adverse reactions; instruct patient regarding medication

Drugs to Treat Ulcers

A. Action
1. Antacids: neutralize gastric hydrochloric acid
2. Anticholinergic drugs: see drugs under the Autonomic Nervous System
3. Antihistamines: block the histamines' receptors and decrease gastric acid production
B. Adverse reactions: constipation, diarrhea; can interfere with absorption of some drugs: tetracycline, digoxin, quinidine
C. Agents (antacids): the following are examples

Aluminum hydroxide (Amphojel)	Aluminum hydroxide / Magnesium hydroxide	(Maalox)
Calcium carbonate (Dicarbosil, Tums)		
Dihydroxyaluminum aminoacetate (Robalate)	Aluminum hydroxide / Magnesium trisilicate	(Trisogel)
Dihydroxyaluminum sodium carbonate (Rolaids)	Aluminum hydroxide gel / Magnesium hydroxide / Simethicone	(Maalox Plus, Mylanta, Gelusil)
Magnesium hydroxide (Milk of Magnesia)		
Aluminum hydroxide / Calcium carbonate / Magnesium hydroxide	(Camalox)	
	Aluminum phosphate gel (Phosphaljel)	
	Magaldrate (Riopan)	

D. Agents (Histamine H$_2$-receptor antagonists): the following are examples

Cimetidine (Tagamet)	Nizatidine (Axid)
Famotidine (Pepcid)	Ranitidine hydrochloride (Zantac)

E. Nursing assessment: obtain baseline data relevant to vital signs, level of consciousness, character and quality of emesis and stool, appropriate laboratory blood studies, abdominal pain, frank bleeding, and occult bleeding
F. Nursing management: monitor vital signs, fluid intake and output, level of consciousness, and character of stools and vomitus; teach that antacids decrease absorption of many drugs including iron, tetracyclines; teach not to take antacids for more than 2 weeks without consulting a physician.
G. Nursing evaluation: observe for therapeutic effects and adverse reactions

Antiemetics

A. Action: control nausea and vomiting by reducing stimulation of labyrinthine receptors; dopamine antagonists, which act on the chemoreceptor trigger zone in the medulla
B. Adverse reactions: drowsiness, blurred vision, dilated pupils, dry mouth, extrapyramidal symptoms
C. Agents: the following are examples

1. Anticholinergics
   Scopolamine hydrobromide

2. Antihistamines
   Dimenhydrinate (Dramamine)
   Diphenhydramine hydrochloride (Benadryl)
   Hydroxyzine pamoate (Vistaril)
   Meclizine hydrochloride (Antivert, Bonine)
   Promethazine hydrochloride (Phenergan)

3. Miscellaneous drugs
   Benzquinamide hydrochloride (Emete-con)
   Diphenidol hydrochloride (Vontrol)
   Trimethobenzamide hydrochloride (Tigan)

4. Dopamine antagonists
   Chlorpromazine hydrochloride (Thorazine)
   Fluphenazine hydrochloride (Prolixin)
   Haloperidol (Haldol)
   Perphenazine (Trilafon)
   Prochlorperazine (Compazine)
   Promazine hydrochloride (Sparine)
   Triflupromazine hydrochloride (Vesprin)

D. Nursing assessment: obtain baseline data regarding vital signs, character and quantity of any emesis, presence of bowel sounds, fluid intake and output
E. Nursing management: monitor vital signs and fluid intake and output
F. Nursing evaluation: observe for therapeutic effects and adverse reactions

Antidiarrhetic Agents

A. Action: decrease tone of small and large bowel; depress smooth muscle contraction; decrease release of acetylcholine; absorb toxins

B. Adverse reactions: respiratory depression, constipation, impaction
C. Agents: the following are examples

Bismuth subsalicylate (Pepto-Bismol)	Loperamide hydrochloride (Imodium)
Codeine phosphate	
Codeine sulfate	
Diphenoxylate hydrochloride with atropine sulfate (Diphenatol, Lomotil, Lofene)	

D. Nursing assessment: obtain baseline data relevant to vital signs, fluid and solid intake and output, nature, and character of stools, skin turgor, fluid and electrolyte balance
E. Nursing management: monitor vital signs, intake and output, frequency and character of stools
F. Nursing evaluation: observe for therapeutic effects and adverse reactions

Laxatives

A. Action: retain water to keep stools large and soft; stimulate motility in large intestine; inhibit reabsorption of water; attract water by osmosis; soften feces
B. Adverse reactions: loss of bowel tone, dehydration, hypokalemia, hyponatremia, malabsorption of fat-soluble vitamins
C. Agents: the following are examples

1. Bulk-forming agents
   Gum karaya
   Plantago seed (psyllium)
   Psyllium hydrocolloid (Effersyllium)
   Psyllium hydrophilic mucilloid (Metamucil)
2. Stimulant cathartics (irritants)
   Bisacodyl (Bisco-Lax, Dulcolax)
   Cascara sagrada
   Castor oil
   Glycerin suppositories
   Phenolphthalein (Ex-Lax, Feen-A-Mint, Phenolax)
   Senna concentrate (Senokot)
   Senna pod
3. Saline cathartics
   Magnesium hydroxide (Milk of Magnesia)
   Magnesium sulfate (Epsom salt)
   Monosodium phosphate (Sal Hepatica)
   Sodium phosphate with sodium biphosphate (Phospho-Soda)
4. Lubricants
   Mineral oil (Agoral Plain, Petrogalar Plain)
5. Fecal softeners
   Docusate calcium (dioctyl calcium sulfosuccinate; Surfak)
   Docusate sodium (dioctyl sodium sulfosuccinate; Colace, Comfolax, D-S-S)
6. Osmotic agents
   Glycerin (Sani-supp)
   Lactulose (Chronulac, Duphalac, Enulose)

D. Nursing assessment: obtain baseline data relevant to vital signs, intake and output, presence of bowel sounds, bowel habits, dietary history, medications
E. Nursing management: monitor diet and fluid intake; instruct patient regarding drugs, and to increase fiber in diet and increase fluid intake

F. Nursing evaluation: observe for therapeutic effects and adverse reactions

ENDOCRINE SYSTEM
Drugs Affecting Pituitary Gland

A. Action
1. Antidiuretic hormone (ADH): increases renal tubule's permeability and thus its ability to reabsorb water
2. Oxytocin: promotes uterine contractions during last stages of labor when cervix is fully dilated
3. Growth hormone: anabolic agent that increases cell size and cell numbers and stimulates linear growth
4. Gonadotropic hormone (GTH): regulates maturation and function of male and female sexual organs
5. Adrenocorticotropic hormone (ACTH): stimulates adrenal cortex to release its hormone
B. Adverse reactions: hyponatremia, water retention, glycosuria, vasoconstriction, nausea
C. Agents

Examples	Clinical Indications
Desmopressin acetate (DDAVP)	Diabetes insipidus
Lypressin (Diapid)	Diabetes insipidus
Posterior pituitary extract (Pituitrin)	Smooth muscle contraction
Vasopressin (Pitressin)	Short-term maintenance of unconscious patient

D. Nursing assessment: obtain baseline data relative to excesses or deficiencies of specific hormone
E. Nursing management: monitor fluid intake and output, laboratory values; instruct patient regarding medications
F. Nursing evaluation: observe for therapeutic effects and adverse reactions

Drugs Affecting Adrenal Glands

A. Action: replace the body's normal amount of hormones; block inflammatory responses; antineoplastic; antagonize autoimmune responses
B. Adverse reactions: impaired glucose tolerance or hyperglycemia; fat deposition; muscle weakness or wasting; peptic ulcer; growth inhibition; mood changes or psychosis; osteoporosis; sodium retention; potassium loss
C. Agents: dosage is individualized to patient and diagnosis; the following are examples

Betamethasone valerate (Valisone)	Methylprednisolone acetate (Depo-Medrol)
Cortisone acetate (Cortone)	Methylprednisolone sodium succinate (Solu-Medrol)
Desoxycorticosterone acetate (Doca, Percorten)	Prednisolone (Delta-Cortef, Paracortol)
Dexamethasone (Decadron, Hexadrol)	Prednisolone sodium phosphate (Hydeltrasol)
Fludrocortisone acetate (Florinef)	Prednisone (Meticorten, Delta-Dome)
Hydrocortisone (cortisol; Cortef, Cortril, Hydrocortone)	Triamcinolone (Aristocort, Kenacort)
Hydrocortisone acetate (Cortef)	Triamcinolone acetonide (Kenalog)
Methylprednisolone (Medrol, Wyacort)	Triamcinolone hexacetonide (Aristospan)

D. Nursing assessment: obtain baseline data relevant to vital signs, weight, glycosuria
E. Nursing management: monitor vital signs, weight, serum electrolyte levels, sugar concentrations in blood and urine, signs of masked infection; instruct patient regarding medications, additive hypokalemia
F. Nursing evaluations: observe for therapeutic effects and adverse reactions

Drugs Affecting Thyroid Gland

A. Action
  1. Hypothyroidism: replace the body's normal amount of hormone
  2. Hyperthyroidism
    a. Control the symptoms of hyperthyroidism
    b. Inhibit the synthesis of thyroid hormones
    c. Inhibit iodine uptake by thyroid gland
    d. Inhibit thyroid hormone release and symptoms
    e. Suppress continued uptake of iodine
    f. Destroy surrounding tissue by emission of low energy radiation
B. Adverse reactions to drugs for hyperthyroidism: agranulocytosis; skin rash, nausea, vomiting, twitching muscles, bronchospasm, iodism, symptoms of hyperthyroidism
C. Adverse reactions to drugs for hypothyroidism: dysrhythmias, hypertension, headache, insomnia, irritability, vomiting, weight loss
D. Agents: the following are examples

1. Hypothyroidism	2. Hyperthyroidism

a. Natural thyroid hormones
  Thyroglobulin (Proloid)
  Thyroid (Delcoid, Thyrar, Thyrocrine)
b. Synthetic thyroid hormones
  Levothyroxine sodium (Eltroxin, Levoid, Synthroid)
  Liothyronine sodium (Cytomel)
  Liotrix (Euthroid, Thyrolar)
c. Adenohypophyseal hormone
  Thyroid-stimulating hormone (TSH) (thyrotropin; Thytropar)
  Protirelin (Thypinone)
	a. Thioamides
	  Methimazole (Tapazole)
	  Propylthiouracil
	b. Beta adrenergic blocker
	  Propranolol hydrochloride (Inderal)
	c. Iodine
	  Potassium or sodium iodide (Lugol's solution)
	d. Radioactive iodine (^{131}I)

E. Nursing assessment: obtain baseline data relevant to vital signs, weight, level of energy, symptoms of hypofunctioning or hyperfunctioning of gland and serum thyroid levels
F. Nursing management: monitor vital signs, weight; instruct patient regarding medications, compliance with therapy
G. Nursing evaluation: observe for therapeutic effects and adverse reactions

Drugs Affecting Parathyroid Gland

A. Action: maintain blood calcium levels in the blood
B. Adverse reactions: nausea, local irritation at injection sites, drowsiness, gastrointestinal complaints, hypertension, facial flushing
C. Agents: the following are examples

Calcitonin (Calcimar)
Calcitriol (Rocaltrol)
Parathyroid hormone

D. Nursing assessment: obtain baseline data relevant to vital signs and blood calcium levels
E. Nursing management: monitor vital signs, blood calcium levels; teach avoidance of spinach, whole grains, and rhubarb and maintaining adequate intake of calcium and vitamin D
F. Nursing evaluation observe for therapeutic effects (i.e., decreased muscle cramping) and adverse reactions; instruct patient regarding medications

FEMALE REPRODUCTIVE SYSTEM
Estrogens

A. Action: replace or supplement natural body hormones; alter cell environment in neoplastic processes
B. Adverse reactions: breast tenderness, increased risk of breast and endometrial cancer, nausea, vomiting, anorexia, malaise, depression, salt and water retention
C. Agents: the following are examples

Chlorotrianisene (TACE)	Estradiol (Estrace)
Diethylstilbestrol (DES) (Stilbestrol)	Estrone (Theelin, Femogen)
Ethinyl estradiol (Estinyl)	Estrogen, conjugated (Premarin)

Progestins

A. Action: suppress endometrial bleeding; withdrawal of drug induces tissue sloughing
B. Adverse reactions: edema, breast tenderness, depression, midcycle bleeding
C. Agents: the following are examples

Medroxyprogesterone acetate (Depo-Provera, Provera)	Megestrol acetate (Megace) Norethindrone (Norlutin, Ortho-Novum)

Fertility Drugs

A. Action: stimulate ovulation by pituitary or ovarian mechanisms
B. Adverse reactions: relatively rare
C. Agents: the following are examples

Clomiphene citrate (Clomid)
Human chorionic gonadotropin (HCG) (Antuitrin S, Follutein)
Menotropins (Perganol)

Contraceptive Drugs

A. Action: suppress ovulation; induce changes in cervical mucus, making uterine entry by sperm difficult; produce changes in endometrium, making implantation difficult

B. Adverse reactions: thromboembolitic diseases, stroke, hypertension
C. Agents: the following examples contain varying amounts of progesterone and estrogen

Brevicon	Ortho-Novum
Depo-provera	Ovrette
Enovid	Ovulen
Norlestrin	

D. Contraceptive effects may be lessened if taken with antibiotics

Oxytocic Drugs

A. Action: induce contraction of the myometrium
B. Adverse reactions: fetal or maternal cardiac dysrhythmias, acute hypertension, nausea, water intoxication, uterine hypertonicity with fetal or maternal injury
C. Agents: the following are examples

Dinoprost tromethamine (Prostin F$_2$ Alpha)	Methylergonovine maleate (Methergine)
Dinoprostone (Prostin E$_2$)	Oxytocin (Pitocin, Syntocinon)
Ergonovine maleate (Ergotrate)	

Uterine Relaxants

A. Action: stimulation of beta-2 adrenergic receptors produces relaxation of uterine muscle
B. Adverse reactions: heart palpitations, nausea, vomiting, trembling, flushing, and headache
C. Agents: ritodrine, terbutaline (Brethine)

Nursing Process

A. Assessment: obtain baseline data relevant to vital signs, weight, current problem; elicit history of previous pregnancies and deliveries, fetal heart tones
B. Management: inform of possible side effects and benefit; monitor vital signs, weight; with oxytocics: maternal and fetal monitoring; infusion monitoring device
C. Evaluation: observe for therapeutic effects and adverse reactions; instruct patient regarding medications

MALE HORMONES
Androgens

A. Action: replace or supplement normal body hormone; relieve postpartum breast engorgement; alter cell environment in neoplastic disease in females
B. Adverse reactions: female masculinization; premature closure of epiphyses in children; nausea, vomiting, diarrhea, mood swing
C. Agents: the following are examples

Danocrine (Danazol)	Testosterone (Delatestryl) (Testaqua, Oreton)
Fluoxymesterone (Halotestin)	
Methyltestosterone (Android)	

Anabolic Steroids

A. Action: increase nitrogen retention and protein formation; stimulate red blood cell formation and increase bone deposition

B. Adverse reactions: increased libido; priapism (continuous erection), female masculinization, precocious sexual development in children, premature epiphyseal fusion
C. Agents: the following are examples

Ethylestrenol (Maxibolin)	Nondrolone phenpropionate (Durabolin)
Methandrostenolone (Dianabol)	Oxandrolone (Anavar)
Methandriol	Stanozolol (Winstrol)

Nursing Process

A. Assessment: obtain baseline data relevant to vital signs, weight, height (children), current problem
B. Management: monitor vital signs, weight, height (children); review possible effects with patient
C. Evaluation: observe for therapeutic effects and adverse reaction; instruct patient regarding medications

THE EYE
Anticholinergic Drugs

A. Action: cause mydriasis (dilated pupils) and cycloplegia (blurred vision)
B. Adverse reaction: dry mouth and skin, fever, thirst, confusion, hyperactivity
C. Agents: the following are examples

Atropine sulfate (Atropisol, Isopto Atropine)	Scopolamine hydrobromide (hyoscine hydrobromide; Isopto Hyoscine)
Cyclopentolate hydrochloride (Cyclogyl)	Tropicamide (Mydriacyl)
Homatropine hydrobromide (Isopto Homatropine, Homatrocel)	

Adrenergic Drugs

A. Action: cause mydriasis
B. Adverse reactions: rare
C. Agents: the following are examples

Phenylephrine hydrochloride (Alconefrin, Mydfrin, Neo-Synephrine Hydrochloride)

Drugs Used to Treat Glaucoma

A. Action: cause miosis (pupil constriction); reduce resistance to outflow of aqueous humor; decrease production of aqueous humor
B. Adverse reactions: blood vessel congestion causing increased intraocular pressure, ocular pain, headache, tachycardia or bradycardia, hypertension, diaphoresis, anorexia, gastrointestinal upset, lethargy, depression, diuresis, dehydration
C. Agents: the following are examples

Acetazolamide (Diamox)	Echothiophate iodide (Phospholine Iodide)
Carbachol (Isopto Carbachol)	Epinephrine bitartrate (Epitrate, Primatene Mist Suspension)
Demecarium bromide (Humorsol)	
Dichlorphenamide (Daranide, Oratrol)	Glycerin (Glyrol, Osmoglyn)
	Isoflurophate (Floropryl)

Isosorbide (Ismotic)
Mannitol (Osmitrol)
Physostigmine sulfate
(Eserine)

Pilocarpine hydrochloride
(Isopto Carpine, Pilocar)
Timolol maleate (Timoptic)
Urea (Ureaphil, Urevert)

Nursing Process

A. Nursing assessment: obtain history of eye-related symptoms such as difficulty in driving or ambulating; examine eyes for signs of infection, exudate, tearing, or drying; assess for eye pain
B. Nursing management: advise patient about effects of drugs such as blurred vision and photophobia; instruct patient regarding drugs (i.e., do not skip doses); teach proper administration of eye medication
C. Nursing evaluation: observe for therapeutic effects and adverse reactions

DRUGS USED TO CONTROL MUSCLE TONE
Acetylcholinesterase Inhibitors (Anticholinergic Agents)

A. Action: allow the accumulation of acetylcholine at neuromuscular junctions and thus ensure muscle contractility; drugs are not used during pregnancy or with patients who have hyperexcitability of muscular symptoms
B. Adverse reactions: muscle cramps, fasciculations (rapid, small contractions), weakness; excessive salivation, perspiration, nausea, vomiting
C. Agents: the following are examples

Ambenonium chloride
(Mytelase)
Edrophonium chloride
(Tensilon)

Neostigmine bromide
(Prostigmin)
Pyridostigmine bromide
(Mestinon, Regonol)

D. Nursing assessment: obtain baseline data relevant to vital signs, ability to swallow, muscle strength, eyelid ptosis, gait, reflexes
E. Nursing management: monitor disease symptoms and vital signs; have suction and intubation equipment at bedside
F. Nursing evaluation: observe for therapeutic effects and adverse reactions

Neuromuscular Blocking Agents

A. Action: produce muscle paralysis
B. Adverse reactions: hypotension, bronchospasm, tachycardia, bradycardia, cardiac dysrhythmias, respiratory distress
C. Agents: the following are examples

Decamethonium bromide
(Syncurine)
Gallamine triethiodide
(Flaxedil)
Pancuronium bromide
(Pavulon)

Succinylcholine chloride
(Anectine Quelicin, Sucostrin)
Tubocurarine chloride
(Tubarine)

D. Nursing assessment: obtain baseline data relevant to pulse, respiration, and blood pressure
E. Nursing management: monitor vital signs; continually assess respiratory status, lung sounds, rate and depth of respirations; have suction and intubation equipment at bedside

F. Nursing evaluation: observe for therapeutic effects: sufficient muscle relaxation to allow procedure to be done; observe for adverse reactions: cough and inability to breathe unassisted and to handle secretions

DIABETES MELLITUS
Insulin

A. Action: restores the cell's ability to use glucose and to correct the metabolic changes that occur with diabetes mellitus
B. Adverse reactions: allergic reactions, insulin resistance, injection site lipoatrophy (Table 3-7)
C. Agents: Table 3-8 lists insulin preparations

Nursing Process

A. Assessment
  1. Obtain baseline data relative to nonfunctioning of the pancreas, vital signs, weight, and blood glucose level
     a. Normal blood glucose level 70 to 120 mg/dl
     b. Glycosylated Hgb may be drawn to evaluate treatment effectiveness; ADA recommends less than 7% for good diabetic control; serious action should be taken when levels rise above 8%
  2. Monitor urine ketones during illness; insulin requirements may increase during stress, infection, or surgery
  3. Assess for signs and symptoms of hypoglycemia and hyperglycemia (see Table 3-7)
B. Interventions
  1. Teach patient to follow recommended diabetic diet and to use exchange system when planning meals
  2. Teach patient techniques for maintaining serum glucose levels, signs and symptoms of hypo- and hyperglycemia, and actions patient should take; physician should be notified if patient unable to eat
  3. Teach patient to carry simple sugar and to wear ID tag describing medication regime
  4. Teach patient the importance of regular exercise, care of feet and nails, self-administration of medications, and rotation of injection sites

ORAL HYPOGLYCEMIC AGENTS
Sulfonylureas

A. Action: stimulate release of insulin from pancreas
B. Adverse reactions: gastrointestinal distress, muscle weakness, parasthesias, skin reactions, hypoglycemia
C. Agents

Examples	Duration of Action
Tolbutamide (Orinase)	6 to 12 hr
Acetohexamide (Dymelor)	12 to 24 hr
Tolazamide (Tolinase)	12 to 24 hr
Glyburide (Micronase)	up to 24 hr
Chlorpropamide (Diabinase)	24 to 72 hr
Glipizide (Glucotrol)	up to 24 hr
Glimepiride (Amaryl)	NA

Biguanides

A. Action: increases the amount of glucose taken up by the muscles and intestinal wall and inhibits hepatic glucose production
B. Adverse reactions: headache, weakness, gastrointestinal distress, thrombocytopenia

TABLE 3-7   Hyperglycemia and Hypoglycemic Reactions

	Hyperglycemia: Ketoacidosis, Diabetic Coma, Too Little Insulin	Hypoglycemia: Insulin Reaction, Too Much Insulin
Onset	Gradual—days	Minutes to hours
Causes	Neglect of therapy, untreated diabetes, intercurrent disease or infection, increase in emotional or psychologic stress	Insulin overdose, omission or delay of meals, excessive exercise before meals
Signs and symptoms	Thirst, headache, excessive urination, nausea, vomiting, abdominal pain, dim vision, coma, flushed face, Kussmaul breathing—rapid, deep—air hunger, dehydration, acetone breath, soft eyeballs, normal absent reflexes	Nervousness, hunger, weakness, cold clammy sweat, nausea, dizziness, double or blurred vision, behavioral changes, stupor, convulsions, pallor, shallow respirations, normal eyeballs, Babinski's reflex may be present
Urine glucose	Positive	Negative or low
Urine acetone	Positive	Negative
Blood glucose	High (above 250 mg)	Low (below 60 mg)
Blood CO_2	Low	Usually normal
Treatment	Insulin, fluid replacement, electrolyte replacement, close observation	Glucose, glucagon, close observation
Response to treatment	Slow	Rapid

C. Agents

Example	Duration of Action
Metformin hydrochloride (Glucophage)	6 to 12 hr

Alpha Glucosidase Inhibitors

A. Action: delays the digestion of ingested carbohydrates; results in a smaller rise in blood glucose after meals; does not increase insulin production
B. Adverse reactions: abdominal pain, diarrhea, flatulence
C. Agents

Examples	Duration
Acarbose (Precose)	4 to 6 hr
Miglitol (Glyset)	4 to 6 hr

Thiazolidinedione

A. Action: Lowers blood glucose by improving tissue response to insulin
B. Adverse reactions: palpitations, increased LDH, nausea, vomiting, diarrhea, anorexia, nephrotoxicity
C. Agents

Example	Duration
Troglitazone (Rezulin)	No data available

Nursing Process Related to All Four Classifications of Oral Hypoglycemic Agents

A. Assessment
   1. Obtain baseline vital signs, weight, blood glucose levels, and other signs and symptoms of the disease
   2. Monitor signs and symptoms of hypo- and hyperglycemia
B. Interventions
   1. Monitor vital signs, blood glucose levels, and other blood levels

   2. Instruct patient on medication administration and how to monitor blood glucose levels; teach that stress, fever, trauma, infection, and surgery may increase requirements for medication or necessitate the need to temporarily switch to insulin
   3. Teach signs and symptoms of hypo- and hyperglycemia and steps to correct
   4. Instruct on the avoidance of alcohol to prevent hypoglycemic reactions
C. Evaluation
   1. Decrease in symptoms associated with diabetes
   2. Blood glucose levels under control

PREVENTION AND TREATMENT OF INFECTIONS (ANTIMICROBIALS/ANTIINFECTIVES)
Penicillins and Cephalosporins

A. Action: bacteriocidal by interfering with the synthesis of the bacterial cell wall
B. Adverse reactions: allergies—rash, anaphylaxis; convulsions with high parenteral doses; gastrointestinal distress—nausea, vomiting, and diarrhea
C. Agents: the following are examples

   1. Penicillins
      Amoxicillin (Amoxil, Larotid, Polymox, Trimox)
      Ampicillin (Amcill, Omnipen, Polycillin, Principen)
      Carbenicillin disodium (Geopen)
      Cloxacillin sodium (Cloxapen, Tegopen)
      Dicloxacillin sodium (Dycill, Dynapen)
      Methicillin sodium (Celbenin, Staphcillin)
      Nafcillin sodium (Nafcil, Unipen)
      Oxacillin sodium (Bactocill, Prostaphlin)
      Penicillin G potassium (Pentids, Pfizerpen)
      Penicillin G benzathine (Bicillin)

TABLE 3-8   Characteristics of Insulin Preparations After Subcutaneous Administration

Insulins*	Onset (hr)	Peak Effect (hr)	Duration of Action (hr)
Rapid Acting			
Insulin injection (Regular Insulin, Humulin R)†	½–1	2–4	5–7
Intermediate Acting			
Isophane insulin suspension (NPH Insulin)	3–4	6–12	18–28
Insulin zinc suspension (Lente Insulin)	1–3	8–12	18–28
Long Acting			
Extended insulin zinc suspension (Ultralente)	4–6	18–24	36
Combinations			
Isophane human insulin (50%) & human insulin (50%) (Humulin 50/50)	½	3	22–24
Isophane human insulin (70%) & human insulin (30%) (Humulin 70/30, Novalin 70/30)	½	4–8	24

From McKenry LM, Salerno E: *Pharmacology in nursing,* ed 20, St Louis, 1998, Mosby.
*Semilente insulin is available in Canada but is no longer available in the United States. Onset of action of Semilente insulin is 1–3 hr, peak effect is in 2–8 hr and duration of action is 12–16 hr.
†These insulins may be administered intravenously. Intravenously, the onset of action is within ⅙ to ½ hr, peak effect within ¼ to ½ hr, and duration of action within ½ to 1 hr.

Penicillin G procaine
(Crysticillin,
Duracillin, Wycillin)
Penicillin V
(Pen Vee K,
V-Cillin, Veetids)
Ticarcillin (Ticar)
Ticarcillin with
Clavulanate
(Timentin)

2. Cephalosporins
Cefaclor (Ceclor)
Cefamandole nafate
(Mandol)
Cefazolin sodium
(Ancef, Kefzol)
Cefoxitin (Mefoxin)
Cephalexin (Keflex)
Cephaloridine
(Loridine)
Cephalothin sodium
(Keflin)
Cephapirin sodium
(Cefadyl)
Cephradrine (Anspor,
Velosef)

D. Clinical indications
  1. Wound and skin infections
  2. Respiratory infections
  3. Prophylaxis for patients with rheumatic fever or congenital heart disease
  4. Gram-positive infections caused by streptococci and some staphylococci
  5. Gram-negative infections caused by *Haemophilus influenza, Escherichia coli,* and *Neisseria gonorrhoeae*
E. Patient teaching
  1. Importance of compliance and completing full therapeutic course
  2. Signs and symptoms of super infection
    a. Vaginal irritation, itching, discharge
    b. Black tongue, furry overgrowth
    c. Loose, foul-smelling stools

Erythromycin, Clindamycin (Penicillin Substitutes)

A. Action: bacteriostatic or bacteriocidal (dosage related) by inhibiting protein synthesis

B. Adverse reactions: abdominal discomfort, cramping, nausea, vomiting, diarrhea, urticaria, anaphylaxis, colitis, liver dysfunction, deafness (vancomycin), permanent kidney damage (systemic bacitracin, vancomycin); Hismanal and Propulsid have the potential to cause fatal dysrythmias when taken with erythromycin
C. Agents: the following are examples

  1. Erythromycins
    Erythromycin (E-Mycin,
    Ilotycin, Robimycin,
    RP-Mycin)
    Erythromycin estolate
    (Ilosone)
    Erythromycin
    ethylsuccinate (E.E.S.)
    Erythromycin stearate
    (Erythrocin)
  2. Clindamycins/lincomycins
    Clindamycin (Cleocin)
    Lincomycin hydrochloride
    (Lincocin)

  3. Penicillin substitutes
    Bacitracin
    Novobiocin sodium
    (Albamycin)
    Spectinomycin hydro-
    chloride (Trobicin)
    Vancomycin
    hydrochloride
    (Vancocin)

D. Clinical indications
  1. See clinical indications for penicillins
  2. Used for patients allergic to penicillin

Tetracyclines and Chloramphenicol

A. Action: bacteriostatic by preventing the start of protein synthesis (tetracyclines) or inhibiting protein synthesis (chloramphenicol)
B. Adverse reactions
  1. Tetracyclines: nausea, vomiting, stomach pain, diarrhea, superimposed infections, impaired kidney functions, jaundice, delayed blood coagulation, brown discoloration of teeth in children under 8 years of age; tetracyclines are known teratogen and should not be given if pregnancy suspected

2. Chloramphenicol: bone marrow toxicity, aplastic anemia, allergies, gastrointestinal irritation, headache, mental confusion, depression

C. Agents: the following are examples

Chloramphenicol (Chloromycetin)	Methacycline hydrochloride (Rondomycin)
Chlortetracycline hydrochloride (Aureomycin)	Minocycline hydrochloride (Minocin, Vectrin)
Demeclocycline hydrochloride (Declomycin)	Oxytetracycline hydrochloride (Terramycin)
Doxycycline hyclate (Vibramycin, Doxychel)	Tetracycline hydrochloride (Achromycin, Panmycin, Sumycin, Tetracyn)

D. Clinical indications
 1. Gram-negative and gram-positive infections
 2. Severe acne vulgaris
 3. Used for patients allergic to penicillin

Aminoglycosides and Polymyxins

A. Action
 1. Aminoglycosides: inhibit early stages of protein synthesis
 2. Polymyxins: alter bacterial cell membrane permeability
B. Adverse reactions: eighth cranial nerve damage, renal damage, respiratory paralysis
C. Agents: the following are examples

1. Aminoglycosides Amikacin sulfate (Amikin) Gentamicin sulfate (Garamycin) Kanamycin sulfate (Kantrex) Neomycin sulfate (Mycifradin, Neobiotic)	Streptomycin Tobramycin sulfate (Nebcin) 2. Polymyxins Colistimethate sodium (Coly-Mycin M) Colistin sulfate (Coly-Mycin S) Polymyxin B sulfate (Aerosporin)

D. Clinical indications: drugs are potentially dangerous and are used only in cases of severe infections, such as gram-negative bone and joint infections and septicemia

Sulfonamides, Trimethoprim, Nitrofurantoins, Nalidixic Acid, Fluoroquinolones

A. Action: block bacterial synthesis of folic acid; inhibit bacterial enzymes required for proper metabolism of sugar; interfere directly with DNA synthesis
B. Adverse reactions
 1. Sulfonamides, trimethoprim, nitrofurantoins: allergies, nausea, vomiting, diarrhea, stomatitis, blood dyscrasias, renal calculi, and hematuria
 2. Nalidixic acid: convulsions, mental instability, headache, dizziness, visual disturbances, photosensitivity
 3. Fluoroquinolones: precautions in children; ciprofloxacin should not be given to children under 18 years of age

C. Agents: the following are examples

1. Sulfonamides Sulfadiazine (microsulfon) Sulfameter (Sulla) Sulfamethizole (Microsul, Thiosulfil, Forte) Sulfamethoxazole (Gantanol) Sulfamethoxazole-phenazopyridine (Azo Gantanol) Sulfamethoxypyridazine acetyl (Midicel) Sulfasalazine (Azulfidine, Salazopyrin) Sulfisoxazole (Gantrisin, Rosoxol, Sulfalar) Sulfisoxazole-phenazopyridine hydrochloride (Azo Gantrisin, SK-Soxazole, Azosul)	2. Sulfonamides: topical agents and solutions Mafenide (Sulfamylon) Silver sulfadiazine (Silvadene) Sulfacetamide sodium (Sulamyd) Sulfisoxazole diolamine (Gantrisin Ophthalmic) 3. Trimethoprim (Proloprim, Trimpex) 4. Nitrofurantoin (Furandantin, Furalan, Nephronex) Nitrofurantoin macro-crystals (Macrodantin) 5. Nalidixic acid (NegGram) 6. Fluoroquinolones Ciprofloxacin hydrochloride (Cipro)

D. Clinical indications
 1. Used to treat acute and chronic urinary tract infections
 2. Other uses include trachoma, chancroid, toxoplasmosis, acute otitis media, and prophylactic therapy in cases of recurrent rheumatic fever
 3. Treatment of ulcerative colitis
 4. Prophylaxis for patients scheduled for bowel surgery (to prevent renal calculi, teach patient to maintain fluid intake of 2000 to 3000 ml/day)
 5. Mafenide and silver sulfadiazine used topically for burn patients; apply Silver sulfadiazine sparingly to a thickness of $\frac{1}{16}$ of an inch
 6. Ciprofloxacin effective against flu, *Staphylococcus, Pseudomonas;* less effective against *Streptococcus*

Drugs Used to Treat Tuberculosis and Leprosy

A. Action: alter several metabolic processes in mycobacteria
B. Adverse reactions: peripheral neuropathies, visual disturbances, gastrointestinal distress, ototoxicity, headache
C. Agents: the following are examples

1. First-line antitubercular drugs Ethambutol hydrochloride (Myambutol) Isoniazid (Isotamine, Niconyl, Nydrazid) Para-aminosalicylic acid (PAS) (aminosalicylic acid, Teebacin acid) Rifampin (Rifadin, Rimactane) Streptomycin	2. Second-line antitubercular drugs Capreomycin (Capastat) Cycloserine (Seromycin) Ethionamide (Trecator S.C.) Pyrazinamide 3. Antileprosy agents Clofazimine (Lamprene) Dapsone (Avlosulfon) Rifampin (Rifadin, Rimactane) Sulfoxone sodium (Diasone)

D. Patient teaching: stress importance of long-term compliance and follow-up visits with the physician; report any adverse reactions promptly; refrain from using alcohol; refrain from taking other medications without the knowledge and permission of the physician; wear a medical identification tag indicating medication being taken

Antifungal Drugs

A. Action: selectively damages the membranes of fungi
B. Adverse reactions: renal damage, anemia, nausea, diarrhea
C. Agents: the following are examples

1. Systemic agents
   Amphotericin B (Fungizone)
   Flucytosine (Ancobon)
   Hydroxystilbamidine isethionate
   Miconazole (Monistat-IV)
2. Topical agents
   Acrisorcin (Akrinol)
   Amphotericin B (Fungizone)
   Candicidin (Vanobid)
   Clioquinol (Vioform)

   Clotrimazole (Gyne-Lotrimin, Lotrimin)
   Griseofulvin (Fulvicin-P/G, Grifulvin V, Grisactin)
   Haloprogin (Halotex)
   Miconazole nitrate (MicaTin, Monistat)
   Nystatin (Mycostatin, Nilstat)
   Tolnaftate (Aftate, Tinactin)
   Undecylenic acid—zinc undecylenate (Desenex, Ting, Cruex)

D. Patient teaching: proper administration of vaginal tablets, use of condom by sexual partner to avoid reinfection

Drugs Used to Treat Viral Diseases

A. Action: selective toxicity in various processes of virus reproduction
B. Adverse reactions: ataxia, slurred speech, lethargy, local irritation, anorexia, nausea, vomiting, diarrhea, dizziness, headache, anemia and bone marrow suppression (zidovudine), bone marrow depression (ganciclovir), visual haze, irritation, burning of eyes, photophobia (idoxuridine)
C. Agents: the following are examples

Acyclovir (Zovirax)
Amantadine (Symmetrel)
Ganciclovir (DHPG)
Idoxuridine (Dendrid, Herplex Liquifilm, Stoxil)

Methisazone
Vidarabine (Vira-A)
Zidovudine (AZT, Retrovir)

D. Clinical indications: zidovudine used in treatment of AIDS; prevents replication of HIV virus, thus delaying disease progression

Antiprotozoal and Anthelmintic Agents

A. Action: destroy the protozoa and helminths at various stages of development
B. Adverse reactions: gastrointestinal distress, flatulence, vision changes, irritability, hemolysis, skin eruptions, blood dyscrasias
C. Agents: the following are examples

1. Amebic infestations
   Chloroquine phosphate (Aralen)
   Diloxanide (Furamide)

   Emetine hydrochloride
   Iodoquinol (Yodoxin)
   Metronidazole (Flagyl)

2. Malaria
   Amodiaquine hydrochloride (Camoquin)
   Chloroquine hydrochloride (Aralen)
   Primaquine phosphate
   Quinine
3. Others
   Povidone-iodine (Betadine, Proviodine)
   Quinacrine hydrochloride

4. Anthelmintics
   Mebendazole (Vermox)
   Niclosamide (Yomesan)
   Piperazine citrate (Antepar)
   Pyrantel pamoate (Antiminth)
   Pyrvinium pamoate (Povan)

Nursing Process

A. Nursing assessment: obtain history of allergies; evaluate baseline data relevant to signs and symptoms of infection, vital signs, pertinent laboratory tests, appearance of wounds, incisions, or lesions, amount and description of drainage, swelling, erythema, subjective symptoms of pain or pressure
B. Nursing management: obtain culture for specimens before starting antibiotics; maintain supportive measures such as rest, comfort, nutrition, fluids and electrolyte balance; maintain proper administration regarding route, time, and dosage; monitor vital signs and laboratory results
C. Nursing evaluation: observe for therapeutic effects and adverse reactions; instruct patient regarding medications to ensure compliance

NEOPLASTIC DISEASES
Specific Antineoplastic Agents

A. Action: selective toxicity during various stages of the cell cycle
B. Agents

Examples	Adverse Reactions
Asparaginase (Elspar)	Central nervous system depression
Bleomycin sulfate (Blenoxane)	Pulmonary toxicity, skin reactions
Busulfan (Myleran)	Bone marrow and kidney toxicity
Calusterone (Methosarb)	Mild virilism, edema, hypercalcemia, nausea, vomiting
Carmustine (BiCNU)	Bone marrow suppression, nausea
Chlorambucil (Leukeran)	Bone marrow suppression
Cisplatin (Platinol)	Renal damage, nausea and vomiting, ototoxicity, neurotoxicity, and anaphylactic reactions
Cyclophosphamide (Cytoxan)	Hemorrhagic cystitis, bladder fibrosis
Cytarabine (Cytosar-U)	Bone marrow suppression
Dacarbazine (DTIC-Dome)	Bone marrow suppression
Dactinomycin (Cosmegen)	Bone marrow suppression, gastrointestinal irritation, skin reactions
Diethylstilbestrol diphosphate (Stilphostrol)	Risk of thromboembolic disease, edema, mood changes

Examples	Adverse Reactions
Doxorubicin hydrochloride (Adriamycin)	Bone marrow suppression, gastrointestinal distress, alopecia
Dromostanolone propionate (Drolban)	Mild virilism, edema, hypercalcemia
Estradiol (Progynon)	Risk of thromboembolic disease, edema, mood changes
Etoposide	Bone marrow suppression
Floxuridine (FUDR)	Gastrointestinal and hematological toxicity
Fluorouracil (5-FU, Adrucil)	Gastrointestinal and hematological toxicity
Hydroxyurea (Hydrea)	Bone marrow suppression
Lomustine (CeeNU)	Myelosuppression, nausea
Mechlorethamine hydrochloride or nitrogen mustard (Mustargen)	Bone marrow suppression
Medroxyprogesterone (Depo-Provera)	Menstrual irregularities, rashes, and thromboembolic diseases
Megestrol acetate (Megace)	Thromboembolic disease
Melphalan (Alkeran)	Leukopenia, anemia, menstrual irregularities
Mercaptopurine (Purinethol)	Hematologic toxicity, immunosuppression
Methotrexate	Gastrointestinal toxicity, bone marrow suppression, immunosuppression
Mitomycin (Mutamycin)	Bone marrow suppression, gastrointestinal irritation, alopecia, renal toxicity
Mitotane (Lysodren)	Gastrointestinal disturbances, skin reactions
Plicamycin (mithramycin; Mithracin)	Gastrointestinal, skin, liver, and kidney toxicity
Polyestradiol phosphate (Estradurin)	Risk of thromboembolic disease, edema, mood changes
Prednisone (Deltasone, Panasol, Meticorten)	Cushing's syndrome
Procarbazine hydrochloride (Matulane)	Bone marrow suppression, gastrointestinal disturbances
Tamoxifen citrate (Nolvadex)	Hot flashes, nausea, vomiting
Teniposide	Bone marrow suppression
Testolactone (Teslac)	Pain and irritation at injection site, hypercalemia
Thioguanine	Hematologic toxicity
Thiotepa	Bone marrow toxicity
Vinblastine sulfate (Velban)	Peripheral neuropathy and bone marrow suppression
Vincristine sulfate (Oncovin)	Alopecia, abdominal pain, peripheral neuropathy

C. Nursing assessment: obtain baseline data regarding possible adverse reactions of drugs; evaluate condition of hair, skin, nails, weight, vital signs and necessary blood laboratory studies (especially WBC, RBC, and platelet count)

D. Nursing management: monitor weight, vital signs, and laboratory studies; institute regular inspection of mouth; maintain good medical asepsis; use infusion monitoring device for IV administration; provide patient/family teaching and psychological support; check hydration status

E. Nursing evaluation: observe for therapeutic effects and adverse reactions

Biological Modifiers

A. Action: stimulates proliferation and differentiation of neutrophils; a glycoprotein; to decrease infection in patients receiving antineoplastics; To increase WBC in patients with drug induced neutropenia

B. Adverse reactions: fever, nausea, diarrhea, anorexia, alopecia, skeletal pain

C. Agent: filigrastin (Neupogen)

D. Nursing assessment: monitor blood studies, check vital signs baseline and during treatment, assess for bone pain

E. Evaluation: absence of infection

Hormones

A. Action: one factor controlling rate of red cell production; anemia caused by reduced endogenous erythropoietin production; primarily end stage renal disease and anemia caused by chemotherapy

B. Adverse reactions: seizures, coldness, sweating, headache, hypertension, bone pain

C. Agent: epoetin alfa (Eprex)

D. Assessment: assess for CNS symptoms, monitor blood studies

E. Evaluation: increased appetite, increase in RBCs in 1 to 2 weeks

NUTRIENTS, FLUIDS, AND ELECTROLYTES

Substances required for human nutrition include water, carbohydrates, proteins, fats, vitamins, and minerals; necessary to maintain health, prevent illness, and promote recovery from illness

Nutritional Products: Oral and Tube Feedings

A. Nutritionally complete formulas
   1. Action
      a. Provide United States Recommended Dietary Allowance for protein, minerals, and vitamins
      b. Provide 1 calorie per milliliter (Sustagen: 1.84 cal/ml)
   2. Agents: the following are examples

Compleat-B	Osmolite
Ensure	Sustacal
Isocal	Sustagen
Meritene	

B. Nutritional agents for limited use
   1. Vital H.N.: contains easily digested forms of protein, carbohydrate, and fat; used for critically ill patients
   2. Lofenalac: a low-phenylalanine preparation used for infants and children with phenylketonuria (PKU)

3. MBF (Meat Base Formula): hypoallergenic infant formula for those who are allergic to milk or have galactosemia
4. Neo-Mull-Soy, Pro Sobee, Isomil: soybean products used as hypoallergenic, milk-free formulas
5. Pregestimil: infant formula containing easily digested protein, fat, and carbohydrate; used in infants with diarrhea or malabsorption syndromes
6. Vivonex: nutritionally complete diet containing amino acids as its protein

C. Nutritionally incomplete supplements
1. Amin-Aid: source of protein for patients with renal insufficiency
2. Casec: carbohydrate calories supplement
3. Lipomul: unsaturated fat supplement
4. Liprotein: high caloric and protein oral supplement for use in burn or debilitated patients
5. Lonalac: milk substitute for sodium-restricted diets
6. Probana: iron-free, high-protein formula for infants and children with diarrhea or malabsorption syndromes

D. Complete infant formulas
1. May be used alone for bottle-fed babies or to supplement breast-fed babies, similar to human breast milk; iron deficient
2. Preparations: Enfamil and Similac are examples

Intravenous Fluids

A. Dextrose injection: contains 2.5%, 5%, 10%, 20%, 40%, 50%, 60%, and 70% dextrose, the 20% to 50% solutions are used for calories in total parenteral nutrition (TPN) and administered through a central or subclavian catheter
B. Dextrose and sodium chloride injection: most commonly used concentrations are 5% dextrose in 0.25% or 0.45% sodium chloride
C. Amino acid solution (Aminosyn): contains essential and nonessential amino acids; most often used with dextrose in TPN
D. Liposyn, Intralipid: concentrated calories and essential fatty acids; most often used as part of TPN

Vitamins

A. General information
1. Group of substances that act as coenzymes to help in the conversion of carbohydrate and fat into energy and to form bones and tissues; necessary for metabolism of fat, carbohydrate, and protein; normally obtained from foods
2. Subclassified as
   a. Fat soluble: A, D, E, K
   b. Water soluble: B complex, C

B. Agents
1. Fat-soluble vitamins: the following are examples

Vitamin A (Alphalin, Aquasol A)
Vitamin E (Tocopherol, Aquasol E)
Vitamin K Menadiol sodium diphosphate (Synkayvite)
Phytonadione (Mephyton, AquaMEPHYTON)

2. Water-soluble vitamins: the following are examples
B-complex

Calcium pantothenate (B$_5$) (Pantholin)
Cyanocobalamin (B$_{12}$) (Rubramin PC, Betalin 12)
Folic acid (Folvite)
Niacin
Pyridoxine hydrochloride (B$_6$) (Hexa-Betalin)
Riboflavin (Riobin-50, B$_2$)
Thiamine hydrochloride (B$_1$) (Betalin S)

2. Vitamin C: ascorbic acid

Minerals and Electrolytes

A. General information: basic constituents of living tissues and components of many enzymes; function to maintain fluid, electrolyte, and acid-base balance; maintain muscle and nerve function; assist in transfer of materials across cell membranes and contribute to the growth process
B. Agents: the following are examples

Deferoxamine mesylate (Desferal)
Ferrous gluconate (Fergon)
Ferrous sulfate (Feosol)
Iron dextran injection (Imferon)
Magnesium sulfate
Potassium bicarbonate—potassium citrate (K-Lyte)
Potassium chloride (Kay Ciel, K-Lor)
Potassium gluconate (Kaon)
Sodium bicarbonate
Sodium polystyrene sulfonate (Kayexalate)

Multiple Mineral-Electrolyte Preparations

Normosol-R
Pedialyte (oral)
Plasma-Lyte 56
Plasma-Lyte 148
Polysal M
Ringer's lactate

Nursing Process

A. Nursing assessment: obtain baseline data with emphasis on presenting signs and symptoms, vital signs, and laboratory blood studies
B. Nursing management: perform nursing actions to foster drug therapy; monitor diet and laboratory blood studies
C. Nursing evaluation: observe for therapeutic effects specific to type of nutrient supplement; instruct patient regarding medications and diet

SUGGESTED READINGS

Clayton BD, Stock YN: *Basic pharmacology for nurses,* ed 11, St Louis, 1997, Mosby.
Edmunds MW: *Introduction to clinical pharmacology,* ed 2, St Louis, 1998, Mosby.
Harkness GA, Dincher JR: *Medical-surgical nursing: total patient care,* ed 10, St Louis, 1999, Mosby.
Lilley LL, Aukers RS: *Pharmacology and the nursing process,* ed 2, St Louis, 1998, Mosby.
McKenry LM, Salerno E: *Mosby's pharmacology in nursing,* ed 20, St Louis, 1998, Mosby.
Physicians' Desk Reference, ed 54, Montvale, 2000, Medical Economics Company.
Potter PA, Perry AG: *Fundamentals of nursing,* ed 4, St Louis, 1997, Mosby.
Skidmore-Roth L: *Mosby's drug guide for nurses,* ed 3, St Louis, 1999, Mosby.

REVIEW QUESTIONS

1. When a patient experiences an effect from a medication that is an unknown effect of the drug, but is considered peculiar to that patient, it is referred to as a(n):
   ① Additive effect
   ● Idiosyncratic effect
   ③ Synergistic effect
   ④ Antagonistic effect

2. To obtain fastest absorption and action from a medication, the nurse knows it should be administered:
   ① By mouth
   ② Intramuscularly
   ③ Subcutaneously
   ● Intravenously

3. The process by which drugs are inactivated by the body is:
   ① Absorption
   ② Distribution
   ● Metabolism
   ④ Excretion

4. In relation to drugs, the term *blood level* refers to the:
   ① Metabolism of the drug
   ② Excretion of the drug
   ● Amount of the drug in the circulating fluids
   ④ Effect of the drug on the red blood cells

5. Drugs absorbed into the bloodstream and circulated to various parts of the body are said to have a:
   ● Systemic effect
   ② Local effect
   ③ Palliative effect
   ④ Curative effect

6. A student nurse questions the nurse as to why the patient has 20 mEq of KCL in his IV. The nurse explains the purpose and then refers the student to which of the following lab tests?
   ● Electrolytes
   ② Glucose
   ③ Hemoglobin
   ④ Arterial blood gases

7. A patient on outpatient anticoagulant therapy asks why he has to have blood drawn every week. The most appropriate answer the nurse should give is:
   ① "The doctor needs to know if the infection is improving."
   ● "The doctor adjusts your dose to help you maintain a therapeutic level."
   ③ "The doctor needs to know if the medication is working."
   ④ "We don't want the medicine to become toxic."

8. A patient asks the nurse why he is receiving patches of nitroglycerin instead of just taking it under the tongue when he needs it. The nurse explains that:
   ● "Given in this manner the medication is absorbed at a slow, steady rate."
   ② "This manner is effective in acute situations."
   ③ "This manner allows for more accurate dosage."
   ④ "Patches administer a day's to a week's worth of medication."

9. A cancer patient has been on high doses of morphine for several days. During an assessment the side effect that the nurse would be likely to see is:
   ● Constipation
   ② Respiratory depression
   ③ Pain relief
   ④ Diarrhea

10. When a mydriatic eye medication is being administered the nurse will observe for:
    ① Decreased drainage
    ② Constriction of the pupil
    ● Dilation of the pupil
    ④ Decreased intraocular pressure

11. A patient is just beginning a drug withdrawal program. Which signs are the nurse likely to observe during the first few days?
    ① Constipation and lethargy
    ● Runny nose and diarrhea
    ③ Back pain and irritability
    ④ Muscle rigidity and headache

12. Which of the following medications would decrease the absorption of cimetidine (Tagamet)?
    ① Heparin
    ② Morphine
    ● Tetracycline
    ● Dilantin

13. The physician has ordered Mycostatin 5 cc swish and swallow bid. The nurse should instruct the patient to do the following:
    ① "Swallow the medication quickly and follow with 8 ounces of water."
    ② "Shake the bottle before administering to help mix the suspension."
    ③ "Brush your teeth carefully before each dose."
    ● "Maintain contact with the mucosa as long as possible before swallowing."

14. The most serious reaction to anticoagulant therapy is:
    ① Rapid fall in blood pressure
    ② Formation of thrombi in major blood vessels
    ● Hemorrhage
    ④ Infection

15. A drug used topically to treat glaucoma is:
    ● Timolol (Timoptic)
    ② Atropine (atropine sulfate)
    ③ Tubocurarine (Tubarine)
    ④ Vasopressin (Pitressin)

16. Toxic effects of digitalis occur more rapidly when body stores of which of the following ions are depleted?
    ① Sodium
    ● Potassium
    ③ Calcium
    ④ Chloride

17. Sublingual administration of drugs:
    ① Is an alternative if medications are irritating to the gastrointestinal tract
    ② Is absorbed primarily in the small intestine
    ③ Allows for a delayed absorption by bypassing the GI tract
    ● Can be used for only a limited number of drugs

18. The patient who understands proper self-administration of cimetidine (Tagamet) will take the medication:
    ① With a liquid antacid preparation
    ● After meals and at bedtime
    ● With meals and at bedtime
    ④ Only when the patient has gastric distress

19. The nurse will know that the patient understands teaching done about self-administration of oral corticosteroids when the patient states she will take the medication:
① Before meals
❷ With or after meals
③ At bedtime
④ With orange juice

20. The patient suffering from salicylate (aspirin) poisoning is most likely to complain that:
① "My head hurts all the time."
② "My stools are hard and tarry."
③ "I'm beginning to have diarrhea."
❹ "I hear ringing in my ears."

21. A patient confides to the nurse that she has been taking Seconal for many years to help her sleep. She wants to stop taking pills and return to a natural sleep. The most important assessment for the nurse at this time is to recognize that:
① The patient is addicted
❷ Discontinuing the drug must be gradual to avoid withdrawal symptoms
❸ Medical supervision is needed at this time
④ Sleeping is difficult for many people when they reach middle age

22. The daughter of a diabetic patient is learning to administer insulin to her mother at home. The nurse will teach the daughter to:
① Give the insulin intramuscularly
② Use a 1½ inch needle
❸ Rotate injection sites
④ Massage insulin into tissues

23. After assessment of lab work the physician orders two units of packed red blood cells for a patient. The nurse knows that the test that the physician used to assess the need for RBCs was:
① Blood glucose
② Electrolytes
❸ Hemoglobin and hematocrit
④ Specific gravity

24. If 7.5 L of a medication is ordered by the physician, the nurse will safely administer:
① 75 ml
② 0.075 ml
③ 750 ml
❹ 7500 ml

25. A physician prescribes 5 ml of cough medicine every 4 hours prn. The nurse explains to the patient that this dose is approximately equal to:
① 2 tablespoons
② 2 teaspoons
③ 1 ounce
❹ 1 teaspoon

26. Foods to avoid when patients are receiving an MAO-inhibitor drug include:
❶ Aged cheese, coffee, chocolate
② Poultry, bananas, eggs
③ Green leafy vegetables, raisins, milk
④ Pork, pickles, whole wheat bread

27. A 19-year-old patient has been given naloxone HCL (Narcan) to overcome a narcotic overdose. The nurse knows that the expected action of the drug is to:
① Induce hypertension
② Induce hypotension
❸ Reverse CNS/respiratory depression
④ Prevent arrhythmias

28. A nurse is making a home visit to care for a patient with COPD. When she arrives at the home, she finds that the couple has a big box of medications that are all mixed together and some of them are outdated. The first priority should be to:
❶ Examine all the labels to determine which ones are still viable
② Question the couple to see what medications they are taking
❸ Report the situation to her supervisor so that she can contact the physician
④ Contact the social worker to begin placement proceedings for the couple

29. Estrogen (Premarin) is contraindicated in patients with a history of:
① Allergies
② Ulcers
❸ Breast cancer
④ Obesity

30. 7.5 mg of iron is ordered every day via a peg tube. The liquid container is labeled 5 mg per 10 cc. How many ml are correctly administered?
① 5 cc
❷ 15 cc
③ 7.5 ml
④ 10 ml

31. An intravenous infusion is ordered at 50 cc per hour with a drip factor of 60. How many drops per minute should be infusing?
① 60
② 25
❸ 50
④ 30

32. A patient in the emergency room is going to be intubated. A medication used to produce muscular relaxation is:
① Epinephrine (Adrenalin)
❷ Pancuronium bromide (Pavulon)
③ Isoproterenol hydrochloride (Isuprel)
④ Propranolol (Inderal)

33. The nurse is going to give a subcutaneous injection to a 42-year-old patient. The needle length and gauge the nurse will use is:
① 19 gauge: 1½ inch
② 22 gauge: 1 inch
③ 24 gauge: 1 inch
❹ 25 gauge: ⅝ inch

34. The doctor has ordered secobarbital (Seconal) 100 mg hs for a 27-year-old patient. The apothecary equivalent for this dose is:
① gr v
❷ gr iss
③ gr iii
④ gr 1/150

35. The nurse will watch a patient receiving a cholinergic drug for which of the following side effects?
❶ Increased peristalsis
② Decreased peristalsis
❸ Increased urine output
④ Decreased urine output

36. Which of the following diagnoses would be a potential contraindication for prescribing amytriptyline (Elavil)?
① Diabetes
② Emphysema
③ Peripheral vascular disease
● Benign prostatic hypertrophy

37. To assess the therapeutic effectiveness of a parkinsonian drug, the nurse will observe the patient's:
① Increased sleep patterns
● Increased ability to ambulate and speak
③ Decreased emotional stability
④ Decreased caloric and nutritional intake

38. An alcoholic is going through withdrawal. Which of the following medications would be the treatment of choice?
● Diazepam (Valium), vitamins B₁ and B₁₂, and folic acid
② Aspirin, calcium, and Tigan
③ Vitamin C, aspirin, and calcium
④ Vitamins B₁ and B₂ and aspirin

39. Spironolactone (Aldactone) is often prescribed for children with congestive heart failure because it is a(an):
● Potassium-sparing diuretic
② Loop diuretic
③ Thiazide carbonic anhydrase inhibitor diuretic
④ Osmotic diuretic

40. A patient with emphysema is taking a bronchodilator. Which of the following instructions/statements would be appropriate for the nurse to give the patient?
● "Increase fluids to 2000–3000 ml every day."
② "Take medication with food."
③ "Slow-release tablets may be chewed."
④ "Antibiotics will decrease action of these drugs."

41. A patient being treated for obesity would use which of the following classifications of medications?
① H₂ histamine blockers
② Tranquilizers
● Amphetamines
④ Antacids

42. When administering a buccal tablet the nurse will tell the patient to:
① Chew the tablet
② Swallow the tablet with water
③ Let the tablet dissolve under the tongue
● Let the tablet dissolve between the cheek and the gum

43. The patient with glaucoma should *not* receive:
● Atropine sulfate
② Morphine sulfate
③ Meperidine hydrochloride (Demerol)
④ Hydroxyzine hydrochloride (Vistaril)

44. A patient has been on phenytoin (Dilantin) for several months and her seizures are well controlled. Which of the following statements indicates the need for further teaching?
① "I understand that I need to continue taking folic acid supplements."
● "I cannot wait to stop taking this medication."
③ "I take my medication with a glass of orange juice every day."
④ "I always wear my identification tag."

45. A 66-year-old patient with pain associated with angina pectoris is given sublingual nitroglycerin. The nurse knows this medication will:
● Dilate blood vessels and increase circulation
② Inhibit the pain sensors in the brainstem
③ Increase respirations and cause drowsiness
④ Dull nerve endings in the myocardium

46. A patient is being treated with methyldopa (Aldomet). A key nursing intervention is:
① Give on a full stomach
② Give early in AM
● Take blood pressure sitting, standing, and lying
④ Take an apical and radial pulse

47. A newly diagnosed diabetic asks why she should not rub the injection site after self-administration. The nurse replies:
① "The insulin is irritating to the tissues."
② "It will delay absorption."
● "It will speed up absorption."
④ "It does not hurt. There is no need to rub."

48. A patient is receiving temazepam (Restoril) 0.015 g po at bedtime for insomnia. The label indicates 15 mg tablets. How many tablets will the nurse give?
● 1
② 1.5
③ 2
④ 2.5

49. A nurse is assessing signs of alcohol withdrawal in one of her patients. These assessments would show:
● Tremors, anxiety, increased blood pressure
② Thirst, excessive sleeping, bradycardia
③ Polyuria, nausea, headache
④ Increased respirations, decreased blood pressure, rigidity

50. While the nurse administers the daily dose of furosemide (Lasix) to the patient, the opportunity arises for patient teaching. Which of the following should the nurse be sure to stress?
① "Take the medicine at bedtime."
② "You may need sodium and potassium supplements."
● "Weigh yourself twice a day."
● "Change positions slowly to prevent dizziness."

51. Early signs of digoxin toxicity are:
① A sustained pulse rate above 60 beats/min
● Nausea and vomiting
③ Diarrhea and rectal bleeding
④ Elevated respiration and blood pressure

52. Which of the following statements by a patient taking phenytoin (Dilantin) indicates the need for further teaching by the nurse?
① "Now that I have been taking my medication for 6 weeks, I should start to see a decrease in seizures."
② "I have to visit the dentist more often."
● "I always take my pill in the morning with a glass of milk."
④ "The doctor says I need blood tests."

53. Decadron is best given:
① On an empty stomach
② With a full glass of water
● With a full glass of milk
④ At night

54. A 9-year-old patient was recently started on methylphenidate (Ritalin) for ADD. On his follow-up office visit his mother reports to the nurse that he is having difficulty sleeping. The nurse knows:
① Ritalin needs to be given early in the day because insomnia is a side effect.
② Children with ADD are frequently hyperactive and this is probably why he can't sleep.
③ The patient may be taking in too much caffeine each day.
④ The patient may need an increase in his Ritalin dose.

55. A child in school is experiencing an acute hypersensitivity reaction after having accidentally ingested a peanut product. The drug treatment that is indicated in this situation is:
① Gentamicin sulfate (Garamycin)
② Prednisone (Deltasone)
③ Epinephrine (Adrenalin)
④ Guaifenesin (Robitussin)

56. Hydroxyzine (Vistaril) is ordered preoperatively for a patient. The assessment that would indicate to the nurse that this medication is effective would be:
① The patient reports decreased anxiety
② The patient complains of thirst
③ The patient is sleeping soundly
④ The patient is able to urinate

57. An 89-year-old male is complaining of urinary retention. During the medication history, which of the following assessments would be a priority to report to the physician?
① Baclofen (Lioresal)
② Diazepam (Valium)
③ Benztropine (Cogentin)
④ Cyclobenzaprine hydrochloride (Flexeril)

58. A patient on morphine is experiencing nausea and vomiting. Which medication might the physician order to alleviate these symptoms?
① Docusate sodium (Colace)
② Loperamide (Immodium)
③ Trimethobenzamide (Tigan)
④ Atropine sulfate (Atropine)

59. Theophylline (Theolair) has been prescribed for a 48-year-old patient with asthma. You are teaching her about the medication. Which of the following statements by the patient indicates she has correct understanding of the medication's action?
① "This medication should relieve the tightness when I breathe."
② "I'm so fortunate to be on a medication that will cure my asthma."
③ "My mucus should be a lot thinner with this medication."
④ "This medication should help my runny nose."

60. A 72-year-old patient with osteoarthritis has been taking nabumetone (Relafen) for 6 weeks. She complains to the nurse that she feels a gnawing feeling in her stomach that doesn't go away for any length of time and that it seems to be getting worse. The nurse calls the doctor and he discontinues the drug. The nurse will:
① Tell the patient that nabumetone (Relafen) can cause ulcers
② Observe the patient for continuance of her symptoms

③ Give the patient other NSAIDs with food
④ Monitor the patient for the presence of occult blood in the stools

61. A postpartum patient is experiencing uterine atony. Which of the following medications would the physician add to the intravenous infusion?
① Depo-provera
② Brevicon
③ Brethine
④ Oxytocin

62. The controlled analgesic most effective for a harsh, nonproductive cough is:
① Codeine
② Ibuprofen (Motrin)
③ Meperidine (Demerol)
④ Dextromethorphan (Romilar)

63. A patient complains to the office nurse that he is experiencing nausea and muscle cramps. He states "I feel like I always have a virus but it never develops." The nurse recognizes that these symptoms might be as a result of which of the following medications that the patient has just started taking?
① Ibuprofen (Motrin)
② Diazepam (Valium)
③ Loratidine (Claritin)
④ Lovastatin (Mevacor)

64. A nurse cautions a student to remain silent during the induction of anesthesia because:
① The physician needs to be able to concentrate
② The physician needs to explain the procedure to a medical student
③ The patient may be able to hear during the procedure
④ Excessive noise may interfere with the induction of the anesthesia

65. The 70-year-old patient is receiving aminophylline. The nurse knows the medication will act to:
① Dilate blood vessels increasing capillary permeability
② Increase contraction of the bronchi and alveoli
③ Decrease contraction of the smooth muscle
④ Decrease the amount of mucous secretion from the bronchi

66. An adverse reaction to atropine sulfate that may be serious for patients with underlying heart disease is:
① Delirium
② Tachycardia
③ Constipation
④ Dry mouth

67. In an attempt to stop a spontaneous abortion, the physician has ordered terbutaline (Brethine), a uterine relaxant for the patient. Adverse reactions the nurse will be alert for are:
① Heart palpitations, nausea, vomiting, headache
② Drowsiness, incoordination, gastrointestinal upset
③ Sedation, dry mouth, blurred vision, urinary retention
④ Anxiety, apprehension, headache, cerebral hemorrhage

68. Diazepam (Valium) is given for treatment of status epilepticus. The nurse knows its expected action is to:
① Decrease anxiety
② Relieve pain
③ Lower neuron excitability
④ Induce sleep

69. A medication used to treat bipolar disorder is:
① Diazepam (Valium)
② Epinephrine (Adrenalin)
❸ Lithium carbonate (Lithium)
④ Propranolol (Inderal)

70. When a nurse is giving dietary instructions appropriate to a person on calcitonin (Calcimar), it would be especially important to include the following:
❶ "Maintain adequate intake of calcium and vitamin D."
② "Increase fiber whole grains and rhubarb."
③ "Increase intake of vitamin C."
④ "Maintain appropriate calories to avoid gaining weight."

71. An athlete asks the school nurse why it is so dangerous to use steroids to increase athletic ability. The nurse explains that the drugs:
① Stimulate red blood cell formation
② Are difficult to withdraw from and a tolerance may develop
③ Are illegal if given without a prescription
❹ Are a risk for many adverse side effects, including cardiac failure

72. It is important to teach patients who are taking sulfonamide to do the following:
① Take the medication early in AM to prevent nocturia
② Take a laxative if constipation develops as an adverse effect
❸ Drink 2000–3000 ml of fluid every day to prevent kidney stones
④ Take at hour of sleep to enhance rest

73. Chloramphenicol (Chloromycetin) is not recommended for long-term use because it has been implicated in the development of:
① Diabetes
② Tuberculosis
❸ Aplastic anemia
④ Acne vulgaris

74. A patient explains to the nurse that she has been taking Sudafed for her allergies for the past several weeks. At first the medication was working very well, but within the past few days her nasal stuffiness and sneezing has returned worse than it was before. The nurse suspects that the patient may have developed which of the following effects?
① Antagonistic effect
② Decreased tolerance
❸ Rebound congestion
④ Worsening allergies

75. A patient in the intensive care unit goes into life-threatening cardiogenic shock. The primary effect that the nurse would look for after a norepinephrine bitartrate (Levophed) drip is initiated on an infusion pump is:
① Decreasing hyperventilation
② Decreasing polyuria
❸ Increasing blood pressure
④ Increasing orientation

76. An evaluation that is of particular importance when a patient is taking ergoloid mesylates (Hydergine) would be:
① Improvement in cardiac rate and rhythm
❷ Improvement in color and temperature of extremities
③ Improvement in labored breathing
④ Increased urinary output

77. A patient has been on lovastatin (Mevacor) for 6 weeks. What is one method that is used to evaluate its effectiveness?
① Monitoring the CBC
② Monitoring blood glucose
③ Monitoring electrolytes
❹ Monitoring cholesterol

78. When a 23-year-old mother asks about giving an antibiotic ordered by the physician for her child after signs and symptoms of the infection have disappeared, the nurse will tell her to:
① Discard what is left
❷ Finish what is left of the drug
③ Save what is left
④ Call the physician

79. An antibiotic used topically in burn treatment is:
① Tetracycline (Achromycin)
❷ Silver sulfadiazine (Silvadene)
③ Claithromyesin (Biaxin)
④ Sulfasoxizole (Gantrisin)

80. A medication is commonly given z-track when it:
❶ Is irritating to surrounding tissues
② Cannot be given intramuscularly
③ Has to be given around the clock
④ Has to be given for a rapid effect

81. A patient being treated for asthma is interviewed by the nurse in a physician's office. He is jittery and complaining of nausea. A statement that might indicate a cause for the jitteriness would be:
① "I have been taking diazepam (Valium) for my nerves."
❷ "I am overdue to have a theophylline level drawn."
❸ "I am taking cimetidine (Tagamet) for my epigastric pain."
④ "I take a laxative when I am constipated."

82. A patient is beginning treatment with isocarboxazid (Marplan) for depression. Which of the following statements should be of most concern to the nurse?
① "I like to take my pills with food so I remember."
② "I am starting to be able to do things again."
❸ "I love to have a glass of red wine with dinner."
④ "I am trying to lose weight."

83. During a postpartum assessment the patient says to the nurse, "I wish I could stop taking a pill every day to prevent having another baby for a while." Which medication should the physician prescribe for the patient?
① Mestranol (Enovid)
② Diethylstilbestrol (DES)
❸ Medroxyprogesterone (Depo-Provera)
④ Oxytocin (Pitocin)

84. A patient who has been on hydrocortisone (Cortisol) for an extended period of time should be monitored for which of the following adverse reactions?
① Hypoglycemia
② Anemia
③ Increased clotting time
❹ Hyperglycemia

85. A patient who has been on phenytoin (Dilantin) for 1 week is very upset and states, "I don't understand why I am still having seizures." The nurse explains:
① "We may need to speak with the physician about changing your medication."
❷ "Therapeutic effectiveness may take several weeks."
③ "Maybe we need to add an additional medication."
④ "Improvement will be gradual."

86. A patient who has been on Claritin for allergy relief for several weeks complains to the nurse that the medication is no longer working. The nurse suspects that the patient may have developed a:
❶ Tolerance
② Cumulation
③ Synergistic reaction
④ Antagonistic effect

87. A child is being treated with Ritalin. How would the therapeutic effectiveness be evaluated?
❶ Less hyperactivity and a more normal attention span
② Decreased irritability and a more normal sleep pattern
③ Decreased headache pain and a more normal appetite
④ Decreased nausea and vomiting

88. A nurse is obtaining the medication history of a newly admitted client. The client has been on Zoloft for 14 days. Which of the following effects would be observed if the drug is therapeutic?
① Absence of diarrhea
② Decreased nausea and vomiting
❸ Decreased depression
④ Decreased insomnia

89. Which of the following signs is the most significant assessment of a possible allergic reaction to a blood transfusion?
① Elevated temperature
② Moist cough
❸ Difficulty breathing
④ Muscular cramping

90. During an admission interview the nurse learns that a patient has been on dipyridamole (Persantine) for several months. This assessment is an indication for:
① Assessing respirations after activity
❷ Monitoring blood pressure sitting, standing, and lying
③ Assessing temperature every 4 hours
④ Monitoring WBCs to check for infection

91. Patients receiving vancomycin (Vancocin) via intravenous infusion should be assessed prior to administration and during the administration for:
① Blurred vision
② Constipation
❸ Hearing damage
④ Muscle cramps

92. A nurse assesses that a diabetic patient is reporting increased episodes of hypoglycemia. Which of the following is the likely explanation?
① Decreasing usual exercise patterns without changing insulin
② Increasing caloric intake without changing insulin
③ Increased exercise patterns with a decreased insulin dose
❹ Decreased caloric intake and increased exercise pattern

93. A troche would most likely be ordered for which of the following assessments?
① An allergic reaction causing respiratory difficulty
❷ A persistent sore throat
③ Complaints of vaginal itching
④ A stomach upset

94. A nurse is interviewing a client concerning her medication history. The patient denies taking any "over-the-counter" medicines. The nurse then asks about dietary habits. The patient removes a bottle of Pepto Bismol from her purse and states she has been taking this "food" for years for her stomach pain. She also has a bottle of vitamin pills, which she takes for her "eyes." The first priority for the nurse at this point is:
① The need to assess the "stomach pain"
② Ask the patient what foods irritate her stomach
③ Investigate what might be wrong with her eyes
❹ Explain to the patient that these are considered medications and investigate further

95. The nurse is taking an admission history for a person being seen by a physician for an initial visit. Which of the following statements most indicates the need for further investigation?
① "Once in a while when I get constipated I take a laxative."
❷ "I have been on aldactone for many years."
③ "I am a fanatic about taking a vitamin every day."
❹ "I have been taking famotidine (Pepcid) almost every day for a month."

96. A patient on digoxin therapy is experiencing a toxic side effect. The nurse recognizes that this would most likely be:
① Tachycardia
❷ Muscle cramps
❸ Green-yellow vision
④ Decreased blood pressure

97. A patient is taking thyroglobulin (Proloid) for the treatment of hypothyroidism. Adverse reactions that the nurse should instruct the client to report include:
① Weight gain and sleeping patterns increased
❷ Headache and insomnia
③ Bronchospasm and iodism
④ Hypotension and lethargy

98. How would the effect of a person being treated with clomiphene citrate (Clomid) be measured?
① Decreased blood pressure
❷ Pregnancy
③ Decreased vaginal bleeding
❹ Decreased menstrual cramps

99. A major adverse reaction the nurse will observe for in a cancer patient receiving antineoplastic drugs is:
❶ Bone marrow depression
② Oliguria
③ Lethargy
④ Photosensitivity

100. A poisonous effect of a drug, either from a regular dose or an overdose, is referred to as a(an):
① Side effect
❷ Untoward effect
❸ Toxic action
④ Idiosyncratic action

101. Which of the following assessments concerning an intravenous infusion would be a priority to report to the charge nurse?
    ① The drops are falling too slowly
    ❷ There is a small, reddened area near the insertion site
    ③ The infusion slows when the patient bends his arm
    ④ The piggyback infusion is complete
102. A student complains to the school nurse about redness and irritation on her toes. After assessment and consulting with the physician, they suspect athlete's foot. The nurse suggests to the student that she apply a topical ointment called Tinactin. The nurse explains to the student that this is:
    ① An antiviral agent and will inhibit the viruses from reproducing
    ② Antibacterial and has a bacteriocidal action
    ❸ Antifungal and selectively damages the membrane of the fungi
    ④ Soothing and will help relieve the itching and irritation
103. A hospitalized patient is being treated for malaria. The drug that the physician uses for treatment is:
    ① Chlorambucil (Leukeran)
    ② Zidovudine (AZT)
    ❸ Quinine sulfate (Quinine)
    ④ Asparaginase (Elspar)
104. A nurse is admitting a patient diagnosed with deep vein thrombosis. He is starting treatment with intravenous coagulation therapy. Which of the following assessments is most important to report to the physician?
    ① The patient takes psyllium (Metamucil) occasionally for constipation
    ❷ The patient uses ketoprofen (Orudis) for the treatment of osteoarthritis
    ③ The patient takes loratidine (Claritin) for the treatment of allergies
    ④ The patient takes nifedipine (Procardia) for the treatment of hypertension
105. Cough medicine should:
    ① Always be given prior to any other medication
    ② Be followed by water to facilitate absorption
    ❸ Be given last and not followed by liquid to increase effect
    ④ Always be given on a scheduled basis
106. A physician orders an intravenous infusion of 3000 cc of D5RL for his patient over the next 24 hours. The drip factor for the tubing is 10. How many drops per minute will deliver the correct amount of fluid?
    ① 10 gtts/min
    ② 28 gtts/min
    ❸ 21 gtts/min
    ④ 60 gtts/min
107. A nurse is administering an antibiotic to an elderly patient at midnight. The patient refuses to take the medication, stating, "I already received my pills before I went to sleep." The most appropriate action for the nurse to take is:
    ① Verify that the medication order is current and correct
    ② Explain to the patient that the physician has ordered the medication to cure his infection

③ Explain to the patient that he received his sleeping pill prior to going to sleep
④ Check previous documentation to be certain that the time of administration was not changed by the previous shift
108. A 1-day postoperative laparotomy patient is quiet, lying on his side splinting his incision with a pillow. He has not had any pain medication in 8 hours. A nurse who has just started her shift asks the patient if he has any pain. The patient says yes and rates it as a 9 on a scale of 1 to 10. The nurse administers the ordered pain medication. What would be the most appropriate action for the nurse to take in 1 hour?
    ❶ Assess the effectiveness of the medication on a scale of 1 to 10
    ② Encourage the patient to ask for medication prior to the pain becoming severe
    ③ Ask the patient why he waited so long and did not request pain medication
    ④ Obtain an order to administer pain medication around the clock and not on a PRN basis
109. A clinic nurse is concerned when a client diagnosed with active TB returns to the clinic after 2 weeks of treatment and reports a worsening cough and reoccurring night sweats. These findings most likely indicate:
    ❶ Noncompliance with medication regimen
    ② Additional exposure to infected individuals
    ❸ The need for additional medication
    ④ The need for follow-up care for family members
110. A dialysis patient is placed on a 1200 cc fluid restriction in 24 hours. The best allocation for the fluid would be:
    ❶ 600 ml on 7-3 shift, 400 ml on 3-11 shift, and 200 ml on 11-7 shift
    ② 500 ml on 7-3 shift, 500 ml on 3-11 shift, and 200 ml on 11-7 shift
    ③ Drink liquids only at mealtimes
    ④ As long as there is 100 ml left for meds, the patient should regulate his or her own fluids
111. The difference between a sedative and a hypnotic is:
    ❶ Dose
    ② Time of administration
    ❸ None
    ④ Length of effect
112. A medication used in the treatment of Parkinson's disease is:
    ① Methylphenidate (Ritalin)
    ② Carbamazepine (Tegretol)
    ❸ Benztropine mesylate (Cogentin)
    ④ Theophylline (Accurbron)
113. A 31-year-old patient who is experiencing nausea and vomiting has an elevated temperature. The nurse will give the antipyretic:
    ① Orally
    ❷ Rectally
    ③ Sublingually
    ④ Topically
114. Patients with increased intracranial pressure are treated with which of the following medications?
    ① Morphine sulfate
    ② Hydrochlorothiazide

❷ Decadron
④ Heparin

115. The nurse expects a placebo to be effective because of the:
❶ Production of endorphins in the brain
❷ Nurturing attitude of the nurse
③ Action of the active drug in the placebo
④ Patient's ability to metabolize the placebo

116. A patient has been on cromolyn (Intal) for 6 weeks. How would the therapeutic effects of this medication be measured?
① Decreased severity of symptoms during asthmatic attacks
❷ Decreased number of asthmatic attacks
③ Improvement in ability to sleep through the night
④ Decreased heart rate during exercise

117. Which of the following statements made during an assessment should indicate to the nurse that the physician may prescribe sulfisoxazole (Gantrisin)?
❶ "I have had urinary frequency and burning for the past 2 days."
② "I am allergic to penicillin."
③ "I have had a runny nose for 3 days."
④ "I have loose, foul-smelling diarrhea."

118. The nurse will do a daily assessment of the integrity of the oral mucosa when the patient is receiving:
① Antibiotics
❷ Cancer drugs
③ Antiparkinsonian drugs
④ Vitamins

119. The law that regulates the manufacture, distribution, advertisement, and labeling of drugs to ensure safety and effectiveness is the:
① Harrison Narcotic Act
② Consumer Protection Act
③ Controlled Substance Act
❹ Federal Food, Drug and Cosmetic Act

120. A patient who had received an overdose of insulin would be exhibiting which of the following symptoms?
① Hyperpnea, drowsiness, fever
② Pallor, fatigability, dizziness
❸ Nervousness, anxiety, diaphoresis
④ Flushed skin, nausea, vomiting

121. The nurse knows that an 80-year-old patient on medication would be prone to which of the following?
① Developing a tolerance to medication
② Metabolizing medications more rapidly
③ Developing more frequent adverse reactions
❹ Experiencing more cumulative effects

122. A 28-year-old patient with hyperthyroidism is placed on phenobarbital to achieve which of the following effects?
❶ Sedation
② Control of seizures
③ Vasoconstriction
④ Vasodilation

123. A pediatric nurse is interviewing a 10-year-old child and her parents. The parents tell the nurse that the child has been irritable and unable to sleep well in recent weeks. Which of the following indications might be a contributing factor?
① Taking amoxicillin (Augmentin) for an ear infection

② Taking Pepto-Bismol for an upset stomach
❹ Taking loratidine (Claritin) for her allergies
④ Taking guaifenesin (Robitussin) for an upper respiratory infection

124. Many drugs have "anticholinergic" side effects. Examples of these effects would include:
❶ Dryness of the mouth and constipation
② Increased salivation and diarrhea
③ Polyuria and thirst
④ Tachycardia and diarrhea

125. A patient is being treated with pyrostigmine (Mestinon) for myasthenia gravis. How would the nurse evaluate the therapeutic effectiveness of this medication?
① Decreased arrhythmias
② Decreased nausea and vomiting
③ Increased perspiration
❹ Increased muscle strength

126. A 62-year-old patient has an attack of acute angina. The nurse knows that the treatment of choice will be:
① Calcium channel blockers
② Beta adrenergic blockers
❸ Nitrates
④ Narcotic analgesics

127. A 3-year-old patient has been receiving high dosages of metaclopramide (Reglan) for side effects associated with chemotherapy. The nurse is reinforcing home care instructions related to adverse medication effects. Which of the following symptoms should be reported to the health care provider immediately?
① Mild sedation and fatigue
❷ Rigidity and tremors
❸ Constipation and dry mouth
④ Headache and insomnia

128. A patient is experiencing hives in an allergic reaction. Which of the following reports would indicate that diphenhydramine (Benadryl) is showing its desired therapeutic effect?
① Improved vision
❷ Decreased pruritis
③ Decreased muscle cramps
④ Decreased headache

129. A medication given as a thrombolytic agent within 4 hours after a witnessed myocardial infarction to dissolve the clot is:
❶ Streptokinase (Streptase)
② Heparin (Heparin Sodium)
③ Phytonadione (Aquamephyton)
④ Aminocaproic acid (Amicar)

130. The drug of choice for the treatment of acute pancreatitis is:
① Morphine (Morphine Sulphate)
❷ Meperidine (Demerol)
③ Erythromycin (E-mycin)
④ Dexamethasone (Decadron)

131. The type of insulin used in emergency situations of hyperglycemia is:
① NPH
❷ Regular
③ Lente
④ Ultralente

132. A nurse is preparing supplies for a TB screening program. She should be certain that which of the following syringes are available in ample supply?
① 22-gauge, 1½-inch needle
② 25-gauge, ⅝-inch needle
❸ 27-gauge, ½-inch needle
④ 20-gauge, 2-inch needle

133. A nurse is administering amoxicillin by mouth to a 3-year-old child diagnosed with an ear infection. The most appropriate approach with the child would be to:
① Give a detailed explanation to the child as to why he needs this medicine
❷ Explain it is time to take your "pink medicine"
③ Have the parent hold the child in his or her arms and inject it quickly into his mouth
④ Administer the medication in 240 cc of apple juice

134. A drug used as a substitute for morphine in the management of addiction is:
① Meperidine
② Narem
❸ Methadone
④ Talwin

135. Doses of warfarin sodium (Coumadin) are ordered on the basis of measurement of the patient's:
① Clotting time
❷ Prothrombin time
③ Bleeding time
④ Capillary fragility testing

136. A patient who is in the 40th week of pregnancy is receiving an IV administration of oxytoxin (Pitocin). The nurse knows the drug is expected to:
❶ Produce rhythmic contractions of uterine muscle fibers
② Relax smooth muscle fibers of the cervix
③ Initiate vigorous sustained contractions of the abdominal muscles
④ Produce relaxation of vaginal walls and perineal muscles

137. A nurse is preparing to administer a vitamin B₁₂ injection IM to an average-weight person. The length and gauge of the needle selected should be:
① 25-gauge, 2-inch needle
② 27-gauge, ½-inch needle
③ 20-gauge needle, 3-inch needle
❹ 22-gauge needle, 1-inch needle

138. Standard precautions are mandatory during the administration of parenteral medications. The nurse knows that this requires:
① That hands must be washed between patients and before procedures
② The need for protection depends on the potential exposure to infected body fluids
❸ The need to wash hands before and to wear gloves during administration
④ The need to wear gloves depends on the patient's diagnosis

139. Enteric-coated medications are ordered for the following purpose:
① Allow the medicine to remain in the stomach longer
❷ Allow for delayed absorption in the small intestine
③ Allow for time-released absorption by having a more gradual release
④ Prevent irritation in the small intestine

140. A patient with diabetes mellitus is being treated with metformin (Glucophage). The nurse understands that the action of this medication is to:
① Improve the breakdown of fats and proteins for use as energy
② Decrease the amount of glucose taken up by the muscles and decreases cellular resistance to insulin
③ Replace insulin not being produced by the pancreas
❹ Increase the amount of glucose taken up by the muscles and intestine and decreases cellular resistance to insulin

141. A patient visits the physician's office for treatment of gastroesophageal reflux disease (GERD). Along with a regimen of antacids an additional prescription that may be prescribed is:
❶ Bethanechol (Urecholine)
② Atropine (Atropine Sulfate)
③ Pilocarpine (Isoptocarpine)
④ Loperamide (Immodium)

142. An asthmatic patient is taking cromolyn sodium (Intal). Monitoring the therapeutic effectiveness would involve:
❶ Observing a decreased severity of symptoms during attack
❷ A decrease in the number and severity of attacks
③ An increase in coughing and sputum production
④ A decrease in the number of upper respiratory infections

143. The patient is to receive an intravenous infusion of lactated Ringer's at 75 m/hr. The drop factor is 20 gtts/ml. The nurse will run the IV at:
① 5 gtt/min
② 15 gtt/min
❸ 25 gtt/min
④ 35 gtt/min

144. A postoperative patient receives 5000 units of heparin (Heparin Sodium) SC bid. The dosage available is 10,000 units per milliliter. The correct amount of medication to be administered is:
① ¼ cc
❷ ½ cc
③ 1 cc
④ 2 ml

145. Atropine ¹⁄₁₅₀ grain is ordered as a preoperative medication. On hand is 0.4 mg per cc. The appropriate amount of fluid to be administered is:
① ½ ml
❷ 1 ml
③ 2 ml
④ ¼ ml

146. A nurse is assisting at a clinic where a 3-month-old infant is required to have an intramuscular injection. The most appropriate site for this injection is:
❶ Vastus lateralis
② Dorsogluteal
③ Deltoid
④ Ventrogluteal

147. Which of the following is effective in the treatment of status epilepticus?
❶ Diazepam
② Hydroxyzine
③ Meprobamate
④ Chlordiazepoxide

148. A patient is being treated in the hospital for an infection that a culture has shown to be positive for MRSA (methycillin-resistant *Staphylococcus aureus*). The nurse knows that the medication most likely to be effective is:
① Penicillin
② Streptomycin
③ Acyclovir
❹ Vancomycin

149. The patient has been taking Reserpine for 12 weeks to treat hypertension. His blood pressure today is 150/92. During the assessment the patient says he has become impotent. He is disturbed and asks what he can do. Which of the following is the *best* nursing response?
① Refer the patient to a psychologist
② Set up a meeting with the wife and husband
❸ Refer the patient to his physician
④ Refer the patient to a discussion group

150. A nurse is caring for a cancer patient undergoing chemotherapy. The patient's white blood cell count is low. The physician would most likely place him on which of the following medications?
① Epoetin alfa (Epogen)
② Vancomycin (Vancocin)
❸ Filgrastim (Neupogen)
④ Vincristine (Oncovin)

151. A nurse is assisting in planning the teaching for a newly diagnosed 15-year-old patient with diabetes. An important consideration for this age group is:
① These individuals need to do things well and develop a sense of self-worth
❷ Adolescents determine identity through role models and peer pressure
③ This group establishes long lasting relationships
④ It is important to allow them to verbalize accomplishments in life

152. Amitriptyline (Elavil) is indicated in the treatment of:
① Euphoria
❷ Depression
③ Confusion
④ Hallucinations

153. A patient with a history of treatment for glaucoma should not be treated with cholinergic blocking agents because:
① This classification of medications decreases intraocular pressure
② They may be absorbed systemically and cause cardiac irregularities
❸ This classification of medications increases intraocular pressure
④ There is a danger of electrolyte imbalances

154. The nurse has been monitoring a patient in his home. Two weeks ago, he was diagnosed with active tuberculosis. Which of these statements would be most indicative that he has an understanding of his treatment?
① "I am so glad that the treatment is over so that I can go back to work."
❷ "I will need support and assistance to take this medication for such a long time."
③ "I have to learn to eat healthier foods."
④ "As long as I am no longer contagious, it is alright for my friends to visit."

155. On a busy surgical unit the common practice is to leave the narcotic keys in a locked utility room where the narcotic box is located. A new graduate is concerned because:
❶ Narcotic keys should be carried with a nurse at all times
② Too many people know the combination to the room
③ All controlled substances have to be signed and accounted for at the end of each shift
④ The pharmacist is responsible for dispensing appropriate medications

156. A patient is being cared for 8 hours after a laminectomy. Morphine sulphate is ordered every 3 hours subcutaneously for moderate to severe postoperative pain. The patient is rating his pain at an 8. It has been 1 hour since his last dose. The first intervention that should be completed by the nurse is:
① Explain to the patient that he will have to wait, because it has only been an hour since his last dose
② Document the pain level at 8 and notify the charge nurse
③ Turn the patient using the log-rolling technique and reposition him on his side
❹ Assess the location and characteristics of the pain

157. A statement that would most indicate that an adolescent is beginning to understand his diagnosis of insulin-dependent diabetes mellitus would be:
① "I am going to hang out with my friends like I always did."
② "Swimming is an important part of my life."
❸ "Watching my diet and taking medication is a drag."
④ "I hate being different from my friends."

158. When teaching self-administration of a diuretic, the nurse will tell the patient to:
① Take the diuretic at bedtime
② Cut down on fluid intake
❸ Take the diuretic after rising
④ Stop taking the diuretic when feeling better

159. When administering an intramuscular injection, the nurse will aspirate after insertion of the needle to:
❶ Avoid injecting the drug directly into the bloodstream
② Ease the patient's discomfort
③ Facilitate absorption into the bloodstream
④ Avoid injuring organs

160. The nurse will administer thyroid drugs:
❶ In a single dose, usually before breakfast
② In divided doses, before meals
③ In divided doses, after meals
④ As the patient's energy level decreases

161. When administering a bulk-forming laxative such as psyllium husk (Metamucil) the nurse will give it:
① At bedtime
② With meals
❸ With a full glass of water
④ With an antacid

162. To instill ear drops in the adult patient, the ear canal is opened by pulling the ear:
❶ Up and back
② Down and back
③ Up and forward
④ Back and forward

163. Emergency treatment of hyperinsulinism consists of administering:
    ① Glucose intravenously
    ② Insulin hypodermically
    ③ Epinephrine (Adrenalin) intramuscularly
    ④ High-caloric liquids by gavage feedings

164. When teaching self-administration of eye drops to a patient, the nurse will stress that the correct method for instilling eye drops is to drop the medication on the:
    ① Eyeball itself
    ② Inner canthus of the eye
    ③ Lower conjunctival sac
    ④ Outermost point of the eye

165. A 72-year-old patient is exhibiting signs of digoxin toxicity. The nurse will:
    ① Give the drug if the apical rate is above 60 beats/min and report to the physician
    ② Omit the drug, take the apical rate, and report to the physician
    ③ Administer an antacid with the digoxin
    ④ Administer oxygen by nasal cannula with the digoxin

166. The physician's order reads to administer 3 L of 5%D/0.45% normal saline IV over 24 hours. The drip factor is 60 gtt/ml. The nurse will regulate the IV at:
    ① 25 gtt/min
    ② 100 gtt/min
    ③ 125 gtt/min
    ④ 150 gtt/min

167. The position of choice for instilling nose drops in an adult patient is:
    ① Lying on the right side
    ② Lying down or sitting with the neck hyperextended
    ③ Lying down or sitting with the neck flexed
    ④ Lying on the left side

168. The process that occurs from the time a drug is taken into the body to the time it enters the circulatory or lymphatic system is called:
    ① Absorption
    ② Distribution
    ③ Metabolism
    ④ Excretion

169. A patient is diagnosed with myasthenia gravis. The following medication is ordered to be administered:
    ① Pancuronium bromide (Pavulon)
    ② Metformin (Glucophage)
    ③ Cimetidine (Tagamet)
    ④ Pyrostigmine (Mestinon)

170. A patient has not voided approximately 12 hours postpartum. Bladder palpation indicates urinary retention. The physician orders the following medication:
    ① Atropine sulfate (Atropine)
    ② Hydroxyzine (Vistaril)
    ③ Bethanechol (Urecholine)
    ④ Trimethobenzamine (Tigan)

171. A patient is starting on phenytoin (Dilantin) for control of his seizures. The nurse explains to the patient that it is very important that he inform his dentist of his new medication. The reason for this is:
    ① This medication can cause nystagmus
    ② This medication can cause gingival hyperplasia
    ③ This medication can cause slurred speech
    ④ He may develop a vitamin D deficiency

172. The official reference book for medications in the United States is:
    ① *United States Pharmacopeia*
    ② *Physicians Desk Reference*
    ③ *American Hospital Formulary*
    ④ Package inserts from the food and drug administration

173. It is dangerous to combine white wine with an analgesic. The effect on the central nervous system when given together is called:
    ① Antagonistic
    ② Synergistic
    ③ Cumulative
    ④ Tolerance

174. A patient is being started on warfarin (Coumadin) in preparation for cardiac tests. Which of the following medications should the patient be instructed to omit while he is on this medication?
    ① Enalapril (Vasotec)
    ② Metformin (Glucophage)
    ③ Ibuprofen (Motrin)
    ④ Digoxin (Lanoxin)

175. A patient on iron treatment for anemia would benefit from which of these medications to prevent constipation?
    ① Loperamide (Immodium)
    ② Docusate sodium (Colace)
    ③ Hydralazine (Apresoline)
    ④ Hydroxyzine (Vistaril)

176. Epinephrine is effective topically during epistaxis because it:
    ① Causes peripheral vasodilation
    ② Causes peripheral vasoconstriction
    ③ Increases intraocular pressure
    ④ Is a cardiac stimulant

177. A patient is being treated for an anticoagulant overdose. The medication prescribed is:
    ① Phytonadione (Konakion)
    ② Warfarin (Coumadin)
    ③ Digoxin (Lanoxin)
    ④ Propranolol (Inderal)

178. A drug used to treat anemia in end-stage renal disease is:
    ① Filgrastim (Neupogen)
    ② Hydrochlorothiazide (Hydrodiuril)
    ③ Furosemide (Lasix)
    ④ Epoetin alfa (Epogen)

179. A nurse is caring for a patient with anorexia as a result of HIV. The medication ordered for this patient to improve his appetite would be:
    ① Megestrol (Megace)
    ② Gentamycin (Garamycin)
    ③ Folic acid (Folate)
    ④ Amantadine (Symmetrol)

180. A nurse is teaching a nutrition class to a group of expectant parents. Which of the following statements may indicate to the nurse that her lecture has been understood?
    ① "Vitamins will protect my baby if I do not eat correctly."
    ② "You can never get too many vitamins and minerals."
    ③ "Adequate folic acid will help to prevent birth defects."
    ④ "I am going to try really hard to eat a lot of vegetables."

181. A nurse has been instructing a person with newly diagnosed diabetes on how to administer a mixed dose of regular and NPH insulin. Which of the following procedures would indicate that the patient had mastered the proper technique?
① The patient cleans the top of both vials, injects air into the NPH vial, withdraws the NPH, and then injects air into the regular insulin vial with a separate syringe. The patient then withdraws the correct amount of regular insulin into the original syringe
❷ The patient cleans the top of both vials, injects air into the NPH vial and withdraws the syringe. The patient then injects air into the regular insulin and withdraws the correct dose. Then the patient goes back to the NPH vial and withdraws the correct dose
③ These medications must be drawn into separate syringes, because they cannot be mixed
④ Using separate syringes put air into each of the vials. Then withdraw the regular insulin and the NPH insulin using a third syringe.

182. A physician has ordered a "gentamycin level" on his patient. The nurse understands that this test is ordered to determine if:
① The patient has developed a tolerance for the medication
② The patient has developed a physical dependence for the medication
❸ The medication is in the therapeutic range
④ The patient has developed any adverse side effects

183. A patient is starting on antihypertensive medications. Which of the following statements would indicate the need for further teaching?
❶ "If I miss a dose I should take two doses the next day."
② "Medications should be taken with a full glass of water."
❸ "If my blood pressure is too high, I should omit a dose."
④ "I should avoid foods high in sodium."

184. A patient with asthma has been placed on a metered dose inhaler. Which of the following statements indicates the need for further teaching?
① "I need to press down on the inhaler to release one puff while inhaling slowly."
② "The inhalers can be used on a multi-dose basis."
❸ "I should inhale both puffs in quick succession."
④ "After each puff I should hold my breath for approximately 10 seconds."

185. The patient receives 32 units of NPH insulin at 8 AM. The most likely time that she would exhibit signs of insulin reaction would be:
① 10 AM
❷ 2 PM
③ 9 AM
④ Midnight

186. A patient is being treated with calcitriol (Rocaltrol) for hypocalcemia. Which report would indicate that the medication is effective?
❶ Calcium levels 9 to 10 mg/dl
② Decreasing blurred vision
③ Hgb level of 14
④ Potassium level of 3.9

187. Which of the following would be a desired or therapeutic effect of loratidine (Claritin)?
① Sedation
② Decreased irritability
❸ Decreased rhinitis
④ Decreased nausea

188. The patient is to receive an IV of 5%D/0.33 normal saline at 1000 ml/8 hr. The drip factor is 10 gtt/ml. The nurse will run the IV at:
① 7 gtt/min
② 14 gtt/min
❸ 20 gtt/min·
④ 28 gtt/min

189. An elderly patient states that his medication costs too much for his fixed income. The nurse will tell him to ask his doctor to write prescriptions for which of the following forms of the medication?
❶ Generic name
② Brand name
③ Chemical name
④ Official name

190. Fluoxetine (Prozac) has been ordered for a 49-year-old man who suffers from depression. In teaching him about his new medicine, the nurse will tell him that:
① It should be taken at bedtime
② A feeling of euphoria will occur within 24 hours
❸ It will take 2 to 3 weeks before the effects of the drug will be felt
④ It should be taken with meals.

191. KCL (potassium chloride) in liquid form is ordered for a 65-year-old patient taking Lasix. Before administering the medication the nurse will:
① Be sure the patient has been NPO since 12 midnight
❷ Dilute it in 3 to 8 oz of cold water or juice
③ Crush the controlled release tablet and mix it with water
④ Partially dissolve the effervescent tablet

192. A 20-year-old male patient is taking ciprofloxacin (Cipro) for a UTI. He also takes theophylline for asthma. In teaching him about his medication, the nurse knows:
① Fluids should be restricted while on Cipro
② The patient should not be started on Cipro until the culture results are obtained
❸ Theophylline levels may be elevated and can become toxic
④ The two medications should be given at alternate times

193. A 29-year-old patient is being discharged on metoclopramide (Reglan). In his discharge teaching the nurse will stress that:
❶ The drug may cause drowsiness
② The drug is best taken after meals
❸ Nausea and vomiting are common side effects
④ If a dose is missed, the patient should skip it and get back on schedule with the next dose

194. A 64-year-old patient with CHF takes a digitalis preparation every day. Before administering the medication the nurse will:
① Weigh the patient
❷ Check the patient's apical pulse
③ Take the patient's blood pressure
④ Monitor the patient's clotting time

195. The patient will be taught to take his iron preparation:
① At bedtime
❷ Before breakfast
❸ With meals
④ Between meals

196. A 76-year-old patient has congestive heart failure (CHF). The patient is on furosemide (Lasix), digoxin, and potassium (Micro-K) and is complaining of abdominal discomfort and visual disturbances described as "people who look like they have yellow-green skin." It is time for all three medications. The nurse will hold the:
❶ Lasix and Digoxin and notify the doctor
② Lasix and Micro-K and notify the doctor
③ Three drugs and notify the doctor
❹ Digoxin and notify the doctor

197. When chest pain is not relieved by nitroglycerin, the dose should be repeated in:
① 1 minute
❷ 5 minutes
③ 10 minutes
④ 30 minutes

198. A nursing measure requiring the use of the anticholinesterase agent neostigmine bromide (Prostigmin) is:
① Inserting a Foley catheter
❷ Inserting a rectal tube
❸ Encouraging oral fluids
④ Assisting the patient to ambulate

199. The nurse will caution a patient on antihypertensive medication to avoid sudden changes in position, especially from a supine to an upright position, because:
① A thrombus might become dislodged
② Severe nausea might result
❸ Postural hypotension might occur
④ Increased diuresis will occur

200. The nurse gives the 59-year-old patient atropine sulfate as a preoperative medication. The nurse will tell the patient that he will not be allowed out of bed because:
① There is depression of the central nervous system
② Vertigo might occur because of dilation of the pupils
❸ One effect of the drug is the development of postural hypotension
④ Diaphoresis may predispose to a chill

ANSWERS AND RATIONALES

1. Knowledge, assessment, pharmacological therapies (a)
   ❷ Idiosyncratic effects (reactions) are not the result of a known pharmacological property of a drug, but are particular to the patient; this type of reaction is a genetically determined abnormal response to ordinary doses of a drug.
   ① An additive effect is when two drugs with similar actions are given together; drugs administered together for an additive effect allow smaller doses of each drug to be given to avoid toxic effects while maintaining appropriate drug action.
   ③ A synergistic effect describes a drug interaction that results in combined drug effects that are greater than those that could have been achieved should either drug have been administered alone.
   ④ An antagonistic effect results when two drugs given in combination produce effects that are less than if the drugs were given separately; antacids given with tetracycline results in decreased absorption of the tetracycline.

2. Comprehension, planning, pharmacological therapies (b)
   ❹ Medication is administered directly into the bloodstream.
   ① Absorption from the stomach is an additional step before entering the bloodstream.
   ② Absorption from muscle is an additional step before entering the bloodstream.
   ③ Absorption from the subcutaneous tissue is an additional step before entering the bloodstream.

3. Knowledge, assessment, pharmacological therapies (a)
   ❸ The question provides the definition of metabolism.
   ① This is the time drug enters the body and time it enters the bloodstream.
   ② This is the transport of drugs in the body.
   ④ Excretion is the elimination of drugs from the body.

4. Knowledge, assessment, pharmacological therapies (a)
   ❸ This is the correct response.
   ① Metabolism or biotransformation involves the biological transformation of a drug into an inactive metabolite, a more soluble compound, or a more potent metabolite.
   ② Excretion is the elimination of the drug from the body.
   ④ This is an adverse reaction of the drug.

5. Knowledge, assessment, pharmacological therapies (a)
   ❶ This is the correct definition.
   ② This means to act at site of application.
   ③ This means to relieve symptoms.
   ④ This means to cure disease.

6. Application, planning, pharmacological therapies (a)
   ❶ Potassium is the primary intracellular electrolyte.
   ②, ③, ④ These are not used to measure potassium.

7. Application, planning, pharmacological therapies (b)
   ❷ The doctor adjusts the dose according to the results of the PTT.
   ① This medication is not used for infection.
   ③ This is true but does not fully answer the question.
   ④ This is true—however rare and induces undue anxiety.

8. Application, implementation, pharmacological therapies (b)
   ❶ After application to the skin the medication is absorbed at a slow, constant rate, allowing for the maintenance of a therapeutic level.
   ② Absorption through the skin is slow and therefore not effective in acute situations.
   ③ Sublingual and transdermal methods both allow for accurate dosage.
   ④ While this is true, it does not answer the patient's question; in addition, dosage and the length of time for administration depends on severity of condition and requires a physician's order; the dosage depends on the patient's condition.

9. Comprehension, assessment, pharmacological therapies (b)
   ❶ Patients need to be on a bowel program. Constipation is the only side effect for which patients do not develop a tolerance.
   ② A patient develops a tolerance to respiratory effects when dose is gradually increased.
   ③ Pain relief is the desired effect.
   ④ Constipation, not diarrhea, is the usual side effect; see rationale for #1.

10. Application, evaluation, pharmacological therapies (a)
    ❸ This is an expected action of a mydriatic agent.
    ① Decreased drainage is an expected action of an antiinfective agent.
    ② Constriction of the pupil is an expected action of a miotic agent.
    ④ This is an expected action of an osmotic agent.

11. Comprehension, assessment, pharmacological therapies (b)
    ❷ These are symptoms of withdrawal; others include gooseflesh, tearing, yawning, muscle twitching and abdominal cramping, insomnia, nausea, and vomiting
    ①, ③, ④ These are not typical symptoms of withdrawal.

12. Knowledge, planning, pharmacological therapies (a)
    ❸ This medication along with antacids, and anticholinergics and others decrease the absorption of Tagamet
    ①, ②, ④ These increase absorption

13. Application, implementation, pharmacological therapies (b)
    ❹ This procedure will allow for maximum contact with impaired oral mucosa.
    ① This is an improper procedure; it minimizes contact with affected area and then rinses away medication.
    ② There is no indication that the medicine is a suspension.
    ③ This is fine; however, it does not answer the question of what "swish and swallow" means.

14. Comprehension, evaluation, pharmacological therapies (a)
    ❸ This is a major adverse reaction.
    ① This is a serious symptom of shock.
    ② Anticoagulants are given to prevent formation of thrombi.
    ④ This is not caused by anticoagulant therapy.

15. Knowledge, planning, pharmacological therapies (a)
    ❶ This is a cholinergic agent that is used to decrease intraocular pressure.
    ② This is a cholinergic blocking agent used during eye examinations. It increases intraocular pressure.
    ③ This is used to induce skeletal muscle paralysis during anesthesia.
    ④ This is a pituitary hormone used in diabetes insipidus.

16. Knowledge, assessment, pharmacological therapies (b)
    ❷ Hypokalemia can increase risk of toxicity.
    ① Sodium intake is usually limited for heart patients.
    ③ Calcium is stored in bone, not depleted by digitalis.
    ④ Chloride depletion has no effect on digitalis toxicity.

17. Comprehension, implementation, pharmacological therapies (a)
    ❹ Only a limited number of drugs can be administered this way. They have to be dissolvable in salivary secretions.
    ①, ② This route bypasses the GI tract.
    ③ This is a very rapid method of absorption because it bypasses the GI tract and directly enters the systemic circulation.

18. Knowledge, planning, pharmacological therapies (a)
    ❸ The medicine inhibits daytime and nocturnal gastric acid secretion as well as gastric acid stimulated by food.
    ① Tagamet *is* an antacid.
    ② After meals gastric acid has already been produced.
    ④ Cimetidine is given to prevent gastric distress.

19. Knowledge, evaluation, pharmacological therapies (b)
    ❷ The medication is considered to be ulcerogenic.
    ① This medication can irritate the stomach and must be taken with meals.
    ③ This medication can irritate the stomach when not taken with meals.
    ④ This medication is taken with antacid, not orange juice, to prevent stomach irritation.

20. Comprehension, assessment, pharmacological therapies (a)
    ❹ Tinnitus is the most common side effect of salicylate poisoning.
    ① This is a symptom of increased intracranial pressure.
    ② This is a side effect of iron ingestion.
    ③ This is a symptom of gastric distress.

21. Comprehension, assessment, pharmacological therapies (b)
    ❸ Medical supervision is required.
    ①, ②, ④ These statements are true; however, they are not a priority.

22. Application, implementation, pharmacological therapies (b)
    ❸ Rotating sites enhances absorption of the drug and prevents lipodystrophy (hardening of the tissue) at the site of injection.
    ① Insulin is given subcutaneously.
    ② This needle is too long for subcutaneous injection.
    ④ Massaging insulin would speed up absorption, therefore affecting onset and peak.

23. Comprehension, assessment, pharmacological therapies (a)
    ❸ This measures RBC volume.
    ①, ②, ④ These are not appropriate measurements.

24. Knowledge, implementation, pharmacological therapies (a)
    ❹ This is the correct equivalent.
    ①, ②, ③ These are incorrect equivalents.

25. Application, implementation, pharmacological therapies (a)
    ❹ One teaspoon equals approximately 5 ml.
    ①, ②, ③ These are incorrect equivalencies.

26. Comprehension, planning, pharmacological therapies (b)
    ❶ These can produce drug-diet interactions.
    ②, ③, ④ These foods are not restricted.

27. Comprehension, assessment, pharmacological therapies (b)
    ❸ This is the desired action of drug for which it is administered.
    ① Hypertension is a possible side effect for which the patient must be monitored.
    ② Hypotension is a possible side effect for which the patient must be monitored.
    ④ Arrhythmias are a possible side effect for which the patient must be monitored.

28. Comprehension, assessment, pharmacological therapies (b)
    ❸ The physician needs to know to verify any needed prescriptions.
    ①, ② These are subsequent steps but not first priorities.
    ④ This is very premature. It is possible that the couple needs education and support.

29. Knowledge, assessment, pharmacological therapies (b)
    ❸ Estrogen increases risk of breast cancer.
    ① Allergies are not affected by Premarin.
    ② Ulcers are not affected by Premarin.
    ④ Obesity is not affected by Premarin.

30. Comprehension, implementation, pharmacological therapies (a)
    ❷ $1 \text{ cc} = 1 \text{ ml} \dfrac{5 \text{ mg}}{10 \text{ cc}} \times \dfrac{7.5 \text{ mg}}{x}$
    $5x = 75$
    $x = 15 \text{ cc}$
    ①, ③, ④ These are incorrect calculations.

31. Knowledge, implementation, pharmacological therapies (a)
    ❸ With a drip factor of 60, cc per hour = drops per minute.
    ①, ②, ④ These are incorrect calculations.

32. Knowledge, planning, pharmacological therapies (b)
    ❷ This is a neuromuscular blocking agent.
    ① This is a cardiac stimulant.
    ③ This is a bronchodilator and cardiac stimulant.
    ④ This is an adrenergic blocking agent used to treat chronic hypertension and prevent angina.

33. Knowledge, planning, pharmacological therapies (a)
    ❹ This is the correct size needle to reach subcutaneous tissue.
    ①, ②, ③ These needles are too long; they could pass through subcutaneous tissue to underlying muscle, bone.

34. Knowledge, implementation, pharmacological therapies (a)
    ❷ This is the correct calculation.
    ①, ③, ④ These are incorrect calculations; review equivalencies.

35. Knowledge, assessment, pharmacological therapies (c)
   ❶ This is a common side effect.
   ② This is a common side effect of abdominal surgery.
   ③ This is an expected effect of a diuretic.
   ④ This is an expected effect of dehydration.

36. Knowledge, assessment, pharmacological therapies (b)
   ❹ Because of the anticholinergic properties of this medication, caution would have to be used with this antidepressant medication.
   ①, ②, ③ These are not contraindications.

37. Application, evaluation, pharmacological therapies (a)
   ❷ This is the therapeutic effect.
   ① Sleep patterns are not affected by antiparkinsonian drugs.
   ③ Emotional stability is not affected by antiparkinsonian drugs.
   ④ Diet and nutrition are not affected by antiparkinsonian drugs.

38. Comprehension, planning, pharmacological therapies (b)
   ❶ A tranquilizer will ease tremors, and vitamins will improve metabolism.
   ② Aspirin and Tigan might be appropriate for an overdose, not for withdrawal. Calcium is not prescribed.
   ③ See #2. Vitamin C is not prescribed.
   ④ See #2.

39. Knowledge, assessment, pharmacological therapies (c)
   ❶ This is the action of the drug.
   ② Loop diuretics deplete potassium.
   ③ This is used for open-angle glaucoma.
   ④ This is used for acute renal failure.

40. Application, implementation, pharmacological therapies (b)
   ❶ Fluids will help to thin secretions and help prevent dehydration. Dehydration is particularly common in elderly and children.
   ② Medication should be taken with water. Food will effect absorption.
   ③ Chewing will speed up absorption.
   ④ Certain antibiotics (particularly erythromycin) will increase action of theophylline.

41. Knowledge, planning, pharmacological therapies (a)
   ❸ These are prescribed with medical supervision for the treatment of obesity.
   ① These are used to treat peptic and duodenal ulcers by decreasing gastric ulcer secretions.
   ② Tranquilizers are used to decrease anxiety.
   ④ Antacids are used to treat indigestion.

42. Comprehension, planning, pharmacological therapies (a)
   ❹ The tablet is prepared to dissolve between the cheek and the gum.
   ① A buccal tablet should not be chewed.
   ② A buccal tablet is not dissolved in the stomach.
   ③ Sublingual tablets are taken this way.

43. Knowledge, assessment, pharmacological therapies (a)
   ❶ Atropine sulfate dilates pupils and increases intraocular pressure.
   ② The patient can receive morphine safely.
   ③ The patient can receive Demerol safely.
   ④ The patient can receive Vistaril safely.

44. Application, assessment, pharmacological therapies (c)
   ❷ It may or may not be possible to discontinue this medication, depending on the cause of the seizure. If it is discontinued, it must be done gradually under the direction of a physician.
   ① Folic acid deficiency is an adverse reaction to this medication. It should be documented by the physician.
   ③ This is fine; the stomach should not be empty.
   ④ This is a safe practice.

45. Application, evaluation, pharmacological therapies (b)
   ❶ This is action of the drug.
   ② Nitroglycerin has no effect on the brainstem.
   ③ Nitroglycerin does not affect respiration or alertness.
   ④ Nitroglycerin acts on the myocardial blood vessels, not nerve endings.

46. Application, implementation, pharmacological therapies (a)
   ❸ Orthostatic hypotension is a side effect of this medication.
   ① The medication should be given before meals.
   ② This is not necessary; the medication is usually given in divided doses.
   ④ This is not necessary.

47. Application, planning, pharmacological therapies (b)
   ❸ Rubbing accelerates absorption into the tissues.
   ① Insulin is not irritating to the tissues.
   ② This is not true.
   ④ This is a judgmental statement.

48. Comprehension, planning, pharmacological therapies (b)
   ❶ This is the correct calculation.
   ②, ③, ④ These are incorrect calculations.

49. Knowledge, assessment, pharmacological therapies (a)
   ❶ These are signs of alcohol withdrawal along with tachycardia, diaphoresis, anorexia, nausea, vomiting and insomnia, hallucinations, and seizures.
   ② These are not signs.
   ③ Polyuria is not a sign; nausea and headache would be signs of an overdose.
   ④ These are not signs.

50. Application, implementation, pharmacological therapies (b)
   ❹ Orthostatic hypotension is a side effect of diuretics.
   ① It is taken in the morning, so it does not disturb sleep.
   ② The patient may require potassium supplements.
   ③ The patient should monitor weight once a week.

51. Comprehension, evaluation, pharmacological therapies (a)
   ❷ Nausea and vomiting is an early sign.
   ① This is the normal range.
   ③ These are possible signs of colitis.
   ④ These are possible signs of stress or other problems.

52. Application, assessment, pharmacological therapies (a)
   ❸ Milk is antagonistic to Dilantin.
   ① It does take several weeks to reach a therapeutic level.
   ② This is a good health practice because of the effect of Dilantin on the gums.
   ③ This does indicate need for explanation of the importance of blood tests but it is not a priority.

53. Knowledge, planning, pharmacological therapies (a)
❸ Giving it this way helps to decrease gastric distress.
①, ② These methods will not help to decrease gastric distress.
④ This medication has to be given around the clock to maintain a therapeutic level.

54. Comprehension, evaluation, pharmacological therapies (b)
❶ Insomnia is a common side effect. Doses are usually administered at breakfast and lunch.
② The patient may be hyperactive, but this is not the best answer.
③ Caffeine is a CNS stimulant and should be limited, but this is not the best answer.
④ Ritalin can be addicting, so dose should not be increased; it would increase his insomnia.

55. Knowledge, planning, pharmacological therapies (b)
❸ Adrenergic agent counteracts the actions of histamines and helps to reverse the pathological condition.
① Antiinfective used in the treatment of gram-negative bacterial infections.
② This is a steroid used systemically in a wide variety of chronic diseases; it is not appropriate in emergency situations.
④ This is an expectorant used for symptomatic relief of dry, unproductive cough.

56. Comprehension, assessment, pharmacological therapies (b)
❶ This is the desired therapeutic effect.
② This is not a therapeutic effect. The anticholinergic medications would cause thirst.
③ The medication would cause drowsiness; sleep would be an overreaction.
④ This is not an effect. The patient should urinate prior to the administration of any medication.

57. Comprehension, assessment, pharmacological therapies (b)
❸ This is a cholinergic blocking agent. Urinary retention is an adverse side effect.
①, ④ This is a skeletal muscle relaxant; a side effect is urinary frequency.
② This is an anti-anxiety agent. Urinary retention is not a side effect.

58. Knowledge, planning, pharmacological therapies (a)
❸ This is an expected action.
① This is a stool softener.
② This is an antidiarrheal.
④ This inhibits gastric secretion and decreases motility.

59. Comprehension, evaluation, pharmacological therapies (c)
❶ Theophylline is a bronchodilator that will relax the smooth muscle of the bronchi; air flow will be enhanced. Subjective complaints of "tightness" will be relieved.
② Theophylline provides symptomatic relief only; it does not cure.
③ Theophylline is not a mucolytic; it does not thin mucus.
④ Theophylline does not dry up secretions; it works on smooth muscle.

60. Comprehension, evaluation, pharmacological therapies (c)
❷ The nabumetone (Relafen) may not be the cause. If the symptoms get worse, another cause must be looked for.
① Nabumetone (Relafen) can irritate the gastric mucosa but this is not the priority; ulcers are more frequently caused by bacteria.
③ Nabumetone (Relafen) and all NSAIDs should be administered with food. The nurse may have given the nabumetone (Relafen) with food and the patient may still have developed the symptoms.
④ Testing for blood could be done but is a medical action; observation of continuance of symptoms is a more important priority.

61. Knowledge, planning, pharmacological therapies (b)
❹ This medication induces uterine contraction.
① This suppresses endometrial bleeding.
② This is a contraceptive agent.
③ This is a uterine relaxant.

62. Knowledge, planning, pharmacological therapies (a)
❶ This controlled agent is effective on the cough center in the brain.
② This is an NSAID; it has no effect on the cough center.
③ This is a controlled substance; side effects are prohibitive to be used for a cough
④ This is an over-the-counter antitussive that can be combined with codeine.

63. Comprehension, assessment, pharmacological therapies (b)
❹ These are side effects of this cholesterol-lowering medication.
① This is an NSAID; nausea may be a side effect at times, but it is generally given to relieve muscle cramps.
② This is a skeletal muscle relaxant. These are not common side effects of this medication.
③ This is an antihistamine given to relieve allergy symptoms. These are not common side effects of this medication.

64. Comprehension, assessment, pharmacological therapies (a)
❸ It has been shown in many studies that patients remember a great deal from what goes on in anesthesia.
① Of course this is true; however, it does not take priority over the patient.
②, ④ These are true; however, #3 takes priority.

65. Comprehension, evaluation, pharmacological therapies (c)
❷ This is the correct action.
① This is an action of histamine.
③ This is an action of beta-antagonist.
④ This is the action of a decongestant.

66. Comprehension, evaluation, pharmacological therapies (b)
❷ Can increase heart rate.
① This is a serious symptom not related to an adverse reaction to atropine.
③ This is caused by lack of bulk in the diet.
④ This is an expected reaction of atropine; would have no effect on heart disease.

67. Application, evaluation, pharmacological therapies (c)
❶ These are adverse reactions of uterine relaxants.
② These are adverse reaction of skeletal muscle relaxants.
③ These are adverse reactions of antihistamines.
④ These are adverse reactions of adrenergic stimulants.

68. Comprehension, evaluation, pharmacological therapies (b)
❸ Diazepam diminishes seizure activity.
① Decreased anxiety is an action Diazepam produces, but not the reason it is given for status epilepticus.
② Pain relief is not an action of Diazepam.
④ Sleep inducement is not an action of Diazepam.

69. Knowledge, planning, pharmacological therapies (a)
❸ This is the correct medication.
① This is a tranquilizer.
② This is a cardiac stimulant.
④ This is used to treat chronic hypertension and angina.

70. Application, planning, pharmacological therapies (c)
❶ Patients being treated with calcitonin require calcium supplements to maintain blood levels.
② Fiber promotes calcium excretion.
③ Vitamin C is not affected by calcitonin.
④ This is true for everyone.

71. Application, planning, pharmacological therapies (b)
❹ Other effects include diabetes, impotence, amenorrhea, and acromegalic syndrome.
①, ③ This is true; however, it does not answer the question.
② This is true; however, it is not the best answer.

72. Comprehension, planning, pharmacological therapies (b)
❸ Renal calculi are an adverse reaction; increasing fluid will help to prevent them.
① This antibiotic must be taken around the clock to maintain blood level.
② Constipation is not an adverse effect of this medication.
④ See #1.

73. Comprehension, planning, pharmacological therapies (b)
❸ This is an adverse reaction.
①, ② These have not shown to be related.
④ Tetracycline has been used to treat acne vulgaris.

74. Comprehension, evaluation, pharmacological therapies (b)
❸ Rebound congestion occurs if the medicine is used too often, too frequently.
① There is no mention of another medicine that could decrease the effect.
② An increased tolerance may be developing.
④ There is no indication of worsening allergies.

75. Comprehension, evaluation, pharmacological therapies (b)
❸ The purpose is to maintain and improve blood pressure.
① Respiration needs to slow down and be more effective. Respiratory depression needs to be avoided.
② Urinary output is decreased in shock. It needs to be maintained to keep circulation adequate.
④ This would not be the first sign. Increasing orientation is a sign of improvement.

76. Comprehension, evaluation, pharmacological therapies (b)
❷ This is the therapeutic effect that is desired with this medication.
①, ③, ④ This is not the reason this medication is given.

77. Comprehension, evaluation, pharmacological therapies (a)
❹ This agent is used to decrease cholesterol.
①, ②, ③ These are not a measure of this medication.

78. Knowledge, implementation, pharmacological therapies (a)
❷ This is important to prevent further infection or superinfection.
① The patient should take what is left to prevent further infection or superinfection.
③ See #1. The medicine should be taken only by the person for whom it was prescribed.
④ The patient should do this only if the infection continues.

79. Knowledge, implementation, pharmacological therapies (a)
❷ This is a clinical indication for this medication.
① This is not a clinical indication for tetracycline.
③ This is not a clinical indication for claithromyesin.
④ This is a PO sulfa-based drug used frequently in the treatment of UTIs.

80. Knowledge, implementation, pharmacological therapies (a)
❶ This is the correct technique to give a deep IM and minimize irritation.
② Z-track is a deep IM.
③ This is not true.
④ This is not a method that allows for rapid effect.

81. Comprehension, assessment, pharmacological therapies (b)
❷ Theophylline can cause these effects. A level is necessary to determine if the medication is in the therapeutic range.
① Valium may be used in an emergency asthmatic situation. It is not used on a routine basis.
③ Tagamet does not cause jitteriness and it is given to decrease nausea.
④ These are not side effects of laxatives.

82. Application, assessment, pharmacological therapies (c)
❸ Red wines contain tyramines and could cause a potentially fatal interaction.
① This medication should be taken with food or fluids to decrease gastric distress.
② If the patient is experiencing less depression, he may be more motivated.
④ As long as it is being done in a healthy manner, this is not a concern.

83. Comprehension, assessment, pharmacological therapies (b)
❸ This provides for 3 months' contraception.
① This is an oral birth control pill and must be taken daily.
② This is a natural body hormone given to replace or supplement.
④ This medication is given to induce contraction of the uterus.

84. Application, assessment, pharmacological therapies (c)
    ❹ This medication causes impaired glucose tolerance and therefore hyperglycemia.
    ① See #4.
    ②, ③ This is not an effect of this medication.

85. Application, evaluation, pharmacological therapies (b)
    ❷ This is the truth and patients need encouragement to comply.
    ① There is no indication of the need to change medication.
    ③ It is not within the scope of practice for the nurse to add a medication. Nor is there any indication that there is a need for the physician to do so.
    ④ This is true; however, it does not answer the question.

86. Comprehension, knowledge, pharmacological therapies (a)
    ❶ This is the correct definition.
    ②, ③, ④ These are incorrect definitions.

87. Comprehension, evaluation, pharmacological therapies (b)
    ❶ These are the therapeutic effects desired in children with hyperactivity.
    ② Irritability is an adverse reaction to the medication. Drug should be given at least 6 hours before bedtime to avoid insomnia.
    ③ Headache is an adverse reaction as is anorexia.
    ④ These are adverse reactions.

88. Comprehension, assessment, pharmacological therapies (b)
    ❸ This is the therapeutic effect. It takes 2 to 3 weeks to reach a therapeutic level.
    ①, ②, ④ Diarrhea, nausea and vomiting, and insomnia are adverse reactions to the drug.

89. Comprehension, assessment, pharmacological therapies (c)
    ❸ This is the sign that an allergic reaction may be occurring.
    ① This would be an indicator of a febrile reaction indicating contamination. It generally occurs late in the transfusion or after completion.
    ② This would be an indication of circulatory overload.
    ④ This would indicate an anticoagulant reaction.

90. Comprehension, assessment, pharmacological therapies (b)
    ❷ This medicine used to treat TIAs; orthostatic hypotension is a common side effect.
    ① This is not a necessary parameter to monitor.
    ③ It does not effect temperature.
    ④ It does not affect WBCs and may increase risk of bleeding.

91. Comprehension, assessment, pharmacological therapies (b)
    ❸ Vancomycin is ototoxic.
    ①, ②, ④ These are not adverse effects of this medication.

92. Application, assessment, pharmacological therapies (b)
    ❹ Less food and more exercise is most likely to cause decreased blood sugar.
    ① Decreasing exercise is more likely to cause hyperglycemia.
    ② This is more likely to cause hyperglycemia.

③ Exercise decreases the need for insulin. Increasing calories is another option.

93. Knowledge, assessment, pharmacological therapies (a)
    ❷ This is the correct use. A troche is a lozenge that should be held in the throat to decrease irritation.
    ① This is not an effect.
    ③, ④ These are not appropriate uses for troches.

94. Application, assessment, pharmacological therapies (c)
    ❹ There may be a cultural influence that causes her to believe these medicines are food; however there definitely is a knowledge deficit.
    ① This is definitely a necessary assessment, but further information on entire pattern of OTC medicines is need.
    ②, ③ See #1

95. Application, assessment, pharmacological therapies (c)
    ❹ Patients should be advised on the danger of taking OTC medicines for more than 2 weeks without consulting a physician. The location and characteristics of the pain need to be investigated.
    ① Occasional use of a laxative is not dangerous, but further dietary teaching may be indicated.
    ② Assessment of blood pressure is called for, but if it is stable this is considered ongoing care.
    ③ Taking a vitamin every day is fine, as long as it is not used as a substitute for good nutrition.

96. Comprehension, evaluation, pharmacological therapies (b)
    ❸ This is a sign of digoxin toxicity.
    ① Digoxin is given to treat elevated heart rate in CHF. A toxic effect would be bradycardia.
    ②, ④ These are not toxic effects.

97. Application, evaluation, pharmacological therapies (b)
    ❷ These are adverse reactions to hypothyroid medication.
    ①, ③ These are adverse reactions to hyperthyroid medications.
    ④ These are the opposite of hypothyroid effects.

98. Comprehension, evaluation, pharmacological therapies (b)
    ❷ This is a fertility drug that stimulates ovulation.
    ① Decreased blood pressure is not an effect.
    ③, ④ These are not therapeutic effects.

99. Knowledge, evaluation, pharmacological therapies (b)
    ❶ This is a major adverse reaction.
    ② This is a sign of kidney disease.
    ③ This is not a major adverse reaction and can be caused by depression.
    ④ This is caused by pupil dilation by medication.

100. Knowledge, evaluation, pharmacological therapies (a)
    ❸ This is the definition of toxic action.
    ①, ② These are undesired effects of a drug.
    ④ This is an unusual or unexpected effect of a drug.

101. Comprehension, assessment, pharmacological therapies (b)
    ❷ This may be indicative of infiltration.
    ① This can be corrected (if the insertion site is still patent) by repositioning and making certain the dial is correctly set.
    ③ This can be corrected with positioning.
    ④ This is important; however, the primary infusion normally begins when the "piggyback" is completed.

102. Application, planning, pharmacological therapies (b)
   ❸ This is caused by a fungus, so an antifungal agent is appropriate.
   ①, ② These are not appropriate.
   ④ This is true, but it does not explain why it is effective.

103. Knowledge, planning, pharmacological therapies (a)
   ❸ This is the first drug indicated in the treatment of malaria.
   ① This is an antineoplastic.
   ② This is antiviral useful in the treatment of AIDS.
   ④ This is also an antineoplastic.

104. Comprehension, assessment, pharmacological therapies (b)
   ❷ Concurrent use of heparin and nonsteroidal antiinflammatory drugs (NSAIDs) may predispose the patient to hemorrhage.
   ① Psyllium is not contraindicated with heparin. It should not be given at the same time as aspirin or digoxin, as it may inhibit absorption.
   ③ This is a CNS depressant and is synergistic with other groups in this classification.
   ④ The need here would be to monitor the cumulative effects of other hypertensive agents.

105. Comprehension, implementation, pharmacological therapies (b)
   ❸ By giving it in this manner the patient receives both local soothing effect and central nervous system effect on the cough center in the brain.
   ① This is not the correct technique.
   ② This method will limit the local effect.
   ③ Cough medicines are normally given on a PRN basis.

106. Comprehension, implementation, pharmacological therapies (a)
   ❷ This is the correct calculation. The formula is

   $$\frac{\text{cc/hr} \times \text{gtt factor}}{60} = \frac{125 \text{ cc/hr} \times 10}{60}$$

   ①, ③, ④ These are incorrect calculations.

107. Comprehension, implementation, pharmacological therapies (b)
   ❹ It is possible that the evening shift obtained permission to give the medication early so that the patient would not be awakened.
   ① This should be done prior to administration.
   ② This is true. It does not answer the question.
   ③ This also may be true, but it does not answer the question.

108. Application, implementation, pharmacological therapies (b)
   ❶ The nurse should observe the effect of analgesics to be certain that pain is relieved and determine if further intervention is needed.
   ② This is true, but it should be done immediately after administration and on a regular, consistent basis.
   ③ Assessing the patient's beliefs is always important; however, it does not take priority at this time.
   ④ For acute pain dosing can be given prn. It requires careful assessment of the pain and documentation of relief by the nurse.

109. Application, implementation, prevention and early detection of disease (b)
   ❶ TB medications must be taken over an extended period of time (6 months–2 years) to be sure of effective treatment.
   ② There is no indication of this and continued exposure would not be a factor if the medication regimen was being followed.
   ③ There may be a need for additional medication in the future, but it would have to be determined if multidrug–resistant TB had developed.
   ④ Family members should have already received follow-up medical care.

110. Comprehension, implementation, physiological integrity (a)
   ❶ This allocation allows for two meals on 7-3, one meal on 3-11, and fluids for meds on 11-7.
   ② There are two meals on 7-3; most patients prefer fluids with meals.
   ③ Fluids must be allowed for medication.
   ④ Patients need to be encouraged to save fluids all during the day to increase comfort.

111. Knowledge, planning, pharmacological therapies (a)
   ❶ Sedatives are given in small doses to decrease anxiety. Hypnotics are given in larger doses to induce sleep.
   ② Sedatives can be given around the clock; hypnotics are given prior to sleep at anytime.
   ③ This is not true.
   ④ Length of effect varies with each drug.

112. Knowledge, planning, pharmacological therapies (a)
   ❸ This is an anticholinergic medication used to treat Parkinson's.
   ① This is a CNS stimulant.
   ② This is an anticonvulsant.
   ④ This is a bronchodilator.

113. Knowledge, planning, pharmacological therapies (b)
   ❷ This would result in optimal absorption.
   ①, ③ Patient is vomiting and would not retain medication.
   ④ This would result in poor absorption.

114. Comprehension, planning, pharmacological therapies (b)
   ❸ This treatment decreases inflammation.
   ① This is used sparingly if at all in head injury patients because it may mask central signs of ICP.
   ② This is used to treat high blood pressure.
   ④ This is used as an anticoagulant.

115. Knowledge, evaluation, pharmacological therapies (a)
   ❶ This is the therapeutic effect.
   ② This is not applicable to the effect of the drug.
   ③ There is no active ingredient in the drug.
   ④ Metabolism of the drug is not necessary to produce the desired effect.

116. Comprehension, evaluation, pharmacological therapies (b)
   ❷ It can only be given preventatively and it does take several weeks to reach a therapeutic level.
   ① Intal does not improve symptoms; if given during an attack it may make symptoms worse.
   ③ Intal does not affect sleeping ability.
   ④ This is not an effect of this medication.

117. Knowledge, assessment, pharmacological therapies (a)
   ❶ This is the most common antibiotic used to treat urinary tract infections.
   ② A penicillin substitute such as erythromycin would be used if the symptoms warranted.
   ③ This may or may not call for an antibiotic, may be viral in nature. If an antibiotic was called for, it would probably be penicillin or a substitute.
   ④ This may be an indication of a super infection.

118. Comprehension, assessment, pharmacological therapies (a)
   ❷ Cancer drugs can affect the integrity of the oral mucosa.
   ① Antibiotics do not affect the oral mucosa.
   ③ Antiparkinsonian drugs do not affect the oral mucosa.
   ④ Vitamins do not affect the oral mucosa.

119. Knowledge, assessment, safety and infection control (a)
   ❹ This is the definition of the law.
   ① This was replaced by Controlled Substance Act.
   ② There is no such act.
   ③ This regulates distribution of narcotics and other drugs of abuse.

120. Application, assessment, pharmacological therapies (a)
   ❸ These are early signs of hyperglycemia.
   ① These are signs of infection.
   ② These are signs of anemia.
   ④ These are signs of gastrointestinal distress.

121. Comprehension, assessment, pharmacological therapies (c)
   ❹ Elderly metabolize drugs more slowly because of declining body function, thus prolonging the half-life of the drug, resulting in drug accumulation.
   ① Age does not make a difference in tolerance.
   ② Elderly metabolize drugs more slowly.
   ③ Age does not cause more frequent adverse effects.

122. Knowledge, assessment, pharmacological therapies (a)
   ❶ Sedation is part of therapy.
   ② This medication does not control seizures.
   ③ This medication does not cause vasoconstriction.
   ④ This medication does not cause vasodilation.

123. Comprehension, evaluation, pharmacological therapies (b)
   ❸ These side effects can occur particularly with children taking this medication.
   ①, ②, ④ These are not common side effects of these medications.

124. Knowledge, evaluation, pharmacological therapies (a)
   ❶ These medications decrease the effects of the parasympathetic nervous system.
   ② These are opposites of what the side effects would be.
   ③ Thirst is a side effect, but polyuria is not.
   ④ These drugs are cardiac stimulants; however, tachycardia is not desirable.

125. Comprehension, evaluation, pharmacological therapies (b)
   ❹ Increased muscle strength would indicate an improvement in the symptoms.
   ① Slowing of the heart rate is an effect. It is not given to treat arrhythmias.
   ② This is a side effect; however, it is not a therapeutic effect.
   ③ See #2.

126. Knowledge, evaluation, pharmacological therapies (b)
   ❸ These dilate coronary arteries in acute angina.
   ① These are used in long-term management.
   ② These are used for chronic angina.
   ④ These are used for severe physical pain.

127. Application, evaluation, pharmacological therapies (c)
   ❷ Children on high doses of Reglan are particularly prone to the extrapyramidal effects of the drug. Presence of these drugs should be reported to the health care provider immediately so that the dose can be adjusted or a new drug prescribed.
   ①, ③, ④ These are common side effects and need not be reported.

128. Comprehension, evaluation, pharmacological therapies (b)
   ❷ Benadryl is an antihistamine that decreases itching.
   ①, ③, ④ These are not common symptoms of hives and Benadryl does not affect these symptoms.

129. Knowledge, planning, pharmacological therapies (b)
   ❶ This is the action of a thrombolytic agent. It must be used only in acute situations.
   ② This is an anticoagulant that may be used for long-term management.
   ③ Vitamin K is an anticoagulant agent.
   ④ Amicar is an anticoagulant agent.

130. Knowledge, planning, pharmacological therapies (c)
   ❷ This is used to relieve pain and does not cause biliary spasms as morphine does.
   ① See #2.
   ③ This is an antibiotic that has GI adverse effects.
   ④ This is an antiinflammatory that causes adverse GI effects.

131. Knowledge, planning, pharmacological therapies (a)
   ❷ This is rapid acting with the fastest onset.
   ① This is intermediate acting. The onset of action would take too long.
   ③, ④ These are long acting; the onset would take too long.

132. Knowledge, planning, pharmacological therapies (a)
   ❸ This is the appropriate length gauge and needle size for intradermal injection.
   ①, ④ Needles are too large and too long for intradermal injections.
   ② This size is appropriate for subcutaneous injections.

133. Application, planning, pharmacological therapies (b)
   ❷ Explanations should be geared to the child's ability to understand.
   ① Long explanations to a child under 5 only increase anxiety.
   ② Of course the parent can hold the child; however, injecting it quickly can cause aspiration.
   ③ It may be appropriate to administer some medication in juice; however, you must be certain that the child will drink all of the juice to receive a correct dose.

134. Knowledge, assessment, pharmacological therapies (a)
   ❸ This is used in addiction management.
   ① This is a narcotic-analgesic used to control pain.
   ② This is a narcotic-antagonist used to reverse CNS and respiratory depression.
   ④ This is a narcotic agonist-antagonist used to control pain.

135. Knowledge, assessment, pharmacological therapies (a)
    ❷ Dosage is individualized according to blood coagulation.
    ① This is the laboratory test for platelet activity.
    ③ This is the laboratory test for time of actual bleeding.
    ④ This is the laboratory test for strength of capillary walls.

136. Comprehension, assessment, pharmacological therapies (a)
    ❶ This stimulates uterine contractions.
    ② This acts on uterine muscle fibers.
    ③ This is an unwanted action.
    ④ This contracts uterine muscle fibers.

137. Comprehension, implementation, pharmacological therapies (a)
    ❹ This is the most common gauge and length for intramuscular injections for normal weight individuals (the larger the number, the finer the needle).
    ① This gauge may be appropriate in the deltoid or with extremely thin persons; however, the length of the needle would be long for an average weight person.
    ② This would be appropriate for an intradermal injection.
    ③ This gauge would be used for oily preparations; the needle length is too long for an average-weight person.

138. Knowledge, implementation, safety and infection control (a)
    ❸ Barrier gloves need to be worn when the nurse can reasonably expect contact with bodily fluids.
    ① This is true; however, it does not answer the question.
    ② This is also true but is nonresponsive to the question.
    ④ Standard precautions apply to all patients.

139. Knowledge, implementation, pharmacological therapies (a)
    ❷ Enteric-coated tablets disintegrate in the small intestine to prevent stomach irritation.
    ① It does not effect the length of stay in the stomach.
    ③ This describes a timed-released or sustained-action tablet.
    ④ It prevents irritation to the stomach, not to the small intestine.

140. Knowledge, planning, pharmacological therapies (b)
    ❹ Increasing the amount of glucose taken up by the muscles decreases glucose level in the blood stream, and if insulin is able to get in the cells, glucose will be used as energy.
    ① Fats being broken down excessively can lead to ketosis. Excess protein is used for energy; however, this is not the primary source for energy.
    ② This is partially true. It does decrease cellular resistance; however, decreasing the amount of glucose used by muscles will increase serum glucose levels.
    ③ Oral hypoglycemics are not oral insulin.

141. Knowledge, planning, pharmacological therapies (b)
    ❶ This cholinergic agent increases lower esophageal sphincter pressure.
    ② This anticholinergic agent is useful in the treatment of spastic conditions of the gastrointestinal condition.
    ③ This miotic agent is useful in the treatment of glaucoma.
    ④ This opiod narcotic is used in the treatment of diarrhea.

142. Application, evaluation, pharmacological therapies (b)
    ❷ Cromolyn sodium is effective only if given prior to an attack in a preventative manner.
    ① It is not effective if given during an attack. It might even make the symptoms worse.
    ③ This would indicate a worsening of the symptoms.
    ④ There is no effect on respiratory infections.

143. Knowledge, implementation, pharmacological therapies (a)
    ❸ This is the correct calculation: $\dfrac{cc/hour \times gtt\ factor}{60}$
    ①, ②, ④ These are incorrect calculations.

144. Knowledge, implementation, pharmacological therapies (a)
    ❷ $1\ cc = 1\ ml\ \dfrac{1\ cc}{10,000} = \dfrac{1/2}{5000\ units}$
    ①, ③, ④ These are incorrect calculations.

145. Knowledge, implementation, pharmacological therapies (a)
    ❷ $0.4\ mg = 1/150\ grain$
    $1\ ml = 1\ cc$
    ①, ③, ④ These are incorrect calculations.

146. Comprehension, implementation, pharmacological therapies (a)
    ❶ This is the preferred site for children under 3, since it is well developed at birth.
    ② This site should not be used for injections at all until the child has been walking for at least 1 year.
    ③ This site can be used with older, larger children.
    ④ This site can be used for children over 3 years who have been walking for a year or two. It has a disadvantage of being visible to the child, however.

147. Knowledge, assessment, pharmacological therapies (a)
    ❶ This is given intravenously to control seizures.
    ② This is an antianxiety agent.
    ③ This is a sedative/hypnotic agent.
    ④ This is used to treat alcohol withdrawal.

148. Knowledge, planning, pharmacological therapies (b)
    ❹ As of this time, this is the most potent antibiotic available.
    ①, ② MRSA is resistent to these antibiotics.
    ② This is an antiviral medication.

149. Knowledge, evaluation, pharmacological therapies (c)
    ❸ The Reserpine may be the cause. Impotence is a common side effect of this drug. The physician can switch the patient to another medication to see if it helps.
    ① If a drug change does not help, the patient may then want to see a psychologist.
    ② This may be an option if the drug change does not work.
    ④ If the drug change does not work, the nurse can discuss other options for the patient.

150. Knowledge, planning, pharmacological therapies (a)
    ❸ This drug is a biological modifier. It stimulates proliferation and differentiation of neutrophils.
    ① Epogen increases the rate of red blood cell production.
    ② This is an antiinfective medication.
    ④ This is used in treatment of cancer. A side effect is immunosuppression.

151. Knowledge, planning, growth and development through the life span (a)
    ❷ This is an appropriate characteristic of adolescents. Activities in the teaching plan should include ways that involve them with their peer group as much as possible.
    ① This is characteristic of a school-age child.
    ③ This is characteristic of young adults.
    ④ This is characteristic of an older adult.

152. Knowledge, planning, pharmacological therapies (a)
    ❷ This is an antidepressant medication.
    ① This is not an effect of Elavil.
    ③, ④ These are undesired effects of Elavil.

153. Comprehension, planning, pharmacological therapies (b)
    ❸ The aim of treatment in glaucoma is to decrease intraocular pressure. This classification of medications will increase pressure and precipitate acute glaucoma in predisposed persons.
    ① Cholinergic agents decrease intraocular pressure.
    ②, ④ This is true; however, it does not respond to the question.

154. Comprehension, evaluation, safety and infection control (b)
    ❷ Follow-up care by health professionals and support of family and friends is vital, because patients may need to be on medications for as long as 2 years.
    ① The treatment may need to go on for anywhere from 6 months to a year.
    ③ This is true to assist in maintaining the immune system. It does not, however, answer the question.
    ④ Patients are contagious in the initial stages of TB. Good health habits should always be maintained to prevent exposure to others.

155. Knowledge, evaluation, coordinated care (a)
    ❶ This is federal law.
    ②, ③, ④ These statements are true; however, they do not answer the question.

156. Application, evaluation, pharmacological therapies (b)
    ❹ This is the first action; the pain could be related to something other than the operation (i.e., urinary retention or cardiac).
    ① This is unacceptable. A patient in pain requires action.
    ② This would be the second action, particularly because the dose of morphine may not be in therapeutic range.
    ③ This would be beneficial after the pain level is decreased.

157. Comprehension, evaluation, growth and development through the life span (b)
    ❸ It may be a "drag," but at least he acknowledges that it has to be done.
    ① This is fine. There is no problem with him hanging out with his friends.
    ② Exercise is fine as long as it is balanced with diet and medication.
    ④ Peers are important to adolescents. This statement does not indicate understanding that he has measures necessary to manage his diabetes, but his activities are not restricted.

158. Comprehension, implementation, pharmacological therapies (b)
    ❸ Major diuresis will occur during waking hours.
    ① Frequent urination caused by the diuretic would disturb the patient's sleep.

② Salt intake, not fluid intake, should be cut down.
④ The medication should be stopped only by physician's order.

159. Comprehension, implementation, pharmacological therapies (b)
    ❶ The medication is not safe for direct intravenous administration.
    ② This action will not relieve any discomfort patient may have.
    ③ This action will not facilitate absorption.
    ④ There are no organs at intramuscular sites.

160. Application, implementation, pharmacological therapies (b)
    ❶ This allows peak drug activity during daytime hours.
    ②, ③, ④ These are not applicable to effect of drug.

161. Knowledge, implementation, pharmacological therapies (a)
    ❸ This prevents possible obstruction as a result of thickening and expansion of the drug.
    ① This will not prevent unwanted side effects.
    ② Fluid, not food, is necessary to prevent undesired effects.
    ④ Gastric distress is not a side effect.

162. Application, implementation, pharmacological therapies (a)
    ❶ This straightens the canal and promotes maximum contact of medication with tissue.
    ② This is proper procedure for children.
    ③ This would block entrance to ear canal.
    ④ This procedure would not allow access to ear canal.

163. Application, implementation, pharmacological therapies (a)
    ❶ Glucose reverses the effect of too much insulin.
    ② This is given for hyperglycemia.
    ③ This facilitates increase in blood glucose but is not an appropriate treatment.
    ④ This is not an emergency treatment.

164. Knowledge, implementation, pharmacological therapies (a)
    ❸ This is the proper procedure.
    ①, ②, ④ Part of dose will be wasted.

165. Application, implementation, pharmacological therapies (b)
    ❷ These are correct actions.
    ①, ③ The drug should be withheld.
    ④ The nurse should withhold drug. Oxygen would not be administered without a physician's order.

166. Knowledge, implementation, pharmacological therapies (b)
    ❸ This is the correct calculation.
    ①, ②, ④ These are incorrect calculations.

167. Knowledge, implementation, pharmacological therapies (a)
    ❷ This is the best anatomical position.
    ① Nose drops would not be retained.
    ③ Flexion of neck prevents administration.
    ④ Nose drops would not be retained.

168. Knowledge, assessment, pharmacological therapies (a)
    ❶ This is the definition.
    ② Distribution is the transport of drugs in the body.

③ Metabolism is the process by which a drug is transformed into an inactive metabolite, a more soluble compound, or a more potent metabolite.

④ Excretion is the elimination of drugs from the body.

169. Knowledge, planning, pharmacological therapies (b)
❹ Mestinon enhances the cholinergic system and increases the accumulation of acetylcholine at nervous system's synapses.
① Pavulon inhibits the transmission of nerve impulses blocking the transmission of acetylcholine.
② This is an oral hypoglycemic.
③ This is an H_2-blocking agent used to treat excessive gastric acid secretion.

170. Application, planning, pharmacological therapies (c)
❸ This is a parasympathetic agent that helps to restore bladder tone.
① This is an anticholinergic agent that would inhibit gastric acid secretion and decrease the tone of the bladder.
② This can be used as a tranquilizer or an antiemetic.
④ This is an antiemetic.

171. Application, planning, pharmacological therapies (c)
❷ This is an overgrowth of the gums, which may require additional dental care.
① Nystagmus is involuntary rhythmic eye movements and is not affected by dental care.
③ This is also true; however, it is not a priority for the dentist.
④ This is true, although rare.

172. Knowledge, planning, pharmacological therapies (a)
❶ This is the official reference book for the United States.
② This is published annually by manufacturers.
③ This is published by the hospital association.
④ This is very useful; however, it is not official.

173. Knowledge, planning, pharmacological therapies (a)
❷ This is the correct definition: the total effect of two drugs when given together is greater than the effects if each is given separately.
①, ③, ④ These are incorrect definitions.

174. Application, planning, pharmacological therapies (b)
❸ This drug will increase anticoagulant effects.
① This drug is used to decrease B/P in hypertension; it is not synergistic with Coumadin.
② This drug is used to decrease blood sugar in NIDDM; it is not synergistic with Coumadin.
④ This drug is used to treat cardiac arrhythmias. It is not synergistic with Coumadin.

175. Knowledge, planning, pharmacological therapies (a)
❷ This is a stool softener.
① This is used to treat diarrhea.
③ This is an antihypertensive medication.
④ This can be used as an antiemetic, or in higher doses, as a tranquilizer.

176. Knowledge, planning, pharmacological therapies (a)
❷ This is an effect of this adrenergic agent.
① This is the opposite effect. Epinephrine causes central dilation and peripheral constriction.
③, ④ This is true; however, it does not answer the question.

177. Knowledge, planning, pharmacological therapies (b)
❶ Vitamin K is the antidote for anticoagulant overdoses.
② This is an anticoagulant.
③ This is used to treat cardiac arrhythmias.

④ This is used to decrease blood pressures and improve cardiac arrhythmias.

178. Knowledge, planning, pharmacological therapies (a)
❹ This medication increases RBC production.
① This is used to increase WBC production
② This is used to treat high blood pressure.
③ This is a diuretic.

179. Comprehension, planning, pharmacological therapies (b)
❶ This medication is prescribed to improve appetite in patients with AIDS.
② This is an antibiotic.
③ This is used to treat nutritional anemias.
④ This is an antiviral medication.

180. Knowledge, evaluation, growth and development through the life span (a)
❸ A deficiency of maternal folic acid has been associated with neural tube defects.
① Vitamins are not a substitute for a well-balanced diet.
② It is not recommended that megadoses of vitamins be taken.
③ This is fine; however, it does not indicate the need for a well-balanced diet, from all of the food levels.

181. Application, evaluation, pharmacological therapies (b)
❷ This methods allows for no contamination of the rapid acting insulin with the NPH, which has been modified.
① This method might lead to potential contamination.
③ These medications can be safely mixed.
④ There is no need to use three syringes.

182. Comprehension, evaluation, pharmacological therapies (b)
❸ The medication must be in the desired range if therapeutic effectiveness is going to be achieved.
① This is not the definition of tolerance. Tolerance means that larger and larger doses need to be given.
② Physical dependence means there is a distinct physical reaction when the drug is discontinued.
④ If the levels came back in the toxic range, there is a possibility that toxic effects could develop. The dosage may need to be decreased.

183. Comprehension, evaluation, pharmacological therapies (b)
❶ Patients should check with their physician on what to do if a dose is missed. They should never double up on a dose.
② It is appropriate to take medicine with water to facilitate absorption.
③ Opposite action should be taken.
④ Foods high in sodium should be avoided by patients with hypertension. This does not answer the question.

184. Application, evaluation, pharmacological therapies (b)
❸ One minute should be allowed between puffs.
① This is the correct procedure; it allows for maximum absorption.
② This is true.
④ This is true—aids in absorption.

185. Cognitive, evaluation, pharmacological therapies (a)
❷ This is correct. NPH insulin peaks in 6 to 12 hours.
① This is too early. Regular insulin peaks in 2 to 4 hours.
③ This is too early.
④ This is too late. This would be within the peak of long-acting insulins.

186. Knowledge, evaluation, pharmacological therapies (b)
❶ This indicates a normal calcium level.
② Vision is not affected with hypocalcemia.
③ This is a normal level and is not used as indicator for hypocalcemia treatment.
④ See #3.

187. Comprehension, evaluation, pharmacological therapies (a)
❸ This is an antihistamine medication that helps to prevent histamines from causing allergic symptoms.
① This is a side effect that is particularly common in the elderly.
② This is not an effect. Older children sometimes have a paradoxical effect of increased irritability when antihistamines are taken.
④ This is not an effect of this medication.

188. Knowledge, implementation, pharmacological therapies (b)
❸ This is the correct calculation.
①, ②, ④ These are incorrect calculations.

189. Comprehension, implementation, basic care and comfort (a)
❶ These are often the least expensive.
② These are often the most expensive.
③, ④ Prescriptions are not written in this form.

190. Application, implementation, pharmacological therapies (b)
❸ The action of the drug takes 2 to 3 weeks while blood levels are building.
① It should be taken in the morning so that the effects of the drug are the strongest during waking hours.
② The action of the drug does not occur in 24 hours; takes 2 to 3 weeks while blood levels are building.
④ This is not necessary.

191. Application, implementation, pharmacological therapies (c)
❷ KCL is diluted to decrease GI upset.
① KCL should be given with or after meals.
③ Never crush controlled-release tablets.
④ Fully dissolve effervescent tablets before administering.

192. Application, implementation, pharmacological therapies (c)
❸ Cipro can increase Theophylline levels.
① Fluids should be forced.
② Cipro should be started while results are pending.
④ The two medications can be given together.

193. Application, implementation, pharmacological therapies (c)
❶ It may cause drowsiness. Machinery should not be operated until the patient's response is known.
② Effectiveness of the drug is not affected by food.
③ It is used to treat nausea.
④ If a dose is missed, it should be taken as soon as that is realized, unless it is time for the next dose.

194. Application, implementation, pharmacological therapies (b)
❷ Check the apical pulse one full minute and hold medication if it is less than 60.

① The patient should be weighed every week.
③ Pulse is more significant.
④ Digitalis level, not clotting time, is monitored.

195. Comprehension, implementation, pharmacological therapies (a)
❸ Drug is irritating to the GI tract; taking the drug with meals decreases irritation.
① Taking the drug at bedtime could irritate the GI tract.
② Taking the drug before breakfast could irritate the GI tract.
④ Taking the drug between meals could irritate the GI tract.

196. Comprehension, implementation, pharmacological therapies (c)
❶ The symptoms are typical of digitalis toxicity. The patient could be dehydrating, so administration of Lasix could complicate the problem.
② The patient could be dehydrating, so administration of Lasix could complicate the problem. The Micro-K is given to replace potassium loss and should be administered.
③ The symptoms are typical of digitalis toxicity. The patient could be dehydrating, so administration of Lasix could complicate the symptoms. The Micro-K is given to replace potassium loss and should be administered.
④ This answer is partially correct, but Lasix needs to be held along with the Digoxin because administration of either will increase symptoms.

197. Knowledge, implementation, pharmacological therapies (a)
❷ This is the correct procedure.
① One minute is not enough time to give the drug to work.
③ Ten minutes is too long to wait to repeat the dose.
④ Thirty minutes is too long to wait to repeat the dose.

198. Application, implementation, pharmacological therapies (b)
❷ This increases gastrointestinal muscle tone and motility.
①, ③ This does not facilitate action of drug.
④ Patient remains in bed with rectal tube.

199. Comprehension, implementation, pharmacological therapies (b)
❸ This is an adverse reaction of antihypertensives.
① This is an adverse reaction of antifibrinolytics.
② This is a side effect.
④ This is an expected action of diuretics.

200. Comprehension, implementation, pharmacological therapies (a)
❸ This could cause patient injury.
① This is not an action of atropine.
② Dilation of pupils does not cause vertigo.
④ This medication decreases diaphoresis.

CHAPTER 4

Nutrition

Nutrition is the combination of processes by which the body uses food for growth, energy, and maintenance. Nutrition is also the study of food and its relation to health and disease. Increasing emphasis is being placed on the role of balanced nutrition in the prevention of many chronic illnesses. The nurse plays an especially important role in the nutritional aspects of patient care. Because of close and continual contact with the patient, the nurse is able to evaluate and monitor the patient's nutritional status and inform the dietician or appropriate dietary person about the patient's nutritional needs and acceptance of the nutritional plan of care. Good nutrition is essential to good health throughout the life cycle, and the nurse is in an excellent position to encourage sound nutritional practice for each patient and the patient's family.

HEALTH PROMOTION

A. Goal: to increase the level of health of individuals, families, groups, and communities, which requires a lifestyle change that will lead to new positive health behaviors
B. In 1990 the U.S. Department of Health and Human Services issued a national report, *Healthy People 2000,* that outlined national health promotion and disease prevention objectives for Americans to be achieved by the year 2000. Nutrition is the key to these goals

PRINCIPLES OF NUTRITION

A. Functions of food
   1. Provides energy
   2. Builds and repairs body tissues
   3. Regulates and controls the body's chemical processes, which are essential for providing energy and building tissues
B. Evidence of good nutrition (Table 4-1); persons receiving less than desired amounts of nutrients have a greater risk of physical illness, are limited in physical work and mental capacity, and have lower immune system function than persons receiving adequate nutrients
C. Primary causes of nutritional deficiency
   1. Dietary lack of specific essential nutrients caused by
      a. Anorexia (resulting from a variety of causes)
      b. Alcoholism (and the resulting lack of proper nutrition)
      c. Poor food habits or eating nutritionally deficient foods
      d. Anorexia nervosa/bulimia
   2. Inability of the body to use a specific nutrient properly as a result of
      a. Diseases of the digestive tract such as ulcerative colitis
      b. Faulty absorption in digestive tract: malabsorption syndrome or excessive use of mineral oil
      c. Metabolic disorders such as diabetes
      d. Drug interactions and/or toxicity
D. Classification of nutrients
   1. Nutrients are chemical substances that are present in food and needed by the body to function
   2. Six prime nutrients
      a. Carbohydrates
      b. Fats
      c. Proteins
      d. Vitamins
      e. Minerals
      f. Water
   3. Individual nutrients have many specific metabolic functions. No nutrient ever works alone. In addition, the

TABLE 4-1   Clinical Signs of Nutritional Status

Features	Good	Poor
General appearance	Alert, responsive	Listless, apathetic; cachexic
Hair	Shiny, lustrous; healthy scalp	Stringy, dull, brittle, dry, depigmented
Neck glands	No enlargement	Thyroid enlarged
Skin, face, and neck	Smooth, slightly moist, good color, reddish-pink mucous membranes	Greasy, discolored, scaly
Eyes	Bright, clear; no fatigue circles	Dryness, signs of infection, increased vascularity, glassiness, thickened conjunctivae
Lips	Good color, moist	Dry, scaly, swollen, angular lesions (stomatitis)
Tongue	Good pink color; surface papillae present; no lesions	Papillary atrophy, smooth appearance; swollen, red, beefy (glossitis)
Gums	Good pink color; no swelling or bleeding; firm	Marginal redness or swelling; receding, spongy
Teeth	Straight, no crowding; well-shaped jaw; clean, no discoloration	Unfilled cavities, absent teeth, worn surfaces; mottled, malpositioned
Skin, general	Smooth, slightly moist; good color; good turgor	Rough, dry, scaly, pale, pigmented, irritated; petechiae, bruises
Abdomen	Flat	Swollen
Legs, feet	No tenderness, weakness, swelling; good color	Edema, tender calf; tingling, weakness
Skeleton	No malformations	Bowlegs, knock-knees, chest deformity at diaphragm, beaded ribs, prominent scapulae
Weight	Normal for height, age, body build	Overweight or underweight
Posture	Erect, arms and legs straight, abdomen in, chest out	Sagging shoulders, sunken chest, humped back
Muscles	Well developed, firm	Flaccid, poor tone; undeveloped, tender
Nervous control	Good attention span for age; does not cry easily; not irritable or restless	Inattentive, irritable
Gastrointestinal function	Good appetite and digestion; normal, regular elimination	Anorexia, indigestion, constipation or diarrhea
General vitality	Endurance; energetic; sleeps well at night; vigorous	Easily fatigued; no energy; falls asleep in school; looks tired, apathetic

From Williams SR: *Essentials of nutrition and diet therapy,* ed 10, St Louis, 1995, Mosby.

lack of one nutrient may inhibit the absorption or utilization of another nutrient

E. Culture and nutrition
1. Food habits are among the oldest and most deeply rooted aspects of many cultures
2. In many cultures foods take on significance in life events
3. If possible cultural preferences should be considered when planning any dietary modifications
4. Many times a religion will greatly influence nutritional practice (Table 4-2)

ASSIMILATION OF NUTRIENTS
Digestion and Absorption

A. Digestion: the process of changing foods to be absorbed and used by cells; mechanical digestion and chemical digestion occur simultaneously
1. Mechanical digestion (chewing, swallowing, peristalsis) breaks food into small pieces, mixes it with digestive juices, and moves it along the digestive tract

TABLE 4-2   Effects of Culture & Religion on Nutrition

Group	Common Dietary Practices
Cultural	
African Americans	Eat foods associated with the Southern United States; milk and dairy foods may be lacking in the diet
Mexican Americans	Liberally season food, many corn products used
Chinese Americans	Include staples of rice, wheat, and soy
Japanese Americans	Include rice, wheat, and seafood
Korean Americans	Include rice, wheat, highly seasoned foods such as cabbage
Italian Americans	Include pasta, breads, sauces, and cheese
Greek Americans	Include lamb, goat milk products, cheese products
Religious	
Jewish–Orthodox	No pork products, meat must be slaughtered and prepared according to ritual, no mixing of meat and milk, only fish with fins and scales are to be eaten
Moslem	Pork and alcohol are strictly prohibited; a month-long period of daylight fasting is observed during Ramadan; children, pregnant women, and ill individuals are exempt from the fasting period
Hindu	Primarily vegetarians; beef is not eaten
Roman Catholic	Restrictions on eating meat on Fridays; special observance from Ash Wednesday through Easter

2. Chemical digestion occurs through the action of enzymes, which break large food molecules into smaller molecules
   a. Carbohydrate digestion begins in the mouth and occurs primarily in the small intestine; carbohydrates are reduced to simple sugars (monosaccharides), such as glucose, for absorption
   b. Protein digestion begins in the stomach and is completed in the small intestine; proteins are broken down into amino acids for absorption
   c. Fat digestion begins in the stomach but occurs primarily in the small intestine; fats are reduced to fatty acids and glycerol for absorption

B. Absorption: the process by which end products of digestion (fatty acids, glycerol, amino acids, and glucose) are absorbed from the small intestine into circulation (blood and lymph) to be distributed to the cells

Metabolism

A. Use of food by the body cells for producing energy and for building complex chemical compounds
B. Consists of two processes
1. Catabolism: the breakdown of food molecules into carbon dioxide and water, which releases energy; carbohydrates are primarily catabolized for energy
2. Anabolism: the process by which food molecules are built up into more complex chemical compounds; proteins are primarily anabolized (used for building)

Energy

A. Energy is required for the metabolic processes of catabolism and anabolism; energy needs of the body are based on three factors
1. Physical activity: the type of activity and how long it is performed
2. Basal metabolism: the energy required for the body to sustain life while in a resting state (1 calorie per kilogram of body weight per hour)
3. Thermal effects of food: energy required for the digestion, absorption, and metabolism of foods
B. Measurement of energy
1. The calorie (or kilocalorie) is the unit used to measure the energy value of food
2. Fuel values of basic nutrients
   a. Carbohydrate: 4 calories per gram
   b. Fat: 9 calories per gram
   c. Protein: 4 calories per gram
3. Total number of calories needed per day
   a. Moderately active man: 20.5 calories per pound (0.45 kg) of ideal weight
   b. Moderately active woman: 18 calories per pound (0.45 kg) of ideal weight

Drugs and Nutrition

A. Drugs affect taste, appetite, intestinal motility, absorption, metabolism, and excretion of nutrients, as well as causing nausea and vomiting. Many of these interactions may compromise nutritional status and health
B. If a nutrient binds with a medication, decreased solubility of both the nutrient and drug can result
C. People at greatest risk of undesirable drug-nutrient interaction are those taking medication for long periods, those tak-

ing two or more medications, and those not eating well. Elderly people fall into the high-risk category

NUTRIENTS
Carbohydrates
A. Classification
1. Monosaccharides: single sugars, which require no digestion and are easily absorbed into the bloodstream (e.g., glucose, fructose, and galactose)
2. Disaccharides: double sugars, which must be broken down before absorption (e.g., sucrose [table sugar], lactose, and maltose)
3. Polysaccharides: complex carbohydrates composed of many sugar units (e.g., starches, glycogen, and dietary fiber)
B. Functions
1. Provide energy (glucose is the only form of energy that can be utilized by the CNS)
2. Protein-sparing effect allows protein to be used for tissue building rather than energy
3. Essential for complete metabolism of fats (incomplete fat metabolism leads to buildup of ketones and acidosis)
C. Sources
1. Polysaccharides (complex carbohydrates): bread, cereal, pasta, rice, corn, baked goods
2. Disaccharides (double sugars): table sugar, sugar cane, molasses
3. Monosaccharides (simple carbohydrates): fruit, honey, milk
D. Digestion and metabolism
1. Carbohydrate digestion primarily occurs in the small intestine. It is acted upon by three enzymes: sucrase, lactase, and maltase
2. Carbohydrates must be broken down into monosaccharides before being absorbed
3. Monosaccharides are carried to the liver, where glucose is released to the cells
4. Excess glucose is stored as glycogen to be used when needed or converted to fat and stored as fat tissue
5. Insulin regulates the use of glucose for use by the cells, thereby lowering blood sugar
6. The hormone glucagon regulates the conversion of glycogen back to glucose, causing an increase in blood glucose
E. Excess carbohydrates in diet may lead to
1. Obesity
2. Tooth decay and gum disease
3. Malnutrition (if empty calorie foods such as candy and soft drinks are eaten/drunk extensively)
F. Dietary considerations
1. Approximately 50% to 60% of total caloric intake may come from carbohydrates (mainly starches)
2. Encourage the intake of whole grain bread and cereal products; if refined cereal products are used, they should be enriched
3. Reduce the dietary intake of simple sugars (which provide empty calories) and substitute starches as sources of carbohydrates
G. Dietary fiber
1. Definition: the total amount of naturally occurring material in foods, mostly plants, that is not digested by the human digestive system and therefore is not absorbed

2. Two categories of dietary fiber: soluble and insoluble, based on the solubility in water

Protein
A. Composed of amino acids
1. Essential amino acids: amino acids the body cannot manufacture and therefore must be supplied in the diet; there are eight essential amino acids
2. Nonessential amino acids: those the body can manufacture and therefore are not as important in the diet
B. Functions
1. Build and repair body tissue (primary function)
2. Furnish energy if there is insufficient carbohydrate or fat for this purpose
3. Maintain normal circulation of tissue and blood vessel fluids through the action of plasma protein
4. Aid metabolic functions by combining with iron to form hemoglobin; used to manufacture enzymes and hormones
5. Aid body defenses by manufacturing lymphocytes and antibodies
C. Digestion and metabolism
1. Digestion of protein begins in the stomach, where it is acted upon by the enzyme pepsin. It is completed in the small intestine by three enzymes: trypsin, chymotrypsin, and carboxypeptidase
2. Protein must be broken down into amino acids to be absorbed and distributed to the cells
3. End products of protein metabolism are hydrogen, oxygen, nitrogen, water, uric acid, and urea
D. Types and sources
1. Complete proteins: foods that contain all eight essential amino acids in amounts capable of meeting human requirements (e.g., mainly animal sources, such as meats, fish, poultry, eggs, milk, and cheese)
2. Incomplete proteins: foods that lack one or more of the essential amino acids (e.g., mainly plant sources, such as cereal grains, nuts, legumes, and lentils)
3. Complementary proteins: foods that, when eaten together, supply the amino acid that is missing or in short supply in the other food (e.g., peanut butter with bread, beans with rice, and baked beans with brown bread) A rule of thumb is that a grain and a legume eaten together supply all the essential amino acids
E. Dietary considerations
1. The recommended daily protein intake for adults is 0.8 g/kg of body weight (15% of total caloric intake)
2. Dietary proteins are not stored in the body as amino acids. Proteins are the main components needed to build and repair body tissues. If the right amount and the right kinds are not available, the nitrogen is broken off and the remainder of the protein is used for energy or stored as fat. The need for cell building and maintenance is continuous. For a supply of proteins to be available on a regular basis, a source of complete proteins should be eaten at every meal
3. Increased protein is necessary during periods of growth, illness, injury, or stress; after surgery; and when bed rest is prescribed (especially for the elderly)
4. Kwashiorkor, a protein deficiency disease, is seen in many underdeveloped countries

5. Marasmus is overt starvation caused by a deficiency of calories from any source

Fats (Lipids)

A. Functions
1. Supply energy for body activities when carbohydrates are not available; all body tissues except brain and nervous cells can use fat for energy; most concentrated form of energy yields 9 calories per gram
2. Act as insulation to maintain body temperature and protect organs from mechanical injury
3. Carry fat-soluble vitamins A, D, E, and K and aid in their absorption
4. Provide a feeling of fullness and satisfaction after eating because of their slow rate of digestion
5. Furnish the essential fatty acid, linoleic acid, which is found primarily in vegetable oils; called essential because it cannot be synthesized in the body and is vital to body functioning
6. Omega-3 fatty acids, (polyunsaturated fat) which are found in fatty fish, may contribute to lower risks of heart disease

B. Types
1. Saturated fats: those whose structure is completely filled with all the hydrogen it can hold; they are usually from animal sources and are usually solid at room temperature (e.g., fats in meat, dairy products, and eggs; coconut oil, palm oil, and chocolate are also highly saturated)
2. Unsaturated fats: those whose chemical structure has one or more places where hydrogen can be added; they are less dense, usually liquid at room temperature, (with the exception of margarine) and are chiefly from plant sources (e.g., vegetable oils such as cottonseed, soybean, corn oil)
   a. Monounsaturated fats have one place for hydrogen to be added
   b. Polyunsaturated fats have two or more places for hydrogen to be added
   c. Hydrogenation: the process of adding hydrogen to a liquid or polyunsaturated fat and changing it to a solid or semisolid state (however, hydrogenation reduces the polyunsaturated fat content and therefore possibly reduces its health value)

C. Digestion and metabolism
1. Digestion of fat begins in the stomach, where gastric lipase acts on emulsified fats
2. Major portions of fat digestion occur in the small intestine, where bile emulsifies fats (breaks it into small droplets); pancreatic lipase changes the emulsified fats into fatty acids and glycerol, the end products of fat digestion
3. Fats are carried as lipoproteins to body cells, where they are either broken down for use as energy or stored as adipose tissue

D. Sources
1. Visible fats: those readily seen (e.g., butter and margarine, salad oils, shortening, and fat in meats)
2. Invisible fats: those in which the fat is less obvious (e.g., milk, avocado, cheese, and lean meat)

E. Cholesterol: a complex fat-related compound
1. A normal component of blood and of all body cells, especially brain and nerve tissue
2. Necessary for normal body functioning as structural material in cells, in the production of vitamin D, and in the production of a number of hormones
3. Supplied by food (mainly animal sources); some synthesized within the body, mainly in the intestinal walls and liver, in response to need
4. Blood cholesterol levels are affected by a variety of factors including diet, heredity, emotional stress, and exercise; saturated fats tend to raise blood cholesterol, whereas polyunsaturated fats are recommended for lowering cholesterol levels
5. Cholesterol is carried to and from body cells by special carriers called lipoproteins
   a. High-density lipoprotein (HDL), or "good" cholesterol, carries cholesterol away from the arteries and back to the liver for removal from the body
   b. Low-density lipoprotein (LDL), or "bad" cholesterol, tends to circulate in the bloodstream and form plaque on the inner walls of arteries
6. Risk is classified according to total cholesterol level as follows
   a. Desirable—below 200 mg/dl
   b. Borderline high—200 to 239 mg/dl
   c. High—above 240 mg/dl
7. If the total cholesterol level is borderline high or high, then the levels and ratio of LDL and HDL should be evaluated
8. High cholesterol levels predispose individuals to atherosclerosis and other serious health problems
9. Foods high in cholesterol: organ meats, animal fat, egg yolk, and shellfish

F. Dietary considerations
1. The Dietary Guidelines for America 1995 recommended that daily intake of fats for adults should not be more than 30% of the total caloric intake; no more than 10% of the intake should be from saturated fat
2. To decrease dietary fat
   a. Use leaner cuts of meat and more poultry; trim fats from all meats
   b. Use fewer eggs or egg substitute products
   c. Use low-fat milk products
   d. Limit use of fat in cooking as much as possible
   e. Decrease frequency of red meat use

G. Effects of excess fat intake
1. Obesity
2. Consumption may predispose to serious conditions such as heart disease, diabetes, and stroke
3. Increased surgical risk

Vitamins

See Table 4-3.

A. Definitions
1. Vitamins: organic compounds needed in small amounts for growth and maintenance of life
2. Precursor (or provitamin): substances that precede and can be changed into active vitamins (e.g., carotene is the precursor of vitamin A)
3. Hypervitaminosis: the excess of one or more vitamins
4. Synthetic: man-made vitamins
5. Enriched: the addition of nutrients to a food often in amounts larger than might be found naturally in that food

TABLE 4-3   Vitamins

Vitamin	Sources	Functions	Deficiency Symptoms
Fat-Soluble Vitamins			
A (retinol) Precursor: carotene	Fish liver oils Liver Green, leafy vegetables Yellow vegetables (corn, carrots, and sweet potatoes) Yellow fruits (apricots and peaches) Egg yolk Whole milk	Regenerates visual purple (necessary for good vision) Formation of bones and teeth Maintains skin and mucous membranes	Night blindness Retardation of skeletal growth Dry, scaly skin Dry mucous membranes Susceptibility to epithelial infection Xerophthalmia (corneal cells become opaque, slough off, could lead to blindness)
D (calciferol)	Sunshine Fish liver oils Fortified milk	Regulates calcium and phosphorus absorption and metabolism Essential for normal formation of bones and teeth	Lowered levels of calcium and phosphorus in blood Soft bones Rickets Malformed teeth
E (tocopherol)	Wheat germ Vegetable oils Dark green, leafy vegetables	Inconclusive at present Preserves integrity of RBCs Antioxidant (protects materials that oxidize easily) Protects structure and function of muscle	Increased hemolysis (breakdown) of red blood cells (RBCs) Anemia Breakdown of vitamin A and essential fatty acids
K (menadione)	Synthesis by intestinal bacteria Green, leafy vegetables Pork liver	Formation of prothrombin (necessary in blood clotting)	Prolonged clotting time (bleeding tendencies) Hemorrhagic diseases
Water-Soluble Vitamins			
C (ascorbic acid)	Citrus fruits Tomatoes Broccoli Strawberries Green peppers Cantaloupes Potatoes	Formation and maintenance of capillary walls and collagen formation Aids in absorption of iron	Scurvy (deficiency disease) Sore gums Tendency to bruise easily Poor wound healing Anemia
B_1 (thiamine)	Wheat germ Whole or enriched grains Legumes Pork and organ meats	Maintains carbohydrate metabolism Maintains muscle and nerve functioning	Beriberi (deficiency disease) Anorexia, fatigue, nerve disorders, irritability
B_2 (riboflavin)	Milk Organ meats Green, leafy vegetables Enriched bread and cereals	Maintains appetite Maintains healthy eyes Maintains color and structure of lips Metabolism of nutrients	Sensitivity to light, dim vision Inflammation of lips and tongue Loss of appetite and weight
B_6 (pyridoxine)	Red meats (especially organ meats) Whole grain cereals Pork, lamb, veal	Synthesis and metabolism of proteins Hemoglobin synthesis Maintenance of muscles and nerves	Nausea and vomiting, anorexia, anemia, irritability, CNS dysfunction, kidney stones, dermatitis
B_{12} (cobalamin)	Found only in animal products Organ and muscle meats Dairy products	Protein metabolism Production of RBCs Normal functioning of nervous system	Pernicious anemia (resulting from lack of intrinsic factor needed for B_{12} absorption)
Niacin (nicotinic acid) Precursor: tryptophan	Meats (especially organ meats) Poultry and fish Peanut butter	Essential for normal functioning of digestive and nervous systems Essential for growth and metabolism	Pellagra (deficiency disease) Nervous disorders Diarrhea and nausea Dermatitis
Folic acid (folacin)		Essential in formation of all body cells, especially RBCs Protein metabolism	Anemia (macrocytic) Gastrointestinal disturbances Glossitis Stomatitis

6. Fortified: the replacement in food of nutrients lost during processing

B. Characteristics
1. Contain no calories
2. Essential to life because they generally cannot be synthesized by the body and are necessary for cell metabolism
3. Functions include tissue building and regulation of body functions
4. Needed in minute amounts (milligrams [mg] or micrograms [mg]); the safety of taking megadoses is debatable
5. Well-balanced diet should provide adequate vitamins to fulfill body requirements

C. Classified on basis of solubility
1. Fat-soluble vitamins: A, D, E, and K
   a. Sufficient fats needed in diet to carry fat-soluble vitamins
   b. Stored in body, so deficiencies are slow to appear
   c. Absorbed in the same manner as fats so anything that interferes with absorption of fats interferes with absorption of fat-soluble vitamins (mineral oil, an indigestible substance, carries fat-soluble vitamins with it out of the body)
   d. Fairly stable in cooking and storage
2. Water-soluble vitamins: C and B complex
   a. Not stored in body; deficiency can occur if vitamins are not consumed in the daily diet
   b. Easily destroyed by air and in cooking

SPECIAL VITAMIN CONSIDERATIONS

A. Current research indicates that the effects of megadoses of vitamin C on the common cold are minimal
B. Effects of vitamin C on cancer still require further study
C. Claims list vitamin E as a "cure-all," especially in prolonging virility in males, preventing miscarriages, and curing muscular weakness
D. Current research has not established the validity of these claims; however, the amounts usually taken in supplements have caused no damage

Minerals

A. Definition: inorganic elements essential for growth and normal functioning (Table 4-4)
B. Types
1. Major minerals, or macrominerals, are found in the largest amounts in the body and are needed in large amounts (100 mg or more per day); they are calcium, phosphorus, potassium, sodium, chlorine, magnesium, and sulfur
2. Microminerals, or trace elements, are needed in small amounts (e.g., iron, zinc, copper, and iodine)
C. Characteristics
1. Found in all body tissues and fluids
2. Occur naturally in foods (especially unrefined foods)
3. Do not furnish energy, but regulate body processes that furnish energy
4. Remain stable in food preparation
D. Functions
1. Constitute bones and teeth (calcium and phosphorus)
2. Transmit nerve impulses and aid in muscle contraction
3. Control water balance (sodium and potassium)
4. Maintain acid-base balance
5. Synthesize essential body compounds (e.g., iodine for thyroxine)

6. Act as catalysts for tissue reactions (e.g., calcium needed for blood clotting)

Water

A. Water makes up 50% to 65% of the weight of an average adult
1. Intracellular: fluid within cells composed of water plus concentrations of potassium and phosphates: contains minerals, potassium, magnesium, and phosphorus
2. Extracellular: all body fluids outside cells including interstitial fluid, plasma, and watery components of body organs and substances; contains minerals, sodium chloride
B. Functions
1. Essential component of all tissues and fluids
2. Transportation of nutrients from the digestive tract to the bloodstream and from cell to cell; also removal of waste products from cells to outside the body
3. Lubrication of joints
4. Maintenance of stable body temperature (as temperature increases, sweating occurs, evaporates, and cools the body)
5. Solvent for all the body's chemical processes
C. Overall water balance in the body
1. Intake: under ordinary conditions, adults need 2 to 3 L of liquid per day—5 to 6 glasses of which should be water
   a. Ingested fluids such as water, soups, and beverages
   b. Water in foods that are eaten
   c. Water formed from cell oxidation (when nutrients are burned)
2. Output: averages 2600 ml daily
   a. Normal routes of excretion: primarily the kidney but also the skin, lungs, and feces
   b. Abnormal and extensive losses can occur from vomiting and diarrhea, open or draining wounds, fever, extensive burns, hemorrhage, and anything that causes excessive perspiration
D. Additional fluids are required
1. By infants
2. During fever or disease process
3. In warm weather
4. During heavy work or extensive physical activity

Cellulose

A. Definition: a polysaccharide that makes up the framework of plants; provides bulk (fiber or roughage) for the diet; cannot be broken down by the human digestive system and therefore is not absorbed
B. Function: to absorb water, provide bulk, and stimulate peristalsis
C. Found in the stalks and leaves of plants, in the skins of fruit and vegetables, and in the outer covering of seeds and cereals (refined cereals have most of the fiber removed and provide little bulk)

NUTRITIONAL GUIDELINES
Recommended Dietary Allowances (RDA)

A. Developed by the Food and Nutrition Board of the National Academy of Science
B. Suggested levels of essential nutrients (proteins, vitamins, and minerals) known from current research to be adequate to meet nutritional needs of most healthy individuals

TABLE 4-4   Major Minerals and Microminerals (Trace Elements)

Vitamin	Sources	Functions	Deficiency Symptoms
Major Minerals			
Calcium (Ca): absorption aided by vitamin D	Milk and milk products Cheese Some green, leafy vegetables (turnips, collards, kale, broccoli)	Bone and tooth formation Blood clotting Muscle (including heart muscle) contraction Nerve transmission Cell wall permeability	Poor bone and tooth formation Rickets (deficiency disease) Stunted growth Osteoporosis Poor blood clotting Tetany
Phosphorus (P): absorption with Ca aided by vitamin D	Milk and cheese Meat Egg yolk Whole grains (Diet adequate in protein and Ca should be adequate in P)	Functions as calcium phosphate in the calcification of bones and teeth Energy metabolism Regulation of acid-base balance Cell structure and enzyme activity	Poor bone and tooth formation Retarded growth Rickets (deficiency disease) Weakness Anorexia
Sodium (Na)	Salt Baking powder and soda Dairy products Meat, fish, and poultry	Regulation of acid-base balance Fluid balance Nerve transmission and muscle contraction Glucose absorption	Nausea and vomiting Apathy Exhaustion Abdominal and muscle cramps
Potassium (K)	Meat, fish, and poultry Whole grain breads and cereals Fruits (oranges, bananas)	Regulates nerve conduction and muscle contraction Necessary for regular heart rhythm Fluid and acid-base balance Cell metabolism	Abnormal heartbeat Muscle weakness Nausea and vomiting
Chlorine (Cl)	Table salt (NaCl)	Formation of hydrochloric acid and maintenance of gastric acidity Maintenance of acid-base balance, osmotic pressure, and water balance	Deficiency results from fluid loss through vomiting, diarrhea, and heavy sweating
Magnesium (Mg)	Green, leafy vegetables Legumes Milk Whole grains	Component of bones and teeth Enzymes essential in general metabolism Conduction of nerve impulses Muscle contraction	Tremors leading to convulsive seizures
Sulfur (S)	Protein foods Meat Milk Eggs Cheese Nuts and legumes	Component of all body cells; important in building connective tissue Component in several B vitamins and several amino acids Energy metabolism	None documented
Microminerals			
Iron (Fe): absorption enhanced by vitamin C	Organ meats (especially liver) Egg yolk Green, leafy vegetables Lean red meats Dried fruits (apricots, raisins)	Synthesis of hemoglobin General metabolic activities	Anemia
Iodine (I)	Iodized salt Saltwater fish	Normal functioning of thyroid gland	Goiter
Zinc (Zn)	Oysters Liver High-protein foods	Component of enzymes Assists in regulation of cell growth Protein synthesis	Impaired wound healing Poor taste sensitivity Retarded sexual and physical development
Copper (Cu)	Liver Cocoa Nuts Raisins	Aids in absorption of iron Component of hemoglobin Component of enzymes	Unknown at present, although secondary conditions may develop

C. Used as a guideline for most federal, state, and local feeding programs but not to be used as requirements for individuals with specific nutritional deficiencies

U.S. Dietary Goals or Dietary Guidelines

A. Developed by the U.S. Department of Agriculture, U.S. Department of Health and Human Services
B. Established in 1980 and are updated every 5 years. The current *Nutrition and Your Health: Dietary Guidelines for Americans,* released in 1995, has a more positive tone that emphasizes health promotion. The following are the seven guidelines:
   1. Eat a variety of foods (for a variety of nutrients)
   2. Balance the food you eat with physical activity; maintain or improve your weight
   3. Choose a diet with plenty of grain products, vegetables, and fruits
   4. Choose a diet low in fat, saturated fat, and cholesterol
   5. Choose a diet moderate in sugars
   6. Choose a diet moderate in salt and sodium
   7. If you drink alcoholic beverages, do so in moderation (alcohol is high in calories but low in nutrients; also heavy drinking contributes to many chronic liver and neurological disorders)

Nutritional Labeling and Education Act of 1990

A. This regulation has increased consumer access to safe products and knowledge of what nutrients are in food.
B. The Nutrition Facts Panel must include the quantities of energy, fat, and other specific nutrients

Nutritional Assessment

A. Two phases: screening and assessment. Purpose: to screen for nutritional risks and apply specific assessment techniques to determine an action plan

B. Components of nutritional assessment; anthropometric measurements, biochemical tests, clinical observations, dietary and personal histories. All components work together to determine the best action plan for the individual in the healthy population and the sick population within the context of their personal, social, and economic background

Food Guide Pyramid

See Figure 4-1.
A. Emphasizes grains, fruits, and vegetables as the foundation of a balanced diet and downplays meats, dairy products, and fats; fats, oils, and sweets are recommended sparingly
B. Specific guidelines
   1. Breads, cereals, rice, pasta: six to eleven servings daily (1 serving equals 1 slice of bread, 1 oz of ready-to-eat cereal, or ½ cup of cooked cereal, rice, or pasta); nutrients primarily supplied are iron, B complex vitamins, and carbohydrates (starches); refined products contain fewer vitamins, whereas the enriched, fortified, or restored products contain many more vitamins
   2. Fruits: two to four servings daily (1 serving equals 1 medium apple, banana, or orange or ½ cup of cooked, chopped, or canned fruit); nutrients primarily supplied are vitamins A and C and fiber
   3. Vegetables: three to five servings daily (1 serving equals 1 cup of raw, leafy vegetables or ½ cup of other vegetables cooked, chopped, or raw); nutrients primarily supplied are vitamins A and C and fiber
   4. Milk, yogurt, cheese: two to three servings daily (1 serving equals 1 cup of milk or yogurt or ½ oz of natural cheese); nutrients primarily supplied are calcium, protein, and riboflavin
   5. Meat, poultry, fish, dry beans, eggs, and nuts: two to three servings daily (1 serving equals 2 to 3 oz of cooked lean meat, poultry, or fish; ½ cup of cooked dry beans, or 1 egg; 2 tbsp of peanut butter equals 1 oz of lean

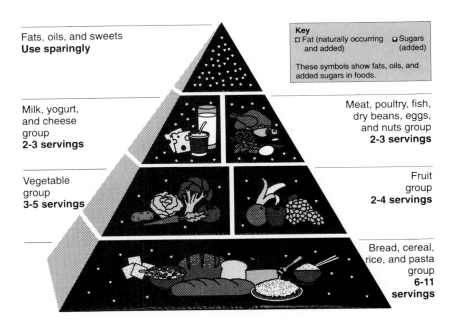

Figure 4-1. Food guide pyramid: a guide to daily food choices. (Courtesy U.S. Department of Agriculture, Washington, DC, 1992.)

meat); nutrients primarily supplied are protein, iron, and B vitamins

FOOD MANAGEMENT
Food Fads and Facts: Meat Eaters Versus Vegetarians

A. Problems exist when too large a portion of the diet consists of meat
1. Excess calories tend to be consumed; meat (and the fat therein) is high in calories; because of the taste the tendency is to eat more than is required
2. When a large portion of the meal is meat, a smaller portion of fruits and vegetables is consumed; therefore, less fiber and fewer of the nutrients in fruits and vegetables are consumed
B. Vegetarians also can have nutritional deficiencies
1. Calories may be insufficient despite large amounts of foods being consumed
2. Protein can be lacking; incomplete protein must be supplemented with complementary proteins
3. Strict vegetarians may need supplements of cobalamin, because it is found only in animal proteins
C. The ideal diet combines both types of diet with a variety of foods
1. Meat eaters should eat smaller servings of leaner meats with more fruits, vegetables, and cereals
2. Vegetarians should improve the quality of their diet by adding dairy products such as eggs and milk (if no dairy products are taken, complementary proteins should be carefully selected)

Economic Considerations in Menu Planning

A. Plan menus in advance
1. Take advantage of specials to prepare balanced meals
2. Shop from a list to avoid impulse buying
B. Choose foods wisely
1. Buy foods in season and in good supply
2. Buy in quantity if adequate storage is available (larger quantities may cost less per unit)
3. Buy sale items only if they can be used
4. Use unit pricing to find the best buys among brands
5. Know grades and brands of foods; grading of canned goods has no bearing on nutritive value; generic labeling can save up to 25% of name brand items
6. Purchase staple and canned goods when on sale
7. Remember that cost per serving rather than per pound is important, especially in buying meat
8. Compare labels for weights and ingredients
9. Buy less expensive forms of food (margarine is less expensive than butter)
10. Limit purchase of empty-calorie foods
11. Decrease the cost of protein in the diet by using small amounts of meats, fish, and poultry and by using lower grades and less expensive cuts of meat; also legumes, peanut butter, eggs, and cheese are good sources of less expensive protein
12. Try to avoid convenience foods (any food bought partially prepared and ready to eat with little home preparation); they are usually more expensive than those prepared entirely at home and are less nutritionally balanced, containing high proportions of fat, calories, and sodium

C. Care for foods after purchase
1. Store foods properly to avoid spoilage and loss of nutrients
2. Consume leftover foods quickly

Storage and Preparation of Basic Foods

A. Milk
1. Store milk refrigerated in covered container; powdered milk should be stored in a cool, dry place; refrigerate powdered milk after reconstituting
2. Cook over low heat; avoid scorching
B. Cheese
1. Refrigerate well wrapped or in tight containers
2. Most palatable if served at room temperature; cook at low temperatures for a short time
C. Eggs
1. Refrigerate promptly; if cracked, use only in foods that will be well cooked
2. Cook at lower temperatures to prevent discoloration, curdling, or toughness
D. Cereals and breads
1. Store in cool, dry place; bread retains freshness best at room temperature but molds faster; bread freezes well
2. Cook cereals according to directions; overcooking reduces vitamin content
E. Meat, fish, and poultry
1. Store in refrigerator for a short time or freeze for longer storage
2. Less expensive meats, although nutritionally equivalent to more expensive ones, require longer cooking at lower temperatures
F. Fruits and vegetables
1. Store ripe fruits and vegetables in the refrigerator (fruits ripen best at room temperature)
2. Cook only until tender, (steaming) using as little water as possible (cooking liquids contain valuable nutrients and should be used if possible); raw fruits and vegetables are especially nutritious

Types of Milk

A. Skim: fat and vitamin A removed (may have vitamins A and D added); contains all other nutrients of whole milk
B. Homogenized: fat particles evenly dispersed so cream does not separate
C. Pasteurized: heated to a specific temperature to destroy pathogenic bacteria (but nutrients are not affected)
D. Condensed: water removed and sugar added so carbohydrate content is increased; low in calcium and vitamins and high in sugar compared with whole milk
E. Evaporated: heated above the boiling point so that more than half the water evaporates
F. Low fat: contains 0.5% to 2% fat; lower in calories than whole milk but comparable in nutrient value
G. Powdered or dry: water removed; least expensive form of milk on the market; when reconstituted, it has the same nutrient value as the milk from which it was made

COMMON TYPES OF FOOD POISONING
Staphylococcal Food Poisoning

A. Caused by *Staphylococcus aureus* bacteria; resistant to heat
B. Involves foods such as custard; potato, macaroni, egg, and chicken salads; cheese; ham; and salami

C. Exhibited by symptoms such as abdominal cramps, diarrhea, and vomiting; lasts 1 to 2 days; usually mild and attributed to other causes

D. Prevented by keeping foods above 140° F (60° C) or below 40° F (4° C); toxin is destroyed by boiling for several hours or heating in a pressure cooker at 240° F (138.5° C) for 30 minutes

Clostridial Food Poisoning

A. Perfringens
   1. Caused by *Clostridium perfringens,* spore-forming bacteria that grow in the absence of oxygen
   2. Involves foods such as stews, soups, and gravies made from poultry and red meat
   3. Exhibited by symptoms such as nausea without vomiting, diarrhea, and acute inflammation of the stomach and intestine; usually lasts 1 day
   4. Prevented by storing foods properly and keeping foods above 140° F (60° C) or below 40° F (4° C)

B. Botulism
   1. Caused by *Clostridium botulinum,* spore-forming bacteria that grow and produce toxins in absence of oxygen (anaerobic)
   2. Involves canned low-acid foods, especially home-canned foods such as meats, corn, peas, green beans, asparagus, and mushrooms
   3. Exhibited by symptoms such as inability to swallow; double vision, and progressive respiratory paralysis; fatality rate is high if untreated
   4. Prevented by pressure cooking canned foods for specified length of time; any can or jar with a bulging top should be discarded

Salmonellosis

A. Caused by Salmonella, bacteria widespread in nature that live in the intestinal tracts of humans and animals; transmitted by eating infected food or by contact with people who are infected or are carriers of the disease; also transmitted by insects or rodents

B. Involves poultry, red meats, dairy products, and eggs

C. Exhibited by symptoms such as severe headache, vomiting, diarrhea, abdominal cramps, and fever; usually last 2 to 7 days

D. Prevented by heating foods to 140° F (60° C) for 10 minutes or higher temperatures for less time

E. coli

A. Caused by pathogenic *Escherichia coli,* some types are normally found in human intestinal system

B. Pathogenic *E. coli* found in raw ground beef

C. Bacteria attacks intestinal wall and spreads to body

D. Exhibited by symptoms such as bloody diarrhea, cramps, fever, chills, dehydration, kidney problems; can be fatal

E. Prevented by using well-cooked meats and sanitary food handling

NUTRITION THROUGHOUT THE LIFE CYCLE
Infant Nutrition

A. Infants require more protein and calories per pound of body weight than adults do because they have more body surface in proportion to weight and because of their growth and activity

B. Breast-feeding is the recommended method of feeding if possible; provides more vitamin C and more easily digested protein and sugar than cow's milk; also provides the infant with antibodies against disease and assists in establishing the mother-child bond; in addition, breastfed babies experience fewer allergies and intolerances, as well as easier digestion

C. Bottle-feeding is an acceptable alternative if close mother-child contact is maintained; most mothers use a commercially prepared formula such as Enfamil; a soy-based product such as Isomil can be used if the infant is allergic to milk products. At no time during the first year of life should an infant be fed regular whole cow's milk. Its concentration may cause GI bleeding or renal discomfort. Skim milk or low-fat milk provides infants with too little energy and linoleic acid

D. The American Academy of Pediatrics recommends breast milk supplemented by vitamin D and fluoride from birth, and iron supplements after 4 months of age

E. Introduction of solid foods varies among pediatricians, most favoring a delay until the infant is at least 6 months of age
   1. Infant cereal is usually given first (often with added iron to supplement a possible lack in the infant's diet; prenatal iron reserves last 5 to 6 months). Rice cereal is given first, it is easy to digest and provokes few allergies
   2. Fruits, vegetables, and egg yolk are frequently given next (because of possible allergic reactions, egg white is delayed until late in the first year)
   3. Solid foods should be introduced one at a time and at 4- to 5-day intervals to observe for any allergic reactions
   4. Adding sugar or salt to infant's food is undesirable
   5. Infants can choke on small foods such as berries, corn, popcorn, or candy
   6. Infants should not receive honey, because honey contains botulism spores, which could harm the infant (even though quantities are too low to harm older children and adults)

Preschool Children

A. Growth rate is slower and more erratic, and food intake will vary accordingly

B. A variety of foods should be offered
   1. "Finger foods" such as carrot sticks are enjoyed
   2. Serve small amounts because too large a serving can discourage a child from eating
   3. Avoid refined sweets
   4. Do not coax a child to eat; if a food is refused, offer it at a later date
   5. Nutritious snacks are a viable alternative for a child who is a poor eater

C. Teach healthy eating habits; avoid rewarding good behavior with food

School Children (5 to 10 Years of Age)

A. Gradual increase in growth at this age (approximately equal for boys and girls)

B. Proper nutrition is important for proper mental and physical development (adequate breakfast is important for alertness during class)

C. Children are usually good eaters at this age and should be encouraged by the examples set at home and at school; promote healthy eating

Adolescents

A. Tremendous growth spurt occurs at puberty (age of sexual maturity)
   1. For girls, usually between 10 and 13 years of age
   2. For boys, between 13 and 16 years of age
B. Diets are influenced by peers, with many empty-calorie foods being consumed
C. Boys gain mostly lean muscle tissue; they consume large amounts of food to meet energy requirements
D. Girls gain more fat tissue; their diets may be more influenced by a desire to remain thin; frequently require iron supplements to meet their needs; adequate nutrition during adolescence helps avoid complications during pregnancy; promote healthy eating along with exercise

Adults

A. Adequate nutrition throughout the life span is important in avoiding many serious illnesses
B. Proper nutrition is based on guidelines set by U.S. government agencies (such as the food pyramid)
C. Persons who consume a balanced diet usually do not need vitamin supplements
D. If a woman of childbearing age is a smoker and has poor dietary intake, a vitamin C supplement of 100 mg/day is recommended

Older Adults

A. Physiological changes affect nutrition of the elderly
   1. Aging slows the basal metabolic rate (BMR); combined with decreased activity the result is decreased energy requirements and decreased number of calories needed
   2. Taste may be adversely affected by gradual diminishment of the senses of smell, sight, and taste
   3. Loss of teeth may affect proper chewing, food intake, or enjoyment
   4. Reduced saliva makes swallowing more difficult and digestion less efficient
   5. Decreased movement of wastes through intestines contributes to constipation
   6. Marginal deficiencies of ascorbic acid, thiamin, riboflavin have occurred in some elderly patients
   7. Decreased absorption and use of nutrients results from decreased digestive juices and gastric motility reduction
B. Economic and social considerations
   1. Decrease in income among the elderly, combined with an increase in the amount spent for medical care, leaves less for adequate nutrition; tendency is to eat less protein (which is expensive) and more carbohydrates (which are cheaper and easier to prepare)
   2. Loss of spouse, friends, or mobility results in isolation, depression, and often decreased will to obtain adequate nutrition
C. Planning diets
   1. Diet should be well balanced in protein, vitamins, and minerals (especially calcium and iron) to allow for diminished absorption
   2. Calories sufficient to maintain energy and activity (reduced from those previously required)
   3. Soft bulk in diet to prevent constipation (cooked fruits and vegetables)

   4. Increased fluid intake required to eliminate metabolic wastes
   5. Meals should be light and easily digested, that is, contain only a small amount of fats; frequent small meals may be easier to digest than three large meals
   6. Individual preferences should be respected and the diet built around them; make changes slowly
   7. Meals eaten with others are often more appetizing than those eaten alone

Pregnancy

A. A well-balanced diet with increased amounts of essential nutrients is important to the well-being of the mother and baby
   1. A protein increase of 20% or 60 g/day over the normal diet is recommended to allow for growth of the baby, placenta, maternal tissues, and increased circulating blood volume, amniotic fluid, and storage
   2. An increase in calories meets increased energy demands and allows protein to be used for tissue building. Calorie needs approximate an extra 300 calories/day, which can be gained by adding a serving of dairy foods
   3. Increased amounts of the following: calcium, phosphorus, and vitamin D are needed both for the mother and for the bones and teeth of the baby; iron for hemoglobin and prenatal storage for the baby; iodine for thyroxine for the mother's increased BMR; and vitamins A, B complex, and C
   4. Weight should not be severely restricted; a gain of 30 lb is considered healthy
   5. Severe restriction of salt is unfounded
B. Vomiting (morning sickness)
   1. Lower fat intake with more high-carbohydrate foods
   2. Fluids between instead of with meals
   3. Dry toast or crackers on awakening

Lactation

A. A baby requires 2 to 2½ oz (60 to 75 ml) of breast milk per pound (488 g) of body weight (1 oz [30 ml] equals approximately 520 calories); there is an increased maternal need for all nutrients during lactation
B. Diet of a lactating mother should be high in protein and calories (approximately 500 extra calories/day)
C. Increased fluids are also required; at least 6 cups (1.5 L) of milk in some form is recommended

DIET THERAPY
Nursing Responsibilities

A. Nutritional assessment: assess physical characteristics of patient; individualize care to allow for patient differences
B. Evaluate the patient's tolerance to diet and provide feedback to other health team members
C. Assist patient in learning about required dietary changes; reinforce information and answer questions
D. If possible, incorporate patient's preferences to increase compliance with the nutritional care plan
E. Prepare the patient for mealtime; assist as necessary
F. See that each person receives the correct tray unless foods are being withheld
G. Serve and remove tray promptly

H. Teach patients the value of proper nutrition and urge compliance with the nutritional care plan

Purposes of Diet Therapy

A. To increase or decrease weight
B. To allow a particular organ or system to rest (e.g., a low-fat diet in gallbladder disease)
C. To regulate the diet to correspond with the body's ability to metabolize a specific nutrient (e.g., diabetes)
D. To correct conditions caused by deficiencies
E. To eliminate harmful substances from the diet (e.g., caffeine, cholesterol, and alcohol)
F. To nourish the body

Diet Modifications

A. Calories may be increased or decreased
B. Nutrients may be adjusted (high or low protein)
C. Certain foods may be omitted or added
D. Modifications in texture (consistency-soft diet)
E. Frequency of meals: more than the standard three

Standard Hospital Diets (Modifications in Consistency)

A. Clear liquid (surgical liquid)
   1. Temporary diet of clear liquids, nonresidue, nonirritating, non–gas-forming; inadequate in protein, vitamins, minerals, and calories
   2. Used postoperatively to replace fluids, before certain tests, and to lessen amount of fecal matter in colon
   3. Includes water, coffee, tea, fat-free broth, pulp-free fruit juices (apple), gelatin, and ginger ale
B. Full liquid diet
   1. Foods liquid at room or body temperatures; may be adequate if carefully planned, although frequently deficient in iron
   2. Used postoperatively as a transition between clear and soft diet, in infections and acute gastritis; in febrile conditions; and for patients unable to chew or swallow or with an intolerance to food for other reasons
   3. Includes all clear liquids, milk, creamed soups, ice creams, sherbets, plain puddings, and thin, strained cereal
C. Soft diet
   1. Normal diet modified in consistency to have limited fiber; easily digested; nutritionally adequate
   2. Used between full liquid and regular, for chewing difficulties, and in gastrointestinal disorders
   3. Includes tender meats and tender, well-cooked vegetables (those with a great deal of fiber should be pureed or omitted); fruits (no fiber) and plain cakes are allowed; no spicy or coarse foods are allowed
D. Regular (general or house) diet
   1. Adequate, well-balanced diet designed to appeal to most people
   2. Used for those not requiring a modified or therapeutic diet
   3. Includes all foods from the four basic food groups

Additional Modified (or Therapeutic) Diets

Table 4-5 lists diets; foods allowed and omitted; and when the diets are used.

DIETS FOR SPECIFIC CONDITIONS
Diabetes Mellitus

A. Classification
   1. IDDM (type I), or insulin dependent: onset is usually before the age of 20; difficult to manage and requires dietary restrictions, insulin injections, and exercise
   2. NIDDM (type II), or maturity onset: usually develops after age 35; frequently controlled by diet alone; insulin or oral hypoglycemics or both may also be needed
B. Diet is determined by age, sex, body build, weight, and activity; maintenance requirements are the same as for a nondiabetic patient
   1. Calories: sufficient to maintain ideal body weight (approximately 30 cal/kg ideal weight)
   2. Protein: 10% to 20% of daily caloric intake
   3. Carbohydrates: 50% to 60% of total calories (obtain greatest portion from complex carbohydrates such as starches, and the least from simple sugars)
   4. Fats: moderately controlled; 30% or less of total calories and 10% from saturated fat
   5. High-fiber foods, which decrease postprandial blood glucose levels, are encouraged
C. Exchange system is used for planning the diabetic diet
   1. Based on simple grouping of common foods according to equivalent nutritional values
   2. Six basic food groups or food exchanges; each food within the group contains approximately the same food value as other foods within the same group
      a. Milk: equal to 1 cup (240 ml) whole milk
      b. Vegetables: variety of low-carbohydrate vegetables
      c. Fruit: fresh or canned without sugar
      d. Bread: starchy items (breads, pasta, cereals, and vegetables equal to 1 slice bread)
      e. Meat: protein food equal to 1 oz (28 g) lean meat
      f. Fat equal to 1 tsp (5 ml) margarine
   3. Total exchanges per day is determined by individual nutritional needs based on nutritional standards (Table 4-6 shows a sample diet based on the exchange system)
   4. Advantages of exchange system
      a. Is easy to understand
      b. Allows diabetic patients more freedom to choose foods they like
      c. Allows choice of foods that fit into their economic status
      d. Can be used for other types of diets
      e. Does not require dietetic or specialized diabetic foods

Surgery

A. Surgery increases the nutritional demands on the body
   1. Protein: increased for tissue repair, to prevent tissue breakdown, and to help replace blood and fluid losses
   2. Carbohydrates: increased to meet body demands for energy and to spare protein for tissue building
   3. Vitamins: especially important in wound healing; vitamin C cements cells, and builds connective tissue and capillaries
B. Types of feeding available postoperatively
   1. Intravenous: immediately administered to supply essential water, electrolytes, and vitamins; intended only as short-term for fluid and electrolytes supplement

TABLE 4-5   Modified or Therapeutic Diets

Diet	Condition	Foods Allowed	Purpose of Diet
High calorie	Underweight (10% or more) Anorexia nervosa Hyperthyroidism	Emphasis on increase in calories Easily digested foods (carbohydrates) recommended Full meals with high-calorie snacks	To meet the increased metabolic needs of the body or provide increased calories for weight gain
Low calorie	Overweight	Fruits and vegetables especially recommended	To reduce the caloric intake below what the body requires so that weight loss will occur
High protein	Children who need additional protein for growth Following surgery Pregnancy and lactation Conditions that cause protein loss Extensive burns	Added amounts of poultry, meat, fish, milk, cheese, and eggs Nonfat dry milk added to soups and baked goods	To increase the intake of high-protein foods for maintaining and rebuilding tissues and correcting protein loss
Low protein	Liver disease Kidney diseases leading to renal failure	Fruits and vegetables Severely limited in amounts of meats, fish, poultry, eggs, and dairy products	To limit the end products of protein metabolism to avoid disturbing the fluid, electrolyte, and acid-base balances
High residue	Constipation (atonic) Diverticulitis (when inflammation has ceased)	Increased whole grain cereals Increased fruits and raw vegetables Fibrous meats	Mechanically stimulates the gastrointestinal tract
Low residue	Before and after bowel surgery Ulcerative colitis Diverticulitis (during inflammatory stage) Diarrhea	Soft cheeses Tender meats Refined cereals and breads Pureed fruits and vegetables Plain puddings	To soothe and be nonirritating to gastrointestinal tract
Low fat	Gallbladder disease Obesity Cardiovascular disease	Vegetables and fruits Skim milk Sherbet Increased carbohydrates and proteins	To lower fat content in diet (may be deficient in fat-soluble vitamins)
Low cholesterol	Cardiovascular disease	Lean meats and fish Poultry without the skin Liquid vegetable oils Skim milk	To decrease the blood cholesterol levels or maintain them at acceptable levels
High iron	Anemias	Regular diet with high-iron foods Liver and organ meats Red meats Dried fruits Egg yolks	To correct an iron deficiency
Sodium restricted	Kidney disease Cardiovascular disease Hypertension	Natural foods without salt Milk and meat in limited quantities	To control or correct the retention of sodium and water in the body by controlling sodium intake
High carbohydrate	Preparation for surgery Liver disease Kidney disease	Emphasis on carbohydrate foods Full meals with high carbohydrate snacks	To provide increased energy and spare protein for tissue building
Low carbohydrate	Dumping syndrome Hyperinsulinism Diabetes mellitus (although severe restriction of carbohydrates is currently considered unwarranted)	Proteins Only enough carbohydrate to maintain health and perform activities	To decrease the amounts of glucose in the bloodstream (increased blood glucose causes increased amounts of insulin to be produced by the body)
Lactose restricted	Lactose intolerance	Avoid foods containing lactose, such as milk, cheese, and ice cream	To eliminate or cut down on lactose—a substance certain individuals cannot metabolize

TABLE 4-6   1800-Calorie Diet With Food Exchanges

Exchange Group	Total Exchanges for the Day
Milk	2
Vegetables	2
Fruit	5
Bread	9
Meat	8
Fat	7

Sample Diet	Exchange List
Breakfast	
Black coffee	Free
2 eggs	2 meat
2 pieces toast	2 bread
with butter	2 fat
Cereal	1 bread
with milk	1 milk
and plain blueberries	1 fruit
Lunch	
Turkey sandwich (3 oz or 84 g)	2 breads
	3 meat
with mayonnaise (2 tsp or 10 ml)	2 fat
with tomatoes	1 vegetable
Sponge cake	1 bread
with strawberries	1 fruit
and whipped cream	2 fat
Supper	
Roast beef (3 oz or 84 g)	3 meat
Mashed potatoes	3 bread
with butter	1 fat
Carrots	1 vegetable
and butter	1 fat
Applesauce	1 fruit
Small apple	1 fruit
Snack	
Raspberries (1 cup or 224 g)	1 fruit
in light cream (2 tbsp or 30 ml)	1 fat
Milk (8 oz or 240 ml)	1 milk

2. Parenteral hyperalimentation (total parenteral nutrition [TPN]): administered through a larger central vein such as the superior vena cava because the TPN solution is hypertonic (high osmolarity) and must enter the body in a region of high blood flow so that the solution is rapidly diluted; provides a higher percentage of water, glucose, amino acids, fats, vitamins, minerals, and electrolytes; requires surgical insertion, careful monitoring, and special care; may also be indicated preoperatively or for debilitated patients whose intake does not meet body requirements
3. Oral feedings: most patients should begin oral feedings as soon as bowel sounds return; provide nutrients essential to recovery; progress from clear liquid onward

Burns

A. Rate of tissue breakdown and loss of other body nutrients is greater with serious burns than with any other disease process
B. Increase of fluids and nutrients is required
   1. Increased energy requires 3000 to 5000 calories
   2. Protein increase of 50% above normal
   3. Vitamin C requirements greatly increased for wound healing
   4. B vitamins increased for higher metabolic rate
   5. Increased fluids to replace lost body fluids and help eliminate waste products
C. Intravenous dextrose, electrolytes, and plasma are given initially; a high-protein, high-calorie diet is given when oral foods can be taken
D. Victims of extensive burns may require parenteral hyperalimentation to meet their extensive nutritional requirements

Cancer

A. The National Cancer Institute and the American Cancer Society have issued the following guidelines for cancer prevention
   1. Eat a variety of foods
   2. Maintain a desirable body weight
   3. Eat a variety of both fruits and vegetables every day
   4. Eat more high-fiber foods, such as whole-grain breads and cereals, legumes, vegetables, and fruits
   5. Reduce fat intake to less than or equal to 30% of total calories
   6. If you drink alcohol, use in moderation
   7. Limit consumption of salt-cured, smoked, and nitrite-preserved foods
B. Diet for the patient with cancer must supply enough protein, fats, carbohydrates, vitamins, minerals, and fluids to meet increased energy demands, prevent weight loss, and rebuild body tissues during treatment; energy and protein needs may increase up to 20%; dietary supplements may be given to supply all necessary nutrients
C. The wasting away that can occur due to the disease itself, or radiation and chemotherapy is termed *cancer cachexia* and can decrease the life of the individual if not prevented and/or treated early
D. When the GI tract cannot be used, nutritional support may be given by total parenteral nutrition (TPN)
E. Nutritional factors most likely are involved in the development of some cancers. Excesses as well as deficiencies have been implicated. Further evaluation is needed
F. No one food causes cancer, and no one food can prevent it. Diet is considered to be one of the most important environmental/lifestyle factors in the etiology and prevention of cancer in the United States

AIDS

A. Nutritional support is vital to the survival of all individuals with acquired immune deficiency syndrome. Weight loss is a major symptom in HIV infection. Malnutrition itself contributes to the suppression of immune function
B. Good nutritional care is essential to preserve lean body mass; maintain weight and strength; improve body's response to medication
C. Nutritional status of individuals with AIDS can be compromised by: decreased oral intake, anorexia, nausea, vom-

iting, dyspnea, fatigue, neurological disease, disorders of mouth and esophagus

D. Techniques to help with food intake: small meals, readily available snacks, ensure adequate hydration, high caloric, high protein diet, nutritional supplements, give drugs after meals

E. General goals of nutrition intervention are the following:
1. Preserve optimal somatic and visceral protein status
2. Prevent nutrient deficiencies or excesses known to compromise immune function
3. Minimize nutrition-related complications that interfere with either intake or absorption of nutrients
4. Enhance the quality of life
5. Educate individuals about the importance of consuming a well-balanced diet

Cardiovascular Disease

A. Cardiovascular diseases are the primary causes of death in the United States; research has shown that diet may be a risk factor in determining whether a person develops heart disease

B. Objectives in dietary treatment of heart disease
1. Provide an adequate diet
2. Prevent gas- and bulk-forming foods from distending stomach and exerting pressure against the heart
3. Maintain patient's weight as near to ideal as possible to reduce workload of heart
4. Prevent edema by lowering sodium intake
5. Reduce the risk of atherosclerosis by reducing circulating blood lipids (low–saturated-fat, low-cholesterol diet)

C. Sodium restriction
1. Component of many diets used in cardiovascular diseases
2. Helps reduce excess edema and is thought to reduce the risk of hypertension
3. Sources of sodium
   a. Naturally present in foods, especially animal products such as meat, poultry, fish, milk, and eggs; fruits have little sodium
   b. Sodium added to foods in the form of table salt and preservatives in processed foods; most canned, packaged, and frozen foods have either monosodium glutamate or sodium added
   c. Water supplies may have a high sodium content; water softeners add a significant amount of sodium to a diet
   d. Nonprescription medicines and home remedies such as baking soda, alkalizers for indigestion, cough

medicines, and laxatives may contain large amounts of sodium
4. Sodium-restricted diets limit the intake of sodium to a level prescribed by the physician
   a. Mild sodium-restricted diet (2 to 3 g) contains about half of the salt previously used; no additional salting of processed foods; no salty foods allowed
   b. 1000 mg sodium diet (moderate)
   c. 500 mg sodium diet (strict)
   d. 250 mg sodium diet (severe)

Peptic Ulcer Disease

A. Current advances in drug therapy to decrease acid secretion and promote healing have decreased the need for a highly restrictive, bland diet

B. These bland diets have been shown to be ineffective and lacking in nutrients to support the healing process. Therapy is based on an individual's response to food choices; avoidance of foods that cause gastric stimulation (such as caffeine) is recommended

Chronic Renal Failure

A. Renal patients require strict monitoring for protein, water, and electrolyte balance. Specific nutritional therapy varies greatly depending on the patient's age and the stage of the disease. Enough protein should be supplied to repair and maintain tissues and avoid the use of protein for energy.

B. The BUN (blood urea nitrogen level) and creatinine clearance level are monitored to assist in regulating protein levels

SUGGESTED READINGS

Eschleman MM: *Introductory nutrition and diet therapy,* ed 3, Philadelphia, 1996, JB Lippincott.

Grodner M, Anderson SL, Hagen-Ansert SL: *Foundations and clinical applications of nutrition: a nursing approach,* St Louis, 1996, Mosby.

Mahan LK, Escott-Stump S: *Krause's food, nutrition and diet therapy,* ed 9, Philadelphia, 1996, WB Saunders.

Physicians' Desk Reference, ed 54, Montvale, 2000, Medical Economics Company.

Pipes PL, Trahms CM: *Nutrition in infancy and childhood,* ed 5, St Louis, 1993, Mosby.

Peckenpaugh NJ, Poleman CM: *Nutrition: essentials and diet therapy,* ed 8, Philadelphia, 1999, WB Saunders.

Williams SR: *Essentials of nutrition and diet therapy,* ed 7, St Louis, 1999, Mosby.

REVIEW QUESTIONS

1. A resident, reading the label on a cereal box, asks the nurse what cellulose does. The nurse knows the main function of cellulose in the diet is to:
   ① Maintain fluid balance
   ② Build and repair body tissues
   ③ Provide a rapid source of energy
   ❹ Absorb water to increase fecal bulk

2. A nurse is presenting a program on nutrition to a group of nursing assistants in an assisted living facility. The nurse states that meal planning at the facility should include the minerals most often deficient in the U.S. diet. Which of the following minerals are most often deficient in the U.S. diet?
   ❶ Calcium and iron
   ② Iodine and fluorine
   ③ Potassium and sodium
   ④ Phosphorus and calcium

3. A nurse is planning refreshments for a community walk-a-thon for diabetes mellitus. When planning refreshments, the nurse is aware that water should be readily available because:
   ① It is the most abundant mineral in the body
   ② It will keep the walkers from getting shin splints
   ③ The diabetic people need it to regulate sugar balance
   ❹ The walkers may need to replace fluids lost from perspiration

4. A nurse working in a school is asked by a third grader why the salt on the table has iodine in it. The nurse responds that iodine is essential to health because it:
   ① Strengthens bone and teeth
   ② Is necessary for blood clotting
   ❸ Helps the body to be able to grow
   ④ Allows oxygen to travel safely to cells

5. A nurse is explaining a discharge plan with an individual who has had surgery. In planning an adequate diet for tissue healing the nurse advises the patient to increase his intake of the vitamins:
   ❶ A and D
   ❷ A and C
   ③ B$_6$ and C
   ④ B$_{12}$ and D

6. A nurse is counseling the mother of a child who has experienced a third-degree burn over 15% of her body. Which of the child's favorite foods would provide necessary foods high in protein and calories?
   ① Potato chips and pizza
   ② Oranges and applesauce
   ③ Green beans and cantaloupe
   ❹ Hamburgers and peanut butter and jelly sandwiches

7. A patient, hospitalized with peptic ulcer disease, is distressed to find he has no coffee on his meal tray. Which of the following statements by the nurse conveys the reason for a caffeine-restricted diet in patients with peptic ulcer disease?
   ① "Caffeine dehydrates the body."
   ② "Caffeine delays gastric emptying."
   ③ "Caffeine buffers milk and antacids."
   ❹ "Caffeine stimulates gastric acid secretions."

8. A patient with liver failure is on the verge of hepatic coma. Which of the following nutrients would the nurse expect to be restricted?
   ① Fats
   ❷ Proteins
   ③ Vitamins
   ④ Carbohydrates

9. A nurse is assisting a patient at a prenatal clinic to plan an adequate diet. The patient states, "I don't want to gain too much weight. When my sister had her baby 10 years ago she gained 20 pounds and her doctor was mad." Which of the following is the nurse's best response?
   ① "Weight gain should not exceed 10 pounds."
   ② "The physician was right to be so concerned."
   ❸ "Acceptable weight gain now averages around 30 pounds."
   ④ "Weight gain should only average approximately 20 pounds."

10. While continuing to plan the diet for the pregnant female, the nurse advises the patient to increase the calories in her diet by:
    ❶ 300 calories/day
    ② 500 calories/day
    ③ 750 calories/day
    ④ 1000 calories/day

11. A pregnant patient has been experiencing morning sickness and is concerned she will be unable to meet the increased caloric needs of pregnancy. To meet the caloric demands of pregnancy, which of the following food groups should the nurse advise the patient to increase by 1 serving?
    ① Meats
    ❷ Starches
    ❸ Milk and dairy
    ④ Fruits and vegetables

12. Which of the following diet modifications would the nurse recommend for a woman suffering from nausea and vomiting during early pregnancy?
    ① Increase fat content
    ❷ Increase protein foods
    ❸ Frequent small meals and snacks
    ④ Increase beverages with meals

13. A patient is concerned with the amount of cholesterol in his bloodstream because he eats a lot of high-fat food. The nurse knows that cholesterol:
    ① Is a derivative of amino acids
    ❷ Can contribute to atherosclerosis
    ③ Supplements should be taken each day
    ④ Is necessary for the body to metabolize vitamin C

14. A nurse is concerned about a teenager with very low-fat diet choices. A diet extremely low in fat may be inadequate in:
    ❶ Vitamin A
    ② Vitamin C
    ③ Minerals
    ④ Carbohydrates

15. Which of the following cardiovascular disorders may require the initiation of dietary sodium restrictions?
    ① Hyperlipidemia and renal failure
    ② Hypercholesterolemia and hypertension
    ❸ Hypertension and congestive heart failure
    ④ Hyperlipidemia and congestive heart failure

16. During a nutrition-related seminar, individuals on a sodium restricted diet are cautioned to read labels to determine the content of added:
    ① Sodium and iron
    ❷ Sodium and MSG
    ③ Monosaccharides
    ④ High-density lipoproteins

17. The most common type of nutritional anemia is:
    ❶ Iron deficiency
    ❷ Pernicious anemia
    ③ Folic acid deficiency
    ④ Vitamin B_{12} deficiency

18. A nurse is instructing a class on safe handling of foods. Which of the following precautions should the nurse advise to minimize the loss of Vitamin C in foods?
    ① Cooking thoroughly to kill any bacteria
    ② Adding baking soda to the cooking water
    ❸ Eating sources of vitamin C raw when possible
    ④ Keeping food in a mesh bag to allow air to circulate

19. The nurse is preparing to give an injection of Vitamin B_{12} to a nursing home resident. The nurse is giving the injection to prevent the disorder:
    ① Scurvy
    ② Pellagra
    ③ Marasmus
    ❹ Pernicious anemia

20. A patient receiving chemotherapy is concerned because she is unable to eat well because of stomatitis. Which of the following interventions should the nurse recommend?
    ① Overeat on good days
    ❷ Eat small, frequent meals
    ❸ Eat foods at room temperature
    ④ Eat protein-rich foods when able

21. To minimize the risk of cancer, most individuals should:
    ① Increase intake of saturated fats
    ❷ Decrease intake of saturated fats
    ③ Decrease intake of raw fruits and vegetables
    ④ Increase intake of smoked and salt-cured meats

22. The prime objective of diet therapy for kidney stones is to:
    ① Decrease calcium intake
    ❷ Dilute the urine by increasing fluids
    ③ Prevent vitamin and mineral deficiencies
    ④ Alleviate the side effects of the drugs involved

23. A middle-aged man comes to the outpatient clinic with complaints of pain in his right great toe. He states he was diagnosed with gout 3 years ago and has been following his diet and medication regimen with no exacerbations until now. Which of the following statements indicates to the nurse that he was following diet therapy for the management of gout?
    ① "I eat a high-calorie diet."
    ❷ "I don't eat foods high in purine."
    ③ "I drink a glass of wine each night."
    ④ "I restrict my fluid intake to 1000 cc/day."

24. A nurse is taking part in an interdisciplinary care meeting. A resident in a long-term care facility is to begin receiving nasogastric tube feedings. Which of the following is important in the selection of the type of feeding?
    ① Feedings are usually hypertonic solutions
    ② Feeding solutions are basically the same for all individuals
    ③ Feedings should be used only if the resident's GI tract is nonfunctional
    ❹ Solutions are chosen on the ability of the resident to absorb nutrients

25. A physician is discussing placing an enteral tube for feeding purposes into an older adult patient with dysphagia. Which of the following types of tubes has the least possibility of aspiration?
    ① Gastrostomy tube
    ❷ Jejunostomy tube
    ③ Duodenostomy tube
    ④ Small bore nasogastric tube

26. Which of the following may be the most important factor for the nurse to consider when planning an adequate diet for healthy persons?
    ① Geographic locale
    ❷ Culture and religion
    ③ Family health history
    ④ Dietary guidelines and recommendations

27. A nurse is attending a cooking class. The chef is discussing the best method for preserving the nutrient content of food. The nurse is aware that the best cooking method to preserve nutrients is:
    ① Frying
    ❷ Steaming
    ③ Microwaving
    ④ Soaking before cooking

28. A patient calls the nurse into his room and explains that he is unable to eat the food because milk and meat are being served on the same tray. Which of the following is the best response by the nurse?
    ① "You need these nutrients to get over your disease."
    ② "Why don't you eat them now, I will note the change later."
    ③ "We need to discuss this with the head dietitian, I will call her."
    ❹ "I will call and notify the dietary department to bring you a kosher tray."

29. A patient of Middle Eastern descent refuses to eat during the day and then asks for a double serving during the evening. The patient is newly diagnosed with IDDM. Which of the following is the best response by the nurse?
    ① "I know that this is Ramadan, but you have to eat during the day."
    ② "We will need to hold your insulin during the day, and then double it at night."
    ③ "I think I should talk with your physician. It is very difficult to manage your diabetes."
    ❹ "We need to find a way for you to observe your religion and manage your diabetes also."

30. A nurse is planning a diet for a patient newly diagnosed with diabetes mellitus. The patient is of the Hindu faith. Which of the following factors is most important to consider when planning this patient's exchange list?
    ① The patient will not eat any fruits or vegetables
    ❷ The protein needs of the patient may be difficult to meet
    ③ The patient will not likely enjoy any of the foods on the plan
    ④ The exchange lists for the ADA diet will need to be modified

31. Which food group is at the base of the food guide pyramid?
    ① Meat and poultry
    ② Fruits and vegetables
    ③ Milk and dairy products
    ❹ Bread, cereals, and grains

32. A nurse's aide is passing out evening snacks to a group of residents. Which of the following snacks should the nurse recommend for the resident with IDDM?
    ① Ice cream
    ② Cookies and milk
    ❸ Cheese and crackers
    ④ Slice of chocolate cake

33. The nurse is counseling a patient with newly diagnosed IDDM concerning preparation for increased exercise or activity. What should the nurse encourage the patient to do before exercise?
    ① Eat a small snack composed of fats
    ② Lower the amount of insulin before activity
    ❸ Eat a small snack composed of carbohydrates
    ④ Increase the amount of insulin before activity

34. Which of the following should the nurse encourage a patient with diabetes to carry on his person at all times?
    ① Gum
    ❷ Candy
    ③ Water
    ④ Crackers

35. A patient is placed on a low-fat diet because of hyperlipidemia. Which of the following foods would be acceptable for this patient?
    ① Whole milk, steak, rice and cake
    ② Liver, fried potatoes, avocado salad
    ❸ Skim milk, fish, tapioca pudding with fruit
    ④ Pork chops, mashed potatoes and gravy, and roll

36. A patient on a sodium-restricted diet is planning his food choices for the next day's menu. Which of the following food choices should the nurse recommend?
    ① Corned beef on rye bread, dill pickles, and pears
    ② Smoked haddock, roll, frozen green beans and an orange
    ❸ Fresh beef, salt-free cottage cheese, roll, small sweet potato.
    ④ Ham and cheese on white bread, hard boiled egg, and an orange

37. A patient presents to the emergency room with pain from acute diverticulitis. Which of the following foods from the patient's 24-hour food history would have aggravated the ulcer?
    ① Broiled fish and rice
    ② Steak and french fries
    ❸ Lettuce salad with raw vegetables
    ④ Baked potato and steamed vegetables

38. When teaching a patient on a sodium-restricted diet, what might the nurse caution the patient against consuming in excessive amounts?
    ① Fruits
    ② Vegetables
    ③ Potatoes and beans
    ❹ Meats and milk products

39. Preoperatively, which diet would be given to a patient scheduled for a cholecystectomy to prevent further recurrence of abdominal discomfort?
    ① Hamburger, french fries, and milkshake
    ② Avocado salad, cookies, and chocolate milk
    ③ Lamb, mashed potatoes, ice cream, and coffee
    ❹ Broiled fish, boiled potatoes, canned peaches, and skim milk

40. Which of the following vegetables would supply a vitamin that might be lacking in a diet used in the treatment of gallbladder disease?
    ① Raisins and prunes
    ② Oranges and bananas
    ③ Oranges and cantaloupe
    ❹ Sweet potatoes and carrots

41. Which of the following meals should the nurse recognize as appropriate for a patient on a moderate sodium restriction?
    ① Macaroni and cheese and cookies
    ② Corned beef, cabbage, bread, and fresh fruit
    ❸ Barbecued chicken, fresh corn, and fresh fruit
    ❹ Lobster, baked potatoes, and canned peaches

42. A postoperative patient will be on intravenous (IV) fluids for the first several days. What remark made by the patient indicates that she is probably ready to be started on oral feedings?
    ① "I can't wait to see some real food rather than this IV bottle!"
    ② "I'm so glad I don't have any more nausea—what a nuisance that was!"
    ❸ "My stomach is really rumbling" I don't know why—there's nothing in it!"
    ④ "My stomach is feeling a little distended. Do you think it's because I haven't had anything in it for so long?"

43. A nurse is teaching a class on proper nutrition to homemakers. One of the students asks the nurse how to supply protein to her family of six when meat is so expensive and they have a limited income. Which of the following menu suggestions should the nurse make to assist this student?
    ① "Pasta is great and it will fill them up."
    ② "Satisfy their appetites with vegetables."
    ❸ "Try peanut butter with bread or beans with rice."
    ④ "Don't worry, we really eat too much protein anyway."

44. A nurse is assisting a physician performing physical exams in a clinic. Which of the following signs should the nurse recognize as a potential clinical sign of poor nutrition?
    ① Feeling of fatigue after exercise
    ② Sleeping 8 to 10 hours every night
    ❸ Complaints of chronic constipation
    ④ Smooth reddish-pink mucous membranes

45. Which of the following menus best meets a postoperative patient's needs for a vitamin especially important in tissue healing?
    ① Liver, mashed potatoes, and carrots
    ② Roast pork, egg noodles, and baked squash
    ③ Baked chicken, white rice, and sliced peaches
    ❹ Swiss steak in tomato sauce, mashed potatoes, and strawberries

46. A patient stops a nurse one day and states her confusion over what she hears about vitamin C. When discussing this vitamin with the patient, the nurse should include:
    ① Vitamin C is fat soluble and readily stored in the body
    ② Deficiency symptoms include night blindness and dry, scaly skin
    ③ Improper storage and cooking can result in food losing its vitamin C
    ④ Vitamin C has been proven to significantly reduce the incidence and severity of colds

47. A home health care nurse is caring for a patient who is recovering from a mild heart attack. His wife says, "He loves to eat milk, meat, and cheese, especially when his family comes for dinner. How am I ever going to get him to change?" The most appropriate response for the nurse should be:
    ① "I will explain all the dangers of not changing his lifestyle."
    ② "His family will understand the importance of his maintaining his health."
    ③ "Make changes gradually; incorporate small portions of favorite foods in moderation."
    ④ "Do the best you can; his heart attack was mild. He does not have to worry too much."

48. Which of the following statements should indicate to the nurse that a mother understands the dietary needs of her teenage diabetic child?
    ① "Lots of fruit is good, because fruit has natural sugar."
    ② "She can eat my baked goods if I use a sugar substitute."
    ③ "I am definitely going to start serving more pasta and whole grains."
    ④ "I am definitely not going to let her hang around with her friends at fast food places anymore."

49. A home health care nurse is interviewing and assessing a family with a newborn. There are also two toddlers living in the household. Which of the following foods on the kitchen counter would be of most concern to the nurse?
    ① Apples
    ② Whole milk
    ③ Chocolate cake
    ④ Bag of popcorn

50. A patient returns to the unit after undergoing a total gastrectomy. After 5 days the patient is placed on total parenteral nutrition (TPN). The nurse should understand that this means:
    ① A short-term supplementation via tube placed in a peripheral vein
    ② Full nutritional support for longer periods of time via a large central vein
    ③ A long-term method of feeding using different points along the gastrointestinal tract
    ④ A short-term supplementation via nasogastric tube until full oral feedings can be resumed

51. A newly diagnosed HIV patient is angry and withdrawn. He verbalizes to the nurse that he does not understand why she is even bothering to tell him about nutrition, when he is going to die anyway. What should the nurse say at this point?
    ① "When you are ready to listen we will talk again."
    ② "I will leave written material here for you to look at."
    ③ "I know you feel you have lost control over your life."
    ④ "Eating well is a way you can maintain your immune system."

52. A patient has been diagnosed with a peptic ulcer and has been placed on medication therapy. Which of the following instructions would be most beneficial concerning diet therapy?
    ① "Include a lot of dairy products in your diet."
    ② "Eat a very bland diet; this means no caffeine or spicy foods."
    ③ "Eat a well-balanced diet and remember to take your medications."
    ④ "Eat 6 small meals a day, because this will decrease stomach discomfort."

53. A patient has had diverticulosis for 5 years. She seems confused about the type of diet to follow. A nurse tells her that current evidence suggests the best diet for diverticulosis is a:
    ① Bland diet
    ② Low-fat diet
    ③ High-fiber diet
    ④ Low-fiber diet

54. An 84-year-old woman is in the health care provider's office complaining of fatigue, anorexia, and indigestion. Which of the following groups of vitamins might be prescribed if the health care provider suspects a deficiency?
    ① C and B_{12}
    ② B_6 and B_{12}
    ③ A, D, and E
    ④ C and B complex

55. A nurse is counseling a 23-year-old woman who is trying to eat a healthier diet. She says she is trying to quit smoking but is having a hard time doing so. Which of the following vitamins should the nurse recommend as a supplement?
    ① Vitamin A
    ② Vitamin K
    ③ Vitamin C
    ④ Vitamin B

56. A patient with a complaint of irregular heartbeat was diagnosed with hypokalemia and advised to increase his dietary intake of potassium. He asks the nurse: "What foods are high in potassium?" The nurse's answer should include:
    ① Dairy products
    ② Apricots, oranges, and bananas
    ③ Fish liver oils and fortified milk
    ④ Wheat germ and dark green, leafy vegetables

57. A patient, whose blood pressure has been elevated, tells the nurse that the physician has recommended that he reduce his intake of dietary sodium. The nurse advises the patient to:
    ① Limit fresh fruits and vegetables
    ② Increase dairy products in his diet
    ③ Increase canned and processed meats in his diet
    ④ Substitute spices, herbs, or lemon juice for salt in seasoning his food

58. A nurse in a prenatal clinic is counseling a patient who wants to lose weight. The patient wants to try a high-protein, high-carbohydrate diet. What should the nurse explain to her to promote a safe weight loss plan?
   ① "This diet is dangerous; you could give yourself serious metabolic problems."
   ② "Fats should be eliminated from the diet as much as possible to prevent heart disease."
   ③ "This is a healthy diet because protein builds new cells and carbohydrates supply energy."
   ❹ "Some fats are needed in any weight loss diet because they perform specific functions in the body."

59. A patient confides to a nurse that she is desperate to lose 10 pounds before she goes to a class reunion in 2 weeks. She says that she is going to try eating a fruit diet with lots of water. The best response for the nurse should be:
   ① "All nutrients are needed to supply a healthy diet."
   ② "It is all right for a short period but be certain to take vitamins."
   ③ "The fruit will supply you with energy, and the water will help circulation."
   ❹ "Eat a variety of foods from all levels of the food pyramid and increase exercise."

60. The patient has been told by her physician that she has a lactose intolerance. In discussing dietary adjustments the nurse advises the patient to avoid:
   ① Citrus fruits
   ② Highly seasoned foods
   ❸ Milk and milk products
   ④ Foods containing seeds and nuts

61. A neighbor asks a nurse for advice on cooking healthy meals for her family. Which of the following should the nurse emphasize?
   ① The more expensive the meat, the more nutrients it contains
   ② The higher the grade on canned goods, the more nutritious the contents
   ③ Refined cereal products are more nutritious than fortified cereal products
   ❹ Raw fruit and vegetables contain more nutrients than cooked vegetables

62. A nurse is working in a prenatal clinic. Which of the following patients should she be most concerned about for the potential of nutritional complications?
   ① A patient in her third trimester who has gained 39 pounds
   ② A woman in her third trimester with complaints of heartburn
   ❸ An underweight adolescent who confesses to eating erratically
   ④ A 36-year-old primigravida in her second trimester who is slightly anemic

63. A high school student asks the school nurse whether or not he should drink a "special electrolyte solution" because he is in training to make the track team. His specialty is the high jump. The best reply for the nurse should be:
   ① "Make certain it has vitamins to increase energy."
   ② "No, you need a sugar solution to add energy for endurance."

③ "Yes. Absolutely. They help to replace minerals lost when you sweat."
   ❹ "For nonendurance events, water is the best solution to prevent dehydration."

64. A patient is recovering from burns over 40% of his total body surface area. A high protein high carbohydrate diet is essential for recovery because:
   ① The vitamins supplied will promote healing and supply energy
   ② Extra calories are needed to allow the person to be active in the rehabilitation process
   ❸ Protein is needed for tissue healing and carbohydrates will assist protein to be used for this purpose
   ④ Extra carbohydrates will assist in counteracting the negative nitrogen balance caused by massive trauma

X **65.** A patient tells the nurse that she is going on a completely vegetarian diet, which includes no meat or dairy products. What nutrient would this patient be particularly deficient in if she continues on this diet?
   ① Iron
   ❷ Protein
   ③ B complex vitamins
   ❹ Fat-soluble vitamins

66. The nutritional requirements of older adults differ from those of younger people. In particular, they will require:
   ① Increased fats
   ❷ Fewer calories
   ③ Decreased fluid intake
   ④ Fewer vitamins and minerals

X **67.** A patient has been taking a diuretic for the past 3 months. Of the following statements made by the patient, which would alert the nurse to a possible dietary deficiency caused by the diuretic?
   ① "I seem to bruise so easily these days."
   ② "My eyes seem especially sensitive to that light."
   ❸ "Every once in awhile my heart feels like it's skipping beats!"
   ❹ "I feel so terribly nervous. Do you think I need a tranquilizer?"

68. A patient tells the nurse that she uses mineral oil as a base for her salad dressing. The nurse's best response to this statement should be:
   ① "That's a good idea! It even fits into your mother's bland diet."
   ② "That's a good idea! Mineral oil doesn't add any calories to your diet."
   ③ "I would use another type of oil. Mineral oil is high in calories with very few vitamins."
   ❹ "Why don't you try a vegetable oil instead? Mineral oil hinders absorption of some important vitamins."

69. A mother of a 2-week-old infant is nervous about his feedings. The nurse's advice to her should include:
   ① "Begin infant cereal at 1 month of age."
   ❷ "Do not give honey to the baby until he is at least 1 year old."
   ③ "Add sugar or salt to foods if he finds something unpalatable."
   ④ "Delay giving egg yolk to the baby until he is 1 year old because this portion of the egg may cause allergic reactions."

70. A patient with a history of family allergies asks what foods she can feed her 4-month-old son that would be least likely to cause an allergic reaction. The nurse's most appropriate response would be to suggest:
① Rice cereal
② Cow's milk
③ Wheat cereal
④ Scrambled eggs

71. A young schoolteacher recently learned she is pregnant and is concerned how she can eliminate morning sickness. The nurse's suggestions to her might include:
① "Drink liquids with your meals."
② "Increase fat products within your diet."
③ "Decrease the carbohydrates within your meals."
④ "Eat crackers when you wake in the morning."

72. A patient has decided to decrease her intake of red meat, but she is concerned that she will also be decreasing her intake of iron. The nurse suggests that she can increase her intake of iron by eating additional:
① Milk and dairy products
② Refined cereal products
③ Dried fruits, such as apricots
④ Yellow vegetables, such as carrots

73. The absorption of iron, especially iron from nonmeat sources, can be enhanced significantly if iron is ingested with:
① Citrus juices
② Fish liver oils
③ Green, leafy vegetables
④ Milk and dairy products

74. The diabetic diet is based on the exchange system. In using this system the patient should be instructed that:
① Only foods listed in the same exchange can be substituted
② Dietetic or diabetic foods should be used as much as possible
③ Substitution within a food exchange for meal planning can only be done by a physician or dietician
④ Food exchanges are not particularly important as long as you stay within your recommended calories

75. When visiting friends, a diabetic patient was offered half a cup of blackberries. Since she does not care for blackberries, what would she be able to substitute for them?
① Pecans
② Ice milk
③ Pineapple juice
④ Cheddar cheese

76. For dinner one evening a diabetic patient fries an egg in 1 teaspoon of margarine, has a biscuit with 1 teaspoon of butter, and drinks a cup of black coffee. Out of which exchange lists has she selected her meal?
① One milk, two bread, and one fat exchange
② One meat, one bread, and two fat exchanges
③ One bread, one meat, and one vegetable exchange
④ One meat, one milk, one fruit, and one fat exchange

77. A diabetic patient remarks that in the late afternoon she frequently becomes shaky and feels very nervous. What would the nurse suggest to her as a readily available source of carbohydrate that could get her over this hypoglycemic episode?
① Cereal
② Oranges
③ Crackers
④ Bread and butter

78. A patient is admitted with a diagnosis of chronic renal failure. Which of the following dinner selections would be best suited for this patient?
① Ground round steak, asparagus, bread and butter, fruit cup, and milk
② Hamburger with tomato on a bun, potato chips, and a glass of chocolate milk
③ Liver, cottage cheese with peach half, deviled eggs, and coffee with cream and sugar
④ Apple juice, 1 oz roasted chicken, asparagus, sliced tomatoes, fruit cup, and tea with sugar

79. A postoperative patient has just begun a clear liquid diet. Which of the following selections would she be allowed?
① Beef bouillon, raspberry ice, and tea
② Cream of mushroom soup, Jell-O, and tea
③ Chicken broth, lime sherbet, and apple juice
④ Beef bouillon, orange juice, and cherry Jell-O

80. A 35-year-old banker is hospitalized with ulcerative colitis. The acute flare-up of his condition has passed, and the nurse should expect him to be placed on a diet:
① Low in fat and calories
② Low in sodium and carbohydrates
③ Low in residue and high in vitamins and protein
④ High in residue and high in vitamins and protein

81. A patient is admitted with a diagnosis of suspected myocardial infarction. He complains about the soft diet ordered by the physician. The nurse explains to the patient that the purpose of this diet is to:
① Reduce the workload on the heart
② Decrease irritation to the digestive tract
③ Reduce the number of calories in his diet
④ Decrease peristalsis within the digestive tract

82. A patient has a problem with atonic constipation probably caused by poor eating habits coupled with his dependence on laxatives. Which of the following menus would be best suited to helping him overcome constipation?
① Ground beef patty, boiled potato, baked squash, and milk
② Baked chicken, macaroni, cooked carrots, custard, and coffee
③ Macaroni and cheese, peach halves, vanilla ice cream, and milk
④ Beef stew with carrots and onions, coleslaw, rye bread, and tea

83. The National Institute of Health, the American Heart Association, and the U.S. Surgeon General have issued similar dietary recommendations. Each has stated that the average person should:
① Decrease total calories in the diet
② Decrease total dietary fats, especially saturated fats
③ Decrease dietary fat, especially polyunsaturated fats
④ Increase carbohydrates to approximately 30% of total caloric intake

84. According to the food pyramid, milk primarily supplies which nutrients?
① Iron and calcium
② Calcium and protein

③ Vitamin C and calcium
④ B complex vitamins and protein

85. A variety of diets have been used over the years to deal with gastrointestinal disorders. Which statement best describes current thinking concerning diet and peptic ulcer disease?
① "Eat what you like but avoid foods that are especially irritating."
② "Milk and milk products should be the foundation of peptic ulcer diets."
③ "Food and drink containing caffeine, chocolate, and alcohol can be taken in unrestricted amounts."
④ "Physicians are strongly encouraging compliance with a bland diet for conditions such as peptic ulcer."

86. Which of the following statements about diabetes mellitus and diet are correct?
① "Include high-fiber foods in menu planning."
② "The food choices available are extremely limited."
③ "The use of any alcoholic beverage is absolutely prohibited."
④ "The best kinds of carbohydrates to include are refined, simple carbohydrates."

87. Which of the following statements is true?
① "Blood cholesterol levels of 250 to 300 mg/dl are considered ideal."
② "Lowering blood cholesterol levels requires both medication and dietary adjustments."
③ "Of the factors an individual can control, diet has the greatest effect on blood cholesterol levels."
④ "A high ratio of low-density lipoprotein (LDL) to high-density lipoprotein (HDL) is considered desirable."

88. A patient asks the nurse what information is available concerning Omega-3 fatty acids. Which of the following statements by the nurse is most correct?
① "No fatty acids are good for you."
② "Why don't I make an appointment for you with the dietician?"
③ "Physicians believe that Omega-3 fatty acids may actually prevent cancer."
④ "Some research suggests that these fatty acids may help to prevent heart disease."

89. A nurse is counseling a group of rural homemakers regarding safe food handling. Which of the following statements made by the nurse is true regarding botulism?
① "It often occurs in home canned, low-acid foods."
② "It can be prevented by keeping hot foods over 140° F."
③ "It can be prevented by keeping cold foods below 40° F."
④ "It is caused by the staphylococci bacteria, which is heat resistant."

90. A condition that would not increase the caloric needs of a patient would be:
① Severe burns
② Healing fracture
③ Surgical infection
④ Hay fever allergies

91. Which group of individuals is most nutritionally compromised?
① Individuals who are vegetarians
② Individuals who are alcoholic
③ Individuals with diabetes mellitus
④ Patients with coronary artery disease

92. The nurse is preparing to administer AquaMEPHYTON to a newborn. AquaMEPHYTON is the pharmacological term for:
① Vitamin A
② Vitamin D
③ Vitamin K
④ Vitamin C

93. A middle-aged female is concerned because her mother has just been diagnosis with osteoporosis. She asks what she can do to limit her chances for getting osteoporosis. Which of the following should the nurse recommend?
① "Increase the potassium in your diet."
② "Try to increase dairy products in your diet."
③ "You should limit the amount of salt you eat."
④ "Increase the amount of protein you consume each day."

94. A patient's sister asks what type of postoperative nutrition her brother will need. The correct response by the nurse should be:
① "All patients need total parenteral nutrition after surgery."
② "It all depends on the location and what kind of surgery was done."
③ "Patients should experience a period of mini-starvation after surgery."
④ "IV fluids and an extremely high protein diet are indicated after surgery."

95. There has been an outbreak of *E. coli*–related illness in the nurse's community. When providing information to the public, the nurse is knowledgeable that *E. coli*–related illness can be prevented by:
① Properly home canning food
② Ensuring that red meats are well done
③ Heating foods to at least 140° F for 10 minutes
④ Making sure that eggs are used quickly after purchase

96. The trace elements in the body are defined as:
① Those minerals that are not essential to health
② Essential nutrients found in very small amounts
③ Only those minerals that are found in the blood
④ Those minerals that are undetectable by blood studies

97. A patient is concerned with edema that develops in her feet throughout the day. Which of the following food choices made by the individual could contribute to the edema formation?
① Eggs and toast
② Tuna fish and cantaloupe
③ Hamburger and french fries
④ Salami sandwich and potato chips

98. A patient with cancer is experiencing anorexia. Which of the following recommendations should assist the client in increasing oral intake?
① "Try to eat three large meals per day."
② "Take pain medication after your meals."
③ "Try to supplement your meals with nutritious milkshakes."
④ "Eat as many fruits and vegetables as you can instead of protein foods."

99. A patient suffering from anorexia nervosa states that even though she is quite thin, she still feels extremely overweight. Which of the following is true concerning anorexia nervosa?
① The individual has a severely altered body image
② There is usually an underlying physical illness involved
③ Treatment programs are short-term in nature and successful
④ Explanation of the need for increased intake will aid in the treatment plan

100. The nurse is planning a diet program for an elderly couple who have both been placed on a low-fat diet. The couple indicate that they really enjoy pastries and sweets, because many other types of foods taste bland to them. Which of the following is the best response by the nurse?
① "Well, we're going to have to find you something else to eat."
② "I will check with the doctor to see if you can still eat mostly pastries."
③ "Other foods are better for you to eat, what protein foods do you like?"
④ "Some sweets are included in the diet. We need to add other foods that are flavorful."

ANSWERS AND RATIONALES

1. Knowledge, implementation, basic care and comfort (a)
   - ❹ The nurse knows that the main function of cellulose is to create bulk in the intestine, aiding in bowel elimination.
   - ① This is not the main function of cellulose, and describes the role of the mineral, sodium.
   - ② This describes the role of protein in the body.
   - ③ Simple sugars provide a rapid source of energy.

2. Application, implementation, coordinated care (b)
   - ❶ Calcium and iron are the minerals most likely to be deficient throughout the life span in the American diet.
   - ② Although deficiencies may arise, these do not constitute the most deficient minerals.
   - ③ Potassium and sodium are readily available in a variety of food sources.
   - ④ For most individuals phosphorous and calcium are readily available by consuming milk products.

3. Application, planning, basic care and comfort (b)
   - ❹ The walkers will need to replace any lost fluids resulting from perspiration.
   - ① Water is the most abundant body component, but this does not explain why it should be available to the walkers.
   - ② Water will assist in the walkers' hydration status but will not prevent shin splints.
   - ③ Water is important to all individuals; however, the diabetic walkers need insulin to regulate glucose utilization in the body.

4. Application, implementation, basic care and comfort (b)
   - ❸ This explanation is short, geared to the child's knowledge level, and accurately condenses what the purpose of iodine is in the body.
   - ① This correctly explains why calcium and phosphorus are necessary for the body.
   - ② Calcium and vitamin K are essential for blood clotting.
   - ④ This explains the role iron plays in hemoglobin.

5. Application, planning, physiological adaptation (b)
   - ❷ Vitamins essential for wound healing include A and C.
   - ① Vitamins A and D can be readily found in fortified milk and assist in the healing of fractures.
   - ② Vitamins B_6 and C, although important in an adequate diet, are not specific for tissue healing.
   - ③ These vitamins are not specific for tissue healing, although important in the diet.

6. Application, evaluation, physiological adaptation (b)
   - ❹ Hamburgers and peanut butter and jelly sandwiches would provide a diet high in protein and calories.
   - ① Although high in calories, these foods are not as high in protein as hamburgers and peanut butter and jelly sandwiches.
   - ② Oranges and applesauce contain vitamins necessary for tissue healing; however, they are low in protein and calories.
   - ③ Although high in vitamin content, these foods are not high in protein or calories.

7. Comprehension, implementation, basic care and comfort (b)
   - ❹ Caffeine stimulates gastric acid secretions, potentially aggravating peptic ulcer disease.
   - ① Caffeine does dehydrate the body, but this is not the reason why it is restricted in peptic ulcer disease.
   - ② This is not the rationale behind a caffeine-restricted diet.
   - ③ Caffeine does not buffer milk or antacids.

8. Comprehension, planning, physiological adaptation (b)
   - ❷ The products of protein metabolism contribute to the accumulation of urea that will further worsen metabolic acidosis.
   - ① Fats are given to provide energy and allow protein to be used for tissue building.
   - ③ Vitamins need to be supplemented in low-protein diets.
   - ④ Carbohydrates are given to provide energy and allow protein to be used for tissue synthesis.

9. Comprehension, implementation, growth and development through the life span (b)
   - ❸ This is the truest statement. In the past weight was restricted, but now focus is on gaining enough weight to safeguard the baby's health.
   - ① This is not true for the majority of pregnant women.
   - ② This does not provide information to the patient and blocks communication
   - ④ Although true in the past, this weight gain is probably not sufficient for the majority of pregnant women.

10. Application, implementation, growth and development through the life span (b)
    - ❶ The caloric needs of the pregnant female increase by 300 calories per day.
    - ② The lactating mother needs to increase her calories to 500 calories per day.
    - ③ Unless severely malnourished, 750 calories is generally too many additional calories.
    - ④ Unless instructed by a physician, 1000 calories is too much of an increase.

11. Comprehension, planning, growth and development through the life span (b)
    - ❷ Frequent small, low-fat meals and snacks consisting of easily digested energy-yielding foods such as carbohydrates (starches) are more easily tolerated by patients experiencing morning sickness.
    - ①, ③, ④ Adding extra servings of these foods would increase foods that are more difficult to digest and therefore not easily tolerated by patients experiencing morning sickness.

12. Comprehension, implementation, growth and development through the life span (b)
    - ❸ Frequent small meals and snacks will not overfill the stomach, causing distension, discomfort, and nausea.
    - ① The feeling of fullness from eating fats may increase nausea and vomiting.
    - ② Increased protein foods will not alleviate the nausea and vomiting associated with pregnancy.
    - ④ Drinking beverages with meals will cause excessive gastric filling, contributing to nausea and vomiting.

13. Knowledge, assessment, basic care and comfort (a)
    ❷ Excessive cholesterol can contribute to the development of fatty plaques in the arteries—atherosclerosis.
    ① Cholesterol is a complex, fat related substance.
    ③ There is no need for supplements to be taken, because cholesterol can be synthesized by the body.
    ④ Cholesterol is a major factor in the manufacture of vitamin D in the body.

14. Application, implementation, basic care and comfort (b)
    ❶ A diet low in fat may lead to a deficiency in the fat-soluble vitamin A.
    ② Vitamin C is water soluble. A low-fat diet would not lead to a deficiency, although a diet that is overall low in calories may.
    ③ Minerals are water soluble and a low-fat diet would not lead to a deficiency.
    ④ Carbohydrates are the food choice most likely for an individual on a low-fat diet.

15. Knowledge, assessment, basic care and comfort (a)
    ❸ Hypertension and congestive heart failure are two pathological conditions that may require sodium restriction.
    ① Hyperlipidemia would require a dietary fat modification. Renal failure may require restriction in water and protein.
    ② Hypercholesterolemia would require restriction of foods high in cholesterol.
    ④ Hyperlipidemia may require a low-fat diet.

16. Comprehension, planning, prevention and early detection of disease (b)
    ❷ Individuals should look for both sodium and monosodium glutamate when reading labels.
    ① Iron is not restricted on a sodium-restricted diet.
    ③ Individuals on a sodium restricted diet may consume monosaccharides.
    ④ High-density lipoproteins, a type of fat in the bloodstream, are not on nutrition labels.

17. Knowledge, assessment, basic care and comfort (a)
    ❶ Iron-deficiency anemia is the most prevalent form of anemia and is due to inadequate absorption of iron or insufficient intake, or increased needs not being met (adolescence, pregnancy, etc.).
    ② Pernicious anemia is caused by a deficiency of B_{12} because of a lack of intrinsic factor.
    ③ Folic acid deficiency is common in perinatal population.
    ④ Anemia from a vitamin B_{12} deficiency is termed pernicious anemia

18. Comprehension, planning, basic care and comfort (b)
    ❸ By eating good sources of vitamin C uncooked, the majority of the vitamin can be preserved.
    ① Excessive cooking will cause vitamin C to evaporate or leech out into the cooking water.
    ② This will not preserve vitamin C.
    ④ Although a good idea, this does not minimize the loss of vitamin C in foods.

19. Application, implementation, pharmacological therapies (b)
    ❹ Vitamin B_{12} injections are given to elderly patients because of the decrease of intrinsic factor in their stomach acid. Vitamin B_{12} cannot be absorbed without intrinsic factor and must be supplemented to prevent pernicious anemia from developing.
    ① Vitamin C prevents scurvy.
    ② Pellagra is caused by a deficiency in niacin.
    ③ Marasmus is a term for general starvation.

20. Comprehension, planning, basic care and comfort (c)
    ❸ Many individuals with stomatitis are able to eat foods that are neither hot or cold and may find it more comfortable if the food is served at room temperature.
    ① This is a dietary recommendation for anorexia.
    ② Anorexia is a common problem for cancer patients, and eating small, frequent meals is one intervention to help this problem.
    ④ This may not be possible and protein-rich foods will not help the problem of stomatitis.

21. Knowledge, planning, prevention and early detection of disease (b)
    ❷ The Dietary Guidelines for Americans recommends that individuals decrease intake of saturated fats.
    ① This is not recommended.
    ③ Studies have shown that raw fruits and vegetables can alleviate some types of cancer.
    ④ The preservatives in smoked and salt-cured meats have been linked to some types of cancer.

22. Knowledge, assessment, basic care and comfort (b)
    ❷ Urine needs to be diluted to prevent the formation of additional kidney stones.
    ① Although the majority of kidney stones are composed of calcium; intake is not restricted.
    ③ There should be no vitamin or mineral deficiencies associated with kidney stones.
    ④ Diet therapy is not aimed in alleviating the side effects of any drugs given. There are very few drugs used in the treatment of kidney stones.

23. Application, evaluation, basic care and comfort (a)
    ❷ Although diet therapy is not as effective in managing gout as are medications, it is generally accepted that a diet low in purines will diminish uric acid in the body.
    ① Usually weight loss is indicated and would require a low calorie diet. Fatty foods precipitate attacks.
    ③ Alcohol precipitates exacerbations and should be avoided.
    ④ A liberal fluid intake is encouraged.

24. Comprehension, planning, basic care and comfort (b)
    ❹ The resident's individual needs are addressed. Some solutions are easier for individuals to digest, making the absorption of nutrients easier.
    ① Hypertonic solutions are not used often, as they pull water into the intestine and cause diarrhea.
    ② Although similar in appearance, there are many solutions tailored to meet the individual needs of individuals.
    ③ Tube feeding solutions can be used only if the GI tract is functional.

25. Application, evaluation, basic care and comfort (b)
    ❷ A jejunostomy tube is the best choice to decrease the possibility of aspiration in a patient with dysphagia, as it is lower in the GI tract. The chance of dumping syndrome and diarrhea are increased.
    ① The chance of aspiration is still quite high with a gastrostomy tube, as reflux in the esophagus could occur.

③ Duodenostomy tubes are not common, however if they were placed, the level of risk would be greater than that of a jejunostomy tube, but less than that of a gastrostomy tube.

④ The chance for aspiration is high when using a nasal feeding tube.

26. Application, assessment, basic care and comfort (c)
❷ Culture and religion shape the food likes and dislikes of the individual, and any plan that did not incorporate foods from culture/religion might not be followed.

① Geographical region is important; however, culture and religion may be the most important.

③ Family health history may cause the nurse to be concerned in planning a diet to prevent certain disorders such as heart disease and cancer; however, these plans may not be complied with if attention is not given to culture and religion.

④ Although important to consider, the individual will more likely comply with the diet plan if personal choices are given consideration.

27. Knowledge, evaluation, basic care and comfort (b)
❷ The best method to preserve the nutrient content of food is steaming.

① Frying causes leeching of nutrients, and the food is less nutritious because of the addition of fat for frying.

③ Steaming could be done in the microwave; however, normal microwave cooking causes some evaporation of water soluble vitamins to take place.

④ Soaking will cause the nutrients to leech out into the water used for soaking.

28. Application, implementation, growth and development through the life span (b)
❹ The patient is most likely an Orthodox Jew. The dietary department will need to be made aware so that subsequent trays can include the appropriate foods.

① This is a block in communication; it will not help to chastise the patient.

② This does not address the patient's concern.

③ As presented, this is a threatening statement, although this may eventually need to be done to satisfy the patient's wishes.

29. Application, implementation, basic care and comfort (c)
❹ This is the only response that preserves the patient's need for religious influence, while recognizing that a solution to this problem must be found.

① This response is condescending to the patient and will likely be met with resistance.

② This is not conducive to the management of diabetes mellitus.

③ This response places the patient in a dependent, passive, role.

30. Application, planning, basic care and comfort (b)
❷ Members of the Hindu faith are vegetarians; meeting protein needs of the patient may be difficult.

① Fruits and vegetables are not restricted in the Hindu religion.

③ If cultural considerations are given, the patient should enjoy his meal plan choices.

④ The exchange lists will not need to be modified, al-

though creative approaches to planning for protein intake will be needed.

31. Knowledge, assessment, basic care and comfort (a)
❹ The base of the food guide pyramid consists of the bread, cereals, and grains group where 6 to 11 servings should be consumed each day.

① Two to three servings of the meat and poultry group should be consumed each day.

② Three to five servings of vegetables are indicated each day and two to four servings of fruits are indicated.

③ Only two to four servings of milk and dairy products are indicated.

32. Application, implementation, coordinated care (b)
❸ The cheese and crackers will provide the patient with IDDM complex carbohydrates, which will be utilized to stabilize blood glucose levels.

① Ice cream would provide too many calories and not enough complex carbohydrates.

② Cookies have too much refined sugar and will raise the person's blood glucose level too high.

④ Although it would depend on the cake's ingredients, generally chocolate cake has too much refined sugar.

33. Application, planning, basic care and comfort (b)
❸ A small snack composed of carbohydrates will fuel the patient's extra activity.

① Fats are incompletely burned for energy and will result in the glucose level increasing too quickly.

② Diet should be modified, not the medication.

④ Once again, medication adjustments are not necessary. This will result in insulin shock.

34. Application, planning, basic care and comfort (b)
❷ The patient with diabetes should carry a fast source of glucose with them at all times. Candy has the most simple sugar content and is easy to carry and use.

① Gum does not have as much sugar as candy and would not work as quickly.

③ Water is important for patients with diabetes to consume but will not correct insulin shock, which is the life-threatening emergency that candy can correct.

④ Crackers are complex carbohydrates and are not a rapid enough source of sugar.

35. Comprehension, evaluation, basic care and comfort (b)
❸ This meal has the lowest fat content.

① Whole milk and cake have a high fat content, and if the steak is not lean, it will also have a lot of fat.

② All of these foods are high in fat.

④ These foods are higher in fat than the fish, skim milk, and pudding with fruit.

36. Application, planning, basic care and comfort (b)
❸ These food choices have the lowest salt content.

① The corned beef and pickles are high in salt content.

② Any smoked or pickled foods are high in salt content.

④ Ham is processed with salt.

37. Application, evaluation, basic care and comfort, (b)
❸ Raw foods such as the vegetables and salad would contribute to the pain the patient is experiencing.

① These foods are generally bland, and when cooked would not aggravate diverticulitis.

② These foods would not stimulate the pain.

④ May contribute to pain but not to the degree that raw, high-fiber foods would.

38. Comprehension, planning, basic care and comfort (b)
❹ Meats and milk products either contain or have salt added.
① Fruits are generally salt-free.
② Most vegetables are salt-free.
③ These vegetables do not contain excessive salt.

39. Knowledge, planning, basic care and comfort (b)
❹ A low-fat diet is recommended to avoid aggravating gallbladder disease. These items are all acceptable on a low-fat diet.
① These are all high-fat foods.
② Avocado and chocolate milk are especially high in fat.
③ Ice cream is high in fat.

40. Comprehension, planning, basic care and comfort (b)
❹ Good sources of vitamin A, which is a fat-soluble vitamin that may be lacking in a low-fat diet.
① These are good sources of iron.
② These are good sources of potassium.
③ These are good sources of vitamin C, a water-soluble vitamin.

41. Comprehension, assessment, basic care and comfort (b)
❸ These foods are low in sodium.
① Macaroni and cheese are high in sodium.
② Corned beef is high in sodium.
④ Lobster and canned peaches are high in sodium.

42. Application, assessment, physiological adaptation (b)
❸ Indicates return of bowel sounds; peristalsis has started and oral feedings may be indicated.
① Hunger is not an accurate predictor of return of bowel sounds.
② Although she may be able to tolerate foods, this does not mean peristalsis has returned.
④ Distension could indicate lack of peristalsis.

43. Comprehension, application, growth and development through the life span (b)
❸ These foods are complementary proteins and are relatively inexpensive.
① Pasta does supply vitamins and energy and is healthy for the diet but does not answer the student's question.
② Does not answer the question.
④ This may be true, but it does not give her any recommendations.

44. Knowledge, assessment, basic care and comfort (b)
❸ Recurrent constipation can indicate a problem with nutrition.
① It is normal to feel fatigue after exercise.
② This is a normal pattern.
④ This is normal for healthy mucous membranes.

45. Comprehension, planning, basic care and comfort (c)
❹ The tomato sauce, mashed potatoes, and strawberries are all good sources of vitamin C, which is the vitamin especially needed for tissue healing.
① Mashed potatoes are the only source of vitamin C.
② None of these foods are a source of vitamin C.
③ None of these foods are a good source of vitamin C.

46. Comprehension, implementation, prevention and detection of disease (b)
❸ Practices such as storing vitamin C foods cut up rather than whole, storing unwrapped, and overcooking in large amounts of water will significantly decrease the amount of vitamin C in a substance.

① This is untrue; it is water-soluble.
② These are the deficiency symptoms of vitamin A.
④ Current research indicates vitamin C has a minor effect on reducing the number and severity of cold symptoms.

47. Comprehension, implementation, basic care and comfort (b)
❸ Food habits are established early and are difficult to change. Incorporating favorite foods will enhance compliance.
① This is closing communication and may not enhance compliance.
② This understanding may exist, but it does not encourage compliance.
④ Attack may have been mild, but behaviors need to change to help prevent a more serious episode.

48. Comprehension, evaluation, basic care and comfort (b)
❸ About 60% of the total calories in the diet should come from carbohydrates. Of this, 40% should come from complex forms such as pastas and whole grains. They break down more slowly than simple sugars, thus providing a steadier blood level.
① About 15% of carbohydrates come from simple sugars such as those found in fruit or milk.
② Artificial sweeteners should be used only in moderation.
④ Teenagers find support with peers and it is important that they spend time with them. Healthy choices can be made at most fast food restaurants.

49. Knowledge, application, safety and infection control (b)
❹ Popcorn is a choking hazard for young children.
① Apples are appropriate for toddlers.
② Toddlers should drink whole milk to help promote growth and energy metabolism.
③ Chocolate cake is not a hazard, although not very nutritious.

50. Knowledge, implementation, pharmacological therapies (b)
❷ TPN is used long term in cases of major surgery, when a patient is unable to obtain sufficient oral nourishment.
① TPN is not given through a peripheral vein, but through a large, central vein.
③ TPN does not utilize the GI tract.
④ TPN is given through a large, central vein.

51. Application, implementation, coping and adaptation (b)
❹ Malnutrition contributes to a compromised immune system. This is one way to have control over his health.
① Closes communication. He may never be ready to talk.
② Written material is appropriate after a discussion as a reinforcement.
③ The nurse has no way of knowing if this is true or not.

52. Application, implementation, basic care and comfort (b)
❸ Newer medications decrease gastric acid secretion. A well-balanced diet provides nutrients for healing.
① Dairy products provide only temporary relief and have a large fat content.
② No longer is indicated.
④ It is better to eat three full meals. Any food intake produces acid.

53. Knowledge, implementation, basic care and comfort (b)
   ❸ A high-fiber diet is recommended for diverticulosis because it helps prevent the development of high-pressure segments and increases the volume and weight of fecal material in the colon.
   ① Bland diets are sometimes recommended following gastric surgery or in peptic ulcer disease.
   ② Low-fat diets may be used in gallbladder, cardiovascular disease, or obesity.
   ④ Low-fiber diets may be required for diverticulitis.

54. Knowledge, assessment, growth and development through the life span (b)
   ❶ These are symptoms of a deficiency of C and B_{12}. The aging process may increase the need for these nutrients because of impaired absorption and decreased intake.
   ② Symptoms are not typical of these deficiencies.
   ③ These are fat-soluble vitamins and are stored in the liver.
   ④ The symptoms are not typical of these vitamin deficiencies.

55. Knowledge, implementation, basic care and comfort (b)
   ❸ It is recommended that smokers increase their vitamin C by 100 mg/day.
   ① Vitamin A is fat soluble and can be toxic in megadoses.
   ② Vitamin K is synthesized by the body.
   ④ Vitamin B has not been shown to be deficient in smokers.

56. Knowledge, planning, basic care and comfort (a)
   ❷ All three are high in potassium.
   ① Good sources of vitamin D but not potassium
   ③ Good sources of calcium and phosphorus, but not potassium.
   ④ Good sources of vitamin C, but not potassium.

57. Knowledge, planning, basic care and comfort (b)
   ❹ Table salt contains a great amount of sodium. Substituting other flavorings for salt can make it easier to cut down on the amount of salt used.
   ① Fresh fruits and vegetables are low in salt and can be used freely on a sodium-restricted diet.
   ② Dairy products contain much salt.
   ③ Canned and processed meats are high in salt.

58. Application, planning, basic care and comfort (b)
   ❹ Fats should be included because they perform specific functions, including providing a feeling of fullness and carrying fat-soluble vitamins.
   ① This is true; however, it causes alarm and does not give any information to make a healthy choice.
   ② Reduction of fat is recommended, not total elimination.
   ③ Although protein does build new cells and carbohydrates supply energy, this does not make this nutrient-restricted diet a healthy diet.

59. Knowledge, implementation, basic care and comfort (b)
   ❹ A healthy weight loss diet should include a variety of foods, as well as exercise.
   ① This is true, but it does not completely answer the question.
   ② A variety of nutrients are needed for a healthy diet.
   ③ This is true, but it does not completely answer the question.

60. Knowledge, planning, basic care and comfort (b)
   ❸ Lactose intolerance refers to the inability to digest milk sugar (lactose) because of a deficiency of the enzyme lactose
   ① Contains no lactose
   ② Does not contain lactose, so does not need to be avoided
   ③ Contains no lactose

61. Knowledge, assessment, basic care and comfort (b)
   ❹ Many nutrients are lost during the cooking process.
   ① There is no correlation between a meal's price and nutrient value.
   ② Grading of canned goods is related to appearance rather than nutritive value.
   ③ Refined products have many of the nutrients removed, fortified foods have added nutritive value.

62. Application, assessment, growth and development through the life span (b)
   ❸ Irregular eating habits and age are two factors that would cause the nurse concern.
   ① This pattern of weight gain is not excessive and should meet the nutrition demands of the baby.
   ② This is typical of this time of pregnancy, caused by the uterus pressing on the diaphragm.
   ④ Physiological anemia in pregnancy is often caused by increased blood volume. True anemia is diagnosed by blood studies and treated by a physician.

63. Application, implementation, basic care and comfort (b)
   ❹ For nonendurance events plain water prevents dehydration. Minerals are obtained in the diet.
   ① Vitamins do not provide energy.
   ② Athletes involved in endurance events may possibly need a 10% sugar solution to replace water and carbohydrates.
   ③ Minerals can be replaced in the diet.

64. Knowledge, implementation, basic care and comfort (b)
   ❸ Extra carbohydrates will assist in counteracting the negative nitrogen balance caused by massive trauma.
   ① Vitamins do not supply energy.
   ② This is true, but it does not answer the question.
   ④ Protein supplies nutrition.

65. Comprehension, assessment, basic care and comfort (a)
   ❷ Meat and dairy products are the main source of protein in our diet.
   ① Green, leafy vegetables and dried fruits can be good sources of iron.
   ③ Bread and cereals can provide many B complex vitamins.
   ④ Many fruits and vegetables can be good sources of vitamins A, D, C, and K.

66. Knowledge, assessment, growth and development through the life span (b)
   ❷ Metabolism slows in the older person; therefore, fewer calories are needed.
   ① Frequently there is less tolerance to fat and it is harder to digest.
   ③ Fluid intake should be increased to help eliminate waste products.
   ④ Vitamin and mineral intake should be maintained and perhaps increased, to account for decreased absorption.

67. Comprehension, evaluation, pharmacological therapies (c)
    ❸ Cardiac arrhythmias are a serious consequence of potassium deficiency. Diuretics can cause hypokalemia.
    ① This can indicate a deficiency in vitamin C.
    ② This can be caused by a deficiency in riboflavin.
    ④ This can indicate a deficiency of niacin or B complex vitamins.

68. Knowledge, planning, basic care and comfort (a)
    ❹ Mineral oil is indigestible and will carry out fat-soluble vitamins with it as it leaves the body.
    ① Mineral oil is not irritating, but it is also not a good idea.
    ② It does not add calories, but it is indigestible and its action on fat soluble vitamins makes it a poor choice.
    ③ Mineral oil has no calories because it is not digested.

69. Application, planning, growth and development through the life span (b)
    ❷ Honey contains botulism spores, which could be a problem for very young babies.
    ① Currently, rice cereal should be started at 4 to 6 months of age.
    ③ It is best not to get the baby used to the taste of additives that have little nutritional value.
    ④ Most allergies to eggs are caused by the white, not the yolk.

70. Knowledge, planning, growth and development through the life span (b)
    ❶ Of the foods listed, rice cereal causes the fewest allergies in children.
    ② Cow's milk is known to cause allergic reactions in certain children.
    ③ Wheat, oats, and barley cereals cause more allergic reactions than does rice cereal.
    ④ Egg whites can cause allergic reactions.

71. Knowledge, planning, growth and development through the life span (b)
    ❹ This is a common suggestion for alleviating morning sickness.
    ① Fluids should be taken between meals.
    ② High-fat foods are a common cause of nausea and should be avoided.
    ③ High-carbohydrate foods help alleviate nausea.

72. Knowledge, planning, basic care and comfort (b)
    ❸ Dried fruits are excellent sources of iron.
    ① Milk and dairy products contain very little iron.
    ② Refined cereals have had much of the valuable nutrients removed.
    ④ Good sources of vitamin A, not iron.

73. Comprehension, planning, basic care and comfort (a)
    ❶ Citrus juices contain vitamin C, which helps in the absorption of iron.
    ② Fish liver oils contain vitamins A and D, not vitamin C.
    ③ Green leafy vegetables contain vitamins A, E, and K, not vitamin C.
    ④ Milk and dairy products contain no vitamin C.

74. Knowledge, assessment, basic care and comfort (b)
    ❶ The exchange system is based on the fact that each food within an exchange is equivalent in nutrients to every other one. Therefore substituting one food for another within an exchange does not significantly alter the diet.

② One advantage of using the exchange system is that specialized foods are not needed.
③ The recommended number of exchanges is set up by a dietician, but substitutions can be done by the individual.
④ Food exchanges are important to space nutrient ingestion over the entire day so that the body is able to metabolize each.

75. Application, planning, basic care and comfort (a)
    ❸ All fruit and fruit juices are on the fruit exchange and so can be substituted for blackberries.
    ① Pecans are on the fat exchange list.
    ② Milk is on the milk exchange.
    ④ Cheese is on the meat exchange.

76. Application, implementation, basic care and comfort (c)
    ❷ The egg is on the meat list, the biscuit on the bread exchange, and the teaspoon of butter and margarine is two fat exchanges.
    ① There is no milk in the breakfast and only one bread and two fats.
    ③ There are no vegetables in the breakfast.
    ④ There is no fruit or milk in the breakfast and there is one meat and two fat exchanges.

77. Knowledge, planning, reduction of risk potential (a)
    ❷ Oranges and orange juice are readily digestible and absorbed.
    ① Cereal is a starch and takes longer to be absorbed.
    ③ Crackers are also a starch and would take longer to be digested and absorbed.
    ④ Bread and butter (starch and fat) both take longer to be absorbed.

78. Application, planning, basic care and comfort (b)
    ❹ The low protein provided on this diet limits end products of protein metabolism—an important consideration in kidney disease.
    ① Steak and milk provide more protein than is desirable for this patient.
    ② Hamburger and milk provide protein not desirable in this case.
    ③ Liver, cottage cheese, eggs and cream provide a high-protein diet.

79. Knowledge, planning, basic care and comfort (a)
    ❶ All are clear liquids.
    ② Cream soups are considered full liquids.
    ③ Sherbet is a full liquid.
    ④ Orange juice is considered a full liquid.

80. Knowledge, planning, basic care and comfort (b)
    ❸ A diet low in residue to avoid irritating the colon, but high in vitamins and proteins will replace nutrients that are frequently lost in ulcerative colitis and provide for tissue repair.
    ① Patients with ulcerative colitis frequently need increased fat and calories.
    ② No reason for low-sodium or low-carbohydrate foods.
    ④ High residue may further irritate the colon.

81. Knowledge, implementation, basic care and comfort (b)
    ❶ Soft diets are easier to digest, thereby reducing the workload of the heart.
    ② Decreasing irritation to the digestive tract is not important in the diet therapy for cardiovascular disease.
    ③ Unless the patient is overweight, no specific reason to reduce calories.

④ This is not the primary reason for the soft diet in this situation.

82. Application, planning, basic care and comfort (b)
❹ A high-fiber diet provides the bulk that stimulates peristalsis, thereby decreasing constipation.
① These provide very little residue.
② All foods in this meal provide very little residue.
③ Once again, little fiber or residue are in these foods.

83. Knowledge, assessment, prevention and early detection of disease (b)
❷ Fats, especially saturated fats, are prime contributors to high blood cholesterol levels and atherosclerotic heart disease.
① Total calories need to be reduced only if the individual is overweight.
③ Polyunsaturated fats should be substituted for saturated fats.
④ Carbohydrates should constitute 60% of total caloric intake.

84. Knowledge, assessment, basic care and comfort (b)
❷ Milk and milk products are excellent sources of calcium and protein.
① Milk is a poor source of iron.
③ Milk and milk products contain very little vitamin C
④ Milk is a poor source of B complex vitamins.

85. Comprehension, planning, prevention and early detection of disease (b)
❶ Currently, medical experts think that the severe restrictions of the past are not warranted and that a diet of omitting only what irritates is healthier.
② Milk increases the secretion of gastric acid more than it buffers it.
③ Caffeine, chocolate, and alcohol are strong stimulants of gastric acid.
④ Use of the bland diet has decreased, because there is no evidence that such a restrictive diet aids the healing process.

86. Knowledge, planning, basic care and comfort (b)
❶ Including high-fiber foods in menu planning lowers blood glucose and blood cholesterol.
② The exchange list system allows a wide variety of food choices.
③ Moderate amounts of alcohol may be consumed with meals.
④ The best carbohydrates are unrefined, high-fiber, complex carbohydrates.

87. Knowledge, planning, basic care and comfort (b)
❸ Diet is the primary controllable factor in regards to cholesterol levels.
① The recommendation is that blood cholesterol levels be maintained below 200 mg/dl.
② Dietary treatment is primarily indicated for high blood cholesterol. Medications are added only if dietary measures fail to bring cholesterol levels down to target amounts.
④ LDL is considered to be "bad cholesterol" and should be lowered in relation to HDL.

88. Application, implementation, basic care and comfort (b)
❹ Research studies have indicated that there may be a link between Omega-3 fatty acids and a low incidence of heart disease.
① This is not a true statement. Fatty acids are essential to the diet.

② There is no evidence that this is necessary. The patient merely requires information from the nurse.
③ There is no evidence to support this.

89. Knowledge, assessment, safety and infection control (b)
❶ Botulism is caused by a spore-forming anaerobic bacteria that grows well in improperly sealed home canned foods that have low acid content.
② This will not prevent the botulism toxin from developing.
③ Botulism normally does not occur in cold foods, but in canned items.
④ Botulism is caused by *Clostridium botulinum.*

90. Knowledge, evaluation, basic care and comfort (b)
❹ Normally the caloric needs of individuals with hay fever do not increase.
① Severe burns require the greatest increase in calories to maintain body weight.
② Healing fractures requires increased calories, also calcium, phosphorus and vitamin D.
③ Any surgery places stress on the body, increasing the body's need for calories.

91. Knowledge, assessment, basic care and comfort (a)
❷ Individuals who are alcoholic are most at risk for malnutrition.
① Vegetarians may have difficulty meeting protein requirements, but alternative sources can be found.
③ By following the ADA exchange program, diabetics should not be nutritionally compromised.
④ Although individuals with coronary artery disease have dietary restrictions, they should not be nutritionally compromised.

92. Knowledge, implementation, pharmacological therapies (b)
❸ Vitamin K is deficient in newborns because of their sterile bowel. AquaMEPHYTON is the pharmacologic term for vitamin K and is given shortly after birth.
① This is not the term for vitamin A.
② Vitamin D is not deficient in newborns and is not the equivalent of AquaMEPHYTON.
④ AquaMEPHYTON is not the pharmacological term for vitamin C.

93. Comprehension, planning, prevention and early detection of disease (b)
❷ Increasing dairy products will increase the female's calcium intake, which could prevent the development of osteoporosis.
① This does not have a significance in preventing osteoporosis.
③ This will not affect the development of osteoporosis.
④ Protein will not prevent osteoporosis, but increasing calcium-rich protein foods will.

94. Application, planning, physiological adaptation (b)
❷ Postoperative nutrition depends on the location and type of surgery involved. This information is not provided in the question.
① Not all patients need TPN after surgery, although it is used commonly after large GI surgeries.
③ The patient will need increased calories, vitamins, and proteins in order to facilitate healing after the surgical experience.
④ Not all surgeries require IV fluids and a high-protein diet.

95. Application, planning, safety and infection control (b)
❷ *E. coli*–related illness is prevented by ensuring that red meats are thoroughly cooked.
① Botulism is prevalent in improperly canned foods.
③ This may prevent infection; however, it is indicated in preventing salmonellosis.
④ Eggs contribute to infections caused by *Salmonella.*

96. Knowledge, assessment, basic care and comfort (b)
❷ This accurately describes the role of trace elements in the body.
① Trace elements are essential to health.
③ This is not accurate.
④ Most of the minerals can be detected in the body's fluids.

97. Comprehension, evaluation, basic care and comfort (b)
❹ The high salt content in the lunchmeat and potato chips would contribute to edema formation.
① Although eggs contain salt, this food choice would not be as likely to contribute to edema.
② Tuna fish and cantaloupe are low-salt food choices that should not contribute to edema.
③ Although the french fries may be salted, this food choice is less likely to contribute to edema than the salami and potato chips.

98. Application, planning, basic care and comfort (b)
❸ Milkshakes, or nutritional supplements, can supply the patient with anorexia additional calories and nutrients without overwhelming them.
① This overwhelms the person, makes him/her feel too full, and is not encouraged for clients with anorexia.

② Taking pain medication before meals will allow a pain-free dining experience that may encourage the patient to eat more.
④ Fruits and vegetables are nutritious but should not be eaten in exclusion of protein or other foods.

99. Comprehension, assessment, psychosocial adaptation (b)
❶ Individuals with anorexia nervosa often feel overweight even though they are very thin. When looking in the mirror, they do not see what the rest of the world sees.
② There is not normally an underlying physical illness involved.
③ Treatment programs are long-term in nature, involve the entire family, and sometimes are not successful.
④ Knowledge of the need for increased intake is not the impetus for causing the individual to begin to eat. A trusting relationship with the therapist, as well as information and family support, are imperative in the treatment plan.

100. Comprehension, planning, growth and development through the life span (b)
❹ This recognizes the couple's needs, but also encourages development of new food choices.
① This is accusatory in nature and will not facilitate communication and planning.
② The doctor has already prescribed the low-fat diet. Efforts should be made to allow some pastry while planning the meal plan.
③ The couple needs a low-fat, varied diet.

CHAPTER 5

Medical-Surgical Nursing

This chapter presents the nursing assessment of medical-surgical patients and is grouped according to the body system affected. Following the nursing process, frequent patient problems and recommended nursing care are identified and discussed. A selected group of major diagnoses, medical management, and nursing care plans is included. Although assessment of each system's functioning and problems is isolated, the student must remember that total patient assessment is necessary each time a patient is given care. The chapter begins with a brief overview of anatomy and physiology before moving on to the anatomy and physiology of the individual body systems, which precede the respective medical diagnoses. Nursing assessment, care, and responsibility for the patient before and after surgery, diagnostic testing, and nursing care procedures are discussed. Medications, the specific nursing responsibilities they entail, and their adverse effects are addressed in Chapter 3.

ANATOMY AND PHYSIOLOGY: AN OVERVIEW

A. Anatomy: the study of the structure of the body, its many parts, and their relationship to one another
B. Physiology: the study of how the body and its many parts function
C. Homeostasis: a state of constancy or dynamic equilibrium within the body
D. Anatomical terminology
   1. Anatomical position: the body is erect, with arms at sides and palms turned forward
   2. Anterior: toward the front of the body
   3. Posterior: toward the back of the body
   4. Cranial: near the head
   5. Superior: toward the head
   6. Inferior: toward the lower aspect
   7. Medial: toward the midline
   8. Lateral: toward the side
   9. Proximal: nearest the origin of a structure (elbows are proximal to the fingers, shoulder is proximal to the elbow)
   10. Distal: farthest from the origin of a structure
E. Body cavities
   1. Dorsal: pertaining to the back; has two subdivisions that are continuous with each other
      a. Cranial: the space inside the skull; contains the brain
      b. Spinal: extends from the cranial cavity nearly to the end of the vertebral column; contains the spinal cord
   2. Ventral: pertaining to the front; contains structures of the chest and abdomen; has two subdivisions
      a. Thoracic: chest cavity; contains the heart, lungs and large blood vessels; separated from the lower cavity by the diaphragm
      b. Abdominopelvic: one large cavity with no separation
         (1) Abdominal: upper portion; contains stomach, liver, gallbladder, pancreas, spleen, kidneys, and most of the intestines
         (2) Pelvic: lower portion; contains urinary bladder, lower part of intestines and internal reproductive organs

Structural Units
CELL

A. Definition: the basic unit of structure and function of all living things; made of protoplasm (meaning "original substance"), which is composed of carbon, oxygen, hydrogen, sulfur, nitrogen, and phosphorus; vary in size and shape
B. Structure and function
   1. Structural parts
      a. Cytoplasmic membrane: keeps cell whole and intact; allows certain substances to pass through and prevents others from entering (semipermeable membrane)
      b. Cytoplasm: area where most cellular activity occurs; the working and storage area
      c. Nucleus: the control center; directs cell activity and is necessary for reproduction; the site of the genetic material, DNA

   2. Characteristics of cells
      a. Irritability: responds to stimuli
      b. Growth and reproduction: gets larger in size and is able to increase in number
      c. Metabolism: chemical reaction consisting of
         (1) Anabolism: forming new substances to build new cell material-constructive
         (2) Catabolism: breaking down of substances into simpler substances and disposing of waste; destructive
      d. Contractility: the ability to shorten and thicken in response to a stimulus
      e. Conductivity: ability to transfer an electrical charge or impulse
   3. Functions
      a. Movement of substances through cell membranes
         (1) Diffusion: movement of dissolved particles through a semi-permeable membrane from an area of high concentration of particles to an area of low concentration of particles. This continues until the particles are evenly distributed
         (2) Osmosis: movement of water through a semipermeable membrane from an area where there is a large amount of water (dilute solution) to an area of a low concentration of water (a concentrated solution). This occurs until the water is evenly distributed
         (3) Filtration: movement of water and particles through a membrane because of a greater pushing force on one side of the membrane
      b. Reproduction mitosis: process of cell division; distributes identical chromosomes (DNA molecules) to each cell formed; enables cells to reproduce their own kind

TISSUES

A. Definition: groups of similar cells having like functions
B. Classifications and functions
   1. Epithelial: cells are packed close together; contain no blood vessels; three main types
      a. Simple squamous: single layer of cells that substances can pass through; function is absorption; lines air sacs of lungs, lines blood vessels, and covers membranes that line body cavity
      b. Stratified squamous: several layers of closely packed cells; protect the body against invasion of microorganisms; outer layer of skin, epidermis
      c. Simple columnar: single layer of cells; lines the stomach, intestines, and respiratory tract; specializes in secreting mucus and in absorption
   2. Connective: cells are separated by intercellular material; located in all parts of the body; various types include areolar, adipose, bone, and cartilage; function is to support and protect
   3. Muscle: three types of muscle tissue
      a. Skeletal or striated (voluntary): cells have striations; attach to bones; contractions are controlled voluntarily; cause movement
      b. Cardiac or striated (involuntary): cells have cross striations; cardiac muscle cells have the inherent power of rhythmic contraction

c. Visceral or nonstriated (smooth involuntary): cells appear smooth; help form walls of blood vessels and intestines; contractions cannot be controlled; cause movement

4. Nerve: composed of cells called neurons; all neurons receive and conduct electrochemical impulses; important in control of the entire body

MEMBRANES

A. Definition: thin, soft sheets of tissue that cover, line, lubricate, and anchor body parts

B. Classification and functions
1. Epithelial: lubricate and protect the body against infection; two types
   a. Mucous: line body cavities that open to the exterior (mouth, nose, intestinal tract, and urinary tract); secrete mucus, which protects against bacterial invasion
   b. Serous: line cavities that do not open to the exterior; cover the lungs, stomach, and heart; secrete thin fluid that prevents friction
2. Connective: cover bone or hold body parts in place
   a. Skeletal: cover bones and cartilage; support the bony structure
   b. Synovial: line joint cavities and secrete synovial fluid, which lubricates
   c. Fascial or fibrous: hold organs in place; superficial, connects the skin to underlying structures; deep, supports the internal organs (the viscera)

ORGANS

Structures composed of several tissues grouped together; they perform a more complex function than a single tissue; their composition and structure depend on their function

SYSTEMS

A. Definition: groups of organs that contribute to the function of the whole; they perform a more complex function than a single organ; no system can function independently of another system

B. Body systems and functions
1. Integumentary (skin): covers and protects the body
2. Musculoskeletal: supports and allows movement; body's framework
3. Circulatory: transports food, water, oxygen, and waste
4. Digestive: processes food and eliminates waste
5. Respiratory: supplies oxygen and eliminates carbon dioxide
6. Urinary: excretes waste
7. Nervous: controls and coordinates body activities
8. Endocrine: regulates body activities
9. Reproductive: increase the number of the species

MUSCULOSKELETAL SYSTEM
Anatomy and Physiology of the Skeletal System (Fig. 5-1)

A. Functions
1. Support: forms framework for body structures and provides shape
2. Protection: protects the internal organs
3. Movement: serves as levers that are activated by the contraction of an attached muscle

4. Mineral storage: stores calcium and minerals used by the body when needed
5. Produces blood cells: forms erythrocytes and thrombocytes and red marrow of bone

B. Bone composition
1. Bone composed of 33% organic material and 67% inorganic mineral salts
2. Collagen: organic part derived from a protein; fibrous material with a jellylike substance between the fibers; gives bone flexibility
3. Inorganic substance consists of large amount of mineral salts, calcium phosphate, calcium carbonate, calcium fluoride, magnesium phosphate, sodium oxide, and sodium chloride; these minerals give bone its hardness and durability

C. Classification of bones
1. Long bone: consists of diaphysis, epiphysis, and medullary cavity (e.g., femur)
2. Short bone: contains more spongy bone than compact; generally cube shaped (e.g., wrist bone)
3. Flat bone: thin and flat; has two thin layers of compact bone with a spongy bone between them; red blood cells are manufactured here (e.g., sternum)
4. Irregular: do not fall into preceding categories; are not symmetrical (e.g., vertebrae)

D. Structure of long bones
1. Similar to other bones in the body as to structure, development, and function
2. Longer than wide; have a shaft with heads at both ends; bones of extremities are long bones
3. Diaphysis or shaft: hollow cylinder of hard compact bone; contains medullary canal, which is filled with yellow bone marrow; in the adult it is primarily a storage area for adipose fat
4. Epiphysis: the ends of the diaphysis composed of spongy bone covered by a thin layer of compact bone; contains red marrow where some red blood cells are manufactured during childhood and adolescence; erythropoietic activity in the adult mainly occurs in flat bones and vertebrae
5. Periosteum: strong fibrous membrane that covers the bone; contains blood vessels, lymph vessels, nerves, and bone cells necessary for growth, repair, and nutrition
6. Epiphyseal disk (flat plate of hyaline cartilage): allows for lengthwise growth of long bones; at puberty when growth stops, it calcifies and becomes the epiphyseal line
7. Haversian canals: run lengthwise through bone matrix, carrying blood vessels and nerves to all areas of the bone; nourish the osteocytes or bone cell

E. Processes: bony prominences that serve as landmarks
1. Acromion: highest point of the shoulder
2. Olecranon: the upper end of the ulna, forms the point of the elbow
3. Iliac crest: curved rim along the upper border of the ilium
4. Ischial spine: lies at the back of the pelvic outlet
5. Acetabulum: the deep socket in the hip bone
6. Greater trochanter: the large protuberance located at the top of the shaft of the femur

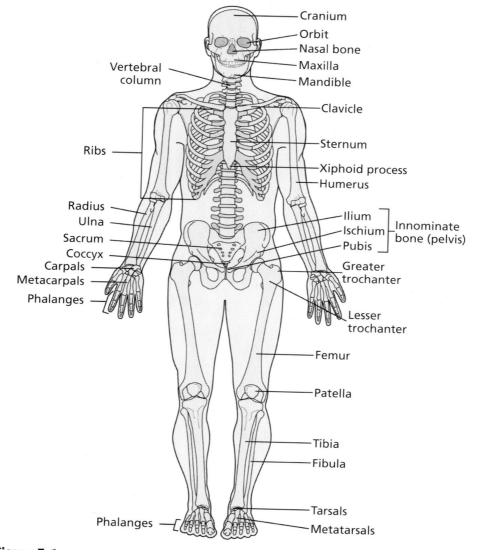

Figure 5-1   Bones of the body. (From Sorrentino SA: *Mosby's textbook for nursing assistants,* ed 5, St Louis, 2000, Mosby.)

F. Factors that affect bone growth and maintenance
   1. Heredity: each person has a genetic potential for height with genes inherited from both parents
   2. Nutrition: nutrients such as calcium, phosphorus, and proteins are raw materials of which bones are made of; without nutrients bones cannot grow properly
   3. Hormones: produced by endocrine glands; help regulate cell division, protein synthesis, calcium metabolism, and energy production
   4. Exercise: bearing weight, such as walking; without exercise bones become thin and fragile
G. Joints: point where bones meet; classification is determined by extent of movement
   1. Synarthroses: fibrous connective tissue holds joining bones close together; no movement (e.g., sutures in skull)
   2. Amphiarthroses: slight movement (e.g., joints between the vertebrae)

   3. Diarthroses: free movement; all have a joint capsule, a joint cavity, and a layer of cartilage
      a. Ball-and-socket joint: ball-shaped head of one bone fits into a concave socket of another bone (e.g., hip joint)
      b. Hinge joint: allows movement in only two directions, flexion and extension (e.g., knee)
      c. Pivot joint: small projection of one bone pivots in an arch of another bone (e.g., vertebrae of the neck)
      d. Saddle joint: exists only between the metacarpal bone and a carpal bone of the wrist (e.g., thumb and wrist)
      e. Gliding joint: bone surfaces slide over one another (e.g., wrist/ankle)
H. Ligaments: connective tissue bands that hold bones together
I. Tendons: connective tissue bands that attach bones to muscles
J. Bursa: a sac or cavity filled with fluid that reduces friction

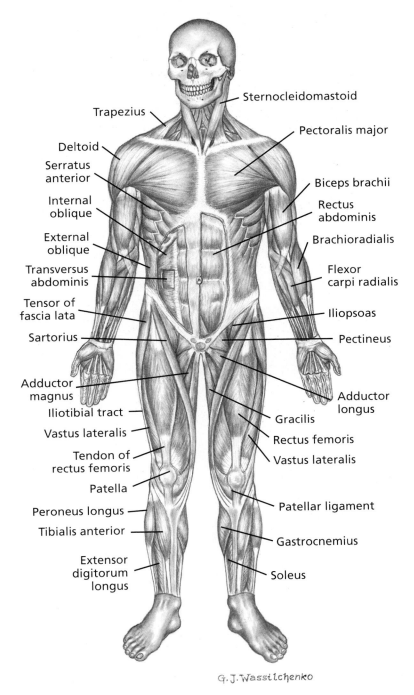

Figure 5-2 Skeletal muscles of the body, anterior view. (From Thompson JM, McFarland GK, Hirsch JE, Tucker SM: *Mosby's clinical nursing*, ed 4, St Louis, 1998, Mosby.) *Continued*

Anatomy and Physiology of the Muscular System (Fig. 5-2)

A. Functions
  1. Produces movement by contraction (Table 5-1)
  2. Maintains posture
  3. Produces heat and energy
B. Structure and types
  1. Striated: skeletal, voluntary muscle; attached to bones and accounts for body movement; controlled consciously

  2. Smooth: visceral, nonstriated, involuntary muscle; found in the walls of internal organs and blood vessels; works automatically
  3. Cardiac: found only in the heart; striated, branched, and involuntary
C. Characteristics
  1. Excitability: capacity to respond to stimulus
  2. Contractility: ability to shorten and thicken in response to a stimulus
  3. Extensibility: ability to stretch

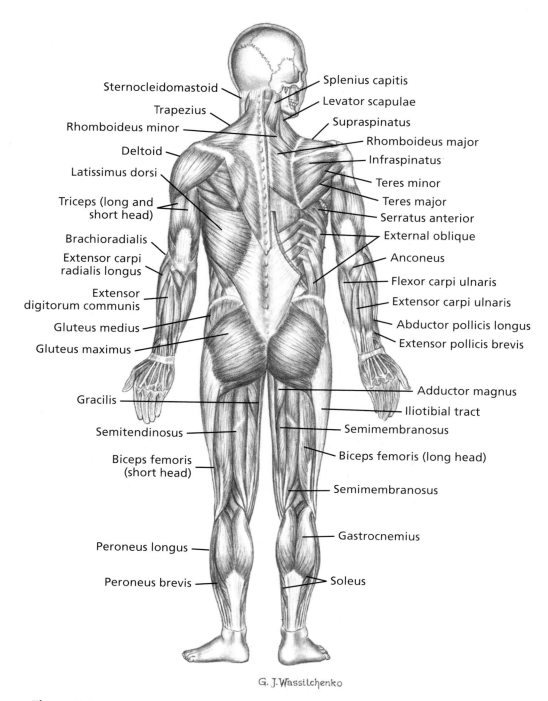

Sternocleidomastoid
Trapezius
Rhomboideus minor
Deltoid
Latissimus dorsi
Triceps (long and
short head)
Brachioradialis
Extensor carpi
radialis longus
Extensor
digitorum communis
Gluteus medius
Gluteus maximus
Gracilis
Semitendinosus
Biceps femoris
(short head)
Peroneus longus
Peroneus brevis

Splenius capitis
Levator scapulae
Supraspinatus
Rhomboideus major
Infraspinatus
Teres minor
Teres major
Serratus anterior
External oblique
Anconeus
Flexor carpi ulnaris
Extensor carpi ulnaris
Abductor pollicis longus
Extensor pollicis brevis
Adductor magnus
Iliotibial tract
Semimembranosus
Biceps femoris (long head)
Semimembranosus
Gastrocnemius
Soleus

G. J. Wassilchenko

Figure 5-2, cont'd   Skeletal muscles of the body, posterior view. (From Thompson JM, McFarland GK, Hirsch JE, Tucker SM: *Mosby's clinical nursing*, ed 4, St Louis, 1998, Mosby.)

4. Elasticity: ability to regain original size and shape
5. Tonicity: ability to maintain steady contraction
D. Contraction and movement
  1. Muscles move bones by pulling on them; as muscle contracts, it pulls insertion bone toward its original bone
    a. Origin: attached to fixed structure of bone
    b. Insertion: attached to movable part
  2. Several muscles contract at the same time to produce movement
    a. Agonist: prime mover; mainly responsible for producing movement

    b. Antagonists: responsible for relaxing when the prime mover is contracting
    c. Synergists: aid the prime mover in producing movement
  3. To contract, muscle must first be stimulated by nerve impulses
    a. Subminimal stimulus: does not cause contraction
    b. Minimal stimulus: does cause contraction
    c. Maximal stimulus: causes all muscle fibers in muscle to contract

TABLE 5-1   The Skeletal Muscles

Muscle	Location	Function
Sternocleidomastoid	Neck	Flexion and rotation of head
Trapezius	Upper Back	Helps hold head erect; also assists in moving the head sideways
Latissimus dorsi	Lower back	Extension and adduction of upper arm
Pectoralis major	Chest	Flexion and abduction of upper arm
Deltoid	Shoulder	Adduction of upper arm
Biceps brachii	Anterior upper arm	Flexion of arm and forearm
Triceps brachii	Posterior upper arm	Extension of arm and forearm
Gluteus maximus	Fleshy part of hips and buttocks	Extension of thigh
Gluteus medius	Lateral part of hips and buttocks	Abduction of thigh when limb is extended
Hamstring group	Posterior thigh	Flexion of lower leg and extension of thigh
Quadriceps femoris	Anterior thigh	Flexion of thigh and extension of lower leg
Gastrocnemius	Calf of leg	Helps in extension of foot and flexion of leg

    d. Supramaximal stimulus: strength of stimulus is above maximal; no effect on strength of contraction
4. Types of contraction
    a. Isometric: increases the tension without causing movement
    b. Isotonic: produces movement
    c. Tonic: does not produce movement but increases firmness of muscles that maintain posture
    d. Twitch: a quick, jerky contraction
    e. Tetanic (tetanus): sustained contraction
5. Types of movement
    a. Flexion: makes angle at joint smaller
    b. Extension: makes angle at joint larger
    c. Abduction: moves part away from midline
    d. Adduction: moves part toward midline

MUSCULOSKELETAL CONDITIONS AND DISORDERS

Musculoskeletal disorders may be acute or chronic. Acute problems are usually related to simple injuries. Chronic disorders may be more distressing to the patient because of loss of mobility and changes in self-image. The nurse needs to possess good skills in observation, positioning the patient safely, and use and care of equipment. The nurse is probably the most important health care provider in preventive care associated with complications of immobility.

Nursing Assessment

A. Nursing observation (objective data)
  1. General appearance
    a. Age
    b. Weight loss or weight gain
    c. Height changes: loss
    d. Abnormal gait
    e. Absence of extremity
    f. Deformity
    g. Malalignment
    h. Use of assistive devices
    i. Spinal curvature
  2. Respirations
    a. Rate
    b. Depth
    c. Character: any difficulty

  3. Pulse
    a. Presence of: check above and below injured/casted part
    b. Rate, quality, character
  4. Neurovascular status
    a. Assessment of skin color and temperature
    b. Pulses, presence of
    c. Intact sensation (noting numbness)
    d. Motor function
    e. Sensation and capillary refill
  5. Motor function
    a. Compare affected and unaffected sides
    b. Limited ability or loss of ability to move body part
    c. Diminished muscle strength to passive resistance
    d. Limited range of motion (ROM)
    e. Degree of ability to perform activities of daily living (ADLs)
  6. Pain and swelling
    a. Location, character, frequency, duration, alleviating/aggravating factors
    b. Bony enlargements or soft tissue swelling
B. Patient description (subjective data)
  1. Pain
    a. Patient's account of location, character, frequency, duration, onset
  2. Stamina
    a. Weakness, fatigue
    b. Changes in ability to perform activities of daily living
  3. Report of recent injury
    a. Description
    b. Evaluation/treatment
  4. Motor function
    a. Pain with movement
    b. Limited movement/difficult gait
  5. General
    a. Maintenance of weight
    b. Changes in appetite
    c. Tolerance of activities of daily living

Diagnostic Tests/Methods

A. Serum laboratory studies
  1. Complete blood count (CBC): an aid in determining anemia or the presence of infection

2. Erythrocyte sedimentation rate (ESR): elevation is evidence of an inflammatory process
3. Rheumatoid factor: a protein found in the blood of most persons afflicted with rheumatoid arthritis
4. Uric acid: high concentration is found in persons who have gout
5. Lupus erythematosus (LE) cell
   a. A cell identified in persons with lupus
   b. Normally there are no LE cells in the blood

B. Procedures
1. Roentgenogram (X-ray): a film to determine the presence of a deformity, fracture, or tumor of the skeletal system
2. Aspiration: withdrawal of fluid from a joint to obtain a specimen for diagnostic purposes
3. Bone biopsy: removal and examination of bone tissue
4. Myelogram: X-ray examination of the spinal cord after injection with radiopaque dye
5. Bone scan: isotope imaging of the skeleton
6. Computerized tomography (CT): use of roentgen rays to provide accurate images of thin cross sections of the body
7. Magnetic resonance imaging (MRI): aid for the diagnosis of musculoskeletal conditions through the clear differentiation of various types of tissue, such as bones, fat, and muscle
8. Arthroscopy: endoscopic examination that allows for direct visualization of a joint
9. Electromyography (EMG): used to evaluate nerve conduction in skeletal muscle
10. Positron emission tomography (PET): using an isotope, scans the brain for evaluation of structure function

C. Nursing intervention for myelogram
1. After procedure, have patient remain flat in bed 12 to 24 hours before allowing him or her to resume usual activities
2. Encourage fluids to 2000 to 3000 ml every 24 hours
3. Observe for alterations in normal motor and sensory states
4. Observe for nausea and vomiting

Frequent Patient Problems and Nursing Care

A. Disturbance in self-concept: body image related to immobility
1. Provide atmosphere of acceptance
2. Express empathy, warmth, and friendliness
3. Encourage acceptance of self-limitations
4. Encourage self-performance

B. Impairment of skin integrity: potential breakdown related to immobility/assistive devices
1. Change the patient's position frequently
2. Keep the skin clean, dry, and lubricated
3. Massage bony prominences
4. Provide sheepskin or polyurethane foam padding

C. Potential for injury: joint contracture related to incorrect body alignment
1. Place hands, feet, and knees in the natural position of function
2. Provide devices to protect against poor alignment of body part
3. Assist in performance of active and passive ROM exercises

4. Provide trapeze over the patient's bed
5. Avoid knee gatch position/pillow under knee

D. Potential respiratory secretion congestion related to ineffective airway clearance
1. Change the patient's position frequently
2. Encourage coughing and deep breathing
3. Observe for coughing, fever, and green-yellow sputum

E. Potential thrombus and emboli related to impaired physical mobility/edema
1. Encourage patient to move lower extremities
2. Encourage adequate hydration
3. Avoid use of knee gatch/pillow under knee
4. To avoid release of emboli, never rub legs
5. Use of elastic stockings
6. Daily calf measurements

F. Bone pain related to bone fracture or disease
1. Inspect and palpate the painful site looking for inflammation, edema, bruising, tenderness, and skin warmth
2. Support the affected body part
3. Apply warm, moist compress to affected body part where prescribed
4. Give prescribed analgesic
5. Evaluate effectiveness of pain relief measures

G. Potential limited ROM related to cast or traction confinement, joint pain, stiffness, or inflammation
1. Explain the reason for and intended effect of ROM exercises
2. Maintain body alignment
3. Provide total exercising of muscles and joints except if severe pain or inflammation is present; contraindicated if recent surgery was performed on or near the joint

H. Alteration in comfort: pain related to cast
1. Massage the area around the cast, except for leg casts
2. Pad rough edges
3. Elevate extremity to reduce swelling
4. Inspect the skin for irritation
5. Observe for cyanosis and assess capillary refill times of the casted extremity
6. Observe for complaints of numbness and tingling of casted extremity
7. Observe cast for indentations

I. Self-care deficits (feeding, bathing, and hygiene) related to impaired physical mobility
1. Assist with ADLs
2. Provide self-care aids/devices
3. Teach self-care activities

Major Medical Diagnoses
RHEUMATOID ARTHRITIS

A. Definition: a chronic, systemic disease in which inflammatory changes occur throughout the body's connective tissue destroying joints internally; joints most involved are hands, wrists, elbows, knees, and ankles
B. Pathology: cause is unknown; related theories include autoimmune, microorganisms, viruses, and genetic predisposition
C. Signs and symptoms
1. Subjective
   a. Sore, stiff, swollen joint(s)
   b. Fatigue
   c. Weakness
   d. Malaise
   e. Loss of appetite

2. Objective
   a. Low-grade fever
   b. Weakened grip
   c. Anemia
   d. Weight loss
   e. Subcutaneous nodes
   f. Enlarged lymph nodes
   g. Joint deformity
   h. Muscle atrophy
   i. Limited ROM
   j. Edema and tenderness of joint
   k. Extraarticular symptoms: lung, heart, blood vessels, muscle, eye, and skin
D. Diagnostic tests/methods
   1. Elevated ESR
   2. Slightly elevated white blood cell (WBC) count
   3. Presence of serum rheumatoid factors
   4. Synovial fluid aspiration
   5. X-ray film reveals joint deformity
   6. Low hemoglobin and hematocrit
E. Treatment
   1. Antiinflammatory agents, analgesics, corticosteroids, gold salts, and immunosuppressive drugs
   2. Heat applications such as paraffin dip, hot packs, and warm tub baths or showers for analgesia or muscle relaxation
   3. Surgical intervention to prevent deformities or remove damaged joints
   4. Physical therapy to maintain optimal function
F. Nursing intervention
   1. Provide undisturbed periods of rest
   2. Use firm mattress, foot boards, splints, and sandbags to maintain proper body alignment
   3. Encourage self-performance activities such as combing hair, feeding self, and brushing teeth
   4. Provide ROM exercises within limits of pain tolerance

OSTEOARTHRITIS

A. Definition: a local joint disorder affecting weight-bearing joints; results in disintegration of the cartilage covering the ends of bones
B. Pathology: cause is unknown; predisposing factors include aging, joint trauma, and obesity
C. Signs and symptoms
   1. Subjective
      a. Pain after exercise; relieved by rest
      b. Morning stiffness
      c. Muscle spasms
      d. Reduced strength
   2. Objective
      a. Limited ROM
      b. Crepitant joint
      c. Prominent bony enlargement
D. Diagnostic tests: X-ray studies reveal joint abnormalities
E. Treatment
   1. Weight reduction to relieve strain
   2. Heat and massage for aching and stiffness
   3. Physical therapy to maintain optimum level of functioning
   4. Drugs to relieve symptoms
      a. Analgesics
      b. Antiinflammatory agents
      c. Steroids

5. Surgical intervention to prevent deformity, relieve inflammation, delay progression, or replace affected joint
F. Nursing intervention
   1. Encourage patient to express feelings concerning disorder
   2. Provide moist heat, massage, and prescribed exercise, if ordered, to relax muscle and relieve stiffness or discomfort

GOUTY ARTHRITIS (GOUT)

A. Definition: a disorder in which excessive amounts of uric acid are retained in the blood
B. Pathology
   1. Cause is related to a disorder of purine metabolism
   2. Uric acid crystals are deposited in the joints and cartilage and form lumps (tophi)
   3. Deposits cause local irritation and an inflammatory response
   4. Men older than 30 years of age are most commonly affected
C. Signs and symptoms
   1. Subjective
      a. Acute pain, swelling, and inflammation of great toe (most affected joint)
      b. Headache
      c. Malaise
      d. Anorexia
      e. Pruritus (local)
   2. Objective
      a. Skin over joint is swollen, warm, and red
      b. Limited ROM
      c. Tophi located in cartilage of ears, hands, and feet
D. Diagnostic tests/methods
   1. Elevated serum uric acid level
   2. Elevated ESR and WBC count
E. Treatment
   1. Dietary restriction of foods high in purine (Box 5-1)
   2. Uricosuric drugs to increase uric acid excretion, Allopurinol to inhibit uric acid formation
   3. Weight loss and periodic blood glucose screening as there may be a relationship between gouty arthritis and insulin resistance.
   4. Colchicine to reduce pain and relieve swelling
   5. Alkaline ash diet to increase urinary pH
F. Nursing intervention
   1. Instruct patient to avoid foods high in purine content

Box 5-1   Foods to Avoid on a Low-Purine Diet

Liver
Kidney
Broth
Mincemeat
Sweetbreads
Sardines
Gravy
Meat extracts
Brains
Anchovies
Goose bouillon

2. Encourage physical activity to promote optimal muscular and skeletal function
3. Use bed cradle (or tent sheets over siderails) to prevent pressure of linen on feet and legs
4. Encourage fluid intake of 2000 to 3000 ml daily to avoid renal calculi unless contraindicated
5. Instruct patient to limit alcohol intake, which may precipitate an acute attack
6. Instruct patient to avoid salicylates because of antagonistic actions of uricosuric drugs

SYSTEMIC LUPUS ERYTHEMATOSUS (SLE)

A. Definition: a chronic multisystem inflammatory disorder involving the connective tissues, such as the muscles, kidneys, heart, and serous membranes; may affect the skin, lungs, and nervous system
B. Pathology
   1. Cause is unknown; is believed to be an autoimmune disorder
   2. Inflammation produces fibroid deposits and structural changes in connective tissue of organs and blood vessels
   3. Results in problems with mobility, oxygenation, and elimination
C. Signs and symptoms
   1. Subjective
      a. Abdominal, joint, and muscle pain
      b. Weakness; fatigue
      c. Depression
   2. Objective
      a. Low-grade fever
      b. Weight loss
      c. Butterfly skin rash over bridge of nose and cheeks, which increases with exposure to the sun
      d. Anemia
      e. Alopecia
D. Diagnostic tests
   1. Positive LE test
   2. Elevated ESR
   3. Increased gamma globulin levels
   4. Positive antinuclear antibody titer
   5. High anti-DNA test
E. Treatment
   1. Corticosteroids, analgesics, and medications for anemia
   2. The drug hydroxychloroquine is indicated in some individuals.
   3. Avoidance of exposure to sunlight
F. Nursing intervention
   1. Provide emotional support to patient and family in coping with poor prognosis
   2. Encourage alternative activity and planned rest periods
   3. Instruct to avoid persons with infections, undue exposure to sunlight, and emotional stress, which can cause exacerbations
   4. Encourage intake of foods high in iron content: liver, shellfish, leafy vegetables, and enriched breads and cereals

SCLERODERMA (PROGRESSIVE SYSTEMIC SCLEROSIS)

A. Definition: fiberlike changes in the connective tissue throughout the body caused by collagen deposits and subsequent fibrosis

B. Pathology
   1. An insidious, chronic, progressive disorder usually beginning in the skin
   2. Skin becomes thick and hard; fingers and toes become fixed in a position
   3. Other disorders that occur are difficulty in swallowing, impaired gastrointestinal (GI) mobility, cardiac and renal problems, and osteoporosis
C. Signs and symptoms
   1. Subjective
      a. Sweating of hands and feet
      b. Stiffness of hands
      c. Muscle weakness
      d. Joint pain
      e. Dysphagia
   2. Objective
      a. Increased pigmentation or dyspigmentation
      b. Dilated capillaries of lips, fingers, face, and tongue
D. Diagnostic tests/methods
   1. Positive LE cell test
   2. False-positive syphilis test
E. Treatment
   1. Skin care to prevent formation of decubiti
   2. Physical therapy
   3. Analgesics for joint pain
   4. Corticosteroids
F. Nursing intervention
   1. Provide emotional support to patient and family in addressing physical and psychological needs
   2. Encourage moderate exercise to promote muscular and joint function
   3. Force fluids
   4. Advise to avoid cold temperatures; use gloves to remove items from freezer
   5. Plan rest periods
   6. Provide assistive devices to help with activities of daily living (eating, grooming)

OSTEOMYELITIS

A. Definition: bone inflammation caused by direct or indirect invasion of an organism
B. Pathology: bacteria enter bloodstream through an open fracture, open wound, or by secondary invasion from blood-borne infection from a distant site such as bone or infected tonsils
C. Signs and symptoms
   1. Subjective
      a. Tenderness over the bones
      b. Painful movement; limited mobility
      c. Malaise
   2. Objective
      a. Fever
      b. Chills
      c. Heat, swelling, and redness of the skin over the bone
      d. Signs of sepsis
      e. Wound drainage
D. Diagnostic tests/methods
   1. Positive blood cultures
   2. Elevated ESR
   3. Elevated WBC count
   4. X-ray film may not reveal abnormalities for 5 to 10 days from onset

E. Treatment
   1. Long-term antibiotic therapy
   2. Drainage from abscess with continuous irrigation of wound
   3. Surgical removal of necrotic bone
F. Nursing intervention
   1. Use strict aseptic technique when changing dressings
   2. Keep affected limb in proper alignment with pillows and sandbags
   3. Maintain drainage and secretion precautions for disposal of dressings
   4. Provide a high-calorie, high-protein diet and adequate hydration
   5. Provide undisturbed rest periods
   6. Move affected body part gently, because of severe pain

OSTEOPOROSIS

A. Definition: metabolic bone disorder in which bone mass is decreased. Bones become weak and brittle. Prevention is crucial; maintain adequate calcium intake throughout life
B. Pathology
   1. Common in postmenopausal women
   2. May be result of deficit of estrogen and androgens, prolonged immobilization, insufficient calcium intake or absorption, or endocrine disorder
   3. Sites usually affected are vertebrae, pelvis, hip, wrist, and femur
C. Signs and symptoms
   1. Subjective: backache that worsens with sitting, standing, coughing, and sneezing
   2. Objective
      a. Kyphosis
      b. Loss of height
      c. Pathological fractures
D. Diagnostic test: X-ray film reveals bone demineralization and compression of vertebrae
E. Treatment
   1. Physical activity and exercise to prevent atrophy
   2. Estrogen replacement to provide calcium balance
   3. Diet high in protein and calcium
   4. Vitamin D supplements
   5. Support of spine with brace or corset
F. Nursing intervention
   1. Encourage use of walker or cane to stabilize balance when ambulating
   2. Encourage fluid intake of 2000 to 3000 ml daily, unless contraindicated, to avoid formation of renal calculi
   3. Give instruction on those foods high in protein and calcium content
   4. Emphasize need to follow prescribed daily activity and exercise
   5. If confined to bed, give passive and active ROM exercises
   6. Teach safety measures to protect from fractures

OSTEOGENIC SARCOMA

A. Definition: a tumor located in the bone composed of cells derived from connective tissue
B. Pathology
   1. Highly malignant tumor that may metastasize to the lungs
   2. Affects children, adolescents, and young adults

   3. Usually occurs in shaft of long bones, especially affecting the femur
C. Signs and symptoms
   1. Subjective: pain
   2. Objective
      a. Restricted ROM
      b. Swelling
      c. Weight loss
      d. Anemia
D. Diagnostic tests/methods
   1. X-ray examination to reveal lesion in the extremity and chest; CT scan
   2. Biopsy examination to evaluate cells
   3. Frozen section for rapid diagnosis of possible malignant lesion
E. Treatment
   1. Chemotherapeutic agents to reduce and retard growth
   2. Radiation therapy to destroy malignant tissue
   3. Amputation of affected limb or resection of tumor
   4. Use of cadaver limb to preserve function after bone removal
F. Nursing intervention
   1. Provide emotional support to patient and family to reduce fear and anxiety
   2. Provide diet high in protein and caloric content
   3. If patient undergoes amputation procedure, follow special nursing actions (refer to amputations)
   4. If patient is receiving radiotherapy
      a. Provide noninfectious environment
      b. Avoid ointments, lotions, powders, and washing of port (treated) areas
      c. Do not remove markings on skin
      d. Observe site for redness, swelling, itching, and drying

OSTEOMALACIA

A. Definition: a disorder in which widespread softening and demineralization of bones occur
B. Pathology
   1. Possible causes
      a. Vitamin D deficiency resulting from poor dietary intake of vitamin D
      b. Body's inability to absorb or use vitamin D
      c. Lack of ultraviolet rays
   2. The effect of parathyroid hormone on bone resorption and calcium absorption is decreased
   3. Most affected bones are spine, pelvis, and lower extremities
C. Signs and symptoms
   1. Subjective
      a. Rheumatic-type pain
      b. Weakness
   2. Objective
      a. Waddling gait
      b. Spontaneous fractures
      c. Bone deformities
D. Diagnostic tests/methods
   1. Reduced calcium and phosphorus serum levels
   2. X-ray examination reveals fracturelike lines of affected bones
E. Treatment
   1. Therapeutic doses of vitamin D
   2. High dietary intake of calcium and phosphorus

F. Nursing intervention
1. Change patient's position gradually
2. Teach good body mechanics
3. Encourage intake of foods high in calcium: meat, shellfish, and dark green, leafy vegetables
4. Emphasize need to maintain weight in normal range
5. Instruct on avoidance of heavy lifting
6. Safety measures to prevent fractures

OSTEITIS DEFORMANS (PAGET'S DISEASE OF BONE)

A. Definition: an inflammatory condition in which certain bones become soft, thick, and deformed
B. Pathology
1. Cause is unknown: occurs mainly in men in middle age or older
2. Disease disturbs new bone tissue with bones becoming enlarged and coarse in texture
C. Signs and symptoms
1. Subjective
a. Bone pain; worsens at night
b. Tenderness on pressure of the bones
c. Back pain
d. Headache from enlarged skull
e. Deafness or blindness caused by pressure from overgrowth of bone
2. Objective
a. Pathological fractures
b. Decrease in height
c. Bowing of femur and tibia
d. Enlarged skull
D. Diagnostic tests/methods
1. Skeletal X-ray film reveals bone enlargement and denseness
2. Elevated serum alkaline phosphate value
3. Urinary excretion of hydroxyproline is increased
E. Treatment
1. Androgen therapy for men; estrogen therapy for women to reverse hypercalciuria, if present
2. Salicylates for pain
F. Nursing intervention
1. Observe for stress fractures
2. Emphasize need for maintenance of normal weight
3. If fracture occurs and patient becomes immobilized
a. Limit calcium intake to avoid renal calculi
b. Provide high fluid intake to avoid hypercalcemia
4. Safety measures to prevent fractures

HERNIATED NUCLEUS PULPOSUS (SLIPPED DISK OR RUPTURE OF INTERVERTEBRAL DISK)

A. Definition: protrusion of the nucleus pulposus, which compresses the nerve roots of the spinal cord
B. Pathology
1. Site usually affected is between L4 and L5, L5 and sacrum, C5 and C6, or C6 and C7
2. Causes may be straining of the spine in an unnatural position, degenerative changes, heavy lifting when bending from the waist, and accidents
C. Signs and symptoms
1. Subjective
a. Cervical disk
(1) Stiff neck

(2) Shoulder pain descending down the arm into the hand
(3) Numbness of arm and hand
b. Lumbosacral disk: low-back pain radiating down the posterior thigh
2. Objective
a. Cervical disk
(1) Sensory disturbances of the hand
(2) Atrophy of biceps and triceps
b. Lumbosacral disk
(1) Difficulty in ambulating
(2) Lasègue's sign: pain in back and leg while raising heel with knee straight
(3) Numbness of leg and foot
(4) Foot drop
D. Diagnostic tests/methods
1. X-ray examination to reveal narrowing disk space
2. Myelogram to localize site
3. Electromyography
4. CT scan of the spine
5. MRI of spine
E. Treatment
1. Cervical traction (cervical disk); traction to lower extremities (lumbosacral disk)
2. Bed rest, heat application, and analgesics
3. Surgical intervention
a. Laminectomy: removal of a portion of the vertebra and excision of the ruptured portion of the nucleus pulposus
b. Spinal fusion: permanent binding of the vertebrae
c. Chemonucleolysis: dissolving of the affected disk through the injection of chymopapain
F. Nursing intervention
1. Encourage patient to verbalize feelings related to immobility, fears, and future impairment
2. Observations for traction
a. Check that it is hanging free and has not fallen or become caught in bed grooves
b. Observe for frayed cords and loosened knots
3. Give back care to promote circulation and relax muscles
4. Maintain proper body alignment
5. Provide diet high in fiber with adequate hydration to avoid constipation and straining
6. Instruct patient on principles of body mechanics
7. If patient has myelogram procedure
a. Position flat for period prescribed by physician
b. Encourage adequate hydration
8. If patient undergoes surgical intervention, follow general postoperative nursing actions
a. Observe for leakage of cerebrospinal fluid on surgical dressing; reinforce dressing until inspected by physician
b. Change position by log rolling to prevent motion of spinal column
c. Provide straight-backed chair for patient to sit in; feet must be on floor
d. Discharge instructions
(1) Avoid heavy lifting and climbing stairs
(2) Avoid riding in car
(3) Avoid forward flexion of head (cervical laminectomy)

FRACTURES

A. Definition: a break in the continuity of bone that may be accompanied by injury of surrounding soft tissue, producing swelling and discoloration

B. Pathology
1. Most fractures are a result of trauma; pathological fractures result from disorders such as osteoporosis, malnutrition, bone tumors, and Cushing's syndrome
2. Types of fractures
   a. Closed (simple): skin is intact over the site
   b. Open (compound): break in skin is present over the fracture site; the ends of the bone may or may not be visible
   c. Complete: fracture line extends completely through the bone
   d. Incomplete (partial): fracture line extends partially through the bone; one side breaks while the opposite side bends
   e. Comminuted: more than one fracture with bone fragments either crushed or splintered into several pieces
   f. Greenstick: splintering of one side of a bone (most often seen in children because of soft bone structure)
   g. Impacted: one bone fragment is driven into another bone fragment

C. Signs and symptoms
1. Subjective
   a. Pain on movement of body part
   b. Tenderness
   c. Loss of function
   d. Muscle spasms
2. Objective
   a. Deformity
   b. Edema
   c. Bruising
   d. Crepitus

D. Diagnostic test: X-ray examination to confirm location and direction of fracture line

E. Treatment
1. Reduction of the fracture consists of pulling the broken bone ends to correct alignment and regain continuity; usually a cast is applied or the part may be placed in a traction device
   a. Closed reduction: manual manipulation to bring ends into contact
   b. Open reduction: surgical intervention to cleanse the area and attach devices to hold the bones in position
2. Cast application to immobilize, support, and protect the part during the healing process
3. Traction to apply a pulling force in two directions to realign the bones
   a. Skin traction is temporarily applied: light weights that are attached to the skin with strips of adhesive tape
      (1) Buck's extension: exerts a straight pull on the limb; used for fractures of upper and lower leg, hip dislocation, and pelvic injuries
      (2) Bryant's traction: vertical extension of lower extremities, hip flexed 90 degrees, knees extended, and buttocks clear of the bed (see Fig. 8-16, p. 477) for reduction of femur or hip dislocation in very young children

      (3) Russell traction: a sling is placed behind the knee to create an upward pull of the knee, and at the same time a horizontal force is exerted on the tibia and fibula; used for fractures of femurs
   b. Skeletal traction provides continuous reduction by the attachment of a device to the bone
      (1) Kirschner wires or Steinmann pins are surgically inserted through the skin and bone; a traction bow or stirrup is attached to the wire or pin to exert a longitudinal pull and control rotation
      (2) Crutchfield tongs are inserted into parietal areas of the skull to obtain hyperextension; used for spinal fractures
      (3) Halo traction-halo loop for alignment of cervical area; loop is attached to a halo vest or cast

F. Nursing intervention
1. Provide emergency nursing care of fractures (see Chapter 10)
2. Provide nursing care for the patient with a cast
   a. Observe for neurovascular impairment of limb (Box 5-2)
   b. Elevate (use palms of hands) extremity in cast on pillow to reduce edema
   c. Promote drying of cast by exposing it to air
   d. Inspect for skin irritation under edges of cast: apply lotion, pad edges, and apply tape to edge of cast
   e. If drainage is present on the cast, measure and note
   f. Observe for possible infection: increased temperature, foul odor from cast, edema, and "hot spots" over the cast
   g. May apply ice for first 24 hours to reduce edema
   h. Observe for complications
      (1) Pulmonary emboli: if emboli lodges in the lungs, patient may experience dyspnea, anxiety, restlessness, chest pain, cough, hemoptysis, and increase in temperature
      (2) Fat emboli: similar to pulmonary emboli, except the emboli is a fat globule, probably arising from central area of the fractured bone
      (3) Compartment syndrome occurs when circulation to the muscles is compromised; look for changes in neurocirculatory status
   i. Educate patient on home cast care
3. Provide nursing care for the patient in traction
   a. Inspect and maintain ropes, knots, and pulleys; taut rope rides easily over pulleys; knots should not slip and should be unobstructed
   b. Inspect and maintain weights: hang freely, off the floor and free of bedding

---

Box 5-2 Signs of Neurovascular Impairment

Compare casted extremity to other extremities when assessing the following:
- Cyanosis
- Slow capillary refill times (greater than 3 seconds)
- Poor pulse
- Lack of sensation
- Complaints of numbness and tingling

c. Observations for skin traction
   (1) Inspect skin condition at distal ends of bandages (wrist and heel) for possible skin breakdown
   (2) Ensure that tapes do not encircle a limb, are applied smoothly, and are applied on skin that is free of irritation
   (3) Assess neurovascular status: color, pulses, warmth, and sensation
d. Observations for skeletal traction
   (1) Inspect insertion points daily for signs and symptoms of infection
   (2) Provide dressing change or wound care aseptically to prevent infection
   (3) Inspect pins, wires, and skeletal apparatus for sharp ends that may catch on bed linen
   (4) Assess neurovascular status
e. Examine and give skin care to all pressure points on which the patient rests
f. Provide foot support to prevent foot drop, especially for patients with Russell traction or Buck's extension
g. Observe for thrombophlebitis, especially for the patient with Russell traction because of pressure to the popliteal space
h. Encourage diet high in protein and vitamins to promote healing
i. Encourage 2000 to 3000 ml fluid intake daily to prevent complications such as constipation, renal calculi, and urinary tract infections
j. Encourage patient to perform ROM and isometric exercises
k. Maintain proper position and good alignment

FRACTURED HIP
A. Definition: fracture of the hip joint
B. Pathology
   1. Site of fracture
      a. Inside the joint (intracapsular or neck of the femur)
      b. Outside the joint (extracapsular or base of the neck of the femur)
   2. Elderly women experience high incidence because of osteoporosis
C. Signs and symptoms
   1. Subjective: pain
   2. Objective
      a. Leg appears shorter than unaffected extremity
      b. Foot points upward and outward on affected side (external rotation)
      c. Edema
      d. Discoloration
D. Diagnostic test: X-ray study confirms discontinuity of the bone
E. Treatment
   1. Russell traction or Buck's extension: before open reduction to prevent muscle spasms if surgery is not contraindicated
   2. Closed reduction with application of hip spica cast if the fracture occurred in the intertrochanteric site
   3. Open reduction and implantation of a prosthesis to replace head and neck of femur or fixation device to secure fragments of the fracture
      a. Austin Moore prosthesis
      b. Thompson prosthesis

c. Neufeld nail and screws
d. Smith-Petersen nail
e. Ziekel nail
F. Nursing intervention
   1. Provide nursing care of the patient in traction as outlined previously in section on fractures
   2. Be aware of coexisting problems such as diabetes or cardiac, vascular, or neurological disorders
   3. Considerations for the older adult patient
      a. Complications of immobility
      b. Reduced tolerance to drugs
      c. Delayed healing because of nutritional problems related to the aging process
   4. Keep side rail up and provide trapeze to facilitate movement
   5. Encourage patient to participate in activities of daily living: eating, bathing, and combing hair
   6. Provide postoperative care
      a. Inspect dressings and linen for drainage and bleeding
      b. Provide trochanter roll to prevent external rotation of legs
      c. Provide and maintain proper alignment. Use of abductor pillow to prevent adduction; adduction, external rotation, or acute flexion of the hip can dislocate hip before it is healed
      d. Encourage quadriceps-setting exercises
      e. Assist the patient to learn to use walker, ambulating with a non–weight-bearing technique
      f. Use of an elevated toilet seat to prevent hip flexion

ARTHROPLASTY
A. Definition: replacement of a joint, which may be necessary to restore function, relieve pain, and correct deformity
B. Pathology: arthritic changes damage the joint, resulting in impaired mobility, pain, and deformity; hip, knee, fingers, elbow, and shoulder are commonly affected
C. Signs and symptoms
   1. Subjective
      a. Pain
      b. Limited ROM
      c. Limited weight-bearing ability
   2. Objective
      a. Limited ROM
      b. Edema and skin character changes around affected joint
D. Diagnostic tests/methods
   1. X-ray studies confirm joint changes and damage
   2. Arthroscopy provides direct visualization and inspection of joint changes
E. Treatment: a prosthetic device used to replace the articulating joint surfaces (hip, knee, shoulder, elbow, and fingers)
F. Nursing intervention
   1. Proper positioning postoperatively (e.g., if hip is replaced, maintain affected leg in abduction)
   2. Wound care: monitor drains, note blood loss, and monitor dressing status
   3. Monitor continuous passive ROM machine, if used for knee replacement
   4. Assist with prescribed activity and encourage prescribed exercise
   5. Monitor pain; provide pain control

6. Assess neuromuscular function
7. Monitor skin integrity

AMPUTATION

A. Definition: surgical removal of part or all of an extremity
B. Pathology
   1. Majority of amputations result from blood vessel disorders causing inadequate oxygen supply to the tissue
   2. Other indications for amputation are gas gangrene, malignant tumors, septic wounds, severe trauma, and burns
   3. Usually a skin flap is constructed for prosthetic equipment
C. Signs and symptoms
   1. Subjective
      a. Gas gangrene and septic wounds: pain
      b. Peripheral vascular diseases
         (1) Pain
         (2) Tingling
   2. Objective
      a. Gas gangrene and septic wounds
         (1) Fever
         (2) Edema
         (3) Foul odor
         (4) Bronze or blackened wound due to necrosis
      b. Peripheral vascular diseases
         (1) Edema
         (2) Pallor
         (3) Shiny, hairless skin
         (4) Hyperpigmentation
         (5) Ulcer formation
      c. Arterial diseases
         (1) Pallor
         (2) Cyanosis
         (3) Diminished pulses
         (4) Pain on pressure
D. Diagnostic tests/methods
   1. Oscillometry
   2. Arteriography
   3. Skin temperature studies
   4. X-ray examination
   5. Doppler flow studies
E. Treatment
   1. Psychological preparation
   2. Rehabilitation preparation
   3. Nutritional status buildup
   4. Prosthetic device
F. Nursing intervention
   1. Provide preoperative care
      a. Encourage expression of feelings by providing honesty concerning loss of limb
      b. Explain to the patient the possibility of experiencing pain in the amputated limb (called phantom limb pain)
      c. Explain to the patient that he or she will undergo a program of exercises that includes strengthening of upper extremities, transferring from bed to chair, and ambulating with a walker or crutches
   2. Provide postoperative care
      a. Provide routine postoperative care
      b. Monitor for hemorrhage; if it occurs apply manual pressure and notify physician
      c. Apply elastic (Ace) bandages in a crisscross or figure-8 pattern only
      d. Elevate the residual limb 8 to 12 hours on a pillow; remove after 12 hours to prevent hip contracture; place in prone position 1 hour out of every 4 hours to prevent hip contracture
      e. Prevent outward rotation by placing trochanter roll along the outer side of the residual limb
      f. Instruct the patient not to hang the residual limb over the edge of the bed, wheelchair, chair, or handrail of his or her crutches to avoid residual limb contracture
      g. When conditioning of the residual limb is ordered, begin by having the patient push the residual limb against a pillow and progress to pushing against a firmer surface
      h. Teach the patient to massage the residual limb to soften the scar and improve vascularity
      i. Use TENS (transcutaneous electrical nerve stimulator) for relief of phantom limb pain
      j. Encourage progressive ambulation and physical therapy

RESPIRATORY SYSTEM
Anatomy and Physiology

A. Respiration: the taking in of oxygen, its use in the tissues, and the giving off of carbon dioxide; has two stages
   1. External: exchange of oxygen and carbon dioxide between body and outside environment; consists of inhalation and exhalation
   2. Internal: exchange of carbon dioxide and oxygen between the cells and the interstitial fluid surrounding the cells
B. Organs (Figs. 5-3 through 5-6)
   1. Nose
      a. Divides into two cavities separated by nasal septum
      b. Ciliated mucosa lines the cavities and traps inhaled foreign particles
      c. Filters, warms, and moistens air
      d. Serves as organ of smell
         (1) Receptors located in olfactory epithelium of upper part of nasal cavity
         (2) Stimulates appetite and flow of digestive juices
         (3) Senses of smell and taste work together to give flavor to food
      e. Paranasal sinuses: lighten skull, act as resonance chamber in speech
   2. Pharynx: passageway for food and air; divided into three parts
      a. Nasopharynx (behind nose): contains adenoids; eustachian tube, which drains the middle ear, opens into the nasopharynx
      b. Oropharynx (mouth): contains tonsils, which are lymphatic tissue
      c. Laryngopharynx: opens into larynx toward front and into esophagus toward back
   3. Larynx (voice box)
      a. Formed by nine cartilages in boxlike formation
      b. Thyroid cartilage forms the Adam's apple
      c. Epiglottis: flap of elastic cartilage that closes off the larynx when swallowing food

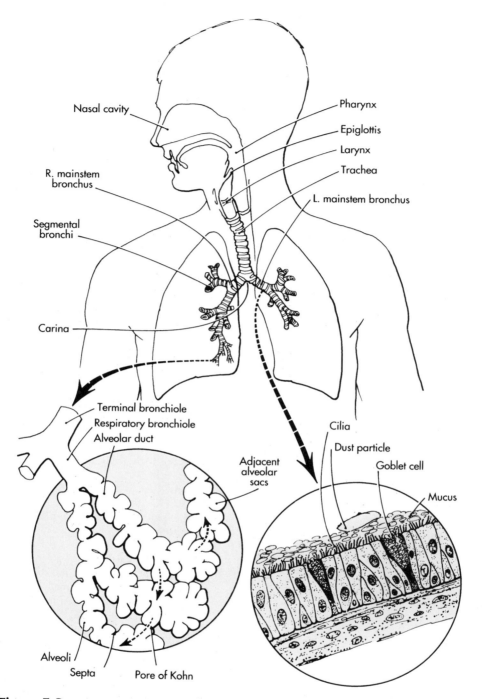

Figure 5-3   Structures of the respiratory tract. **A,** Pulmonary functional unit. **B,** Ciliated mucous membrane. (From Price SA, Wilson LM: *Pathophysiology: clinical concepts of disease processes,* ed 5, St Louis, 1997, Mosby.)

d. Produces sound; vocal cords vibrate with expelled air
e. Passageway for air to the trachea
4. Trachea (windpipe): tube reinforced by **C**-shaped rings; open ends of rings face posteriorly toward the esophagus and allow esophagus to expand when swallowing food; solid portion keeps the trachea open for the passage of air
5. Bronchi
   a. Formed by the division of the trachea into two branches; distribute air to the lungs' interior; called bronchial tree

b. Right main bronchus is larger and more vertical; aspiration is more common by this route
c. Bronchi divide into smaller branches called bronchioles
d. Bronchioles divide into smaller tubes and terminate in the alveoli
e. Alveoli: microscopic air sacs that resemble bunches of grapes; composed of a single, thin layer of squamous epithelium; external surface surrounded with spider webbed pulmonary capillaries; here the gas ex-

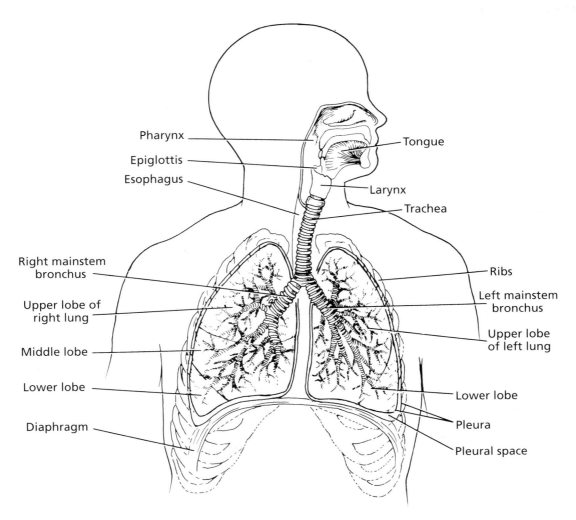

Figure 5-4 Anatomy of the thorax and lungs. (From Phipps WJ, Sands JK, Lehman MK, Cassmeyer VL: *Medical-surgical nursing: concepts and clinical practice*, ed 5, St Louis, 1995, Mosby.)

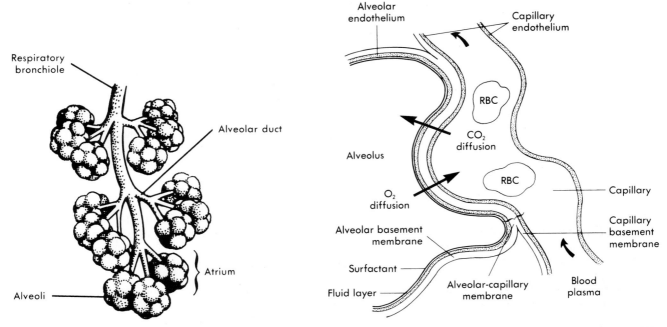

Figure 5-5 Respiratory unit. (From Phipps WJ, Sands JK, Lehman MK, Cassmeyer VL: *Medical-surgical nursing: concepts and clinical practice*, ed 5, St Louis, 1995, Mosby.)

Figure 5-6 Alveolar-capillary membrane. (From Long BC, Phipps WJ, Cassmeyer VL: *Medical-surgical nursing: a nursing process approach,* ed 3, St Louis, 1993, Mosby.)

changes occur, oxygen passes from the alveoli into the capillary blood, and carbon dioxide leaves the blood to enter the alveoli

6. Lungs
   a. Cone shaped; upper part is the apex; broad lower part is the base; base is concave and rests on diaphragm
   b. Tissue is porous and spongy
   c. Pleura: thin, moist, slippery membrane covering lungs; prevents friction during breathing movement

C. Physiology
   1. Two phases of breathing: inspiration and expiration
   2. Respiration controlled by respiratory center in medulla oblongata
   3. Carbon dioxide stimulates respiration
   4. Muscles of respiration
      a. Diaphragm: dome shaped; separates thoracic and abdominal cavities; contracts and relaxes
      b. Intercostals: between the ribs; elevate the ribs and enlarge the thorax during inspiration
   5. Mechanism of inspiration
      a. Contraction of diaphragm causes thorax to expand
      b. The lungs cling to the thoracic wall as a result of the attachment of the pleural membranes
      c. Intrathoracic pressure decreases
      d. The volume within the lungs (intrapulmonary) increases, and gases in the lungs spread out to fill the space
      e. Result is a decrease in gas pressure, and a partial vacuum sucks air into the lungs; air continues to move into the lungs until intrapulmonic pressure equals atmospheric pressure
   6. Mechanism of expiration
      a. Respiratory muscles relax and thorax decreases in size
      b. Intrathoracic and intrapulmonary volumes decrease
      c. As volume decreases, gases are forced closer together, and intrapulmonary pressure rises higher than atmospheric pressure
      d. Gases flow out of lungs and equalize pressure inside and outside the lung
   7. Volumes of air exchanges
      a. Total lung capacity (TLC): total volume of air present in the lungs after maximum inspiration
      b. Vital capacity (VC): volume of air that can be expelled after maximum inspiration
      c. Tidal volume (TV): volume of air exhaled after normal inspiration
      d. Residual volume (RV): amount of air remaining in lung after maximum expiration

RESPIRATORY CONDITIONS AND DISORDERS

All cells of the body depend on adequate oxygenation and removal of carbon dioxide for health. The respiratory system is dependent on central nervous system regulation and on the cardiovascular system for blood supply. Respiratory distress or dysfunction may be secondary to disease in another system. Many pulmonary diseases are chronic. Therefore it is essential that the nurse make a complete respiratory assessment of all patients and include this in nursing care planning, even when the primary diagnosis is unrelated to the respiratory system.

The following are terms used to describe respirations:
bradypnea: slow respirations
Cheyne-Stokes: periods of apnea alternating with rapid respirations
DOE: dyspnea on exertion
dyspnea: difficulty breathing; may be subjective or objective
Kussmaul breathing: fast, deep, and labored respirations
orthopnea: difficulty breathing in a supine position; relieved by sitting up
paroxysmal: nocturnal dyspnea transient episodes of acute dyspnea that occur a few hours after falling asleep
SOB: short of breath
tachypnea: rapid respirations
wheeze: sound as air moves out through bronchi and bronchioles that have been narrowed by spasm, swelling, and secretions

Nursing Assessment

A. Nursing observations (objective data)
   1. Respirations
      a. Rate
      b. Depth
      c. Characteristics (wheezing); any difficulty breathing; dyspnea on exertion
   2. Oxygen deprivation (note any)
      a. Restlessness
      b. Yawning
      c. Anxiety
      d. Drowsiness
      e. Confusion
      f. Disorientation
      g. Flaring nostrils
      h. Retractions
   3. Cough
      a. Frequency
      b. Relationship to activity and precipitating factors
      c. Production of sputum
      d. Describe completely (e.g., dry, productive, nonproductive, hoarse, barking, moist, or hacking)
   4. Lung sounds (adventitious)
      a. Crackles
      b. Wheezes
      c. Friction rub
      d. Stridor
   5. Sputum (note the following)
      a. Consistency (e.g., thick, tenacious, watery, or frothy)
      b. Amount (e.g., scant, moderate, or copious)
      c. Color (e.g., white, yellow, pink, rust, blood tinged, or green)
      d. Odor
   6. Skin color
      a. Pallor, ashen, or ruddy
      b. Cyanosis (bluish discoloration): observe lips, nail beds, and mucous membranes
   7. Skin
      a. Temperature
      b. Diaphoresis
   8. Vital signs
      a. Pulse: note rate, quality, and characteristics
      b. Blood pressure
      c. Temperature (rectal; tympanic)
      d. Pulse oximetry

9. Nasal discharge
10. Voice: huskiness
B. Patient description (subjective data)
   1. Cough
   2. Pain
   3. Difficulty breathing
   4. Fatigue or weakness, dizziness or fainting
   5. Sputum
C. Patient history
   1. Use of extra pillows needed to sleep
   2. Respiratory illness or difficulty
   3. Injuries
   4. Use of medications or respiratory aids
   5. Smoking
   6. Seasonal exacerbations
   7. Exposure to environmental irritants
   8. Known allergies
   9. Coexisting, chronic illness, i.e., HIV, diabetes, immunocompromised conditions, and therapies

Diagnostic Tests/Methods

A. Chest X-ray examination: a picture of lung tissue from different angles; based on a knowledge of normal anatomy and usual changes in disease, diagnosis of many conditions can be made (e.g., tumors, pneumonia); there is no preparation and no special care or observations after X-ray examination
B. Bronchoscopy
   1. Direct inspection of the trachea and bronchi through a scope passed via the nose or mouth; with this procedure specimens are obtained for biopsy and culture; foreign bodies can be removed (e.g., fish bones)
   2. Nursing responsibilities: provide general preparation as that for a surgical procedure (see Chapter 2); after procedure monitor vital signs, provide oral hygiene, and observe for cough and blood-streaked sputum; do not allow patient to eat or drink until gag reflex returns
C. Bronchogram
   1. Visualization of bronchial tree through X-ray examination after introducing radiopaque dye; patient is given sedative and antispasmodic
   2. Nursing responsibilities: provide postural drainage to aid in removal of dye; encourage deep breathing and coughing; do not allow patient to eat or drink until gag reflex returns
D. CT scan: produces clear, anatomic images of the chest cavity
E. Ultrasound: image of area is created by high-frequency sound; used for specific data relative to lung capacities
F. MRI: image created by magnetic resonance, a noninvasive procedure
G. Thoracentesis
   1. Needle aspiration of fluid from pleural cavity (space); local anesthesia is used
   2. Nursing responsibilities: maintain proper positioning; support and reassure patient during the procedure; monitor vital signs during and after the procedure
H. CBC: WBC count changes from normal values may indicate infection
I. Arterial blood gases
   1. Measurement of the partial pressure of oxygen and carbon dioxide in the blood; arterial puncture is performed
   2. Nursing care: once the blood sample is obtained, apply constant pressure to the site for 5 minutes; apply pressure dressing; inspect site frequently for hematoma and pain; distally for skin temperature, color
J. Culture and sensitivity
   1. Throat or nasopharynx
   2. Sputum
      a. Identifies organisms and specific medication to which patient will respond
      b. Nursing responsibilities: obtain before starting antibiotics; first sputum in the morning usually has the most organisms
K. Sputum analysis
   1. Acid-fast bacillus (AFB): determines presence of mycobacterium tuberculosis
   2. Cytology: assists in the diagnosis of lung carcinoma
L. Pulmonary function tests: determine extent of respiratory difficulty and evaluate function of respiratory system; no special preparation or nursing care after testing; a spirometer is used to diagram air movement, lung volumes, and airflow; the computer determines the actual value, predicted value, and percentage of the predicted value; examples of these tests are:
   1. Volumes: tidal volume, expiratory reserve volume, residual volume, and inspiratory reserve volume
   2. Capacities: total lung capacity, functional residual capacity, vital capacity, inspiratory capacity
M. Lung scan/positron emission tomography (PET): radioisotopes are inhaled or administered intravenously; a scanning device records the pattern of radioactivity; used in diagnosing vascular diseases (e.g., pulmonary embolism); no special preparation or nursing care
N. Biopsy examination
   1. Removal of a small amount of tissue to identify disease; biopsy may be of a lymph node to determine if the disease has spread into the lymphatic system
   2. Nursing care: provide general preoperative and postoperative care (see Chapter 2)

Frequent Patient Problems and Nursing Care

A. Activity intolerance related to fatigue and weakness: body cells' demand for oxygen is not met; the patient tires easily and becomes short of breath
   1. Protect from exertion; provide care; space activities appropriately
   2. Plan care to include rest periods
   3. Leave bed in low position
   4. Leave call bell and all personal belongings within easy reach
   5. Provide oxygen with humidity as ordered
   6. Limit conversation
B. Risk for injury related to dizziness: caused by diminished oxygen to the brain cells
   1. Provide all care as in preceding list
   2. Maintain safety; use side rails
   3. Perform neurological assessment every 4 hours (q4h)
   4. Assist when patient is out of bed
C. Altered oral mucous membrane related to mouth breathing
   1. Encourage fluids if allowed
   2. Provide oral hygiene q2h
   3. Lubricate lips with nonpetroleum base product

D. Altered breathing pattern related to orthopnea
  1. Place a pillow longitudinally under back
  2. Provide table with pillow for headrest in extreme difficulty
  3. Use footboard to prevent slipping down in bed
  4. Semi- to high-Fowler's position

E. Ineffective airway clearance; impaired gas exchange related to dyspnea and coughing
  1. Oxygen therapy: maintain safety of equipment and proper care and observations
  2. Organize care and work efficiently to conserve patient's energy
  3. Plan rest periods
  4. Position in semi- to high-Fowler's position; use two pillows
  5. Provide soft diet and small, frequent feedings
  6. Avoid gas-forming foods
  7. Prevent constipation and straining
  8. Use rectal thermometer; take tympanic temperature
  9. Make accurate observations about cough and sputum
  10. Obtain specimens as needed
  11. Provide tissues and bag for disposal within easy reach for infection control
  12. Provide sputum cup if specimen needed
  13. Change position q2h
  14. Encourage deep breathing
  15. Encourage fluids q2h
  16. Provide oral hygiene q2h
  17. Provide postural drainage if ordered (see Chapter 2)
  18. Give expectorants as ordered (see Chapters 2 and 3)
  19. Suction prn

F. Anxiety related to dyspnea, fatigue, and weakness
  1. Maintain quiet environment
  2. Remain calm
  3. Explain everything slowly and carefully
  4. Provide physical and mental rest
  5. Answer call lights promptly
  6. Provide frequent contacts
  7. Offer realistic encouragement
  8. Provide restful diversion (e.g., music)
  9. Encourage patients to express feelings and concerns

G. Alteration in nutrition, less than body requirements, related to dry mouth from mouth breathing, foul taste and odor from sputum, and fatigue; may affect desire for food
  1. Make mealtime pleasant
  2. Provide oral hygiene before each meal
  3. Remove used tissues and sputum cups
  4. Request food preferences
  5. Give small, frequent, attractively served meals

Major Medical Diagnoses
SINUSITIS
A. Definition: inflammation of one or more of the sinuses of the frontal, ethmoid, sphenoid, or maxillary bones; secretions become infected; is acute but becomes chronic if not treated or leads to complications: septicemia, meningitis, brain abscess
B. Cause: results from the spread of organisms from the nose or trapped secretions interfering with drainage (e.g., nasal polyps or edema from allergy)
C. Signs and symptoms
  1. Subjective: pain and headache

2. Objective
   a. Nasal secretions, possibly purulent and blood tinged
   b. Elevation of temperature; mild leukopenia
D. Diagnostic tests/methods
  1. Patient history and physical assessment
  2. X-ray examination, transillumination
E. Treatment
  1. Irrigation and inhalation of steam
  2. Antibiotics and decongestants (see Chapter 3)
  3. Surgery (e.g., Caldwell-Luc [infected maxillary sinus is removed through an incision under the upper lip] or ethmoidectomy)
F. Nursing intervention
  1. Administer nonnarcotic analgesics or nasal constrictors (see Chapter 3)
  2. Provide moist steam; a hot, dry environment will increase congestion; a vaporizer may thin secretions and soothe passages
  3. Provide hot wet pack; this may relieve pain and congestion of over-involved sinus
  4. Give general preoperative and postoperative care (see Chapter 2); note specific orders for care or observations

EPISTAXIS (NOSEBLEED)
A. Definition: bleeding from the nose
B. Cause: may be spontaneous, related to direct trauma, or a result of a systemic diseases (e.g., hypertension or blood dyscrasias); may be caused by local irritation from chronic infections or low-humidity environment
C. Sign: bleeding; shock if profuse
D. Diagnostic tests/methods: patient history and physical examination; platelet, HCT, HGB if profuse
E. Treatment (only if bleeding cannot be stopped)
  1. Nasal packing
  2. Cauterization of site with 10% silver nitrate stick
  3. Epinephrine spray
  4. Treatment of systemic disease
  5. Hemostatic agents
F. Nursing intervention
  1. Maintain patent airway (direct patient to breathe through mouth); have suction available
  2. Control bleeding: pinch nose firmly with fingers on soft part of nose; position in high-Fowler's with head forward
  3. Instruct patient to expectorate blood (swallowing will cause vomiting)
  4. Apply ice or cold compresses to nasal area to constrict blood vessels
  5. Monitor vital signs
  6. Avoid hot liquids
  7. Provide oral hygiene
  8. Reassure patient and family

DEVIATED SEPTUM
A. Definition: airway obstruction caused by deflection of bone and cartilage in the nasal septum
B. Causes
  1. Trauma
  2. Congenital
C. Diagnostic test/methods
  1. Patient history
  2. Physical assessment
  3. X-ray examination

D. Treatment: surgery-submuclous resection (SMR), performed through the mucous membrane within the nares; bone and cartilage are removed

E. Nursing intervention
1. Provide general preoperative and postoperative care (see Chapter 2)
2. Before surgery inform patient that nasal packing will be in place 24 to 48 hours; nasal breathing will not be possible; there will be a temporary loss of smell; sneezing must be avoided; and there will be pain, discoloration, and swelling around the eyes
3. Maintain airway; place patient on side or in semi-Fowler's position; monitor respirations
4. Provide oral hygiene every 1 to 2 hours
5. Provide ice compresses; note bleeding on dressing; inspect back of throat for trickle of blood
6. Use rectal or tympanic thermometer
7. Provide liquid diet when tolerated; encourage fluids; prevent constipation
8. Discourage forceful coughing

POLYPS

A. Definition: grapelike swellings of tissue; nasal polyps obstruct breathing and block sinus drainage (see sinusitis)
B. Treatment: surgical removal
C. Nursing intervention
1. Surgical preparation
2. Close check on bleeding postoperative

LARYNGITIS

A. Definition: an inflammation and swelling of the mucous membrane lining of the larynx
B. Cause: local irritation (e.g., smoking, spread of infection from elsewhere in the upper respiratory tract, or abuse of vocal cords)
C. Signs and symptoms
1. Subjective: pain
2. Objective
   a. Hoarseness
   b. Loss of voice
   c. Cough
D. Diagnostic tests/methods
1. Physical assessment
2. Patient history
3. Indirect laryngoscopy
E. Treatment and nursing intervention
1. Rest voice; provide alternate means of communication
2. Removal of cause
3. Provide steam inhalations
4. Administer astringent or antiseptic spray (see Chapter 3)

CARCINOMA OF THE LARYNX

A. Description: squamous cell carcinoma grows, spreads, and metastasizes; the rate of growth is determined by location of the lesion in the larynx
B. Causes: related to heavy smoking, chronic laryngitis and vocal abuse, and alcohol consumption
C. Signs and symptoms
1. Subjective: anxiety (i.e., concerning surgery; confirmation of diagnosis; disfigurement)

2. Objective
   a. Hoarseness
   b. Signs of metastasis: pain, lump in throat, difficulty swallowing, dyspnea, and enlarged, painful lymph nodes
D. Diagnostic tests/methods
1. Patient history
2. Visual examination (laryngoscopy)
3. Biopsy examination
4. Laryngeal tomography
E. Treatment: Surgery
1. Removal of larynx (laryngectomy) (partial or complete)
2. Radical neck dissection: wide excision including lymph nodes, epiglottis, thyroid cartilage, and muscle tissue; a permanent tracheostomy is performed
3. Radiotherapy with surgery
F. Nursing intervention
1. Provide general preoperative and postoperative care (see Chapter 2)
2. Immediate postoperative care
   a. Maintain patent airway; patient may have a permanent tracheostomy (see Chapter 2); there will be a shorter tube (laryngectomy tube); place patient in semi-Fowler's position; frequent mouth care
   b. Observe dressing qh; connect wound drains to suction as ordered; prevent movement of head
3. Continued postoperative care
   a. Provide method of communication (e.g., magic slate), leave call bell close to hand, and answer promptly in person
   b. Assist and be supportive as alternate methods of speech are learned (e.g., esophageal speech or use of mechanical voice box)
   c. Provide high-calorie, high-protein diet (may require tube feedings at first)
   d. Arrange for a visit from someone who has had a similar operation and satisfactory rehabilitation
   e. Investigate lifestyle changes (i.e., smoking, alcohol consumption) to decrease further risk of complications

PNEUMONIA

A. Definition: an inflammation of the lungs or part of the lung (e.g.; left lower lobe [LLL] pneumonia); secretions fill the alveolar sacs, which is a good medium for bacterial growth; the inflammation spreads to adjacent sacs; spaces of the lung consolidate with thick exudate; irritation may cause bleeding, and sputum has the characteristic rusty color; exchange of air is difficult and, in advanced conditions, not possible
B. Causes: bacterial infections and viruses are spread by respiratory secretions (droplets); chemical irritation; fungi and other organisms; aspirations; patients with poor health and low natural resistance to infection are more susceptible (e.g., the elderly, those with chronic illness, and immunocompromised individuals should consider receiving Pneumovax vaccine as a preventative measure for the most common type of bacterial pneumonia)
C. Signs and symptoms
1. Subjective
   a. Dyspnea, shortness of breath
   b. Pain on inspiration

c. Shallow breathing, signs of air hunger, orthopnea, and oxygen deprivation

2. Objective
   a. Marked elevation in temperature
   b. Cough: painful and dry at first, then productive with copious amounts of thick sputum (color according to organism)
   c. X-ray results
D. Diagnostic tests/methods
   1. Patient history
   2. Physical assessment with auscultation of chest
   3. Chest X-ray examination
   4. Sputum culture and sensitivity
   5. CBC
E. Treatment
   1. Specific and broad-spectrum antibiotics (see Chapter 3)
   2. Antipyretics, analgesics (codeine), expectorants, and bronchodilators (see Chapter 3)
   3. Intravenous (IV) fluids; encourage oral fluids
   4. Oxygen with humidity; incentive spirometer
F. Nursing intervention
   1. Provide optimum rest: provide care; help patient conserve energy; schedule rest periods; limit conversation; keep personal items and call bell within easy reach; alleviate anxiety
   2. Maintain oxygen with humidity
   3. Isolate as indicated, especially patients with oral and nasal secretions; provide for proper disposal (see Chapter 2)
   4. Liquefy secretions: force fluids (3000 ml daily or more); observe and document production of sputum; suction as necessary
   5. Provide oral hygiene q2h
   6. Monitor vital signs q4h; use rectal thermometer; monitor lung sounds
   7. Assist with loosening of secretions: have patient turn, cough, and deep breathe q2h (splint chest if painful); observe and document cough; may need aerosol treatment
   8. Maintain adequate nutrition: provide liquid-to-soft diet high in protein and calories
   9. Maintain IV fluids and medication schedule to ensure continued blood levels
   10. Position for comfort (high-Fowler's or lying on affected side)

PLEURISY

A. Definition: inflammation of the pleural membranes (local or diffuse); may or may not have fluid exudate; when fluid is present, the condition is pleural effusion, when purulent, the condition is empyema
B. Cause: infections (e.g., pneumonia, lung abscess, trauma, fungus, tuberculosis, lung cancer, congestive heart failure, or ascites)
C. Signs and symptoms
   1. Subjective
      a. Sharp pain on inspiration (referred to shoulder, abdomen, or affected side)
      b. Dyspnea
      c. Anxiety

2. Objective
   a. Cough
   b. Elevation of temperature
   c. Decreased breath sounds
   d. Pleural rub
D. Diagnostic tests/methods
   1. Chest X-ray examination
   2. Patient history
   3. Physical assessment including auscultation of chest
   4. Examination of pleural fluid obtained via thoracentesis and laboratory analysis
E. Treatment (according to cause)
   1. Analgesics and antibiotics
   2. Drainage of fluid: thoracentesis, then chest tubes to underwater seal drainage with suction
   3. Oxygen if dyspnea is severe; alleviate pain by turning patient to affected side
F. Nursing intervention: see plan for patient with chest tubes (the box to the right); provide diet high in protein, calories, minerals, and vitamins; alleviate anxiety

PNEUMOTHORAX/HEMOTHORAX

A. Definition
   1. Pneumothorax: air in pleural space allowing for partial or complete collapse of the lung
   2. Hemothorax: blood in pleural space
B. Causes
   1. May be spontaneous
   2. Trauma (e.g., knife wound or fractured rib that punctures lung)
   3. Postoperative (e.g., where the thoracic cavity has been entered)
   4. Diagnostic (e.g., CVP line, thoracentesis, pleural biopsy)
C. Signs and symptoms
   1. Subjective
      a. Sudden, sharp chest pain (when spontaneous)
      b. Vertigo
   2. Objective
      a. Diaphoresis, rapid pulse, and rapid respirations
      b. Decreased blood pressure
      c. Decreased breath sounds
      d. Dyspnea
D. Diagnostic tests/methods
   1. Patient history and physical assessment
   2. Chest X-ray examination
   3. Auscultation
   4. Observation
E. Treatment
   1. Closure of wound with airtight dressing
   2. Aspiration of fluids and air; water-seal drainage
   3. Analgesics
   4. Thoracentesis
F. Nursing intervention
   1. Provide nursing care and observations as necessary for primary diagnosis
   2. Place patient in high-Fowler's position
   3. Monitor vital signs
   4. Administer oxygen
   5. Provide nursing care for a patient with chest tubes as described in Box 5-3

Box 5-3   Patient With Chest Tubes

Description
Drainage tubes are inserted between the ribs into the pleural cavity to allow for drainage of secretions, blood, or air; the tube(s) is attached to an underwater seal system to allow for expansion of the lung and to prevent air from entering the pleural cavity; the drainage system may or may not be attached to suction

Indications
Chest surgery
Stab wounds to the chest
Pleural effusion
Spontaneous pneumothorax

Nursing Intervention
Do complete assessment of the respiratory system q2h; place patient in semi-Fowler's position; provide oxygen with humidity

Prevent complications of immobility; have patient turn, deep breathe, and cough q2h; encourage patient to ambulate as ordered and as condition allows; splint chest to cough

Encourage fluids to liquefy secretions; provide tissues and bag for proper disposal; provide sputum cup

Provide oral hygiene q2h

Anticipate pain; medicate as needed; observe respirations 30 minutes after administration of sedative or analgesic

Observe underwater seal system qh:
Drainage color and amount
Rise and fall of water in bottle (or suction) going to patient
Bubbling (if connected to suction)
Alleviate anxiety
Pace activities to allow for periods of rest
Monitor chest tube drainage

6. Provide instructions on tube/dressing care if discharged with chest tube in place

INFLUENZA
A. Definition: acute disease that may occur as an epidemic; recovery is usually complete; no permanent immunity results; complications and death may occur in patients with chronic or debilitating conditions, especially cardiac or pulmonary
B. Cause: virus
C. Signs and symptoms
   1. Subjective
      a. Headache, chest pain, muscle ache
      b. Dry throat
   2. Objective
      a. Nuchal rigidity
      b. Elevated temperature
      c. Coughing, sneezing, nasal discharge, and herpetic lesions
   3. Gastrointestinal symptoms; nausea, vomiting, and anorexia
   4. Weakness

D. Diagnostic tests/methods: patient history and physical assessment
E. Treatment
   1. Prevention with vaccines; influenza vaccine recommended on a yearly basis
   2. Symptomatic
   3. Antiviral therapy: amantadine hydrochloride for the prophylaxis and treatment of influenza A virus
F. Nursing intervention
   1. Provide rest, assist with care; provide quiet environment and dim lighting
   2. Encourage fluids
   3. Relieve symptoms: provide antipyretics, analgesics

PULMONARY TUBERCULOSIS
A. Definition: a chronic, progressive infection; alveoli are inflamed, and small nodules are produced called primary tubercles; the tubercle bacillus is at the center of the nodule (these become fibrosed); the area becomes calcified and can be identified on X-ray film; the person who has been infected harbors the bacillus for life; it is dormant unless it becomes active during physical or emotional stress
B. Cause: *Mycobacterium tuberculosis*, Koch's bacillus, an acid-fast bacillus (AFB) spread by droplets from an infected person
C. Signs and symptoms
   1. Subjective
      a. Malaise; patient is easily fatigued
      b. Chest pain
      c. Anorexia and weight loss
      d. Anxiety (i.e., fear of chronic disease, fear of public rejection)
   2. Objective
      a. Cough and hemoptysis (coughing up blood from the respiratory tract)
      b. Elevation of temperature and night sweats
D. Diagnostic tests/methods
   1. Patient history and physical assessment, coexisting chronic illness
   2. Chest X-ray examination
   3. Sputum specimen for AFB; aspiration of gastric fluid for AFB if unable to obtain specimen
   4. Tuberculin skin testing (e.g., Mantoux test)
E. Treatment
   1. Antituberculin drugs for 18 to 24 months (see Chapter 3)
   2. Rest (physical and emotional)
   3. Diet high in carbohydrates, proteins, and vitamins (especially B_6)
   4. Surgical resection of affected lung tissue or involved lobe (only when necessary)
F. Nursing intervention
   1. Provide rest; assist with or provide care; plan rest periods; limit conversation; leave personal items in easy reach
   2. Prevent transmission: ensure proper isolation (AFB; tuberculosis); provide tissues and bag for disposal; encourage proper use of tissues; insist on patient covering mouth and nose when coughing or sneezing; provide mask for patient if necessary; room must be equipped with special means of ventilation

3. Provide frequent, small meals and nutritious snacks; mouth care after meals
4. Avoid chills; keep skin dry and clean; protect from drafts, especially at night
5. Allay fears of patient and family about transmission: encourage proper adherence to drug maintenance; explain how organism is carried, transmitted, and destroyed (nurse must be aware that a tuberculin test is recommended for all contacts with a person with tuberculosis [TB]); a positive test result does not mean the disease has manifested but indicates that the organism has entered the body and that the body has produced antibodies at some point; explain need for multiple, long-term drug therapy

CHRONIC OBSTRUCTIVE PULMONARY DISEASE

Chronic obstructive pulmonary disease (COPD) includes chronic and frequently progressive pulmonary disorders that affect expiratory air flow; asthma, chronic bronchitis, and pulmonary emphysema may occur independently or together.

ASTHMA

A. Definition: spasms of the bronchial muscle occur; edema and swelling of the mucosa produce thick secretions; air flow is obstructed; air enters and is trapped; a characteristic wheeze accompanies attempts to exhale through narrowed bronchi; breathing is labored; coughing is attempted, but patient fails to expectorate satisfactory amounts; patient experiences great anxiety; the attacks last 30 to 60 minutes, often with normal breathing between attacks; if attack is difficult to control, and is resistant to all forms of treatment, it is called status asthmaticus
B. Causes
   1. Recurrent respiratory infection
   2. Allergic reaction
   3. Physical or emotional stress may provoke attack in a person with asthma
C. Signs and symptoms
   1. Subjective: Anxiety or feeling of suffocation, dyspnea
   2. Objective
      a. Shortness of breath, expiratory wheeze, labored respirations, diaphoresis, use of accessory muscles, and flaring nostrils
      b. Thick, tenacious sputum (after acute attack)
D. Diagnostic tests/methods: patient history and physical examination, ABGs, allergy testing, pulmonary function; peak flow meter
E. Treatment
   1. Removal of cause (source of allergy) or desensitization
   2. Low-flow, humidified oxygen
   3. Bronchodilators, mast cell inhibitors, corticosteroids, or sedatives (see Chapter 3); metered dose inhalers
F. Nursing intervention
   1. Reduce anxiety: provide time to listen; do not leave patient alone during attack
   2. Remove cause: keep environment free from dust and other allergens
   3. Provide continuous humidity as ordered
   4. Encourage fluids; maintain IV as ordered
   5. Position for maximum comfort and breathing: have patient sit in high-Fowler's position with arms supported by over-bed table

6. Prevent secondary infections: avoid staff and visitors with upper respiratory infections
7. Teach abdominal breathing
8. Do not allow smoking; refer patient for help in quitting
9. Avoid exposure to cold, wet weather
10. Instruct on preventive treatment for exertional asthma
11. Instruct on medications, use of inhalers

CHRONIC BRONCHITIS

A. Definition: chronic, progressive infection accompanied by hypersecretion of mucus by the bronchioles; without treatment and prevention of acute attacks, the alveolar sacs and capillaries will extend and destruct
B. Causes
   1. Asthma
   2. Acute respiratory tract infections (e.g., pneumonia, influenza, smoking, and air pollution contribute to incidence)
   3. Familial tendency
C. Signs and symptoms
   1. Subjective
      a. Worsening dyspnea
      b. Exertional dyspnea
   2. Objective
      a. Results of diagnostic tests
      b. Cough, productive with thick, white sputum; sputum is blood tinged as disease progresses (cough is greatest on arising)
      c. May progress to wheezing, prolonged expiratory time, use of accessory muscles
D. Diagnostic tests/methods
   1. Patient history
   2. Pulmonary testing to rule out other disease (e.g., tuberculosis or malignancy)
   3. Chest X-ray
E. Treatment
   1. Prevent irritation of bronchial mucosa: encourage patient to discontinue smoking and change aggravating conditions in occupation or home environment
   2. Prevent upper respiratory tract infection: maintain optimum health, adequate rest, and high-protein, high-vitamin diet
   3. Provide bronchodilators, antibiotics, corticosteroids, and influenza vaccine during epidemics (see Chapter 3)
F. Nursing intervention
   1. Provide care to relieve patient problems (see discussion on frequent patient problems and nursing care outlined earlier in this chapter)
   2. Loosen, liquefy, and remove secretions: provide postural drainage and chest percussion as ordered; encourage fluids
   3. Involve patient and family in care and care planning
   4. Do not allow smoking; refer patient for help in quitting

EMPHYSEMA

A. Definition: a chronic, progressive condition in which the alveolar sacs distend, rupture, and destroy the capillary beds; the alveoli lose elasticity, inspired air is trapped; inspiration is difficult and expiration is prolonged; the lung tissue becomes fibrotic; exchange of gases is not possible; anxiety increases; signs of oxygen deprivation are evident

B. Cause (see bronchitis)
C. Signs and symptoms
   1. Subjective
      a. Dyspnea on exertion (later, dyspnea on slightest exertion and orthopnea)
      b. Anorexia and weakness
   2. Objective
      a. Results of diagnostic tests
      b. Wheezing, prolonged expiratory time
      c. Chronic cough; productive, purulent sputum in copious amounts
      d. Speaks in short, jerky sentences
      e. Cerebral anoxia: is drowsy and confused; may become unconscious and go into coma
      f. Barrel chest
      g. Weight loss
D. Diagnostic tests/methods
   1. Patient history and physical examination
   2. Chest X-ray examination
   3. Pulmonary function tests
   4. Arterial blood gases; CBC
   5. Sputum analysis
E. Treatment (see bronchitis)
F. Nursing intervention
   1. Loosen, liquefy, and remove secretions: provide postural drainage and chest percussion as ordered; encourage fluids; administer expectorants as needed
   2. Promote respiratory function: breathing exercises and coughing
   3. Administer oxygen; oxygen is administered in low concentrations only (1 to 2 L); oxygen can be dangerous when the carbon dioxide level of the blood is high; the respiratory center of the brain becomes accustomed to the low blood oxygen level; if oxygen increases, respiratory rate will slow significantly
   4. Prevent and control infections: administer antibiotics; avoid contact with people with upper respiratory tract infections; avoid smoking
   5. Provide rest: limit exertion of any type; provide care; minimize conversation; assist with all movements (e.g., turning and getting into chair)
   6. Include family in care and care plan; be understanding that this condition is chronic
   7. Teach pursed-lip breathing; abdominal breathing
   8. Encourage small, frequent meals

CANCER OF THE LUNG

A. Definition: primary or secondary (from metastasis [e.g., from prostate]) malignant tumor; bronchogenic carcinoma is the most common primary tumor; is usually without symptoms until late stages when metastasis has occurred to brain, spinal cord, or esophagus; treatment is difficult in late stages and treatment is based on symptoms; prognosis is poor unless detected and treated early
B. Cause: strongly related to smoking, air pollution, and chemical irritants
C. Signs and symptoms (occur in late stages)
   1. Subjective
      a. Dyspnea and chest pain
      b. Fatigue, anorexia
   2. Objective
      a. Results of diagnostic tests

b. Productive cough with blood-streaked sputum
      c. Weight loss
D. Diagnostic tests/methods
   1. CT scan; MRI
   2. Examination of sputum for cells (cytology)
   3. Bronchial biopsy examination
E. Treatment
   1. Surgery: procedure depends on size and location of tumor (lobectomy, pneumonectomy, or laparoscopic thoracotomy)
   2. Radiation
   3. Chemotherapy
   4. Photodynamic therapy with laser
F. Nursing intervention
   1. Provide nursing care for symptoms (see discussion on frequent patient problems and nursing care earlier in chapter)
   2. Provide preoperative and postoperative nursing care (see Chapter 2)
      a. Maintain patent airway; administer oxygen; have patient turn, cough, and deep breathe q2h; a patient with a pneumonectomy must not cough; do not turn on operative side until physician orders (prevent mediastinal shift)
      b. Provide special care for a patient with chest tubes (rarely used, but still a possibility)

CARDIOVASCULAR, PERIPHERAL, AND HEMATOLOGIC SYSTEMS
Anatomy and Physiology of the Circulatory System

A. Functions
   1. Major function: transports oxygen, carbon dioxide, cell wastes, nutrients, enzymes, and antibodies throughout the body
   2. Secondary function: contributes to the body's metabolic functions and maintenance of homeostasis
B. Heart (Fig. 5-7)
   1. Hollow, cone-shaped muscular organ the size of a man's fist; functions as pump
   2. Positioned in thoracic cavity between the sternum and thoracic vertebrae
   3. Apex extends slightly to the left and rests on the diaphragm, approximately at the level of the fifth rib; point where apical pulse is assessed
   4. Layers
      a. Pericardium: outer covering; consists of two layers of serous membrane that is lubricated and prevents friction when the heart beats
      b. Myocardium: dense fibrous connective tissue; the wall of the heart
      c. Endocardium: a thin, serous lining that helps the blood flow smoothly through the heart; lines the heart chamber
   5. Chambers
      a. Atria: upper chambers: primarily receiving chambers; mostly receiving chambers, do not exert the major pumping force of the heart
         (1) Right atrium: receives deoxygenated blood from the coronary sinus and the superior and inferior vena cava

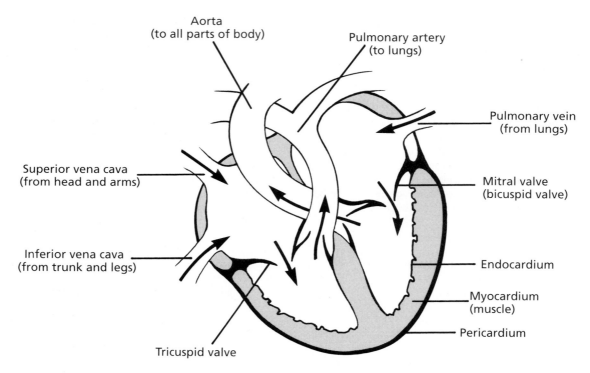

Figure 5-7   Structures of the heart.

(2) Left atrium: receives oxygenated blood from the lungs by way of the four pulmonary veins
  b. Ventricles: lower chambers; the pumping chambers; have the major responsibility of forcing blood out into large arteries
    (1) Right ventricle: receives blood from right atrium and pumps blood to lungs by way of the pulmonary artery
    (2) Left ventricle: does the major work of the heart; has the thickest muscular wall; pumps blood to all parts of the body by way of the aorta
    (3) Interventricular or interatrial septum: divides the heart longitudinally
6. Valves: permit flow of blood in only one direction
  a. Atrioventricular valves
    (1) Tricuspid: allows blood to flow from right atrium into right ventricle
    (2) Mitral or bicuspid: allows blood to flow from left atrium to left ventricle
  b. Semilunar valves
    (1) Pulmonary semilunar: allows blood to flow out of right ventricle into pulmonary artery
    (2) Aortic semilunar: allows blood to flow out of left ventricle into aorta
7. Physiology
  a. Cardiac cycle: refers to one complete heartbeat, consisting of contraction or systole and relaxation or diastole of the atria and ventricles
  b. Auscultatory sounds: heard through a stethoscope; the first sound, systolic, is longer and louder because of the closure of the cuspid valves; the second sound, diastole, is shorter and softer because of the closure of the semilunar valves

  c. Conduction system
    (1) Functions: initiates heartbeat; conducts electrical impulses around heart; coordinates heartbeat
    (2) Components
      (a) Sinoatrial (SA) node: the pacemaker of the heart, sets and regulates the beat by sending electrical impulses to the atria and the AV node
      (b) Atrioventricular (AV) node: receives impulses from SA node; transmits electrical impulses by way of bundle of His to the ventricles
      (c) Bundle of His: fibers that begin at AV node and follow the interventricular septum; divides into Purkinje's fibers
      (d) Purkinje's fibers: conducting fibers; stimulate the ventricles to contract
  d. Heart rates: controlled by internal and external factors
    (1) Bradycardia: slower than normal rate, less than 60 beats/min
    (2) Tachycardia: faster than normal rate, more than 100 beats/min
    (3) Extrasystole: premature beat
    (4) Sinus arrhythmia: a deviation from the normal pattern of the heartbeat resulting from changes in the rate and depth of breathing or other benign causes
C. Blood vessels
  1. Arteries: elastic, muscular-conducting tubes; carry blood away from the heart and to the capillaries; all arteries (except pulmonary) carry oxygenated blood
    a. Aorta: the largest artery, from which all other arteries branch out and become smaller and smaller

b. Arterioles: extremely small arteries; branch into the capillaries

2. Veins: thin-walled tubes that have one-way valves to prevent backflow of blood; transport blood back to the heart; all veins (except pulmonary) carry deoxygenated blood
   a. Venae cavae: largest veins; enter the right atrium
      (1) Superior vena cava: returns blood from the head, arms, and thoracic region
      (2) Inferior vena cava: returns blood from body regions below the diaphragm
   b. Venules: extremely small veins; collect blood from the capillaries
3. Capillaries: microscopic vessels; carry blood from arterioles to venules; exchange of nutrients and waste products occurs in capillaries

D. Types of circulation
1. Systemic: blood flows from the left ventricle into the aorta, through the body, and back to the right atrium; provides oxygen-rich, nutrient-laden blood to body organs
2. Pulmonary: blood flows from the right ventricle into the pulmonary artery, to the lungs, and then back to the left atrium through the pulmonary vein; its function is to carry blood to the lungs for gas exchange and return it to the heart
3. Portal: detour of venous blood from stomach, pancreas, intestines, and spleen through the liver, where it is processed, and returned by way of the inferior vena cava; excess glucose is removed and stored in the liver as glycogen; poisonous substances are removed and detoxified

E. Blood
1. Functions
   a. Transports oxygen and carbon dioxide to and from lungs
   b. Transports nutrients, hormones, and waste products
   c. Helps maintain acid-base balance, electrolyte balance, and fluid balance
   d. Carries substances that help fight infection
   e. Acts to maintain homeostasis
2. Composition
   a. Plasma: liquid, straw-colored portion of blood
      (1) Approximately 90% water
      (2) Contains blood proteins (fibrinogen, prothrombin, albumin, gamma globulin)
      (3) Contains mineral salts (electrolytes), hormones, nutrients, oxygen, carbon dioxide, and waste products (urea, lactic acid, and uric acid)
   b. Formed elements
      (1) Erythrocytes: red blood cells (RBCs)
         (a) Contain hemoglobin, which carries oxygen to cells and carbon dioxide from cells
         (b) Originate in red bone marrow
         (c) Life span is 100 to 120 days
         (d) Destroyed by the spleen, liver, and bone marrow
         (e) Normal range: male, 4.5 to 6.2 million per cubic millimeter; female, 4 to 5.5 million per cubic millimeter
      (2) Leukocytes: white blood cells (WBCs)
         (a) Principal function is to fight infection
         (b) Able to multiply rapidly
         (c) Classified according to whether they contain visible granules in their cytoplasm
            Granulocytes: include neutrophils, eosinophils, and basophils
            Agranulocytes: include lymphocytes and monocytes
         (d) Formation is in red bone marrow and by lymphatic tissue in lymph nodes, thymus, and spleen
         (e) Normal range: 5000 to 10,000 per cubic millimeter
      (3) Thrombocytes: platelets
         (a) Aid in clotting process
         (b) Originate in bone marrow
         (c) Normal range: 200,000 to 400,000 per cubic millimeter

3. Blood types
   a. Every person belongs to one of the four groups: type A, type B, type AB, or type O; and is classified as either Rh positive or Rh negative
   b. Type A blood: A antigens in RBCs, anti-B antibodies in plasma
   c. Type B Blood: type B antigens in RBCs, anti-A antibodies in plasma
   d. Type AB blood: has type A and type B antigens in RBCs; no anti-A or anti-B antibodies in plasma; type AB called universal recipient
   e. Type O blood; no type A or type B antigens in RBCs; both anti-A and anti-B antibodies in plasma; type O is called universal donor blood
   f. Rh-positive blood: Rh-factor antigen in RBCs
   g. Rh-negative blood: no Rh factor in RBCs; no anti-Rh antibodies in plasma
   h. Harmful effects can result from a blood transfusion if donor's RBCs become agglutinated by antibodies in the recipient's plasma

F. Lymphatic system: represents an accessory route for return of fluid from interstitial spaces to cardiovascular system; consists of lymphatic vessels, lymph nodes or glands, and spleen
1. Lymph: transparent fluid in surrounding spaces between tissue cells; made of water and end products of cell metabolism; referred to as intercellular or interstitial fluid
2. Function of system
   a. Lymphatic vessels: return fluid and proteins to blood
   b. Lymph nodes: filter injurious particles such as microorganisms and cancer cells
   c. Tonsils: filter and remove bacteria or pathogens entering the throat
   d. Thymus: most active during early life; relates immune reaction through puberty; atrophies at adulthood
3. Spleen: consists of lymphoid tissue
   a. Forms lymphocytes and monocytes
   b. Destroys old RBCs
   c. Stores blood until needed and then releases it into circulation

G. Immunity: the body's defense system against diseases and substances interpreted as nonself; mediated by T- and

B-lymphocytes of the circulatory system; the functions of lymphocytes in immunity by cell type are

1. T-lymphocytes: originate from stem cells in thymus; responsible for cellular immunity (a slow response) to an antigen; act against most bacteria, viruses, tumor cells, and foreign organs or grafts; clone into types of regulatory cells-helper and suppressors
   a. Helper T-cells: interact directly with B-cells by stimulating activity of B-cells on killer T-cells
   b. Killer T-cells: directly attack virus-infected cells, promote lysis
   c. Suppressor T-cells: terminate normal immune response
2. B-lymphocytes: originate mainly in fetal liver and lymphoid tissue during first few months of life; responsible for humoral immunity (a rapid response) to an antigen
   a. Clone antibody producing plasma cells
   b. Protect against toxin
3. Naturally acquired immunity
   a. Active: acquired through contact with disease
   b. Passive: acquired from antibodies obtained through placenta and mother's milk
4. Artificially acquired immunity
   a. Active: immunization with vaccines
   b. Passive: administration of immune serum

CARDIOVASCULAR CONDITIONS AND DISORDERS

Diseases related to the cardiovascular system are the leading cause of death in the United States. Cardiovascular health problems occur across the age continuum. To reduce death and disability, three major objectives include early detection of the disease, appropriate treatment to control the disease progression, and reduction of predisposing factors by promoting screening, education, and patient care of cardiovascular health.

Nursing Assessment

A. Nursing observations
   1. Vital signs
      a. Temperature
      b. Pulse: character, rate, rhythm, and any irregularities
      c. Respiration: character, rate; note abnormalities
   2. General appearance
      a. Note skin temperature, character, and color (jaundice, cyanosis, pallor); note clamminess
      b. Distended neck veins
      c. Dyspnea on exertion
      d. Limited or reduced ability to perform activities of daily living
      e. Clubbing of fingers
      f. Presence of edema; pedal, pulmonary, ascites, or sacral (if supine)
   3. Heart sounds
      a. Note bruits (whooshing sounds caused by turbulent blood flow) in carotids
      b. Abnormal heart sounds/dysrhythmias/murmurs
      c. Precordial movements/thrills
B. Patient description (subjective data)
   1. Chest pain
      a. Onset, location, frequency, duration, radiation
      b. Alleviating/aggravating factors

c. Chest pain may occur during periods of physical and emotional stress (emotions, eating, exercise, environment); pain may radiate to arm or jaw, or may occur at rest
2. Easily fatigued
   a. Can no longer perform usual activities without frequent rest periods
   b. Intolerance of exercise/exertion
3. Palpitations
4. Dizziness/fatigue feeling, especially when arising or standing
5. Cough
   a. Frothy or blood tinged (hemoptysis)
   b. Nocturnal cough
6. Family history of heart disease and hypertension
7. Dyspnea on exertion

Diagnostic Tests/Methods

A. Electrocardiogram (ECG)
   1. Tracing of the electrical activity of the heart
   2. Tool used to identify abnormal cardiac rhythms (dysrhythmias) and coronary atherosclerotic heart disease
   3. Reassure the patient that the ECG is recording the electrical impulses of the heart and is not delivering any electrical impulses to the body
   4. May be done on ambulatory patients through the use of telemetry units, signals from a box that the patient carries on them is conveyed to a monitor at a nurse's station
B. Stress test
   1. A procedure designed to detect cardiac ischemia that develops during exercise or exertion
   2. A heart tracing (ECG) is recorded and monitored while a patient performs an activity such as stair climbing, pedaling a stationary bicycle, or walking on a treadmill
C. Blood tests
   1. Complete blood count (CBC): analyzes components of the blood
      a. Low hemoglobin and hematocrit indicate anemia
      b. Elevated WBC count indicates inflammation/infection
   2. Erythrocyte sedimentation rate (ESR): may indicate inflammation
   3. Blood urea nitrogen (BUN) and creatinine: to detect the effects of heart disease on the kidneys
   4. Serum enzymes and isoenzymes (serum glutamic oxaloacetic transaminase [SGOT], creatine phosphokinase [CPK], and lactate dehydrogenase [LDH]): will elevate in a myocardial infarction
   5. Serum lipids: elevated blood lipids have been associated with coronary disease
   6. Blood cultures: if bacterial endocarditis is suspected
   7. Coagulation studies: PT/PTT-useful in monitoring anticoagulant therapy
   8. Serum electrolytes: detect imbalances in sodium, potassium, and calcium
   9. Arterial blood gases: monitor oxygenation and acid-base balance
D. Urinalysis: to determine the effects of heart disease on the kidney

E. Holter monitoring
1. Portable monitor designed and equipped to record the patient's heartbeat during a 24-hour period; a written record of the patient's activity is kept simultaneously; helpful in determining dysrhythmias
2. Assist the patient in the recording of activity
F. Coronary angiography
1. A roentgenogram of the coronary circulation facilitated by the introduction of contrast medium into the artery to outline the vessel and determine the extent of the disease process
2. After the study the patient must be observed for bleeding from the puncture site and have a cardiovascular status check of the involved area (pulses and skin temperature)
G. Chest X-ray examination: a standard chest roentgenogram is used to determine heart size and shape
H. Echocardiography (ultrasound cardiography)
1. Echoes from sound waves are used to study the movements and dimensions of cardiac structures; determines abnormalities
2. Information derived includes size of cardiac structures
I. Radionuclide studies
1. Tracing material is injected intravenously, and the radioactivity concentration over a body part is recorded
2. Size, shape, and filling of the heart chambers can be recorded; heart damage as well as cardiac circulation can also be evaluated
J. Cardiac catheterization
1. A cardiac catheter is introduced through a vein or artery and is advanced through the system; pressures of the heart chambers and pulmonary arteries are recorded and blood is analyzed; a contrast dye can be injected for visualization of certain structures to detect defects
2. Patient may feel a warm flushing sensation on injection of the dye; some patients experience chest pain
3. Patient observations after examination: monitor bleeding at the insertion site, check pulses and skin warmth in the involved area, and check heart rate and rhythm
K. Oscillometry: a noninvasive test that measures the amplitude of pulsations over an artery

Frequent Patient Problems and Nursing Care

A. Pain related to decreased cardiac output; overactivity
1. Evaluate and record onset, duration, and intensity
2. Note any associated symptoms (nausea, vomiting, dyspnea, etc.)
3. Monitor vital signs and record
4. Give vasodilators as prescribed; monitor for effectiveness and observe for side effects
5. If pain is unrelieved in 15 minutes by drugs or rest, notify physician
6. Reinforce patient teaching regarding diet, drugs, planned exercise, and stress management
7. Administer oxygen as prescribed
8. Record reactions to treatment and nursing care
B. Ineffective breathing pattern related to dyspnea
1. Monitor vital signs and record
2. Note character and rate of respirations
3. Elevate the head of the bed at least 30 degrees
4. Help patient assume an orthopneic position when necessary
5. Auscultate chest and note the presence of abnormal lung and heart sounds
6. Monitor oxygen therapy
7. Monitor intake and output
8. Record reactions to treatment and nursing care
9. Give diuretics, cardiotonics, and bronchodilators as prescribed and monitor for side effects
10. Note color, character, and amount of sputum
C. Decreased cardiac output related to dysrhythmias
1. Monitor vital signs and record
2. Note and report any changes in the vital signs
3. Auscultate chest, noting any abnormal heart sounds and report abnormalities
4. Give antidysrhythmic drugs as prescribed and monitor for side effects
5. Monitor for and report any associated symptoms
D. Impaired tissue perfusion related to edema
1. Note and record location and degree of edema
2. Elevate legs
3. Change positions when in bed
4. Note degree of pitting
5. Note "weeping" of skin areas
6. Monitor for skin breakdown
7. Give prescribed diuretics and cardiotonics
8. Note the presence of tenderness in the upper quadrant of the abdomen
9. Note the presence of ascites
10. Note daily weight
11. Record intake and output
12. Limit fluid intake as prescribed
13. Reinforce teaching for reduction of dependent edema
E. Fatigue/activity intolerance related to reduced cardiac reserve
1. Encourage progressive ambulation
2. Encourage progressive resuming of activities of daily living
3. Provide for planned activity and rest periods
4. Monitor for signs of fatigue
5. Stop activity at the first sign of intolerance
6. ROM exercises
7. Provide prescribed diet
8. Reinforce patient instruction of planned exercise
F. Alteration in tissue perfusion related to decreased cardiac output
1. Observe for presence of postural hypotension-orthostatic vital signs (note if blood pressure drops when standing)
2. Assist patient to dangle legs over the side of the bed before standing to reduce dizziness.
3. Instruct patient to get up slowly
4. Assess patient's pulse when standing
G. Fluid volume excess related to decreased cardiac output
1. Daily weight; report weight changes
2. Record intake and output
3. Monitor serum electrolytes
4. Limit fluids as indicated
5. Provide salt-restricted diet if ordered
6. Give diuretic medication as prescribed

7. Reinforce instructions regarding diet, drugs, and weight control

H. Alteration in tissue perfusion related to hypertension
1. Monitor vital signs and report changes
2. Provide sodium-restricted diet as prescribed
3. Provide cholesterol-controlled diet if prescribed and monitor for side effects
4. Instruct in the avoidance of risk factors (smoking, stress, and obesity)
5. Reinforce teaching in the areas of diet, weight control, avoidance of risk factors, and home monitoring of blood pressure

Major Medical Diagnoses

ARTERIOSCLEROSIS AND ATHEROSCLEROSIS

A. Definition
1. Arteriosclerosis: a process in which the arterial walls harden, thicken, and lose their elasticity, resulting in restricted blood flow
2. Atherosclerosis: one form of arteriosclerosis; fatty plaques form on the intima (inner layer) of the arteries

B. Pathology
1. The underlying mechanism is the formation of fatty plaque deposits in the arteries
2. The plaque increases in size and ultimately obstructs blood flow to vital areas

C. Arteriosclerosis is associated with the following health problems
1. Coronary artery disease
2. Angina pectoris
3. Myocardial infarction
4. Hypertension
5. Peripheral vascular disease
6. Cerebrovascular accidents (strokes)

D. Signs and symptoms vary, depending on the arteries affected by the sclerosing process
1. Extremity involvement
   a. Cramping pain (intermittent claudication)
   b. Numbness and tingling
   c. Reduced circulation, causing ulceration or pain
   d. Outward changes: skin pallor, cool skin, reduced or absent pulses, loss of leg hair, and skin ulceration
2. Coronary involvement
   a. Chest pain
   b. Dyspnea
   c. Palpitations
   d. Fainting (syncope)
   e. Fatigue

E. Diagnostic tests/methods
1. Patient history and physical examination
2. Arteriograms
3. ECG
4. Oscillometry

F. Treatment
1. Dietary restriction of fat and cholesterol
2. Vasodilating drugs
3. Cholesterol-lowering drugs
4. Elimination or reduction of risk factors (Box 5-4)
5. Weight management
6. Planned exercise
7. Prevention of pressure in extremities
8. Use of special devices such as bed cradles

Box 5-4	Risk Factors in the Development of Atherosclerosis

Obesity
Sedentary lifestyle
Smoking
Stress
High-fat diet

9. Bypass surgery or removal of plaques may be considered

G. Nursing intervention
1. Assess and document signs and symptoms
2. Protect the extremity from trauma
3. Monitor protective devices (bed cradles, pads, etc.)
4. Provide skin care to ulcerated areas or areas affected by reduced circulation
5. Monitor pulses and skin character of involved extremities
6. Report changes in the involved extremities
   a. Absence of pulse
   b. Cyanosis
   c. Increased pain
   d. Temperature change (coldness)
7. Monitor for signs and symptoms of infection in ulcerated areas
8. Provide slow, progressive physical activity as prescribed
9. Administer prescribed diet
10. Administer prescribed drugs
11. Relieve pain from ischemia
12. Avoid cold and provide adequate warmth to prevent vasoconstriction
13. Avoid constrictive clothing
14. Educate patient and family regarding avoidance of risk factors, dietary management, medication, and activity

ANGINA PECTORIS

A. Definition: episodes of acute chest pain resulting from insufficient oxygenation of myocardial tissue, caused by decreased blood flow to the area (ischemia)
1. Episodes occur most frequently during periods of physical or emotional exertion
   a. Exercise
   b. Eating a heavy meal
   c. Environmental temperature extremes
2. Episodes seldom last more than 15 minutes

B. Causes
1. The major cause is atherosclerosis
2. Narrowed coronary arteries obstruct blood flow; thus oxygen carried by the blood cannot sufficiently meet tissue demands, particularly during periods of exertion

C. Signs and symptoms
1. Substernal chest pain, usually brought on by exertion
2. Radiation of pain to the jaw or an extremity
3. Dyspnea
4. Anxiety or feeling of impending doom
5. Tachycardia
6. Diaphoresis
7. Sensation of heaviness, choking, or suffocation
8. Indigestion

D. Diagnostic tests/methods
1. Patient history and physical examination
2. ECG
3. Holter monitoring
4. Coronary angiography
5. Stress testing
6. Chest X-ray examination
7. Serum lipid and enzyme values
E. Treatment
1. Relief of chest pain through the use of vasodilating drugs (e.g., nitrates, beta blockers, calcium channel blockers), sedatives, and analgesics
2. Dietary restriction of fat and cholesterol
3. Planned exercise
4. Weight management
5. Stress management
6. If conservative measures are unsuccessful, coronary by-pass surgery or an angioplasty may be considered
F. Nursing intervention
1. Assess and document signs and symptoms and reactions to treatment
2. Administer vasodilating medication and monitor for side effects
3. Instruct patient to inform the nursing staff at the onset of an anginal attack
4. Provide emotional support and assurance
5. Provide prompt relief of pain
6. Monitor vital signs, particularly during an attack
7. Educate patient and family regarding diet, activity, drug therapy, and avoidance of risk factors

HYPERTENSION (HIGH BLOOD PRESSURE)

A. Definition: characterized by persistent elevation of blood pressure in which the systolic pressure is above 140 mm Hg and the diastolic pressure is above 90 mm Hg
1. Primary hypertension (essential): a persistent elevation of blood pressure without an apparent cause
   a. Actual cause is unknown
   b. Primarily, small blood vessels are affected; peripheral resistance increases; and blood pressure rises
   c. Constricted blood vessels eventually cause damage to organs that rely on a blood supply from these vessels
2. Secondary hypertension: a persistent elevation of blood pressure associated with another disease state
   a. Renal disease
   b. Toxemia
   c. Adrenal dysfunction
   d. Atherosclerosis
   e. Coarctation of the aorta
B. Predisposing factors
1. Smoking
2. Obesity
3. Heavy salt and cholesterol intake
4. Heredity
5. Aggressive, hyperactive personality
6. Age: develops between 30 and 50 years of age
7. Sex: primarily men over 35 years of age and women over 45 years of age
8. Race: blacks have twice the incidence of whites
9. Birth control pills and estrogens

> **Box 5-5 Foods High in Sodium**
>
> Processed meats (luncheon meats)
> Processed cheese
> Shellfish
> Canned vegetables
> Milk
> Snack foods such as potato chips and french fries
> Salted nuts

C. The heart brain, kidney, and eyes can be damaged if the hypertensive state continues without correction
D. Signs and symptoms may be insidious and vague; a person can have the disorder and not know it
1. Tinnitus
2. Light-headedness
3. Blurred vision
4. Irritability
5. Fatigue
6. Tachycardia and palpitations
7. Occipital, morning headaches
8. Nosebleeds (epistaxis)
9. Dyspnea on exertion
E. Diagnostic tests/methods
1. Patient history and physical examination
2. Series of resting blood pressure readings
3. Routine urinalysis, BUN, and serum creatinine to screen for renal involvement
4. Serum electrolytes to screen for adrenal involvement
5. Blood sugar levels to screen for endocrine involvement
6. Lipid profile
7. Chest X-ray examination
8. ECG
9. Holter monitoring
10. Funduscopic eye examination
F. Treatment
1. Lowering blood pressure through the use of antihypertensive drugs
2. Sodium-restricted diet (Box 5-5)
3. Cholesterol-controlled diet
4. Weight management
5. Stress management
6. Reduction or elimination of smoking
7. Planned exercise
G. Nursing intervention
1. Assess and document signs and symptoms and reactions to treatments
2. Administer prescribed medication
3. Observe for and report drug-related side effects
4. Monitor weight every day (qd) to evaluate initial diuretic therapy
5. Monitor intake and output to evaluate initial diuretic therapy
6. Monitor vital signs, particularly blood pressure, under the same conditions qd
7. Provide planned activity and rest periods
8. Provide prescribed diet
   a. Calorie controlled
   b. Sodium restricted
   c. Cholesterol controlled

9. Educate patient and family
   a. Drug therapy and side effects
   b. Dietary restrictions; weight management
   c. Elimination of risk factors, such as smoking
   d. Activity
   e. Blood pressure monitoring
   f. Need for participation in and compliance with the prescribed regimen

MYOCARDIAL INFARCTION (HEART ATTACK)

A. Definition: the obstruction of a coronary artery or one of its branches
   1. The obstruction results in the death of the myocardial tissue supplied by that vessel
   2. The myocardial tissue dies because of oxygen deprivation (infarction or necrosis)
   3. The heart's ability to regain or maintain its function depends on the location and size of the area of infarction
B. A myocardial infarction can occur whenever a coronary artery or branch of the artery becomes occluded by a thrombus, emboli, or the atherosclerotic process
C. Signs and symptoms
   1. "Crushing" chest pain lasting longer than 15 minutes and unrelieved by rest or drugs
   2. Shortness of breath
   3. Nausea and vomiting
   4. Tachycardia
   5. Diaphoresis and pallor
   6. Temperature rise after 48 hours
   7. Elevation of the cardiac enzymes
   8. Dysrhythmias
   9. Anxiety
D. Diagnostic tests/methods
   1. Patient history and physical examination
   2. ECG
   3. Cardiac enzyme studies (SGOT, LDH, CPK-MB)
   4. Chest X-ray examination
E. Treatment
   1. Analgesic drugs to relieve pain
   2. Oxygen to relieve respiratory distress
   3. Vasopressor drugs to prevent circulatory collapse (cardiogenic shock)
   4. Cardiac monitoring to detect dysrhythmias
   5. Hemodynamic monitoring: internal monitoring of the blood pressure and pulmonary artery pressure
   6. Bed rest with progressive activity to allow the damaged myocardium to heal
   7. Intravenous (IV) fluids to provide for IV drug administration
   8. Cardiopulmonary resuscitation in the event of cardiac standstill (arrest)
   9. Pacemaker insertion
   10. Anticoagulant therapy
   11. Thrombolytic therapy to dissolve blood clot and restore blood flow
   12. Nitrates
F. Nursing intervention
   1. Provide pain relief
   2. Provide ongoing assessment and documentation of symptoms and reactions to treatment
   3. Administer and monitor oxygen
   4. Record vital signs qh during the acute period

5. Record intake and output qh during the acute period
6. Provide bed rest during the acute period and progressive activity as prescribed
   a. Apply antiembolism stockings
   b. Allow patient out of bed to use bedside commode (less taxing to the cardiovascular system)
   c. Monitor pulse during periods of activity
7. Avoid activities that produce straining (Valsalva's maneuver) to avoid stimulation of the vagus nerve, which will induce bradycardia
   a. Administer stool softeners as prescribed
   b. Caution patient against straining when attempting a bowel movement
8. Provide diet as prescribed
   a. May start out on liquids and then progress
   b. Sodium and cholesterol may be restricted
   c. Caffeine may be restricted
9. Give prescribed antidysrhythmics and monitor for side effects
10. Give prescribed cardiotonics and diuretics and monitor for side effects
11. Monitor for complications
    a. Cardiogenic shock: circulatory collapse caused by decreased cardiac output; the vital organs are not being perfused
       (1) Monitor vital signs q 15 min
       (2) Record intake and output qh
       (3) Report changes in rate, rhythm, and conductivity
       (4) Observe and report signs and symptoms of restlessness, diaphoresis, pallor, low blood pressure, and tachycardia
       (5) Administer and monitor prescribed vasopressors and antidysrhythmics
       (6) Administer oxygen as prescribed
       (7) Provide cardiac and hemodynamic monitoring (hemodynamic monitoring refers to the internal monitoring of blood pressure and pulmonary artery pressure)
    b. Pulmonary edema: left ventricle failure (pumping mechanism) caused by strain on a diseased heart; cardiac output (the amount of blood pumped out by the heart to the body per minute) is reduced, resulting in lung congestion
       (1) Observe and report symptoms of anxiety, dyspnea, orthopnea, frothy, pink-tinged sputum, crackles in the lungs, decreased urine output, and dependent edema
       (2) Record vital signs q 15 min
       (3) Record intake and output qh
       (4) Place bed in high-Fowler's position
       (5) Administer cardiotonics and diuretics as prescribed and monitor for side effects
       (6) Administer and monitor oxygen therapy
       (7) Be prepared to administer analgesics to allay anxiety and reduce respiratory rate
       (8) Provide emotional support to patient and family

HEART FAILURE

A. Definition: failure of the pumping mechanism of the heart resulting in an insufficient blood supply to meet the body's needs

B. Causes
1. The underlying mechanism in heart failure (HF) involves the failure of the pumping mechanism of the heart to respond to the metabolic changes of the body
2. The result is a heart that cannot supply a sufficient amount of blood in relation to the body's needs and to the amount of blood returning to the heart (venous return); pressure builds up in the vascular beds on the affected side of the heart
C. HF is described in terms of left-sided or right-sided failure, depending on which ventricle is affected
D. Signs and symptoms are divided into left-sided failure and right-sided failure, although both sides may be affected
1. Left-sided failure leads to pulmonary congestion
   a. Dyspnea
   b. Orthopnea
   c. Nonproductive cough that worsens at night
   d. As severity of failure increases, frothy, blood-tinged sputum is noted (pulmonary edema)
   e. Anxiety and restlessness
   f. Fatigue
2. Right-sided failure may follow left-sided failure and results in systemic venous congestion
   a. Weight gain caused by fluid accumulation in the tissues
   b. Dependent edema in the form of ankle edema or sacral edema
   c. Ascites caused by the collection of fluid in the abdominal cavity; ascites may also hinder respiration
   d. Fatigue
   e. Gastrointestinal symptoms such as nausea, vomiting, and anorexia
   f. Decreased urine output
   g. Distended neck veins
E. Diagnostic test/methods
1. Patient history and physical examination including the findings of edema, abnormal heart sounds, and the presence of crackles with dyspnea
2. Chest X-ray examination
3. ECG
4. Arterial blood gas studies
5. Liver function studies
6. Renal function studies
F. Treatment
1. Drug therapy: digitalization, diuretics, and sedatives
2. Recording of weight qd
3. Monitoring intake and output
4. Oxygen therapy
5. Hemodynamic monitoring
6. Restricting fluids
7. Restricting dietary sodium
8. Bed rest with progressive activity
9. Elevate the head of the bed on blocks
10. Monitor vital signs
G. Nursing intervention
1. Provide ongoing assessment and documentation of signs, symptoms, and reactions to treatment
2. Monitor oxygen therapy
3. Record vital signs every 15 minutes to 2 hours during the acute phase
4. Record intake and output qh during the acute phase
5. Weigh patient qd
6. Administer and monitor prescribed cardiotonics, diuretics, and sedatives; observe for side effects
7. Determine the amount of activity that produces the least discomfort to the patient
8. Monitor for dependent edema
   a. Ankle edema when sitting upright
   b. Sacral edema when in supine position
9. Raise the head of the bed as prescribed
10. Observe for complications of bed rest
    a. Have patient turn, cough, and take deep breaths
    b. Apply antiembolism stockings
11. Provide emotional support to the patient and family
12. Provide a diet low in sodium if prescribed
13. Educate the patient and family concerning dietary management, drug therapy, and activity
14. Restrict fluids as ordered

VALVULAR CONDITIONS

A. Valvular dysfunction results in either stenosis or insufficiency of the heart valves
1. Valvular stenosis results from cardiac infections; the valve leaflets (cusps) become fibrotic and thicken and may even fuse together, thus hindering blood flow
2. Valvular insufficiency occurs in much the same way as valvular stenosis; after repeated infections the valve leaflets (cusps) become inflamed and scarred and no longer close completely; the incomplete closure allows blood to leak from the left ventricle into the left atrium during systole
B. Blood flow through the heart is altered, resulting in decreased cardiac output, systemic and pulmonary congestion, and dilation of the heart chambers
C. Causes
1. Rheumatic heart disease is the primary cause of valvular dysfunction
2. Other causes include syphilis, bacterial endocarditis, and congenital malformations
D. Signs and symptoms
1. Mitral stenosis
   a. Dyspnea on exertion
   b. Orthopnea
   c. Pink-tinged sputum
   d. Fatigue
   e. Palpitations
   f. Heart murmur
2. Mitral insufficiency
   a. Fatigue
   b. Dyspnea or exertion
   c. Heart murmur
   d. Orthopnea
   e. Pulmonary congestion
3. Aortic stenosis
   a. Fatigue
   b. Angina
   c. Syncope
   d. Heart murmur
   e. Heart failure
4. Aortic insufficiency
   a. Palpitations
   b. Dyspnea
   c. Fatigue

d. Orthopnea
e. Anginal pain occurring even at rest
E. Diagnostic tests/methods
  1. Patient history and physical examination; a murmur is a common finding of the examination
  2. ECG
  3. Chest X-ray examination: to determine heart size
  4. Cardiac catheterization: may reveal pressure changes
  5. Echocardiogram: provides information concerning structure and function of valves
  6. Laboratory studies
F. Treatment
  1. Mitral stenosis
    a. Antibiotics administered prophylactically to prevent recurrences of causative agents
    b. Drug therapy: diuretics, cardiotonics, and antidysrhythmics
    c. Restricted sodium diet
    d. Planned activity and avoidance of symptom-producing activity
    e. Surgical correction of the defect
      (1) Mitral commissurotomy: the fused valve leaflets are separated, and the mitral opening may be dilated
      (2) Valve replacement: diseased valve is replaced with a prosthetic valve
  2. Mitral insufficiency
    a. Planned exercise and avoidance of symptom-producing activity
    b. Sodium-restricted diet
    c. Drug therapy; diuretics, cardiotonics, antidysrhythmics, and vasodilators
    d. Surgical correction
      (1) Valvuloplasty: repair of the existing valve
      (2) Valve replacement
  3. Aortic stenosis
    a. Prevention of infective endocarditis
    b. Treatment of symptoms
    c. Drug therapy: diuretics, nitrates, and cardiotonics
    d. Sodium-restricted diet
    e. Valve replacement
G. Nursing intervention
  1. Assess and document signs and symptoms and reaction to treatments
  2. Administer prescribed medication and observe patient for side effects
  3. Provide a calm, quiet environment
  4. Allow patient and family to verbalize their anxieties and fears
  5. Monitor vital signs and report changes
  6. Weigh the patient qd
  7. Provide the prescribed diet
    a. Nutritionally well balanced
    b. Sodium restricted to prevent fluid retention
  8. Progressive activity as prescribed
    a. Consider the patient's limitations
    b. Provide rest periods
  9. Monitor intake and output if diuretics are used
  10. Educate patient and family concerning diet, drugs, activity, and need for compliance
  11. Vocational counseling may be needed if the patient has a demanding job

INFLAMMATORY DISORDERS OF THE HEART

A. Definition: diseases resulting from acute or chronic inflammation of the lining of the heart and valves caused by bacteria or viruses, trauma, or other factors
  1. Pericarditis: an inflammation of the pericardium
    a. The result is a loss of elasticity or fluid accumulation within the pericardial sac
    b. Heart failure and cardiac tamponade may result
  2. Myocarditis: an inflammation of the myocardium
    a. The result is impairment of contractility
    b. Myocardial ischemia and necrosis may result
  3. Endocarditis: an inflammation of the inner lining of the heart and valves associated with a streptococcal infection
  4. Rheumatic heart disease
    a. Usually associated with rheumatic fever
    b. Rheumatic fever is an inflammatory process that can affect all the layers of the heart
    c. Cardiac impairment results from swelling and scarring of valve leaflets, leading to valvular changes (mitral insufficiency, aortic insufficiency, and pericarditis)
B. Signs and symptoms
  1. Chest pain
  2. Dyspnea
  3. Chills and intermittent fever
  4. Weakness and fatigue
  5. Diaphoresis
  6. Anorexia
  7. Dysrhythmias
  8. Elevated cardiac enzymes
  9. Friction rubs (auscultatory sound created by the rubbing together of two serous surfaces)
  10. Presence of Aschoff bodies (collection of cells and leukocytes in the interstitial layers of the heart)
  11. New heart murmur or an abnormal heart sound
  12. Existing streptococcal infection
  13. Cardiac enlargement
  14. Joint involvement
C. Diagnostic tests/methods
  1. Patient history and physical examination
    a. History of recent infections
    b. History of heart disease
  2. ECG
  3. Chest X-ray examination
  4. Cardiac enzyme studies
  5. Blood cultures
  6. Echocardiogram: to assess valvular disease and vegetation (growth of scar tissue)
  7. Laboratory studies: CBC, electrolytes, ESR
  8. Radionuclide studies: to assess heart structure and heart damage
D. Treatment
  1. Identification and elimination of the infecting agent
  2. Drug therapy: antibiotics, cardiotonics, antiinflammatory agents, analgesics, and corticosteroids
  3. Blood cultures
  4. Oxygen
  5. Rest and planned activity
  6. Well-balanced diet
  7. Prevention of exposure to other infectious agents

E. Nursing intervention
1. Assess and document signs and symptoms and reactions to treatment
2. Maintain a calm, quiet environment
3. Administer prescribed drugs and monitor for side effects
4. Evaluate the patient's understanding of the disease process and the need for compliance
5. Alleviate pain
6. Allay patient's and family's fears and anxieties
7. Monitor vital signs and report changes
8. Observe for signs and symptoms of complications (tachycardia, dyspnea, and orthopnea)
9. Educate patient concerning the illness, diet, drugs, activity, avoidance of infections, dental care, vocational counseling, and compliance to the regimen

PERIPHERAL VASCULAR CONDITIONS AND DISORDERS

Peripheral vascular disease refers to vascular disorders exclusive of those affecting the heart. The underlying factor in peripheral vascular disease is the arteriosclerotic process. Blood flow is slowed because of vessels that are narrowed or obstructed. The lack of normal blood flow causes tissue changes (see section on arteriosclerosis). Vascular disease related to the lower extremities is discussed in this section.

Nursing Assessment

A. Nursing observation
1. Skin of the lower extremities
   a. Redness (hyperemia) of the leg when in a dependent position
   b. Cold or blue feet
   c. Varicose veins
   d. Sparse hair distribution
   e. Lesions or stasis ulcers
   f. Edema
   g. Dermatitis or brown pigmentation of the skin
2. Delayed capillary filling
3. Diminished or absent pulses
   a. Rigidity (hardness) of the vessels
   b. Palpable vibration of the vessels (thrill)
4. Assess major arteries for bruits (an auscultatory sound taking the form of a whooshing, buzzing, or humming sound caused by turbulent blood flow)
5. Differences in leg circumference
6. Thickening of nail beds
B. Patient description (subjective data)
1. Leg cramps
2. Aching calves
3. Leg numbness
4. Leg pain occurring during exercise (claudication)
5. Loss of sensation in the leg(s)
6. Past or present history
   a. Alcohol excess
   b. Diabetes mellitus
   c. Hypertension
   d. Thrombophlebitis

Diagnostic Tests/Methods

A. Chest X-ray examination for abnormalities
B. Oscillometry: a noninvasive test that measures the amplitude of pulsations over an artery

C. Doppler ultrasonography: a device that emits sound waves that can be used to measure the amount of blood flow through a vessel
D. Arteriography: used to determine the location and extent of the disease process
E. Venography: radiographic study used to determine the location and size of a blood clot, vessel distention, and development of collateral circulation
F. Trendelenburg test
1. Used to determine valvular competency
2. The leg is elevated to 90 degrees, and a tourniquet is placed around the thigh
3. The patient stands, and the vein-filling pattern is observed
4. Normally the veins fill slowly from below in 20 to 30 seconds; the rate of filling should not greatly accelerate when the tourniquet is removed
G. Lung scan
1. Used to assess the presence of pulmonary embolism and lung damage
2. An intravenous, radiographic isotope is injected into the patient
3. Pulmonary circulation is assessed with a scanning device
4. The patient also inhales a radioactive gas and is scanned to determine lung distribution of this gas
H. Arterial blood gas analysis: used to assess the adequacy of ventilation
I. X-ray examination of the abdomen: may show evidence of an aneurysm
J. Blood tests
1. CBC: for routine evaluation
2. ESR: used to determine the presence of an inflammatory process
3. Coagulation studies (platelet count, bleeding time, prothrombin time [PT], and partial thromboplastin time [PTT]): used to determine the existence of blood disorders

Frequent Patient Problems and Nursing Care

A. Pain related to intermittent claudication
1. Evaluate and record onset, duration, and intensity
2. Provide rest during the episode
3. Determine the amount of exercise the patient can tolerate before claudication occurs
4. Assess for and report claudication occurring without activity
5. Educate the patient to avoid exposure to cold and maintain warmth
B. Fluid volume excess as evidenced by edema of the lower extremities/decreased cardiac output
1. Note and record location and degree
2. Instruct patient to avoid activity that places the legs in a dependent position for prolonged periods
3. Instruct patient to avoid wearing constricting clothing around the legs
4. Monitor for skin breakdown
5. Elevate legs
C. Impaired skin integrity related to stasis ulcers
1. Note location and character of ulceration
2. Maintain bed rest with leg elevation
3. Perform prescribed wound care
4. Instruct patient to avoid trauma to the legs

5. Instruct patient in proper skin care measures
6. Reinforce patient teaching in the area of drugs, diet, activity, and skin care

Major Medical Diagnoses
ARTERIOSCLEROSIS OBLITERANS
A. Definition: a chronic arteriooclusive disease
   1. Progresses slowly and insidiously
   2. The medial and intimal layers of arteries become inflamed and thrombosed
   3. There is loss of vessel elasticity, and plaques obstruct blood flow
   4. Vessels primarily affected are the femoral and carotid arteries
B. Causes
   1. Associated with atherosclerotic process
   2. Predisposing factors include hypertension, smoking, hyperlipidemia, obesity, and a positive family history
C. Signs and symptoms
   1. Intermittent claudication
   2. Pain in the legs at rest
   3. Impotence
   4. Paresthesia
   5. Pallor or blanching on elevation of leg
   6. Hyperemia (redness) or dusky appearance of the leg(s) when dependent
   7. Loss of hair on extremities
   8. Absent or diminished pulses
D. Diagnostic tests/methods
   1. Patient history and physical examination
   2. Oscillometry
   3. Doppler ultrasonography
   4. Arteriography
   5. Laboratory studies
E. Treatments
   1. Protection of extremity from injury
   2. Prevention and control of infection
   3. Drug therapy: vasodilators, analgesics, and antibiotics
   4. Weight-reduction diet if patient is obese
   5. Bed rest
   6. Avoidance of smoking
   7. Surgical management: endarterectomy (removing the obstructing plaque) or a bypass graft
F. Nursing intervention
   1. Assist the patient in obtaining body warmth and warmth to the extremity
      a. Warm room
      b. Warm bath
      c. Warm clothes such as socks
   2. Avoid applying direct heat to the affected part
   3. Protect the affected part from trauma and pressure
      a. Use bed cradle
      b. Assess skin lesions and monitor for signs of infection
      c. Caution patient against wearing anything that constricts
   4. Give prescribed drugs and monitor for side effects
   5. Assess the affected part qd
      a. Assess skin color, temperature, and circulation
      b. Monitor for pain
   6. Provide emotional support
   7. Educate the patient and family regarding
      a. Hygiene and avoidance of infection
      b. Rest and planned exercise
      c. Protection from injury
      d. Diet
      e. Drugs
      f. Improvement of circulation

BUERGER'S DISEASE (THROMBOANGIITIS OBLITERANS)
A. Definition: an inflammatory process primarily affecting arteries that causes occlusion, thrombosis, and ultimately ischemia
   1. Medium-sized distal arteries of the legs are primarily affected
   2. Veins can also be affected
B. Causes
   1. Exact cause is unknown
   2. Associated with smoking
   3. Men in the 25- to 40-year age group who smoke are at risk
   4. Familial tendency
C. Signs and symptoms
   1. Coldness of the extremities
   2. Diminished or absent pulses
   3. Numbness and tingling
   4. Cramping pain (intermittent claudication)
   5. Pain at rest, not associated with activity
   6. Skin ulceration
   7. Aggravation of symptoms by exposure to cold environment
   8. Change in appearance of extremities
   9. Muscle atrophy
   10. Slow-healing cuts
   11. Gangrene
   12. Sensitivity to cold
D. Diagnostic tests/methods
   1. Patient history and physical examination
   2. Oscillometry
   3. Doppler ultrasonography
   4. Arteriography
   5. Laboratory studies
   6. ECG
   7. Chest X-ray examination
E. Treatment
   1. Restricting smoking
   2. Drug therapy: vasodilating drugs, analgesics, and anticoagulants
   3. Moderate exercise
   4. Avoidance and treatment of infection
   5. Protection from trauma
   6. Sympathectomy (disruption of nerve impulses to a particular area)
   7. Nerve blocks (use of drug injections to block nerve impulses)
   8. Amputation, as a last resort
F. Nursing intervention
   1. Support the patient in his effort to stop smoking
   2. Give prescribed vasodilators, analgesics, and anticoagulants; monitor for side effects
   3. Document location and character of pain
   4. Assist the patient in maintaining warmth
   5. Educate the patient and family concerning drug therapy, activity, and avoidance of smoking, exposure to cold, constricting clothing, and trauma

RAYNAUD'S DISEASE

A. Definition: a peripheral vascular disease affecting digital arteries
   1. Disease occurs primarily in women
   2. Exposure to environmental cold, emotional stress, or tobacco use produces spasms of the arteries
   3. Hands and arms are usually affected
B. Cause
   1. Exact cause is unknown
   2. Associated with collagen diseases in women
C. Contributing factors
   1. Pressure to the fingertips such as that encountered by typists and pianists
   2. Use of hand-held vibrating equipment on a regular basis
D. Signs and symptoms
   1. Numbness and tingling
   2. Blanching of digits and cyanosis
   3. Hyperemia
   4. Coldness
   5. Dryness and atrophy of the nails
   6. Pain
   7. Punctate (small hole) lesions of the fingertips
   8. Eventual gangrene of the fingertips
E. Diagnostic tests/methods
   1. Patient history and physical examination
   2. Doppler ultrasonography
   3. Arteriography
   4. ECG
   5. Chest X-ray examination
F. Treatment
   1. Drug therapy with vasodilators
   2. Sympathectomy: in advanced cases
   3. Elimination of smoking
   4. Avoidance of stressful situations
   5. Avoidance of exposure to cold
G. Nursing intervention
   1. Document location and characteristics of pain
   2. Observe affected areas qd
   3. Administer prescribed vasodilators and analgesics; monitor for side effects
   4. Instruct patient to avoid activities that precipitate spasms
   5. Instruct patient to avoid exposing the hands to the cold without proper protection
   6. Support patient's effort to give up smoking
   7. Offer emotional support and allay anxiety
   8. Educate patient and family concerning drug therapy, avoidance of cold, protection from trauma/infection, and prevention of spasms

ANEURYSMS

A. Definition: the enlargement or ballooning of an artery, usually caused by trauma, congenital weakness, arteriosclerosis, or infection; aorta is most frequently affected artery
B. Causes
   1. Causes are varied, but the prime culprit is arteriosclerosis; plaque formation causes degenerative changes leading to loss of vessel elasticity, weakness, and dilation
   2. Syphilis
   3. Infections
   4. Congenital disorder
   5. Trauma

   6. Risk factors: obesity, smoking, hypertension, stress, high blood cholesterol levels
C. Signs and symptoms
   1. Abdominal
      a. Increased blood pressure
      b. Visible or palpable pulsating mass
      c. Pain or tenderness in the abdominal area
   2. Thoracic
      a. Dyspnea
      b. Dysphagia
      c. Hoarseness or cough
      d. Severe chest pain
   3. Ruptured aneurysm
      a. Anxiety
      b. Restlessness
      c. Pain
      d. Diminished pulses
      e. Hypotension and shock
D. Diagnostic tests/methods
   1. Patient history and physical examination
   2. Chest X-ray examination
   3. Abdominal X-ray examination
   4. Ultrasonography
   5. Angiography/arteriography
   6. Routine ECG
   7. Laboratory studies
E. Treatment
   1. Conservative measures
      a. Drug therapy: antihypertensives, pain relievers, and negative inotropic agents
      b. Correct hydration and electrolyte imbalances
      c. Decreased activity
   2. Surgical repair
      a. Resection and replacement with a prosthesis of Teflon or Dacron
      b. Resection and replacement with a graft
F. Nursing intervention
   1. Provide immediate postoperative care
      a. Assess vital signs and peripheral pulses every 15 minutes; then decrease the frequency as ordered
      b. Record intake and output qh
      c. Compare extremities for warmth and color
      d. Administer IV fluids at prescribed rate
      e. Relieve pain with prescribed analgesic
      f. Monitor oxygen therapy
      g. Give prescribed prophylactic antibiotics as ordered
      h. Assess level of consciousness q1h to q2h
      i. Auscultate lung sounds and bowel sounds at least q4h
      j. Monitor for dysrhythmias
      k. Have patient turn, cough, and deep breathe at least q2h
   2. Other postoperative considerations
      a. Provide antiembolism stockings
      b. Provide emotional support and allay anxiety
      c. Encourage early ambulation as prescribed
      d. Instruct patient to observe for changes in the extremities such as color and warmth
      e. Instruct patient on assessments of peripheral pulses

PHLEBITIS AND THROMBOPHLEBITIS

A. Definition: inflammatory disorders of the veins
   1. Phlebitis: inflammation of a vein

2. Thrombophlebitis: inflammation of a vein with clot formation
B. Causes
1. The inflammation and clot formation are associated with venous stasis, vessel damage, and enhanced blood coagulability
2. Situations that produce venous stasis include immobility, prolonged periods of standing, wearing confining clothing, and increased abdominal pressure
C. Signs and symptoms
1. Redness and pain along vein path
2. Elevation of temperature
3. Swelling
4. Positive Homans' sign (pain on dorsiflexion of the foot)
5. Area is sensitive to the touch
D. Diagnostic tests/methods
1. Patient history and physical examination
2. Doppler ultrasonography
3. Venography
4. Laboratory studies: CBC, ESR, and coagulation studies
5. Lung scan to rule out pulmonary embolism
E. Treatment
1. Bed rest
2. Anticoagulant therapy
3. Thrombolytic therapy
4. Vasodilators
5. Warm, moist packs to the affected leg (some physicians prefer ice packs to the area)
6. Antiembolism stockings
7. Elevation of affected extremity
8. Surgical intervention is required in only a small percentage of patients
F. Nursing intervention
1. Assess and document signs and symptoms
2. Administer analgesics as ordered and monitor for side effects
3. Elevate leg as ordered; avoid the use of a knee gatch or pillow under the affected knee; avoid crossing legs
4. Apply warm, moist heat as ordered
5. Assess thigh and calf measurements qd
6. Monitor vital signs q4h
7. Maintain bed rest as ordered
8. Apply antiembolism stockings on unaffected leg
9. Avoid massaging calf of affected leg
10. Avoid constrictive clothing
11. Monitor anticoagulant therapy
12. Monitor for bleeding tendencies
    a. Bleeding gums
    b. Epistaxis
    c. Bruising easily
    d. Melena
    e. Petechiae
13. Monitor hemoglobin and hematocrit levels
14. Educate patient and family concerning drug therapy, avoiding activities that aggravate the existing state, and monitoring for signs and symptoms of complications
15. Monitor patient for complications such as an embolism

EMBOLISM
A. Definition: a blood clot circulating in the blood
B. Causes
1. The clot may be a fragment of an arteriosclerotic plaque, or it may have originated in the heart
2. If large, an embolism may lodge in a vessel bifurcation and obstruct the flow of blood to vital organs or tissues
3. Most emboli arise from deep vein thrombi; the embolus travels in the bloodstream until it lodges in a narrowed area, usually the lungs
C. Signs and symptoms: depend on the area involved
1. Pain at the site
2. Shock
3. Areas supplied by the involved vessel evidence pallor, coldness, numbness, tingling, and cyanosis
4. Sudden onset of dyspnea
5. Cough and hemoptysis
6. Chest pain
7. Tachycardia
8. Tachypnea
D. Diagnostic tests/methods
1. Patient history and physical examination
2. Lung scan
3. Chest X-ray examination
4. Arterial blood gases
E. Treatment
1. Oxygen therapy
2. IV fluids
3. IV anticoagulants
4. Analgesics
5. Thrombolytic agents
F. Nursing intervention
1. Assess and document signs and symptoms and reactions to treatments
2. Monitor vital signs
3. Monitor arterial blood gas reports
4. Administer prescribed analgesic and monitor for side effects
5. Administer anticoagulants as prescribed and monitor for bleeding tendencies
6. Monitor oxygen therapy
7. Give ROM exercises
8. Provide antiembolism stockings
9. Educate patient and family concerning drug therapy, monitoring for bleeding tendencies, and restriction of activities

VARICOSE VEINS
A. Definition: dilated, tortuous leg veins resulting from blood backflow caused by incomplete valve closure; this leads to congestion and further enlargement
B. Causes
1. Basic cause of varicosities is unknown
2. Predisposing factors: heredity, pregnancy, obesity, and aging
C. Signs and symptoms
1. Leg fatigue and aching
2. Leg cramping and pain
3. Heaviness in the legs
4. Dilated veins
5. Ankle edema

D. Diagnostic tests/methods
  1. Patient history and physical examination
  2. Venography
  3. Trendelenburg test
E. Treatment
  1. Rest with elevation of legs
  2. Exercise
  3. Support stockings
  4. Avoid prolonged standing, sitting, and crossing the legs
  5. Weight management
  6. Surgical vein stripping/ligation; vein sclerosing
  7. Laser
F. Nursing intervention
  1. After surgery check legs for color, movement, temperature, and sensation
  2. Provide leg exercises as prescribed
  3. Reinforce the importance of weight management
  4. Instruct the patient to avoid prolonged sitting and standing
  5. Avoid constrictive clothing

HEMATOLOGIC CONDITIONS AND DISORDERS

Disorders of hemopoiesis refer to problems of the blood-forming tissues. These include the blood cells, bone marrow, spleen, and lymph system. This discussion includes descriptions of the anemias, leukemia, and acquired immunodeficiency syndrome.

Nursing Assessment

A. Nursing observations
  1. Pulse
    a. Character, rate, rhythm
    b. Note tachycardia or periods of palpitations
  2. Respirations
    a. Character, rate, rhythm
    b. Tachypnea
    c. Dyspnea on exertion
    d. Shortness of breath (SOB)
  3. Blood pressure: Hypotension, perhaps orthostatic
  4. Temperature: Unexplained occurrences of elevation, sometimes accompanied by chills and sweating
  5. Skin
    a. Color: pallor, cyanosis
    b. Pruritus
    c. Bruising
    d. Slow to heal cuts
    e. Bleeding from nose or mouth
  6. Oral mucosal changes
    a. Mouth ulcerations
    b. Bleeding gums
    c. Smooth tongue
  7. Motor
    a. Uncoordination
    b. Loss of usual stamina
    c. Changes in ability to perform activities
    d. Intolerance to exertion (climbing stairs, usual housework, walking)
B. Patient description (subjective)
  1. Changes in ability to perform activities of daily living
  2. Self-reported increase in weakness and fatigue
  3. Dyspnea on exertion
  4. Changes in appetite
    a. Weight loss
    b. Anorexia
    c. Nausea and vomiting
  5. Skin
    a. Easily bruises
    b. Bleeding from gums, nose
  6. Mood changes: irritable
  7. Progressive symptoms
    a. Onset of headaches
    b. Onset of fatigue
    c. Numbness, tingling, burning feet
    d. Intermittent swollen, tender lymph nodes

Diagnostic Tests/Methods

A. Red blood cell (RBC) count
  1. The blood study is used in routine screenings and provides information about the hematologic system
  2. Circulating RBC counts elevate in conditions such as anemia and hypoxia
B. Erythrocyte indexes (mean cell volume, mean cell hemoglobin concentration, and mean cell hemoglobin)
  1. Aid in describing the anemias
  2. Provide a relationship between the number, size, and hemoglobin content of the RBCs
C. Hemoglobin and hematocrit levels
  1. Provide an index to the severity of the anemia
  2. Hematocrit refers to the number of packed RBCs found in 100 ml of blood
  3. Hemoglobin is the oxygen-carrying component of the RBC and is more reliable in determining the severity of the anemia
D. Reticulocyte count-number of newly formed RBCs
  1. Provides information concerning the cause of the anemia
  2. Indicates whether the anemia is a result of diminished production or excessive loss or destruction of RBCs
E. Erythrocyte sedimentation rate (ESR)
  1. Not specific to anemias
  2. Elevated ESR suggests the presence of an underlying disease process; therefore further studies may be indicated
F. Serum iron
  1. Helpful in classifying the anemia
  2. Useful in differentiating an acute from a chronic disorder
G. Total iron-binding capacity (TIBC): helpful in classifying the anemia and differentiating between an acute and a chronic disorder
H. Serum bilirubin
  1. Useful in evaluating the degree of RBC hemolysis
  2. Bilirubin is formed from the hemoglobin of destroyed RBCs
  3. Elevations may indicate the increased destruction of RBCs caused by a particular disease process
I. Schilling test
  1. Used in classifying anemias, particularly a vitamin B_{12} disorder
  2. Helps differentiate between an intrinsic factor deficiency and an intestinal absorption disorder

3. Patient preparation
   a. The patient may be instructed to take nothing by mouth (NPO) before the test
   b. Oral radioactive vitamin B_{12} is administered
   c. Nonradioactive parenteral dose is given 2 hours later
   d. Urine collection follows
   e. A third of the vitamin appears in the urine; little or no radioactivity in the urine suggests a gastrointestinal malabsorption problem
   f. Procedure may be repeated with the addition of intrinsic factor to the oral vitamin B_{12}
   g. Nonabsorption of B_{12} without intrinsic factor but absorption with the intrinsic factor is suggestive of pernicious anemia
4. Nursing intervention
   a. Explain the basic procedure to the patient
   b. Maintain NPO
   c. Collect the urine at the specified time
J. Vitamin B_{12} level
   1. Used to help identify pernicious anemia
   2. Provides an index for determining the adequacy of B_{12} levels and the need for further evaluation
   3. Vitamin B_{12} is important for normal hematopoiesis
K. Serum folate level
   1. Folic acid is another important factor in hematopoiesis
   2. Useful in folic acid deficiency anemia
L. Gastric analysis
   1. Nasogastric tube is inserted and then histamine is injected to stimulate gastric secretions
   2. Gastric contents are aspirated and analyzed
   3. Achlorhydria (absence of hydrochloric acid) is a feature of pernicious anemia because of a lack of intrinsic factor in the stomach
M. Sickle cell preparation
   1. The reaction of the blood specimen in hypoxia is observed
   2. Sickling of cells in hypoxia suggests sickle cell trait or sickle cell anemia
N. Hemoglobin electrophoresis
   1. An electric field separates the specimen into the various types of hemoglobin present
   2. Hemoglobins S and A suggest sickle cell anemia or trait
   3. Hemoglobin F suggests thalassemia
O. Bone marrow biopsy
   1. Bone marrow aspiration provides information about blood cell production
   2. Test may be used in patients suspected of having leukemia, aplastic anemia, and other hematologic disorders
   3. Sample of marrow may be obtained from the sternum, iliac crest, vertebrae, or vertebral body
   4. Procedure
      a. The skin over the designated area is prepared and anesthetized
      b. The needle is inserted into the center of the bone, and a small amount of marrow is aspirated
   5. Nursing intervention
      a. Allay patient's anxiety before examination
      b. Assist with the marrow as instructed
      c. Place patient in a comfortable position after the procedure
      d. Monitor pain status (soreness remains for several days)
      e. Monitor puncture site for bleeding

P. WBC count and differential
   1. Determines the total number of leukocytes
   2. The differential helps analyze each type of WBC and determine if the amount present is in proper proportion
   3. Aids in the diagnosing of infection and blood disorders such as leukemia
Q. Platelet count
   1. Evaluates adequacy of platelet levels
   2. If platelet levels drop below a certain level, spontaneous hemorrhage is possible
R. Serum for HIV: determines the presence of the HIV antibodies
S. Lymphangiography: radiologic examination used to detect lymph node involvement

Frequent Patient Problems and Nursing Care

A. Activity intolerance related to weakness and fatigue
   1. Provide planned activity and rest periods
   2. Monitor for signs of fatigue
   3. Reinforce patient teaching of planned activity and exercise
   4. Assist patient with activities of daily living
   5. Assess vital signs as ordered
B. Potential alteration in tissue perfusion related to hypotension
   1. Observe for evidence of postural hypotension
   2. Assist patient to dangle legs over the side of the bed before standing
   3. Instruct patient to get up slowly
   4. Assess patient's pulse when standing
C. Ineffective breathing pattern related to dyspnea on exertion
   1. Note the degree or kind of activity that causes dyspnea
   2. Note character and rate of respirations during the episodes
   3. Instruct the patient to stop the activity and relax when dyspnea is experienced
   4. Assist the patient in planning activities so that dyspnea will not occur
   5. Reinforce patient teaching regarding planned exercise and rest periods
D. Impaired swallowing caused by ulcerations of the mouth and tongue
   1. Assess the ulcerated areas qd
   2. Provide mouth care with a soft-bristle brush or cotton swab
   3. Offer soothing mouthwashes every 2 to 4 hours
   4. Instruct the patient to avoid ingesting food or drink that may aggravate the ulcers
E. Fluid volume deficit related to hemorrhage
   1. Assess for signs of bleeding
      a. Tarry stools
      b. Hematuria
      c. Bleeding gums
      d. Bleeding tendency
      e. Petechiae
      f. Epistaxis
   2. Protect from trauma and injury
   3. Avoid parenteral injections
   4. Have patient use soft-bristle brush for mouth care
   5. Monitor vital signs at least q4h
   6. Monitor hemoglobin and hematocrit values
   7. Encourage intake of fluids and the prescribed diet

F. High risk for infection related to interference with the immune system
　1. Prevent exposure to others with infection
　2. Monitor for signs and symptoms of infection
　3. Give prescribed drugs and monitor for side effects
　4. Place in protective isolation if ordered

Major Medical Diagnoses
ANEMIA CAUSED BY DECREASED RBC PRODUCTION
A. Normally there is a balance between RBC production and RBC destruction; however, alterations do occur that significantly affect RBC production
　1. Iron deficiency anemia
　　a. Results from insufficient dietary intake of iron, which is needed for the formation of hemoglobin and RBCs
　　b. Other causes: malabsorption, blood loss, and hemolysis
　2. Pernicious anemia
　　a. Caused by a lack of intrinsic factor in the GI tract
　　b. Intrinsic factor is needed for the absorption of vitamin B_{12}
　　c. Anemia usually results from a loss of the mucosal surface of the GI tract, which secretes intrinsic factor
　　d. Patients undergoing total gastrectomies and small bowel resections are at risk
　3. Folic acid deficiency anemia
　　a. Folic acid is required in the synthesis of DNA, which in turn is necessary for the production of RBCs
　　b. Common causes: poor diet (lacking in green, leafy vegetables, citrus fruits, liver, grains, and dried beans), malabsorption, and drugs that interfere with the absorption of folic acid
　4. Thalassemia
　　a. Unlike the other three anemias, thalassemia is a genetic disorder resulting in abnormal hemoglobin synthesis
　　b. The main problem is an inadequate production of normal hemoglobin; hemolysis is a secondary problem
　　c. People of Mediterranean ancestry are at risk
　　d. Mild forms of this anemia (thalassemia minor) may be asymptomatic
　　e. Patients with a more severe hemolytic form (thalassemia major) may experience hepatomegaly, splenomegaly, jaundice, and bone marrow hypertrophy
B. Signs and symptoms
　1. Skin changes
　　a. Pallor
　　b. Jaundice
　　c. Pruritus
　　d. Dermatitis
　2. Eye and visual disturbances
　　a. Blurred vision
　　b. Scleral icterus
　3. Mouth
　　a. Glossitis
　　b. Smooth tongue
　　c. Ulcerations of the mucosa
　4. Cardiovascular
　　a. Tachycardia
　　b. Murmurs
　　c. Angina
　　d. Congestive heart failure (CHF)
　　e. Hypotension
　5. Respiratory
　　a. Tachypnea
　　b. Dyspnea on exertion
　　c. Orthopnea
　6. Neurological
　　a. Dizziness
　　b. Headaches
　　c. Irritability
　　d. Depression
　　e. Incoordination
　　f. Impaired thought processes
　7. Gastrointestinal (GI)
　　a. Nausea and vomiting
　　b. Anorexia
　　c. Hepatomegaly
　　d. Splenomegaly
　8. General
　　a. Weight loss
　　b. Weakness and fatigue
　　c. Bone pain
　　d. Numbness, tingling, and burning of the feet
C. Diagnostic tests/methods
　1. Patient history and physical examination
　2. Routine chest X-ray examination
　3. Routine ECG
　4. Schilling test
　5. Gastric analysis
　6. CBC/red blood cell indexes
　7. Bone marrow aspiration or biopsy
　8. Serum iron level
D. Treatment
　1. Iron therapy
　2. Increase dietary iron intake
　3. Vitamin B_{12} replacement (pernicious anemia)
　4. Folic acid replacement
　5. Use of hematinics
　6. Blood transfusions (thalassemia)
E. Nursing intervention
　1. Assess and document signs and symptoms and reactions to treatments
　2. Provide planned activity alternated with rest periods
　3. Assist patient with activities of daily living to avoid fatigue
　4. Monitor supplemental oxygen therapy in use
　5. Administer prescribed drugs and monitor for side effects
　6. Monitor blood transfusions
　7. Provide oral hygiene, particularly if mouth ulcers are present
　8. Provide the prescribed diet
　9. Instruct patient to get up from bed or chair slowly to avoid dizziness
　10. Instruct patient on avoiding and preventing exposure to infection
　11. Support patient and allay anxiety
　12. Educate patient and family concerning drugs, diet therapy, and planned activity

ANEMIA CAUSED BY RBC DESTRUCTION

A. Definition: a process in which RBCs are destroyed faster than they are produced
B. Known causes of RBC destruction
1. Snake venom
2. Infections
3. Drugs or chemicals
4. Heavy metals or organic compounds
5. Antigen antibody reaction
6. Splenic dysfunction
7. Congenital causes
   a. Thalassemia: a group of hereditary hemolytic anemias characterized by a defect or defects in one or more of the hemoglobin polypeptide chains
   b. Sickle cell anemia: see Chapter 8
   c. Spherocytosis: A hemolytic anemia characterized by spherocytes (small, globular erythrocytes without the characteristic central pallor) in the blood; the abnormal cells are destroyed by the spleen
   d. Glucose-6-phosphate dehydrogenase (G6PD) deficiency: a hemolytic disorder brought on by stressors such as infection, certain drugs, acidosis, and toxic substances; individuals with this genetic disorder are relatively symptom free until they experience the stressor that initiates the hemolytic process
C. Signs and symptoms
1. Anemia
2. Jaundice
3. Splenomegaly
4. Hepatomegaly
5. Weakness and fatigue
6. Skin pallor
7. Anorexia
8. Weight loss
9. Dyspnea
10. Tachycardia
11. Tachypnea
12. Hypotension
13. Cholelithiasis (gallstones): caused by excessive bilirubin
D. Diagnostic tests/methods
1. Patient history and physical examination
2. Laboratory studies
3. Routine chest X-ray examination
4. Routine ECG
5. Bone marrow biopsy
6. Renal studies to monitor kidney status
E. Treatment
1. Identify the causative agent
2. Blood or blood product replacement
3. Supportive care
4. Genetic counseling
5. Splenectomy to halt the destruction of abnormal RBCs by the spleen
6. Maintain renal function
7. Maintain fluid and electrolyte balance
F. Nursing intervention
1. Assess and document signs and symptoms and reactions to treatment
2. Monitor vital signs as ordered and report abnormalities
3. Allay fears and anxieties
4. Provide planned exercise and rest periods
5. Caution patient to get up slowly from the bed or chair to avoid postural hypotension
6. Assist patient with activities of daily living
7. Monitor intake and output
8. Monitor laboratory studies
9. Encourage intake of fluids
10. Provide prescribed diet
11. Administer prescribed drugs and monitor for side effects
12. Educate patient and family concerning drugs, diet, activity, and compliance to the prescribed regimen

APLASTIC ANEMIA (HYPOPLASTIC)

A. Definition: a failure of the bone marrow to produce adequate amounts of erythrocytes, leukocytes, and platelets
B. Exact cause is unclear (idiopathic)
1. May be congenital
2. Related to radiation exposure
3. Results from a disorder that suppresses bone marrow (cancer)
4. Exposure to toxic substances may be a contributing factor
C. Signs and symptoms
1. General symptoms of anemia; refer to the preceding outlines in this section
2. Susceptibility to infection
3. Fever
4. Bleeding tendencies
D. Diagnostic tests/methods
1. Patient history and physical examination
2. Laboratory studies, particularly WBC count and platelet count; a reduced WBC count predisposes patient to infection; a low platelet count predisposes patient to a bleeding disorder
3. Bone marrow biopsy examination to evaluate blood cell production
4. Routine chest X-ray examination
5. Routine ECG
E. Treatment
1. Identify the causative agent
2. Supportive care
3. Administration of blood or blood products
4. Hydration with IV fluids
5. Protect from injury and infections
6. Prevent hemorrhage
7. Splenectomy
8. Bone marrow transplant
F. Nursing intervention
1. Assess and document signs and symptoms and reactions to treatment
2. Monitor vital signs at least q4h
3. Monitor for and report signs of bleeding
4. Give prescribed medication and monitor for side effects
5. Avoid fatiguing the patient; provide planned exercise and rest periods
6. Prevent injury and exposure to infection
7. Neutropenic precautions may be necessary
8. Monitor supplemental oxygen if ordered
9. Provide and encourage the prescribed diet
10. Allay fears and anxiety
11. Provide oral hygiene, avoiding aggravation of bleeding gums

12. Provide skin care using protective devices and frequent repositioning
13. Educate patient and family concerning drug therapy, diet, planned activity, avoidance of injury and infection, monitoring for bleeding tendencies, and compliance with the regimen

LEUKEMIA

A. Definition: a disorder of the hematopoietic system characterized by an overproduction of immature WBCs
   1. As the disease progresses, fewer normal WBCs are produced
   2. The abnormal cells continue to multiply and eventually infiltrate and damage the bone marrow, spleen, lymph nodes, and other organs
B. Classification of leukemias
   1. Two major categories: acute and chronic
     a. Acute leukemia has a rapid onset; cells in this phase are young, undifferentiated, and immature
     b. Chronic leukemia has a gradual onset; cells are mature and differentiated
   2. Further classification: identifying the type of WBC involved
     a. Acute granulocytic leukemia: the myeloblasts proliferate; myeloblasts are the precursors of granulocytes
     b. Acute lymphoblastic leukemia: immature lymphocytes proliferate in the bone marrow
     c. Chronic granulocytic leukemia: excessive neoplastic granulocytes are found in the bone marrow
     d. Chronic lymphocytic leukemia: characterized by inactive, mature-appearing lymphocytes
C. Leukemia is considered a neoplastic process; cause is unknown
D. Predisposing factors
   1. Familial tendency
   2. Viral origin
   3. Exposure to chemicals
   4. Exposure to radiation
E. Once leukemia is diagnosed, the aim of therapy is to prolong survival by attaining a state of remission
   1. Management of acute leukemia aggressive
   2. Management of chronic leukemia aims to control the disorder and maintain remission
   3. All forms of leukemia are fatal if untreated
F. Signs and symptoms
   1. General symptoms of anemia
   2. Decreased resistance to infection
   3. Fever
   4. Bleeding tendencies
   5. Enlarged lymph nodes
   6. Splenomegaly
   7. Hepatomegaly
   8. Elevated WBC count
   9. Low platelet count and low hemoglobin and hematocrit levels
   10. Poor appetite
   11. Mouth ulcers
   12. Diarrhea
G. Diagnostic tests/methods
   1. Patient history and physical examination
   2. Laboratory studies to evaluate peripheral blood
   3. Bone marrow biopsy
   4. Routine chest X-ray examination
   5. Routine ECG
   6. Lymph node biopsy examination
H. Treatment
   1. Drug therapy: chemotherapeutic agents, analgesics, sedatives, and antibiotics
   2. Radiation therapy (prophylactic measure)
   3. Bone marrow transplants are still under investigation
   4. Hydration with IV fluids
   5. Replacement of blood and blood products
   6. Monitoring renal status
   7. Protection against infection (neutropenic precautions if needed)
   8. Prevention of hemorrhage
I. Nursing intervention
   1. Assess and document signs and symptoms and reactions to treatment
   2. Prevent patient from being exposed to infection
     a. Screen visitors
     b. Monitor WBC counts
     c. Good hand washing
   3. Avoid fatigue
     a. Provide planned exercises and rest periods
     b. Assist patient with activities of daily living
   4. Monitor for bleeding tendencies
   5. Administer blood or blood components as ordered and monitor for side effects
   6. Monitor intake and output
   7. Encourage intake of fluids
     a. Keep fluids at the bedside
     b. Provide patient with favorite fluids
   8. Administer prescribed medication as ordered and monitor for side effects
     a. Analgesics and sedatives
     b. Antiemetics
   9. Monitor IV fluids
     a. Monitor the IV site for infiltration
     b. Monitor rate
   10. Allay anxieties and fears
   11. Monitor vital signs at least q4h and report abnormalities (an elevated temperature may be the only sign of infection in an immunocompromised patient)
   12. Monitor supplemental oxygen if ordered
   13. Provide and encourage the prescribed diet
   14. Provide oral hygiene, which avoids aggravation of bleeding and drying of the mouth; carefully monitor oral status
   15. Provide skin care to include the use of protective devices and frequent repositioning
   16. Educate patient and family concerning drug therapy, diet, activity, monitoring for bleeding tendencies, avoidance of injury and infection, and compliance with the regimen

ACQUIRED IMMUNODEFICIENCY SYNDROME (AIDS)

A. Definition: a viral disorder that disrupts the balance of T-lymphocytes and ultimately destroys them, rendering the body incapable of defending itself against infection; course is progressive and fatal
B. Cause: infection with HIV (human immunodeficiency virus)
   1. The virus is spread by sexual contact; sharing of infected needles; and infected blood and blood products

2. Infected mothers can pass the virus to the unborn baby during the gestational period, the birth process, or breast-feeding
3. The virus may also enter the body when contaminated blood or body fluids come in contact with broken skin surfaces

C. Signs and symptoms (vary with each patient; may harbor the virus, but be asymptomatic for months and/or years)
1. Swollen lymph glands
2. Recurrent fever; night sweats
3. Weight loss; diminished appetite
4. Chronic diarrhea
5. Fatigue
6. White patches or lesions in the mouth
7. Presence of opportunistic infections such as *Pneumocystis carinii* (pneumonia) and Kaposi's sarcoma (purplish skin lesions)
8. Dry cough; shortness of breath
9. Centers for Disease Control clinical categories (Table 5-2)
   a. Category A: categories B and C have not occurred; asymptomatic HIV infection; persistent, generalized lymphadenopathy; acute HIV infection
   b. Category B: category C has not occurred; presence of conditions commonly associated with HIV
   c. Category C: once in this category, person remains in this category; all clinical conditions listed as associated with advanced HIV disease or AIDS
10. Symptoms may occur as early as 2 to 6 weeks after exposure, or individual may be asymptomatic for months or years; seroconversion (when the bloodwork changes from a "negative" to a "positive" for HIV antibodies) may not occur for 8 to 12 weeks or longer; retesting is advisable 6 months after exposure, then at 1 year; further testing is left up to the health care provider

D. Diagnostic tests/methods
1. Patient history and physical examination
2. Serum for HIV antibodies
3. Presence of opportunistic infections
   a. *Pneumocystis carinii* pneumonia
   b. Kaposi's sarcoma
4. Bronchial biopsy (tests for presence of opportunistic infections)
5. Lumbar puncture (tests for neurological evidence of infections)
6. CT scan
7. Enzyme-linked immunosorbent assay (ELISA); detects antibodies for HIV; false positives may occur
8. Western blot test: used to confirm the results of a positive ELISA test; detects HIV antibodies

TABLE 5-2 **1993 Revised Classification System for HIV Infection and Expanded AIDS Surveillance Case Definition for Adolescents and Adults**

	Clinical Categories*		
CD4 Cell Categories	**(A) Asymptomatic or PGL**	**(B) Symptomatic, Not (A) or (C) Conditions**	**(C) AIDS-Indicator Conditions**
>500/mm³	A1	B1	C1
200-499/mm³	A2	B2	C2
<200/mm³ AIDS-indicator cell count	A3	B3	C3

Centers for Disease Control and Prevention: Impact of the expanded AIDS surveillance case definition on AIDS case reporting–US first quarter, 1993, *MMWR* 42(16):308-310, 1993a.

*Description of Clinical Categories

A: One or more of the conditions listed below with documented HIV infection. Conditions listed in categories B and C must not have occurred.
  —Asymptomatic HIV infection
  —Persistent generalized lymphadenopathy (PGL)
  —Acute (primary) HIV infection with accompanying illness or history of acute infection

B: Symptomatic conditions that meet at least one of the following criteria: (a) the conditions are attributed to HIV infection and/or are indicative of a defect in cell-mediated immunity; or (b) the conditions are considered by physicians to have a clinical course or management that is complicated by HIV infection. Examples of conditions in clinical category B include, but are not limited to the following:
  —bacterial endocarditis, meningitis, pneumonia, or sepsis
  —candidiasis, vulvovaginal that is persistent (greater than one month duration) or poorly responsive to therapy
  —candidiasis, oropharyngeal (thrush)
  —cervical dysplasia, severe; or carcinoma
  —constitutional symptoms, such as fever (38.4° C) or diarrhea lasting more than one month
  —hairy leukoplakia, oral
  —herpes zoster (shingles), involving at least two distinct episodes or more than one dermatome
  —idiopathic thrombocytopenic purpura
  —listeriosis
  —*Mycobacterium tuberculosis,* pulmonary
  —nocardiosis
  —pelvic inflammatory disease
  —peripheral neuropathy

C: Any condition listed in the 1993 surveillance case definition for AIDS. The conditions in clinical category C are strongly associated with severe immunodeficiency, occur frequently in HIV-infected individuals, and cause serious morbidity or mortality.

Adapted from Harkness G, Dincher JR: *Medical surgical nursing: total patient care,* ed 9, St Louis, 1996, Mosby.

9. CD-4 cell counts: if less than 200 there is an increased risk for opportunistic infections (see Table 5-2)
E. Treatment
   1. Treatment is instituted according to the symptoms
   2. Protect the patient from opportunistic infections
   3. Zidovudine (AZT, Retrovir)
   4. Didanosine
   5. Zalcitabine
   6. Nutritional support
   7. Treatment of opportunistic infections
F. Nursing care
   1. Assess and document signs and symptoms and reactions to treatment
   2. Monitor vital signs
   3. Monitor arterial blood gas, CBC, and platelet count
   4. Administer prescribed medication and monitor for side effects
   5. Employ blood and body fluid precautions (Note: this should be followed when caring for all patients)
      a. Wear protective clothing (gloves, masks, goggles, gowns, etc.) as needed for the procedure
      b. Wash hands thoroughly
      c. Label specimens accordingly
      d. Dispose of contaminated articles properly
   6. Plan activity followed by rest periods
   7. Encourage physical independence
   8. Monitor oxygen therapy
   9. Monitor pain status and provide analgesia and comfort measures
   10. Support patient and allay anxiety
   11. Educate the patient and family concerning mode of spread, protective measures, and home care

LYMPHOMA

A. Definition: a group of malignancies originating in the stem cell of the bone marrow
B. Causes: unknown, possibly linked to viruses, genetics, environmental exposures, and possibly autoimmune links
C. Two main types
   1. Hodgkin's disease
   2. Non-Hodgkin's lymphoma
D. Signs and symptoms
   1. Swollen, painless lymph nodes
   2. Fever, chills
   3. Weight loss
   4. Night sweats
   5. Fatigue
   6. Loss of usual stamina; changes in ability to perform ADLs
E. Diagnostic tests/methods
   1. History and physical exam
   2. Complete blood count/RBC indices
   3. Blood chemistry: alkaline phosphatase, gamma globulin
   4. Serum protein electrophoresis
   5. Urine electrophoresis
   6. Lymph node biopsy
   7. Bone marrow biopsy
F. Treatment
   1. Staging laparotomy with splenectomy (to improve response to chemotherapy)
   2. Chemotherapy
   3. Radiation therapy

G. Nursing care
   1. Assess and document signs and symptoms and reactions to treatment
   2. Monitor vital signs
   3. Monitor lab studies
   4. Prevention of infection and recognition of early signs
   5. Planned activity; rest periods
   6. Monitor oxygen therapy if ordered
   7. Monitor pain status and provide comfort measures
   8. Give support and allay anxiety
   9. Maintain hydration

GASTROINTESTINAL SYSTEM
Anatomy and Physiology

A. Organs (Fig. 5-8)
   1. Mouth (buccal cavity)
      a. Receives food; aids in digestion; aids in speaking
      b. Consists of hard and soft palate, teeth, tongue, and salivary glands
         (1) Teeth
            (a) Deciduous: baby teeth
            (b) Permanent: appear at approximately 6 years of age
            (c) Incisors: cut food
            (d) Canines: tear food
            (e) Molar: grind food
         (2) Salivary glands, parotid, submandibular, submaxillary; manufacture saliva, which contains ptyalin to begin the chemical breakdown of starches
         (3) Tongue: also organ of taste
            (a) Receptors (taste buds, located in tongue): stimulated only if substance is in solution
            (b) Four kinds: sweet (tip of tongue); sour (side of tongue); salty (tip of tongue); bitter (back part of tongue)
            (c) Stimulates appetite and flow of digestive juices
      c. Functions
         (1) Ingestion of food
         (2) Mastication of food
         (3) Lubrication of food
         (4) Digestion of starch with salivary amylase
   2. Pharynx: transports food
   3. Esophagus: muscular tube; uses peristalsis to conduct food from pharynx to stomach
   4. Stomach
      a. J-shaped pouch; varies in size depending on contents; stores food and changes it into chyme
      b. Three divisions
         (1) Fundus: upper portion; the cardiac sphincter between the esophagus and fundus; controls the entrance of food
         (2) Body: the largest, central portion
         (3) Pylorus: lower portion above the small intestine; the pyloric sphincter controls the passage of food into the duodenum
      c. Special cells in the stomach secrete gastric juices and enzymes (including hydrochloric acid): the chemical breakdown of protein begins in the stomach
         (1) Pepsin: begins digestion of protein
         (2) Lipase: acts on emulsified fat

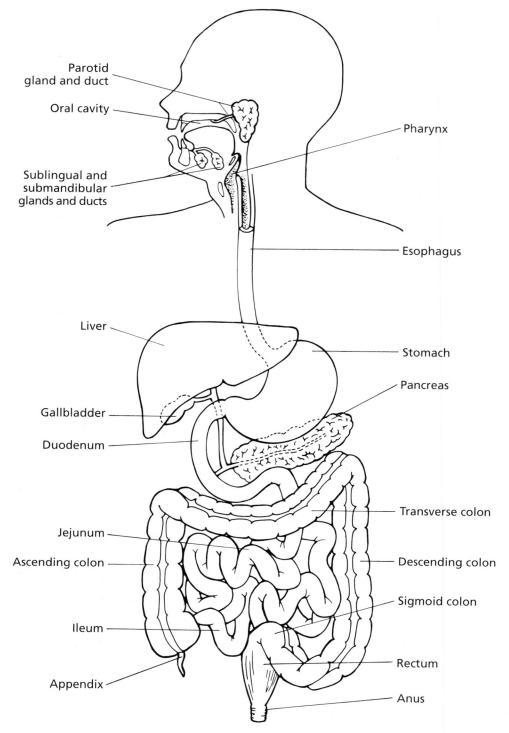

Figure 5-8   Digestive system. (Modified from Phipps WJ, Sands JK, Lehman MK, Cassmeyer VL: *Medical-surgical nursing: concepts and clinical practice*, ed 5, St Louis, 1995, Mosby.)

(3) Renin: acts on casein (a protein) in milk

(4) Gastrin (hormone): related to the control of gastric secretions; not an enzyme

(5) Hydrochloric acid: makes stomach content acid and activates enzymes

d. Chyme: the semiliquid contents of the stomach, consisting of partially digested food and gastric enzymes

e. Functions

(1) Storage of food

(2) Breakdown of food by churning

(3) Liquefying of food with hydrochloric acid
(4) Digestion of protein with enzyme, pepsin
5. Small intestine: extends from the pyloric sphincter to the ileocecal valve, which prevents backflow of material and regulates forward flow
  a. Size: approximately 20 ft (600 cm) long and 1 inch (2.5 cm) in diameter
  b. Three major divisions
    (1) Duodenum: approximately 10 inches (25 cm) long; curves around head of the pancreas; pancreatic and common bile duct enter below pyloric sphincter
    (2) Jejunum: approximately 8 ft (240 cm) long
    (3) Ileum: approximately 12 ft (360 cm) long; terminal part
  c. Functions
    (1) Digestion of food
    (2) Absorption of food
  d. Intestinal glands, pancreas, liver, and gallbladder secrete digestive enzymes that complete the chemical breakdown of food
    (1) Bile (formed in the liver and stored in the gallbladder): not an enzyme; emulsifies fat
    (2) Trypsin (pancreas): digests proteins into amino acids
    (3) Amylase (pancreas): digests starches into sugars
    (4) Lipase (pancreas): digests fat into simplest forms (fatty acids and glycerol)
    (5) Erepsin (intestine): digests proteins into amino acids
    (6) Lactose, maltose, sucrose (secretions of the small intestine): digest sugar into simplest forms (glucose, fructose, galactose)
6. Large intestine
  a. Size: approximately 5 to 6 ft (150 to 180 cm) long and $2\frac{1}{2}$ inches (6 cm) in diameter
  b. Divisions
    (1) Cecum: a blind pouch approximately 3 inches (7.5 cm) long; appendix attaches to distal end; located in right lower quadrant
    (2) Colon: ascending, continues up right side; transverse, extends across to the left; descending, descends on left side of pelvis
    (3) Sigmoid: S-shaped portion; extends to rectum
    (4) Rectum: approximately 8 inches (20 cm) long
    (5) Anus: terminal opening: guarded by internal and external sphincters
  c. Functions
    (1) Reabsorption of fluids
    (2) Temporary storage of fecal matter; defecation
B. Accessory organs (see Fig. 5-8)
1. Liver: largest organ in body; lies below diaphragm in upper right quadrant of abdominal cavity
  a. Metabolizes carbohydrates, fats, and proteins
  b. Detoxifies harmful substances
  c. Produces and stores heparin and fibrinogen
  d. Stores glycogen and vitamins A, B, B_{12}, and K
  e. Manufactures bile; hepatic duct drains bile into gallbladder

2. Gallbladder: small sac embedded in the interior surface of the liver
  a. Concentrates and stores bile
  b. Releases bile through the common bile duct into the duodenum when fat enters the small intestine
3. Pancreas: long, triangular gland; lies behind the stomach; produces enzymes that break down food particles; secretes enzymes into the duodenum; has two functions
  a. Exocrine gland; secretes digestive enzymes that neutralize chyme
  b. Endocrine gland: islets of Langerhans; secretes insulin for utilization of glucose; secretes glucagons to regulate blood sugar level
C. Functions
1. Digestion: two processes
  a. Mechanical: chewing, swallowing, and peristalsis of food; ends with elimination
  b. Chemical: breakdown of food into simpler compounds by the action of enzymes on food
2. Absorption
  a. Occurs in small intestine
  b. Most water absorbed in large intestine
3. Metabolism: the sum of all body functions to convert simple compounds into living tissue
  a. Catabolism: process in which substances are broken down into simpler substances, resulting in the release of heat and energy
  b. Anabolism: the building phase in which simpler substances are combined to form more complex substances (conversion of food into living tissues)
  c. Basal metabolism: the amount of energy (calories) used by the body when at rest

GASTROINTESTINAL CONDITIONS AND DISORDERS

The GI system provides a means by which food and fluids enter the body and are converted into elements that help maintain the human organism. It is important to note that other systems of the body influence this system. The endocrine system, central nervous system, and autonomic nervous system all serve as regulators to the GI system.

Nursing Assessment

A. Nursing observations (objective data)
1. Vital signs
2. Skin and mucous membrane character/color
  a. Gingivitis
  b. Stomatitis
  c. Jaundice
3. Hematemesis: emesis is like coffee grounds in appearance, signifying digested blood
4. Stool changes
  a. Melena (tarry stool)
  b. Clay-colored (lack of bile pigment)
  c. Frothy, foamy, foul-smelling (seen in pancreatitis)
  d. Constipation
  e. Diarrhea
  f. Changes in size and/or shape (may indicate colon lesion)
5. Urine color: dark urine (tea-colored)
6. Hemorrhoids

7. Abdominal distention
8. Edema
9. Bowel sounds
B. Patient description (subjective data)
   1. General
      a. History of GI-related problems
      b. Family history of GI-related problems
   2. Weight
      a. Loss or gain
      b. Appetite changes: increase or decrease
   3. Dietary/eating changes
      a. Presence of nausea/vomiting
      b. Difficulty chewing
      c. Dysphagia
      d. Occurrence of indigestion or dyspepsia
      e. Intolerance to certain foods
      f. Presence of pain: relationship to meals/eating
   4. Changes in bowel habit
      a. Diarrhea
      b. Constipation
      c. Alternating diarrhea and constipation
      d. Gas formation
   5. Easily bruised

Diagnostic Tests/Methods

A. Patient history and physical examination
B. Examination of stool
   1. Examination of stool for occult (hidden) blood
   2. Fecal analysis: analysis of stool for mucus, pus, blood, parasites, and fat content
   3. Stool for ova and parasites must be taken to the lab while it is still warm.
   4. Nursing intervention
      a. Instruct the patient in the proper collection of the specimen
      b. Take the specimen to the laboratory promptly
C. Radiographic examination
   1. Upper GI series
      a. Patient ingests contrast medium (barium)
      b. Movement of the medium through the esophagus and into the stomach is observed by fluoroscopy; X-ray films are also taken
         (1) Aids in identification of esophageal and stomach pathology
         (2) Nursing intervention
            (a) Explain procedures to the patient
            (b) Patient is usually NPO before the examination
            (c) Enemas or cathartics may be given before and after the examination
            (d) Allay patient's anxiety
   2. Lower GI series (barium enema)
      a. The filling of the colon with barium is observed by fluoroscopy; X-ray films of the colon are also taken
      b. Aids in the detection of abnormalities or defects in the colon such as lesions, polyps, tumors, and diverticula
      c. Nursing intervention
         (1) Explain procedures to the patient
         (2) Patient is usually NPO before the examination

(3) Enemas or cathartics may be given before and after the examination
(4) Allay patient's anxiety
   3. Gallbladder series (oral cholecystography)
      a. Patient is given an oral radiographic dye to ingest the evening before the examination
      b. The gallbladder is visualized to detect gallstones and obstruction of the biliary tract
      c. Nursing intervention
         (1) Explain procedures to the patient
         (2) Administer the radiographic dye as prescribed
         (3) Maintain NPO after the dye is given
         (4) Allay patient's anxiety
   4. Cholangiography
      a. Aids in the visualization of the biliary duct system
      b. Three methods
         (1) Intravenous cholangiography (IVC): a radiographic dye is administered intravenously, and X-ray films are taken
         (2) Percutaneous transhepatic cholangiography: under fluoroscopy a cannula is inserted into the liver and bile duct; a radiographic dye is injected into the duct, and filling is observed
         (3) Operative or T-tube cholangiography: contrast medium is instilled into the common bile duct, cystic duct, or gallbladder using a fine needle or catheter during surgery or via an existing T-tube postoperatively
      c. Nursing intervention
         (1) Explain procedures to the patient
         (2) Maintain NPO as ordered
         (3) Monitor the patient for bleeding or bile leakage if the percutaneous approach was used
   5. Barium swallow: barium contrast study used to detect esophageal abnormalities and reasons for dysphagia
D. Endoscopy
   1. Endoscopy of the upper GI tract (esophagoscopy, gastroscopy, gastroduodenoscopy, esophagogastroduodenoscopy)
      a. Visualization of the esophagus, stomach, or duodenum with a lighted scope
      b. Useful in detecting inflammation, ulceration, tumors, and other lesions
      c. Nursing intervention
         (1) Explain procedures to the patient
         (2) Obtain signed consent
         (3) Maintain NPO as ordered
         (4) Administer preoperative medication as ordered
         (5) After the examination, maintain NPO until the gag reflex returns
   2. Colonoscopy/sigmoidoscopy
      a. Visualization of the internal structures of the colon with a fiberoptic scope
      b. Lesions, tumors, and polyps may be visualized, and a biopsy may be performed
      c. Nursing interventions
         (1) Explain procedures to the patient
         (2) Prepare patient with enemas and cathartics as ordered

(3) After the examination, observe for rectal bleeding and signs of perforation (malaise, distention, and tenesmus)
E. Ultrasonography
1. Noninvasive test that uses echoes from sound waves to visualize deep structures of the body
2. No special preparation is needed
3. Useful in detecting masses, fluid accumulation, cysts, tumors, etc.
F. Scans (liver and pancreas)
1. Assessment of size, shape, and position of the organ
2. Radionuclide is injected intravenously, and a scanning device picks up the radioactive emissions, which are recorded on paper
3. Nursing intervention
a. No preparation is required for liver scanning
b. Fasting and dietary preparation may be ordered for pancreatic scanning
c. Explain procedures to the patient
d. Allay patient's anxiety
G. Computerized tomography (CT scan)
1. Noninvasive, radiological imaging technique that takes exposures of the body or body part at different depths
2. No special preparation is necessary
H. Liver biopsy
1. Invasive procedure in which a needle is inserted into the liver through a small incision in the skin and a sample of liver tissue is obtained
2. The incision is usually made on the right side, at the sixth, seventh, eighth, or ninth intercostal space
3. Nursing interventions
a. Obtain signed consent
b. Explain procedure to the patient
c. Take baseline vital signs
d. Provide assistance during the procedure
e. After the procedure monitor the vital signs every 15 minutes to 1 hour; carry out prescription for bed rest (position flat or on the right side), assess the site and monitor for complications
I. Laboratory studies
1. Serum amylase
a. Measures the secretion of amylase by the pancreas
b. Useful in diagnosing pancreatitis
2. Serum lipase
a. Measures the secretion of lipase by the pancreas
b. Useful in diagnosing pancreatitis
3. Serum bilirubin and spot urine amylase: indicates the liver's ability to conjugate and excrete bilirubin
4. Coagulation studies (PT and PTT): useful in analyzing hemostatic functions
5. Liver enzyme studies (SGOT, serum glutamic-pyruvic transaminase [SGPT], and LDH): elevations usually indicate liver damage
6. Hepatitis-associated antigen (HAA): presence suggests hepatitis
7. Ammonia levels: elevated in advanced liver disease
8. Urine amylase: elevated amylase levels indicate pancreatic dysfunction
J. Gastric analysis
1. Gastric contents are analyzed primarily for hydrochloric acid content

2. Acidity (pH), volume, and cytology may also be determined
K. D-xylose tolerance test
1. This study evaluates absorption
2. Xylose in water is given orally
3. A urine collection of several hours follows; the amount of D-xylose in the urine is measured
4. Abnormal amounts of D-xylose in the urine indicate a malabsorption problem
5. Nursing interventions
a. Explain procedure to the patient
b. Maintain NPO before the examination
c. Give patient instructions on collecting the urine

Frequent Patient Problems and Nursing Care

A. Pain related to stomatitis (inflammation of the mucous lining of the mouth)
1. Give soft, bland foods
2. Encourage intake of fluids that do not aggravate the condition
3. Encourage the use of soothing mouth rinses
4. Administer topical medication as prescribed
B. Impaired swallowing related to gingivitis
1. Give mouth irrigations as prescribed
2. Offer soft, bland foods and liquids
3. Instruct the patient in the benefit of good oral hygiene and professional dental cleaning
C. Potential fluid volume deficit related to nausea and vomiting
1. Observe character and quantity of emesis
2. Observe for associated symptoms
3. Observe for precipitating factors
4. Administer antiemetics as prescribed
5. Offer ice chips
6. Maintain cool environment
7. Apply a cool compress to the neck and forehead for comfort
8. Offer sips of clear liquids such as 7-Up, ginger ale
9. Reduce environmental stimuli such as noise, unpleasant odors, and unpleasant sights
10. Encourage rest and deep breathing
11. Serve patient's favorite foods
12. Limit food servings
13. Provide mouth care after episodes of emesis
D. Impaired swallowing related to dysphagia
1. Provide patient with favorite foods arranged attractively
2. Provide soft, bland foods that can easily be chewed
3. Provide small, frequent feedings
4. Avoid irritating food and fluid
5. Monitor intake
6. Administration topical medication as ordered
E. Alteration in nutrition, less than body requirements, related to anorexia
1. Assess status of the anorexia
2. Monitor intake of food and fluid
3. Determine patient's food likes and dislikes
4. Prepare patient for meals
a. Relieve pain
b. Provide mouth care

c. Assist patient to a comfortable position

d. Use patient screen for privacy

e. Remove unpleasant stimuli from patient's view

5. Prepare food tray

a. Serve food at the proper temperature

b. Make the tray attractive

c. Serve appropriate quantities (large quantities may reduce the appetite)

F. Potential fluid volume deficit related to diarrhea

1. Document character, consistency, number, and appearance of stools

2. Assess for associated symptoms

3. Monitor intake and output

4. Administer antidiarrheals as prescribed and monitor for side effects

5. Avoid milk and milk products

6. Increase fluid intake to at least 3000 ml daily

7. Monitor vital signs at least q4h

8. Identify symptoms of electrolyte imbalance

9. Monitor laboratory reports for electrolyte values

G. Constipation related to decreased peristalsis/activity

1. Administer enemas, stool softeners, and cathartics as ordered

2. Encourage fluids to at least 3000 ml daily

3. Provide hot drinks to stimulate peristalsis

4. Encourage a diet high in fiber

5. Check for an impaction

6. Encourage exercises

7. Instruct patient concerning proper diet, increased fluid intake, exercise, and avoidance of laxative abuse

Major Medical Diagnoses

ESOPHAGITIS

A. Definition: an inflammation of the esophagus; more common in middle age

B. Causes

1. Inflammation of the esophagus may be brought on by irritants (food and tobacco), bacteria, or trauma (also see hiatal hernia)

2. Fungal: Candida

3. Reflux esophagitis: an incompetent lower esophageal sphincter allows a reflux of gastric contents into the esophagus

4. Malignancy

5. Prolonged nasogastric intubation

6. Repeated vomiting

C. Signs and symptoms

1. Heartburn (epigastric distress)

2. Pain with eructation or regurgitations

3. Dysphagia

4. Pain associated with ingestion of citrus liquids, alcohol, or hot or cold fluid

5. Symptoms aggravated by lying down after meals

6. Bleeding

D. Diagnostic tests/methods

1. Patient history and physical examination

2. Barium swallow

3. Esophagoscopy and biopsy

4. Routine chest X-ray examination

E. Treatments

1. Avoid food and fluids that aggravate the symptoms

2. Administer antacids, analgesics, and sedatives

3. Elevate head of bed on shock blocks

4. Maintain bland diet

5. Surgery may be necessary if conservative measures fail

a. Fundoplication: plication (making tucks) in the fundus of the stomach around the lower end of the esophagus

b. Vagotomy and pyloroplasty: interruption of the impulses carried by the vagus nerve to reduce gastric secretions; the pylorus is also surgically manipulated to provide a larger conduit between the stomach and the duodenum

F. Nursing intervention

1. Assess signs and symptoms and reactions to treatments

2. Provide small, frequent feedings of bland, low-roughage foods

3. Discourage intake of food close to bedtime

4. Administer medication as prescribed and monitor for side effects

5. Place in semi-Fowler's position

ESOPHAGEAL VARICES

A. Definition: dilated vessels that occur at the lower end of the esophagus

B. Causes

1. Dilation of these vessels is usually a complication arising from cirrhosis of the liver

2. Veins in the lower esophagus become distended as a result of increased portal pressure; the varices may rupture, causing hemorrhage and subsequent shock

C. Signs and symptoms

1. Usually no signs and symptoms appear until the varices become ulcerated

2. Hematemesis and coffee-ground emesis

3. Melena

4. Tachycardia

5. Hypotension

6. Low hemoglobin and hematocrit levels

D. Diagnostic tests/methods

1. Patient history and physical examination: history of alcoholism may exist

2. Fiberoptic endoscopy

3. Laboratory studies: hemoglobin, hematocrit, and liver function studies

4. Angiography

5. Barium swallow

6. CT scan

7. Ultrasound

E. Treatment

1. Blood and blood product replacement

2. Control of bleeding through ice water lavages, insertion of Sengstaken-Blakemore tube, and vitamin K therapy

3. Laboratory studies to monitor bleeding status and effectiveness of treatments

4. Hydration with IV fluids

5. Monitor intake and output

6. Surgery if needed to control bleeding

7. Injection of the bleeding varices with a sclerosing agent to control the bleeding

F. Nursing intervention

1. Provide ongoing assessment of signs and symptoms and reactions to treatment

2. Monitor vital signs at least q4h and monitor vital signs q1/2h if bleeding is occurring
3. Record intake and output qh if varices are bleeding
4. Monitor fluids: assess the site and monitor flow rate
5. Give prescribed medication as ordered and monitor for side effects
6. Allay patient's anxieties and fears
7. Assess all emesis and stool for the presence of blood
8. Monitor laboratory studies and inform physician of incoming laboratory test values
9. Keep head of bed elevated
10. Monitor the Sengstaken-Blakemore tube if in use; keep scissors taped to the head of the bed in case of emergency
11. Note the character of respirations

HIATAL HERNIA

A. Definition: a protrusion of the proximal area of the stomach through a weakened area of the diaphragm into the thoracic cavity (Fig. 5-9)
B. Causes
   1. Congenital weakness
   2. Increased abdominal pressure
   3. Trauma
   4. Relaxation of the musculature
   5. Gastric reflux may flow into the esophagus, causing inflammation and ulceration
C. Signs and symptoms
   1. Heartburn (pyrosis)
   2. Sternal pain after a heavy meal
   3. Regurgitation
   4. Feeling of fullness
   5. Dysphagia
   6. Dyspnea
D. Diagnosis tests/methods
   1. Patient history and physical examination
   2. Upper GI series (barium swallow)
   3. Esophagoscopy
   4. Routine chest X-ray examination
E. Treatment
   1. Conservative
      a. Elevation of the head of the bed on shock blocks
      b. Bland diet with frequent small feedings
      c. Avoidance of caffeine, alcohol, and chocolate
      d. Drug therapy with anticholinergics and antacids
      e. Weight management
      f. Avoidance of activities that increase intraabdominal pressure
   2. When conservative measures fail, surgery is indicated: fundoplication—"wrapping" the upper part of the stomach around the esophageal sphincter to prevent reflux
      a. Nasogastric tube
      b. IV therapy
      c. Drug therapy with analgesics and antiemetics
      d. Monitor vital signs
      e. Monitor intake and output
F. Nursing intervention
   1. Assess and document signs and symptoms and reactions to treatments
   2. Administer prescribed drugs and monitor for side effects
   3. Monitor vital signs at least every shift and more often if surgery was performed
   4. Monitor intake and output if surgery was performed
   5. Provide the prescribed diet
   6. Inform the physician if gastric reflux is reported by the patient after surgery
   7. Educate patient and family concerning drug therapy, diet, activities to avoid, and the need for compliance

GASTRITIS

A. Definition: an inflammation in the mucosal lining of the stomach; the condition may be acute or chronic
B. Gastritis may be caused by bacteria, alcohol, drugs, or toxins that cause the lining of the stomach to become inflamed and edematous
C. Signs and symptoms
   1. Nausea and vomiting
   2. Anorexia
   3. Epigastric tenderness
   4. Feeling of fullness
   5. Cramping
   6. Diarrhea
   7. Fever

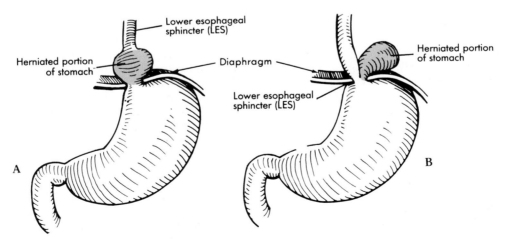

Figure 5-9   Hiatal hernia. **A,** Sliding hernia. **B,** Paraesophageal hernia. (From Phipps WJ, Sands JK, Marek JR: *Medical-surgical nursing: concepts and clinical practice,* ed 6, St. Louis, 1999, Mosby.)

D. Diagnostic tests/methods
1. Patient history and physical examination
2. Identification of a causative agent
3. Laboratory studies
4. Stool culture
5. Endoscopy with biopsy
6. Gastric analysis

E. Treatment
1. Supportive care
2. Bed rest
3. NPO if nausea or vomiting is severe
4. Hydration with IV fluids
5. In severe cases a nasogastric tube is inserted
6. Drug therapy: antiemetics, antacids, and H_2 receptor antagonists
7. Progressive diet when acute symptoms subside
8. Restriction of smoking

F. Nursing intervention
1. Assess and document signs and symptoms and reactions to treatments
2. Monitor vital signs at least q4h
3. Monitor intake and output
4. Provide the prescribed diet
5. Administer medication as prescribed and monitor for side effects
6. Note amount and character of emesis and diarrhea
7. Monitor IV fluids
8. Educate patient and family concerning drug therapy, diet, activities, and any restrictions

CANCER OF THE STOMACH

A. Cancer can develop anywhere in the stomach
B. Causes
1. Exact cause is unknown
2. Familial tendency is suspected
3. Predisposing conditions: chronic gastric ulcers and gastritis

C. Signs and symptoms
1. Loss of appetite; early satiety
2. Weight loss
3. Weakness and fatigue
4. Pain
5. Melena
6. Anemia
7. Hematemesis
8. Dizziness
9. Indigestion or dysphagia
10. Constipation

D. Diagnostic tests/methods
1. Patient history and physical examination
2. Laboratory studies
3. Stool analysis
4. Gastric analysis
5. Barium studies
6. Gastroscopy

E. Treatment
1. Preoperative therapy
   a. Correct nutritional deficiencies
   b. Treat anemias
   c. Blood replacement
   d. Gastric decompression with a nasogastric tube
2. Surgery: removal of the cancerous lesion or tumor along with a margin of normal tissue

3. Radiation therapy and chemotherapy may be used if the patient is not expected to undergo surgery
   a. Combination therapy has a better response rate
   b. Single-agent therapy has proved to be of little value

F. Nursing intervention
1. Preoperative care
   a. Support the patient and family
   b. Assess and document signs and symptoms and reactions to treatments
   c. Provide and encourage the prescribed diet
   d. Monitor vital signs at least q8h
   e. Monitor blood and fluid replacement therapy
   f. Provide preoperative teaching
2. Postoperative care (immediate)
   a. Have patient turn, cough, and breathe deeply
   b. Monitor nasogastric suctioning and tube patency
   c. Monitor vital signs as ordered
   d. Record intake and output
   e. Administer prescribed medication and monitor for side effects
   f. Assess dressing
   g. Assess for bowel sounds
   h. Encourage early ambulation and ROM exercises to prevent thrombosis
   i. Provide antiembolism stockings
   j. Relieve pain with drugs and supportive measures
3. Postoperative period
   a. Provide six to eight small feedings
   b. Weigh patient qd while in hospital to monitor weight loss
   c. Reduce fluids taken with meals if not tolerated
   d. Educate patient and family concerning drug therapy, dietary restrictions, activity, wound care, and compliance with the regimen

PEPTIC ULCERS

A. Definition: ulcerations in the mucosal lining of the distal esophagus, stomach, or small intestine (duodenum or jejunum); duodenal ulcers are more common than gastric ulcers, and men are more prone to ulcers than women
B. Cause: exact cause is unknown; recurrent or refractory ulcers linked with *Helicobacter pylori* infections
C. Predisposing factors
1. Stress
2. Smoking
3. Heavy caffeine ingestion
4. Ingestion of certain drugs (ASA, steroids, NSAIDs)
5. Infection of the mucosa by *H. pylori*

D. Signs and symptoms
1. Loss of appetite
2. Weight loss or gain
3. Pain (gnawing, burning)
4. Melena
5. Anemia
6. Hematemesis; coffee-ground emesis
7. Occasional nausea or vomiting
8. Dark, tarry stools

E. Diagnostic tests/methods
1. Patient history and physical examination
2. Gastroscopy and duodenoscopy
3. Barium studies
4. Gastric analysis
5. Laboratory studies

F. Treatment
   1. Conservative
      a. Rest
      b. Drug therapy: antacids, anticholinergics, histamine receptor antagonists, sedatives, and analgesics
      c. Elimination of smoking and caffeine
      d. Reduction of stress
      e. Bland diet with small, frequent feedings
      f. In acute situations the patient may be NPO and have nasogastric tube inserted
   2. Surgical intervention
      a. Closure if perforation has occurred
      b. Pyloroplasty and vagotomy if the gastric outlet is obstructed
      c. Total or partial resection of the stomach to remove the ulcerated area(s)
G. Nursing intervention
   1. Conduct ongoing assessment of signs and symptoms and reactions to treatments
   2. Monitor vital signs at least q4h
   3. Administer the prescribed medication and monitor for side effects
   4. Provide the prescribed diet
   5. Provide physical and emotional rest
   6. Monitor for signs and symptoms of complications (perforation, hemorrhage, and obstruction)
   7. Instruct patient regarding elimination of smoking, avoidance of certain foods, and reduction of stress
   8. Educate patient and family concerning drug therapy, diet and dietary restrictions, avoidance of stress, and the need for compliance with the prescribed regimen

OBSTRUCTION

A. Definition: a mechanical or neurological abnormality inhibiting the normal flow of gastric or intestinal contents
B. Obstructions may result from scar tissue formation, cancer, or strangulated hernias; all are mechanical barriers to the normal flow of gastric or intestinal contents
C. A neurological obstruction, in the form of a paralytic ileus, causes interference with innervation, thus hindering normal peristaltic activity
D. Signs and symptoms
   1. Abnormal pain and distention
   2. Projectile vomiting
   3. Nausea
   4. Possible absence of bowel sounds or increase in bowel sounds
   5. Cramping
   6. Abdomen may be tense (distended)
   7. Obstipation (chronic constipation)
E. Diagnostic tests/methods
   1. Patient history and physical examination
   2. Flat plate of the abdomen
   3. Laboratory studies
F. Treatment
   1. Surgery is the treatment for mechanical obstructions
   2. Gastric or intestinal decompression to decrease nausea and vomiting
   3. Hydration with IV therapy
   4. Prophylactic antibiotics
   5. Monitor intake and output
   6. Supportive care

G. Nursing intervention
   1. Assess and document signs and symptoms and reactions to treatments
   2. Monitor vital signs at least q4h
   3. Record intake and output
   4. Monitor the decompression tube and assess quantity and character of drainage
   5. Provide mouth care while patient is intubated
   6. Administer prescribed medication and monitor for side effects
   7. Maintain NPO
   8. Monitor the states of distention and hydration
   9. Provide routine postoperative care if patient undergoes surgery

CROHN'S DISEASE (REGIONAL ENTERITIS)

A. Definition: an inflammatory disease affecting primarily the small bowel and also possibly the large bowel; the intestinal lining ulcerates, and scar tissue forms; bowel becomes thick and narrow
B. Cause is unknown; stricture, obstruction, and perforation can occur as a result of this disorder; malabsorption of fluid and nutrients is also associated with this disorder
C. Signs and symptoms (aggravated by illness/stress)
   1. Abdominal pain and cramping
   2. Diarrhea
   3. Weight loss
   4. Fever
   5. Anemia
   6. Weakness and fatigue
   7. Anorexia
   8. Abdominal tenderness
D. Diagnostic tests/methods
   1. Patient history and physical examination
   2. Laboratory studies: CBC, electrolytes, clotting studies
   3. Stool examination
   4. Endoscopy
   5. Proctosigmoidoscopy and biopsy examination
   6. Barium studies
E. Treatment
   1. Drug therapy: sedatives, antidiarrheals, antibiotics, steroids, hematinics, anticholinergics, and analgesics
   2. Hydration with IV therapy
   3. Correct nutritional deficiencies
   4. Provide symptomatic relief
   5. In severe cases the patient may be NPO, have a nasogastric tube, and require blood transfusions
   6. High-calorie, high-protein, low-residue diet
   7. Surgery is indicated if there is fistula formation, bleeding, perforation, or obstruction
F. Nursing intervention
   1. Assess and document signs and symptoms and reactions to treatments
   2. Monitor vital signs q4h
   3. Record intake and output
   4. Provide and encourage the prescribed diet
   5. Assist with activities of daily living
   6. Monitor the number, amount, and character of stools
   7. Monitor hydration status
   8. Assess for abdominal distention
   9. Maintain skin integrity and monitor for anal excoriation
   10. Provide support to the patient

11. Administer prescribed medication and monitor for side effects
12. Educate patient and family concerning drug therapy, dietary restrictions, and compliance; ostomy care if applicable

ULCERATIVE COLITIS

A. Definition: an inflammatory disorder of the large bowel; the inflammatory process begins in the distal segments of the colon and ascends
   1. The mucosa ulcerates, bleeds, and becomes edematous and thickens
   2. Perforations and abscesses can occur
   3. The colon eventually loses its elasticity, and its absorptive ability is reduced
B. Cause is unknown, although it has been associated with stress, autoimmune factors, and food allergies
C. Signs and symptoms
   1. Abdominal cramping pain with diarrhea
   2. Nausea
   3. Dehydration
   4. Cachexia
   5. Weight loss
   6. Anorexia
   7. Bloody diarrhea
   8. Anemia
D. Diagnostic tests/methods
   1. Patient history and physical examination
   2. Laboratory studies reveal anemia and electrolyte imbalance: CBC, electrolytes
   3. Stool examination
   4. Proctosigmoidoscopy
   5. Barium studies
E. Treatment
   1. Drug therapy: sedatives, antidiarrheals, antibiotics, steroids, hematinics, anticholinergics, and analgesics
   2. Correction of malnutrition
   3. Hydration with IV therapy
   4. Colectomy with ileostomy if other medical treatment fails
   5. Provide symptomatic relief
   6. Monitor weight
   7. Monitor intake and output
   8. Parenteral hyperalimentation may be necessary
   9. Psychotherapy
F. Nursing intervention
   1. Assess and document signs and symptoms and reactions to treatments
   2. Provide emotional as well as physical rest
   3. Monitor number, amount, and characteristics of stools
   4. Provide skin care measures to avoid anal excoriation
   5. Monitor intake and output
   6. Monitor vital signs q4h
   7. Weigh patient qd
   8. Increase intake of fluids
   9. Provide the prescribed diet
   10. Administer prescribed medication and monitor for side effects
   11. Assess bowel sounds q4h
   12. Assist with activities of daily living
   13. Provide emotional support
   14. Educate patient and family concerning drug therapy, dietary restrictions, avoidance of stress, and compliance with the prescribed regimen

DIVERTICULOSIS/DIVERTICULITIS

A. Definition: diverticulum—an outpouching of the mucosa of the colon
   1. Diverticulosis: the existence of diverticula in the large intestine
   2. Diverticulitis: an inflammation of the diverticulum
B. Cause of diverticulosis is unknown; theories include a congenital weakness of the colon, colon distention, constipation, and inadequate dietary fiber
C. Signs and symptoms
   1. Abdominal cramps
   2. Lower-quadrant tenderness
   3. Constipation or constipation alternating with diarrhea
   4. Fever
   5. Occult bleeding
   6. Elevated WBC count
D. Diagnostic tests/methods
   1. Patient history and physical examination
   2. Laboratory studies
   3. Stool examination for occult blood
   4. Sigmoidoscopy
   5. Colonoscopy
   6. Barium studies
E. Treatment
   1. High-residue diet
   2. Drug therapy: bulk laxatives, antibiotics, stool softeners, and anticholinergics
   3. In more severe cases the patient may be NPO and require IV therapy
   4. Surgery: colon resection for obstruction and hemorrhage
F. Nursing intervention
   1. Assess and document signs and symptoms and reactions to treatments
   2. Provide increased roughage in the diet
   3. Increase intake of fluids
   4. Administer prescribed medication and monitor for side effects
   5. Instruct patient to avoid activity that increases intraabdominal pressure (straining at stool, lifting, bending, and wearing restrictive clothing)
   6. Educate patient and family concerning drug therapy, dietary restrictions, and avoidance of constipation and activity that increases intraabdominal pressure

COLON/RECTAL CANCER AND POLYPS

A. Definition: the cancerous process can invade the large intestine; cancer of the colon and rectum may take the form of well-defined tumor or cancerous polyp: a polyp is a pouchlike structure projecting from the wall of the bowel; polyps may be cancerous or benign
B. Cause of colon cancer is unknown; persons with colon polyps, lesions, diverticula, or ulcerative colitis are monitored closely for malignant changes in the bowel
C. Signs and symptoms
   1. Changes in bowel pattern
   2. Rectal bleeding
   3. Changes in the shape of stool

4. Weakness and fatigue
5. Weight loss
6. Rectal pain
7. Abdominal pain
8. Anemia
D. Diagnostic tests/methods
  1. Patient history and physical examination
  2. Laboratory studies
  3. Barium studies
  4. Proctosigmoidoscopic examination
E. Treatment
  1. Surgical resection of the affected area/creation of a colostomy if necessary
  2. Chemotherapy
  3. Radiation therapy
  4. Supportive therapy
F. Nursing intervention (also see nursing care plan for cancer of the stomach)
  1. Assess and document signs and symptoms and reactions to treatments
  2. Monitor vital signs at least q4h and more often during the postoperative periods
  3. Record intake and output
  4. Monitor dressings and wound drainage
  5. Relieve pain
  6. Administer prescribed medication and monitor for side effects
  7. Provide psychological support
  8. Monitor colostomy site
  9. Monitor perineal area if drain or packing has been inserted
  10. Assist patient with sitz baths if ordered
  11. Assist patient with activities of daily living as needed
  12. Monitor hydration status
  13. Encourage increased fluid intake
  14. Educate patient and family concerning drug therapy, diet, activities, colostomy care, and adaptation to everyday activity

HEMORRHOIDS

A. Definition: varicosities or dilated vessels in the rectal and anal area
B. Cause: hemorrhoids result from increased abdominal pressure such as that during pregnancy and from prolonged periods of sitting and standing; constipation and obesity are also predisposing factors
C. Signs and symptoms vary from no symptoms at all to pain, itching, and bleeding
D. Diagnostic tests/methods
  1. Patient history and physical examination
  2. Digital examination
  3. Proctoscopy
E. Treatment
  1. Symptomatic relief in mild cases
    a. Topical medication to shrink the mucous membrane
    b. Stool softeners and laxatives to keep stool soft and avoid straining
    c. Sitz baths to relieve pain
    d. High-fiber diet to keep stools soft
  2. Rubber-band ligation of internal hemorrhoids: the constriction impairs circulation; the tissues become necrotic and slough off

3. Hemorrhoidectomy: the surgical excision of hemorrhoids
    a. Removal may be by clamp, excision, or cautery
    b. Postoperative treatments are similar to those identified previously for symptomatic relief
F. Nursing intervention
  1. Assess and document signs and symptoms and reactions to treatments
  2. Alleviate pain with analgesics, positioning, and sitz baths
  3. Administer prescribed medication and monitor for side effects
  4. Monitor vital signs at least q4h
  5. Monitor dressings for drainage
  6. Monitor voiding after surgery
  7. Assist with gradual return to activity
  8. Encourage increased fluid intake
  9. Provide patient with rationale for avoiding constipation and prolonged sitting and standing
  10. Educate patient and family concerning drug therapy, high-fiber diet, activity, and avoidance of constipation

CHOLELITHIASIS/CHOLECYSTITIS

A. Definition
  1. Cholelithiasis: the presence of gallstones in the gallbladder or biliary tree
  2. Cholecystitis: an inflammation of the gallbladder usually associated with the presence of gallstones
B. Cause
  1. Cholelithiasis is believed to be precipitated by chemical changes in bile
    a. Bile stasis, infections of the gallbladder, and metabolic changes can precipitate stone formation
    b. Stones may lodge in the biliary tree, causing obstruction and biliary colic (Fig. 5-10)
  2. Cholecystitis: may be brought on by cholelithiasis or the presence of an organism in the gallbladder
C. Signs and symptoms
  1. Indigestion after a meal high in fat
  2. Nausea and vomiting
  3. Flatulence
  4. Belching
  5. Right upper-quadrant pain radiating to the back or shoulder
  6. Fever
  7. Jaundice
  8. Clay-colored stools
  9. Dark-colored urine
  10. Elevated WBC count
D. Diagnostic tests/methods
  1. Patient history and physical examination
  2. Laboratory studies
  3. Oral cholecystography
  4. IV cholangiography
  5. Ultrasound of gallbladder
E. Treatment
  1. Hydration with IV fluids
  2. Drug therapy: analgesics, antibiotics, and antispasmodics
  3. Drug therapy to dissolve stones has been effective in certain patients
  4. Low-fat diet

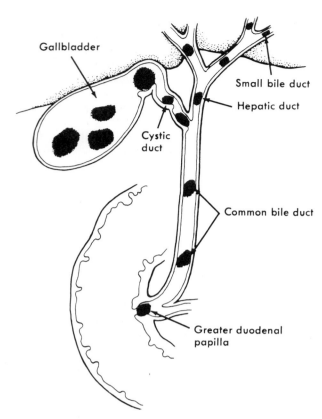

Figure 5-10 Common sites of gallstones. (From Phipps WJ, Sands JK, Marek JR: *Medical-surgical nursing: concepts and clinical practice*, ed 6, St Louis, 1999, Mosby.)

5. Lithotripsy (use of shock waves to disintegrate gallstones) has been attempted in patients having few stones
6. Surgical removal of the gallbladder (cholecystectomy) or gallstones (cholecystostomy)
7. Laparoscopic cholecystectomy (removal through an endoscope inserted through the abdominal wall)

F. Nursing intervention
1. Assess and document signs and symptoms and reactions to treatments
2. Administer prescribed medication and monitor for side effects
3. Alleviate pain and promote comfort
4. Monitor IV therapy
5. Provide the prescribed diet
6. Monitor the state of hydration
7. Assess vital signs at least q4h
8. Provide postoperative care: monitor dressing, nasogastric tube, and T tube (tube is inserted into the common bile duct during surgery if the common bile duct is explored) (Fig. 5-11)
9. Educate patient and family concerning drug therapy, dietary restrictions, and wound care if surgery was performed

HEPATITIS

A. Definition: inflammation of the liver
B. Causes
1. Drugs or chemicals (toxic hepatitis)

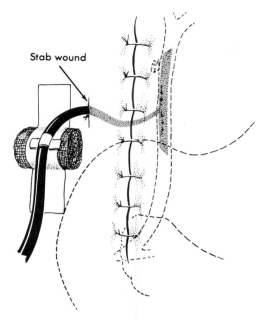

Figure 5-11 Section of T-tube emerging from stab wound may be placed over roll of gauze anchored to skin with adhesive tape to prevent its lumen from being occluded by pressure. (From Phipps WJ, Sands JK, Marek JR: *Medical-surgical nursing: concepts and clinical practice*, ed 6, St Louis, 1999, Mosby.)

2. Viral origin (hepatitis A [HAV] and B [HBV])
3. Multiple blood transfusions (hepatitis non-A or non-B)

C. The most common forms of HAV and HBV
1. HAV: infectious hepatitis
a. Transmitted by the fecal-oral route
b. Incubation period is approximately 2 to 7 weeks
c. May be spread by contaminated food, water, milk, and shellfish
2. HBV: serum hepatitis
a. Associated with contaminated needles and syringes
b. Transmitted through blood or blood products and pricking of the skin with contaminated equipment
c. May also be spread through feces, urine, saliva, and semen
d. Patients are prone to exacerbations and complications (cirrhosis) from the disease
e. Incubation period is approximately 6 to 26 weeks
f. Immunization available: given to newborn, then again at 2 and 6 months of age
3. Hepatitis C (HCV; formerly known as non-HAV and non-HBV) and hepatitis E
a. Name given to forms of hepatitis caused by a virus genetically different from hepatitis A or B
b. Associated with blood transfusions, particularly from paid donors; previous IV drug use
c. No specific antigen is associated with the form
d. Similar to hepatitis B in characteristics but course is insidious in the beginning
e. HCV now tested on all blood donors

D. Signs and symptoms: (early symptoms of HAV may be more severe)
1. Fever and chills
2. Headache

3. Respiratory symptoms
4. Anorexia
5. Nausea and vomiting
6. Liver tenderness
7. Jaundice and itching
8. Elevated liver enzymes
9. Elevated prothrombin time (PT) values
10. Elevated bilirubin levels
11. Presence of HAV in feces and serum
12. Presence of the hepatitis surface antigen HBsAg
13. Clay-colored stools and dark-colored urine

E. Diagnostic tests/methods
1. Patient history and physical examination
2. Laboratory studies: hepatitis-associated antigen (HAA); liver profile
3. Stool examination
4. Urinary bilirubin and urobilinogen
5. Liver biopsy
6. Serum ammonia levels-protein is restricted if ammonia levels are elevated.

F. Treatment
1. Monitor liver function studies
2. Bed rest with bathroom privileges
3. High-calorie, high-carbohydrate, high-protein, moderate-fat diet
4. Topical lotions to alleviate dry, itchy skin
5. Hydration with IV therapy
6. Administration of vitamin K preparations
7. Monitor for bleeding tendencies and progression of the illness
8. Blood and body fluid precautions
9. Passive immunity

G. Nursing intervention
1. Assess and document signs and symptoms and reactions to treatments
2. Monitor skin, stool, and urine color
3. Promote balanced activity and rest periods
4. Maintain blood and body fluid precautions
5. Monitor IV therapy
6. Assess intake and output
7. Monitor vital signs at least q4h
8. Provide and encourage the prescribed diet
9. Support the patient and family
10. Administer prescribed medication and monitor for side effects
11. Monitor for bleeding tendencies
12. Educate patient and family concerning drug therapy, the prescribed diet, activity level, and monitoring for complications

CIRRHOSIS

A. Definition: cell degeneration occurring in the liver wherever scar tissue replaces normally functioning tissue
B. Cirrhosis is a complication of alcoholism, hepatitis, biliary disease, and certain metabolic disorders
C. Whatever the cause of the liver destruction, the course of cirrhosis is the same
1. Liver parenchyma dies and regenerates, and fibrous tissue (scarring) occurs
2. This alteration in structure progresses in the liver, causing problems in hepatic blood flow and normal liver function; in time the liver fails

D. Major complications of cirrhosis
1. Portal hypertension: hypertension resulting from the obstruction of normal blood flow through the portal system; the obstruction is caused by changes in the liver from the cirrhotic process
2. Esophageal varices (see esophageal varices)
3. Ascites: the accumulation of fluid in the peritoneal or abdominal cavity, which is a later symptom in cirrhosis
4. Hepatic coma (encephalopathy): a condition of advanced liver disease; blood enters the general circulation without being properly detoxified by the liver

E. Signs and symptoms
1. Headache
2. Nausea and vomiting
3. Weight loss
4. Anorexia
5. Jaundice
6. Abdominal pain
7. Fatigue and weakness
8. Liver enlargement and fibrosis
9. Bleeding disorders caused by disruption in the manufacture of vitamin K-dependent factors
10. Edema
11. Telangiectasis (blood vessels develop a spiderlike appearance)
12. Ascites
13. Esophageal varices
14. Hepatic coma

F. Diagnostic tests/methods
1. Patient history and physical examination
2. Laboratory studies to assess liver function
3. Liver scan
4. Liver biopsy

G. Treatment
1. Rest with activity as tolerated
2. Nutritious diet with protein level determined by liver functioning
3. If ascites is present, restrict fluid and sodium, monitor weight, and monitor intake and output
4. Monitor for complications such as ascites, esophageal varices, and hepatic coma
5. Drug therapy to reduce ammonia levels, prevent bleeding, reduce edema, and provide comfort

H. Nursing intervention
1. Assess and document signs and symptoms and reactions to treatments
2. Administer prescribed medication and monitor for side effects
3. Provide and encourage the prescribed diet
4. Promote comfort
5. Monitor vital signs at least q4h and report abnormalities
6. Monitor status of ascites
   a. Record weight
   b. Assess measurements of extremities and abnormal girth
   c. Monitor intake and output
7. Provide planned exercise and rest periods
8. Assist patient with activities of daily living
9. Monitor skin status and take measures to prevent skin breakdown

10. Protect against infection
11. Provide diversional activity
12. Offer emotional support
13. Provide ongoing assessment for evidence of hepatic encephalopathy
    a. Monitor for symptoms of lethargy, confusion, twitching, tremors, sweetish breath odor, fever, and increasing somnolence
    b. Eliminate dietary protein
    c. Administer prescribed drugs and enemas to reduce ammonia levels
    d. Monitor IV fluids
    e. Give narcotics and sedatives cautiously
14. Also see care of patient with esophageal varices at the beginning of this section
15. Educate patient and family concerning home-bound care

PANCREATITIS

A. Definition: an acute or chronic inflammation of the pancreas
B. Pancreatitis is associated with biliary disease, infections, drug toxicity, nutritional deficiencies, and ingestion of alcohol
C. The digestive enzymes of the pancreas are released into the pancreatic tissue, causing inflammation
   1. As the condition progresses, ischemia, duct obstruction, and necrosis may occur
   2. Bleeding occurs if tissue necrosis affects vessels
   3. Pancreatic abscesses may occur if bacteria invade the necrotic tissue
   4. In chronic pancreatitis the tissue becomes fibrotic and normal function is compromised
D. Signs and symptoms
   1. Acute pancreatitis
      a. Epigastric pain that radiates to the back
      b. Eating tends to aggravate pain
      c. Patient may assume a side-lying position with knees bent for comfort
      d. Nausea and vomiting
      e. Low-grade fever
      f. Hypotension
      g. Tachycardia
      h. Jaundice
      i. Elevated WBC count
      j. Shock: if there is blood vessel or tissue erosion
   2. Chronic pancreatitis
      a. Abdominal pain
      b. Weight loss
      c. Steatorrhea (foul-smelling, foamy stool)
      d. Diabetes mellitus if beta cell function is affected
E. Diagnostic tests/methods
   1. Patient history and physical examination
   2. Laboratory tests, particularly electrolytes, amylase, lipase, and liver enzymes
   3. Pancreatic scan and sonography
   4. Visualization of the pancreatic duct (endoscopy)
   5. X-ray studies
F. Treatment
   1. Control of pain
   2. Hydration with IV fluids

3. Correction of any bleeding
4. Nasogastric tube and NPO to reduce pancreatic secretions
5. Drug therapy: analgesics, antibiotics, steroids, vitamins, and pancreatic extracts
6. Diet that does not stimulate pancreatic secretions
7. Control of blood glucose levels if beta cells are affected
G. Nursing intervention
   1. Assess and document signs and symptoms and reactions to treatments
   2. Administer prescribed medication and monitor for side effects
   3. Provide the prescribed diet
   4. Explain dietary restrictions to patient
   5. Monitor vital signs at least q4h
   6. Monitor IV therapy
   7. Promote comfort and relieve pain
   8. Provide emotional support
   9. Assess intake and output
   10. Relieve nausea and vomiting if present
   11. Note color, character, and amount of urine and stool
   12. Monitor jaundice if present
   13. Monitor the nasogastric tube and secretions
   14. Educate patient and family concerning drug therapy, diet and dietary restrictions, avoidance of alcohol, monitoring steatorrhea, blood glucose monitoring (glucometer), and compliance with the regimen

CANCER OF THE PANCREAS

A. Cancer of the pancreas can affect any portion of the pancreas, including the beta cells; metastasis readily occurs to adjacent structures
B. Cancerous tissue impairs normal pancreatic function, primarily by causing obstruction and hindering the flow of pancreatic secretions
C. Signs and symptoms
   1. Early symptoms may be vague
      a. Nausea and vomiting
      b. Anorexia
      c. Weight loss
      d. Weakness and fatigue
   2. Later symptoms
      a. Pain
      b. Jaundice
      c. Diabetes mellitus
D. Diagnostic tests/methods
   1. Patient history and physical examination
   2. Laboratory studies
   3. Pancreatic scan and sonography
   4. X-ray studies
   5. Visualization of the pancreatic duct
E. Treatment
   1. Supportive therapy
   2. Surgical excision: Whipple's procedure may be performed removing the head of the pancreas, lower portion of the common bile duct, distal portion of the stomach, and the duodenum
   3. Palliative surgery: to restore bile and pancreatic output
   4. Chemotherapy
F. Nursing intervention: see cancer of the stomach

APPENDICITIS

A. Definition: inflammation of the appendix
B. Signs and symptoms
   1. Right lower-quadrant pain
   2. Nausea and vomiting
   3. Anorexia
   4. Fever
   5. Elevated WBC count
C. Diagnostic tests/methods
   1. Patient history and physical examination
   2. Laboratory tests, particularly a WBC count
D. Treatment
   1. Supportive therapy
   2. Immediate surgical removal (appendectomy)
E. Nursing intervention
   1. Assess and document signs and symptoms and reactions to treatments
   2. Monitor IV fluids
   3. Provide comfort measures such as an ice pack to the abdomen and analgesia
   4. Administer prescribed drugs and monitor for side effects
   5. Monitor vital signs as ordered
   6. Encourage progressive ambulation after surgery
   7. Monitor the dressing and operative site after surgery
   8. Educate patient and family concerning drug therapy, activity restrictions, and care of the operative site

PERITONITIS

A. Definition: infection and subsequent inflammation of the peritoneal membrane by trauma or bacterial invasion
B. The inflammation may be localized or widespread and may affect the organs of the abdominal cavity; adhesions, abscesses, and obstructions may occur
C. Signs and symptoms
   1. Nausea and vomiting
   2. Abdominal pain
   3. Abdominal rigidity and distention
   4. Fever
   5. Paralytic ileus
   6. Fluid and electrolyte imbalance
   7. Elevated WBC count
   8. Constipation; diarrhea
D. Diagnostic tests/methods
   1. Patient history and physical examination
   2. Laboratory tests including a WBC count, electrolytes, and blood cultures
E. Treatment
   1. Identification of the causative agent
   2. Intestinal decompression
   3. Hydration with IV therapy
   4. Pain control
   5. Drug therapy: analgesics and antibiotics
   6. Monitoring vital signs
   7. Monitoring intake and output
   8. Controlling the spread of infection
F. Nursing intervention
   1. Assess and document signs and symptoms and reactions to treatment
   2. Assess vital signs every 1 to 2 hours during the acute period

3. Monitor intake and output
4. Administer prescribed medication and monitor for side effects
5. Provide comfort and relief of pain
6. Assess bowel sounds
7. Maintain NPO during the acute period
8. Maintain nasogastric tube and monitor output during the acute period
9. Support patient and allay anxieties
10. Place patient in semi-Fowler's position
11. Have patient turn, cough, and deep breathe at least q2h

HERNIA

A. Definition: a protrusion of an organ or structure through the muscle wall of the containing cavity
B. Hernias may occur around the umbilical area, inguinal area, diaphragm, femoral ring, and at the site of an incision
C. Hernias are categorized as
   1. Reducible: can be returned to the normal position
   2. Irreducible: cannot be returned to the normal position
   3. Incarcerated: obstruction of intestinal flow
   4. Strangulated: blood supply is cut off (occluded)—surgical emergency
D. Causes
   1. Congenital weakness in the containing wall
   2. Weakness in containing wall is related to straining and the aging process
   3. Trauma
   4. Increased intraabdominal pressure (obesity or pregnancy)
E. Signs and symptoms
   1. Protrusion of a structure without symptoms
   2. Appearance of a protrusion when straining or lifting
   3. In certain instances there may be pain
   4. If the intestine is obstructed, there may be distention, pain, nausea, and vomiting
F. Diagnostic methods: patient history and physical examination
G. Treatment
   1. Surgery is the treatment of choice
      a. Herniorrhaphy: surgical repair of the hernia
      b. Hernioplasty: the surgical reinforcement of the weakened area
   2. Use of a truss (a support worn over the hernia to keep it in place)
H. Nursing intervention
   1. Assess and document signs and symptoms and reactions to treatments
   2. Assess vital signs every shift before surgery
   3. Report any symptoms of coughing, sneezing, or upper respiratory tract infection noted before surgery because this will weaken the surgical repair
   4. Apply ice packs as ordered to control pain and swelling
   5. Monitor voidings following inguinal hernia repair
   6. Educate patient and family concerning care of the operative site, activity restrictions, and avoidance of constipation

NEUROLOGIC SYSTEM
Anatomy and Physiology

The nervous system acts as a coordinated unit both structurally and functionally

A. Functions
1. Regulates system; responsible for coordinating body functions and responding to changes in or stimuli from the internal and external environment
2. Controls communication among body parts
3. Coordinates activities of body system

B. Divisions
1. Central nervous system (CNS): brain and spinal cord; interprets incoming sensory information and sends out instruction based on past experiences
2. Peripheral nervous system (PNS): cranial and spinal nerves extending out from brain and spinal cord; carry impulses to and from brain and spinal cord
3. Autonomic nervous system: functional classification of the PNS; regulates involuntary activities
4. Somatic nervous system: functional classification of the PNS; allows conscious or voluntary control of skeletal muscles

C. Structure and physiology
1. Neurons or nerve cells: respond to a stimulus, connect it into a nerve impulse (irritability), and transmit the impulse to neurons, muscle, or glands (conductivity), consists of three main parts
   a. Cell body: contains nucleus and one or more fibers or processes extending from cell body
   b. Dendrites: conduct impulses toward cell body; neuron has many dendrites
   c. Axons: conduct impulses away from cell body; neuron has one axon

2. Types of neurons
   a. Motor (efferent): conduct impulses from CNS to muscle and glands
   b. Sensory (afferent): conduct impulses toward CNS
   c. Connecting (interneuron): conduct impulses from sensory to motor neurons
3. Synapse: chemical transmission of impulses from axon to dendrites
4. Myelin sheath: protects and insulates the axon fibers; increases the rate of transmission of nerve impulses
5. Neurilemma: sheath covering the myelin; found in PNS; function is regeneration of nerve fiber
6. Neuroglia: connective or supporting tissue, important in reaction of nervous system to injury or infection
7. Ganglia: clusters of nerve cells outside CNS
8. White matter: bundles of myelinated nerve fibers; conducts impulses along fibers
9. Gray matter: clusters of neuron cell bodies; fibers not covered with myelin; distributes impulses across selected synapses

D. Central nervous system
1. Brain (Fig. 5-12)
   a. Cerebrum: largest part of brain; outer layer called cerebral cortex; cortex composed of dendrites and cell bodies; controls mental processes; highest level of functioning (Table 5-3)
   b. Cerebellum: controls muscle tone coordination and maintains equilibrium
   c. Diencephalon: consists of two major structures located between cerebrum and midbrain
      (1) Hypothalamus: regulates the autonomic nervous system; controls blood pressure; helps maintain

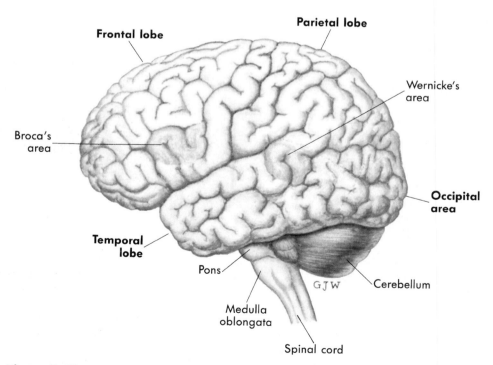

Figure 5-12   Lateral view of the brain. (From Chipps E, Clanin N, Campbell V: *Neurological disorders*, St Louis, 1992, Mosby.)

normal body temperature and appetite; controls water balance and sleep
  (2) Thalamus acts as a relay station for incoming and outgoing nerve impulses; produces emotions of pleasantness and unpleasantness associated with sensations
 d. Brainstem: connects the cerebrum with the spinal cord
  (1) Midbrain: relay center for eye and ear reflexes

TABLE 5-3   Specific Functions of Cerebral Cortexes

Frontal cortex	Conceptualization Abstraction Judgment formation Motor ability Ability to write words Higher level centers for autonomic functions
Parietal cortex	Highest integrative and coordinating center for perception and interpretation of sensory information Ability to recognize body parts Left versus right Motor movement
Temporal cortex	Memory storage Auditory integration Hearing
Occipital cortex	Visual center Understanding of written material

From Phipps WJ, Sands JK, Marek JR: *Medical-surgical nursing: concepts and clinical practice,* ed 6, St Louis, 1999, Mosby.

  (2) Pons: connecting link between cerebellum and rest of nervous system
  (3) Medulla oblongata: contains center for respiration, heart rate, and vasomotor activity
2. Spinal cord
 a. Inner column composed of gray matter, shaped like an H, made up of dendrites and cell bodies; outer part composed of white matter, made up of bundles of axons called tracts
 b. Function: sensory tract conducts impulses to brain; motor tract conducts impulses from brain; center for all spinal cord reflexes
3. Protection for CNS
 a. Bone: vertebrae surround cord; skull surrounds brain
 b. Meninges: three connective tissue membranes that cover brain and spinal cord
  (1) Dura mater: white fibrous tissue; outer layer
  (2) Arachnoid: delicate membrane, middle layer; contains subarachnoid fluid
  (3) Pia mater: inner layer, contains blood vessels
 c. Spaces
  (1) Epidural between dura mater and the vertebrae
  (2) Subdural space: between dura mater and arachnoid
  (3) Subarachnoid space: between arachnoid and pia mater, contains cerebrospinal fluid
 d. Cerebrospinal fluid: acts as a shock absorber; aids in exchange of nutrients and waste materials
E. Peripheral nervous system
1. Carries voluntary and involuntary impulses
2. Cranial nerves (Table 5-4)
3. Spinal nerves: 31 pairs; conduct impulses necessary for sensation and voluntary movement; each group named for the corresponding part of the spinal column

TABLE 5-4   Cranial Nerves

Cranial Nerves		Conducts Impulses	Function
I	Olfactory	From nose to brain	Sense of smell
II	Optic	From eye to brain	Vision
III	Oculomotor	From brain to eye and eye muscles	Contraction of upper eyelid; maintain position of eyelid; pupillary reflexes
IV	Tochlear	From brain to external eye muscles	Eye movements
V	Trigeminal	From skin and mucous membranes of head and teeth to chewing muscles	Sensations of head and teeth; muscles of chewing
VI	Abducens	From brain to external eye muscles	Eye movements
VII	Facial	From taste buds of the tongue and facial muscles to muscles of facial expression	Taste; facial expression
VIII	Acoustic	From organ of Corti to brain	Hearing
	Vestibular branch	From semicircular canals to brain	Balance
IX	Glossopharyngeal	From pharynx and posterior to third of tongue to brain; also from brain to throat muscles and salivary glands	Sensations of tastes, sensations of pharynx; swallowing; secretion of saliva
X	Vagus	From throat and organs in thoracic and abdominal cavities to brain; to muscles of throat and abdominal cavities	Important in swallowing, speaking, peristalsis, and production of gastric juices
XI	Accessory	From brain to shoulder and neck muscles	Rotation of head and raising shoulders
XII	Hypoglossal	From brain to muscles of tongue	Movement of tongue

F. Autonomic nervous system
1. Part of PNS; controls smooth muscle, cardiac muscle, and glands
2. Two divisions
   a. Sympathetic: "fight or flight" response; increases heart rate and blood pressure; dilates pupils
   b. Parasympathetic: dominates control under normal conditions; maintains homeostasis

NEUROLOGICAL CONDITIONS AND DISORDERS

Pathology of the central nervous system (CNS) arises from injuries, new growths, vascular insufficiency, infections, and as complications secondary to other diseases. Patient problems are related to interference with normal functioning of the affected tissue.

The following terms are used in describing the patient with a neurological impairment.

anesthesia: complete loss of sensation

aphasia: loss of ability to use language

auditory/receptive aphasia: loss of ability to understand

expressive aphasia: loss of ability to use spoken or written word

ataxia: uncoordinated movements

coma: state of profound unconsciousness

convulsion: involuntary contractions and relaxation of muscle

delirium: mental state characterized by restlessness and disorientation

diplopia: double vision

dyskinesia: difficulty in voluntary movement

flaccid: without tone, limp

neuralgia: intermittent, intense pain along the course of a nerve

neuritis: inflammation of a nerve or nerves

nuchal rigidity: stiff neck

nystagmus: involuntary, rapid movements of the eyeball

papilledema: swelling of optic nerve head

paresthesia: abnormal sensation without obvious cause, with numbness and tingling

spastic: convulsive muscular contraction

stupor: state of impaired consciousness with brief response only to vigorous and repeated stimulation

tic: spasmodic, involuntary twitching of a muscle

vertigo: dizziness

Nursing Assessment

A. Nursing observations
1. Mental status: drowsiness or lethargy, ability to follow commands
2. Level of consciousness (LOC): ability to be aroused in response to verbal and physical stimuli; ranges from awake and alert to "coma"; Glasgow Coma Scale (Table 5-5) is the usual guide for assessing and describing the degree of conscious impairment, based on three determinants:
   a. Eye opening
   b. Motor response
   c. Verbal response
3. Orientation
   a. Time: knows month or year
   b. Place: has general knowledge of where patient is (e.g., hospital)
   c. Person: knows own name; able to name relative or friend
4. Behavior: is it appropriate for the situation

TABLE 5-5   Glasgow Coma Scale

	Stimuli	Score
Eyes open	Spontaneously	4
	To speech	3
	To pain	2
	None	1
Best verbal response	Oriented	5
	Confused	4
	Inappropriate words	3
	Incomprehensible	2
	None	1
Best motor response	Obeys commands	5
	Localizes to pain	4
	Flexes to pain	3
	Extends arm to pain	2
	None	1

Adapted from Phipps WJ, Sands JK, March JR: *Medical-surgical nursing: concepts and clinical practice,* ed 6, St Louis, 1999, Mosby.

5. Emotional response: is it appropriate for the situation
6. Memory: capability for early and recent recall, remote, recent, and new learning ability
7. Speech: presence of aphasia, appropriate speech, words distinct or slurred, quality, rate, loudness, fluency
8. Vital signs: temperature, pulse, respirations, and blood pressure; note pulse pressure
9. Ability to follow simple directions
10. Eyes
    a. Pupillary reaction to light: the pupils are periodically assessed with a flashlight to evaluate and compare size, configuration, and reaction. Differences between both eyes and from previous assessments are compared for similarities and differences
    b. Movement of lids and pupils
11. Motor function: coordination, gait, balance, posture, strength, functioning, muscle tone
12. Bladder and bowel control
13. Ears for drainage (may indicate CSF leak)
14. Facial expression for symmetry
15. Sensation for
    a. Pain
    b. Light touch, pressure
    c. Smell
16. Rancho Los Amigos Scale: A scale of cognitive functioning that was developed to aid in assessment and treatment after traumatic brain injury (TBI)
    a. No response: patient is completely unresponsive to any stimuli
    b. Generalized response: reacts inconsistently and nonpurposefully to stimuli
    c. Localized response: reacts specifically yet inconsistently to stimuli
    d. Confused-agitated: in agitated state yet has decreased ability to process information
    e. Confused-inappropriate: appears alert, able to respond to simple commands fairly consistently
    f. Confused-appropriate: has goal-directed behaviors, needs cues

g. Automatic-appropriate: oriented, does daily routine, has shallow recall of actions
h. Purpose-appropriate; aware and oriented, able to recall and integrate past and recent events
17. Grooming, personal hygiene
18. Thoughts, perceptions, attention span
B. Patient description (subjective data)
1. History of head injury, loss of consciousness, vertigo, weakness, headache, sleep problems, paralysis, seizures, or diplopia
2. Complains of pain, numbness, problems with elimination, memory loss, difficulty concentrating, drowsiness, or visual problems
3. Medications taken
C. History from family
1. Medical
2. Activities of daily living (ADLs)
3. Behavior

Diagnostic Tests/Methods

A. Computerized tomography (CT; CAT scan): computer analysis of tissues as X-rays pass through them; has replaced many of the usual tests; no special preparation or care after test
B. Lumbar puncture (spinal tap)
1. Description: under local anesthesia a puncture is made at the junction of the third and fourth lumbar vertebrae to obtain a specimen of cerebrospinal fluid; cerebrospinal fluid pressure can be measured; this procedure is also used to inject medications (e.g., spinal anesthesia) and in diagnostic X-ray examination to inject air or dye (e.g., myelogram)
2. Nursing intervention
a. Monitor vital signs
b. Keep patient supine 4 to 8 hours
c. Observe for headache and nuchal rigidity
d. Monitor site for leakage
C. Cerebral angiography
1. Description: intraarterial injection of radiopaque dye to obtain an X-ray film of cerebrovascular circulation
2. Nursing intervention after procedure
a. Related to dye: observe for allergic reaction: urticaria, decreased urinary output, respiratory distress, and difficulty swallowing; have tracheostomy set available
b. Related to injection site
(1) Provide ice pack and bed rest
(2) Monitor vital signs
(3) Observe for pain, tenderness, bleeding, temperature, color
D. Electroencephalography (EEG)
1. Description: electrodes are placed on unshaven scalp with tiny needles and electrode jelly
2. Nursing intervention
a. Anticipate patient's fears about electrocution; do not give stimulants/depressants before test
b. No smoking or caffeinated beverages; patient needs to eat a full meal before the test; fasting may cause hypoglycemia and alter brain waves
c. Stress need for restful sleep before test; sleep deprivation may cause abnormal brain waves
d. Wash hair and scalp after procedure to remove jelly
e. Patient may resume all previous activities

E. Brain scan
1. Description: after an IV injection of a radioisotope, abnormal brain tissue will absorb more rapidly than normal tissue; this can be detected with a Geiger counter to diagnose brain tumors
2. Nursing intervention
a. No observations
b. Patient may resume all previous activities
F. Magnetic resonance imaging (MRI)
1. Description: MRI uses a combination of radio waves and a strong magnetic field to view soft tissue (does not use X-rays or dyes); produces a computerized picture that depicts soft tissues in high-contrast color
2. Nursing intervention
a. Before the procedure, instruct the patient to remain perfectly still in the narrow cylinder-shaped machine
b. Inform the patient that there will be no pain or discomfort, but there is no room for movement during the MRI
c. No specific care or observations are necessary after the procedure
G. Myelography (MEG)
1. Description: injection of a radiopaque dye into the subarachnoid space via a lumbar puncture; performed to locate lesions of the spinal column or ruptured vertebral disk
2. Types of agents used: metrizamide and Pantopaque; if metrizamide is used, the patient should not take phenothiazines, tricyclic antidepressants, CNS stimulants, or amphetamines for 24 to 48 hours before test; after the procedure is completed, pantopaque dye is removed; leaving it in would cause meningeal irritation; metrizamide is water soluble and does not need to be removed
3. After procedure with pantopaque, the patient lies flat in bed for 6 to 8 hours; after procedure with metrizamide patient's head must be elevated 30 to 50 degrees for 6 to 8 hours; fluids are encouraged; common side effects include nausea, vomiting, and possibly seizures; check with physician when medications withheld prior to test may be given; with both types of agents observe site for leakage of CSF; strength and sensation in lower extremities should be assessed; encourage fluids; maintain bed rest; monitor vital signs; observe for headache, pain, and dizziness
H. Positron emission tomography (PET scan)
1. The patient inhales or is injected with a radioactive substance
2. The computer can diagnose and determine level of functioning of an organ
3. Exposure to radiation is minimal and no special care is indicated
I. Skull X-ray examination: no preparation; no nursing care or observations indicated afterward

Frequent Patient Problems and Nursing Care

A. Impaired physical mobility related to progression of primary disease
1. Give specific care and perform assessment as required (see Chapter 2)
2. Perform neurological assessment every 2 to 4 hours

3. Initiate nursing care measures to prevent complications of immobility
4. Use of assistive devices

B. Risk for injury/infection related to "fixed eyes" (no blinking)
   1. Protect with eye shields
   2. If needed remove dried exudate with warm saline solution and mineral oil
   3. Close eyes
   4. Inspect for inflammation

C. Ineffective breathing pattern related to neuromuscular impairment
   1. Maintain patent airway, suction as needed, and elevate head 20 to 30 degrees
   2. Have tracheostomy set available
   3. Provide oxygen with humidity
   4. Monitor vital signs q2h
   5. Provide oral hygiene q2h
   6. Lubricate lips

D. Risk for alteration in body temperature related to neuromuscular impairment
   1. Assess rectal temperature q2h
   2. Use external heating and cooling, (e.g., hypo-hyperthermia machine)

E. Risk for aspiration related to neuromuscular impairment
   1. Maintain NPO
   2. Position patient on side; turn q2h
   3. Provide nasogastric tube feedings
   4. Monitor IV fluids

F. Risk for injury related to restlessness, involuntary motions, or seizures
   1. Maintain safety (e.g., padded side rails, bed in low position)
   2. Follow precautions, care, and observations for a patient with seizures (see convulsive disorders, pp. 245-246)

G. Altered patterns of urinary elimination related to neuromuscular impairment
   1. Oliguria (urinary retention)
      a. Provide indwelling catheter care
      b. Monitor intake and output qh
   2. Incontinence
      a. Wash, dry, and inspect skin as needed
      b. Implement measures to prevent skin breakdown
      c. Implement bladder training

H. Bowel incontinence/constipation related to neuromuscular impairment
   1. Incontinence
      a. Wash, dry, and inspect skin as needed
      b. Implement measures to prevent skin breakdown
      c. Implement bowel training
   2. Constipation
      a. Record bowel movements
      b. Provide stool softeners, laxatives, and enemas as ordered
      c. Check for impaction; disimpact as needed
      d. Encourage fluids as tolerated
      e. Encourage activity as tolerated
      f. Increase fiber in the diet

I. Fear/anxiety related to pain; complications; surgery; possible disfigurement, disability, or dependency; fatal prognosis
   1. Explain everything (actions) carefully

2. Encourage patient to express feelings
3. Report to health team
4. Involve family/significant others in care

J. Other possible patient problems include
   1. Self-care deficit: perform own ADLs related to sensory-motor impairments
   2. Altered nutrition: less than body requirements related to dysphagia and fatigue
   3. Grieving related to actual/perceived loss and/or uncertain future
   4. Impaired swallowing related to chewing difficulties, muscle paralysis
   5. Activity intolerance related to fatigue and difficulty in performing ADLs
   6. Fatigue related to weakness, spasticity, fear of injury, and stressors
   7. Risk for social isolation related to spasticity, change in body image
   8. Risk for injury related to visual field, motor, or perception deficits
   9. Altered family processes related to physiological deficits, role disturbances, uncertain future
   10. Sensory-perceptual alterations specifically related to hypoxia secondary to trauma, progression of disease process
   11. Impaired communication related to dysarthria and/or aphasia secondary to physiological changes
   12. Risk for fluid volume deficit related to vomiting secondary to increased intracranial pressure (IICP)

SPECIAL SITUATIONS

A. The patient in coma
   1. Unconscious state in which the patient is unresponsive to verbal or painful stimuli; this occurs with many primary diseases; the patient depends on the nurse for maintenance of all basic human needs, nourishment, bathing, elimination, respiration, prevention of complications, and assessment and provision of care for problems (see the preceding section)
   2. Nursing intervention
      a. Include family in nursing care and care planning as much as possible
      b. Note level of consciousness (LOC) (see nursing assessment of the neurological patient) every 15 minutes if LOC decreases; assess every 1, 2, or 4 hours as LOC improves
      c. Demonstrate respect in patient's presence
      d. Provide a quiet, restful environment
      e. Speak to patient; use proper name; introduce self, and explain all care before starting
      f. Provide privacy

B. The patient with paralysis
   1. Paraplegia: paralysis of the lower extremities from sudden injury (e.g., automobile accident) or progressive degenerative disease (e.g., multiple sclerosis) to the spinal cord; there may be no motion or sensory function or reflexes; there may be uncontrollable muscle spasms; perspiration ceases and then becomes profuse; there is a loss of bladder and bowel control; sexual dysfunction, anxiety, fear, depression, anger, and embarrassment are major patient problems; patient may be totally dependent

2. Quadriplegia (tetraplegia): paralysis of all four extremities from sudden injury (e.g., diving accident) or progressive degenerative disease (e.g., amyotrophic lateral sclerosis [ALS]); symptoms and patient problems include those encountered with paraplegia, as well as autonomic dysreflexia
3. Nursing intervention
   a. Take measures to prevent complications of immobility
   b. Provide bowel and bladder training
   c. Prevent deformity: maintain joint mobility and correct alignment
   d. Encourage fluid intake
   e. Provide high-protein diet
   f. Encourage independence according to ability
   g. Communicate and work closely with the physiatrist, physical therapist, occupational therapist, and other members of the rehabilitation team
   h. Include family in nursing care and planning

Major Medical Diagnoses
INCREASED INTRACRANIAL PRESSURE (IICP)

A. Description: fluid accumulation or a lesion takes up space in the cranial cavity, producing IICP; the brain is gradually compressed, or life-sustaining functions cease; may be sudden or progress slowly
B. Causes: tumors, hematoma, edema from trauma, and abscesses from infections
C. Signs and symptoms: related to primary diagnosis
   1. Headache, restlessness, and anxiety
   2. Vomiting: recurrent, projectile, and not related to nausea or meals
   3. Change in pupil response to light
   4. Seizures
   5. Respiratory difficulty: irregular, Cheyne-Stokes, or Kussmaul breathing
   6. Blood pressure elevates, with wide pulse pressure
   7. Pulse increases at first then slows to 40 to 60 beats/min, regular and strong
   8. Altered LOC: becomes lethargic, speech slows, becomes confused, and shows decreased level of response
   9. Visual disturbances: diplopia and blurred vision
   10. Progressive weakness or paralysis
   11. Loss of consciousness, coma, and death
D. Diagnostic tests/methods: neurological assessment by physician and nurse
E. Treatment: depends on cause
   1. Surgical intervention (craniotomy)
   2. Steroids, anticonvulsants, mannitol, dexamethasone (Decadron), or urea to decrease edema
F. Nursing intervention
   1. Elevate head to semi-Fowler's position; never place in Trendelenburg position
   2. Monitor vital signs every 15 minutes
   3. Prevent aspiration; place patient on side
   4. Maintain airway; O_2 therapy as necessary
   5. Observe pupillary response (usually unequal and may not react to light)
   6. Report any change in LOC immediately
   7. Provide special care and observation when a patient has a seizure
   8. Provide care and safety for an unconscious patient
   9. Monitor IV fluids closely to prevent overhydration

CONVULSIVE DISORDERS

A. Description: frequently a convulsion or seizure is not a disease but a symptom of a neurological disorder; epilepsy is a disease characterized by a disposition for seizures; the following are types of seizures
   1. Generalized or grand mal: there may be a premonition or sign (aura); the individual cries out, loses consciousness, and enters a tonic phase (the body is rigid, and the jaw is clenched); then there is a clonic phase, with jerking movements of muscles, cessation of respirations, and fecal and urinary incontinence; lasts 1 to 2 minutes followed by a short period of unresponsiveness
   2. Partial or petit mal: loss of consciousness that lasts 5 to 30 seconds, during which time normal activities may or may not cease; there may be amnesia concerning this time
   3. Jacksonian (motor): a focal seizure that may be limited to jerky movements of one extremity; may precede a grand mal seizure
B. International Classification of Epileptic Seizures (Box 5-6)
C. Causes
   1. May be secondary to another condition: cerebrovascular accident (CVA), head injury, brain tumor, markedly elevated temperature, toxins, or electrolyte imbalance
   2. Epilepsy may have no known cause; onset usually is in childhood, before 30 years of age
D. Patient problems
   1. Related to primary disease
   2. Fear of injury
   3. Anxiety related to a chronic disease
   4. Embarrassment
   5. Fear of public rejection
   6. Side effects of drug therapy
E. Diagnostic tests/methods
   1. Specific tests to identify lesions
   2. EEG, CT scan, MRI, and brain mapping
   3. Serum chemistries
F. Treatment
   1. Treat and remove cause, if known
   2. Anticonvulsant drugs (see Chapter 3)
   3. Surgery-stereotactic (electrical stimulation to locate and resect [destroy] epileptogenic focus)

Box 5-6 International Classification of Epileptic Seizures

Partial (focal) seizures (consciousness may not be impaired): with motor symptoms, with special sensory symptoms, with autonomic symptoms, with psychic symptoms. May become complex partial seizures. May evolve to generalized seizures.

Generalized seizures (involve the entire brain; consciousness is lost): may last from several seconds to minutes. Types: absence seizures, tonic-clonic seizures, atonic seizures

Unclassified seizures: unable to classify because of incomplete or inadequate data

G. Nursing intervention
1. Provide accurate observation and documentation including: aura, time of onset, whether seizure is generalized or focal, specific parts of body involved, progression of seizure; duration of seizure, eye movement, loss of consciousness, loss of bowel and bladder control, condition after seizure, memory loss, weakness, and any injury caused by seizure
2. Encourage patient to wear medical identification tag
3. Have suction available
4. Secure airway for easy accessibility
5. During generalized (grand mal) seizure
   a. Insert airway between teeth before seizure (do not force)
   b. Maintain airway
   c. Prevent head injury
   d. Place patient on side if possible
   e. Protect extremities from injury by guiding movements
   f. Do not restrain
   g. Loosen clothing
   h. Remove pillows
   i. Maintain safety until fully conscious

TRANSIENT ISCHEMIC ATTACKS (TIAs)

A. Definition: altered cerebral tissue perfusion related to a temporary neurological disturbance
1. Manifested by sudden loss of motor or sensory function
2. Lasts for a few minutes to a few hours
3. Caused by a temporarily diminished blood supply to an area of the brain
4. Patient is at high risk for developing a stroke
B. Medical management is indicated (control of hypertension, low-sodium diet, possible anticoagulant therapy, stop smoking)
C. Nursing care would include close observation and assessment; specific care based on treatment

CEREBROVASCULAR ACCIDENT (CVA, STROKE) AND CEREBROVASCULAR DISRUPTIONS

A. Description: decreased blood supply to a part of the brain caused by rupture, occlusion, or stenosis of the blood vessels; onset may be sudden or gradual; symptoms and patient problems depend on location and size of area of brain with reduced or absent blood supply (left CVA results in right-sided involvement often associated with speech problems; right CVA results in left-sided involvement often associated with safety/judgment problems)
B. Causes: increased incidence with aging
1. Atherosclerosis
2. Embolism
3. Thrombosis
4. Hemorrhage from a ruptured cerebral aneurysm
5. Hypertension
C. Signs and symptoms
1. Subjective
   a. Change in mental status: decreased attention span, decreased ability to think and reason, difficulty following simple directions
   b. Headaches
2. Objective
   a. Altered level of consciousness

b. Communication: motor or sensory aphasia, difficulty reading, writing, speaking, or understanding
c. Bowel or bladder dysfunction: retention, impaction, or incontinence
d. Seizures
e. Limited motor function: paralysis, dysphagia, weakness, hemiplegia, loss of function, or contractures
f. Loss of sensation/perception
g. Loss of temperature regulation and elevated temperature, pulse, and blood pressure
h. Absent gag reflex (aspiration)
i. Unusual emotional responses: depression, anxiety, anger, verbal outbursts, and crying; emotional lability
j. Problems related to immobility (see Chapter 2)
D. Diagnostic tests/methods
1. Physical assessment and patient or family history
2. EEG, CT scan, lumbar puncture, cerebral angiography, or carotid ultrasonography, Doppler flow studies
E. Treatment
1. Remove cause, prevent complications, and maintain function; rehabilitation to restore function
2. Provide antihypertensives, anticoagulants, antiplatelet aggregation, antifibrinolytics, and stool softeners (see Chapter 3)
3. Surgical removal of clot, repair of aneurysm, carotid endarterectomy, balloon angioplasty, stents
F. Nursing intervention
1. Maintain bed rest; provide complete care; use turning sheet, foot board, firm mattress, pillows; and trochanter rolls to maintain proper body alignment; anticipate needs and leave things within reach (e.g., call bell)
2. Reposition patient q2h; provide passive and active ROM exercises; place patient in chair as soon as allowed; use flotation mattress or sheepskin
3. Provide bath, inspect, and provide nursing measures to prevent decubitus ulcers
4. Provide oxygen with humidity; have patient cough and take deep breaths q2h if possible; maintain airway; suction as needed; prevent aspiration; keep head turned to side; place in semi-Fowler's position
5. Ensure adequate nutrition and fluid and electrolyte balance; provide nasogastric/gastrostomy tube feeding; maintain IV fluids; provide soft diet when tolerated; use total parenteral nutrition (TPN); aspiration precautions
6. Establish means of communication: call bell, pad and pencil, and nonverbal gestures; use simple commands; speak slowly, explain all care; provide speech therapy
7. Be nonjudgmental about personality changes; encourage family participation; provide diversional activities; praise accomplishments realistically
8. Assess LOC; maintain safety in environment; use side rails; restrain only as necessary
9. Observe for IICP
10. Monitor vital signs q4h
11. Ensure elimination; check bowel sounds; monitor bowel movements; monitor intake and output; provide indwelling catheter care; then conduct bowel and bladder training
12. Provide care, safety, and precautions for a patient with seizures

13. Provide support for family
14. Schedule physical and occupational therapy as soon as possible
15. Provide nursing measures to prevent complications of immobility (see Chapter 2)
16. Encourage self-care

BRAIN TUMOR

A. Definition: a benign or malignant growth that grows and exerts pressure on vital centers of the brain, depressing function and causing increased pressure
B. Cause: unknown
C. Signs and symptoms: individual, depending on location and size
   1. Personality changes, fear, and anxiety
   2. Headaches, dizziness, and visual disturbance (e.g., double vision)
   3. Seizures
   4. Pituitary dysfunction
   5. Signs of IICP
   6. Local paresthesia or anesthesia
   7. Aphasia
   8. Problems with coordination, gait
D. Diagnostic tests/methods
   1. Patient history and physical examination
   2. Neurological assessment including EEG, CT scan, angiography, MRI, PET scan
E. Treatment: surgical removal if possible (craniotomy), frequently combined with radiotherapy and chemotherapy
F. Nursing intervention
   1. Perform timely neurological assessment and documentation
   2. Provide safety and assist with care as needed
   3. Be nonjudgmental about personality changes; encourage the patient to express feelings
   4. Provide postoperative care
      a. Anticipate and provide care as needed to maintain airway
      b. Provide safety and observation during a seizure
      c. Regulate body temperature
      d. Position on unoperated side
      e. Elevate head only under medical order
      f. Inspect dressing every 30 minutes for hemorrhage or drainage (leakage of cerebrospinal fluid)
      g. Make neurological assessment qh until patient is stable and then q4h; observe for IICP
      h. Provide care for the patient in coma as indicated earlier in this section

HEAD INJURIES

A. Definition: trauma to scalp, skull, or brain; a fracture to the skull may result, either a simple break in the bone or bone fragmentation that penetrates the brain tissue; can also cause hemorrhage, concussion, or contusion
   1. Cerebral concussion: injury to the head; patient may be dazed or unconscious for a few minutes; some functions (e.g., memory) may be impaired for as long as several weeks
   2. Cerebral contusion: head injury causing bruising of brain tissue; person experiences stupor, confusion, or loss of consciousness; if severe, may go into coma
   3. Cerebral laceration: a break in continuity of brain tissue

B. Cause: blow to the head (e.g., from a fall or automobile accident)
C. Signs and symptoms: individual, according to location and extent of blow
   1. Nausea and vomiting, dizziness, vertigo
   2. Lethargy: increasing loss of consciousness to impending coma
   3. Disorientation
   4. Drainage of cerebrospinal fluid from ear or nose (Battle's sign)
   5. Convulsions
   6. Problems related to IICP
D. Diagnostic tests/methods
   1. Patient history and physical/neurological assessment
   2. X-ray examination
   3. Angiography, Doppler studies
   4. CT scan, MRI
   5. PET
E. Treatment
   1. Anticonvulsants, corticosteroids, mannitol—if cerebral edema
   2. Maintenance of fluid balance
   3. Surgery
F. Nursing intervention
   1. Provide care as discussed for a patient with IICP (see p. 245)
   2. Neurological assessment qh
   3. Maintain airway
   4. Give care as required for the unconscious patient if necessary
   5. Take precautions for a patient with seizures
   6. Observe for serous or bloody discharge from ears/nose

MULTIPLE SCLEROSIS

A. Description: a chronic, progressive disease of the brain and spinal cord; lesions cause degeneration of the myelin sheath and interfere with conduction of motor nerve impulses; there are periods of remissions and exacerbations; onset occurs in young adults; it has an unpredictable progression
B. Cause: unknown, exacerbates with stress
C. Signs and symptoms vary with individual
   1. Ataxia
   2. Paresthesia, numbness, tingling
   3. Weakness and loss of muscle tone, fatigue
   4. Loss of sense of position
   5. Vertigo
   6. Blurred vision, diplopia, nystagmus, patchy blindness that may progress to total blindness
   7. Inappropriate emotions: euphoria/apathy/depression
   8. Dysphagia
   9. Slurred speech
   10. Bladder and bowel dysfunction: incontinence or retention
   11. Sexual dysfunction: impotence, diminished sensation
   12. Spasticity as disease progresses
D. Diagnostic tests/methods
   1. Patient history and physical/neurological assessment
   2. CT Scan
   3. MRI
   4. Examination of cerebrospinal fluid (CSF)
   5. PET scan
   6. Evoked responses

E. Treatment: symptomatic; corticosteroids during acute exacerbations

F. Nursing intervention
1. Provide care to prevent complications of immobility (see Chapter 2)
2. Encourage patient to maintain independence
3. Encourage patient to participate in care plan
4. Encourage high-caloric, high-vitamin, high-protein diet; provide nutrition that can be swallowed easily
5. Provide bowel and bladder training (may have indwelling catheter)
6. Provide diversional activities
7. Provide safety
8. Allow time for patients to express concerns about disabilities and dependencies: be supportive
9. Avoid precipitating factors that cause exacerbations (fatigue, cold, heat, infections, stress)
10. Patient/family education

PARKINSON'S DISEASE

A. Definition: a progressive, degenerative disease causing destruction of nerve cells in the basal ganglia of the brain caused by a deficiency of dopamine; limbs become rigid, fingers have characteristic pill-rolling movement, and head has to-and-fro movement; the patient has a bent position and walks in short, shuffling steps; facial expression becomes blank with wide eyes and infrequent blinking (Parkinson's mask); intelligence is not affected

B. Cause: unknown

C. Signs and symptoms
1. Tremor
2. Voluntary movement is slow and difficult; coordination is poor (ataxia)
3. Impaired chewing and eating; excessive salivation and drooling
4. Speech is slow and patient is soft spoken; written communication is difficult
5. Excessive sweating
6. Emotional changes: depression, paranoia, and eventually confusion
7. Dependency
8. Results of diagnostic tests
9. Side effects of drugs
10. Autonomic manifestations, such as urinary incontinence, constipation, hypotension

D. Diagnostic tests/methods
1. Patient history and physical assessment
2. Neurological assessment, CSF, CT scan

E. Treatment: many patients respond to drug therapy, and the disease is controlled with medication for the remainder of their lives; others have no response, and the disease progresses to a state of invalidism and immobility (usually treated with a combination of drugs) (see Chapter 3); surgeries: stereotaxic, fetal dopamine transplant, adrenal medullary transplant

F. Nursing intervention
1. Encourage patient to maintain independence as much as possible in hygiene and dressing; include patient in planning all aspects of care as much as possible
2. Encourage participation in previous work and social and diversional activities (avoid social withdrawal)
3. Help patient avoid embarrassment while eating; use straws, wipe drooling saliva, use bib, and keep cloth-

ing clean; use utensils with large handles for easy grip
4. Recommend a soft diet or one of a consistency the patient is able to chew
5. Provide diversion (activity therapy)
6. Encourage daily exercises as tolerated, especially walking; take safety measures
7. Encourage patient to avoid fatigue
8. Help patient to avoid frustration; emphasize capabilities rather than limitations
9. Reinforce speech, physical, and occupational therapy treatment protocols
10. Administer stool softeners to avoid constipation
11. Provide bowel and bladder training
12. Be patient when patient is slow or clumsy
13. Establish a means of communication
14. Enhance cognitive skills (reorient frequently)
15. Prevent pneumonia; force fluids; turn patient when in bed and encourage patient to be out of bed as much as possible
16. Provide mouth care q4h
17. Encourage family participation in all aspects of rehabilitation

AMYOTROPHIC LATERAL SCLEROSIS (ALS)

A. Definition: also known as Lou Gehrig's disease, ALS is a degenerative disease that affects the upper or lower motor neurons of the brain, the spinal cord, or both

B. Cause: unknown; a genetic link or a slow-moving viral infection is suspect

C. Signs and symptoms
1. Fatigue, weight loss
2. Difficulty doing fine motor tasks (buttoning a shirt)
3. Progressive muscle weakness; muscle wasting; atrophy
4. Dysphagia (difficulty swallowing)
5. Dysarthria (difficult speech)
6. Tongue fasciculation (twitching)
7. Jaw clonus (involuntary tightening/relaxing of muscles)
8. Spasticity of flexor muscles
9. Respiratory difficulty
10. Involvement of upper/lower extremities; one side of body affected more than other (late in disease process)
11. No sensory loss; patient remains alert
12. Death usually occurs 5 to 10 years from onset; caused by respiratory or bulbar paralysis

D. Diagnostic tests/methods: no specific test is available to diagnose ALS; an electromyography (EMG) may be done initially to rule out other neuromuscular diseases

E. Treatment: symptomatic relief as disease progresses; surgery may be necessary to insert a gastrostomy tube during the latter stages of the disease

F. Nursing intervention
1. Provide care to prevent complications of immobility
2. Promote adequate nutrition; implement safety measures
3. Provide adequate rest periods; avoid hot baths or traveling in hot weather
4. Provide alternative means of communication
5. Prevent bowel and bladder problems with adequate diet; medications to prevent urinary tract infections/constipation; bowel and bladder training programs may be necessary
6. Promote skin integrity

7. Assist in maintaining activities of daily living
8. Assist in maintaining a clear airway; encourage use of a tucked chin position when eating or drinking; use of a suction machine; ventilator may be used for respiratory assist during latter stages of disease
9. Patient/family education
10. Facilitate coping/adjustment; be supportive and allow patient and family to express their concerns; refer to local support group

Spinal Cord Impairment

The vertebral column houses the spinal cord. A small cartilage disk acts as a cushion between the vertebrae. All sensory and motor nerves to the neck, trunk, and extremities branch out from the spinal cord. The degree of disability and patient problems is related to the part of the body controlled by the injured or diseased nerves. For herniated intervertebral disk, see musculoskeletal conditions.

SPINAL CORD LESION

A. Definition: a growth compressing the spinal cord; may be benign or malignant; interferes with nerve function
B. Cause: unknown
C. Signs and symptoms: individual, according to area involved
D. Diagnostic tests/methods
   1. Patient history
   2. Myelography, CT, MRI
   3. Neurological assessment
E. Treatment: surgical removal
F. Nursing intervention: see Care of a patient with a laminectomy, p. 192

SPINAL CORD INJURIES

A. Description: trauma to spinal cord may cause complete or partial severing of the spinal cord; if severing is complete, there is permanent paralysis of body parts below site of injury; when there is partial damage, edema may cause a temporary paralysis
B. Cause: accident (e.g., automobile, shooting, or diving)
C. Signs and symptoms: individual, according to level of spinal cord involved (signs of spinal shock)
   1. Respiratory distress
   2. Paralysis
D. Diagnostic tests/methods: physical examination
E. Treatment
   1. Immobilization: Crutchfield tongs, halo traction, back brace, or body cast
   2. Surgery, corticosteroids, mannitol
F. Nursing intervention
   1. See Care of a patient with paralysis, pp. 244-245; observe for complications of spinal shock
   2. Maintain airway and respiratory function
   3. See Emergency care of a patient with a spinal cord injury, Chapter 10, pp. 542-543

ENDOCRINE SYSTEM
Anatomy and Physiology

A. Classification and secretions
   1. Exocrine glands: have ducts (tubes); secretions carried to an external or internal surface of the body by ducts (e.g., lacrimal gland)
   2. Endocrine glands: ductless; secretions by glands (hormones) carried to body tissue by blood and lymph

B. Endocrine glands and hormones (Fig. 5-13 and Table 5-6)
   1. Pituitary: located at base of the brain in a saddle-like depression of the sphenoid bone at the base of brain; called the master gland, approximately the size of a grape; composed of two parts
      a. Anterior lobe: secretes many hormones
      b. Posterior lobe: secretes two hormones
   2. Thyroid: located in the neck inferior to the Adam's apple; easily palpated; the largest of the endocrine glands; consists of two lobes joined by a narrow band (isthmus)
   3. Parathyroid (four glands): located on posterior surface of the thyroid; regulates calcium level in the blood
   4. Adrenal
      a. Two small glands; curve over the top of the kidneys
      b. Each gland has two separate parts: inner area (medulla) and outer area (cortex); produces different hormones
      c. Medulla: mimics the action of the sympathetic nervous system
      d. Cortex: outer part of the adrenals: produces three major groups of steroid hormones
   5. Gonads (sex glands)
      a. Ovaries in female: located in pelvic cavity; produce ova and two hormones, estrogen and progesterone; do not function until puberty
      b. Testes in male: suspended in a sac called the scrotum outside the pelvic cavity; produce sperm and sex hormone, testosterone
   6. Islets of Langerhans: located within the pancreas; consist of alpha and beta cells
      a. Alpha cells: produce glucagon
      b. Beta cells: secrete hormone insulin
   7. Pineal: lies just above midbrain; secretes melatonin, which inhibits gonadotropic hormone (GTH) secretion; exact function in man unclear
C. Functions: regulators of body functions
   1. Growth and development
   2. Reproduction
   3. Metabolism
   4. Fluid and electrolyte balance

ENDOCRINE SYSTEM CONDITIONS AND DISORDERS

The endocrine system is composed of numerous glands and hormones. These hormones are chemical messengers for other target glands or cells. A disturbance in one of the secreting glands may affect the regulation of another gland; therefore the patient may experience multiple problems and have varying needs. Some of the hormonal disturbances may affect patient appearance, personality, and stamina. Part of the nursing intervention is aimed at providing support and education for the patient and the family. Some patients must undergo lifelong hormonal therapy as the result of the endocrine disorder that affects them.

Nursing Assessment

A. Nursing observations
   1. General appearance
   2. Vital signs
   3. Weight

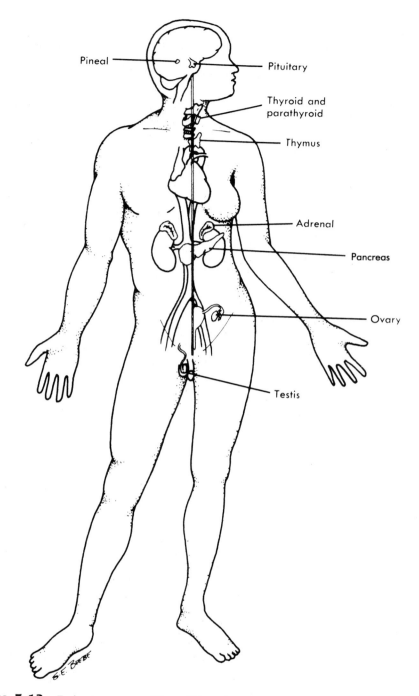

Figure 5-13 Endocrine system. (From Phipps WJ, Sands JK, Lehman MK, Cassmeyer VL: *Medical-surgical nursing: concepts and clinical practice*, ed 5, St Louis, 1995, Mosby.)

4. Skin
   a. Color
      (1) Pallor
      (2) Flushed
      (3) Yellow pigmentation
      (4) Bronze pigmentation
      (5) Purple striae over obese areas
   b. Temperature
   c. Dry
   d. Moist
   e. Excess diaphoresis
   f. Poor wound healing

5. Hair
   a. Dry
   b. Brittle
   c. Thin
6. Nails
   a. Dry
   b. Thin
   c. Thick
7. Musculoskeletal
   a. Muscle mass distribution
   b. Fat distribution
   c. Change in height

TABLE 5-6 Endocrine Glands, Hormones, and Actions

Endocrine Glands and Hormones	Actions of Hormones
Anterior Pituitary	
Corticotropin (andrenocorticotropic hormone [ACTH])	Stimulates the adrenal cortex to produce and secrete glucocorticoid hormones
Somatotropic hormone (STH)	Stimulates growth of body cells
Thyroid-stimulating hormone (TSH)	Stimulates the thyroid gland to produce and release thyroid hormone
Gonadotropic hormones (GTH)	Affect growth, maturity, and function of primary and secondary sex organs
Luteinizing hormone (LH)	
Follicle-stimulating hormone (FSH)	
Lactogenic hormone (prolactin)	
Posterior Pituitary	
Antidiuretic hormone (ADH)	Promotes sodium and water retention in the kidney; increases blood pressure
Oxytocin	Initiates and maintains labor; influences the breasts to release milk
Thyroid	
Thyroxine	Regulates the metabolic rate of all body cells
Pancreas	
Insulin	Promotes glucose use by the cell and decreases blood sugar level
Glucagon	Promotes glucose release from the liver and increases blood sugar level
Adrenal Cortex	
Glucocorticoids (includes cortisol and cortisone)	Assist the body to respond to stress; concerned with carbohydrate, fat, and protein metabolism; reduces inflammation
Mineralocorticoids (includes aldosterone)	Promote sodium and water retention in the kidney and potassium excretion
Sex hormones (androgens, estrogen, and progesterone)	Mainly affect development of secondary sex characteristics
Adrenal Medulla	
Epinephrine (adrenaline) and norepinephrine (noradrenaline)	Constrict blood vessels and channel the blood to vital internal organs to prepare the body for emergency situations
Ovaries	
Estrogen	Promotes development of female sex characteristics, growth of female sex organs, and development of the uterine wall for implantation of the fertilized ovum; regulates menstruation
Progesterone	Prepares the uterine wall for implantation of the fertilized ovum; maintains the placenta and pregnancy; regulates menstruation
Testes	
Androgens (includes testosterone)	Stimulates development of the secondary male sex characteristics; essential for normal functioning of male sex organs

    d. Changes in body proportions: enlarged ears, nose, jaws, hands, and feet
    e. Diminished muscle strength
  8. Central nervous system
    a. Personality changes
    b. Alterations in consciousness
      (1) Listlessness
      (2) Slowed cognitive ability
      (3) Stupor
      (4) Seizures
      (5) Confusion
      (6) Coma
    c. Slowed, hoarse speech
    d. Reflexes
      (1) Trousseau's sign
      (2) Chvostek's sign

  9. Eyes
    a. Periorbital edema
    b. Protruding eyeball (exophthalmos)
    c. Drooping eyelids (ptosis)
 10. Gastrointestinal system
    a. Anorexia
    b. Polyphagia
    c. Polydipsia
    d. Constipation
    e. Diarrhea
    f. Nausea and vomiting
 11. Cardiovascular system
    a. Hypertension
    b. Hypotension
    c. Tachycardia
    d. Bradycardia

12. Respiratory system
    a. Tachypnea
    b. Acetone breath
    c. Kussmaul-Kien respirations
13. Renal system
    a. Polyuria
    b. Oliguria
14. Reproductive system
    a. Menstrual disturbances
    b. Libido disturbances
    c. Galactorrhea (excess mammary gland secretion in females)
    d. Gynecomastia (increased breast tissue in males)
B. Patient description (subjective data)
    1. Pain
       a. Headache
       b. Skeletal pain
       c. Back pain
       d. Muscle spasms
    2. Appetite
       a. Anorexia
       b. Polyphagia
    3. Weakness
    4. Numbness
    5. Tingling
    6. Mood swings
    7. Nausea
    8. Intolerance to heat or cold
    9. Polydipsia
    10. Polyuria, nocturia, and dysuria
    11. Decreased libido and impotence
    12. Frequent infections

Diagnostic Tests/Methods

A. Serum laboratory studies
    1. Protein-bound iodine (PBI)
       a. The thyroid hormone, thyroxine, contains iodine that binds itself to blood proteins; therefore the function of the thyroid gland is evaluated by measuring the amount of this iodine
       b. Factors that may alter test findings
          (1) Ingestion of drugs or administration of dyes containing iodine
          (2) Mercurial diuretics or estrogen
          (3) Pregnancy
    2. Iodine 131 uptake (radioactive iodine thyroid uptake)
       a. Measures the amount of radioactive iodine that has concentrated in the thyroid gland after ingestion of the iodine preparation
       b. Test findings may be altered by recent ingestion of iodides or use of radiographic dyes
       c. A normal thyroid gland removes 15% to 50% of iodine from the bloodstream
    3. Basal metabolic rate (BMR): measures the amount of oxygen consumed by the body while the patient is in a state of complete mental and physical rest
    4. T_3 (triiodothyronine): measures thyroid function indirectly by evaluating whether radioactive triiodothyronine binds to a serum specimen
    5. T_4 (thyroxine): measures the amount of thyroxine in the circulation
    6. Thyroid-stimulating hormone (TSH) radioimmunoassay: indicator of thyroid-stimulating hormone production based on pituitary function; measures TSH levels
    7. Fasting blood sugar (FBS)
       a. Measures the amount of glucose in the bloodstream during a fasting period
       b. No food is permitted for 12 hours before the test
       c. Normal value: 80 to 120 mg/dl
    8. Postprandial blood sugar
       a. Evaluates the patient's ability to dispose of blood glucose after a meal
       b. Normal value: 80 to 120 mg/dl serum
    9. Glucose tolerance test (GTT)
       a. Determines patient response to a measured dose of glucose
       b. Normal value: blood glucose climbs to a peak of 140 mg/dl serum in the first hour and returns to normal by the second or third hour
    10. Serum potassium
        a. Measures the amount of K in the bloodstream
        b. Normal range: 3.5 to 5.0 mEq/L
    11. Serum sodium
        a. Measures the amount of Na in the bloodstream
        b. Normal range: 135 to 145 mEq/L
    12. Total serum calcium
        a. Measures the amount of Ca in the bloodstream
        b. Normal range: 4.8 to 5.2 mEq/L (9 to 11 mg/dl)
    13. Serum ketones: determines the amount of ketones produced by the metabolism of fat
    14. Blood pH
        a. Measures the acid-base status of the blood
        b. Normal arterial blood findings: pH 7.35 to 7.45
        c. Normal venous blood findings: pH 7.31 to 7.41
    15. Serum phosphorus: measures the amount of serum phosphorus in the bloodstream
    16. Adrenocorticotropic hormone (ACTH) stimulating test (or glucocorticoid-stimulating test)
        a. Evaluates the changes in adrenocortical function produced by the administration of ACTH
        b. ACTH is administered intramuscularly (IM) or intravenously (IV)
        c. For the IM methods a blood specimen is obtained 1 hour after the administration of ACTH
        d. For the IV method a 24-hour urine specimen is collected and analyzed
    17. Cortisone suppression test: used to differentiate between Cushing's syndrome and Cushing's disease
    18. Plasma cortisol
        a. Hormonal study of the adrenal cortex
        b. Low levels are seen in Addison's disease
        c. Elevated levels indicate Cushing's syndrome
    19. Plasma cortisol response to ACTH
        a. Hormonal study of the adrenal cortex
        b. Patient's blood specimen is drawn in a fasting state and examined for plasma cortisol levels
        c. Next ACTH is administered IM, and a second blood sample is withdrawn
        d. Rise in the plasma cortisol level in the second specimen is normal
    20. Urine 17-ketogenic steroids
        a. Measures adrenocortical function
        b. Urine specimen is collected for a 24-hour period and should be kept cold

B. Urine laboratory studies
   1. 24-hour quantitative sugar specimen
      a. Evaluation of the patient's glucose loss over a 24-hour period
      b. Normally the urine is free of sugar
      c. Nursing implications
         (1) Have the patient void and discard the specimen at the beginning of the 24-hour period
         (2) Save all urine voided in a container provided by the laboratory
         (3) At the end of the 24 hours, have the patient void again and save the specimen in the container
   2. Urine pH
      a. Measures the acid-base balance of the urine
      b. Normal range: pH 4.8 to 7.5
   3. Quantitative urinary calcium: measures the amount of Ca in a 24-hour urine specimen after a period of Ca deprivation
   4. Vanillylmandelic acid (VMA) test
      a. Determines the amount of urinary excretion of the end product of catecholamine metabolism
      b. Factors that may alter test findings
         (1) Ingestion of coffee, tea, chocolate, bananas, vanilla-containing food, or aspirin
         (2) Stress
C. Scans
   1. Thyroid scan: radionucleotide study of the thyroid to determine function
   2. CT scan: used to visualize cross sections of tissue

Frequent Patient Problems and Nursing Care

A. Self-esteem disturbance related to body image
   1. Observe the patient for loss of appetite, insomnia, disinterest in self, and unwillingness to discuss alteration in body image
   2. Encourage patient to express feelings
   3. Encourage communication with significant other
B. Altered nutrition, less than body requirements, related to noncompliance with therapeutic diet
   1. Observe the patient for diet intolerance such as refusal to eat, complaints of foods, and eating of foods that are contraindicated
   2. Explain to the patient and family the reason for and intended effect of therapeutic diet and necessity of maintaining it until discontinued by physician
   3. Instruct the patient and family on prescribed food selection
C. Knowledge deficit related to prescribed medication
   1. Explain to the patient and family the dosage and method of administering prescribed drugs
   2. Provide information about the purpose of the drug and potential side effects
   3. Describe symptoms that should be reported to the physician
   4. Explain where therapeutic supplies may be obtained
   5. Evaluate the patient's response to teaching
D. High risk for injury related to toxic effects of iodine preparations. Discontinue iodides if evidence of the following exists
   1. Swelling of buccal mucosa
   2. Excessive salivation
   3. Swelling of neck glands
   4. Skin eruptions
E. High risk for injury related to hypoglycemia
   1. Observe for complaints of headache, nervousness, hunger, dizziness, pallor, and sweating (diaphoresis)
   2. Assess vital signs
   3. Give quick-acting carbohydrate
      a. Orange juice
      b. Cola
      c. Granulated sugar
      d. Crackers
      e. Hard candy
   4. If patient is unconscious: give instant glucose (buccally); glucagon (SC); IV glucose
   5. Have laboratory withdraw serum specimen for glucose assessment
   6. Assess reason for reaction after situation has been controlled
      a. Length of time since last meal
      b. Correct amount of food eaten or meal omitted
      c. Correct dosage of insulin
      d. Kinds of activities or situation before reaction
F. High risk for injury (seizures) related to hypocalcemia
   1. Observe for complaints of numbness, tingling, cramping, or spastic movements of extremities
   2. Emergency treatment requires administration of IV calcium
   3. Prevent airway obstruction
      a. Keep airway (seizure stick) at bedside
      b. Provide suction machine at bedside
      c. Provide tracheostomy set at bedside
   4. Prevent injury by putting padding along side rails, easing patient to floor, or removing constrictive clothes
   5. Monitor and record vital signs
   6. Note frequency, time, level of consciousness, and length of seizure

Major Medical Diagnoses
HYPERPITUITARISM

A. Definition: overproduction of growth hormone by the anterior pituitary gland
B. Pathology
   1. Increased activity of the gland usually results from a secreting pituitary tumor
   2. Two major disorders arise from hypersecretion
      a. Gigantism: develops in children; hypersecretion before the growth plate closes, results in bone and tissue growth
      b. Acromegaly: a disorder in adults caused by hypersecretion after closure of the epiphyses of the long bones
C. Signs and symptoms
   1. Subjective
      a. Headache
      b. Visual disturbances
      c. Weakness
   2. Objective
      a. Coarse facial features: enlarged ears, nose, lips, tongue, and jaws
      b. Broad hands, fingers, and feet
      c. Palpable, enlarged visceral organs
      d. Disturbances in carbohydrate metabolism, menstruation, and libido

e. Gynecomastia in the male; galactorrhea in the female
f. Symmetrical bone overgrowth (gigantism)
g. Increased heights; 8 to 9 ft (gigantism)
D. Diagnostic tests/methods
1. X-ray studies of jaws, sinuses, hands, and feet
2. Changes in physical appearance
3. CT scan to identify tumor
4. Cerebral arteriography to identify tumor
5. Growth hormone assay
E. Treatment
1. Surgical intervention: hypophysectomy (excision of the pituitary gland); excision of tumor with laser
2. Irradiation of the pituitary gland
3. Medication to treat symptoms related to other hormonal disturbances as a result of hypersecretion
F. Nursing intervention
1. Assist the patient to accept altered body image emphasizing person's value as an individual
2. Explain the basis for altered sexual functioning
3. Emphasize need for lifelong medical follow-up
4. If the patient has undergone hypophysectomy
a. Follow nursing care as for the patient who has undergone intracranial surgery
b. Observe for potential postoperative complications
(1) Adrenal insufficiency
(2) Hypothyroidism
(3) Diabetes insipidus

HYPOPITUITARISM (SIMMONDS' DISEASE)

A. Definition: total absence of all pituitary secretions
B. Pathology: occurs after destruction of the pituitary gland by surgery, infection, injury, hemorrhage, or tumor
C. Signs and symptoms
1. Subjective
a. Lethargy
b. Loss of muscle strength
c. Weakness
d. Menstrual irregularities
2. Objective
a. Emaciation
b. Pallor
c. Dry, yellow skin
d. Diminished axillary and pubic hair
e. Decreased muscle size
f. Increased susceptibility to infection
D. Diagnostic tests/methods
1. T_3 and T_4
2. Urine 17-ketogenic steroids
E. Treatment
1. Replacement hormones
2. Surgical ablation if tumor is present in pituitary gland
F. Nursing intervention
1. Emphasize need for lifelong medical follow-up
2. Teach the patient self-administration of drug: purpose, proper dosage, and potential side effects
3. Follow nursing care as for the patient who has undergone intracranial surgery

HYPERTHYROIDISM (GRAVES' DISEASE AND THYROTOXICOSIS)

A. Definition: overactivity of the thyroid gland with hypersecretion of T_4

B. Pathology
1. Metabolic rate is increased, resulting in a high amount of energy and oxygen expenditure
2. May be caused by decreased production of thyroid-stimulating hormone (TSH) by malfunctioning pituitary gland, which results in high T_4 serum concentration
3. May be attributed to enlarged thyroid gland caused by decreased iodine intake
C. Signs and symptoms
1. Subjective
a. Polyphagia
b. Hyperexcitability/personality changes
c. Heat intolerance
d. Insomnia
e. Amenorrhea
f. Diarrhea/constipation
g. Increased appetite
h. Fatigue/weakness
2. Objective
a. Weight loss
b. Exophthalmos
c. Excessive sweating
d. Increased pulse rate
e. Fine hand tremors
f. Warm, flushed skin
g. Elevated blood pressure
h. Bruit over thyroid
D. Diagnostic tests: increased laboratory values of T_3, T_4, ^{131}I uptake, PBI, and BMR confirm hyperthyroidism; thyroid scan
E. Treatment
1. Medication to inhibit T_4 production
2. Radioactive iodine to destroy thyroid gland cells to decrease T_4 secretion
3. Drugs to control tachycardia and hyperexcitability
4. Subtotal or total thyroidectomy
F. Nursing intervention
1. Teach the patient and family signs and symptoms of hypothyroidism when patient is receiving thyroid-inhibiting drugs
a. Increased body weight
b. Sensitivity to cold
c. Fatigue
d. Dry skin, hair, and nails
e. Slow, hoarse speech
f. Constipation
2. Encourage adequate nutrition for increased energy expenditure
a. High-calorie, high-vitamin, and high-carbohydrate intake
b. Between-meal snacks
c. Increased fluid intake
d. Avoidance of caffeine
3. Plan undisturbed rest periods to restore energy: provide cool, quiet, nonstressful environment
4. Advise the patient to elevate the head of bed while recumbent to improve eye drainage
5. If the patient has undergone surgery
a. Place patient on back in a low-Fowler's or semi-Fowler's position to avoid strain on sutures
b. Observe dressing for hemorrhage or constriction of

the throat; examine back of neck for pooling of blood

    c. Keep tracheostomy set at bedside in event of respiratory obstruction caused by hemorrhage, edema of glottis, laryngeal nerve damage, or tetany

    d. Encourage patient to cough and expectorate secretions from throat and bronchi

    e. Observe for signs of thyroid storm (may occur as a result of gland manipulation during surgery): fever, tachycardia, and restlessness

    f. Observe for signs of tetany (may occur if parathyroids are accidentally removed); numbness and tingling around mouth, carpopedal spasms, convulsions

HYPOTHYROIDISM

A. Definition: absence or decreased production of T_4 by the thyroid gland

B. Pathology
1. The disorder causes a depression of metabolic activity, resulting in physical and mental sluggishness
2. There are three classifications of hypothyroidism
    a. Cretinism: total absence of T_4 from birth
    b. Hypothyroidism without myxedema: mild thyroid failure in older children and adults
    c. Hypothyroidism with myxedema: a severe form of gland failure in adults

C. Signs and symptoms
1. Subjective
    a. Lethargy
    b. Fatigues easily
    c. Cold intolerance
    d. Constipation
2. Objective
    a. Increased body weight with loss of appetite
    b. Coarse facial features
    c. Slow, hoarse speech
    d. Dry skin, hair, and nails
    e. Bradycardia
    f. Impaired memory
    g. Slowed thought process
    h. Personality changes

D. Diagnostic tests: decreased laboratory values of T_3, T_4, ^{131}I uptake, PBI, and BMR confirm hypothyroidism; thyroid scan

E. Treatment: thyroid-replacement drugs

F. Nursing intervention
1. Educate the patient on self-administration of drug: purpose, proper dosage, and potential side effects
2. Emphasize need for lifelong medical follow-up
3. Teach the patient and family signs and symptoms of hyperthyroidism when receiving thyroid-replacement drugs: chest pain, tachycardia, nervousness, headache, excessive sweating, heat intolerance, and weight loss
4. Encourage decreased caloric intake to avoid weight gain
5. Encourage application of emollients to soothe dry skin

HYPERPARATHYROIDISM

A. Definition: oversecretion of parathormone by the parathyroid gland(s)

B. Pathology
1. Results in calcium loss from the bones and an increased secretion of calcium and phosphorus by the kidneys

2. Usually the result of a parathyroid tumor

C. Signs and symptoms
1. Subjective
    a. Fatigue
    b. Thirst; poor appetite
    c. Nausea
    d. Back pain
    e. Skeletal pain
    f. Pain on weight bearing
    g. Constipation
    h. Visual disturbances
2. Objective
    a. Pathological features
    b. Vomiting
    c. Kidney stones composed of calcium phosphate

D. Diagnostic tests
1. Quantitative urinary calcium
2. Total serum calcium
3. Serum phosphorus
4. X-ray film to reveal skeletal changes

E. Treatment: surgical resection of parathyroid gland

F. Nursing intervention
1. Observe for postoperative conditions (refer to postoperative nursing intervention under diseases of the thyroid gland: hyperthyroidism)
2. Observe for tetany: tingling of hands and feet, facial muscle spasms, and muscle twitching
3. Protect from accidents: position carefully, keep bed low, keep side rails up, and assist to ambulate
4. Explain rationale for low-calcium, low-phosphorus diet
5. Encourage adequate hydration and dietary fiber to avoid constipation

HYPOPARATHYROIDISM

A. Definition: undersecretion of parathormone by the parathyroid glands

B. Pathology
1. Insufficiency of parathormone causes a decrease of the serum calcium level and slows bone resorption
2. Serum phosphorus value rises
3. Increased neuromuscular irritability results in tetany

C. Signs and symptoms
1. Subjective
    a. Lethargy
    b. Painful muscle spasms
    c. Tingling of hands and feet
    d. Visual disturbances
2. Objective
    a. Dry skin, hair, and nails
    b. Respiratory distress caused by laryngeal spasms
    c. Convulsions

D. Diagnostic tests/methods
1. Quantitative urinary calcium
2. Total serum calcium
3. Positive Trousseau's sign (spasms of fingers and hands after application of blood pressure cuff to arm)
4. Presence of Chvostek's sign (hyperactivity of facial muscle in response to tapping near the angle of the jaw)
5. X-ray studies reveal increased bone density

E. Treatment
1. Calcium replacement in chronic cases
2. Calcium gluconate IV for emergency treatment

3. Diet high in calcium and low in phosphorus
4. Vitamin D preparation
F. Nursing intervention
  1. Keep endotracheal tube and tracheostomy set at bedside at all times when caring for patients with acute tetany
  2. Promote rest with a quiet, calm, and low-lit environment
  3. Explain need for diet high in calcium but low in phosphorus: avoid milk, cheese, and egg yolks
  4. Emphasize importance of lifelong medical follow-up; serum calcium level should be assessed at least three times a year

DIABETES MELLITUS

A. Definition: insufficiency or absence of insulin production by pancreatic islets, creating a disturbance in carbohydrate metabolism as well as a deficiency in protein and fat conversion
B. Pathology
  1. Develops when there is a persistent deficiency of insulin
  2. May be caused by trauma, infection, or tumor of the pancreas or increased insulin requirements attributable to obesity, pregnancy, infection, or stress
  3. Those at risk: women over 40 years of age and individuals who are obese or who have a familial tendency to diabetes
  4. Two classifications
     a. Type I: insulin dependent diabetes mellitus (IDDM) (formerly juvenile diabetes): rapid onset with no production of insulin; affects children and adolescents; is controlled with insulin
     b. Type II: noninsulin-dependent diabetes mellitus (NIDDM) (formerly adult onset): gradual onset; may be controlled by diet, oral hypoglycemic drugs, or insulin injection
  5. Lack of insulin disrupts transportation of glucose into cells, and cells become energy exhausted; cells must use proteins and fats as a compensatory mechanism
  6. Blood sugar level becomes elevated because of lack of insulin in the cells
  7. Cellular dehydration occurs because blood sugar pulls water from the cells into the bloodstream
  8. Glucose builds up in urine, creating osmotic pull; kidneys cannot reabsorb water
C. Signs and symptoms
  1. Subjective
     a. Polyuria and nocturia
     b. Polydipsia
     c. Polyphasia
     d. Weakness
     e. Blurred vision
  2. Objective
     a. Hyperglycemia
     b. Glycosuria
     c. Polyuria
     d. Ketosis
     e. Weight loss
     f. Retarded wound healing
D. Diagnostic tests/methods
  1. Presence of polyuria, polydipsia, and polyphagia
  2. Family and medical history

3. Laboratory studies: FBS, postprandial blood sugar, GTT, and glycosylated hemoglobin
4. 24-hour urine quantitative sugar specimen
E. Treatment
  1. Drug therapy for hyperglycemia; refer to Chapter 3 for indicated nursing actions
  2. Therapeutic diet with controlled calories to correct and avoid obesity
     a. American Diabetes Association (ADA) food exchange list widely prescribed by physicians
     b. Identifies calorie intake of protein (15% to 20%), carbohydrates (50% to 60%), fats (no more than 30%)
F. Nursing intervention
  1. Assist patient in adjusting to condition: allow verbalization of feelings, offer reassurance, and give support at patient's own pace
  2. Emphasize need to comply with diet and eat meals at prescribed times
  3. Instruct the patient and family on signs of impending hypoglycemia: diaphoresis, pale, cold, and clammy skin, nervousness, hunger, mental confusion; give orange juice, sugar, or hard candy
  4. Encourage prompt treatment of minor injuries or irritation to skin
  5. Emphasize importance of continued medical follow-up, regular vision examinations, and foot care
  6. Patient teaching should include
     a. Self–blood-glucose-level monitoring
     b. Self-injection of insulin: selection of equipment, sites of injection, rationale for rotation, accurate withdrawal of insulin, injection technique, and peak action time of insulin
     c. How to use food substitution
     d. Instructions on foot care: hygiene, proper trimming of toenails, proper fit of shoes and stockings, and treatment of minor abrasions
     e. Relationship between exercise and blood glucose
  7. Instruction to patient and family on signs and symptoms of impending ketoacidosis: hot, dry, flushed skin, polydipsia, fruity odor of breath, nausea, and abdominal pain
  8. Administration of insulin by way of pump
     a. Method of needle insertion and filling of syringe
     b. Instruction on site rotation and needle change q48h
     c. Remove pump and cover needle and tubing for bathing

DIABETIC COMA (KETOACIDOSIS)

A. Definition: excess glucose and acid (ketones) in the bloodstream
B. Pathology
  1. A response to insufficient insulin levels
  2. Fats are mobilized for energy; fatty acids are rejected by muscles, resulting in buildup of acids in the bloodstream
  3. Body's buffer system becomes exhausted
C. Signs and symptoms
  1. Subjective
     a. Weakness
     b. Polydipsia

c. Abdominal pain
d. Nausea
e. Headache
f. Polyphagia
2. Objective
a. Hot, dry, flushed skin
b. Listlessness and drowsiness
c. Kussmaul's respirations
d. Sweet or acetone breath
e. Hypotension
f. Confusion
g. Polyuria
h. Nausea/vomiting
i. Coma
D. Diagnostic tests
1. Elevated serum glucose level
2. Elevated serum and urinary ketones
3. Lowered blood pH
E. Treatment
1. Insulin replacement
2. Correct electrolyte and pH imbalance
3. Fluid replacement
F. Nursing intervention
1. Give insulin as ordered; have another person check to prevent error
2. Monitor and record vital signs and intake and output
3. Test for glucose and acetone levels; record on diabetic flow sheet
4. Position patient with head of bed elevated 30 degrees
5. Maintain patent airway
6. Give oral care q4h and when required (prn); keep lips and mouth moist
7. Assess level of consciousness
8. Observe patient for signs of hypoglycemia: pale, cool, clammy skin, lethargy, and hypotension
9. Instruct patient and family on factors and signs of impending ketoacidosis
10. Explain importance of balance among diet, exercise, and insulin
11. Before discharge provide diabetic alert band or chain

HYPERGLYCEMIC HYPEROSMOLAR NONKETOTIC COMA (HHNC)

A. Definition: similar to ketoacidosis, but occurs in non–insulin-dependent diabetes mellitus (NIDDM); ketosis does not develop
B. Pathology: high serum glucose levels increase osmotic pressure; this leads to polyuria, and dehydration occurs at the cellular level
C. Signs and symptoms
1. Subjective
a. Polyuria
b. Polydipsia
c. Drowsiness
d. Confusion
2. Objective
a. Dry, hot skin
b. Flushed skin
c. Hyperglycemia
d. Glycosuria
e. Hypotension

D. Diagnostic tests (see ketoacidosis)
E. Treatment (see ketoacidosis)
F. Nursing intervention (see ketoacidosis)

HYPOGLYCEMIA (INSULIN SHOCK)

A. Definition: abnormally low level of glucose in the bloodstream
B. Pathology
1. Accelerated glucose is removed from the serum
2. May be caused by overproduction or overdosage of insulin
3. Omission of a meal or too little food eaten by a patient receiving insulin
4. Too much exercise without extra food; rapid onset
C. Signs and symptoms
1. Subjective
a. Hunger
b. Weakness
c. Visual disturbances
d. Tingling lips and tongue
e. Nervousness
2. Objective
a. Pale, moist skin
b. Tremors
c. Tachycardia
d. Hypotension
e. Muscle weakness
f. Disorientation
g. Coma
D. Diagnostic test: lowered serum glucose level
E. Treatment
1. Sweetened fluids or sugar given orally; oral glucose preparations
2. Glucagon SC or IM
3. Glucose IV
F. Nursing intervention
1. Give medications as ordered
2. Monitor and record vital signs and intake and output
3. Patient teaching should include
a. Always carry and ingest quick-acting carbohydrate when initial signs appear; fruit juices, sweetened sodas, granulated sugar, or hard candy
b. Prevent medication error by having another person check dosage
c. Record each administration of medication to avoid duplication
d. Always wear medical identification tag
e. Remember to eat a regular meal after raising glucose level to prevent a rebound effect

DIABETES INSIPIDUS

A. Definition: water metabolism disorder related to hyposecretion of antidiuretic hormone (ADH) by the posterior pituitary lobe
B. Pathology
1. Renal tubules are unable to reabsorb water, resulting in elimination of large amounts of water
2. Hyposecretion may occur in conjunction with lung cancer, head injuries, pituitary tumor, myxedema, or encephalitis

3. Other causes may result from malfunctioning, surgical removal, or atrophy of the pituitary gland

C. Signs and symptoms
  1. Subjective
    a. Polydipsia
    b. Polyuria
  2. Objective
    a. Signs of dehydration (loss of skin turgor, dry skin and mucous membranes, and cracked lips)
    b. Low specific gravity (sp gr) (1.001 to 1.006)
    c. Increased fluid intake (5 to 40 L/24 hr)
    d. Increased urine output (5 to 25 L/24 hr)
    e. Electrolyte imbalance

D. Diagnostic method: restriction of fluid intake to observe changes in urine volume and concentration

E. Treatment: vasopressin replacement

F. Nursing intervention
  1. Monitor and record intake and output
  2. Monitor specific gravity
  3. Weigh patient daily

PRIMARY HYPERALDOSTERONISM (CONN'S SYNDROME)

A. Definition: hypersecretion of aldosterone by the adrenal cortex

B. Pathology
  1. Usually caused by a tumor(s), which results in renal retention of sodium and excretion of potassium
  2. Leads to inability of kidneys to concentrate urine (acidify)

C. Signs and symptoms
  1. Subjective
    a. Headache
    b. Polyuria and polydipsia
    c. Paresthesia
  2. Objective
    a. Hypertension with postural hypotension
    b. Signs of kidney damage: flank pain, chills, fever, and increased frequency of voiding
    c. Low specific gravity

D. Diagnostic tests
  1. Low serum potassium level
  2. Elevated serum sodium value
  3. Elevated urinary aldosterone level
  4. Increased urine pH
  5. X-ray study reveals cardiac hypertrophy caused by chronic hypertension

E. Treatment: surgical removal of adrenal tumor

F. Nursing intervention
  1. Monitor and record blood pressure, specific gravity, and intake and output
  2. Identify and explain diet high in potassium and low in sodium
  3. Provide fluids to meet excessive thirst
  4. If the patient has undergone adrenalectomy
    a. Protect the patient from exposure to infections
    b. Follow general postoperative nursing actions
  5. Once patient is convalescent, teach the patient self-administration of drugs: purpose, proper dosage, and potential side effects
  6. Before discharge, obtain medical identification tag

CUSHING'S SYNDROME

A. Definition: hyperactivity of the adrenal cortex

B. Pathology
  1. Excessive cortisol is secreted
  2. Disorder results from abnormal growth of cortices or tumor to one of the glands
  3. May occur because of pituitary gland dysfunction, causing excessive production of adrenocorticotropic hormone (ACTH)

C. Signs and symptoms
  1. Subjective
    a. Weakness
    b. Bruises easily
    c. Amenorrhea
    d. Decreased libido
    e. Changes in secondary sex characteristics
  2. Objective
    a. Fat deposits to face, back of neck, and abdomen
    b. Decreased muscle mass on limbs
    c. Unusual growth of body hair
    d. Purple striae over obese areas
    e. Impaired wound healing
    f. Hypertension
    g. Mood lability

D. Diagnostic tests
  1. Increased plasma cortisol levels
  2. ACTH stimulating test
  3. Cortisone suppression test

E. Treatment
  1. Drugs to inhibit cortisol production
  2. Bilateral adrenalectomy
  3. Resection of pituitary gland
  4. Potassium supplements
  5. Diet with sodium restriction

F. Nursing intervention
  1. Assist patient in adjusting to altered body image
  2. Place in noninfectious environment
  3. Maintain diet low in calories, carbohydrates, and sodium and high in potassium
  4. Weigh patient daily
  5. Monitor glucose and acetone levels
  6. Follow general postoperative nursing actions if patient undergoes adrenalectomy
  7. Once the patient is convalescent, instruct on self-administration of replacement hormones and drugs: proper dosage, purpose, and potential side effects

ADDISON'S DISEASE

A. Definition: hypofunction of adrenal cortex

B. Pathology
  1. As a result of dysfunction, adrenal cortex shrinks and atrophies
  2. Disorder usually originates within itself or may result from destruction of the adrenal cortex
  3. Results in disturbances of sodium and potassium

C. Signs and symptoms
  1. Subjective
    a. Weakness and fatigue
    b. Anorexia and nausea
    c. Depression
    d. Diarrhea
    e. Abdominal pain

2. Objective
   a. Weight loss
   b. Hypotension
   c. Hypoglycemia
   d. Bronze or tan skin pigmentation
   e. Susceptibility to infection
   f. Dysrhythmias
D. Diagnostic tests
   1. 8-hour IV ACTH test
   2. Plasma cortisol response to ACTH
   3. Low serum sodium level
   4. High serum potassium level
E. Treatment
   1. Replacement of adrenal cortex hormones
   2. Restoration of sodium and potassium balance
   3. Diet high in sodium and low in potassium, with adequate fluids
F. Nursing intervention
   1. Monitor and record vital signs and intake and output
   2. Weigh patient daily
   3. Observe for sodium imbalance: increased body weight, pitting edema, puffy eyelids, coughing, and diaphoresis
   4. Observe for potassium imbalance: lethargy, flaccid muscles, anorexia, hypotension, and dysrhythmias
   5. Provide small, frequent feedings
   6. Observe for hypoglycemia: weakness, clammy skin, tremors, and mental confusion
   7. Before discharge, obtain medical identification tag
   8. Emphasize need for compliance to diet and medication regimen
   9. Observe for addisonian crisis (causes: stress, surgery, trauma, infection, withdrawal of medication): hypotension, asthenia, abdominal pain, confusion, shock, and vascular collapse
   10. Teach patient to avoid infections and stressful situations

PHEOCHROMOCYTOMA

A. Definition: hyperactivity of the adrenal medulla
B. Pathology: caused by tumor in adrenal medulla, resulting in increased secretion of epinephrine and norepinephrine
C. Signs and symptoms
   1. Subjective
      a. Headache
      b. Visual disturbances
      c. Nervousness
      d. Heat intolerance
   2. Objective
      a. Hypertension (blood pressure may be as high as 220/140)
      b. Orthostatic hypotension
      c. Tachycardia
      d. Hyperglycemia
      e. Blanching of skin
      f. Weight loss
      g. Dysrhythmias
      h. Diaphoresis
D. Diagnostic tests
   1. Chemical and pharmacological drug tests to differentiate from hypertension or hyperthyroidism
   2. X-ray studies to reveal adrenal medullary tumor

3. 24-hour urine collection for vanillylmandelic acid (VMA) and metanephrines
   4. Arteriography
   5. CT scan
   6. Intravenous pyelogram
E. Treatment
   1. Surgical excision of tumor
   2. Drugs to control hypertension and dysrhythmias
F. Nursing intervention
   1. Monitor blood pressure q4h and record
   2. Plan undisturbed rest periods: cool, quiet, nonstressful environment
   3. Encourage adequate hydration: record intake and output
   4. If patient undergoes adrenalectomy, follow general postoperative nursing actions: observe for adrenal crisis—falling blood pressure, tachycardia, elevated temperature, restlessness, convulsions, and coma
   5. Patient teaching should include
      a. Self-administration of medications: purpose, proper dosage, and potential side effects
      b. Signs of impending adrenal crisis
      c. Avoidance of exposure to infection; report symptoms of infections to physician
      d. Avoidance of stressful situations
      e. Emphasize need for adequate rest and good nutrition
   6. Provide medical identification tag

RENAL (URINARY) SYSTEM
Anatomy and Physiology

A. Organs (Figs. 5-14 and 5-15)
   1. Kidneys: bean shaped and reddish brown; lie against posterior abdominal wall; right kidney is slightly lower than the left
      a. External structure
         (1) Hilus: concave notch; blood vessels, nerves, lymphatic vessels, and ureters enter the kidneys at this point
         (2) Renal capsule; protective fibrous tissue surrounding kidneys
      b. Internal structure
         (1) Cortex: outer portion; the greater portion of the nephron is located here
         (2) Medulla: inner portion; consists of 12 cone-shaped structures (pyramids); tip of pyramid points toward renal pelvis and drains waste and excess water into pelvis
         (3) Pelvis: funnel shaped; forms upper end of ureter and receives waste and water
      c. Nephron: basic unit of function; microscopic structure composed of capillaries; approximately 1 million per kidney; control the processes of filtration, reabsorption, and secretion (Fig. 5-16)
         (1) Glomerulus: filtering unit; process of urine formation begins
         (2) Renal tubules: reabsorption occurs in the proximal convoluted tubules, through Henle's loops, and the distal convoluted tubules; then the collecting tubules pass the final urine product into the pelvis
   2. Ureters: two long, narrow tubes; transport urine from kidney to bladder by peristalsis

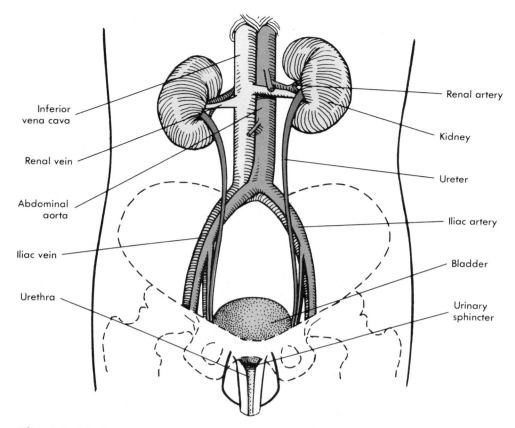

Figure 5-14 Organs and other structures of the urinary system. (From Phipps WJ, Sands JK, Lehman MK, Cassmeyer VL: *Medical-surgical nursing: concepts and clinical practice,* ed 5, St Louis, 1995, Mosby.)

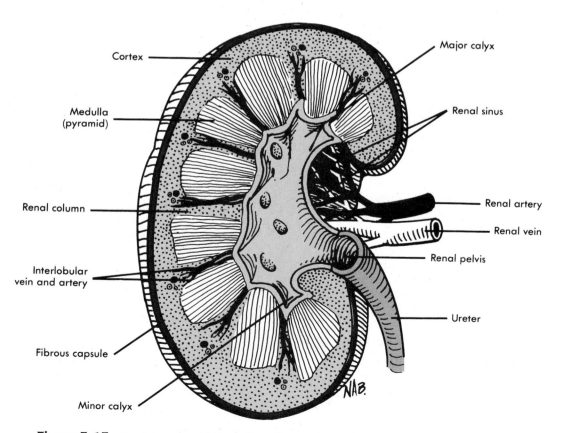

Figure 5-15 Frontal section of kidney. (From Phipps WJ, Sands JK, Lehman MK, Cassmeyer VL: *Medical-surgical nursing: concepts and clinical practice*, ed 5, St Louis, 1995, Mosby.)

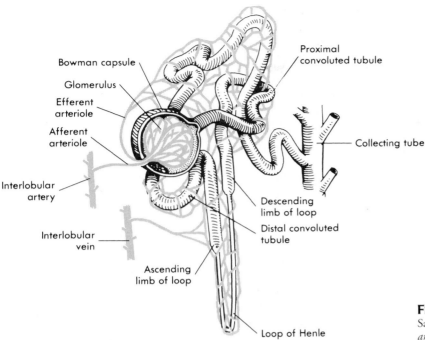

Bowman capsule
Glomerulus
Efferent arteriole
Afferent arteriole
Interlobular artery
Interlobular vein
Ascending limb of loop
Loop of Henle
Proximal convoluted tubule
Collecting tube
Descending limb of loop
Distal convoluted tubule

Figure 5-16 Nephron. (From Phipps WJ, Sands JK, Marek JR: *Medical-surgical nursing: concepts and clinical practice,* ed 6, St Louis, 1999, Mosby.)

3. Bladder: elastic, muscular organ, capable of expansion; stores urine; assists in voiding (micturition: the release of urine or voiding)
4. Urethra: narrow, short tube from bladder to exterior; exterior opening called the meatus
   a. Female: approximately 1¼ to 2 inches (3 to 5 cm) long; transports urine
   b. Male: approximately 8 inches (20 cm) long; transports urine and is a passageway for semen
B. Functions
   1. Excretion: nitrogen-containing waste (urea, uric acid, and creatinine) is excreted; normal daily output is 1200 to 1500 ml; primary function is to regulate the volume and composition of extracellular fluid
   2. Maintenance of water balance: absorbs more or less water depending on intake; normally, intake is approximately equal to output
   3. Other major functions include renin secretion and blood pressure control, erythropoietin production, vitamin D activation and acid-base balance
C. Urine composition
   1. Clear, yellowish, slightly aromatic, and slightly acid
   2. Contains 95% water and 5% solids, which includes urea, uric acid, creatinine, ammonia, sodium, and potassium; specific gravity (sp gr) indicates amount of the dissolved solids; normal range: 1.05 to 1.03 sp gr
   3. Abnormal substances: glucose, blood protein, RBC, bile, and bacteria

RENAL (URINARY) SYSTEM CONDITIONS AND DISORDERS

The urinary system regulates the composition and volume of the blood. It excretes metabolic wastes and fluids and maintains fluid and electrolyte balance and acid-base balance. Malfunction of this system has generalized effects on the body's normal physiology. Frequently patients are older and have chronic medical problems (e.g., cardiac); these must be considered when nursing care is planned (e.g., many diagnoses and procedures require additional fluids as a natural irrigation; increased fluids might be contraindicated in the patient with a cardiac condition). Problems of the male reproductive system are discussed in this section.

The following terms are used to describe urine output:
anuria: absence of urine output
bacteriuria: bacteria in the urine
costovertebral angle tenderness: examiner strikes one or more light blows to the area where the lower ribs meet the vertebrae (flank); tenderness in this area may indicate renal disorders
dribbling: voiding without stream, in small amounts, frequently or constantly
dysuria: painful or difficult urination
enuresis: involuntary voiding while asleep
frequency: voiding often and in small amounts
hematuria: blood in the urine
hesitancy: cannot immediately empty full bladder when the desire is present
hydronephrosis: dilation of the pelvis and calices of one or both kidneys, resulting from obstruction to the flow of urine
incontinence: partial or complete inability to control urine output
micturition: voiding, urination
nocturia: awakening to void
overflow incontinence: leakage of urine in small amounts while bladder remains full and distended
polyuria: excessive production and excretion of urine
residual urine: urine remaining in the bladder after voiding
retention: inability to excrete urine from bladder
urgency: an intense stimulus to void (may cause incontinence)
voiding: micturition, elimination of urine

Nursing Assessment

A. Nursing observations
   1. Observe bladder for distention: lower abdominal area

will be rigid, tense, swollen, and sensitive to the touch
2. Assess urine: amount, color, odor, opacity (clear or cloudy), presence of sediment, mucus, or clots
3. Check catheter (if indwelling) for drainage and meatus for irritation or secretions
4. Check genitals (scrotum, labia, and anal area) for irritation, rashes, and lesions
5. Monitor fluid and electrolyte balance
6. Check eyes, extremities, presacral area, and scrotum for edema
7. Monitor vital signs: note elevation of temperature and blood pressure
8. Note problems related to aging (i.e., urgency, stress incontinence)

B. Patient description (subjective data)
1. Change in voiding habits
2. Problems with elimination or changes in patterns of urination
    a. Frequency
    b. Nocturia
    c. Hesitancy of stream
    d. Urgency
    e. Retention
    f. Incontinence
    g. Enuresis
    h. Dribbling
3. Urethral discharge
4. Burning on voiding
5. Pain: suprapubic or flank

C. Obtain patient history regarding
1. Normal urinary and bowel elimination habits
2. Medical problems with the urinary system (e.g., stones or sexually transmitted diseases [STDs])
3. Medical problems with other body systems (i.e., cardiac); trauma
4. Medications
5. Diet
6. Food or medication allergies
7. Decreased urinary stream
8. Pain or spasms: what precipitated this and what relieved it
9. Discharge
10. Edema

Diagnostic Tests/Methods

A. Blood studies
1. Blood urea nitrogen (BUN): normal level 10 to 20 mg/dl; urea is an end product of protein metabolism and is excreted by the kidneys in urine; an increase indicates impaired renal function
2. Creatinine: normal level 0.5-1.3 mg/dl; elevation indicates decreased renal function
3. Acid and alkaline phosphatase: normal value varies with laboratory; increase may indicate metastasis to bone or liver from the kidney; nurse must assess for bone fracture or liver pathology
4. Albumin: globulin ratio is usually 2:1; a change indicates damage to nephron and loss of albumin in the urine; patient retains fluid and has edema

B. Urine studies
1. Routine urine: a single voided specimen to observe and compare to known normal specimens; results give information about renal function and systemic health

2. Specific gravity (sp gr): normal value 1.010 to 1.030; change indicates dehydration or inadequate kidney function; a single voided specimen is required
3. Urine culture and sensitivity (see Chapter 2)
4. Creatine: 24-hour urine collection to measure creatinine excreted; oral fluids are encouraged (see Chapter 2)

C. X-ray procedures, radiographic studies
1. Kidneys, ureter, bladder (KUB): an abdominal X-ray study that gives baseline information about size, shape, and placement of organs; flatus and stones are visualized; no preparation or care after procedure is required
2. Intravenous pyelogram (IVP): an IV injection of a radiopaque dye that is rapidly excreted by the kidney; this tests renal function, and the X-ray films outline renal pelvis, ureters, bladder, and urethra; nursing responsibilities: maintain NPO status before procedure; after procedure observe for allergic reaction to dye; note voiding
3. Retrograde pyelogram: visualization of upper genitourinary (GU) tract by injecting radiopaque dye through ureteral catheters to locate obstruction (e.g., stone or tumor); nursing implications: preparation is the same as for preoperative preparation (see Chapter 2); after procedure monitor vital signs, anticipate pain, and administer analgesics, note voiding, and observe urine
4. Cystoscopy: a direct visualization of the bladder and urethral orifices; a cystoscope is inserted through the urethra into the bladder; the bladder is distended with sterile solution; stones, tumors, and polyps can be diagnosed; urine can be observed entering the bladder from each ureter to evaluate renal function; instruments may be passed through the cystoscope to crush stones, take biopsy specimens, or pass catheters into ureters; nursing responsibilities: provide general preoperative and postoperative care (see Chapter 2); after procedure determine what was done during procedure; assess urinary function; observe urine; provide care and observation of a patient with indwelling catheter (see Chapter 2)
5. Renogram: also called renal angiogram; for pre and post procedure, see pyelogram
6. CT scan

D. Other procedures
1. MRI
2. Urodynamic studies

Frequent Patient Problems and Nursing Care

A. Incontinence (types: urge, total, stress, reflex, and functional) related to catheter use, infection, tissue damage, immobility
1. Minimize embarrassment; provide privacy
2. Wash, dry, and inspect skin and take measures to prevent decubitus ulcers (pressure sores)
3. Provide bladder training

B. Impaired skin integrity related to retention of metabolic wastes and resulting toxicity (uremia)
1. Urea is excreted through the skin, causing odor and pruritus: provide frequent and thorough skin care; wash and pat dry
2. Confusion and disorientation; may progress to state of unconsciousness and coma; provide all care; maintain safety (see comas)

3. Nausea and vomiting: provide mouth care q2h
4. Renal failure: see Nursing care for patient with chronic renal failure, pp. 267-268
C. Pain related to bladder spasms: bladder spasms caused by catheter irritation are intermittent in the suprapubic area, radiating to the urethra
   1. Assess type, location, and severity of pain
   2. Check catheter for obstruction; irrigate as ordered
   3. Administer medication as ordered (see Antispasmodics, Chapter 3)
   4. Reassure patient that spasms are not abnormal
D. Fluid volume deficit related to dehydration
   1. Use hydration methods (encourage fluids)
   2. Monitor intake and output
E. Risk for infection/injury (hematuria) related to surgery and/or pathogens
   1. Monitor signs and symptoms; vital signs
   2. Administer medication as ordered
   3. Note characteristics or urine at each voiding
   4. Encourage fluids if not contraindicated
   5. Report and document clots noted in urine
   6. Maintain patency and gravity drainage of catheters
   7. Assess for signs of anemia (weakness and fatigue)
   8. Provide nursing care and safety as indicated
   9. Reassure patient that blood-tinged urine is not unusual after instrumentation or surgery
F. Urinary retention related to surgery
   1. Take nursing measures to assist patient with voiding (see Chapter 2)
   2. Monitor intake and output
   3. Encourage fluids if not contraindicated
G. Anxiety related to sexual dysfunction, impending surgery, and/or possible change in body image and/or function
   1. Provide time to listen to patient express feelings
   2. Explain all care and procedures; reassure often
   3. Be honest; provide privacy; avoid embarrassing situations
   4. Praise patient's progress toward discharge goals
H. Potential fluid excess
   1. Assess deep skin (i.e., sacral, feet)
   2. Monitor lung sounds

Major Medical Diagnoses

CYSTITIS

A. Definition: inflammation of the bladder mucosa; is difficult to cure; recurs and may be chronic
B. Pathology: is usually a bacterial infection
   1. May be secondary to infection elsewhere in urinary system (e.g., urethritis)
   2. Contamination during catheterization or instrumentation
   3. An obstruction causing urinary stasis in the bladder (e.g., enlarged prostate or urethral stricture)
C. Signs and symptoms
   1. Subjective
     a. Burning, dysuria, urgency, frequency, nocturia, hematuria, and pyuria
     b. Low-back pain and bladder spasms
   2. Objective: elevation of temperature
D. Diagnostic tests/methods
   1. Patient history and assessment
   2. Urine culture, IVP, voiding cystoureterogram

E. Treatment: systemic medications, urinary antiseptics, antibiotics, sulfonamides, and antispasmodics (see Chapter 3)
F. Nursing intervention
   1. Encourage fluids: 3000 ml daily over that of dietary intake unless contraindicated
   2. Provide and supervise proper perineal care
   3. Provide diet that acidifies urine (e.g., cranberry juice)
   4. Monitor temperature and administer antipyretics as ordered
   5. Provide sitz baths
   6. Teach preventive measures
     a. Taking full course of antibiotic therapy as prescribed
     b. Empty bladder completely
     c. Maintain a consistent fluid intake of 2 liters per day
     d. Void after sexual intercourse

URETHRITIS

A. Definition: inflammation of the urethra; may develop scar tissue and stricture, causing obstruction, cystitis, and nephritis
B. Pathology
   1. Prostatitis; injury during instrumentation or catheterization
   2. Gonococcus infection; chlamydial infection
C. Signs and symptoms
   1. Subjective
     a. Urgency
     b. Frequency
     c. Dysuria
     d. Burning on urination
   2. Objective
     a. Purulent discharge
     b. Results of urine culture
D. Diagnostic tests/methods
   1. Patient history and physical examination
   2. Culture of discharge
E. Treatment
   1. Antibiotics
   2. Dilatation for stricture
F. Nursing intervention
   1. Sitz baths
   2. Demonstrate and supervise thorough hand washing
   3. Care of Foley catheter
   4. Avoid unnecessary catheterization and instrumentation

PYELONEPHRITIS

A. Definition: infection of the kidney; may be acute or become chronic; kidney becomes edematous, mucosa is inflamed, and multiple abscesses may form; the kidney will become fibrotic, and uremia may develop
B. Pathology
   1. Ascending infection from an infection lower in the GU tract
   2. Staphylococcal or streptococcal infection carried in the blood
C. Signs and symptoms
   1. Subjective
     a. Nausea
     b. Chills
     c. Dysuria, burning, frequency
     d. CVA tenderness

2. Objective
   a. Markedly elevated temperature (102° F to 105° F)
   b. Vomiting
   c. Pyuria, hematuria
   d. Increased WBC count
   e. Results of urine cultures and IVP
D. Diagnostic tests/methods
  1. Urine culture and sensitivity
  2. Patient history and physical examination
  3. IVP
E. Treatment: urinary antiseptics and specific antibiotics (see Chapter 3); follow-up care for at least 1 year
F. Nursing intervention
  1. Prevent dehydration: encourage fluids and maintain IV therapy
  2. Provide rest and conserve energy
  3. Prevent chill; keep skin dry and clean
  4. Provide mouth care q2h
  5. Provide soft diet
  6. Provide and assist with pericare; demonstrate proper technique and hand washing
  7. Anticipate pain: administer analgesics and local heat
  8. Administer antiemetic as needed
  9. Control temperature: administer antipyretics

CALCULI (LITHIASIS)

A. Definition: formation of stones in the urinary tract caused by deposits of crystalline substance that normally remain in solution and are excreted in the urine; may be found in the kidney, ureters, or bladder; vary in size from renal calculi that can be as large as an orange or as small as grains of sand; can obstruct urine flow, causing chronic infection, backflow, hydronephrosis, and gradual destruction of kidney; many small stones pass spontaneously
B. Cause
  1. Infection
  2. Urinary stasis
  3. Dehydration and concentration of urine
  4. Metabolic diseases (e.g., gout, hyperparathyroidism)
  5. Immobility (see Dangers of immobility, Chapter 2)
  6. Familial tendency
  7. Elevated uric acid
  8. Excessive calcium intake
C. Signs and symptoms
  1. Subjective
   a. Pain (can be extreme) radiates down flank to pubic area
   b. Frequency and urgency
  2. Objective
   a. Hematuria and pyuria
   b. Diaphoresis, nausea, vomiting, and pallor (related to pain)
   c. Results of diagnostic tests
D. Diagnostic tests/methods: X-ray studies—KUB, IVP; urine studies—ultrasonography, cystoscopy, serial blood calcium and phosphorus levels
E. Treatment: depends on location—stones are removed; normal urine production and elimination are restored; recurrence is prevented
  1. Cystoscopy and crushing of stones (lithotripsy)
  2. Dislodging ureteral stone by passing ureteral catheter; laser lithotripsy

3. Surgery to remove ureteral or kidney stone
   a. Pyelolithotomy: removal of stones from renal pelvis
   b. Nephrolithotomy: incision through kidney and removal of stone
   c. Ureterolithotomy: removal of ureteral calculus
   d. Transcutaneous shock wave lithotripsy: ultrasonic waves used to disintegrate renal calculi
   e. Percutaneous stone dissolution: chemical agents are injected into a nephrostomy tube to dissolve the stone
F. Nursing intervention
  1. Provide general preoperative and postoperative nursing care (see Chapter 2)
  2. Supervise and explain diet restrictions as ordered according to type of stone
  3. Provide analgesics as ordered
  4. Observe, describe, and strain all urine
  5. Maintain gravity drainage: never clamp ureteral or nephrostomy catheters
  6. Observe patency of catheters: usually never irrigate renal or ureteral catheters
  7. Record output from each catheter separately; immediately report scanty output from one tube
  8. Encourage fluids (but keep NPO if there is nausea, vomiting, or abdominal distention)

HYDRONEPHROSIS

A. Definition: an accumulation of fluid in the renal pelvis; there is distention of the renal tubules, calyces, and pelvis; renal tissues are destroyed from pressure; leads to uremia (azotemia)
B. Pathology
  1. Congenital defective drainage; blockage from stones or scar tissues
  2. Reflux (backup) from obstructed bladder neck in benign prostatic hypertrophy
C. Signs and symptoms
  1. Subjective
   a. Related to cause; in some patients, no symptoms, or mild pain
   b. Severe colicky renal pain
   c. Flank pain radiating to groin
   d. Dysuria
   e. Oliguria to anuria
   f. Nausea
   g. Abdominal fullness
   h. Dribbling, hesitancy
  2. Objective
   a. Hematuria, pyuria
   b. Results of diagnostic tests
D. Diagnostic tests/methods
  1. Patient history and physical examination
  2. Blood serum tests (urea/creatinine)
  3. IVP, ultrasonography
E. Treatment
  1. Remove cause
  2. Provide for adequate urinary drainage (e.g., bladder catheter or nephrostomy tube)
  3. Antibiotics
F. Nursing intervention
  1. Provide rest
  2. Provide medication and care as needed for symptoms (e.g., elevation of temperature or pain)

3. Assess for and provide care as indicated for patient with uremia

BLADDER TUMORS

A. Definition: benign or malignant lesions that ulcerate into the mucous membrane; bladder capacity is decreased; benign tumors tend to recur and become malignant
B. Pathology
   1. Related to cigarette smoking and exposure to dyes (environmental—nitrates, benzene, rubber, petroleum)
   2. Chronic bladder irritation (e.g., stones or infection)
   3. Related to aging
C. Signs and symptoms
   1. Subjective: signs of bladder infection: dysuria, frequency, urgency, and chills
   2. Objective
      a. Painless, gross hematuria
      b. Anemia
D. Diagnostic tests/methods
   1. Patient history and physical examination
   2. X-ray studies: IVP, KUB, and retrograde pyelogram
   3. Cystoscopy and biopsy examination
   4. Renoscan, ultrasonography, CT, MRI
E. Treatment
   1. Removal of the tumor through cystoscopy if benign
   2. Surgery
      a. Partial cystectomy
      b. Cystectomy: total removal of the bladder and provision for urinary diversion
      c. Radiation, intravesicular, external
      d. Chemotherapy, intravesicular
      e. Fulguration (coagulation)
      f. Experimental therapy (photodynamic therapy—use of photosensitivity agent and laser destruction of tumor cells)
      g. Interferon (Roferon-A)
F. Nursing intervention: give according to method of treatment (see specific sections)
   1. Be supportive of patient concerns expressed
   2. General pre- and postoperative care (see Chapter 2)

URINARY DIVERSION

A. Definition: surgical intervention to allow for urinary elimination; the bladder is removed; the procedure is permanent
   1. Ileal conduit (ileal passageway): a small segment of ilium is separated from the intestine and the distal end is brought out of the abdomen to form a stoma; the ureters are implanted into this ileal pouch; urine flows continuously from the renal pelvis through the ureters into the ileal pouch and into a collecting bag
   2. Ureterointestinal implant: the ureters are anastomosed into the sigmoid colon or rectum; urine is mixed with feces, and evacuation is controlled from the anal sphincter
   3. Cutaneous ureterostomies: the ureters are implanted on the abdomen, forming one or two stomas that drain urine continuously into drainage bags
   4. Continent ileal urinary reservoir (Koch pouch): the ureters are anastomosed to an isolated segment of ileum, which has a one-way valve; urine is drained by periodic insertion of a catheter
   5. Nephrostomy (may be long-term): tubes are inserted

in the pelvis of each kidney, brought through the skin, and connected to a closed drainage system
B. Indication: cancer of the bladder
C. Patient problems (depends on procedure)
   1. Susceptibility to infection
   2. Anxiety or depression about diagnosis and change in body image
   3. Inability to control elimination
   4. Embarrassment
   5. Odor if urine leaks onto skin; risk for impaired skin integrity
   6. Impaired skin integrity due to incision/ostomy
   7. Pain from surgical incision and/or urinary obstruction
D. Nursing intervention (varies with procedures)
   1. Provide general preoperative and postoperative care (see Chapter 2)
   2. Provide time to listen to patient fears and anxieties
   3. Assess fluid and electrolyte imbalance
   4. Maintain integrity of the skin: clean, inspect, and change drainage bag as needed
   5. Monitor temperature
   6. Monitor urine output from each catheter/tube; maintain separate output records for each; if nephrostomy tubes—contact physician if tube fails to drain urine, if urine is grossly bloody, or if patient complains of sudden severe flank pain
   7. Stoma care (see ileostomy, colostomy); may need to have stoma dilated in postoperative period
   8. Monitor fluid and electrolyte balance
   9. Prevent infection: maintain asepsis; encourage fluids; patient must know when to seek medical attention for pain or elevation of temperature
   10. Do not give patient laxatives or enemas (rectal implant)
   11. Arrange a visit from a person who has undergone a similar procedure (with permission of physician and patient)
   12. Elimination of odor in drainage bags; use weak solution of vinegar or a liquid appliance deodorant
   13. Empty or change pouch when one third to one half full
   14. Avoid odor-producing foods such as onions, fish, eggs, cheese; drink cranberry juice

KIDNEY TUMOR

A. Definition: most tumors of the kidney are malignant; no early symptoms are presented
B. Cause: unknown
C. Signs and symptoms (only in late stages)
   1. Hematuria with no pain
   2. Low-grade temperature
   3. Weight loss
   4. Anemia
   5. Symptoms related to metastasis (e.g., bone pain)
D. Diagnostic tests/methods
   1. Renal arteriogram: IVP and KUB
   2. Renal biopsy examination
E. Treatment
   1. Surgery: radical nephrectomy
   2. Radiation
   3. Chemotherapy
   4. Biological response modifiers (interferon)
F. Nursing intervention

1. Provide nursing care for individual symptoms
2. Provide general nursing care: before and after surgery, during radiation (see Chapter 2), and for a patient receiving chemotherapy (see Chapter 3)

ACUTE RENAL FAILURE (RENAL SHUTDOWN)

A. Definition: sudden damage to the kidneys causing cessation of function and retention of toxins, fluids, and end products of metabolism; patient may recover, or disease may become chronic or be fatal; may be prerenal, intrarenal, postrenal
B. Causes: blood transfusion reaction, shock, toxins, burns, renal ischemia, nephrotoxins, trauma, or reaction to chemotherapy
C. Signs and symptoms
   1. Subjective
      a. Nausea, weakness
      b. Metallic taste in mouth
   2. Subjective
      a. Lethargy, headache, and drowsiness; convulsion; may go into coma
      b. Vomiting and diarrhea
      c. Sudden oliguria or anuria
      d. Increased bleeding time
      e. Electrolyte imbalance
      f. Abnormal BUN and creatinine levels
      g. Paresthesia
      h. Hypotension
D. Diagnostic tests/methods
   1. Patient history and physical examination
   2. Blood serum tests, especially potassium
   3. Renal scan, renal biopsy, KUB
   4. Nephrotomography
   5. Retrograde pyelogram
   6. Ultrasonography, CT, MRI
   7. Urinalysis, CBC
E. Treatment
   1. Removal of cause
   2. Peritoneal dialysis
   3. Hemodialysis
F. Nursing intervention
   1. Provide nursing observations and care as indicated for primary problem
   2. Provide care and observations as indicated for patient with chronic renal failure (see chronic renal failure)
   3. Provide nursing care as indicated for patient receiving peritoneal dialysis (see peritoneal dialysis)
   4. Provide nursing care as indicated for patient receiving hemodialysis (see hemodialysis)
   5. Offer emotional support

CHRONIC RENAL FAILURE (END-STAGE RENAL DISEASE)

A. Definition: progressive kidney damage; the nephron deteriorates; the kidneys stop functioning; this is the final stage of many chronic diseases (e.g., hypertension)
B. Causes
   1. Glomerulonephritis, pyelonephritis, polycystic kidney, or urinary tract obstruction, diabetes
   2. Essential hypertension
   3. Lupus erythematosus
   4. Toxic agents
   5. Vascular disorders

C. Signs and symptoms (Fig. 5-17)
   1. Subjective
      a. Malaise
      b. Nausea
      c. Headaches and visual disturbances
   2. Objective
      a. Anemia
      b. Oliguria
      c. Hyperkalemia
      d. Twitching (from low serum calcium and increased phosphorus levels); pathological fracture
      e. Hypertension (from fluid retention)
      f. Very susceptible to infection: delayed wound healing and ulcers in the mouth
      g. Bleeding tendency
      h. Uremic frost: urea is excreted in perspiration onto the skin, and small crystals can be seen; this causes severe pruritus
      i. Vomiting
      j. Decreased erythropoietin
      k. Disorientation, convulsions, coma
      l. Results of diagnostic tests
D. Diagnostic tests/methods
   1. Patient history and physical examination
   2. Serum blood tests
   3. Kidney function tests; BUN; creatinine level
   4. X-ray studies
   5. Renal arteriograms, renal ultrasound
   6. Nephrotomograms
   7. Kidney biopsy
E. Treatment
   1. Remove (treat) cause
   2. Hemodialysis
   3. Peritoneal dialysis
   4. Kidney transplant
F. Nursing intervention
   1. Monitor fluid balance: weigh patient daily; record intake and output
   2. Maintain asepsis: provide catheter care, prevent infections, and encourage frequent hand washing; do not expose patient to staff or visitors with upper respiratory tract infections
   3. Conserve energy: provide care, maintain rest periods
   4. Provide safety (see care of patient in coma)
   5. Relieve pruritus: wash patient frequently with tepid water; do not use soap; handle skin gently; use skin lotion; cut nails; apply calamine lotion
   6. Assist with administration of transfusion; biologic response modifiers; epoetin alfa (erythropoietin)
   7. Provide oral hygiene every 1 to 2 hours; use cotton swabs and soft toothbrush; hard candy and mouthwash minimize bad taste in mouth and alleviate thirst
   8. Provide soft, high-carbohydrate, low-potassium, low-sodium, low-protein diet in small feedings
   9. Restrict fluids as ordered
   10. Anticipate cardiac arrest: monitor vital signs
   11. Assess LOC: orient as necessary
   12. Provide nursing care and precautions as indicated for a patient with seizures (see convulsive disorders)
   13. Provide nursing measures to prevent dangers of immobility (see Chapter 2)

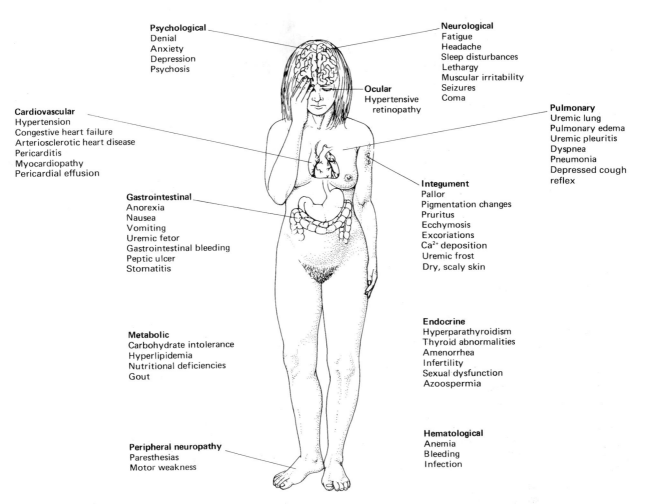

Psychological
Denial
Anxiety
Depression
Psychosis

Neurological
Fatigue
Headache
Sleep disturbances
Lethargy
Muscular irritability
Seizures
Coma

Ocular
Hypertensive
retinopathy

Cardiovascular
Hypertension
Congestive heart failure
Arteriosclerotic heart disease
Pericarditis
Myocardiopathy
Pericardial effusion

Pulmonary
Uremic lung
Pulmonary edema
Uremic pleuritis
Dyspnea
Pneumonia
Depressed cough
reflex

Gastrointestinal
Anorexia
Nausea
Vomiting
Uremic fetor
Gastrointestinal bleeding
Peptic ulcer
Stomatitis

Integument
Pallor
Pigmentation changes
Pruritus
Ecchymosis
Excoriations
Ca^{2+} deposition
Uremic frost
Dry, scaly skin

Metabolic
Carbohydrate intolerance
Hyperlipidemia
Nutritional deficiencies
Gout

Endocrine
Hyperparathyroidism
Thyroid abnormalities
Amenorrhea
Infertility
Sexual dysfunction
Azoospermia

Hematological
Anemia
Bleeding
Infection

Peripheral neuropathy
Paresthesias
Motor weakness

Figure 5-17   Clinical manifestations of chronic uremia. (Modified from Lewis SM, Heitkemper MM, Dirksen SR: *Medical-surgical nursing: assessment and management of clinical problems,* ed 5, St Louis, 2000, Mosby.)

14. Anticipate and prevent bleeding
    a. Observe stool, urine, sputum, and vomitus
    b. Monitor vital signs, lab values
    c. Use soft swab for mouth care
    d. Avoid injections if possible
15. Reinforce instructions for kind of drug therapy (i.e., erythropoietin, iron, minerals, antihypertensives, phosphate binders, and ion-exchange resins)

PERITONEAL DIALYSIS (FIG. 5-18)

A. Description: toxins, end products of metabolism, and fluids are removed from the blood through the peritoneal membrane; a catheter is passed into the peritoneal cavity; dialyzing fluid, which is similar to plasma, is instilled by gravity into the abdominal cavity, and the catheter is clamped; toxins and electrolytes, which are in greater concentration in the blood vessels of the peritoneal membrane, pass into the dialyzing fluid; after a specified dwell time the catheter is unclamped, and the fluid drains out by gravity
B. Types
   1. Intermittent peritoneal dialysis (IPD)
   2. Continuous ambulatory peritoneal dialysis (CAPD)
   3. Continuous cycling peritoneal dialysis (CCPD)

4. Access devices may be temporary or permanent
C. Patient problems
   1. Risk for infection related to dialysis procedure
   2. Self-care deficit related to discomfort and immobility
   3. Fluid volume excess or deficit
   4. Body image disturbance
D. Nursing intervention
   1. Record baseline vital signs; complete assessment; carefully measure fluid instilled/drained
   2. Maintain surgical asepsis; prevent peritonitis
   3. Assist patient with self-care activities
   4. Observe for complications (hypotension, pain, respiratory distress, hypovolemia, peritonitis, atelectasis)

HEMODIALYSIS

A. Description: blood leaves the patient through an arterial cannula and travels through coils placed in a solution; dialysis takes place, and the detoxified blood returns to the patient's venous circulation; a surgically created arteriovenous fistula (connection) is necessary for repeated dialysis
B. Patient problems
   1. Self-esteem disturbance related to threatened self-image
   2. Powerlessness related to dependency on machine

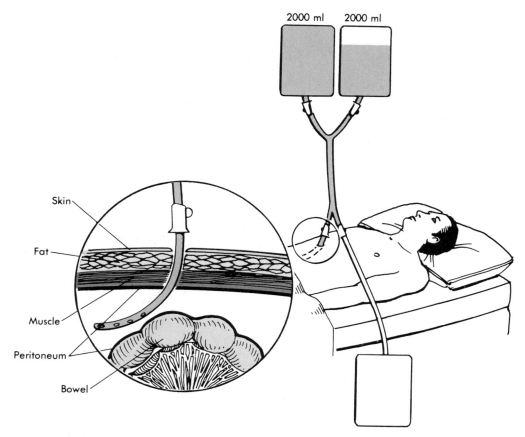

Figure 5-18 Patient receiving peritoneal dialysis. Dialysis fluid is being infused into the peritoneal cavity. (From Phipps WJ, Sands JK, Lehman MK, Cassmeyer VL: *Medical-surgical nursing: concepts and clinical practice*, ed 5, St Louis, 1995, Mosby.)

3. Risk for infection related to the hemodialysis procedure
4. Anxiety related to lifelong, life-threatening disease
5. Fluid volume excess related to fluid accumulation/inadequate dialysis
6. Fluid volume deficit related to rapid removal of body fluid during treatment

C. Nursing intervention
1. Maintain surgical asepsis
2. Assess AV fistula, graft, or shunt for patency; normally a thrill can be felt by palpating the area of anastomosis and a bruit can be heard with a stethoscope; the bruit and thrill is created by arterial blood rushing into the vein
3. Provide emotional support; alleviate anxiety
4. Provide patient teaching

KIDNEY TRANSPLANT

A. Removal of the diseased kidney and transplantation of a normal kidney is sometimes performed for patients with advanced renal failure; restores normal function; less expensive than dialysis after first year

B. Patient problems
1. Risk for infection related to altered immune system secondary to medications
2. Anxiety related to possibility of organ rejection
3. Fear of pain/rejection

4. Body image disturbance
5. Knowledge deficit (surgery, drug therapies, nutrition, activities, follow-up care)

MALE REPRODUCTIVE SYSTEM
Anatomy and Physiology (Fig. 5-19)

A. External genitals
1. Scrotum: skin-covered pouch; lies outside of pelvic cavity; contains testes, epididymis, and lower part of vas deferens; lower body temperature here is necessary for reproduction
2. Penis: erectile tissue; organ of coitus (sexual intercourse); serves as passageway for urine and semen

B. Testes: small oval glands in scrotum; produce spermatozoa; secrete testosterone

C. Ducts
1. Seminiferous tubules: formation of sperm
2. Epididymis: narrow, tightly coiled tubes; provides temporary storage space for immature sperm
3. Vas deferens: continuation of the epididymis; lies near surface of scrotum; called the spermatic cord
4. Ejaculatory: pass through prostate; ejaculate semen into urethra

D. Accessory glands
1. Seminal vesicles: located on each side of the prostate; empty secretion into the prostatic ampulla

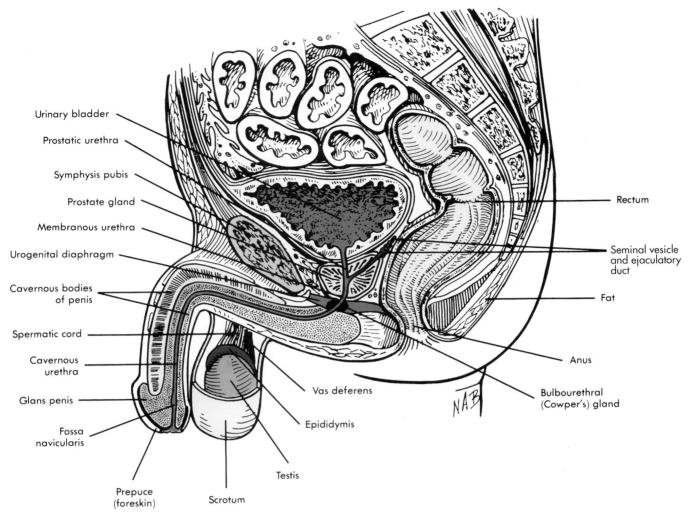

Figure 5-19 Male organs of reproduction. (From Phipps WJ, Sands JK, Lehman MK, Cassmeyer VL: *Medical-surgical nursing: concepts and clinical practice,* ed 5, St Louis, 1995, Mosby.)

Labels on figure:
- Urinary bladder
- Prostatic urethra
- Symphysis pubis
- Prostate gland
- Membranous urethra
- Urogenital diaphragm
- Cavernous bodies of penis
- Spermatic cord
- Cavernous urethra
- Glans penis
- Fossa navicularis
- Prepuce (foreskin)
- Scrotum
- Testis
- Epididymis
- Vas deferens
- Rectum
- Seminal vesicle and ejaculatory duct
- Fat
- Anus
- Bulbourethral (Cowper's) gland

2. Prostate: encircles the upper area of the urethra; secretes alkaline fluid; increases sperm motility
3. Cowper's gland: located below prostate; produces an alkaline secretion that is primarily a lubricant during sexual intercourse

E. Semen: alkaline fluid (pH 7.5); the major bulk (60%) is secreted by the seminal vesicles; the remaining 40% is secreted by other accessory organs

F. Function
  1. Reproduction
  2. Production of testosterone

MALE GENITOURINARY SYSTEM CONDITIONS AND DISORDERS
Benign Prostatic Hypertrophy/ Hyperphasia (BPH)

A. Description: the prostate gland slowly enlarges (hypertrophies) and extends upward into the bladder; outflow of urine is obstructed; the urinary stream is smaller, and voiding is difficult; a pouch is formed in the bladder as the gland continues to enlarge; stasis of urine occurs; obstruc-

tion causes gradual dilation of ureters and kidneys; may cause hydronephrosis; when obstruction is complete, there is acute urinary retention

B. Cause: unknown; increased incidence with age, usually over 50 years of age; related to smoking

C. Signs and symptoms
  1. Subjective
    a. Dysuria, frequency, nocturia, urgency, retention, hesitancy
    b. Burning on urination, decreased force of stream, end stream dribbling
  2. Objective
    a. Urinary tract infection
    b. Acute urinary retention
    c. Hematuria
    d. Enlarged prostate gland
    e. Results of diagnostic tests

D. Diagnostic tests/methods
  1. Patient history and assessment; palpation through rectal examination
  2. IVP, cystoscopy, and retrograde pyelography

3. Urine culture
4. BUN, CBC
5. Serum creatinine
6. Transrectal ultrasonography

E. Treatment
1. Immediate
   a. Bladder drainage with indwelling catheter
   b. Decompression
   c. Antibiotics as indicated
   d. Suprapubic cystotomy and insertion of catheter for long-term drainage
2. Surgery: type depends on patient's age and size of enlargement (open approaches)
   a. Transurethral resection of the prostate (TURP): an instrument is passed through the urethra to the prostate; under direct visualization, small pieces of the obstructing gland are removed with electric wire; the bleeding points are cauterized; there is no incision; bleeding is a common postoperative problem
   b. Suprapubic (transvesical) prostatectomy: a low incision is made over the bladder; the bladder is opened, and the prostatic tissue is removed through an incision into the urethral mucosa; two drainage tubes are inserted (a cystotomy tube and a Foley catheter); these are connected to a continuous bladder irrigation setup
   c. Retropubic prostatectomy: a low abdominal incision is made; the bladder is not entered
   d. Perineal prostatectomy: the gland is removed through an incision in the perineum; the entire gland and capsule are removed
   e. Bilateral vasectomy may be performed with a prostatectomy to reduce risk of epididymitis
3. Other treatment methods
   a. Finasteride (Proscar), an androgen hormone inhibitor, can be used to decrease symptoms; may arrest prostate enlargement
   b. Transcystoscopic urethroplasty: balloon dilatation of prostatic urethra
   c. TUIP: transurethral incision at bladder neck
   d. Short-term effects treatment involving microwaves
   e. Implantation of intraurethral prostatic stent

F. Nursing intervention
1. On admission, complete assessment related to
   a. Aging
   b. Possible infection
   c. Anxiety
   d. Medical problems associated with aging: diabetes, cardiovascular, hearing, sight, and gastrointestinal
2. Encourage fluids if not contraindicated; monitor intake and output
3. Maintain gravity drainage of indwelling catheter
4. Provide general preoperative and postoperative care (see Chapter 2)
5. Provide specific postoperative care; depends on the procedure performed
   a. Continue to maintain gravity drainage of indwelling catheter
   b. Keep irrigation flowing (note clots); maintain a closed, continuous irrigation; ensure drainage not obstructed

c. Maintain asepsis; change dressing when wet (may need physician's order); there may be fecal incontinence if a perineal prostatectomy was performed
d. Monitor vital signs; hematuria is expected; report frank bleeding or clots
e. Use oral thermometer (no rectal treatments)
f. Encourage patient to avoid straining; encourage fluids; provide stool softeners
g. Observe for bladder spasms; note if catheter is draining freely; irrigate by syringe as ordered; administer antispasmodics
h. Administer analgesic as needed for postoperative pain
i. Monitor intake and output; record all drainage tubes separately
j. Sitz bath for pain and inflammation if perineal prostatectomy
k. Provide care instructions if patient is discharged with indwelling catheter

CANCER OF THE PROSTATE

A. Definition: a malignant tumor; it has no symptoms until it has become large or metastasized
B. Cause: unknown; increased incidence with age (all men older than 40 years should have rectal examinations yearly)
C. Signs and symptoms
1. Early tumor has no symptoms
2. Subjective
   a. Back pain
   b. Frequency, nocturia, dysuria, and urinary retention
3. Objective: symptoms from metastasis
D. Diagnostic tests/methods
1. Rectal examination
2. Biopsy examination
3. Acid phosphatase
4. Transrectal ultrasonography
5. Prostate-specific antigen level (PSA)
6. Serum alkaline phosphatase level (elevated in bone metastasis)
7. Bone scan to assess metastasis
8. MRI, CT
E. Treatment surgery
1. Radical perineal prostatectomy (removal of prostate, capsule, and seminal vesicles)
2. Bilateral orchiectomy (removal of both testicles)
3. TURP
4. Estrogen therapy
5. Agonists of luteinizing hormone–releasing hormone
6. Radiation (external, interstitial, spot)
F. Nursing intervention
1. See nursing intervention for a patient with BPH
2. Be supportive as concerns are expressed about a malignancy and feminization from estrogens; answer questions; refer problems to physician
3. Pain control for terminally ill patient; may consider hospice care

HYDROCELE

A. Definition: a cystic mass filled with fluid that forms around the testicle
B. Causes
1. Infection
2. Trauma

C. Signs and symptoms
   1. Swelling of testicle
   2. Discomfort in sitting and walking
D. Diagnostic tests/methods: assessment by physical examination
E. Treatment
   1. Aspiration (usually only in children)
   2. Injection of a sclerosing solution
   3. Surgical removal of the sac (hydrocelectomy)
F. Nursing intervention
   1. Provide usual preoperative and postoperative care (see Chapter 2)
   2. Scrotal support (elevation) may be necessary during postoperative period
   3. Be supportive to concerns expressed by patient

CANCER OF THE TESTES

A. Definition: an uncommon malignancy; usually no systemic symptoms are present until metastasis occurs; can be diagnosed early only by examination and finding a hard, non-tender mass (testicular self-examination should be done monthly); age of incidence is usually in early 30s
B. Treatment
   1. Surgery: orchiectomy
   2. Radiotherapy
   3. Chemotherapy
   4. Possibly radical: lymph node dissection

C. Nursing intervention: related to treatment selected
D. Teach monthly preventative testicular self-exam

FEMALE REPRODUCTIVE SYSTEM
Anatomy and Physiology

A. External genitals
   1. Vulva
      a. Labia majora: two long folds of skin on each side of the vaginal orifice outside of the labia minora
      b. Labia minora: two flat, thin, delicate folds of skin that are highly sensitive to manipulation and trauma; enclose the region called the vestibule, which contains the clitoris, the urethral orifice, and the vaginal orifice
      c. Clitoris: very sensitive erectile tissue; becomes swollen with blood during sexual excitement
      d. Vaginal orifice: opening into vagina; hymen, fold of mucosa, partially closes orifice and generally is ruptured during first sexual intercourse
      e. Bartholin's glands: located on each side of vaginal orifice; secrete lubrication fluid
   2. Perineum: between vaginal orifice and anus; forms pelvic floor
B. Internal organs (Fig. 5-20)
   1. Ovaries: main sex glands
      a. Located on either side in pelvic cavity
      b. Produce ova, which form in the graafian follicles

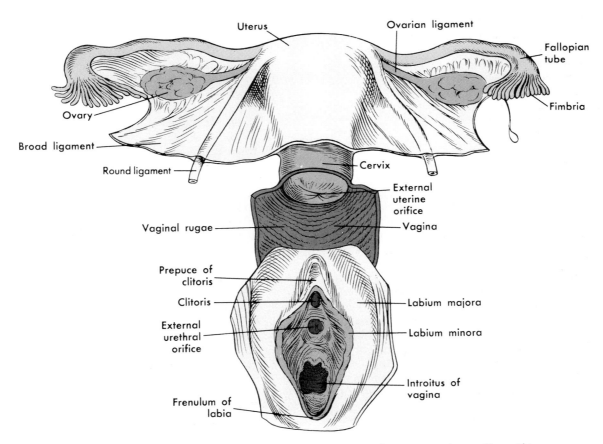

Figure 5-20 Female internal organs of reproduction. Major ligaments are shown. (From Phipps WJ, Sands JK, Lehman MK, Cassmeyer VL: *Medical-surgical nursing: concepts and clinical practice,* ed 5, St Louis, 1995, Mosby.)

c. Graafian follicle produces estrogen

d. Rupture of a follicle releases an ovum (ovulation)

e. Ruptured follicles become glandular mass called corpus luteum

f. Corpus luteum secretes estrogen, but mainly progesterone

2. Fallopian tubes

 a. Extend from point near ovaries to uterus; no direct connection between ovaries and tubes

 b. Fimbriae: fingerlike extensions on tubes; pick up ova and transport into fallopian tubes

 c. Fertilization occurs in outer one third of the fallopian tubes

3. Uterus

 a. Upper portion rests on upper surface of bladder; the lower portion is embedded in pelvic floor between the bladder and the rectum

 b. Pear-shaped, hollow organ that expands tremendously to accommodate a fetus

 c. Divisions

  (1) Body: upper main part

  (2) Fundus: bulging upper surface of the body

  (3) Cervix: neck of the uterus

 d. Endometrium: uterine lining; sloughs off during menstruation

 e. Functions

  (1) Menstruation

  (2) Pregnancy

  (3) Labor

4. Vagina

 a. Located between rectum and urethra

 b. Structure: wrinkled mucous membrane (rugae); capable of great distention

 c. Functions

  (1) Lower part of birth canal

  (2) Receives semen from male

  (3) Passageway for menstrual flow

C. Breasts (mammary glands)

1. Located over pectoral muscles

2. Size depends on adipose tissue rather than glandular tissue

3. Consists of lobes, lobules, and milk-secreting cells (acini)

4. Ducts lead to the opening called the nipple

5. Areola: pigmented area surrounding the nipple

D. Function

1. Reproduction

2. Production of estrogen and progesterone

E. Menstrual cycle (Fig. 5-21)

1. Phases: regulated primarily by the hormonal control of pituitary gland, ovaries, and uterus

 a. One ovum discharged each month from an ovary; ripens in the graafian follicle; follicle-stimulating hormone (FSH) from anterior lobe of pituitary stimulates the formation of the follicle

 b. Estrogen produced by the follicle builds up the endometrium in expectation of a fertilized ovum

 c. Ovum is discharged into the fallopian tube by luteinizing hormone (LH) from the anterior lobe pituitary; follicle is converted into the corpus luteum

 d. Postovulation: corpus luteum secretes progesterone and estrogen for final preparation of the endometrium

 e. Premenstrual: the gradual drop in progesterone and estrogen leads to menses

2. Length of cycle: usually 28 days; highly variable; ovulation occurs midway

3. Menopause (climacteric) the gradual cessation of menstrual cycle; the ability to bear children ends; occurs at approximately 45 years of age

 a. Ovaries lose their ability to respond to hormones

 b. Decrease in levels of estrogen and progesterone

  (1) Failure to ovulate

  (2) Monthly flow is less, is irregular, and gradually ceases

  (3) Reproductive organs atrophy

FEMALE REPRODUCTIVE SYSTEM CONDITIONS AND DISORDERS

Childbearing is the major physiological function of the female reproductive system. Disorders of this system are distressing to the patient because of interference with sexuality, conception, and self-image. The nurse plays an important role by clearly providing information to the concerned patient.

Nursing Assessment

A. Nursing observations (objective data)

1. General appearance

2. Vital signs

3. Weight

4. Breasts

 a. Contour

 b. Skin dimpling

 c. Nodules

  (1) Size

  (2) Consistency

  (3) Mobile or fixed

 d. Nipples

  (1) Asymmetry

  (2) Retraction

  (3) Rash

  (4) Ulceration

  (5) Discharge

5. External genitalia

 a. Irritation

 b. Redness

 c. Excoriation

 d. Bulge

6. Introitus

 a. Irritation

 b. Redness

 c. Excoriation

 d. Nodules

7. Discharge

 a. Color

 b. Malodorous

 c. Consistency

B. Patient description (subjective data)

1. Lower abdominal pain and cramping

2. Backache

3. Stress incontinence

4. Urinary frequency and urgency

5. Urine or fecal material draining from vaginal tract

6. Breasts

 a. Tenderness

 b. Burning

 c. Swelling

 d. Pain

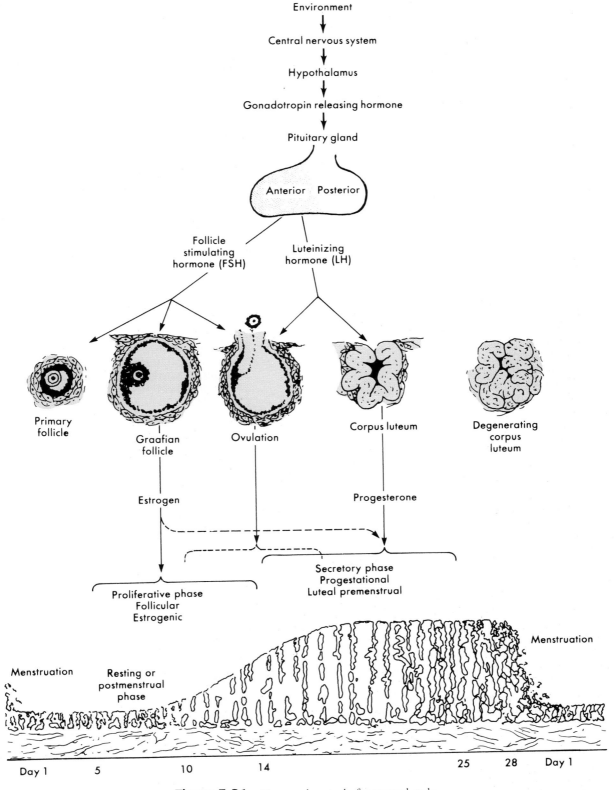

Environment

↓

Central nervous system

↓

Hypothalamus

↓

Gonadotropin releasing hormone

↓

Pituitary gland

Anterior   Posterior

Follicle stimulating hormone (FSH)

Luteinizing hormone (LH)

Primary follicle

Graafian follicle

Ovulation

Corpus luteum

Degenerating corpus luteum

Estrogen

Progesterone

Proliferative phase
Follicular
Estrogenic

Secretory phase
Progestational
Luteal premenstrual

Menstruation

Resting or postmenstrual phase

Menstruation

Day 1   5   10   14   25   28   Day 1

Figure 5-21   Hormonal control of menstrual cycle.

e. Nipples
   (1) Tenderness
   (2) Burning
7. External genitalia
   a. Itching
   b. Burning
8. Introitus
   a. Burning
   b. Itching
   c. Tenderness
   d. Dyspareunia (painful intercourse)
9. Menstrual cycle
   a. Duration of cycles
   b. Number of days between cycles
   c. Associated symptoms
      (1) Pain
      (2) Headache
      (3) Irritability
      (4) Depression
      (5) Insomnia

Diagnostic Tests/Methods

A. Serum laboratory studies
1. Luteinizing hormone (LH)
   a. Stimulates progesterone secretion
   b. Diminished levels may relate to prolonged, heavy menses
   c. Elevated levels may result in short, scanty menses
2. Follicle-stimulating hormone (FSH)
   a. Stimulates estrogen secretion
   b. Diminished levels may relate to bleeding between cycles
   c. Elevated levels may result in excessive uterine bleeding
3. Thyroid function tests
   a. Used to rule out menstrual abnormality secondary to thyroid dysfunction
   b. Diminished thyroid hormone secretion may result in bleeding between cycles, irregular menses, or absence of menstrual flow
4. Adrenal function tests
   a. Used to rule out menstrual abnormality secondary to adrenal dysfunction
   b. Elevated or decreased production of adrenal cortex hormone secretion may result in amenorrhea
B. Procedures
1. Pelvic examination: to inspect and assess the external genitalia, perineal and anal areas, introitus, vaginal tract, and cervix
   a. Have patient empty bladder
   b. Place patient in the lithotomy position
   c. Flex and abduct patient's thighs
   d. Place patient's feet in stirrups
   e. Extend patient's buttocks slightly beyond the edge of the examining table
2. Laparoscopy: visualization of the pelvic structures with a lighted laparoscope inserted through the abdominal wall
3. Culdoscopy: visualization of the ovaries, fallopian tubes, and uterus with a lighted instrument inserted through the vaginal tract
   a. After procedure, position patient on abdomen to expel air

b. Monitor for vaginal bleeding
c. Instruct patient to abstain from intercourse, douching, and use of tampons until advised by physician
4. Colposcopy: visualization of the cervix with an instrument that magnifies tissue
5. Papanicolaou smear test (Pap smear): a sample of cervical scrapings is obtained for study under a microscope for evidence of malignant cell changes
   a. Follow nursing actions as in a pelvic examination
   b. Write patient's name on the frost side of the slide, handling edges only
   c. Smear the specimen on a glass slide
   d. Place a drop of a fixative, dry, and send to laboratory
   e. Reinforce importance of Pap smears as recommended by the American Cancer Society
6. Cervical biopsy examination: removal of tissue to examine for presence of malignancy
   a. After procedure, advise patient to rest and avoid strenuous activity for 24 hours
   b. Leave packing in place until physician permits removal (usually 12 to 24 hours)
   c. Monitor for vaginal bleeding
   d. Instruct patient to abstain from intercourse, douching, and use of tampons until advised by physician
   e. Explain that there will be a malodorous discharge that may last 3 weeks; daily bath should help control this
7. Conization
   a. Removal of cone-shaped tissue of the cervix for analysis of cancerous cells
   b. Indicated for removal of diseased cervical tissue
   c. Nursing intervention
      (1) Maintain packing 12 to 24 hours
      (2) Monitor for bleeding
      (3) Instruct patient to abstain from intercourse, douching, and use of tampons until advised by physician
8. Schiller's test
   a. Application of a dye to the cervix to aid in detecting cancerous cells
   b. Normal vaginal cells will stain a deep brown
   c. Abnormal cells with not absorb the dye
   d. Nursing intervention: recommend to patient that a perineal pad be used to protect clothes from stain
9. Ultrasonography
   a. A sound frequency that reflects an image of the pelvic structures
   b. An aid in confirming ovarian and uterine tumors
10. Culture and sensitivity
   a. The culture of a specimen of exudate suspected of infection
   b. The sensitivity of an antibiotic to the microorganism
11. Dilatation and curettage (D & C)
   a. A diagnostic and therapeutic procedure
   b. The cervix is dilated to scrape the lining of the uterine cavity with a curet
   c. Nursing intervention
      (1) After procedure, provide sterile perineal pads and record amount of drainage
      (2) Encourage voiding to prevent urinary retention

(3) Instruct patient to abstain from intercourse, douching, and use of tampons until advised by physician

12. Mammography: an X-ray examination of the breasts to detect tumors; screening test done yearly for women over 40 years of age
13. Thermography: infrared photography used to detect breast tumors
14. Xerography: an X-ray examination of the breasts and skin that provides good definition of the tissue
15. CT; MRI

Frequent Patient Problems and Nursing Care

A. Anxiety related to modesty
1. Keep the patient's body covered at all times
2. Provide privacy
3. Speak with the patient during the examination or procedure

B. Knowledge deficit related to understanding of menstruation
1. Provide factual information related to the process of menstruation
2. Describe abnormalities associated with menstruation
3. Describe emotional changes associated with menstruation
4. Teach menstrual hygiene
   a. Change perineal pad or tampon every 3 to 4 hours
   b. Remove napkin front to back
   c. Alternate sanitary napkins and tampons qd to prevent toxic shock syndrome or backflow of menstruation

C. Knowledge deficit related to menstrual abnormalities: explain which menstrual symptoms are considered abnormal
1. Flow occurring more frequently than every 21 days
2. Flow occurring less frequently than every 35 days
3. Duration of less than 3 days
4. Duration of more than 7 days
5. Use of 12 or more perineal pads per 24 hours

D. Pain related to menstruation
1. Assess location, duration, onset, and quality of pain
2. Apply heating pad to the abdomen
3. Provide warm liquids of patient's choice
4. Provide massage to lumbar area
5. Provide pain relief medication as ordered by physician

E. Knowledge deficit related to breast self-examination (BSE)
1. Recommend that breasts be examined 7 days after onset of menstruation every month (Fig. 5-22)
2. Instruct patient on technique of breast self-examination
   a. Inspect breasts in front of mirror with arms at sides
   b. Observe breasts with arms raised above the head
   c. With hands on hips, lean forward and contract chest muscles
3. Lying supine, palpate each breast with flat part of fingers and continue in a circular movement to nipple
4. Observations of the breasts
   a. Size
   b. Symmetry
   c. Skin texture
   d. Color
   e. Nipple position
   f. Nipple discharge

F. Knowledge deficit related to menopause
1. Describe accompanying symptoms associated with menopause
   a. Irregular menses
   b. Hot flashes
   c. Night sweats
   d. Insomnia
   e. Depression
   f. Anxiety
2. Onset is usually after age 40 years
3. Explain that menopause does not interfere with sexuality
4. Recommend use of lubricant before intercourse
5. Recommend use of contraception for 6 months after the last menstrual period

Major Medical Diagnoses
MENSTRUAL ABNORMALITIES
DYSMENORRHEA

A. Definition: intense pain at the time of menses
B. Cause: uterine spasms cause cramping of the lower abdomen
C. Signs and symptoms
1. Subjective
   a. Headache, backache
   b. Abdominal pain
   c. Chills
   d. Nausea
2. Objective
   a. Fever
   b. Vomiting
D. Diagnostic method: pelvic examination to rule out other physical disorders
E. Treatment
1. Analgesics, such as nonsteroidal antiinflammatory agents
2. Local application of heat
3. Pelvic exercises
4. D & C
F. Nursing intervention
1. Instruct patient on avoidance of fatigue and overexertion during menstrual period
2. Instruct patient on ingestion of warm beverages before onset of pain to prevent attack

PREMENSTRUAL TENSION SYNDROME (PMS)

A. Definition: a number of symptoms occurring a few days before menstruation
B. Cause: cause is unclear; may be related to fluid retention combined with emotional tension; usually disappears with onset of menstruation
C. Signs and symptoms
1. Subjective
   a. Breast tenderness
   b. Headache
   c. Nausea
   d. Depression
   e. Insomnia
   f. Irritability
   g. Fatigue
2. Objective: weight gain 2 to 10 days before onset of menstruation
D. Diagnostic method: assessment of specific symptoms and psychological health

How to do BSE

1. Lie down and put a pillow under your right shoulder. Place your right arm behind your head.
2. Use the finger pads of the three middle fingers on your left hand to feel for lumps or thickening. Your finger pads are the top third of each finger.

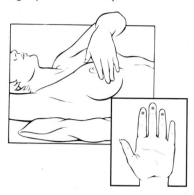

3. Press hard enough to know how your breast feels. If you're not sure how hard to press, ask your health care provider. Or try to copy the way your health care provider uses the finger pads during a breast exam. Learn what your breast feels like most of the time. A firm ridge in the lower curve of each breast is normal.

4. Move around the breast in a set way. You can choose either the circle (A), the up and down line (B), or the wedge (C). Do it the same way every time. It will help you to make sure that you've gone over the entire breast area and to remember how your breast feels each month.

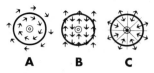

A   B   C

5. Now examine your left breast using right hand finger pads.
You might want to check your breasts while standing in front of a mirror right after you do your BSE each month. You might also want to do an extra BSE while you're in the shower. Your soapy hands will glide over the wet skin making it easy to check how your breasts feel.

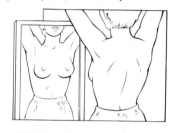

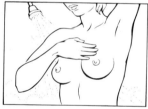

Figure 5-22   Breast self-examination. (Courtesy American Cancer Society.)

E. Treatment
  1. Diuretics
  2. Mild sodium restriction
  3. Mild tranquilizers
  4. Well-balanced diet
  5. Exercise
F. Nursing intervention
  1. Assist patient in working out a diet with decreased sodium content
  2. Instruct patient to decrease consumption of coffee, alcohol, and nicotine during latter half of menstrual cycle

AMENORRHEA

A. Definition: absence of menstrual periods
B. Causes
  1. Diabetes
  2. Debilitating illness
  3. Malnutrition
  4. Obesity
  5. Extreme anxiety
  6. Anemia
  7. Oral contraceptives
  8. Chronic nephritis
  9. Tumors of the endocrine glands
C. Signs and symptoms
  1. Subjective: anxiety
  2. Objective
    a. Absence of menses by age 17 years (primary amenorrhea)
    b. Failure of a menstrual period (secondary amenorrhea)
D. Diagnostic tests/methods
  1. Pelvic examination
  2. LH level
  3. FSH level
  4. Thyroid function test
  5. Adrenal function test
E. Treatment: according to cause
F. Nursing intervention
  1. Encourage patient to follow prescribed orders to ensure success of therapeutic plan

2. Provide clear explanations related to cause of disorder to decrease anxiety

MENORRHAGIA (HYPERMENORRHEA)
A. Definition: excessive menstrual flow (amount or duration)
B. Causes
   1. Uterine tumors
   2. Pelvic inflammatory disease
   3. Endocrine disturbances
C. Signs and symptoms
   1. Subjective
      a. Feeling of pelvic heaviness
      b. Fatigue
   2. Objective
      a. Profuse menstrual bleeding with clots
      b. Pale, tired appearance
D. Diagnostic tests/methods
   1. Pelvic examination
   2. LH level
   3. FSH level
   4. Thyroid function test
   5. Adrenal function test
   6. RBC count
E. Treatment
   1. According to cause
   2. D & C
F. Nursing intervention
   1. Encourage intake of foods high in iron content
   2. Encourage planned rest periods
   3. Instruct the patient to count number of pads used during an abnormal period
   4. Weigh each pad before and after use to estimate blood loss

METRORRHAGIA
A. Definition: bleeding between menstrual intervals
B. Pathology
   1. Causes are similar to those of menorrhagia
   2. Breakthrough bleeding may occur with use of contraceptive pills
   3. May be early symptom of cervical cancer
C. Signs and symptoms
   1. Subjective
      a. Feeling of pelvic heaviness
      b. Fatigue
   2. Objective
      a. Spotting or bleeding between menstrual periods
      b. Tired appearance
D. Diagnostic tests/methods
   1. Pelvic examination
   2. LH level
   3. FSH level
   4. Thyroid function test
   5. Adrenal function test
   6. RBC count
   7. Pap smear
E. Treatment: according to cause
F. Nursing intervention
   1. Instruct the patient on how to keep accurate records of bleeding episodes
   2. Encourage continued medical follow-up because of possible cervical changes associated with cancer

VAGINITIS
A. Definition: inflammation of the vaginal mucosa
B. Pathology
   1. Invasion of virulent organisms permitted by changes in normal flora; pH becomes alkaline
   2. Causes:
      a. Trichomoniasis: parasitic organism
      b. Candida albicans (moniliasis): fungal organism
      c. Atrophic (senile): occurs in postmenopausal women because of atrophy of vaginal mucosa
      d. Bacterial: invasion by staphylococci, streptococci, *Escherichia coli*, Chlamydia, or *Gardnerella vaginalis*
      e. Foreign body
      f. Allergens or irritants
C. Signs and symptoms
   1. Trichomoniasis: thick, white or yellow, frothy, malodorous discharge causing itching, burning, and excoriation of vulva
   2. Monilial: thick or watery, white or yellow, curdlike discharge; mucosa becomes reddened
   3. Atrophic: blood-flecked discharge with burning and itching of the vagina and dyspareunia
   4. Bacterial: profuse, yellow mucoid discharge with irritation to vulva and urethra; fishy or foul odor
   5. Foreign body: blood-tinged serosanguineous or purulent discharge; foul odor; may be thin or thick
   6. Allergens/irritants: increase in usual secretions, itching, burning, rash
D. Diagnostic tests/methods: culture and sensitivity; pelvic exam
E. Treatment
   1. Trichomoniasis: metronidazole (Flagyl), Floraquin tablets administered vaginally, and carbarsone suppositories administered rectally; sitz baths to relieve itching
   2. Candidiasis: nystatin (Mycostatin) or miconazole (Monistat) creme daily for 14 days; sitz baths to relieve itching
   3. Atrophic: antibiotics and estrogen therapy
   4. Bacterial: antibiotics and sulfonamide creams
   5. Foreign body: removal of object; use of antibiotics
   6. Allergens or irritants: removal of cause; use of topical steroid ointment if necessary
F. Nursing intervention
   1. Reassure patient during vaginal examination to decrease anxiety
   2. Instruct patient on perineal hygiene: cleansing front to back
   3. In the event of trichomoniasis, instruct patient to abstain from intercourse or have partner wear a condom, because this infection can be transmitted
   4. Advise patient to use perineal pads because of increased discharge
   5. Teach patient importance of compliance with treatment

UTERINE CANCER (ENDOMETRIUM)
A. Definition: new growth of abnormal cells in the uterine lining
B. Pathology
   1. Spreads to cervix, fallopian tubes, ovaries, bladder, and rectum

2. Associated factors are women over 50 years of age, obesity, diabetes, and hypertension
3. Prognosis is good if identified in early stages
C. Signs and symptoms
   1. Subjective
      a. Postmenopausal bleeding
      b. Bleeding between cycles
      c. Bleeding after intercourse
      d. Watery vaginal discharge
   2. Objective
      a. Uterine enlargement
      b. Suspicious Pap test results
D. Diagnostic tests/methods
   1. D & C
   2. Tissue biopsy examination
E. Treatment
   1. Surgical intervention
      a. Panhysterectomy (removal of uterus and cervix)
      b. Oophorectomy (removal of ovaries)
      c. Salpingectomy (removal of fallopian tubes)
   2. Chemotherapy
   3. Radiation
F. Nursing intervention: see cancer of the cervix

UTERINE FIBROID TUMORS

A. Definition: a benign tumor located in the uterus
B. Pathology
   1. Develops slowly, symptoms occur only in relation to size, location, and number of tumors present
   2. Occurs in 25% of women over 35 years of age
C. Signs and symptoms
   1. Subjective
      a. Menstrual disturbances
      b. Backache
      c. Frequent urination
      d. Constipation
   2. Objective; uterine enlargement
D. Diagnostic tests/methods
   1. Pelvic examination
   2. Laparoscopy
E. Treatment
   1. Excision of the myoma is indicated for small tumors
   2. Hysterectomy (removal of uterus) with preservation of ovaries is indicated for large tumors
F. Nursing intervention
   1. Explain to patient that tumors may decrease in size after menopause
   2. Encourage patient to verbalize concerns
   3. If patient undergoes myomectomy, follow general postoperative nursing measures related to abdominal surgery
   4. If the patient undergoes a hysterectomy, follow nursing interventions, cancer of the cervix

ENDOMETRIOSIS

A. Definition: tissue resembling the endometrial membrane grows in another location in the pelvic cavity
B. Pathology
   1. During menstrual period, endometrial cells are stimulated by ovarian hormone
   2. Bleeding into surrounding tissue occurs, causing inflammation

3. Condition may result in adhesions, fusion of pelvic organs, bladder dysfunction, stricture of bowel, or sterility
C. Signs and symptoms: symptoms usually appear in women over 30 years of age
   1. Subjective
      a. Discomfort of pelvic area before menses, becoming worse during menstrual flow, and diminishing as flow ceases
      b. Dyspareunia
      c. Fatigue
   2. Objective: infertility
D. Diagnostic tests/methods
   1. Laparoscopy
   2. Culdoscopy
E. Treatment
   1. Hormonal therapy to suppress ovulation
   2. Surgical intervention: hysterectomy, oophorectomy, or salpingectomy
F. Nursing intervention
   1. Provide emotional support
   2. If patient is young, advise not to delay family because of risk of sterility
   3. Explain that hormonal drug may cause pseudopregnancy and irregular bleeding
   4. If patient is middle aged, advise her that menopause may stop progression of condition
   5. Follow general postoperative nursing actions if the patient undergoes surgical procedure
      a. Observe for vaginal hemorrhage, malodorous vaginal discharge, or vaginal discharge other than serosanguineous discharge
      b. Observe for urine retention, burning, frequency, or urgency to void
      c. Listen for renewed bowel sounds
   6. Patient teaching on discharge
      a. Heavy lifting, prolonged standing, walking, and sitting are contraindicated
      b. Sexual intercourse should be avoided until approved by physician

PELVIC INFLAMMATORY DISEASE (PID)

A. Definition: inflammation of the pelvic cavity
B. Pathology
   1. Pathogenic organisms are introduced into the cervix
   2. PID may be confined to one or more structures: fallopian tubes, ovaries, pelvic peritoneum, pelvic veins, or pelvic tissue
   3. May result in adhesions, strictures, or sterility
   4. Most common causative organism: gonococcus
   5. Also caused by staphylococci or streptococci
C. Signs and symptoms
   1. Subjective
      a. Abdominal pain
      b. Pelvic pain
      c. Low-back pain
      d. Nausea
   2. Objective
      a. Malodorous, purulent discharge
      b. Fever
      c. Vomiting
D. Diagnostic tests/method: culture and sensitivity test and CBC; pelvic exam; laparoscopy

E. Treatment
  1. Antibiotic therapy
  2. Analgesics
F. Nursing intervention
  1. Provide nonjudgmental, accepting attitude
  2. Place patient in semi-Fowler's position to provide dependent pelvic drainage
  3. Apply heat to abdominal area if ordered to improve circulation and provide comfort
  4. Patient teaching should include
    a. Take shower instead of tub bath
    b. Perineal hygiene: wipe from front to back
    c. How to recognize if sexual partner is infected with gonococcus: discharge from penis of whitish fluid with painful urination (not all males are symptomatic)
    d. Importance of routine physical examinations, because gonococcal infection is asymptomatic in females
    e. Reinforce "safe sex" guidelines

VAGINAL FISTULA

A. Definition: tubelike opening between two internal organs
B. Pathology
  1. Causes include radiation therapy, gynecological surgery, or traumatic childbirth
  2. Results in impaired blood supply and sloughing of tissue, leading to abnormal opening
  3. Four types affect female reproductive organs
    a. Ureterovaginal: between ureter and vagina; urine leaks into vagina
    b. Vesicovaginal: between bladder and vagina; urine leaks into vagina
    c. Urethrovaginal: between urethra and vagina; urine leaks into vagina
    d. Rectovaginal: between rectum and vagina; flatus and fecal matter leak into vagina
C. Signs and symptoms
  1. Subjective
    a. Leakage of urine, flatus, and fecal matter
    b. Pain in affected area
  2. Objective
    a. Excoriation
    b. Malodor
D. Diagnostic methods
  1. Symptoms and physical examination
  2. Patient history of radiation therapy
  3. Intravenous pyelogram (IVP)
  4. Cystoscopy
E. Treatment
  1. Small fistula may heal spontaneously
  2. Surgical excision
  3. Temporary colostomy for rectovaginal fistula
F. Nursing intervention
  1. Provide psychological support: offer reassurance and acceptance
  2. Encourage patient to verbalize feelings; express empathy
  3. Observe vaginal discharge and record
  4. Change perineal pad q4h and prn
  5. Instruct on perineal hygiene
  6. Provide sitz bath and irrigation solutions for hygiene if ordered

  7. Follow general postoperative nursing actions if patient undergoes surgery
    a. Observe Foley catheter for drainage at all times
    b. Caution patient not to strain when having a bowel movement

PROLAPSED UTERUS

A. Definition: downward displacement of the uterus through the vaginal orifice
B. Pathology
  1. A result of weakened supporting muscles and ligaments of the pelvis
  2. Causes include childbirth injuries, repeated pregnancies with short intervals between, menopausal atrophy, and congenital weakness
C. Signs and symptoms
  1. Subjective
    a. Pain in lower abdomen
    b. Feeling of pressure within pelvis
    c. Stress incontinence
    d. Dyspareunia
    e. Backache
  2. Objective
    a. Urinary stasis
    b. Elongated cervix
D. Diagnostic methods
  1. Signs and symptoms
  2. Pelvic examination
E. Treatment
  1. Placement of a pessary in the vagina to support uterus
  2. Surgical suspension of the uterus
  3. Hysterectomy if condition is postmenopausal
F. Nursing intervention
  1. Approach unhurriedly, demonstrate calmness, and encourage expression of feelings to decrease anxiety
  2. Explain all procedures
  3. Follow general postoperative nursing actions
    a. Chart number of perineal pads used during 8-hour period
    b. Observe for hemorrhage
    c. Observe for vaginal discharge other than serosanguineous fluid
    d. Listen for renewed bowel sounds
    e. Observe for urinary retention and pelvic congestion

CYSTOCELE AND RECTOCELE

A. Definition
  1. Cystocele: abnormal protrusion of the bladder against the vaginal wall
  2. Rectocele: abnormal protrusion of part of the rectum against the vaginal wall
B. Pathology
  1. Result of weakened supporting muscles and ligaments of the pelvis
  2. Causes include childbirth injuries, repeated pregnancies with short intervals between, menopausal atrophy, and congenital weakness
C. Signs and symptoms
  1. Subjective
    a. Pelvic pressure; backache
    b. Stress incontinence and dysuria (cystocele)

c. Constipation or incontinence of feces and flatus (rectocele)
   2. Objective
      a. Residual urine after voiding (cystocele)
      b. Hemorrhoids (rectocele)
D. Diagnostic methods
   1. Signs and symptoms
   2. Pelvic examination
E. Treatment
   1. Anterior colporrhaphy to adjust cystocele
   2. Posterior colporrhaphy to adjust rectocele
F. Nursing intervention
   1. Administer catheter care twice a day (bid) and prn
   2. Splint abdomen when coughing
   3. Place in low-Fowler's position or flat in bed to avoid pressure on suture line
   4. Explain to patient that she should respond to bowel stimuli to avoid suture strain
   5. After each bowel movement, clean perineum with warm water and soap; pat dry anterior to posterior
   6. Apply heat lamp, anesthetic spray, or ice packs if ordered to relieve discomfort
   7. Patient teaching
      a. Heavy lifting and prolonged standing, walking, and sitting are contraindicated
      b. Sexual intercourse should be avoided until approved by physician
      c. Pelvic exercises

OVARIAN TUMORS

A. Definition: a mass of tissue growing on the ovary; is usually asymptomatic until large enough to cause pressure
B. Pathology: two classifications
   1. Ovarian cyst: a benign condition but may transform to a malignancy; may be small, containing clear fluid, or may be filled with a thick, yellow fluid; size varies
   2. Malignant tumors: a cancerous growth found on the ovary; can be the primary site of the cancer or secondary site caused by metastasis from the GI tract, breast, pancreas, or kidneys
C. Signs and symptoms
   1. Subjective
      a. Pelvic pain
      b. Menstrual disturbances
      c. Abdominal distention
      d. Constipation
      e. Dyspareunia
   2. Objective: palpable mass
D. Diagnostic tests/methods
   1. Culdoscopy
   2. Ultrasonography
   3. Biopsy examination
E. Treatment
   1. Cyst may be observed for regression in size
   2. Oophorectomy (removal of ovaries)
   3. Removal of all reproductive organs
   4. Estrogen replacement therapy
   5. X-ray therapy and chemotherapy
   6. Radiation therapy
F. Nursing intervention
   1. If patient undergoes oophorectomy, follow general postoperative nursing care related to abdominal surgery
   2. If the patient undergoes surgery for removal of all abdominal reproductive organs, follow nursing intervention covered below under cancer of the cervix
   3. Assist the patient in dealing with changes of body image

CANCER OF THE CERVIX

A. Definition: new growth of abnormal cells in the neck of the uterus
B. Pathology
   1. Early stage is confined to epithelial cervical layer
   2. Will continue to invade surrounding area such as bladder and rectum
   3. Metastasizes to lungs, bones, and liver
C. Signs and symptoms
   1. Subjective
      a. Asymptomatic in early stage
      b. Menstrual disturbances
      c. Postmenopausal bleeding
      d. Bleeding after intercourse
      e. Watery discharge
   2. Suspicious Pap test result
D. Diagnostic tests/methods
   1. Pap smear
   2. Cervical biopsy examination
   3. Colposcopy
   4. Schiller's test
   5. Conization
E. Treatment
   1. Panhysterectomy (excision of uterus and cervix)
   2. Radiation in advanced case
   3. Chemotherapy
F. Nursing intervention
   1. Reassure patient and family that adjustment to illness can be slow
   2. Acknowledge that patient must adapt to illness according to her age, developmental stage, and past life experiences
   3. If patient is to receive internal radium implant
      a. Provide isolation
      b. Instruct patient to maintain supine or side-lying position
      c. Explain to patient and visitors that the amount of time spent with patient will be limited to avoid overexposure to radiation
      d. Provide high-protein, low-residue diet to avoid straining of bowels, which may dislodge implant
      e. Maintain high fluid intake: 2000 to 3000 ml daily
      f. Insert Foley catheter to prevent bladder distention
      g. Administer antiemetics as ordered
   4. If the patient undergoes surgery, follow general postoperative nursing actions
      a. Observe for vaginal hemorrhage, malodorous vaginal discharge, or any vaginal discharge other than serosanguineous discharge
      b. Observe for urinary retention
      c. Change perineal pads every 3 to 4 hours and prn
      d. Listen for renewed bowel sounds

BARTHOLIN CYSTS

A. Definition: a tumorlike capsule formed of retained secretions

B. Pathology
   1. May develop as a consequence of an earlier bacterial infection of these structures
   2. Formation of these cysts results from obstruction in the outlet of these glands
C. Signs and symptoms
   1. Subjective
      a. Pain on walking
      b. Dyspareunia
   2. Objective: mobile nodule
D. Diagnostic methods
   1. Pelvic examination
   2. Palpable nodule
E. Treatment
   1. Incision and drainage
   2. Antiseptic wound packing
F. Nursing intervention
   1. Reassure the patient that normal function of the gland will be regained after the procedure
   2. After surgery provide a sterile perineal pad q4h and prn
   3. Provide sterile wound care as ordered
   4. Instruct on perineal hygiene
   5. Provide sitz baths for increased circulation and comfort
   6. On patient's discharge from the hospital explain that the surgical wound is susceptible to bacterial infection until healing has taken place

FIBROCYSTIC BREAST DISEASE

A. Definition: fiberlike tumors of the breast tissue with cyst formation
B. Pathology
   1. Cause is unknown; possible hormonal imbalance
   2. Condition occurs during reproductive years and disappears with menopause
   3. A benign condition affecting 25% of women over 30 years of age
C. Signs and symptoms
   1. Subjective: breast tenderness and pain
   2. Objective: small, round, smooth nodules
D. Diagnostic tests/methods
   1. Mammography
   2. Thermomastography
   3. Xerography
E. Treatment: conservative
   1. Aspiration
   2. Biopsy examination to rule out malignancy
F. Nursing intervention
   1. Explain importance of monthly breast self-examination
   2. Encourage patient to seek medical evaluation if nodule forms, because cystic disease may interfere with early diagnosis of breast malignancy

CANCER OF THE BREAST

A. Definition: small, painless, fixed lump most frequently located in the upper, outer portion of the breast
B. Pathology
   1. Risk factors increase with age
   2. Influenced by heredity
   3. Sites of metastasis: lymph nodes, lungs, liver, bone, brain
   4. Other risk factors
      a. Obesity
      b. Diet high in fat and protein
      c. Nulliparity
      d. Parity after age 35
      e. Menarche before 11 years of age
      f. Menopause after 55 years of age
      g. History of cancer in one breast
C. Signs and symptoms
   1. Subjective: nontender nodule
   2. Objective:
      a. Enlarged axillary nodes
      b. Nipple retraction or elevation
      c. Skin dimpling
      d. Nipple discharge
D. Diagnostic tests/methods
   1. Mammography
   2. Thermography
   3. Xerography
   4. Breast biopsy examination
E. Treatment
   1. Lumpectomy: removal of the lump and partial breast tissue; indicated for early detection
   2. Mastectomy
      a. Simple mastectomy: removal of breast
      b. Modified radical mastectomy: removal of breast, pectoralis minor, and some of adjacent lymph nodes (the pectoralis major is preserved)
      c. Radical mastectomy: removal of the breast, pectoral muscles, pectoral fascia, and nodes
   3. Oophorectomy, adrenalectomy, or hypophysectomy to remove source of estrogen and those hormones that stimulate the breast tissue
   4. Radiation therapy to destroy malignant tissue
   5. Chemotherapeutic agents to shrink, retard, and destroy cancer growth
   6. Corticosteroids, androgens, and antiestrogens to alter cancer that is dependent on hormonal environment
F. Nursing intervention
   1. Provide atmosphere of acceptance, frequent patient contact, and encouragement in illness adjustment
   2. Introduce a person who has successfully undergone the same experience: arrange contact from Reach to Recovery representative
   3. Encourage grooming activities such as hair, nails, teeth, and skin
   4. Arrange attractive environment
   5. If the patient is receiving radiation or chemotherapy, explain and assist her with potential side effects
      a. Nausea and vomiting
      b. Anorexia
      c. Diarrhea
      d. Stomatitis
      e. Malaise
      f. Itching
      g. Hair loss (alopecia)
   6. If the patient has undergone surgical intervention, follow postoperative nursing actions
      a. Elevate affected arm above level of right atrium to prevent edema
      b. Drawing blood or administering parenteral fluids or taking blood pressure on affected arm is contraindicated
      c. Monitor dressing for hemorrhage; observe back for pooling of blood

d. Empty Hemovac and measure drainage q8h
e. Assess circulatory status of affected limb
f. Measure upper arm and forearm, bid, to monitor edema
g. Encourage exercises of the affected arm when approved by physician; avoid abduction
    (1) Brushing hair
    (2) Squeezing ball
    (3) Feeding self
7. Patient teaching on discharge
    a. Exercise to tolerance
    b. Sleep with arm elevated
    c. Elevate arm several times daily
    d. Avoid injections, vaccinations, and taking of blood pressure in affected arm
    e. Never allow blood to be drawn from or IV started in affected arm

PAGET'S DISEASE OF THE BREAST

A. Definition: cancer of the nipple
B. Pathology
    1. Rare occurrence affecting women over 40 years of age
    2. Spreads from nipple to areola to part of the breasts; ulcerates
C. Signs and symptoms
    1. Subjective
        a. Itching
        b. Swelling
    2. Objective
        a. Blistering
        b. Discharge
        c. Nipple retraction
D. Diagnostic method: biopsy examination
E. Treatment: mastectomy
F. Nursing intervention: see nursing intervention, cancer of the breast

SEXUALLY TRANSMITTED INFECTIOUS DISEASES (STDs)

SYPHILIS

A. Description: caused by a spirochete, *Treponema pallidum*; appears in three stages; transmitted through sexual contact or warm blood
    1. Primary stage: after an incubation period of 10 to 60 days (usually 3 weeks), during which there are no symptoms, an ulcer or chancre appears at the site of entry; it contains many organisms and is highly infectious; there may be minor local discomfort or mild generalized symptoms (e.g., headache or lymph node enlargement); without treatment it heals in 3 to 5 weeks
    2. Secondary stage: 3 weeks later it appears as a mild rash on skin (usually palms of hands and soles of feet) and as papules on mucous membranes; all lesions contain organisms and are highly contagious; symptoms may be mild or generalized (e.g., bone pain, sore throat, hair loss in patches, or lymph node changes); lasts a few weeks and becomes dormant if not treated; patient is infectious for about 1 year
    3. Third or latent stage: 10 to 30 years later the spirochetes, which have been deposited in tissues and organs are in lesions (gummas); these destroy the tissue; common sites are the CNS, eyes, and the aorta

B. Signs and symptoms: relate to organ involved (e.g., aortic aneurysm)
C. Diagnostic tests/methods
    1. Primary stage: microscopic examination of smear
    2. Second and third stages: blood serum tests (e.g., VDRL and RPR)
D. Treatment: penicillin or tetracycline (patient and partner)

GONORRHEA

A. Definition: a highly communicable disease; there is inflammation of the urethra and spread to other organs of the genital tract; incubation period is 3 to 4 days
B. Cause: *Neisseria gonorrhoeae*, transmitted by sexual contact
C. Signs and symptoms
    1. Female patients may have no early symptoms or purulent vaginal discharge, dysuria, or urgency; untreated, it may spread to other organs in the pelvic cavity (see pelvic inflammatory disease [PID])
    2. Male patients have purulent urethral discharge and burning on urination; may develop urethral stricture; epididymitis, prostatitis
D. Diagnostic tests/methods
    1. Patient history and physical examination
    2. Smear or culture
E. Treatment: penicillin or tetracycline; ceftriaxone (a cephalosporin) for penicillinase-resistant strains

HERPES GENITALIS

A. Description: fluid-filled vesicles on genitalia form crusts, causing generalized symptoms such as elevated temperature; pain; may have no symptoms; there are recurrent episodes; problems arise in pregnancy; is believed to predispose to cervical cancer
B. Cause: *Herpesvirus hominis* type 2 HSV
C. Treatment: symptomatic; topical or oral antiviral agents (acyclovir [Zovirax]); no cure
D. Recommend use of barrier forms of contraception

CHLAMYDIA TRACHOMATIS

A. Definition: most common STD in the United States; causes symptoms similar to gonorrheal infections
B. Cause: *Chlamydia trachomatis*
C. Signs and symptoms
    1. Males: urethritis, dysuria, frequency, watery mucoid discharge; complications include epididymitis, prostatitis, infertility
    2. Females: often asymptomatic; mucopurulent cervicitis, dysuria, frequency, local soreness; complications include salpingitis, PID, ectopic pregnancy, and infertility
D. Diagnostic tests/methods: urogenital smear analysis for enzyme or antibody
E. Treatment: antibiotic therapy (doxycycline, tetracycline, erythromycin)

CONDYLOMATA ACUMINATA

A. Definition: also referred to as genital/venereal warts; often seen with other STDs such as gonorrhea and trichomoniasis; highly contagious
B. Cause: human papilloma virus (HPV)
C. Signs and symptoms: initially single, small papillary growths that grow into large cauliflower-like masses, profuse foul-smelling vaginal discharge, bleeding; may progress to genital and cervical dysplasia, cancer

D. Diagnostic tests/methods: inspection of urinary meatus, vulva, labia, vagina, cervix, penis, scrotum, anus, perineum; culture and biopsy

E. Treatment
1. Cryotherapy with liquid nitrogen or cryoprobe
2. Laser therapy
3. Acid treatments
4. Surgery
5. Chemotherapy (5FU)

TRICHOMONIASIS/CANDIDIASIS

A. Definition: very common STD; symptoms frequently seen only in women

B. Cause: *Trichomonas vaginalis* and *Candida albicans*, respectively

C. Signs and symptoms: itching; discharge

D. Diagnostic tests/methods: culture and inspection of affected tissues

E. Treatment: antifungals; antiprotozoal drugs (metronidazole [Flagyl])

INTEGUMENTARY SYSTEM
Anatomy and Physiology

A. Structure of skin: (Fig. 5-23) includes epithelial, connective, and nerve tissue; consists of sweat and oil glands; is soft and has elasticity
1. Epidermis: outermost layer; cells are flat and tough; no blood supply
   a. Cells undergo constant cellular change by mitosis

b. Contains pigment (melanin); amount of pigment varies among races and individuals

2. Dermis: "true skin," the inner layer, composed of living cells
   a. Connective tissue framework
   b. Contains blood vessels, nerves, hair roots, and oil and sweat glands
   c. The ridges and grooves form the pattern for fingerprints, unique to each individual
   d. Nerve endings provide sensation (touch)
      (1) Receptors: small, round bodies (tactile corpuscles)
      (2) Located in dermis; numerous in tips of fingers, toes, and tongue
      (3) Allows perception of heat, cold, and pain

3. Subcutaneous tissue: lies under dermis
   a. Contains fat cells, which give the skin its smooth appearance
   b. Serves as a shock absorber and insulates deeper tissues

4. Glands
   a. Sebaceous (oil glands)
      (1) Excrete oily substance (sebum)
      (2) Keep skin soft and moist
   b. Sudoriferous (sweat glands)
      (1) Secrete perspiration
      (2) Part of the body's heating and regulating equipment

5. Appendages
   a. Hair: covers the skin except on the palms of the

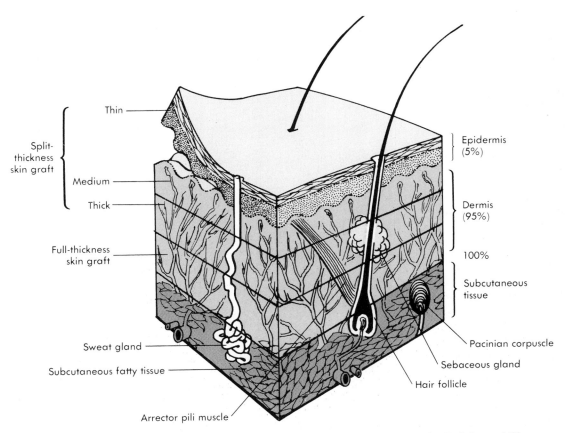

Figure 5-23   Structures of the skin and skin layers. (From Phipps WJ, Sands JK, Lehman MK, Cassmeyer VL: *Medical-surgical nursing: concepts and clinical practice,* ed 5, St Louis, 1995, Mosby.)

TABLE 5-7 Changes from Aging in Skin, Hair, and Nails

Parameters	Observable Changes	Cause
Skin		
Color	Paleness in white skin	Decreased vascularity of dermis; loss of melanocytes
	Brown spots (senile lentigines)	Hyperpigmentation
	Purple patches (senile purpura)	Blood leaking from poorly supported, fragile capillaries
Moisture	Dry skin, decreased perspiration	Decreased sebaceous and sweat gland activity
Elasticity, turgor	Decreased elasticity	Loss of collagen and elastic fibers
	Loose folds and wrinkles	
	Decreased turgor	
Texture	Some rough areas	Environmental effects over time and decreased moisture
	Thinner, more transparent skin	Thinning of epidermis from decreased vascularity of dermis; loss of underlying tissue
Hair		
Color	Grayness	Decreased number of melanocytes in hair
Consistency	Thinner on head and body	Decreased density and rate of hair growth
	Coarser in nose of men	Increased density of nasal hair
Distribution	Loss of hair on head and body	Decreased rate of hair growth; decreased hormones; decreased peripheral circulation
	Increased hair on face of women	Higher androgen-to-estrogen ratio
Nails	More brittle	Slowing of nail growth; decreased peripheral circulation
	Longitudinal ridges	
	Thickening and yellowing of toenails	

From Phipps WJ, Sands JK, Marek JF: *Medical-surgical nursing: concepts and clinical practice,* ed 6, St Louis, 1999, Mosby.

hands and the soles of the feet; composed of dead keratinized cells
  (1) Shaft: the hair above the skin
  (2) Follicle: a tiny sac from which the hair root grows
  b. Nails: tightly packed cells of scaly epidermis
  (1) Roots are living cells; visible ends are dead cells
  (2) They protect the tips of the fingers and toes
  (3) The pink coloring comes from the blood supply in the nail bed
B. Functions
  1. Protection: protects deeper tissues from pathogenic organisms and harmful chemicals
  2. Excretion: limited to water and urea; only a small amount of waste products are eliminated
  3. Regulation: helps regulate body temperature and fluid content
  4. Sensory: contains millions of nerve endings that provide sensory reception to pressure, touch, pain, and temperature
  5. Vitamin D production—effect of sunlight
C. Effects of aging: skin, hair, nails (Table 5-7)

INTEGUMENTARY SYSTEM CONDITIONS AND DISORDERS

The skin is the body's barrier and protection from the environment. It prevents loss of body fluids and protects tissues and organs from external injury and organisms. Temperature regulation, sensation, and excretion of small amounts of water and sodium chloride are functions of the skin. Maximum health and healing of the skin are maintained by proper nutrition, hydration, electrolyte balance, exercise, and rest. Problems arise from systemic allergies (e.g., food and medication, exposure to exter-

nal irritants such as chemicals, plants, and cosmetics, exposure to sun, parasites, microorganisms, injury, and new growths).
  The following terms are used to describe skin lesions:
atheroma: fatty patch or thickening on skin
bleb: blister filled with fluid
bulla: large blister filled with fluid, as occurs with burns
comedo: blackhead or acne
cyst: sac or capsule containing fluid or semisolid material (e.g., sebaceous cyst of scalp)
erythema: red area (e.g., sunburn)
excoriation: abrasion of the outer layer of skin (e.g., friction trauma)
exudate: fluid, usually containing pus, bacteria, and dead cells (e.g., fluid from infected wound)
fissure: groove, crack, or slit as occurs with ulceration
furuncle: painful erythematous raised lesion (e.g., boil)
hive: solid, raised, and itchy area (wheal), usually the result of allergy
macule: small, flat discolored area (e.g., freckle)
maculopapular: multiple lesions consisting of both macules and papules (e.g., early chickenpox)
mole: flat or raised pigmented growth (e.g., birthmark)
nevus: congenital raised, pigmented growth (e.g., birthmark or mole)
nodule: small, solid mass (e.g., swollen lymph node)
papule: small, red, raised elevation (e.g., measles)
petechia: red pinpoint hemorrhage; seen in some blood diseases
pustule: small elevation on the skin containing purulent fluid (e.g., acne)
ulcer: depression (e.g., open lesion on skin)
urticaria: hives (e.g., blood transfusion reaction)
vesicle: small sac containing serous or sanguineous fluid (e.g., pimple)

wheal: raised lesion, usually accompanied by itching (e.g., mosquito bite)

Nursing Assessment

A. Nursing observations
   1. Skin
      a. Color: any deviation from normal (e.g., pallor, cyanosis, jaundice, or blanching), general pigmentation, vascularity, bruising
      b. Turgor: evaluate hydration, elasticity, and mobility
      c. Lesions and rashes: size, location, color, drainage, crusts, pattern or shape, distribution
      d. Skin temperature for inconsistency: areas cool or warm to the touch
      e. Cleanliness and hygiene
      f. Odor
      g. Pressure areas for existing or potential decubitus ulcers
   2. Hair and scalp
      a. Unusual distribution or absence of scalp and body hair; lesions
      b. Texture: smooth or coarse
      c. Parasites: scalp and pubic
   3. Nails
      a. Cleanliness
      b. Brittleness
      c. Length
      d. Pitting
      e. Shape, contour, clubbing
      f. Color, splinter hemorrhages
B. Patient description (subjective data)
   1. History to include onset, changes, and presence of itching, pain, or burning
   2. Factors that make condition worse/better
   3. Allergies
   4. Recent changes in environment and diet
   5. Medications taken
   6. Concerns about appearance, change in body image, and disfigurement
   7. Changes in activities or life-style caused by disease
   8. Environmental or occupational hazards (sun exposure, toxic chemicals, insect bites)
   9. History of systemic disorders

Frequent Patient Problems and Nursing Care

A. Body image disturbance related to disfigurement
   1. Show acceptance by being nonjudgmental
   2. Plan time to allow patient to express feelings
B. Pain related to pruritus (itching)
   1. Administer antipruritics and antihistamines (see Chapter 3)
   2. Keep nails short
   3. Use cotton bedding and clothing; avoid rough fabrics
   4. Encourage use of cotton gloves when sleeping
   5. Bathe with tepid water; use minimal soap; pat dry using no friction
   6. Give oil, medicated, or starch baths
C. Risk for infection/injury related to open lesions
   1. Use aseptic technique in cleaning, teach hand washing
   2. Monitor for redness, swelling, elevated temperature
   3. Use dressings only when necessary and apply loosely with gauze and nonallergenic tape

D. Impaired skin integrity related to seborrhea: oily scalp with shedding of greasy scales
   1. Give frequent shampoos
   2. Use medicated shampoos; rinse thoroughly

Major Medical Diagnoses

CONTACT DERMATITIS

A. Definition: an inflammatory response of the skin with redness, edema, thickening of the skin, and frequent scaling; there may be vesicles and papules
B. Cause: an allergic reaction or unusual sensitivity when a substance comes in direct contact with the skin (e.g., poison ivy, soaps, cleaning agents, and fabrics)
C. Symptoms: pruritus; erythema
D. Diagnostic test/methods
   1. Allergy testing
   2. Patient history and assessment
E. Treatment
   1. Systemic medication: antihistamines, antipruritics, and corticosteroids (see Chapter 3)
   2. Topical medication: corticosteroids (see Chapter 3)
   3. Remove cause
F. Nursing intervention
   1. Prevent scratching
   2. Give tepid baths
   3. Cut nails
   4. Administer prn medications as soon as possible

PSORIASIS

A. Definition: a chronic condition in which there are patches of inflammation that are red and covered with silvery scales that shed; these usually occur on elbows, knees, lower back, and scalp; they may cover the entire body
B. Cause: unknown, may be a family tendency, symptoms increase during stress and high anxiety; other related factors are alcoholism, trauma, and infection
C. Signs and symptoms
   1. Subjective
      a. Pruritus, mild to severe
      b. Depression related to appearance
   2. Objective
      a. Scratching
      b. Sharply demarcated scaling plaques
D. Diagnostic methods: patient history and physical appearance
E. Treatment (individual)
   1. Topical medication: coal tars and corticosteroids (see Chapter 3)
   2. Systemic medication: corticosteroids and methotrexate (in severe cases) (see Chapter 3)
   3. Exposure to ultraviolet light; photochemotherapy
   4. Anxiolytics
   5. Antimetabolites
F. Nursing intervention
   1. During bath gently remove scales with cloth or brush
   2. Occlusive dressing may be wrapped in plastic

HERPES SIMPLEX (COLD SORE/FEVER BLISTER) TYPE I (HSV-I)

A. Definition: a group of blisters on a reddened base usually on or near mouth or genitalia
B. Cause: a viral infection precipitated by an upper respiratory tract infection or elevation of temperature from systemic

TABLE 5-8   Classification of Common Tumors of the Skin

Classification	Description	Treatment
Benign	Nevus, brown or black mole	Observe for changes: remove only if irritated or changes are observed
Premalignant or potentially malignant	Actinic keratosis: common, sun-induced, premalignant (precancerous) lesions; often on the face and backs of hands; ill-marginated, increased vascularity, and rough-textured surface; becomes reddish and scaly	Cryosurgery; topical medication
	Senile keratosis; brownish scaly spots on face and hands of aging persons	Surgical removal or topical medication or cryosurgery
	Leukoplakia: shiny white patches on mucous membranes of mouth and female genitalia	Removal of irritating teeth; oral hygiene. For genitalia: surgical excision; biopsy
	Moles (nevi) that bleed, grow, or are irritated or crusted	May become malignant and are surgically removed
	Black, smooth moles	
Malignant	Squamous cell carcinoma: begin as a warty growth and grow and become ulcerated; found on exposed surfaces of the body (tongue and lip)	Early surgical removal
	Basal cell carcinoma: a slow-growing tumor; results from exposure to the sun	Chemosurgery, electrosurgery, or surgical removal
	Malignant melanoma: black tumor that metastasized	Widespread excision

infection; frequently related to emotional upset, menstrual cycle, or general immunosuppression
C. Signs and symptoms
 1. Pain and local discomfort
 2. Distress about appearance
D. Diagnostic methods: physical assessment; viral isolation by tissue culture
E. Treatment: lasts about 1 week; antiviral agents (acyclovir) administered topically or systemically
F. Nursing intervention: none indicated

HERPES ZOSTER (SHINGLES)

A. Definition: crops of vesicles and erythema following sensory nerves on face and trunk; higher incidence in the elderly
B. Cause: varicella zoster virus (chickenpox)
C. Signs and symptoms
 1. Subjective
  a. Severe pain
  b. Malaise
  c. Anorexia
  d. Pruritus
 2. Objective
  a. Elevation of temperature
  b. Results of diagnostic tests
D. Diagnostic methods: physical examination; vesicles follow sensory nerve paths
E. Treatment: no specific treatment (symptomatic only); analgesics may be used for pain; usually subsides in 3 weeks (pain may last for months); antivirals, corticosteroids, capsaicin (Zostrix) for temporary relief of pain
F. Nursing intervention
 1. Keep patient in isolation while vesicles are present
 2. Apply topical lotions to lesions for itching
 3. Give baths or compresses for cooling and soothing
 4. Prevent scratching and secondary infection
 5. Anticipate pain: medicate as needed
 6. Provide small, frequent, well-balanced meals
G. Varicella vaccine (Varivax)

NEOPLASMS

A. Definition: any new and abnormal growth; may be of varied size and location
B. Cause
 1. Benign: unknown
 2. Malignant: related to exposure to the sun and chemical and physical irritants, such as pipe smoking
C. Signs and symptoms: anxiety related to diagnosis and change in physical appearance; appearance of lesions
D. Diagnostic test: biopsy examination: high cure rate with early detection
E. Treatment: see Table 5-8
F. Nursing intervention
 1. Assess all patients for skin lesions
 2. Discuss with patient the importance of reporting any changes in moles
 3. Give preoperative and postoperative instructions (see Chapter 2); surgery is usually outpatient
 4. Provide general care for patient receiving radiotherapy (see Chapter 2)
 5. Give general care for patient receiving chemotherapy (see Chapter 3)
G. Classification of common skin tumors (Table 5-8)

BURNS

A. Definition: a wound in which the skin layers and underlying tissue is destroyed
B. Causes
 1. Heat: dry or moist (e.g., fire)
 2. Chemical (e.g., acids)
 3. Electrical (e.g., lightning or electrical wires)
 4. Radiation (e.g., sun)
 5. Mechanical (e.g., friction from rope)
C. Signs and symptoms: depend on depth (Table 5-9) and area involved
 1. Infection: there is destruction of the body's first line of defense and time postburn (hypovolemic and diuretic stage)

TABLE 5-9   Description of Burns

Classification	Depth	Description	Possible cause
Superficial or shallow partial thickness	Epidermis	Red and dry; painful; may have edema; no scarring	Sunburn
Deep partial thickness	Epidermis and some dermis	Mottled, pink to red blisters; painful; leave scar	Hot oil
Full thickness partial	Epidermis, dermis, and subcutaneous tissue	Black or bright red eschar forms leathery covering; leaves scar; may have no pain	Fire
Full thickness deep	All of the above plus subcutaneous fat, fascia, muscle, and bone (nerve endings, hair follicles, and sweat glands are destroyed)	Black; there is no pain	Fire

2. Loss of body tissue (protein)
3. Loss of fluid and electrolytes (edema)
4. Pain
5. Respiratory distress
6. Immobilization
7. Disfigurement
8. Impending shock

D. Diagnostic methods: physical assessment

E. Treatment
  1. Respiratory evaluation, maintenance of airway, and possible tracheostomy; edema of lung tissue from smoke inhalation may cause increased secretions
  2. Replacement of fluids and electrolytes with IV solutions: plasma, blood, dextran, and electrolytes
  3. Emergency wound care: removal of foreign material; avoidance of contamination
  4. Prevention of infection: tetanus immune globulin and antibiotics
  5. Analgesics for pain (see Chapter 3)
  6. Prevention of shock: plasma expanders; keep patient warm; monitor vital signs, urine output
  7. Wound treatment method
    a. Open method exposure; wound heals by epithelialization of eschar; this method requires reverse isolation; eschar must be removed by debridement (cutting away), whirlpool baths, and escharotomy (incision into eschar)
    b. Topical medications (see Chapter 3)
    c. Grafts: to minimize infection and fluid loss; may be temporary because they are frequently rejected; this method allows for growth of new tissue underneath the protection of the graft
      (1) Autograft: transplantation of skin from patient's own body; care must also be given to donor site; can also grow skin in test tube, then do graft procedure
      (2) Homograft (allograft): transplantation of tissue from living human
      (3) Heterograft: transplantation from animal (pig or cow xenograft)
      (4) Synthetic material used in grafting
    d. Cosmetic surgery may be performed during recovery phase

F. Nursing intervention
  1. Anticipate and prevent respiratory distress; maintain airway, monitor breathing qh then q4h (see Chapter 2); keep tracheostomy equipment available
  2. Maintain fluid balance: monitor IV fluids; monitor urine output qh through indwelling catheter; monitor sp gr qh; weigh patient qd
  3. Anticipate infection: maintain asepsis and reverse isolation; administer antibiotics; monitor temperature q2h; keep patient warm
  4. Anticipate pain: give frequent sedation as ordered, especially before dressing change (administered intravenously during early phase of treatment)
  5. Prevent dangers of immobilization (see Chapter 2); provide proper alignment to prevent deformities (may be uncomfortable or painful); prevent skin surfaces from touching; use turning frames and cradles
  6. To enhance tissue repair, diet must be high in calories (6000 calories qd) and high in protein; tube feeding or total parenteral nutrition may be necessary
  7. Anticipate shock: assess level of consciousness and mental status; monitor pulse rate and blood pressure
  8. Anticipate Curling's ulcer (stress ulcer): at the end of the first week assess for gastrointestinal distress or bleeding
  9. Be aware of anxiety: provide diversional activities; allow time for patient to verbalize feelings; encourage contact with family; involve patient as much as possible with planning and self-care; administer tranquilizers and sedation as necessary

SENSORY SYSTEMS
Visual System
ANATOMY AND PHYSIOLOGY (FIGS. 5-24 AND 5-25)
A. Lies in a protective bony orbit in the skull
B. Eyebrows, eyelids, and lashes also protect the eye
C. Sphere consists of three layers of tissue
  1. Sclera: thick, white fibrous tissue (white of eye); a transparent section over the front of the eyeball, the cornea, permits light rays to enter
  2. Choroid: the middle vascular area: brings oxygen and nutrients to the eye: choroid extends to ciliary body (two smooth muscle structures), which helps control shape of the lens; the front is a pigmented section (iris),

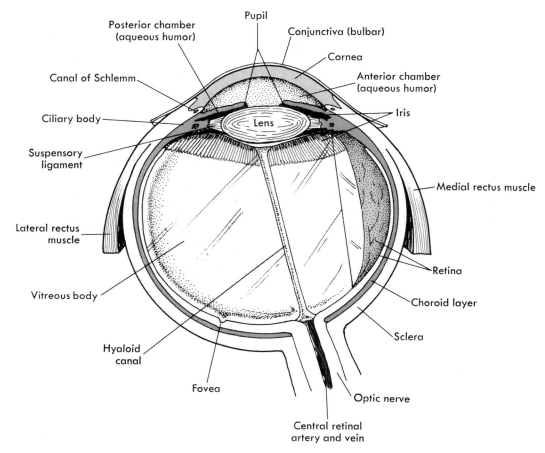

Figure 5-24 Horizontal section through left eyeball. (From Phipps WJ, Sands JK, Marek JR: *Medical-surgical nursing: concepts and clinical practice*, ed 6, St Louis, 1999, Mosby.)

which gives the eye color; in the center of the iris lies the pupil, the "window of the eye" (allows light to pass to lens and retina)

3. Retina: inner layer; physiology of vision takes place; contains receptors of optic nerve; neurons are shaped like rods and cones; cones permit perception of color, rods permit perception of light and shade

D. Chambers
 1. Anterior: contains aqueous humor, maintains slight forward curve in cornea
 2. Posterior: contains vitreous humor: maintains spherical shape of eyeball

E. Conjunctiva: mucous membrane that covers eyeball and eyelid; keeps eyeball moist

F. Lens: transparent structure behind iris; focuses light rays on retina

G. Lacrimal apparatus: gland located in upper, outer part of eye; produces tears to lubricate and cleanse; nasolacrimal duct is located in nasal corner, tears drain into nose

H. Normal intraocular pressure: 10 to 21 torr (mm Hg)

CONDITIONS AND DISORDERS OF THE EYE

Sight is the most important sense to most people. Visual acuity is dependent on general good health, CNS regulation of movement and conduction, and condition of the structures of the eye. Changes in vision are frequently indicative of systemic disease; routine examination of the eye can provide information about diseases in other systems. The nurse must assess the eyes of each patient under his or her care. Although the incidence of blindness and visual impairment increases with age, problems are seen in patients of all ages.

NURSING ASSESSMENT

A. Nursing observations
 1. Glasses, contact lenses, or false eyes
 2. Tearing, discharge (clear or purulent), and color of sclera (white, yellow, or pink)
 3. Accuracy and range of vision
 4. Edema of eyelids; crusting; blinking, rubbing; redness
 5. Clouded appearance over pupil; protrusion or bulging of eye(s); pupil response to light; PERRLA
 6. Squinting or drooping (ptosis) of lid
 7. Symmetry

B. Patient description (subjective data)
 1. Double vision (diplopia), decreased or absent vision in one or both eyes, or blurred or clouded vision
 2. Sensitivity to light (photophobia), spots, halos around lights, flashes of light, or problems seeing in the dark
 3. Eye fatigue, itching, pain, tearing, burning, headache, dryness

C. Note patient history of
 1. Stumbling
 2. Trauma of face or eyes
 3. Contact lenses or eye medication

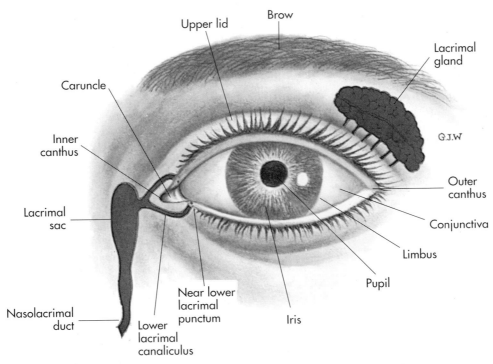

Figure 5-25   External eye structures. (From Thompson JM, McFarland GK, Hirsch JE, Tucker SM: *Mosby's clinical nursing*, ed 4, St Louis, 1998, Mosby.)

4. Changes in vision and any related circumstances
5. Any systemic medications taken

DIAGNOSTIC TESTS/METHODS

A. Ophthalmoscope: assessment of the interior of eye
B. Tonometer: measurement of intraocular pressure; increased pressure may indicate early glaucoma; recommended every 3 years for individuals between 35 and 40 years of age and on a yearly basis for individuals over 40
C. Fields of vision: testing to measure sight on one or both sides (peripheral vision); perimetry
D. Refraction: measurement of light refraction and lenses required for visual acuity
E. Slit lamp: examination of intraocular structures with a high-intensity light beam (corneal abrasions, iritis)
F. Snellen chart: assessment of visual acuity (3 times OS, OD, OU)
G. Retinal angiography: retinal vessels

EYE CARE PROFESSIONALS

A. Ophthalmologist (also called oculist): a medical doctor who specializes in diagnosis, treatment, and surgery of the eyes, including the prescribing of glasses
B. Optometrist: educated and licensed to test for refractive problems; may prescribe and fit glasses; may, within limits, diagnose disease, prescribe medication, or treat eye diseases (laws vary among states)
C. Optician: fills prescription for corrective lenses as prescribed by physician; fits glasses properly

FREQUENT PATIENT PROBLEMS AND NURSING CARE

A. Anxiety/fear related to concerns about loss of vision, altered lifestyles, ability to function, employment, plans for the fu-

ture, and altered body image: allow time for the patient to express feelings
B. Risk for infection related to drainage, use of eye drops
   1. Clean as necessary with normal saline solution
   2. Gently apply compresses to loosen if necessary
   3. Use aseptic technique; wipe from inner canthus to outer canthus
   4. If drainage is purulent, dispose of properly
C. Risk for injury related to need for corrective lenses
   1. Glasses must be kept clean and in a protective case
   2. Contact lenses are kept in a case with *R* and *L* to designate which eye the lens fits; obtain directions for soaking from patient
   3. If patient is dependent on lenses, obtain permission for patient to wear glasses or lenses when going for diagnostic tests
D. Risk for injury related to photophobia
   1. Keep room dim and evenly lighted
   2. Keep blinds adjusted to avoid glare

MAJOR MEDICAL DIAGNOSES
LOW VISION

A. Definition: defects that cannot be corrected with lenses
B. Cause: disease of the eye itself, in the visual pathways to the brain, or in the receptors in the brain; macular degeneration
C. Signs and symptoms: vision may be blurred and images distorted; vision may be clear only at close range; shades of color may not be distinguishable

TOTAL OR LEGAL BLINDNESS

A. Definition: legal blindness is the ability to see at no more than 20 feet (6 m) what normally should be seen at a distance of 200 feet (60 m) (20/200); this may also refer to severe restrictions in peripheral fields of vision (after corrective lenses are used)

B. Pathology
1. Macular degeneration, glaucoma, detached retina, or diabetic retinopathy
2. Trauma or laceration
3. Inflammation or optic neuritis
4. Vascular or hypertensive retinopathy
5. Neoplasms of the brain or eye
6. Cataract

C. Patient problems
1. Inability to care for self (dependency)
2. Frustration
3. Occupational hazards
4. Boredom

D. Nursing diagnoses
1. Anxiety related to degree of visual impairment
2. Risk for injury/trauma related to degree of visual impairment
3. Body image disturbance

E. Nursing intervention
1. Allow as much independence as possible; help make use of existing vision; encourage use of any visual aids recommended by physician (e.g., special lenses, large-type books, and cane); provide reading material in braille for the patient who has learned this method
2. Do not touch patient without talking; always address patient by name; introduce yourself; and tell patient when you are leaving the room
3. Explain all care and treatments; encourage patient to participate in planning care
4. At mealtime, indicate position of utensils and placement of food on dish by comparing it to numbers on a clock (e.g., "the potato is at 3 o'clock")
5. Orient patient to room and entire unit; point out hazards and obstacles (doors and windows); explain location of furniture, bathroom, call bell, and telephone; keep things in the same place
6. Leave bedside table, call bell, and personal items in close reach
7. Maintain safety; keep unit uncluttered, floor clean and dry, bed in low position, and side rail(s) up as necessary; tell patient position of bed and side rails
8. Guide the ambulatory patient by placing patient's arm on yours while walking slowly
9. Provide diversion: radio and books on tapes; be aware of local agencies in your community; many libraries have braille books or tapes available
10. Be mindful of patient confidentiality and security

REFRACTIVE DISORDERS

A. Definition: inability of the refractory media to converge light rays and focus on retina
1. Myopia (nearsightedness): the eyeball is too long; light rays focus at a point before reaching the retina
2. Hyperopia (farsightedness): the eyeball is shorter than normal; light rays focus beyond the retina
3. Presbyopia: a gradual loss of elasticity of the lens; there is decreased ability to focus on near objects
4. Astigmatism: unequal curve in the shape of the cornea or lens; vision is distorted

B. Cause: unknown; may be inherited
C. Symptoms: diminished or blurred vision
D. Diagnostic tests/methods
1. Patient history
2. Refraction
E. Treatment: corrective lenses (glasses or contact lenses); keratorefractive surgery
F. Nursing intervention
1. Encourage proper care of lenses
2. Encourage follow-up checkups as indicated

CONJUNCTIVITIS

A. Definition: infection or inflammation of the conjunctiva
B. Causes: bacteria, usually staphylococci, allergens, chemical reactions, and chlamydial or viral infections
C. Patient problems
1. Very contagious (especially in young children); spread by direct contact with organisms
2. Purulent drainage and itching
3. Photophobia
4. Tearing
D. Diagnostic method: physical assessment; culture and sensitivity of conjunctival scrapings
E. Treatment: ophthalmic antibiotics (see Chapter 3)
F. Nursing intervention
1. Prevent transmission to others: encourage frequent hand washing
2. Provide warm compresses; cleanse eyelids; remove crusts before administering ophthalmic medications
   a. Discourage rubbing of eyes
   b. Isolate personal items (towels, washcloths, and pillowcases)

CATARACT

A. Definition: the crystalline lens becomes clouded and opaque (not transparent)
B. Causes
1. Trauma
2. Congenital
3. Related to diabetes
4. High incidence in the elderly (senile cataracts)
5. Heredity
6. Infections
7. Long time exposure to the sun; ultraviolet rays
C. Signs and symptoms
1. Loss of vision
2. Progressive blurring
3. Haziness with eventual complete loss of sight
D. Diagnostic tests/methods
1. Examination with ophthalmoscope
2. Patient history
3. Ultrasonography
E. Treatment: surgical removal of opaque lens, usually on an outpatient basis; after surgery, corrective lenses are necessary (glasses, contact lenses, or surgical implantation of an artificial lens [IOL])
F. Nursing intervention
1. Give general preoperative care (see Chapter 2)
2. Provide nursing care as for the patient with low vision
3. Postoperative management depends on surgical procedure; be careful to adhere to physician's order; general principles: have patient avoid coughing, bending, or

rapid head movements; provide bed rest for a specified time (usually 2 hours); keep patient flat or in low-Fowler's position; have patient deep breathe (avoid coughing); be sure patient avoids straining (give stool softener); help patient avoid vomiting (an antiemetic will be ordered; administer as needed); observe dressing; report pain or bleeding; position patient with unoperated side down

GLAUCOMA

A. Definition: intraocular pressure increases because of a disturbance in the circulation of aqueous humor; there is an imbalance between production and drainage as the angle of drainage closes
   1. Acute (closed-angle) glaucoma: dramatic onset of symptoms; immediate treatment is required, usually surgery
   2. Chronic (open-angle) glaucoma: symptoms progress slowly and are frequently ignored; if disease is not detected early, it may lead to permanent loss of vision
B. Pathology
   1. Familial tendency
   2. Related to age; incidence increases over 40 years of age
   3. Secondary to injuries and infections
C. Signs and symptoms
   1. Subjective
      a. Loss of peripheral vision (tunnel vision), halos around lights, and permanent loss of vision (a leading cause of blindness)
      b. Pain, malaise, nausea
      c. Reduced visual acuity at night
   2. Objective
      a. Pupils fixed and dilated
      b. Vomiting
      c. Results of diagnostic tests
D. Diagnostic tests/methods
   1. History of symptoms
   2. Measurement of visual fields
   3. Measurement of intraocular pressure
   4. Gonioscopy: measures angle of the anterior chamber
   5. Tonometry
E. Treatment
   1. Miotics to decrease intraocular pressure (see Chapter 3)
   2. Surgery: iridectomy (an incision through the cornea to remove part of the iris to allow for drainage); laser trabeculoplasty (relieves excess intraocular pressure); trabeculectomy (new opening made to bypass obstruction and facilitate flow of aqueous humor); laser iridotomy
   3. Continued medical supervision
F. Nursing intervention
   1. Encourage patient to wear medical identification tag
   2. Administer eye medications on schedule
   3. Inform the patient to avoid drugs with atropine; discourage straining and lifting
   4. Give preoperative and postoperative care according to that for a patient with a cataract; pay careful attention to specifics in physician's orders

DETACHED RETINA

A. Definition: the sensory layer of the retina pulls away from the pigmented layer, vitreous humor may leak into the space occupying the position the retina normally assumes

B. Cause: usually unknown and spontaneous; may be related to sudden blow to the head or follow eye surgery (e.g., removal of cataract)
C. Signs and symptoms
   1. Subjective
      a. Loss of vision in affected area (may be complete loss)
      b. Painless
      c. Visual disturbance (blurring)
      d. Spots and flashes of light
   2. Objective: results of diagnostic tests
D. Diagnostic tests/methods
   1. Patient history and physical assessment
   2. Retinal examination with ophthalmoscope
   3. Ultrasonography
   4. Slit lamp
E. Treatment: depends on area of detachment
   1. Bed rest
   2. Prevention of extension of detachment by restricting eye movements
   3. Mydriatics
   4. Surgical intervention: laser photocoagulation; cryopexy; diathermy; scleral buckling; pneumatic retinopexy, and vitrectomy
F. Nursing intervention
   1. Provide individual care according to location of detachment; physician's orders will be specific
   2. Maintain absolute rest; restrict activity; patch eye to limit eye movement; may use eye shield; patient position based on location of retinal detachment
   3. Prepare patient for postoperative care: inform patient that both eyes may be patched and he or she may be unable to see
   4. Postoperative care: position patient exactly as ordered; maintain eye patch(es); have patient deep breathe and avoid coughing; administer medication for pain; provide care as needed for a person with limited sight
G. Patient problems/nursing diagnoses
   1. Anxiety related to possibility of permanent vision loss
   2. Self-care deficit related to imposed activity restrictions
   3. Pain related to surgical correction and unusual positioning

Auditory System
ANATOMY AND PHYSIOLOGY (FIGS. 5-26 and 5-27)

A. External ear (pinna or auricle): outer, visible portion, shaped like a funnel; gathers sound and sends it into the auditory canal, which is lined with tiny hairs and secretes cerumen, a waxy substance; canal extends to the eardrum, also called the tympanic membrane
B. Middle ear: small, flattened space; contains three small bones called ossicles: malleus (hammer), incus (anvil), and stapes (stirrup); bones are mobile and vibrate; conduct sound waves; the eustachian tube extends into nasopharynx and equalizes the pressure in the middle ear to that of atmospheric pressure
C. Internal ear (labyrinth): vestibule; cochlea, snail-shaped bony tube, contains organ of Corti (organ of hearing); semicircular canals are the receptors for equilibrium and head movements
D. Function
   1. Transmission of sound waves; result is hearing
   2. Maintenance of equilibrium

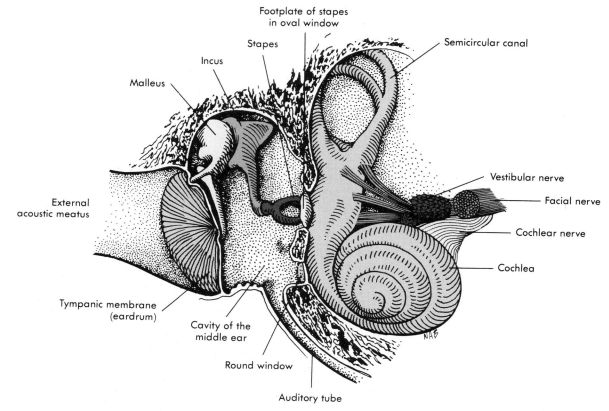

Figure 5-26 Structures of the ear. (From Phipps WJ, Sands JK, Lehman MK, Cassmeyer VL: *Medical-surgical nursing: concepts and clinical practice*, ed 5, St Louis, 1995, Mosby.)

Conditions and Disorders of the Ear

Hearing problems are not as obvious initially during assessment as are many other problems. Hearing loss may be misinterpreted. Many people associate hearing aids with dependency or disfigurement or signs of aging and refuse to wear them. However, the sense of hearing contributes to well-being and safety. This assessment (hearing) must be made for each patient.

NURSING ASSESSMENT

A. Nursing observations
 1. Difficulty hearing or understanding verbal communication
 2. Not responding to loud or sudden noises
 3. Use of hearing aid, lip reading, or sign language
 4. Drainage, dried secretion, or deformities of the ear
B. Patient description (subjective data)
 1. Earache or headache
 2. Difficulty hearing (or lack of hearing) in one or both ears
 3. Itching, drainage, pressure or full feeling
 4. Ringing, buzzing, popping, or echoes
 5. Vertigo
 6. Medications taken
C. Note history of
 1. Ear infections
 2. Ear surgery
 3. Head injury
 4. Medication taken

DIAGNOSTIC TESTS/METHODS

A. Audiometry: a hearing test to determine ability to discriminate sounds, voices, and degrees of loudness and pitch
B. Otoscopy: visual examination of the ear canal and tympanic membrane
C. Weber's test: a tuning fork is struck and placed midline on the patient's forehead; the patient is asked where the sound is heard; in this test of conduction, sounds should be heard equally well in each ear
D. Rinne test: the tuning fork is struck and placed on the mastoid process of the skull behind the ear; the fork is removed, and the patient indicates when the sound can no longer be heard; the still vibrating fork is then placed near the external ear canal; normally the sound will be heard longer through air conduction than through bone conduction
E. Caloric stimulation test (CST): tests vestibular reflexes of the inner ear that control balance
F. Electronystagmography: monitors eye movements; done with CST

PATIENT WITH IMPAIRED HEARING

A. Definition
 1. Conductive hearing loss occurs when injury or disease interferes with the conduction of sound waves to the inner ear (e.g., cerumen in canal)
 2. Sensory hearing loss occurs when there is malfunction of the inner ear, auditory nerve, or auditory center in

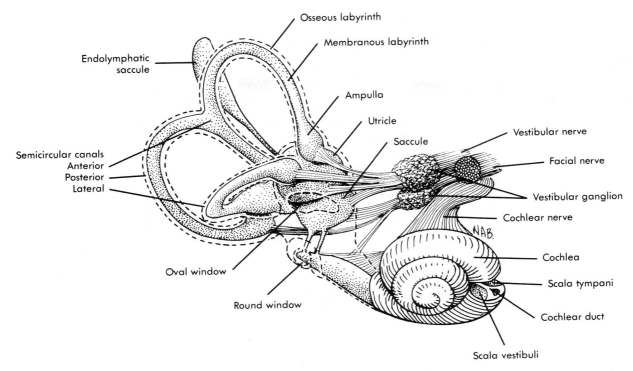

Figure 5-27 Structures of the inner ear. (From Phipps WJ, Sands JK, Marek JR: *Medical-surgical nursing: concepts and clinical practice*, ed 6, St Louis, 1999, Mosby.)

the brain (e.g., toxic effect to eighth cranial nerve from drugs [aspirin])

B. Patient problems
 1. Inability to communicate
 2. Inability to hear hazards in the environment (e.g., automobiles)
 3. Frustration, anxiety, anger, and insecurity
 4. Misinterpretation of communication

C. Treatment: according to cause (cochlear implants, stapedectomy); frequently none

D. Nursing intervention
 1. Find out if a hearing aid can be fitted
  a. Encourage patient to wear it
  b. Test batteries for function
  c. Make sure hearing aid is turned on
  d. Protect hearing aid from breakage; ask patient or family about usual care and storage
 2. Attract patient's attention before speaking
 3. Do not touch patient until he or she is aware that you are in the room
 4. Speak face to face; articulate clearly but not too slowly; move close to patient; avoid covering mouth with hand
 5. Provide alternate methods of communication
  a. Find out if patient lipreads or uses sign language
  b. Provide magic slate or pad and pencil
 6. Nursing intervention after surgery
  a. Give general preoperative and postoperative care (see Chapter 2)
  b. Report drainage immediately
  c. Observe for facial nerve injury: inability to close eyes or pucker lips
  d. Anticipate vertigo: provide safety

e. Be sure patient avoids blowing nose
f. Note specific instructions from physician for positioning, activity, and diet

MAJOR MEDICAL DIAGNOSES
MÉNIÈRE'S SYNDROME

A. Definition: a chronic disease with sudden attacks of vertigo and tinnitus (ringing in the ear) with progressive hearing loss; attacks last a few minutes to a few weeks; usually occurs in women over 50 years of age

B. Cause: unknown; related to fluid in cochlea, either increased production or decreased absorption

C. Signs and symptoms
 1. Vertigo
 2. Nausea and vomiting
 3. Ringing in the ears and hearing loss
 4. Disequilibrium

D. Diagnostic tests/methods: patient history; physical examination; neurological assessment; CST; radiography; electronystagmography; audiogram

E. Treatment
 1. Diuretics, low sodium diet, vasodilators, antihistamines, antiemetics, vestibular depressants, adrenergic agents
 2. Surgery: endolymphatic shunt (reduces pressure and controls vertigo); destruction of the labyrinth as a last resort

F. Nursing intervention
 1. Bed rest; position of comfort
 2. Maintain quiet and safety
 3. Low-sodium diet
 4. Provide specific nursing care as that for patient with impaired hearing

5. Provide general preoperative and postoperative care (see Chapter 2)
6. Provide nursing care for patient after ear surgery

MASTOIDITIS

A. Definition: infection of the mastoid process; may be acute or chronic; not common because of antibiotics
B. Cause: extension of middle ear infection that was inadequately treated
C. Signs and symptoms
   1. Subjective: headache, ear pain, tenderness over mastoid process
   2. Objective
      a. Elevation of temperature
      b. Drainage from ear
D. Treatment
   1. Antibiotics
   2. Surgery
      a. Simple mastoidectomy: removal of infected cells
      b. Radical mastoidectomy: more extensive excision resulting in some degree of hearing loss
E. Nursing intervention
   1. See care of patient with impaired hearing
   2. Provide general preoperative and postoperative care (see Chapter 2)
   3. Provide nursing care for patient after ear surgery (see section on patient with impaired hearing)

OTOSCLEROSIS

A. Definition: a progressive formation of new bone tissue around the stapes preventing transmission of vibrations to the inner ear
B. Cause: unknown
C. Signs and symptoms
   1. Loss of hearing
   2. Ringing or buzzing (tinnitus)

D. Treatment
   1. Hearing aid
   2. Surgery; stapedectomy (removal of diseased bone and replacement with prosthetic implant)
E. Nursing intervention
   1. Provide general care for patient who is hearing impaired
   2. Give general preoperative and postoperative care (see Chapter 2)
   3. Follow specific orders from physician
   4. Provide general nursing care for patient after ear surgery (see section on patient with impaired hearing)

SUGGESTED READINGS

Cole G: *Fundamental nursing concepts and skills*, ed 2, St Louis, 1996, Mosby.

Dirksen SR, Lewis SL, Heitkemper MM: *Clinical companion to medical-surgical nursing,* ed 2, St Louis, 2000, Mosby.

Elkin MK, Perry AG, Potter PA: *Nursing interventions and clinical skills*, ed 2, St Louis, 2000, Mosby.

Harkness GA, Dincher JR: *Medical-surgical nursing: total patient care*, ed 10, St Louis, 1999, Mosby.

Mosby's medical, nursing and allied health dictionary, ed 5, St Louis, 1998, Mosby.

Phipps WJ, Sands JK, Marek JM: *Medical-surgical nursing: concepts and clinical practice,* ed 6, St Louis, 1999, Mosby.

Physicians' desk reference, Montreal, NJ, Medical Economics (published annually).

Thibodeau GA, Patton KP: *Structure and function of the body*, ed 10, St Louis, 1997, Mosby.

Thompson JM et al: *Mosby's clinical nursing*, ed 4, St Louis, 1998, Mosby.

Tucker SM, et al: *Patient care standards: collaborative practice planning guides*, ed 6, St Louis, 1996, Mosby.

REVIEW QUESTIONS

1. Which of the following are the formed elements in the blood that aid in blood clotting?
   ① Antibodies
   ② Leukocytes
   ③ Erythrocytes
   ④ Platelets

2. The body's continual response to changes in the external and internal environment is called:
   ① Homeostasis
   ② Diffusion
   ③ Osmosis
   ④ Filtration

3. The ability of a cell to reproduce is called:
   ① Lysis
   ② Mitosis
   ③ Osmosis
   ④ Crenation

4. The immunity that occurs when a person is given a substance containing antibodies or antitoxins is called:
   ① Active
   ② Passive
   ③ Permanent
   ④ Autoimmune

5. The part of the cell necessary for reproduction is the:
   ① Nucleus
   ② Cytoplasm
   ③ Protoplasm
   ④ Cytoplasmic membrane

6. The hormone that regulates the metabolic rate of body cells is:
   ① Thyroxine
   ② Oxytocin
   ③ Cortisone
   ④ Aldosterone

7. The ovaries produce the hormones:
   ① Estrogen and testosterone
   ② Estrogen and progesterone
   ③ Progesterone and prolactin
   ④ Progesterone and testosterone

8. A greater amount of body heat is lost when surface blood vessels:
   ① Dilate
   ② Contract
   ③ Help the skeletal muscles relax
   ④ Increase the production of sweat

9. The pigmented area surrounding the nipple is the:
   ① Areola
   ② Urochrome
   ③ Cowper's gland
   ④ Bartholin's gland

10. The hormone produced by the testes is:
    ① Estrogen
    ② Progesterone
    ③ Testosterone
    ④ Aldosterone

11. Connective tissue that attaches muscles to bones is called:
    ① Osseous
    ② Tendons
    ③ Cartilage
    ④ Ligaments

12. Which of the following is the major function of the lymphatic system?
    ① Destroys enzymes
    ② Manufactures erythrocytes
    ③ Filters and aids in blood clotting
    ④ Localizes infections and filters foreign cells

13. A patient with a low hemoglobin level would be deficient in which of the following essential minerals:
    ① Iron
    ② Copper
    ③ Calcium
    ④ Magnesium

14. Bile is important in the digestive process because it:
    ① Digests simple fats and sugars
    ② Changes complex sugars to glucose
    ③ Dissolves meat fibers and makes them easier to digest
    ④ Breaks down fat globules so that they can be more easily digested

15. Which of the following is the tissue that forms a protective covering for the body and lines the intestinal and respiratory tract?
    ① Epithelial
    ② Periosteum
    ③ Pericardium
    ④ Connective

16. Which of the following prevents food from flowing back into the esophagus?
    ① Rugae
    ② Chyme
    ③ Cardiac sphincter
    ④ Pyloric sphincter

17. Which of the following structures absorbs most of the nutrients that are used by the body?
    ① Liver
    ② Stomach
    ③ Small intestine
    ④ Large intestine

18. Which of the following are muscles whose functions are to close off body openings?
    ① Flexors
    ② Abductors
    ③ Sphincters
    ④ Extensors

19. Tears drain into the nose through the:
    ① Ciliary body
    ② Lacrimal gland
    ③ Eustachian tube
    ④ Nasolacrimal duct

20. The first eight deciduous teeth to appear through the gums of a baby are the:
    ① Molars
    ② Incisors
    ③ Canines
    ④ Eye teeth

21. A patient is admitted with a brainstem infarction. The nurse is aware that the respiratory and cardiac centers are found in the brainstem, specifically in the:
    ① Pons
    ② Medulla
    ③ Cerebrum
    ④ Cerebellum

22. The main function of the large intestine is to:
    ① Absorb digested food
    ② Produce digestive enzymes
    ③ Secrete digestive enzymes
    ④ Absorb water from waste material
23. The movement that propels food down the digestive tract is called:
    ① Rugae
    ② Peristalsis
    ③ Mastication
    ④ Pylorospasm
24. The end product of protein metabolism is:
    ① Ptyalin
    ② Glucose
    ③ Amino acids
    ④ Hydrochloric acid
25. The completion of digestion occurs in the:
    ① Stomach
    ② Sigmoid
    ③ Small intestine
    ④ Large intestine
26. Which of the following is a function of the liver?
    ① Emulsify fats
    ② Absorb nutrients
    ③ Manufacture trypsin
    ④ Produce fibrinogen
27. Which of the following minerals would the nurse encourage a patient with hypothyroidism to increase consumption of?
    ① Iron
    ② Iodine
    ③ Calcium
    ④ Phosphorus
28. The exchange of nutrients and waste products occurs in the:
    ① Veins
    ② Venules
    ③ Arterioles
    ④ Capillaries
29. The chamber of the heart that receives venous blood from body tissues is:
    ① Left atrium
    ② Right atrium
    ③ Left ventricle
    ④ Right ventricle
30. The hormone released by the adrenal medulla during a body emergency is called:
    ① Insulin
    ② Aldosterone
    ③ Epinephrine
    ④ Testosterone
31. The reabsorption of water from the kidney tubules is promoted by:
    ① Oxytocin
    ② Prolactin
    ③ Calcitonin
    ④ Antidiuretic hormone (ADH)
32. The exchange of oxygen and carbon dioxide in the lungs occurs in the:
    ① Bronchi
    ② Alveoli
    ③ Trachea
    ④ Bronchioles
33. The pacemaker of the heart is the:
    ① AV node
    ② SA node
    ③ Bundle of His
    ④ Purkinje fibers
34. Which of the following arteries carries deoxygenated blood?
    ① Aorta
    ② Carotid
    ③ Coronary
    ④ Pulmonary
35. Immunity occurring in the early months of an infant's life results from the functioning of which gland?
    ① Pineal
    ② Thymus
    ③ Thyroid
    ④ Pituitary
36. Which of the following describes the rounded portion at the upper and lateral portion of the femur that is most often involved in fractures?
    ① Acromion
    ② Acetabulum
    ③ Greater trochanter
    ④ Olecranon process
37. Which of the following is the major function of the periosteum?
    ① Produce RBCs
    ② Produce storage for adipose fat
    ③ Provide for yellow bone marrow
    ④ Provide a structure for blood, lymph, and nerves
38. The muscular structure that forms the floor of the pelvis is the:
    ① Perineum
    ② Peritoneum
    ③ Mons pubis
    ④ Rectus abdominis
39. Which of the following assessment data would be included in an integumentary assessment?
    ① Blood sugar levels
    ② Blood pressure and pulse
    ③ Rashes, bruises, and decubitus
    ④ Rashes, bruises, and blood sugar levels
40. A teenager inquires of the nurse why he has so many pimples and blackheads. Which of the following would be the best response by the nurse?
    ① "The blackheads are caused by a blockage of the lacrimal gland."
    ② "Sometimes the ceruminous glands will become blocked and cause blackheads."
    ③ "Why don't I see if I can't get you a dermatology consult? I'll ask your doctor."
    ④ "The blackheads are caused by blockage of the sebaceous glands and become pimples when they are infected."
41. Which of the following is a normal assessment finding in urine?
    ① Lack of odor
    ② Clear, yellow liquid

③ Presence of a high specific gravity

④ Presence of red blood cells in the urine

42. Grooves and ridges that make up fingerprints are located in the:
    ① Elastic skin tissue
    ② Subcutaneous layer of tissue
    ③ Upper surface of the dermis
    ④ Upper surface of the epidermis

43. The hormone that regulates blood composition and blood volume by acting on the kidney is:
    ① Oxytocin
    ② Antidiuretic
    ③ Aldosterone
    ④ Parathormone

44. Which of the following provide energy for skeletal muscle contraction?
    ① Oxygen and glycogen
    ② Oxygen and acetylcholine
    ③ Glycogen and acetylcholine
    ④ Carbohydrates and lactic acid

45. A nurse is caring for a patient who has an injury to the left motor area of the cerebrum. Where would the nurse expect to see paralysis?
    ① Both arms and legs
    ② The left side of the body
    ③ The right side of the body
    ④ No paralysis should be observed

46. The large, flat, dome-shaped muscle that assists in breathing is the:
    ① Diaphragm
    ② Gastrocnemius
    ③ Latissimus dorsi
    ④ Sternocleidomastoid

47. Which of the following is the part of the nervous system that directs the digestion of food and the circulation of blood?
    ① Sensory
    ② Sympathetic
    ③ Interneurons
    ④ Parasympathetic

48. Which of the following parts of the brain is responsible for the regulation of body temperature?
    ① Medulla
    ② Cerebellum
    ③ Hypothalamus
    ④ Cerebral cortex

49. Which of the following is considered the organ of hearing?
    ① Malleus
    ② Organ of Corti
    ③ Tympanic membrane
    ④ Semicircular canal

50. The equalizing of pressure in the middle ear with atmospheric pressure is the function of the:
    ① Ossicles
    ② Labyrinth
    ③ Oval window
    ④ Eustachian tube

51. Which of the following structures is chiefly responsible for fluid and electrolyte balance?
    ① Gonads
    ② Kidney
    ③ Bladder
    ④ Islets of Langerhans

52. Insulin is produced by the:
    ① Liver
    ② Duodenum
    ③ Pineal gland
    ④ Islets of Langerhans

53. A patient who is HIV positive asks the nurse what the T-cells have to do with immunity. Which of the following statements would best answer the patient's question?
    ① T cells clone into helpers and suppressors
    ② T cells are responsible for humoral immunity
    ③ T cells clone antibody-producing plasma cells
    ④ T cells act against bacteria, viruses, tumor cells, and foreign organs

54. The primary function of the fluid within the eyeball is to:
    ① Produce tears
    ② Dilate the pupil
    ③ Regulate the thickness of the lens
    ④ Give and maintain shape of the eyeball

55. A nurse is caring for a patient in skin traction. Which of the following tasks of the nurse would be most important?
    ① Assess neurovascular status
    ② Encourage liberal fluid intake
    ③ Encourage a diet high in carbohydrates and vitamins
    ④ Limit patient's activities to maintain effectiveness of traction

56. A patient is admitted with bile duct obstruction. The nurse alerts the patient that the stools may appear:
    ① Tarry
    ② Very watery
    ③ Clay colored
    ④ Full of mucus

57. A patient with diabetes is being managed on a split dose of 70/30 isophane insulin suspension (NPH insulin) at 7:30 AM and 4:30 PM. At 2:30 PM one afternoon, the patient calls the nurses' station stating that she is not feeling well. On assessment, the nurse notes her skin is cool and clammy, her hands are shaking, and she appears very apprehensive. The glucometer blood sugar is 45 mg/dl. The most appropriate nursing intervention for the patient's current symptoms is to provide:
    ① A cube of sugar
    ② A large candy bar
    ③ Four ounces of fruit juice
    ④ Twelve ounces of diet drink

58. A patient diagnosed with insulin-dependent diabetes mellitus (IDDM) is receiving regular insulin (Humulin R) by sliding scale. Glucometer readings show a blood sugar of 250 mg/dl. Based on this finding the patient will receive 6 units of Humulin R at 3 PM. When should the nurse be particularly alert to a possible hypoglycemic episode?
    ① 5 PM
    ② 7 PM
    ③ 8 PM
    ④ 10 PM

59. A patient is recovering from a comminuted fracture of the patella. On the second postoperative day the surgeon is concerned that the patient may have developed osteomyelitis. Which of the following assessment data may indicate this osteomyelitis?
   ① Chest pain and dyspnea
   ② Edema, pain, and drainage
   ③ Numbness and delayed capillary refill
   ④ Paresthesia and bluish skin around the knee

60. A patient has undergone a craniotomy for removal of a meningioma. Which of the following questions would be the most appropriate in assessing a possible complication of this patient's surgery?
   ① "Have you noticed any salty or sweet-tasting drainage coming from your incision?"
   ② "Do you have any headache when you turn to your left side?"
   ③ "Are you hungry or thirsty yet?"
   ④ "Do you feel that you need to sleep more?"

61. The nurse is preparing to suction the tracheostomy of a patient with AIDS. Which of the following personal protective equipment should be worn by the nurse?
   ① Mask and gown
   ② Mask and gloves
   ③ Gloves and gown
   ④ Mask with eyeshield and gloves

62. A nurse is caring for a patient who has had chemotherapy. The patient's WBC count is 0.2 mm/cm^3. The primary concern of the nurse caring for this patient would be to:
   ① Protect the patient from infection
   ② Instruct the patient to wear a face mask
   ③ Implement contact isolation precautions
   ④ Encourage participation in group activities to build the immune system

63. A patient with suspected muscular dystrophy has been assigned to your unit. Which of the following observations would be characteristic of this disease?
   ① Pillrolling
   ② Waddling gait
   ③ Shuffling gait
   ④ Tardive dyskinesia

64. An active patient who has been complaining of difficulty dressing, weight loss, fatigue, and progressive muscle weakness is diagnosed with amyotrophic lateral sclerosis (ALS). When planning care for a patient with ALS, a priority nursing intervention would include:
   ① Increased periods of exercise
   ② Alternative means of communication
   ③ Clear airway maintenance
   ④ Facilitating coping/adjustment to diagnosis

65. An elderly patient who states that she has "always been healthy" is being treated for a respiratory tract infection. The nurse observes that the patient uses her diaphragm during inspiration and plans to teach her to pursed-lip breathe, based on the understanding that:
   ① Older persons need to consciously think about taking deep breaths
   ② The older one becomes, the more likely one will develop COPD
   ③ Age-related changes of loss of elastic recoil of the lungs occur
   ④ Older people lose the use of their intercostal muscles

66. A patient with severe degenerative joint disease has been scheduled for an arthroscopy of the left knee. The patient asks the nurse what to expect after the surgery. Which of the following is the nurse's best response?
   ① "You may need to ask your surgeon that question."
   ② "You should not need a knee replacement in the future."
   ③ "You should have less pain and improved joint function."
   ④ "The procedure will virtually cure your degenerative joint disease."

67. A nurse caring for a patient with amyotrophic lateral sclerosis (ALS) must continually assess for signs and symptoms of disease progression. Which of the following signs and symptoms would indicate disease progression?
   ① Aphasia, flexor muscle spasticity, and jaw clonus
   ② Flexor muscles flaccid, dysarthria, and respiratory difficulty
   ③ Dysphagia, dysarthria, and spasticity of flexor muscles
   ④ Sensory loss, jaw clonus, and dysarthria

68. A nurse is caring for an overweight patient with osteoarthritis. Which of the following would the nurse suggest to the patient to help control joint strain?
   ① Exercising the involved joint
   ② Weight reduction and maintenance
   ③ Applying intermittent heat application
   ④ Taking medication at the first sign of pain

69. A nurse is caring for a patient with a suspected diagnosis of osteoarthritis. Which of the following are common characteristics of osteoarthritis?
   ① Tenderness and crepitus
   ② Bilateral inflammation and immobility
   ③ Pain resulting from destruction of supportive structures
   ④ Fluid within the joint along with inflammatory tissue changes

70. A 60-year-old with a history of osteoarthritis presents to a clinic for a short-stay cataract removal. An important piece of information for the nurse to obtain in planning his care is:
   ① Hobbies and interests
   ② Food likes and dislikes
   ③ Use of alcohol and tobacco
   ④ Use of a cane, walker, or crutches

71. A nurse is caring for a patient with IDDM. The nurse finds the patient unconscious 2 hours after administering 12 units of regular insulin. A blood glucose reading reads 30 mg/dl. What is the nurse's next course of action?
   ① Administer IV insulin
   ② Sit the patient up and place small amount of orange juice in her mouth
   ③ Place crushed crackers in the patient's mouth and assist her to swallow
   ④ Place concentrated glucose between the cheek and the gum and allow it to absorb

72. A patient has been diagnosed with acromegaly. The nurse is aware that this condition is caused by an overproduction of:
   ① Prolactin
   ② Cortisol
   ③ Growth hormone
   ④ Thyroid hormone

73. The nursing assistant asks the nurse about the turning schedule for a patient who had a right pneumonectomy yesterday. The nurse explains that the patient should be turned every hour from:
    ① Back to left side to right side
    ② Back to left side to back
    ③ Left side to right side to left side
    ④ Back to right side to back

74. A nurse is administering pulse oximetry to a patient receiving oxygen therapy. The patient inquires what the purpose of the test is. Which of the following is the nurse's best response?
    ① "This measures how much energy your body uses."
    ② "This determines how fast or slow your heart is beating."
    ③ "This test let's us know how much fluid is in your lungs."
    ④ "This determines how much oxygen your tissues are receiving."

75. A patient is admitted to the hospital with the diagnosis of cirrhosis of the liver related to alcohol abuse and malnutrition. He is jaundiced, has ascites, and has recently experienced dyspnea. A nursing assistant asks the nurse what causes the ascites. Which of the following is the most correct statement by the nurse?
    ① The fluid is caused by cardiovascular hypertension
    ② Low levels of albumin causes fluid to collect in the abdomen
    ③ The fluid is accumulating because of a large obstruction of the patient's common bile duct
    ④ The patient is producing large amounts of ammonia, which cause the fluid collection

76. A nurse is assisting a physician with a thoracentesis. Upon completion of the procedure, the physician applied a dressing over the puncture site. A student asks the nurse the type of dressing and why it was needed. The nurse's most appropriate response is:
    ① "A clean dressing is used to prevent the patient from infecting the puncture site."
    ② "The physician has his special way of doing things. A Band-Aid would do."
    ③ "A sterile occlusive dressing is done because of the needle placement."
    ④ "A wet-to-dry dressing is used in case there is any leakage."

77. A patient had a right lower lobectomy at 10 AM. It is now 2 PM. The nurse knows that the best turning schedule for the patient is:
    ① Right side to back to left side to right side
    ② Left side to back to left side to back
    ③ Back to left semiprone to back
    ④ Back to right semiprone to back

78. A patient with cholelithiasis is experiencing right upper quadrant pain after eating a meal that was high in fat and asks the nurse for an explanation of how his diet can precipitate pain. The most appropriate response by the nurse would be:
    ① "Foods high in fat are harder to digest."
    ② "The ducts from the liver and pancreas become obstructed."
    ③ "Obstructed bile flow limits the amount of bile available to emulsify fat."
    ④ "There is an inadequate absorption of both fat and soluble vitamins."

79. The nurse is caring for a patient who has had a subtotal thyroidectomy. The nurse is aware that accidental removal of the parathyroid glands could occur and will closely monitor the patient for:
    ① Tetany
    ② Seizures
    ③ Renal shutdown
    ④ Loss of the gag reflex

80. The patient with a hiatal hernia and reflux syndrome is having discomfort lying in a supine position and is having trouble sleeping. An appropriate suggestion by the nurse would be:
    ① Removing high-acid food from the diet
    ② Suggesting a hot cup of cocoa before retiring for the night
    ③ Suggesting that the head of the bed be raised up on blocks
    ④ Recommending a glass of milk and a sandwich just before going to bed

81. The nurse is to prepare a patient for a proctoscopic exam that is to be performed in the treatment room of the nursing unit. Which of the following positions should the nurse assist the patient in achieving?
    ① Sims'
    ② Prone
    ③ Supine
    ④ Dorsal recumbent

82. When reviewing patient histories, which of the following patients would the nurse consider to be at greater risk for developing an oral form of cancer?
    ① Alcohol abuse
    ② Poor dental hygiene
    ③ Frequent bouts of tonsillitis
    ④ Chain smoker

83. The nurse is teaching a patient newly diagnosed with diabetes mellitus about reducing the risk of hypoglycemia. Which of the following will be included in the health teaching?
    ① "Exercise by running each day."
    ② "Space your meals 5 to 6 hours apart."
    ③ "Take your diabetes medicine in early afternoon."
    ④ "Carry a form of rapid-acting sugar with you at all times."

84. When instructing a female patient about antibiotic therapy, the nurse should alert the patient concerning the possibility of getting candidiasis as a secondary infection. For which of the following symptoms should the nurse tell the patient to be alert?
    ① High fever and swollen lymph nodes
    ② Itching and cream cheese–like white discharge
    ③ Chancres that develop on the outside of the vagina
    ④ Excessive bleeding occurring in the absence of a period

85. In planning the nursing care of a patient with Addison's disease, a priority of nursing care is:
    ① Providing diversional activities
    ② Protecting the patient from stress and exertion
    ③ Planning a well-balanced diet and nourishing snacks
    ④ Permitting all activity as desired by the patient

86. A patient with Addison's disease is being regulated with medication. The nurse knows that the primary goal of medication therapy is:
   ① Restoring electrolyte balance
   ② Reducing the white blood cell count
   ③ Increasing bone marrow functioning
   ④ Maintaining the red blood cell count level

87. A patient awakens and states that she is having difficulty breathing. The nurse can provide relief to the patient by first:
   ① Remaining calm
   ② Elevating the head of the bed
   ③ Suctioning her
   ④ Medicating for pain

88. A patient who recently returned to the unit after a bronchoscopy starts to wheeze and appears frightened. The nurse's most appropriate response to the patient's obvious concern is:
   ① "Wheezing frequently occurs after this type of test."
   ② "This is a sign that the local anesthetic is wearing off."
   ③ "This means that your gag reflex is returning."
   ④ "I will notify your physician that this is occurring."

89. A neighbor comes to your house after falling on an icy sidewalk. You note that the right lower arm is angulated, but the skin is intact. First-aid measures would include:
   ① Call 911
   ② Splint the affected area
   ③ Wrap the area in a warm compress
   ④ Keep the affected area below the level of the heart

90. Following a lobectomy a patient has difficulty doing deep breathing and productive coughing exercises. The use of an incentive spirometer hasn't helped the situation. Nursing notes indicate the patient's cough is weak and dry and that he tires easily. The most appropriate plan of action the nurse should consider is to:
   ① Encourage the patient to drink 8 to 10 glasses of water a day
   ② Ask the physician for PRN throat lozenges and cough demulcent orders
   ③ Report to the physician and ask if aerosol treatments may help
   ④ Increase the room temperature to 70° F and humidity to 70%

91. A patient's sputum has suddenly become pink and frothy. The nurse has gathered the following data during her assessment. Which of the data is significant and needs to be reported and documented?
   ① Decreased appetite
   ② Respirations 16, regular, easy
   ③ Complaints of dull headache
   ④ Coughing when supine

92. A nurse is caring for a patient with hypertension and states that he fails to see why he should go on medication when he feels fine. Which of the following is the nurse's best response to the patient's statement?
   ① "I will need to call your doctor if you refuse treatment."
   ② "Your symptoms will get worse and you should take your pills."
   ③ "If hypertension is not managed it can affect many other organ systems."

   ④ "An ounce of prevention is worth a pound of cure, and you would be wise to take care of this problem now."

93. A patient is scheduled for a pulmonary angiogram and wants to know what will happen. The nurse explains that:
   ① She will receive a local anesthetic and a tube will be inserted through her nose
   ② She will be placed in a big hollow tube and must remain completely still
   ③ She will wear a clip on her nose and breathe into a machine
   ④ A dye will be injected through an IV and an X-ray will be taken

94. A patient wants to know why she must have a chest X-ray now, since the physician just performed a thoracentesis on her 15 minutes ago. The nurse's most appropriate response to the patient's concern is:
   ① "This test is a double-check to see that the physician removed all the fluid."
   ② "This test should have been done before the procedure, but the physician wouldn't wait."
   ③ "The chest X-ray is routinely done after this type of procedure to make sure everything is all right."
   ④ "The chest X-ray is done to make sure the physician didn't nick your lung."

95. A patient is scheduled for a CAT scan of the thorax using contrast medium. The nurse is preparing the patient as per standard procedure for this type of diagnostic test. Which of the actions by the nurse indicates proper protocol is being followed?
   ① Restricting fluids to 1000 cc 4 hours before the test
   ② Placing the patient on NPO status for at least 4 hours before the test
   ③ Allowing the patient to have her usual meal
   ④ Telling the patient she will be on bed rest for 4 hours after the test

96. A patient experienced an acute episode of sharp chest pain, breathing difficulty, and change in breath sounds. She is scheduled for a ventilation/perfusion lung scan. When explaining the reason for the procedure to staff the nurse explains that it:
   ① Was scheduled because the patient may have had a pulmonary embolus
   ② Was ordered to rule out acute myocardial infarction
   ③ Measures vital lung capacity to rule out a pulmonary tumor
   ④ Involves a contrast dye injected IV to check circulation of blood flow through the heart

97. A patient scheduled for a thoracentesis to instill medication wants to know where the needle will be placed. The nurse shows her by placing her hand:
   ① Below the patient's diaphragm
   ② Between the patient's second and third rib
   ③ Between the patient's fifth and sixth rib
   ④ Between the patient's eighth and ninth rib

98. The physician has ordered oxygen at 6 L per nasal cannula for his patient. While the nurse is preparing the necessary equipment, the patient asks about the bottle of water and cannister, stating she didn't have all that stuff the last time she needed oxygen. The nurse's most appropriate response would be which of the following?
   ① "Apparently they had different equipment when you were here last."

② "Based on the ordered rate, humidification is necessary to keep your nose from becoming too dry."

③ "Most patients feel more comfortable when the oxygen is humidified."

④ "Humidity decreases the fire hazard of using oxygen."

99. A nurse is caring for a patient with cirrhosis. Which of the following measures would help to prevent the development of hepatic coma?
① Give soapy enemas
② Perform iced saline lavages
③ Eliminate protein from the diet
④ Eliminate carbohydrates from the diet

100. The nurse is caring for a patient in diabetic ketoacidosis. Which of the following insulins should the nurse expect to administer in the acute phase of this condition?
① Lente
② NPH
③ Regular
④ Glucotrol

101. Which of the following would be the reason that glucose is used by the cell?
① Protoplasm
② Repair material
③ A protein source
④ An energy source

102. A nurse is cautioning a patient with diabetes mellitus about the dangers of developing diabetic ketoacidosis. Which of the following situations should the nurse alert the patient as a possible cause of diabetic ketoacidosis?
① Stress
② Infection
③ Excess insulin
④ Insufficient calories in the diet

103. A patient is admitted with a diagnosis of mitral stenosis or mitral insufficiency. Which of the following symptoms would be found in either condition?
① Angina
② Murmur
③ Syncope
④ High blood pressure

104. The nurse is monitoring a patient on bed rest for symptoms of fluid retention. Where would the nurse best assess for edema in this patient?
① Feet
② Hands
③ Knees
④ Sacrum

105. Uncontrolled hypertension over time can affect the heart, brain, kidney, and eyes. The patient wants the nurse to tell him the name of the recommended annual eye exam he is to have. The best response by the nurse would be to explain the examination called a:
① Vision screen
② Tonometer test
③ Funduscopic exam
④ Visual fields exam

106. A patient who had a CVA has paresis of her left side and weighs 90 kg, is incontinent of urine and perspires heavily. The nurse instructs the nursing assistant to:
① Pull the patient up in bed at least once a shift

② Keep the patient off the affected side when positioning the patient
③ Get help to move and reposition the patient
④ Lower the temperature in the room

107. Because of pneumonia, a dark-skinned patient has spent most of the day in bed. Which of the following might cause the nurse the most concern during skin assessment rounds?
① A productive cough when she moves
② A dark, almost purple area over her right scapula
③ Complaints of feeling cool
④ Complaints of feeling "stiff"

108. The nurse notes that the edges of her patient's incisional area are not healing properly. The patient had a thoracotomy a week ago and has not been eating well. Which of the following actions would be most appropriate for the nurse to pursue?
① Sit down and help the patient with menu selection
② Encourage the patient to exercise more
③ Ask the physician for an antidepressant order
④ Offer mouth care before each meal

109. A patient who has had frequent bouts of pneumonia spends most of her time in bed, insisting that the head of her bed remain at 90 degrees. Because she has reddened areas on her coccyx, the nurse teaches her that:
① She needs to stay off her back for the next 24 hours
② The head of the bed should be kept at 15 to 30 degrees
③ She keeps getting pneumonia because of the moisture that forms on her skin
④ Her buttocks hurt because the skin over the bones is dying

110. A patient complained of dizziness immediately after receiving eardrops. This may indicate that:
① The eardrops were administered too quickly
② The auditory canal is occluded
③ The ear drops were very warm
④ He is having an allergic reaction

111. Symptoms of hypertension are vague and subtle. In assessing hypertensive patients, the nurse may observe symptoms of:
① Nausea, vomiting, and nosebleeds
② Increased urination, fatigue, and blurred vision
③ Chest pain, shortness of breath, and nervousness
④ Blurred vision, irritability, and occipital headaches

112. Your patient with multiple sclerosis requires intermittent catheterizations and is apprehensive. When she asks why this is necessary, the nurse's best response is:
① "You need to discuss this with your physician."
② "It will empty your bladder completely at certain times each day."
③ "It guarantees that you will not be incontinent."
④ "It relieves any pressure on your bowels so you will not become constipated."

113. A patient who has been receiving high doses of oxygen is suspected of developing oxygen toxicity. Besides observing for hallucinations and confusion, which of the following should the nurse assess for in this patient?
① Halos around lights
② Loss of peripheral vision
③ Increased shallow respirations
④ Uncontrolled muscular twitching

114. A patient diagnosed with chronic renal failure is becoming more confused. Because all previous laboratory test results were within normal range, which of the following would be of concern to the nurse and should be reported at once?
① Potassium of 5.5 mEq/L
② Glucose of 90 mg/100 ml
③ Platelet count of 150,000/mm³
④ Leukocyte count of 5500/mm³

115. A patient refuses to cough and deep breathe or to use the incentive spirometer. Besides assessing respirations and laboratory results, which of the following data would indicate beginning respiratory acidosis?
① Warm, flushed skin
② Numbness of fingers
③ Peripheral cyanosis
④ Facial twitching

116. In the acute phase of treatment for a myocardial infarction, the nurse administers supplemental oxygen to the patient. The main goal of oxygen therapy is to:
① Prevent ventricular fibrillation
② Decrease anxiety and restlessness
③ Prevent the complications of shock
④ Increase oxygen supply to myocardial tissue

117. A patient who had a CVA 3 years ago has been admitted with blisters and tiny open areas on her buttocks. No drainage is present at this time. The most appropriate dressing for the nurse to use for this patient is:
① Hydrophilic
② Steri-Strips
③ Hydrophobic
④ Wet-to-dry

118. A patient was recently admitted because of a motor vehicle accident. Which of the following observations would cause the nurse to monitor intake and output closely?
① Capillary refill less than 3 seconds
② Elastic skin turgor
③ Crackles in lower lobes
④ Amber aromatic urine

119. During routine AM rounds, the nurse notes that a patient with chronic pulmonary disease is more forgetful today. The nurse also notes an unusual odor on the patient's breath while assessing lung sounds. It is essential that the nurse evaluate the patient within the hour because the patient:
① May need to be oriented to her environment more today
② May be developing a respiratory infection
③ May need more encouragement to eat today
④ Is at risk for developing acidosis

120. A nurse is caring for a patient who has undergone arthroplasty of the left knee. Which of the following data, observed in the immediate postoperative period, must be reported immediately?
① Nausea and vomiting
② Slow capillary refill to left foot
③ Infiltration of intravenous fluids
④ Inability to cough productively

121. A patient being treated for kidney failure complains of nausea, diarrhea, and postural dizziness. Her pulse is rapid, thready, and regular. The most appropriate action by the nurse would be to:
① Monitor her output hourly
② Assess her level of consciousness twice/shift
③ Make her NPO until the diarrhea clears
④ Notify the RN or physician of these complaints

122. The nurse is caring for the stomal area of a patient who had a urinary diversion 2 weeks ago. Which of the following actions is most appropriate?
① Massaging the area 2 to 3 times per day
② Applying baby oil to the area and stoma
③ Moistening the stoma and area with aloe lotion
④ Cleansing the area with soap and water and patting dry

123. Your patient with multiple sclerosis has a neurogenic bladder. When evaluating the patient's response to medical therapy, which of the following medications would you expect to be therapeutic for this bladder problem?
① Oxybutynin chloride (Ditropan)
② Bethanechol (Urecholine)
③ Propantheline bromide (Pro-Banthine)
④ Trimethoprim sulfamethoxazole (Bactrim, Septra)

124. To best prepare the patient for a cystoscopy where no X-rays will be taken, the nurse:
① Administers enemas until clear
② Shaves the pubic area
③ Inserts an indwelling catheter
④ Encourages fluid intake

125. A patient returns to the unit following a TURP with a continuous bladder irrigation and is complaining of bladder spasms. Which of the following interventions can the nurse implement to help relieve this problem?
① Increase the flow rate of the irrigating solution
② Raise the collecting drainage bag to the level of the bladder
③ Encourage relaxation techniques to avoid straining to pass urine
④ Elevate the scrotum on towels

126. During a patient's annual physical an enlarged boggy prostate is noted by the physician. Based on this information, which of the following data is most important?
① Hesitancy, change in urine stream
② Color and odor of urine
③ Constipation and smoking history
④ Type and amount of fluids taken daily

127. A patient diagnosed with hyperthyroidism and exhibiting signs of exophthalmus has been complaining of dry eyes. Which of the following physician's orders would the nurse expect to implement to meet the patient's comfort needs?
① Artificial tears
② Mydriatic eye drops
③ Antibiotic ointment
④ Prone position for sleep and rest

128. In a patient with myasthenia gravis, which one of the following drugs would the nurse question if they were ordered?
① Neostigmine (Prostigmin)
② Neomycin (Mycifradin)

③ Prednisone (Deltasone)

④ Pyridostigmine (Mestinon)

129. A patient with a ureterostomy is to adhere to an acid ash diet. Which of these menu selections should the nurse question?
① Cereal with cranberries, bowl of prunes
② Fish, buttered noodles, peanuts for dessert
③ Chicken with rice, cheese slices
④ Steak, creamed vegetables, glass of milk

130. When a patient returns from dialysis she is diaphoretic, restless, vomiting, and has tachycardia. Which of the following actions by the nurse is most appropriate initially?
① Apply a cool washcloth to the patient's forehead and monitor vital signs
② Encourage frequent sips of water and elevate foot of bed
③ Lower the head of the bed, elevate the foot of the bed, turn the patient on her side
④ Decrease the temperature in the room and turn the patient on her side

131. When assessing a patient's range of motion, the nurse notices that the patient has trouble extending his right arm out from his side. Moving a body part away from the midline is called:
① Flexion
② Abduction
③ Adduction
④ Pronation

132. A nurse is preparing to administer an injection to a patient who has been on bed rest and has muscle atrophy to both upper and lower extremities. Where should the nurse administer the intramuscular injection?
① Deltoid
② Abdomen
③ Ventrogluteal
④ Gluteus maximus

133. The nurse is caring for a patient with a possible diagnosis of Cushing's syndrome. When evaluating the lab reports on the patient, which of the following would indicate a diagnosis of Cushing's syndrome?
① Elevation of cortisol levels
② Elevation of growth hormone
③ Large amounts of TSH, T_3, and T_4
④ Serum elevation of the hormone epinephrine

134. A nurse is caring for a patient who is 2 days postoperative appendectomy. The patient complains of incisional pain upon ambulation. The nurse suggests splinting the wound with a pillow based on the understanding that:
① Splinting allows for deeper respirations and coughing
② Persons with abdominal incisions are hesitant to ambulate
③ An abdominal binder would restrict the patient's movements
④ Sustained stress disrupts wound layers and may impede tissue repair

135. A patient with hypertension is upset that he is having to undergo treatment and states, "I don't feel bad. Why is the doctor making such a fuss?" The best reply by the nurse is:
① "I will ask the doctor to see you in the morning."

② "Why do you question our care? We are only trying to help you."
③ "What could I do to help you understand the seriousness of your disease?"
④ "What questions do you have regarding your care? Maybe I can answer them."

136. The nurse is assessing a patient for evidence of a hypoglycemic reaction. Which assessments indicate this reaction?
① Polyuria, dysuria, and fever
② Glycosuria, hematuria, and tachypnea
③ Pale, clammy skin and confusion
④ Ketonuria, fruity odor to the breath, and hot/dry skin

137. An individual who is donating blood is found to be of the type that is considered the "universal donor." The patient's blood type is:
① A
② B
③ O
④ AB

138. A patient who has diabetes mellitus fell on the ice and sustained a skin abrasion. She asks the nurse to apply an ice wrap to her ankle. The nurse hesitates based on the understanding that:
① The open area will become infected
② She will first have to get an X-ray of her ankle
③ Rebound swelling may occur once the ice is removed
④ Diabetics have a greater potential for injury related to cold

139. A stroke patient continues to complain of numbness and discomfort in her right knee. The most appropriate nursing intervention to ensure her comfort is to:
① Administer the PRN heat wrap ordered for joint stiffness
② Administer the PRN medication ordered for temperature over 101° F
③ Secure an order for an ice wrap to the right knee
④ Visit with the patient and reposition her

140. A patient admitted 6 days ago with a chest wound was transferred to the subacute unit and is complaining of increased pain at the wound site, which is covered with a dry 4 x 4 dressing. Based on the information given by the patient, the nurse knows this may mean that:
① The pain medication is no longer effective
② An infection is developing
③ The dressing is too tight
④ The dressing needs to be changed

141. A patient, who is 3 days postpneumonectomy, develops an infection of the surgical site. When securing supplies for the wet-to-dry dressing changes, the nurse orders Montgomery straps, based on the understanding that these:
① Are more cost effective
② Are less likely to cause additional infection
③ Will cause less trauma to the skin
④ Will decrease the need for frequent dressing changes

142. A patient who had chest surgery has a taped, windowed, sterile dressing covering the surgical site. A nursing goal is to maintain skin integrity of the surrounding tissues. To meet this goal, when removing the dressing the nurse needs to:
① Explain each step of the procedure
② Soak the old dressing with normal saline before attempting removal
③ Apply sterile gloves, loosen all tape first and lift up, bringing the edges toward her
④ Loosen tape by pulling toward the incision and, using the thumb, gently pull skin away from tape

143. A dark-skinned patient is at high risk for a pressure ulcer. The nurse assesses the patient's pressure points for blanching. The color that describes blanching in patients with dark skin is:
① Pale, like someone who is anemic
② Grayish, like ashes in a fireplace
③ Hyperemic, like the color of a plum
④ Pinkish, like circles of red blush makeup

144. When assessing a patient who is in kidney failure, the nurse suspects electrolyte imbalance based on her symptoms. Which of the following are signs of electrolyte imbalance and should be reported to the physician?
① Nausea, vomiting, increased depth of respirations
② Anxiety, abdominal cramps, irregular heartbeat
③ Crackles, nausea, excessive thirst
④ Dry lips, loss of weight, dark amber urine

145. A patient receiving chemotherapy has just received a rapid infusion of 3 units of whole blood and is complaining of numbness in his fingertips, lips, and tongue. While taking his blood pressure, the nurse noted a twitching of the patient's wrist and fingers. The nurse promptly reports the finding to the team leader because:
① These are signs of hypocalcemia
② These signs may signal an impending seizure
③ These are symptoms that the cancer has spread
④ These signs are adverse effects of chemotherapy

146. A patient who has cancer of the lung started receiving TPN yesterday. The patient's wife asks you to explain what the TPN feeding is doing for her husband. The best response would be:
① "These feedings are the safest type of feeding for debilitated persons."
② "These feedings contain all the essential nutrients that can't be given through small veins."
③ "These tube feedings place the necessary nutrients directly into the stomach."
④ "These feedings make eating unnecessary. This keeps your husband from tiring so easily."

147. The nurse is assisting a physician in the performance of a paracentesis to reduce the discomfort associated with ascites. Which of the following nursing actions would the nurse anticipate in assisting with the procedure?
① Record amount and color of fluid removed
② Place patient in right lateral position to facilitate drainage
③ Assist with the application of a simple sterile dressing after the procedure
④ Prepare the area by cleansing with warm, soapy water and drape with sterile towels

148. Nursing observations of a patient with severe liver dysfunction with accompanying jaundice would include which of the following?
① Dark stools, yellow sclera, and dark urine
② Clay-colored stools, pruritus, and dark urine
③ Dark stools, pruritus, and straw-colored urine
④ Clay-colored stools, yellow sclera, and blood-tinged urine

149. A patient who is very weak secondary to her lung cancer requires frequent suctioning of her nasopharynx. Based on the standards of care, the nurse checks the suction machine and adjusts the pressure setting to:
① 50 to 95 mm Hg
② 95 to 110 mm Hg
③ 10 to 115 mm Hg
④ 135 to 150 mm Hg

150. A patient who has a thoracotomy tube in his left thorax is apprehensive and afraid to move. The tube is attached to water-seal chest drainage. The appropriate teaching for this patient is to:
① Comb his hair with his left arm every 4 to 6 hours
② Avoid any sudden movements or turning
③ Apply lotion around the tube after his bath
④ Keep the side rails up while in bed

151. The water seal chamber of the patient's chest drainage set-up has stopped fluctuating. The suction control is working properly. The chest tube has been in place for 2 days. The most appropriate first action for the nurse to do is to:
① Notify the physician or RN of this development
② Ask the patient to bear down and perform a Valsalva maneuver
③ Check the tubing for dependent loops
④ Add reinforcing tape around the tube insertion site

152. The nurse is instructing the patient on how to prevent most upper airway infections. She/he should stress frequent good hand washing and encourage the patient to:
① Maintain proper dental hygiene
② Stay in air conditioning as much as possible
③ Use more disposable Kleenex
④ Take megadoses of vitamin C daily

153. During a care conference, the head nurse asks if the nursing diagnosis of ineffective clearance related to bronchial secretions is still appropriate for the patient. The nurse caring for this patient can best evaluate this by:
① Taking the patient's temperature
② Checking the rate and strength of the patient's pulse
③ Counting the patient's respirations for 1 full minute
④ Listening for clear breath sounds

154. The position a majority of patients with respiratory tract infections find to be the most comfortable is:
① Low-Fowler's
② High-Fowler's
③ Left lateral
④ Semiprone

155. A patient with influenza has ineffective airway clearance related to bronchial secretions. To assist the patient in bringing up bronchial secretions, the nurse should plan to:
① Monitor intake and output
② Limit visitors
③ Increase room humidity to 60%
④ Encourage liberal fluid intake of 2000 cc/day

156. The patient's left thoracotomy tube is connected to water-seal drainage. When the patient is sitting in a chair, the nurse should make sure that the tube and drainage system remains:
① Connected on the bed frame
② Even with the level of the patient's heart
③ On a towel sitting on the floor
④ Below her chest

157. The patient has severe pharyngitis and has developed an elevated temperature, chills, and a skin rash. A sputum specimen for culture and sensitivity has been ordered. The nurse reports the skin rash based on the understanding that:
① Medicated creams need to be ordered
② Antibiotics need to be started
③ The patient may be developing scarlet fever
④ The rash may be very painful

158. The patient who had a right lower lobectomy 5 days ago is being discharged. The instructions the patient is given should include:
① Avoiding soft or low chairs
② Avoiding lifting items over 5 pounds until the incision is healed
③ Taking sponge baths until his follow-up physician appointment
④ Staying indoors until outdoor activities are approved by the physician

159. A patient begins to complain of pruritus and the nurse notices that she has been scratching and has excoriated areas. The plan is to make her comfortable and her skin pliable. This can best be achieved by:
① Cutting her fingernails to the top of her fingertips
② Keeping the environment cool and at 40% humidity
③ Checking to see what medication she is receiving
④ Administering a PRN nonsteroidal antiinflammatory drug (NSAID)

160. Damage to the laryngeal nerve may occur following a thyroidectomy. Which of the following assessment data may indicate that the nerve has been damaged?
① Hoarseness
② Frothy sputum
③ Choking sensation
④ Positive Chvostek's sign

161. A nurse is caring for a patient who had a complete thyroidectomy, including the parathyroid glands. Which of the following data would indicate tetany, a possible complication of having the parathyroids removed?
① Hypertension and somnolence
② Blood-tinged urine and frequency
③ Unrelenting headache and blurred vision
④ Painful muscle spasms of the hands and face

162. A nurse is caring for a patient diagnosed with hyperthyroidism. The patient is extremely nervous and anxious and her family constantly hovers over her bed. Which of the following would the nurse include in this patient's plan of care?
① Maintaining a calm, relaxed environment
② Encouraging visitors to help stimulate patient interactions
③ Providing for frequent interactions between the patient and staff
④ Placing her in a semiprivate room or ward to foster interaction and release tension

163. A patient who is being evaluated for heart failure is scheduled for an X-ray and asks why a chest X-ray is necessary. The best reply by the nurse is:
① "Ask your doctor to explain this to you."
② "You can ask to speak to the radiologist once you are in X-ray."
③ "This study will be useful in determining the size of your heart."
④ "This study will outline the vessels of your heart and show any heart damage."

164. A 73-year-old black male with a history of hypertension and arteriosclerosis was admitted from a nursing home for observation. The nursing home attendant reported noticing that the patient had become more withdrawn, had trouble using his right hand, and that the right side of his mouth sagged. The nurse would be alert for progressive signs of:
① Angina
② Hypertension
③ Myocardial infarction
④ Cerebrovascular accident

165. Which of the following might a patient undergoing a gastrectomy develop postoperatively?
① Diabetes mellitus
② Esophageal reflux
③ Pernicious anemia
④ *Helicobacter pylori* infection

166. The nurse is preparing to educate a group of students regarding measures in preventing the spread of hepatitis B. Which of the following does the nurse include in lecture?
① Testing blood donors
② Avoiding blood donations.
③ Adding bleach to the water
④ Avoiding consumption of all shellfish

167. A young patient with a diagnosis of Crohn's disease has had a recent ileostomy. The patient asks the nurse what sports he should avoid when returning to school. In which of the following would the nurse caution the patient against participating?
① Track
② Football
③ Shot put
④ Swimming

168. A patient is admitted with the diagnosis of ruptured appendix. The nurse is alert for the development of the complication of peritonitis. Which assessment findings would support the diagnosis of peritonitis?
① Fever and nervousness
② Fever and reduced urine output
③ Increased bowel motility accompanied by fever
④ Abdominal muscular rigidity accompanied by fever

169. A nurse is preparing to educate a group of individuals who are at high risk for developing diabetes mellitus due to family history. Which of the following cardinal symptoms of diabetes mellitus will the nurse include in her notes?
① Clammy skin, tremors, confusion
② Polyuria, polydipsia, and polyphagia
③ Headache, high blood pressure, and nosebleeds
④ Lethargy, slowed mental processes, and hypotension

170. A patient presents to the emergency room with bleeding esophageal varices. For which of the following treatments should the nurse prepare the patient?
① Administration of platelets and refrigerated blood
② Gastric lavage with room-temperature saline solution
③ Administration of vasodilators, antibiotics, and antacids
④ Use of Sengstaken-Blakemore tube and iced saline lavages

171. A patient has long-standing stasis dermatitis of the legs. The nurse's main concern is to:
① Keep her from bathing with soap
② Maintain skin integrity on her legs
③ Administer antiinflammatory drugs as ordered
④ Wear gloves when applying ointments to her legs

172. A nurse is assigned to do medications and treatments on a patient who received a skin graft 5 days ago. Which of the following orders for the donor site on the left thigh should the nurse question?
① Wet-to-dry dressing changes every 6 hours
② Out of bed ad lib
③ Give analgesics as necessary for discomfort
④ Apply bed cradle to the foot of the bed

173. A patient has allergies. He has redness and itching of his eyelids. Warm compresses to the eyes are ordered. The most appropriate nursing action would be to:
① Wear sterile gloves and use sterile technique
② Wear clean gloves and use clean technique
③ Tape compresses in place
④ Warm the solution in a microwave

174. The nurse is to administer an antibiotic eye ointment to a patient with a bacterial infection of his right eye. The nurse would:
① Place an eye pad on the eye after administering the ointment
② Wear gloves to administer the ointment
③ Place the ointment on the eyeball
④ Use the unit's stock supply of ointment

175. The patient returning home after a right cataract extraction with an intraocular lens implant needs to be instructed to:
① Sleep on his left side
② Restrict fluid intake to 1000 cc/day
③ Shower and shampoo every other day
④ Avoid watching television

176. The nurse is to administer eye medications for a group of six patients, all of whom have glaucoma and are receiving cholinergic agents (miotics) such as Pilocarpine. The nurse knows it is vital that these medications be given as ordered. This is based on the understanding that:
① Giving medications on time is part of your job
② These medications keep the pupil constricted to permit better aqueous humor drainage
③ Glaucoma is a leading cause of blindness
④ The patient will experience severe eye pain if a dose is late

177. A patient, who has noticed that she tends to bump into objects, is being tested for glaucoma. The nurse explains to her that with glaucoma:
① Circulation to the brain is decreased
② Blindness is an eventual result
③ Her sense of balance is disturbed
④ A decrease in peripheral vision is a first symptom

178. A patient who has been treated for glaucoma for 4 months recently had a CVA. As the nurse cares for her in the rehabilitation unit, the patient questions her about difficulty seeing after she receives her eyedrops. The nurse explains that:
① The blurred vision after receiving the drops will decrease with prolonged use
② Bright lights are to be avoided
③ The room should be dark right after the eyedrops are inserted
④ Smoking while receiving these drops is contraindicated

179. The nurse just learned that her patient is suspected of having a retinal detachment. The patient is presently in bed and it is important that the nurse:
① Explain and show that her call light is within easy reach
② Tell her that she will receive antiemetics to prevent acid reflux
③ Remind her that she will remain on bed rest for 3 to 4 weeks
④ Assure her that she will receive eye drops for the ocular pain

180. A 5-year-old patient has an upper respiratory infection. When teaching him how to blow his nose, the nurse tells him to:
① Blow with both nostrils open
② Blow one side of his nose at a time
③ Keep his mouth open when blowing one side at a time
④ Shut his eyes while blowing hard

181. A patient with the diagnosis of heart failure is being with furosemide (Lasix). The patient has begun to experience tinnitus. The nurse advises her that:
① She will not be able to drive
② The sounds she hears are normal
③ This symptom is caused by nerve deafness
④ This may be related to her diuretic medication

182. Which of the following is a postoperative measure following a hemorrhoidectomy that the nurse should anticipate?
① Encouraging warm showers
② Changing occlusive rectal dressings
③ Using fecal tube to reduce gas pain
④ Administering laxatives and stool softeners

183. The nurse is assessing a nursing home resident admitted to the ER with the tentative diagnosis of "probable right femoral neck fracture." Which assessment finding would support the diagnosis?
① The leg is pronated and internally rotated
② The leg is supinated and internally rotated
③ The right leg is longer than the left and is laterally rotated
④ The right leg is shorter than the left and is externally rotated

184. A patient is diagnosed with Cushing's syndrome. Which of the following is the patient at risk for developing due to the overproduction of hormones?
① Hyperkalemia
② Hypocalcemia
③ Hyperglycemia
④ Hypoinsulinemia

185. An important nursing assessment of a patient in hypovolemic shock is:
① Assessing pedal pulses
② Checking urine output
③ Monitoring bowel movements
④ Checking for the presence of jugular vein distention

186. The physician will periodically order a complete blood count on a patient with lymphoma, who is undergoing chemotherapy. For what condition is the physician monitoring?
① Thalassemia
② Cancer in remission
③ Bone marrow depression
④ Increasing platelet counts

187. Which of the following diets would be best for a patient with hyperthyroidism?
① Low-purine, high-fat, 1000-calorie diet
② Clear liquids in the form of 6 small feedings
③ 2-gram low-sodium diet with an evening snack
④ High-protein, high-calorie, high-carbohydrate diet with snacks

188. A patient entered the clinic with symptoms of nervousness and weight loss. A tentative diagnosis of hyperthyroidism was made. Which of the following additional assessment data would support the diagnosis?
① Constipation, depression, and brittle hair
② Increased sweating, hand tremors, and palpitations
③ Urinary frequency, blurred vision, frequent infections
④ Dry skin, intolerance to cold, and slowed response time

189. A patient with hypertension is being managed by medication, including a diuretic. In regards to diet, the nurse would educate the patient to:
① Maintain a high-potassium diet
② Drink at least a quart of liquids a day
③ Avoid spicy and high-fat, high-cholesterol foods
④ Refrain from caffeine and caffeine-containing products

190. A patient has been diagnosed with primary hypertension. Which one of the following medications is designed to lower blood pressure?
① Digoxin (Lanoxin)
② Ibuprofen (Motrin)
③ Cimetidine (Tagamet)
④ Hydrochlorothiazide (HydroDIURIL)

191. The nurse needs to obtain a sterile urine specimen for culture and sensitivity. The best way to obtain this specimen in a patient with an indwelling Foley catheter is to:
① Disconnect the catheter from the drainage tubing and let the urine drip into the sterile bottle
② Use a needle and syringe to withdraw urine from the tubing port and inject the specimen into the sterile bottle
③ Place a towel under the bag and open the drainage valve at the bottom of the drainage bag
④ Remove the old Foley, using a straight catheter, and recatheterize

192. The patient's wife is concerned because her husband, who suffered a CVA 3 days ago, laughs and cries inappropriately. The nurse's best reply is:
① "This is a normal healing sign for someone who has had a CVA."
② "I ignore him when he starts acting like that."
③ "He has what is called 'emotional lability.' This may occur after a stroke."
④ "Men your husband's age like to tease us by acting this way."

193. A head trauma patient has impaired speech but seems to understand what is said to him. The nurse needs to include which of the following in his plan of care?
① Keep the room dimly lighted
② Allow extra time for communication
③ Avoid the use of gestures
④ Keep voice level, soft, and low

194. A patient who had a CVA 2 weeks ago has dysphagia. Based on these data the nurse tells the aide to:
① Keep the patient in bed
② Speak loudly when talking
③ Allow extra time for him to answer her
④ Make sure he swallows his food

195. The patient requires nasopharyngeal suctioning. The nurse places the suction catheter into sterile solution. The underlying principle for this action is to:
① Maintain sterile technique
② Prevent tissue trauma
③ Check patency of the tube
④ Check the suction's pressure

196. The nurse performing nasopharyngeal suctioning applies suction for a maximum of 10 seconds at a time. The underlying principle for this action is that it:
① Maintains catheter tube patency
② Prevents contamination of the catheter
③ Allows patient to breathe normally
④ Prevents improper tube placement

197. The nurse observes that her patient, age 60, has stress incontinence each time she coughs or gets out of bed. The nurse understands that:
① Hormonal changes place older women at risk for stress incontinence
② Her patient is not emptying her bladder completely
③ The nerves controlling the bladder are affected
④ Her patient's bladder is displaced in her pelvic cavity

198. A patient who grows her own fruits and vegetables is concerned that her urine, which is red in color, indicates that she is bleeding. The most appropriate response from the nurse is:
① "You must increase your milk intake to about 8 to 10 glasses a day."
② "This is nothing to be concerned about. Let me know if it is still happening next week."
③ "Tell me, do you feel any pain or pass flatus when you urinate?"
④ "Tell me, what types of vegetables and fruits have you been eating?"

199. A patient sustained an injury to his spinal cord at the C5 level. Based on a spinal cord injury at this level, the nurse would most likely expect the patient to have loss of:
① His emotions
② Movement of all extremities
③ His sexual desires
④ Speaking ability

200. In a patient with chronic bronchitis, which of the following early signs of hypoxemia should the nurse watch for?
① Dyspnea, hypotension, bradycardia
② Bradycardia, wheezing, confusion
③ Capillary refill > 3 seconds, SOB, confusion
④ Restlessness, tachycardia, yawning

201. A patient is being transferred to the unit where he is to be observed following a 2-day stay in coronary care for a possible myocardial infarction. He is receiving several medications and is complaining of a headache. Which of the following medications taken by the patient commonly causes the side effect of headache?
① Tylenol
② Lanoxin
③ Nitroglycerin
④ Potassium chloride

202. A 36-year-old female has been experiencing intermittent episodes of mild chest pain and shortness of breath, particularly with exertion but also at rest. The physician wants to assess if the symptoms are aggravated or precipitated by activity. The nurse will anticipate counseling the patient in the use of:
① A glucometer
② Urine collection
③ A Holter monitor
④ A Doppler flow study

203. Which of the following risk factors for hypertension is not under the control of the individual?
① Obesity
② Smoking
③ Lack of exercise
④ Genetic predisposition

204. A patient is transferred to an intermediate care unit from a coronary care unit four days after having a myocardial infarction. Because he has been on extended bed rest, the nursing care plan includes monitoring for thrombophlebitis. Which of the following assessment data may indicate the complication of thrombophlebitis?
① Numbness and tingling of an extremity
② Absence of pulses and reduced sensation
③ Edema and pain along the course of the vein
④ Coldness and paleness of the involved extremity

205. A patient with a diagnosis of myocardial infarction has been admitted to the coronary care unit. The nurse assesses the patient's breath sounds and hears fine crackles in the lower lung bases. This symptom may indicate:
① Pneumonia
② Dysrhythmias
③ Lung congestion from heart failure
④ An extension of the myocardial infarction

206. When ambulating a patient with right hemiparesis, the nurse should stand on the patient's:
① Right side and hold one arm on the gait belt on the patient's waist
② Left side and hold one arm around the patient's waist
③ Right side and 12 inches behind the patient
④ Left side and hold the patient's right hand

207. A patient is very anxious about going home, and the nurse needs to give her discharge teaching, remembering that her:
① Anxiety is hidden anger at being discharged too soon
② Feelings are based on fear of the unknown
③ Concerns are self-centered
④ Anxiety may interfere with her ability to understand or remember the instructions

208. A patient has chronic respiratory disease and is newly-diagnosed with Alzheimer's disease. In planning his care, the nurse should prioritize his care as:
① Safety, physiological assessment, comfort
② Psychological care, personal integrity, comfort
③ Safety, pain relief, cueing
④ Physiological assessment, reorientation, cueing

209. A patient has started receiving bronchodilators (theophylline). When checking for toxic and side effects, the nurse should observe for:
① Hypotension, abdominal cramping, diarrhea
② Urticaria, nausea and vomiting, dehydration
③ Restlessness, tachycardia, insomnia
④ Anorexia, blurred vision, cramps

210. A patient has had emphysema for 3 years and has dyspnea even at rest. Which of the following observations is characteristic of the disease?
① Dry, hacking cough
② Elevated body temperature
③ Use of accessory muscles of respiration
④ Hemoptysis

211. A patient with bilateral hearing aids complains of ear pressure and is subsequently diagnosed with right ear otitis media. The nurse instructs the aide in his care, which includes:
① Turning the hearing aids' sensitivity levels higher
② Wiping off the right hearing aid with an alcohol sponge after removal
③ Making sure the patient receives his ear drops before putting in his hearing aid
④ Leaving the right hearing aid out of the patient's ear

212. A patient is to receive 1000 cc of 5% dextrose in water plus 40 mEq KCL in 12 hours. In checking the flow rate, how many ccs should the patient receive per hour?
① 42 cc/hr
② 83 cc/hr
③ 100 cc/hr
④ 125 cc/hr

213. A patient is at risk for a pulmonary embolism secondary to deep vein thrombosis. Which one of the following expected outcomes is appropriate for the patient?
① No pain with respiratory effort
② Participates in ADL
③ Maintains stable weight
④ Demonstrates effective coughing techniques

214. The nurse is determining an asthmatic patient's achievement of the goals for the nursing diagnosis: Activity intolerance related to imbalance between oxygen supply and demand. Which of the following expected outcomes is appropriate?
① No evidence of anxiety
② Demonstrated knowledge of disease process
③ Able to perform ADLs
④ Clear breath sounds

215. A patient scored 5 on the Rancho Los Amigos Scale, meaning that she is confused-inappropriate. The nurse expects this patient to:
① React inconsistently and nonpurposefully to stimuli
② Appear alert and be able to respond to simple commands fairly consistently
③ Show goal-directed behavior but depend on external input for direction
④ Be in a heightened state of activity with decreased ability to process information

216. Following a myocardial infarction a patient receives Coumadin. Which of the following symptoms would alert the nurse to a possible adverse effect to the Coumadin?
① Vomiting
② Epistaxis
③ Back pain
④ Blurred vision

217. A patient is being evaluated because of complaints of cervical neck pain. As part of the evaluation, the intent is to rule out the possibility of a ruptured disc. Which of the following is a common symptom of cervical disc involvement?
① Stiff neck
② Difficulty walking
③ Numbness of the lower extremities
④ Atrophy of the gastrocnemius muscle group

218. Which of the following interventions will the nurse anticipate implementing for a patient with a diagnosis of a myocardial infarction?
① Adjusting the bed to Trendelenburg position
② Maintaining prescription of complete bed rest for at least 5 days
③ Providing clear, room-temperature liquids throughout hospitalization
④ Administering a stool softener to prevent straining with bowel movements

219. A concern for a patient having experienced a recent myocardial infarction is the development of cardiogenic shock. Which of the following are signs of cardiogenic shock?
① Bounding pulses, clammy skin, and fever
② Hypotension, weak pulses, and clammy skin
③ Hypertension, shallow respirations, and chest pain
④ Hot, dry skin, rapid respirations, and mental confusion

220. Building construction is going on next to the hospital. The nurse is concerned about the noise level and plans to encourage her patients to:
① Keep their TVs off so as not to add to the noise
② Wear temporary ear protectors during the hours construction is going on
③ Request a transfer to another unit
④ Practice distraction techniques during the construction hours

221. A diabetic patient is being treated for pneumonia. She received 22 units of regular insulin at 6:30 AM and was unable to eat her breakfast. The nurse should be alert for signs of:
① Polydipsia
② Somnolence
③ Diaphoresis
④ Increased urine output

222. The nurse is determining how well a patient with tuberculosis has achieved the goals for the nursing diagnosis: Ineffective breathing pattern related to sputum production. Which of the following expected outcomes is appropriate?
① Stable weight
② Clear breathing sounds
③ Negative sputum culture
④ Verbalizes need for Isoniazid (INH)

223. A patient has Ménière's disease and is taking medication for the vertigo. The nurse is with the patient during a severe attack. Which of the following helps reduce the vertigo?
① Encourage the patient to move slowly to a chair
② Take an additional dose of meclizine (Antivert)
③ Increase fluid intake to 2000 cc/day
④ Darken the room

224. A patient suffers from presbycusis. Based on an understanding of this condition, which of the following best states nursing concerns for the patient?
① At risk for alteration in comfort (physical)
② At risk for injury: falls
③ At risk for alteration in family roles
④ At risk for increasing alteration in sensory perception, auditory

225. A patient fell in the bathroom, hitting her head on the commode. In monitoring her vital signs, which of the following blood pressures would indicate that the patient is experiencing an increase in intracranial pressure?
① Systolic decreasing, diastolic decreasing
② Systolic decreasing, diastolic increasing
③ Systolic increasing, diastolic decreasing
④ Systolic increasing, diastolic increasing

226. A patient, who wears a hearing aid in her left ear, has sensory perceptual alteration: Auditory, related to decreased hearing secondary to cerumen buildup. The most appropriate plan is to:
① Encourage chewing motions and daily washing of the external ears
② Encourage periodic ear washing in the clinic
③ Encourage increasing fluid intake to 2000 cc/day
④ Encourage cleaning the hearing aid with hydrogen peroxide

227. The nurse is watching for any early, untoward effects in a patient who just had a lumbar puncture done. The nurse should be assessing for:
① Delayed capillary refill of the lower extremities
② Complaints of headache
③ Difficulty with bladder control
④ Change in blood pressure

228. The nurse is evaluating her patient's ability to demonstrate correct technique in doing an ear irrigation. The pinna in an adult is pulled:
① Up, back, and out
② Up, forward, and in
③ Down, back, and in
④ Down, forward, and in

229. A nurse is presenting a class on hearing difficulties of the elderly to the aides. Behavioral clues indicating difficulty in hearing and the need for evaluation by an otolaryngologist include:
① Complaining of ringing in the ears
② Avoiding face-to-face contact
③ Changing body positions frequently
④ Speaking while others are talking

230. In a patient who has a stage 2 decubitus ulcer and pneumonia, the nurse makes the following observations. Which one is the priority?
① Temperature of 99.6° F (37.5° C)
② Facial flushing
③ Tachypnea
④ Productive cough

231. In distinguishing between a sprain and a fracture, the nurse would be more suspicious of a fracture if which of the following signs were present on assessment?
① Edema
② Deformity
③ Limited movement
④ Tenderness to palpation of the area

232. An adult patient is placed in Buck's extension traction to the left leg. The nurse is aware that this type of traction can be useful in which of the following injuries?
① Neck sprains
② Spinal fractures
③ Shoulder dislocations
④ Lower extremity and hip fractures

233. There are several complications associated with Russell's traction. Which of the following symptoms may indicate a complication?
① Drainage at the cast site
② Signs of compartment syndrome
③ Pressure under the popliteal space
④ Evidence of undue skin pressure from under the boot

234. Which one of the following special precautions will the nurse incorporate into the plan of care for an 82-year-old patient who has undergone an open reduction and internal fixation of the hip?
① Monitor for nutritional problems
② Maintain proper extremity alignment
③ Keep the side rails in an elevated position
④ Frequent inspection of linen and dressings for drainage

235. In planning preoperative care for a patient about to undergo a below-the-knee amputation, the nurse may focus on postoperative care by explaining:
① Elements of the exercise program
② Postoperative measures to control pain
③ Visiting hours immediately after surgery
④ Turning, coughing, and deep breathing maneuvers

236. A 42-year-old male fractured his right tibia and fibula and arrives on the unit following an open reduction and application of a long plaster cast. Two hours after arriving on the unit, the patient complains of severe pain in his right leg. The best nursing action would be to:
① Administer the oral pain medication as ordered
② Turn the patient, rub his back, and straighten the linen
③ Evaluate the neurocirculatory status of the affected leg
④ Check the right leg to make sure that it is elevated and externally rotated

237. A patient is being instructed on postlumbar puncture care and is apprehensive about getting "sick with a terrible headache like her neighbor did when she had that test done." The nurse's most appropriate response is:
① "Moving about after the test is the best way to prevent a headache."
② "You will need to remain flat on your stomach after the test. This will prevent the headache."
③ "You will be able to drink fluids after the test. That, as well as lying flat, helps most people."
④ "With all the advances in medicine, these types of headaches are not common anymore."

238. In a patient with emphysema, the priority nursing diagnosis is: Alteration in nutritional status related to fatigue secondary to work of breathing. In planning to instruct the patient, which of the following instructions refers to the nursing diagnosis?
① Eat several small meals each day
② Keep the oxygen between 1 and 2 L/min
③ Increase fluid intake to 8 glasses/day
④ Increase hours of sleep throughout the day

239. The nurse noticed that her patient has new areas of ecchymosis. Based on his understanding that some skin lesions may result from toxic, metabolic, or allergic reactions to drugs, which of these newly ordered drugs would the nurse suspect?
① Mafenide acetate (Sulfamylon)
② Warfarin (Coumadin)
③ Penicillin G (Bicillin)
④ Salicylates (Trilisate)

240. The nurse on the previous shift charted that the patient was drowsy. Which of the following behaviors would support this description of the patient's level of consciousness?
① Appropriate response when aroused
② Absence of response even to painful stimuli
③ Incomplete arousal to painful stimuli
④ Response to verbal command is inconsistent, vague

241. A patient is being observed for increased intracranial pressure. Which classification of drugs, besides anticonvulsants and corticosteroids, would you expect to be ordered?
① Narcotic analgesics
② Antiemetics
③ Osmotic diuretics
④ Antibiotics

242. The nurse is distributing health literature on prostate cancer. Which of the following blood tests is recommended by the American Cancer Society as a screening test for this type of cancer?
① CEA (carcinogenic embryonic antigen)
② PSA (prostate-specific antigen)
③ DRE (digital rectal exam)
④ ELISA (enzyme-linked immunoabsorbent assay)

243. In a head trauma patient being treated for increased intracranial pressure, which of the following would be least likely to cause complications?
① Isometric exercises
② Aerobic exercises
③ Passive range of motion exercises
④ High-Fowler's position

244. A patient has just returned to his room after undergoing a myelogram using Pantopaque (iodine-based) dye. What position is most therapeutic for this patient?
① Up ad lib
② Supine for at least 6 to 8 hours
③ Head of bed elevated 15 degrees
④ Head of bed elevated 60 degrees

245. When teaching a patient who is experiencing migraine headaches, which of these behaviors indicates that the patient teaching has been successful?
① The patient states that she needs to exercise daily
② The patient states that she will wear sunglasses when outdoors

③ The patient states that she will take an aspirin daily to prevent the headache

④ The patient identifies the factors that trigger her headaches

246. The nurse is teaching a health class to adolescent men about the testicular self-exam and testicular cancer. Which of the following would the nurse stress as a warning sign that needs to be reported to a physician?
① A tight prepuce that cannot be retracted
② Urinary urgency and frequency
③ A dull ache in the lower abdomen
④ Pain upon urination

247. A nurse is caring for a patient with heart failure who has the symptoms of dyspnea, pedal edema, and increased abdominal girth. Which part of the heart is most likely failing?
① Mitral valve
② Aortic valve
③ Left ventricle
④ Right ventricle

248. A patient with diabetes has developed an elevated temperature, cough, and congested breath sounds. The physician orders a complete blood count (CBC) "stat." When the results are received, the nurse will focus on what part of the CBC to help guide her care of the patient?
① White blood cells
② Red blood cell indices.
③ Hemoglobin and hematocrit
④ Platelet count and morphology

249. The nurse is assessing a patient who is in a long-leg cast. The nurse is aware that this patient had an abraded area of the involved leg and has been in this cast for 7 days. A very warm spot is noted in a particular area of the cast. This finding most likely indicates:
① Swelling under the cast
② The cast is too tight
③ Inflammation under the cast
④ A foreign body under the cast

250. A hypertensive patient has been started on a medication that can cause orthostatic hypotension. The nurse can explain to the patient that this side effect can be minimized by:
① Resting on the edge of the bed
② Wearing antiembolic stockings
③ Limiting the sodium in the diet
④ Sitting on the edge of the bed momentarily before arising

251. A patient reports that he has chest pain that increases with exertion. The nurse is aware that this may indicate:
① A myocardial infarction
② A thrombosed cerebral artery
③ Problems with the mitral valve
④ Insufficient blood supply to the heart muscle

252. A patient's injuries sustained in a car accident have resulted in cerebral edema. Which of the following is the most appropriate position for this patient?
① Supine
② Prone
③ Low- to mid-Fowler's
④ Mid- to high-Fowler's

253. In a patient receiving continuous bladder irrigations following a transurethral prostatectomy, the nurse assesses that the catheter may be blocked. The most appropriate instruction the nurse should give the patient is to:
① Try to void around the catheter
② Deep breathe, cough, and remain perfectly still until the doctor arrives
③ Notify the nurse if he notices a change in the color of the drainage in the bag
④ Increase fluid intake to 4000 cc/day

254. A patient has returned from having a myelogram using metrizamide (water-based) dye. Which of the following postprocedure actions is most appropriate?
① Encourage fluids
② Secure a bedside commode
③ Spray the room with a room deodorizer
④ Administer all drugs withheld before the procedure

255. A patient, diagnosed with a seizure disorder, is being treated with phenytoin (Dilantin) and valproic acid (Depakene). Which of the following statements should the nurse consider the priority teaching need for this patient?
① Must use good oral hygiene
② Must increase intake of green, leafy vegetables
③ Must carry a padded tongue blade at all times
④ Must sleep 6 to 8 hours each night

256. In a patient with cerebral edema, which of the following nursing plans is most appropriate?
① Administer stool softeners as ordered
② Encourage a full glass of water with each medication
③ Keep the room dark and quiet
④ Medicate for pain before ambulation

257. Patients with sensory dysfunction, such as persons with paraplegia, have many teaching needs. Which one of the following is a high-priority teaching need?
① Importance of doing own weight shifts for 5 minutes qh
② Importance of decreasing calcium intake
③ Importance of avoiding cold or very hot foods
④ Importance of adequate fluid intake of 2000 cc/day

258. The patient has been maintaining an acid ash diet and has been instructed to avoid certain medications and foods. Which of the following may the patient have?
① Salt substitutes
② Antacids
③ Sulfa drugs
④ NutraSweet

259. The patient has chronic renal failure. The nurse is evaluating his knowledge of the dietary restrictions. Which of the following statements by the patient reflects his understanding of the dietary restrictions?
① "I never did eat much meat."
② "I eat a lot of bread and potatoes."
③ "I'd better watch how many pickles and olives I eat."
④ "Bananas give me gas, so I avoid them."

260. A patient just underwent a cystoscopy. Immediately following this procedure, which of the following nursing actions is most appropriate?
① Taking vital signs
② Administering the PRN narcotic ordered for pain
③ Applying cool towels to the lower abdomen
④ Assisting the patient off the table to the wheelchair

261. A patient has had a cutaneous ureterostomy performed and has catheters (stents) inserted through the ureters to drain the renal pelvis. One of the nurse's main concerns is:
① Irrigating the stents
② Maintaining patency of the stents
③ Testing urine for protein, blood, and glucose
④ Preventing contamination of the stents with stool

262. A patient has Parkinson's disease and takes the following medications: amantadine (Symmetrel) and trihexyphenidyl HCl (Artane). In evaluating the effectiveness of these medications, which of the following therapeutic responses would the nurse expect?
① Decreased salivation, less tremor of head/hands at rest
② Expressions of depression and thoughts of suicide
③ Normal vital signs, propulsive gait
④ Less visual blurring and mental confusion

263. A concern of the nurse who is caring for an HIV-positive patient is to provide education. The nurse should explain how the patient can prevent:
① AIDS
② Pneumonia
③ Hypotension
④ Opportunistic infections

264. The nurse is aware that oral hypoglycemic agents may be used for patients with diabetes mellitus who have:
① Obesity
② Liver disease
③ Type I diabetes
④ Some insulin production

265. A patient is admitted to the unit in diabetic ketoacidosis. The most common cause of DKA is:
① Stress
② Infection
③ Not enough food
④ Too much insulin

266. What type of insulin would the nurse expect to give to a patient in diabetic ketoacidosis?
① NPH
② Lente
③ Regular
④ Ultra-Lente

267. A 76-year-old patient with severe arthritis is taking large doses of an antiinflammatory medication that has a side effect of gastric irritation. Patient teaching should include instructions to:
① Avoid driving
② Take with food
③ Discontinue if CNS effects develop
④ Take on an empty stomach to enhance absorption

268. When preparing for a new patient with the diagnosis of rheumatoid arthritis, the nurse should be aware that the disease is a:
① Local joint disease
② Self-limited illness
③ Disease of striated muscles
④ Chronic and systemic disease

269. Which of the following is a first-line pharmacological medication used in the treatment of rheumatoid arthritis?
① Muscle relaxants
② Narcotic analgesics
③ Antiinflammatory agents
④ Calcium channel-blocking agents

270. In the patient who has a cystostomy drain in place following a suprapubic prostatectomy, the nurse should:
① Assess the perineal dressing for drainage
② Take vital signs more frequently
③ Catheterize the patient if he complains of bladder fullness
④ Assess the abdominal dressing and change PRN

271. In the patient suspected of having benign prostatic hypertrophy, the common, most frequent, and disturbing signs to assess for are:
① Dysuria, nocturia
② Hematuria, groin discomfort
③ Flank pain, chills
④ Bladder stones, malaise

272. The patient with a cervical spinal injury exhibits spasticity of the extremities. Which of the following types of medications will assist in decreasing the spasticity for the patient?
① Muscle relaxants such as baclofen (Lioresal)
② Vasodilators such as terazosin HCl (Hydrin)
③ Narcotic analgesics such as morphine sulfate (Roxanol)
④ NSAIDs such as tolmetin sodium (Tolectin)

273. The patient with an arteriovenous fistula and graft in the left forearm receives hemodialysis 3 times a week. The nurse should plan to:
① Keep the patient on bed rest
② Irrigate the fistula every 4 hours
③ Take the blood pressure on the right arm
④ Monitor I and O hourly

274. In a patient with the nursing diagnosis of knowledge deficit related to TURP, the expected outcome is that the patient will describe activity restrictions. Which of the following teaching points is most appropriate?
① "Avoid straining at stool for 4 to 6 weeks by using stool softeners as necessary."
② "Do Kegel perineal exercises every 4 to 6 hours for the next 2 weeks."
③ "Report any dribbling that occurs in the next 2 weeks."
④ "Monitor appearance of urine and report if urine becomes persistently bright red."

275. During the fifth day in coronary care, a patient with a diagnosis of myocardial infarction develops dyspnea, has blood-tinged, frothy sputum, and becomes very anxious. These symptoms may indicate:
① Emphysema
② Pulmonary edema
③ Pulmonary embolism
④ Chronic obstructive pulmonary disease

276. A nurse is providing care to a patient with a sprained ankle. Which of the following instructions should be given to the patient in regard to decreasing swelling in the ankle?
① Instruct the patient to dangle the foot over the edge of the bed
② Tell the patient to elevate the foot and ankle on a pillow
③ Tell the patient to request help in performing active range of motion to the foot
④ Instruct the patient to soak the foot in a cold water bath

277. A patient with rheumatoid arthritis complains to the nurse that she is in a great deal of pain and all the doctor did was "give me some stupid aspirin." Which of the following responses would best increase the knowledge base of the patient?
① "The physician wants to start you on a low-dose pain reliever."
② "I am sure that the doctor put you on salicylates because of their ability to relax skeletal muscles."
③ "The aspirin interrupts the nerve transmission of pain and will reduce your pain."
④ "The antiinflammatory properties of the aspirin will reduce the inflammation in your joints."

278. A patient is 6 hours post-op for an open-reduction, internal fixation of a fractured femur. Which of the following symptoms would alert the nurse to a possible fat embolism?
① Shortness of breath and restlessness
② Dysphagia and aspiration pneumonia
③ Abdominal distension and clay colored stools
④ Complaints of abdominal pain and absent bowel sounds

279. A nurse is assisting a physician in the application of a plaster cast to a foot and calf. Which of the following is the correct way for the nurse to handle the extremity?
① Instruct the patient to elevate the extremity
② Place a pillowcase under the cast to move the extremity
③ Pick up the casted extremity, supporting it with the palms of the hands
④ Instruct a nursing assistant to elevate the extremity by pulling up on the patient's toes

280. A nurse is providing dietary instruction to a patient with gouty arthritis. Which of the patient's favorite foods would the nurse recommend he eliminate from his diet?
① Chicken and rice
② Liver and onions
③ Beef and potatoes
④ Veal parmesan and garlic bread

281. A patient with osteomyelitis of the right knee is admitted to an orthopedic unit. Which of the following statements would indicate to the nurse that further teaching may be necessary?
① "I should only be in the hospital overnight."
② "I guess this infection could have came from the accident I had a few weeks ago with the staple gun."
③ "I need to stay in bed for a while."
④ "I guess I should expect my knee to hurt when I move it around."

282. A nurse is bathing a patient who is 1 day post-op total hip replacement. Which of the following statements made by the patient would indicate understanding of the positioning required after this surgery?
① "I know I shouldn't point my toes."
② "I need to have lowered chairs."
③ "It will be hard for me not to cross my legs."
④ "I will have trouble not walking for a long time."

283. A nurse is caring for a patient with a diagnosis of possible rheumatoid arthritis. Which of the following elevated lab values would support the patient's diagnosis?
① WBCs and hematocrit
② Uric acid and hemoglobin
③ ESR and rheumatoid factor
④ LE and rheumatoid factor

284. A nurse is caring for a patient who has been immobilized for 6 days because of the presence of skeletal traction. Which of the following assessment findings might indicate the patient has developed a thrombosis?
① Shortness of breath
② Distended neck veins
③ Calf pain and swelling
④ Pain at the skeletal pin sites

285. A nurse is assisting a patient with an above the knee amputation into a prone position. Which of the following statements made by the patient would indicate that the patient understands the need for this positioning?
① "Lying prone will alleviate my phantom limb pain."
② "I have to lay this way to make sure I have good circulation to my stump."
③ "This position will allow me greater comfort than lying on my back."
④ "I have to do this to make sure my hip doesn't get a flexion contracture."

286. A patient who has undergone a hemigastrectomy has been diagnosed with pernicious anemia. The patient asks the nurse what could have caused her problem. Which the following should be the nurse's best response?
① "You are no longer able to absorb vitamin B_{12} because of your surgery."
② "You are most likely not receiving enough folic acid in your low-fat diet."
③ "Because you have less hydrochloric acid since your surgery, you will have difficulty absorbing vitamin B_{12}."
④ "You can no longer utilize iron adequately in your body because of your surgery."

287. A nursing assistant is assessing on an unconscious patient with acute lymphoblastic leukemia. Which of the following modes of temperature assessment should the nurse instruct the nursing assistant to use?
① Oral
② Rectal
③ Tympanic
④ Axillary

288. A patient with a diagnosis of iron deficiency anemia has had a series of dyspneic episodes. The patient asks the nurse why this has occurred. Which of the following is the nurse's best response?
① "Your disease has decreased blood flow to your lungs."
② "You don't have as much oxygen circulating in your bloodstream because of your low red blood cell count."
③ "You may have had some damage to your brain cells because of your chronic low red blood cell count."
④ "The anemia that you have causes you to become short of breath when exercising."

289. A patient presents to the emergency department with a history of epistaxis and black tarry stools. When evaluating the patient's lab reports, which of the following conditions might indicate a reason for the patient's symptoms?
① Leukopenia
② Leukocytosis
③ Thrombocytosis
④ Thrombocytopenia

290. A patient with chronic heart failure inquires why he does not become short of breath until he exercises or takes a shower. Which of the following statements made by the nurse would best answer his question?
    ① "The shortness of breath is caused by your lung constricting."
    ② "You need to condition your heart to be able to tolerate exercise."
    ③ "When you exercise your heart can no longer meet the oxygen needs of your body."
    ④ "The blood vessels of your lungs constrict as you exercise, causing the shortness of breath."

291. A nurse is assessing a patient who has just returned to a telemetry unit after a cardiac catheterization. Which of the following nursing interventions would be the *most* important in the immediate postoperative period?
    ① Cough, deep breath, and leg exercises
    ② Urinary output, early ambulation, and cardiac monitoring
    ③ Monitoring for cardiac arrhythmias, bleeding, and shortness of breath
    ④ Vital signs, physical therapy and ambulation, and monitoring intake and output

292. A nurse is educating a patient with heart failure regarding a low-sodium diet. Which of the following dietary practices may the patient need to eliminate from his routine?
    ① Corned beef sandwiches with canned broth each day
    ② Shredded wheat and fruit for breakfast each morning
    ③ Crispy chicken sandwich and cheesy broccoli once per week
    ④ Hamburgers and french fries for lunch three times per week

293. A patient is 2 days post myocardial infarction. Which of the following data might suggest that the patient may be experiencing left-sided heart failure?
    ① Nausea
    ② Heart murmur
    ③ Crackles in lungs
    ④ Edema in feet and legs

294. A nurse is obtaining a history from a patient who has been admitted with a diagnosis of probable mitral insufficiency. Which of the following facts in the patient's history would be most significant?
    ① Appendectomy 1 year ago
    ② One-pack-a-day smoker for 20 years
    ③ History of rheumatic fever as a child
    ④ History of a pacemaker insertion 5 years ago

295. A nurse is assessing a patient with complaints of pain and swelling of the left calf. Which of the following recent histories may be significant in this situation?
    ① Atrial fibrillation
    ② Fractured femur
    ③ Narrow angle glaucoma
    ④ New-onset diabetes mellitus

296. The family of a patient who has just returned from an exophagogastroduodenostomy attempts to feed the patient a milkshake. Which of the following should be the nurses first course of action?
    ① Check the patient's diet order to see if a full liquid diet is ordered
    ② Explain that the patient must wait at least 6 hours before eating

③ Monitor the procedure to ensure that the patient swallows the liquid
④ Ask the family to wait until you have checked the patient's gag reflex

297. A resident in long-term care has a diagnosis of elevated ammonia levels related to cirrhosis. Which of the following foods would the nurse advise the nursing assistant to eliminate as a possible snack for the resident?
    ① Pretzels
    ② Crackers and cheese
    ③ Chicken salad sandwich
    ④ A bowl of vanilla ice cream

298. Which of the following assessment data would indicate that a patient may be suffering from appendicitis?
    ① Hematemesis
    ② Sharp back pain
    ③ Severe abdominal distention
    ④ Rebound abdominal tenderness

299. A patient, recently diagnosed with cholecystitis arrives at an outpatient clinic complaining of severe, right upper quadrant pain. Which of the following data, obtained from the patient history, may have precipitated this problem?
    ① Spent 3 hours mowing the lawn
    ② Had a hamburger and french fries for lunch
    ③ Took three acetaminophen for complaints of a headache
    ④ Had three beers and a bowl of pretzels after mowing the lawn

300. Which of the following nursing orders would the nurse expect to find in the chart of a patient with advanced liver failure?
    ① Force fluids
    ② Low-glucose diet
    ③ Measure abdomen daily
    ④ High-calorie, high-protein diet

301. A patient is admitted to the hospital with a diagnosis of hepatitis A. The patient asks the nurse how he could have possibly caught the virus. Which of the following is the nurse's most appropriate response?
    ① "Did you come into contact with a person who has it?"
    ② "You may have ingested some contaminated food or water."
    ③ "Have you had a transfusion of whole blood or platelets lately?"
    ④ "You might have inhaled some of the virus in your respiratory tract."

302. A nurse is teaching a patient regarding the proper method for administering pancreatic enzymes. Which of the following methods would the nurse advise?
    ① "Take the enzymes between meals."
    ② "Take the enzymes only if eating a fatty meal."
    ③ "Take the enzymes at the same time you eat the meal."
    ④ "Take the enzymes before you retire to bed each night."

303. A patient is scheduled for an elective, herniorrhaphy. The nurse notes that the patient has a cold. The nurse reports the cold to the surgeon because:
    ① The cold will increase the chance of a postoperative infection
    ② The patient may have an increased chance of peritonitis because of the cold

③ Coughing and sneezing may compromise the integrity of the surgical incision

④ The patient may have a prolonged, more expensive hospital stay because of the cold

304. A nurse notes that a patient's nasogastric tube has not been draining as much as usual. The patient complains of nausea, and abdominal distention is noted. Which of the following is the patient's next course of action?
① Remove the nasogastric tube
② Call the physician immediately
③ Assess the patency of the tube
④ Call for a portable abdominal X-ray

305. A patient has a diagnosis of diverticulitis. Which of the following of the patient's daily activities may need to be restricted as a result of the patient's diagnosis?
① Driving for 3 to 4 hours/day
② Teaching bible study classes
③ Typing during the evening hours
④ Stocking shelves in a grocery store

306. A nurse is counseling a patient with hypothyroidism concerning drug therapy. Which of the following statements by the patient would indicate that additional teaching may be needed?
① "I should discontinue the medicine when I feel better."
② "I should call the doctor if I have a headache or am nervous."
③ "I should try to take the medicine at the same time each day."
④ "I should let the doctor know if I experience weight loss or sweating."

307. Which of the following positions should a nurse assist the patient into after a thyroidectomy?
① Supine
② Left Sims'
③ Trendelenberg's
④ Semi-Fowler's

308. Which of the following would be most important in the teaching of a patient that has undergone an adrenalectomy?
① "Weigh yourself daily."
② "Avoid stressful situations."
③ "Maintain a diet high in potassium."
④ "Avoid drinking large amounts of water."

309. Which of the following assessment data may indicate that a patient has the disorder of diabetes insipidus?
① Bounding pulse and low urine output
② Increased blood pressure and tachycardia
③ Decreased fluid intake and high specific gravity of urine
④ Increased fluid intake and low specific gravity of urine

310. A patient has been admitted to the hospital with the diagnosis of Addisonian crisis. Which of the following medications when stopped abruptly can precipitate an Addisonian crisis?
① Insulin
② Cardizem
③ Prednisone
④ Diltiazem

311. Which of the following measures would assist in ensuring that a patient with diabetes mellitus would receive proper care outside of the hospital or clinic?
① Wearing a medical alert tag

② Carrying a rapid source of glucose with them
③ Carrying a syringe full of insulin with them all times
④ Reporting their condition to the local ambulance service

312. A nurse is caring for a patient with hyperpituitarism. Which of the following nursing diagnoses may be appropriate for this patient?
① Alteration in comfort
② Alteration in body image
③ Alteration in fluid and electrolyte balance
④ Altered nutrition, less than body requirements

313. A patient is admitted with a diagnosis of HHNK. The nurse is aware that HHNK differs from DKA in that:
① HHNK is more different to treat.
② DKA includes the complication of metabolic acidosis.
③ DKA is mostly found in patients who are not insulin dependent.
④ HHNK includes elevated serum levels of glucose and ketones.

314. A patient has just returned from a thyroidectomy. Which of the following assessment data would be of priority in the immediate post-op period?
① No bowel sounds
② Blood pressure of 160/100
③ Swelling in the neck region
④ Dime-sized area of blood on the operative dressing

315. A patient with diabetes mellitus is going to engage in a strenuous physical activity. Which of the following snacks would the nurse suggest that the patient consume before engaging in the activity?
① An orange
② A candy bar
③ A can of soda
④ Cheese and crackers

316. A nurse is caring for a female patient who has had a conization. Which of the following nursing interventions should the nurse expect to carry out for this patient?
① Instruct patient to replace tampon every 3 hours
② Maintain vaginal packing for the first 12 to 24 hours
③ Assist the patient in using a sitz bath twice per day
④ Instruct patient in the use of a medicated, vaginal douche

317. A 47 year-old female patient who works as a nursing assistant comes to an outpatient clinic for a routine physical. The nurse collects the following group of data. Which of the following needs to be addressed by the nurse?
① Gynecological exam 6 months ago
② Hepatitis B vaccine 4 months ago
③ Last mammogram was 8 years ago.
④ Last TB test was 3 months ago after starting a new job

318. The nurse is educating a group of females on the correct technique for breast self-examination. Which of the following methods should the nurse recommend?
① "Examine your breasts when your period first starts."
② "Palpate your breasts for lumps while sitting at a table."
③ "Use the palms of your hands to feel for lumps in your breasts."
④ "Palpate the breasts while lying, sitting, and standing each month."

319. A patient complains of excessive pain during menstruation. Which of the following interventions might the nurse suggest to alleviate discomfort?
① "Drink cold beverages early in the morning."
② "Drink warm beverages before pain begins."
③ "Exercise rigorously to counteract the uterine contractions."
④ "Recommend that the patient ask her doctor for a narcotic prescription."

320. The nurse is caring for a patient who has developed a possible rectovaginal fistula after delivery of her fifth child. Which of the following symptoms would suggest that the patient had developed a rectovaginal fistula?
① Leakage of urine from the vagina
② Extreme pain following a bowel movement
③ Passage of stool and flatus from the vagina
④ White creamy discharge and extreme pruritus

321. A female patient presents to an outpatient clinic because she is concerned that she may have gonorrhea. The patient states her male partner was diagnosed but she hasn't had any symptoms. Which of the following is the best response by the nurse?
① "I am sure there is no reason to worry if you have no symptoms."
② "I think we should test you, because gonorrhea can be asymptomatic in women."
③ "You can return to the clinic whenever you have burning on urination or get a fever."
④ " I think we can prescribe you an antibiotic without even doing a culture, because your partner is infected."

322. A nurse is assisting a physician in a gynecological examination. Which of the following interventions would increase the comfort of the patient during the procedure?
① Allow the patient to keep her undergarments on
② Have the patient void before positioning on the exam table
③ Ensure that the patient is menstruating when the exam is done
④ Leave the room when the exam begins to reduce embarrassment to the patient

323. A nurse is preparing a patient for an upcoming panhysterectomy. Which of the following should the nurse caution the patient to expect following the surgery?
① The patient will have a catheter after surgery
② The patient should expect to be on bed rest at least 4 days
③ It is unlikely that the patient will resume a normal diet for a few days
④ Physical therapy will be an integral part of her rehabilitation process

324. A nurse is caring for a patient who has an internal radium implant in her uterus for treatment of cervical cancer. Which of the following statements made by the patient would indicate that further teaching may be necessary?
① "I should be taking stool softeners everyday."
② "I can either lay on my back or side when I sleep."
③ "I should expect to get sick to my stomach with this type of treatment."

④ "I can have my daughter come in and sit with me if I get bored being hospitalized."

325. A nurse is educating a group of women on premenstrual tension. The nurse has the participants complete a survey of favorite foods. Which of the following favorite foods of the participants could aggravate PMS?
① Pizza
② Mineral water
③ Pasta and sauce
④ Raw fruits and vegetables

326. A patient has shallow respirations at 8 to 10 times a minute. This hypoventilation results in acidosis by:
① The retention of CO_2
② Excreting needed CO_2
③ Excreting O_2
④ Retaining too much O_2

327. A patient in the clinic has been diagnosed with asthma. Lab studies have been done and returned. The nurse knows that the primary antibody affected in asthmatic patients is:
① International Normalized Ratio (INR)
② Immunoglobulin E (IgE)
③ Hepatitis C Virus Antibody (HCV)
④ Carcinoembryonic Antigen (CEA)

328. Persons with active TB disease are usually no longer infectious after being on therapy for how long?
① 1 to 2 days
② 2 to 3 weeks
③ 3 to 4 months
④ They will remain infectious for life

329. A new admission has asthma and uses inhalers. He takes metaproterenol (Alupent), albuterol (Proventil), and beclomethasone (Vanceril). He complains that he doesn't like the side effects these inhaled medications cause. The nurse will instruct him that he:
① Must sit down when using inhalers
② Is overdosing himself if he uses all three inhalers within 1 hour
③ Needs to use the Alupent and Proventil inhalers before the Vanceril
④ Needs to stop using the inhalers until his next scheduled clinic appointment

330. A coworker was exposed to active tuberculosis last week. She had a PPD test done as soon as she found out. She will need to have another PPD test done to see if she has developed a positive test for the infection. This should be done when?
① 1 week later
② 1 month later
③ 3 months later
④ 12 months later

331. The patient tells the nurse that the reason he came to the clinic is because he has been having difficulty breathing, especially at night. The nurse would be most correct in documenting this information under which section of the admission sheet?
① Chief complaint
② Psychosocial history
③ Past medical history
④ Review of systems

332. A case of active TB has been confirmed in the nurse's neighborhood and a neighbor asks how she might have been exposed. The nurse's reply states how TB is transmitted. This includes:
① By using the same door handle as the infected person
② By an airborne route; the infected person coughing, sneezing, laughing
③ By touching a tissue that a person infected with TB used
④ By riding the bus after the person infected with TB was on it

333. A patient has a medical diagnosis of respiratory acidosis. His nursing diagnosis is activity intolerance. Which of the following activities is most directly aimed at his nursing diagnosis?
① Encouraging fluid intake by offering fluids every 2 hours
② Suctioning him every 2 hours and prn
③ Doing postural drainage with cupping every 2 to 4 hours
④ Planning activities to provide rest periods in between

334. A patient was seen and treated for obstructive urinary retention as a result of an enlarged prostate gland. The nurse is preparing him for discharge from the clinic following a cystourethroscopy with balloon dilation. He has a prescription for trimethoprim/sulfamethoxazole (Bactrim). She informs him to:
① Limit fluid intake to 1000 ml/day to prevent bladder distention
② Rest the bladder by urinating every eight to ten hours
③ Avoid using caffeine and alcohol because they irritate the bladder
④ Stop the Bactrim once he feels better

335. The nurse in the clinic is gathering data from a new patient. The nurse documents the data gathered. Vital signs are an example of data that should be recorded as:
① Subjective data
② Routine data
③ Objective data
④ Graphic data

336. A 48-year-old patient has COPD and is overweight. She has a chronic cough, brings up copious amounts of mucopurulent sputum, and at times experiences bronchospasms. These are all assessment findings of:
① Emphysema
② Asthma
③ Lung cancer
④ Chronic bronchitis

337. A patient being seen in the clinic has a history of glaucoma. When gathering data related to chronic glaucoma, which of the following complaints would the nurse expect to hear?
① Seeing flashes of light and floaters
② Having attacks of double vision
③ Experiencing sudden onset of eye pain with nausea and vomiting
④ Bumping into objects

338. A patient is admitted to the clinic for a complete physical exam. To prevent injury during the otoscopic exam, which of the following actions should the nurse avoid?
① Inserting the otoscope until it touches the eardrum
② Tipping the patient's head away from the examiner
③ Bracing the examining hand against the patient's head
④ Pulling the ear being examined up and back

339. A patient is admitted for possible obstructive urinary retention, possibly because of an enlarged prostate gland. The nurse is preparing him for a cystourethroscopy with balloon dilation. In planning his care, the nurse should inform him to expect:
① An indwelling catheter after the procedure
② Mild impotence
③ General anesthesia for the procedure
④ Quite significant pain

340. In a morning report the nurse learns her patient has an upper urinary tract infection. In assessing the patient, the nurse listens for complaints of:
① Chills, nausea, flank pain
② Burning on urination, urgency
③ Frequency, suprapubic pain
④ Pain at the end of urination

341. The nurse is making a home visit on her patient who has nephrotic syndrome. The most recent lab results show hypoalbuminemia and hyperlipidemia. Loss of which element is the major pathophysiological factor in this syndrome?
① Protein
② Potassium
③ Calcium
④ Sodium

342. The patient has received a prescription for an antimicrobial drug for his upper urinary tract infection. Usually this therapy is prescribed for:
① 1 day
② 3 to 5 days
③ 5 to 7 days
④ 10 to 14 days

343. A male patient is being evaluated for chlamydia. Which of the following symptoms would cause the physician to suspect a chlamydia infection?
① Urethritis, mucocutaneous lesions
② A chancre
③ Anal itching
④ Papular warts

344. The nurse is gathering objective data about her patient who is experiencing "kidney problems." The nurse looks at the lab results. The glomerular filtration rate (GFR) can be measured by evaluating the:
① Hemoglobulin
② Blood area nitrogen
③ White blood cells
④ Creatine clearance

345. The patient returns to the unit from a prostatic suprapubic resection. He has an IV and three-way Foley catheter connected to a continuous bladder irrigant. There is light red drainage with a few red clots in the drainage tubing. Four hours after returning to the unit, the patient states his bed is wet. The nurse finds the linen under him is pink-tinged and wet. The tubing is not kinked. The nurse should further assess for:
① Bowel sounds
② Atonic bladder
③ Bladder spasms
④ Elevated temperature

346. A 23-year-old patient seen in the clinic has been diagnosed with prostatitis. He is started on antibiotics. Which of the following should the nurse include in her teaching plan?
① This cannot be spread to his sexual partner, so it isn't necessary to wear a condom
② He should avoid having bowel movements for at least 3 days
③ He should take antibiotics until he feels better
④ He should avoid sexual arousal during acute inflammation

347. The patient sustained a gashing head wound when he was hit by a car. The wound required cleansing and 24 sutures. The nurse is assessing the wound status. Three key factors that affect the rate of wound healing are:
① Condition of the patient, type of wound, degree of contamination
② Age of the patient, type of wound, skill of closure
③ General nutritional status, age of wound, mental awareness of patient
④ Location of wound, degree of cleansing, type of suture used

348. The nurse inspects the abdominal incision of a patient who has returned to the skilled nursing facility. Which type of exudate should be reported to the physician?
① Serosanguineous
② Serous
③ Clear
④ Purulent

349. A patient had a CVA 2 days ago. He has been receiving nutrients by IV and has progressed to diet as tolerated. The nurse assesses that he has an intact gag reflex, although he does cough when you provide water for him to drink. The best approach to help him swallow is to:
① Make sure suction equipment is available during feedings
② Ensure that the patient is in a semi-Fowler's position with his head hyperextended during meals
③ Place patient in a semi-Fowler's position with head flexed slightly forward, provide soft textured food
④ Insist that his food be pureed, liquefied, and bland

350. Autonomic hyperreflexia may occur after a spinal cord injury. It is critical that the nurse observe for signs of this state. What are the manifestations of increased sympathetic stimulation that are not mediated by the parasympathetic system?
① Sweating, hypertension, flushed skin
② Pallor, hypotension, dehydration
③ Tachycardia, pallor, hypotension
④ Thirst, muscle spasticity, goose flesh

351. A patient is unable to respond appropriately and clearly. He is also disoriented to time and demonstrates an inability to follow commands. Which of the following best describes his level of consciousness?
① Oriented, arousable, and difficult
② Confused
③ Having periods of lethargy
④ In a stuporous state

352. Autonomic hyperreflexia may occur after a spinal cord injury. Which of the following is the most common stimuli that can cause the manifestation of autonomic hyperreflexia?
① Visitors
② Full bladder
③ Taking tympanic temperatures
④ Taking an apical pulse

353. The nurse is assigned to a newly admitted patient who was burned in an apartment fire. The patient quickly develops edema. Which statement best addresses why the nurse is concerned about the edema?
① Edema means the patient's kidneys have shut down
② Edema means frequent skin care is necessary
③ Edema may lead to hypovolemic shock
④ Edema indicates that the IV is being infused too rapidly

354. A patient has asthma and has been using an inhaler. He takes beta-adrenergic agonists metaproterenol (Alupent) or albuterol (Proventil). He complains that he doesn't like the side effects these inhaled medications cause. The common side effects he is complaining about are:
① Itching, peripheral edema
② Nervousness, dizziness
③ Nausea, vomiting
④ Bruising, increased appetite

355. A nurse is administering PPD tests to the residents on the assisted living wing of a retirement facility. The nurse should assess the injection sites of these residents:
① Within 12 to 24 hours
② Within 24 to 36 hours
③ Within 48 to 72 hours
④ Within 96 hours to a week

356. A patient has gastroesophageal reflux (GERD) and emphysema. She has a nursing diagnosis of ineffective airway clearance related to expiratory airflow obstruction. Based on this nursing diagnosis, you plan to observe for:
① Retained secretions
② Pitting edema of the lower extremities
③ Chronic fatigue
④ Dyspnea on exertion

357. A patient has been receiving vancomycin hydrochloride (Vancocin) for a methicillin-resistant *Staphylococcus aureus* (MRSA) infection following a craniotomy. With regard to vancomycin hydrochloride, the nurse should report which of the following lab results to the physician?
① Hemoglobin 12.4 g
② Sodium 137 mEq/L
③ Potassium 4.2 mEq/L
④ Creatinine 26 mg/dl

358. There are new medications and combinations of medications used to treat active TB disease. The most predominant side effect the nurse needs to look for with the use of TB drugs such as Isoniazid (INH) is:
① Changes in liver enzymes
② Sores in the mouth
③ Increased urination
④ Decreased saliva

359. A patient with COPD and pneumonia is unable to walk 20 feet without becoming dyspneic. His pulse oximeter reading drops to 79% with activity. His nursing diagnosis is activity intolerance related to insufficient oxygen to meet body requirements. Which of the following would be an appropriate goad for activity intolerance?
① Lips are cyanotic after ambulation
② Pulse returns to baseline within a half hour after walking
③ Oxygen saturation remains greater than 90% after walking
④ Respiratory rate returns to baseline within a half hour of ambulating

360. A 65-year-old patient is to have chest physiotherapy performed by the respiratory therapist. The nurse should plan to:
① Administer her albuterol nebulization treatments after the respiratory therapist finishes
② Serve her tray just before this treatment and offer to take her to the bathroom
③ Assess her tolerance to dependent positions required for lower lobe drainage
④ Take vital signs 1 hour after the treatment is completed

361. The nurse is gathering data from a patient who has a history of cataracts. which of the following complaints would the patient relate to the nurse?
① Floaters
② Eye pain
③ Eye dryness
④ Blurred vision

362. A patient returns to the unit from a suprapubic prostatic resection. He has an IV and three-way Foley catheter connected to a continuous bladder irrigation. At the end of the shift, he had an intake of 725 cc IV fluid, 150 cc PO fluids, 3200 cc of irrigation fluid, and 4000 cc output. His intake for the shift was:
① 150 cc
② 725 cc
③ 875 cc
④ 3200 cc

363. A patient is admitted for possible obstructive urinary retention possibly because of an enlarged prostate gland. In planning his care, the nurse would expect him to have which of the following complaints?
① Diminished force of urinary stream
② Nocturia
③ Increased thirst
④ Dysuria

364. A patient has a history of UTIs. The nurse is doing patient education and should stress the need to:
① Avoid sexual intercourse
② Avoid perfumed feminine hygiene products
③ Take tub baths daily
④ Increase her daily orange juice to eight 8-oz glasses

365. Assessment of a patient's current and past use of medications, including over-the-counter drugs and herbs, is important. The nurse might expect a change in the ability to control voiding if the patient, during a patient assessment, said he was taking:
① Calcium channel blockers
② Anticoagulants
③ Nonsteroidal antiinflammatory drugs
④ Antiemetics

366. A patient has a history of UTIs. The nurse is doing patient education and should stress the need to:
① Empty her bladder when she feels the urge to void
② Make sure she uses protection during sexual activities
③ Test her urine with a dipstick after each voiding
④ Drink milk before retiring

367. A patient has chronic renal failure. Which of the following would the nurse anticipate being low?
① Calcium levels
② White blood cells
③ Creatinine
④ Blood urea nitrogen

368. When providing care to a patient taking sulfa drugs for a urinary tract infection, the nurse should offer fluids frequently during the day to:
① Prevent crystals from forming in the urine
② Provide comfort from the burning sensation
③ Maintain constant blood levels of the medication
④ Maintain sufficient urine output

369. A patient is admitted for obstructive urinary retention due to prostatic hyperplasia. The nurse begins preparation for surgery. Which of the following surgical procedures for this condition causes the most bladder trauma?
① Perineal resection
② Retropubic resection
③ Suprapubic resection
④ Balloon dilation

370. When caring for a patient with a history of metabolic acidosis, the nurse should assess for:
① Increased urine output
② Decreased urine output
③ Increasing respirations
④ Decreasing respirations

371. A 35-year-old patient is admitted following an automobile accident with a Glasgow Coma Score ranging between 13 and 15 since the accident. The nurse knows that these scores indicate:
① Coma
② Mild head injury
③ Moderate head trauma
④ Optimum cerebral functioning

372. The nurse is planning her care for a patient who has edema of his legs following extensive burns to both lower extremities. The nurse knows that intracellular swelling after a severe burn is related to:
① Decreased circulating immunoglobulin
② Increased cardiac output
③ Increased metabolic demands
④ Disruption in sodium-potassium at the cellular level

373. It is reported that a patient has suffered a stroke. He has right brain damage with middle cerebral artery involvement. Which of the following behaviors are typical of this type of stroke?
① Aphasia
② Dysphasia
③ Inability to remember words
④ Right-sided paralysis

374. The nurse is watching a patient for the possibility of seizures. He is not known to have epilepsy. Besides a head trauma, what is a secondary cause for seizures?
① Weight loss of 5% in the last month
② Chemical changes, such as during drug administration
③ Obesity with a sedentary life style
④ History of cigarette smoking

375. The nurse in the assisted living facility has been assisting a patient who has a lower motor neuron disorder similar to multiple sclerosis. The nurse is aware that in giving care she must remember that dysfunction in the lower motor neuron pathways result in:
① Spasticity
② Hypertonia
③ Hypertrophy
④ Flaccidity

376. In the postoperative period for cranial surgery, a variety of drugs may be used to control cerebral edema. Which of the following statements best describes how these drugs act in this postoperative phase?
① Dexamethasone (Decadron) increases kidney output by acting as a thiazide diuretic
② Phenytoin (Dilantin) increases the cerebral metabolic rate, decreasing cerebral blood flow and ICP.
③ Furosemide (Lasix) is a diuretic that also reduces the rate of CSF production
④ Mannitol (Osmitrol) induces deep sedation, thereby decreasing cerebral metabolic rate

377. The patient has been admitted with deep partial-thickness (second-degree) burns to both arms. Which of the following best describes a second-degree deep partial-thickness burn?
① Erythema of intact skin
② Blister formation that may have ruptured
③ Loss of subcutaneous tissue down to the bone
④ Tissue destruction possibly involving the entire dermis

378. A patient with asthma tells the nurse that he does not use his albuterol (Ventolin) inhaler because it is the same thing as his ipratropium (Atrovent). The nurse needs to teach him that both inhalers contain:
① Medications that cause bronchodilation but in different ways. He should wait 5 minutes after using the one inhaler before using the next
② Medications that cause bronchoconstriction but in different ways. He should wait 15 minutes after using one inhaler before using the next
③ Medications that are used for bronchospasms. He can use either one if he feels an attack coming on
④ The same medication. The names are different because they are made by a different company. He is acting correctly

379. A patient has COPD. He has signs of both emphysema and chronic bronchitis. Which one of the following assessment findings is usually present in these two categories of COPD?
① Diminished breath sounds
② Bronchospasm
③ Cardiac enlargement
④ Increased residual lung volume

380. Which situation best describes the potential of contracting a TB infection from a person who has active tuberculosis?
① Lack of frequent hand washing practices in the work setting
② Close, frequent, or extended contact
③ Sharing a computer at work
④ Sharing the same bathroom in a restaurant

381. The patient has had nasal surgery with the insertion of posterior and packing. The nurse should watch for signs of possible bleeding by:
① Observing for frequent swallowing
② Checking for stools for occult blood
③ Observing for discoloration about the eyes
④ Checking capillary refill

382. The lab results for a patient who is being treated for asthma have just arrived. Which of the following results indicate the therapeutic blood level for theophylline?
① 10-20 mcg/ml
② 20-30 mcg/ml
③ 30-40 mcg/ml
④ 40-50 mcg/ml

383. A patient has gastroesophageal reflux (GERD) and emphysema. She is very thin. The nurse questions her about her usual diet at home and she says that she is so short of breath that she hasn't eaten very much. The diet the nurse should plan to order for her is a:
① Low-fat diet with six small feedings a day
② Regular diet with juice between meals and at bedtime
③ High-calorie, high-protein diet
④ High-carbohydrate, bland diet

384. During assessment, the nurse should be alert for cardinal signs and symptoms of respiratory dysfunction, including:
① Complaints of headache
② Skin turgor
③ Red, burning eyes
④ Dyspnea

385. A patient comes in to the clinic concerned about his infected foot. He has had emphysema for the past 5 years. The physician believes that this patient is in acidosis and orders ABGs. The patient can develop acidosis as a result of:
① CO_2 retention
② Hyperventilation
③ Malnourishment
④ Decreased activity

386. The nurse is caring for a patient who has nosocomial pneumonia. According to the CDC, the single most effective way to prevent the spread of disease is:
① Using antibiotics
② Using protective isolation technique
③ Frequent hand washing
④ Using standard precautions

387. The patient has come into the clinic with complaints of repeated episodes of Ménière's disease. The chief symptom this patient experiences during an acute episode is:
① Sudden hearing loss
② Ear pain
③ Vertigo
④ Headache

388. A patient has cataracts. Patient education that is appropriate for this patient is to:
① Teach him to avoid bright light or bright sunlight
② Tell him that special glasses will help him see better
③ Tell him that over-the-counter medications will help to reduce eye pain
④ Tell him to wear sunglasses at night to reduce glare from the headlights

389. A patient has a lower urinary tract infection. The nurse should advise her to avoid beverages that may irritate the bladder. These beverages are:
① Milk and dairy products
② Caffeine and carbonated drinks
③ Bottled water products
④ Fruit-flavored drinks

390. The nurse is instructing the patient with asthma about the importance of measuring peak flow rates. Which of the following statements about the purpose for measuring peak flow rates is correct?
① Help to wean him off his bronchodilator
② Measure his response to bronchodilator therapy
③ Eliminate the need for blood test monitoring of the drug level
④ Determine when he may return to work

391. Which of the following data should the nurse be most concerned with during assessment of a patient with pneumonia?
① The patient's capillary refill is greater than 3 seconds and buccal cyanosis
② A Hct of 47% and WBCs of 5500/ml
③ Nonproductive cough and clear lung sounds
④ Potassium level of 3.7 mEq/L and clear, amber urine

392. Drugs affect the urinary tract in several ways. During patient assessment, the nurse would expect a change in the normal characteristics and quantity of urine if the patient stated he was taking:
① Calcium channel blockers
② Anticoagulants
③ Diuretics
④ Antihistamines

393. Which of the following interventions is appropriate for a patient who has urolithiasis?
① Ambulation
② Diuretic medications
③ Restricting fluids to 1000 cc per day
④ Low-protein diet

394. The nurse has been told in report that her patient has an upper urinary tract infection. In assessing the patient, the nurse knows that the infection is in her:
① Bladder
② Urethra
③ Kidney
④ Blood stream

395. A patient has a urinary tract infection and the nurse encourages her to void every 2 to 3 hours to:
① Train the bladder
② Reduce the possibility of reflex incontinence
③ Reduce urinary stasis and the risk of infection
④ Prevent fluid retention with overflow

396. A patient is admitted for obstructive urinary retention. He is newly diagnosed with adult onset diabetes mellitus. The nurse checked his blood glucose level before dinner. It was 45 mg/dL. The best action is to:
① Give 6 oz of orange juice to drink immediately
② Administer regular insulin according to the sliding scale orders
③ Call the physician immediately
④ Call the dietary department to have them deliver his dinner as soon as possible

397. A patient was admitted with second- and third-degree burns over 40% of her body after her house burned down yesterday. The nurse is monitoring her condition. Which of the following would the nurse want to report immediately?
① Urine output of 200 cc in the past 6 hours
② Decrease of body temperature to 98.4° F in the last hour
③ Edema formation in the upper airway
④ Complaints of pain during dressing changes

398. When planning care for a patient with an infection, it is important for the nurse to remember that fever and profuse perspiration:
① Increase the body's need for fluids
② Increase urinary output
③ Result in a rise is serum electrolytes
④ Decrease the respiratory rate

399. The nurse needs to assess for the signs of hypocalcemia in a patient who:
① Has been taking high doses of vitamin C
② Is on hydrochlorothiazide (Esidrix) medication
③ Is diagnosed with hyperparathyroidism
④ Is being treated for chronic renal failure

400. A 42-year-old patient is recovering from cranial surgery. It is important to plan nursing interventions to prevent an increase in intracranial pressure. Which of the following actions best helps to decrease the possibility of the intracranial pressure from increasing?
① Encouraging her to do deep breathing and coughing
② Doing endotracheal suctioning every 4 hours are prn
③ Maintaining her bed in a high-Fowler's (90-degree) position
④ Spreading interventions evenly throughout the day

ANSWERS AND RATIONALES

1. Knowledge (a)
   ❹ Platelets stick together and form a plug that seals the wound. They release chemicals that eventually result in formation of a clot.
   ① Antibodies are produced in response to a specific antigen.
   ② Leukocytes are WBCs, which aid in infection control.
   ③ Erythrocytes are RBCs, which carry oxygen from lungs to tissues.

2. Knowledge (a)
   ❶ The body is constantly stabilizing and equalizing its environment to prevent any sudden or severe change.
   ② Diffusion is the process of dissolved particles being distributed evenly throughout a fluid.
   ③ Osmosis is the movement of water through a permeable membrane.
   ④ Filtration is the movement of water and solutes through a membrane because of a greater pushing force on one side of the membrane.

3. Knowledge (a)
   ❷ The DNA molecules in the nucleus of a cell duplicate themselves, and the cell divides, forming two identical cells.
   ① Lysis is the swelling of red blood cells placed in a hypotonic salt solution.
   ③ Osmosis is the movement of water through a permeable membrane.
   ④ Crenation is the shrinking of red cells placed in a hypertonic solution.

4. Knowledge (a)
   ❷ In acquiring passive immunity, the body of the recipient plays no active part in response to an antigen.
   ① In active immunity the resistance to a disease results from the development of antibodies within the body.
   ③ Newborn babies receive a short-term immunity as a result of the antibodies of their mother, but it is not considered permanent.
   ④ Autoimmune immunity occurs by the body's producing antibodies to its own tissues.

5. Knowledge (a)
   ❶ This functional unit is suspended near the center of the cell and has the property of division.
   ② Cytoplasm is the portion of the protoplasm of a cell outside the nucleus.
   ③ Protoplasm is a thick, viscous substance that exists only in cells.
   ④ The cytoplasmic membrane that encloses the cytoplasm.

6. Knowledge (a)
   ❶ Produced by the thyroid, thyroxine controls the rate at which glucose is burned and converts it to heat and energy.
   ② Oxytocin initiates and maintains labor.
   ③ Cortisone assists the body to respond to stress and reduce inflammation.
   ④ Aldosterone promotes sodium and water retention in the kidney.

7. Knowledge (a)
   ❷ Estrogen and progesterone promote development of the female sex characteristics and sex organs and regulate menstruation for the purpose of reproduction.
   ① Testosterone is produced by the testes of males.
   ③ Prolactin is produced by the pituitary gland.
   ④ Although progesterone is produced by the ovaries, testosterone is produced by the testes.

8. Knowledge (a)
   ❶ Dilation of the blood vessels brings more blood to the surface so that heat can be dissipated.
   ② Contraction of blood vessels will preserve body heat.
   ③ An increase in blood supply constricts muscles, rather than relax them.
   ④ The production of sweat is increased by dilation if blood vessels but is not the primary cause of lost body heat.

9. Knowledge (a)
   ❶ The area is located slightly below the center of the breast and contains slightly raised areas.
   ② Urochrome gives urine its color.
   ③ Cowper's glands are located on either side of the urethra and just below the prostate gland in the male.
   ④ Bartholin's glands lie on either side of the vagina.

10. Knowledge (a)
    ❸ The testes produce testosterone, which gives males their secondary sex characteristics.
    ① Estrogen is produced by the ovaries.
    ② Progesterone is produced by the ovaries.
    ④ Aldosterone is produced by the adrenal cortex.

11. Knowledge (a)
    ❷ The connective tissue is made of dense fibrous tissue in the shape of a cord and has great strength.
    ① Osseous is another term for bone tissue.
    ③ Cartilage makes a slick surface for rotation and shock absorption at joints.
    ④ Ligaments attach bone to bone.

12. Knowledge (a)
    ❹ The lymphatic system drains excess fluids through a series of filters, lymph nodes, where bacteria and foreign bodies are trapped and destroyed.
    ① The lymphatic system destroys bacteria.
    ② Erythrocytes are manufactured in the red bone marrow of long bones.
    ③ Clotting of blood is aided by platelets.

13. Knowledge (a)
    ❶ Iron is an essential mineral in the formation of hemoglobin.
    ② Copper assists in the use of iron.
    ③ Calcium is essential in bone and tooth formation.
    ④ Magnesium is essential in general metabolism.

14. Knowledge (a)
    ❹ The primary purpose of bile is to emulsify fats so that they can be more easily digested.
    ① The liver converts glycogen to glucose.
    ② Bile does not act on sugars, only fats.
    ③ Trypsin is the enzyme primarily responsible for digesting meats.

15. Comprehension (a)
    ❶ Epithelial tissue has many forms that are arranged in single or several layers to form a protective covering and lining for the internal organs of the body.
    ② Periosteum is a connective tissue covering of bone.
    ③ Pericardium is a fibrous sac lined with serous membrane that surrounds the heart.
    ④ Connective tissue supports and connects other tissues and parts of the body.

16. Comprehension (b)
    ❸ The cardiac sphincter prevents regurgitation of stomach contents back into the esophagus.
    ① Rugae are the folds in the stomach lining that allow for its expansion.
    ② Chyme is the semi-liquid in the stomach that is formed from the combination of hydrochloric acid and food.
    ④ The pyloric sphincter separates the stomach and duodenum. It determines how long food will stay in the stomach.

17. Comprehension (a)
    ❸ The small intestine contains villi that absorb most of the nutrients that are derived from the digestion of food.
    ① Absorbed nutrients travel by way of the portal vein to the liver.
    ② The stomach absorbs very little nutrients, as most food has not been digested into small enough particles for absorption.
    ④ By the time the food reaches the large intestine, most of the nutrients have been absorbed and all that is left is the undigestible wastes left from the food.

18. Knowledge (a)
    ❸ Sphincters are circular muscles that contract, closing a body opening.
    ① Flexors are muscles that cause an angle of a joint to become smaller.
    ② Abductors move body parts away from the midline.
    ④ Extensor muscles contract and cause the angle of a joint to become larger.

19. Knowledge (a)
    ❹ The nasolacrimal duct is a small opening into the nose at the inner corner of the eye that allows the fluid to drain through.
    ① The ciliary body is a smooth muscle structure to which the lens is attached.
    ② The lacrimal gland releases tears into the anterior face of the eyeball.
    ③ The eustachian tube connects the middle ear chamber with the throat.

20. Knowledge (a)
    ❷ Incisors are the four top and bottom front teeth.
    ① Molars are the last to appear, usually by 2-2½ years.
    ③ Canines are another name for eye teeth and appear after the incisors.
    ④ Eye teeth, or canines, appear later in a baby.

21. Comprehension (b)
    ❷ Many gray matter areas that form the cranial nerves are located in the medulla and control the vital functions of the body.
    ① The pons carries messages between the cerebrum and medulla.
    ③ The cerebrum controls the highest level of functioning, sensation, memory, reasoning, and intelligence.
    ④ The cerebellum controls muscle tone, coordination, and equilibrium.

22. Knowledge (a)
    ❹ As peristalsis moves content along, water is absorbed through the walls into the circulation, and the remaining cellulose passes on to the rectum.
    ① Absorption of food occurs in the small intestine.

② Enzymes are produced in the mouth, stomach, pancreas, and small intestine.
③ Enzymes are secreted from the mouth, stomach, pancreas, and small intestine.

23. Knowledge (a)
    ❷ The progressive, wavelike movement that occurs involuntarily forces food in a forward motion.
    ① Rugae are the folds that are found in the stomach that allow for expansion.
    ③ Mastication is the action of chewing.
    ④ This is a spasm of the pyloric sphincter.

24. Knowledge (a)
    ❸ Amino acids are the digestible form of protein.
    ① Ptyalin is an enzyme found in saliva that begins the breakdown of starches.
    ② Glucose is the end product of carbohydrate digestion.
    ④ Hydrochloric acid is a solution found in the stomach.

25. Comprehension (a)
    ❸ Most of the digestion and absorption of food occurs in the small intestine.
    ① The stomach digests some food, but the primary site for digestion and absorption is the small intestine.
    ② The sigmoid is part of the large intestine.
    ④ Digestion is complete by the time the food comes into the large intestine.

26. Comprehension (b)
    ❹ The liver is responsible for the production of fibrinogen, which aids in the clotting process.
    ① Bile is responsible for emulsifying fats, and is produced by the liver.
    ② The small intestine is responsible for the absorption of nutrients.
    ③ The pancreas manufactures and secretes trypsin, which aids in the digestion of proteins.

27. Application (b)
    ❷ Iodine is an element that aids in the formation of thyroxine, which is the hormone produced by the thyroid gland; a lack of it causes hypothyroidism.
    ① Iron is essential in the manufacture of hemoglobin.
    ③ Calcium is essential to the clotting process, muscular function, and bone growth and development.
    ④ Phosphorus is also essential for bone growth and development.

28. Knowledge (a)
    ❹ Capillaries are one cell layer deep and provide for the exchange of nutrients and wastes.
    ① Veins transport blood back to the heart.
    ② Venules carry blood from capillaries to veins.
    ③ Arterioles carry blood from arteries to capillaries.

29. Knowledge (a)
    ❷ The right atrium receives deoxygenated blood from all the body tissues via the superior and inferior vena cava.
    ① The left atrium receives oxygenated blood from the four pulmonary veins.
    ③ The left ventricle receives oxygenated blood from the left atrium and pumps blood to all the body's tissues.
    ④ The right ventricle receives deoxygenated blood from the right atrium and pumps that blood to the lungs to be oxygenated.

30. Knowledge (a)
    ❸ Epinephrine is a hormone manufactured in the adrenal medulla and increases blood pressure and heart rate.
    ① Insulin is manufactured in the pancreas and decreases blood sugar levels.
    ② Aldosterone is produced in the adrenal cortex and aids in regulating electrolytes and water balance.
    ④ Testosterone is produced by the testes and stimulates growth and development of the sex organs.

31. Comprehension (b)
    ❹ Antidiuretic hormone is produced in the posterior pituitary and promotes reabsorption of water in the kidney.
    ① Oxytocin is produced in the posterior pituitary and causes uterine muscle contraction.
    ② Prolactin is produced by the anterior pituitary and promotes milk formation.
    ③ Calcitonin is produced in the thyroid and assists in decreasing serum calcium levels.

32. Comprehension (a)
    ❷ The diffusion of gas occurs across the thin epithelial lining of the alveoli.
    ① The bronchi carry air to the right and left lung.
    ③ The trachea conducts air down toward the bronchi.
    ④ Bronchioles are the smallest branches of the bronchi.

33. Knowledge (a)
    ❷ The SA node, located in the right atrium, sets and regulates the rate of the heart rate.
    ① The AV node conducts the electrical impulse of the heartbeat down toward the Bundle of His.
    ③ The Bundle of His receives the electrical impulse of the heartbeat from the AV node and conveys it to the Purkinje fibers.
    ④ The Purkinje fibers are the terminal branches of the conduction system of the heart.

34. Knowledge (a)
    ❹ The pulmonary artery carries deoxygenated blood from the heart to the lungs.
    ① The aorta carries oxygenated blood from the heart to all body tissues.
    ② The carotid artery carries oxygenated blood to the brain.
    ③ The coronary arteries carry oxygenated blood to the heart muscle itself.

35. Knowledge (a)
    ❷ The thymus gland produces T cells which protect the infant during the first few months of life.
    ① The pineal secretes melatonin, which may regulate sexual development.
    ③ The thyroid influences body metabolism.
    ④ The pituitary secretes many substances that affect growth and development, protect the body in stressful situations, and promote reabsorption of water.

36. Comprehension (a)
    ❸ The greater trochanter closely articulates with the hip joint and is involved in many fractures.
    ① The acromion process is the highest point of the shoulder.
    ② The acetabulum is the hollowed out area of the hip joint.
    ④ The olecranon process forms the point of the elbow.

37. Knowledge (b)
    ❹ The periosteum is a tough covering that provides structure for blood, lymph, and nerve channels.
    ① Red bone marrow produced red blood cells.
    ② Adipose tissue is stored in the diaphysis or shaft.
    ③ Yellow bone marrow provides a site for storing fatty material.

38. Knowledge (a)
    ❶ The perineum is the external region between the vulva and anus in a female or between the scrotum and anus in the male. The perineum forms the pelvic floor.
    ② The peritoneum lines the abdominal cavity and provides protection to the internal organs.
    ③ The mons pubis is the fatty rounded area overlying the pubic symphysis.
    ④ The rectus abdominis is an abdominal muscle.

39. Comprehension (a)
    ❸ Rashes, bruises, and decubitus are all data that are derived from assessing the skin and its appendages—the integumentary system.
    ① Blood sugar levels would be an assessment of the endocrine system.
    ② Blood pressure and pulse are considered part of the respiratory and cardiovascular system.
    ④ Blood sugar levels are not part of the assessment of the integumentary system.

40. Application, assessment, coping and adaptation (b)
    ❹ Sebaceous glands produce an oily secretion that, combined with dirt, can give the appearance of blackheads; once infected, the bump is now termed a pimple.
    ① The lacrimal gland produces tears.
    ② The ceruminous glands secrete cerumen, or ear wax, in the ear canal.
    ③ This does not address the teen's question.

41. Application, assessment, basic care and comfort (b)
    ❷ Normal urine should be a clear, yellow liquid. Differences in color and clarity may signify body imbalance.
    ① Normally, urine is slightly aromatic.
    ③ The specific gravity of urine is normally low.
    ④ The presence of RBCs in a urine sample would signify kidney disease.

42. Knowledge (a)
    ❸ The upper surface of the dermis have raised and depressed areas that are unique to each individual and thus provide a means for identification.
    ① Elastic connective tissue is found in the subcutaneous layer, not on the surface of the skin.
    ② The subcutaneous layer is below the level of the dermis.
    ④ The upper surface of the epidermis consists of epithelial cells that are constantly being shed.

43. Comprehension (b)
    ❸ Aldosterone is released by the adrenal cortex in response to decreased blood volume, decreased blood sodium ions or increased potassium ions.
    ① Oxytocin stimulates uterine muscles during birth.
    ② ADH prevents excess water loss in the urine.
    ④ Parathormone regulates calcium ion homeostasis of the blood.

44. Knowledge (b)
❶ Oxygen prevents the formation of lactic acid and glycogen is the form of energy that the skeletal muscles use.
② Acetylcholine is important in the transmission of nerve impulses.
③ Although oxygen prevents lactic acid buildup, acetylcholine is a neurotransmitter.
④ Lactic acid is a waste product caused by anaerobic metabolism in the muscles.

45. Comprehension, assessment, physiological adaptation (b)
❸ The left motor control center in the brain controls the right side of the body because of the crossing of the nerve tracts within the brain.
① Only one side of the body is affected if an injury is to only one side of the brain.
② The left side of the body is controlled by the right side of the brain.
④ Normally, some paralysis is observed when there is damage to the motor control center of the brain.

46. Knowledge (a)
❶ The diaphragm separates the abdomen from the thoracic cavity. It contracts with inspiration and relaxes with expiration.
② The gastrocnemius is located in the calf of the leg.
③ The latissimus dorsi is located in the back and produces arm movement.
④ The sternocleidomastoid is alongside the neck and assists in turning and rotating the head.

47. Comprehension (b)
❹ The parasympathetic division of the autonomic nervous system maintains homeostasis by regulating digestion and circulation.
① The sensory neurons carry impulses towards the CNS.
② The sympathetic nervous system controls the "fight or flight" response.
③ Interneurons conduct impulses from the sensory neurons to the motor neurons.

48. Knowledge, assessment, coordinated care (a)
❸ The hypothalamus is an important autonomic nervous system center and controls body temperature.
① The medulla controls heart rate, blood pressure, breathing, and swallowing.
② The cerebellum controls muscle tone and coordination and coordinates action of the voluntary muscles.
④ The cerebral cortex is the outer layer of the cerebrum.

49. Knowledge (a)
❷ The snail-like cochlea contains the organ of Corti, which contains the hearing receptors.
① The malleus is an ossicle in the middle ear.
③ The tympanic membrane is the eardrum.
④ The semicircular canal controls equilibrium.

50. Comprehension (b)
❹ The eustachian tube connects the middle ear with the throat; swallowing or yawning equalizes the pressure, which allows the eardrum to vibrate easily.
① The ossicles are the three tiny bones of the middle ear.
② The labyrinth is the internal ear.
③ Sound waves are passed through the oval window to the internal ear.

51. Knowledge (b)
❷ When water intake is excessive, the kidneys excrete generous amounts of urine. If water intake is lost, they produce less urine, the process is regulated by hormones.
① The gonads are the sex glands and are not directly involved in fluid and electrolyte balance.
③ The bladder is the storage center for urine but does not affect fluid and electrolyte balance.
④ The islets of Langerhans are the functional cells of the pancreas that secrete insulin and glucagon.

52. Knowledge (a)
❹ The beta cells of the islets of Langerhans manufacture insulin.
① The liver does not produce the hormone insulin, however does manufacture bile, heparin, and fibrinogen.
② The duodenum is the first part of the small intestine.
③ The pineal gland is found in the brain and atrophies at an early age.

53. Comprehension (b)
❹ The primary responsibility of T cells is to destroy any foreign related protein in the body.
① Although correct, this statement does not explain the T cells role in the immune response.
② This is incorrect; B cells are responsible for humoral immunity.
③ B cells are responsible for cloning antibody-producing plasma cells.

54. Knowledge (a)
❹ The primary function of the humors, or fluids of the eye, is to maintain the shape of the eyeball.
① The production of tears is regulated by the lacrimal gland.
② Dilation of the pupil is the responsibility of the intrinsic muscles of the eye.
③ The ciliary body regulates the thickness of the lens.

55. Application, planning, reduction of risk potential (b)
❶ This action takes priority. If the patient's neurovascular status is compromised the patient may lose a limb.
② Although important, this is not the most important nursing intervention.
③ Maintenance of diet is important, but is not the most important in this list.
④ Activity, within the limits of the patient's traction, should be encouraged.

56. Comprehension, implementation, basic care and comfort (b)
❸ With blockage of the bile duct, little bile enters the small intestine, causing the stool to appear clay colored as bile gives stool its characteristic color.
① Tarry stools are a sign of GI bleeding.
② This is common in individuals having food poisoning, or the flu.
④ This is not a common finding in gallbladder disease.

57. Application, implementation, physiological adaptation (c)
❸ This should raise the blood sugar to the desired level. The patient is alert and is able to consume the juice.
① This will not be a sufficient amount to raise the glucose level.
② This could cause the blood sugar to rise quickly, and then fall quickly again.
④ Diet drinks do not contain sugar and will not alter the blood sugar level.

58. Comprehension, assessment, coordinated care (a)
- ❶ The peak action for regular insulin is 2-4 hours after administration, so the nurse should be particularly alert around 5 or 6 PM for any hypoglycemic episodes.
- ② The peak action will most likely occur before this time.
- ③ Regular insulin should have left the patient's bloodstream by this hour.
- ④ By this time the patient will not have any effect from the regular insulin.

59. Application, assessment, physiological adaptation (b)
- ❷ These are the classic symptoms of osteomyelitis.
- ① These symptoms could signal a pulmonary emboli.
- ③ These symptoms may indicate neurovascular impairment.
- ④ These are symptoms of neurological impairment.

60. Application, assessment, reduction of risk potential (c)
- ❶ Salty or sweet-tasting drainage from the operative area may indicate cerebral spinal fluid is leaking.
- ② Headache is frequent after craniotomy, usually caused by stretching or irritation of nerves of the scalp during the operation. Position shouldn't affect headache unless the left is the operative side.
- ③ Neither hunger nor temporary anorexia would indicate a possible complication. You would anticipate thirst postoperatively.
- ④ The patient has had general anesthesia so sleepiness is expected but level of consciousness changes are critical.

61. Comprehension, planning, safety and infection control (b)
- ❹ A mask with an eyeshield and gloves are needed to protect the caregiver's hands and eyes from direct contact or spraying of infected secretions.
- ① A plain mask will not offer adequate protection against spraying of material.
- ② Gloves are mandatory, however the mask without an eyeshield will not be adequate.
- ③ A mask with eyeshield is indicated, gown and gloves are not adequate protection.

62. Application, planning, safety and infection control (b)
- ❶ A WBC count of 0.2 is indicative of immunosuppression. The immunocompromised patient is unable to resist foreign agents and is susceptible to overwhelming infection.
- ② The nursing staff wears face masks to prevent spread of microorganisms to the patient.
- ③ Protective isolation precautions are indicated.
- ④ Patients with immunosuppression are encouraged not to be around groups of people, because this increases the risk of infection.

63. Comprehension, assessment, physiological adaptation (b)
- ❷ The pelvis of a patient with muscular dystrophy widens, causing a waddling gait.
- ① Pillrolling is a common behavior associated with Parkinson's disease.
- ③ Patients with Parkinson's disease also have a shuffling gait.
- ④ Tardive dyskinesia is an irreversible condition of involuntary muscle movements seen in patients taking antipsychotic medications.

64. Application, planning, coping and adaptation (b)
- ❹ A patient newly diagnosed with ALS needs support from family and health care professionals. Of all the responses, this is a priority at this time.
- ① Periods of exercise are necessary, but they would not be increased. Adequate periods of rest are a necessity for this patient.
- ②, ③ These are unrelated to situation at this time; they are a priority during later stages of the disease.

65. Comprehension, planning, basic care and comfort (a)
- ❸ It is true that it takes longer to inspire or expire air because of age-related physiological changes.
- ① This is not a proven fact for the elderly.
- ② This is not a proven correlation.
- ④ Overall respiratory muscle structure and function decrease in the elderly.

66. Comprehension, implementation, coping and adaptation (b)
- ❸ The purpose of an arthroscopy is to improve joint function and limit the amount of pain.
- ① This does not alleviate the patient's anxiety, and although a surgeon may need to speak to the patient, the nurse should answer the patient's question to the best of her/his ability.
- ② Having an arthroscopy will most likely postpone the need for a knee replacement but may postpone it.
- ④ This procedure will not cure degenerative joint disease but will alleviate some of the symptoms.

67. Comprehension, assessment, physiological (b)
- ❸ These are signs noted during later stages of the disease; others include jaw clonus and respiratory difficulty.
- ① Aphasia is not a symptom noted in ALS; the patient can speak but has difficulty doing so.
- ② Flexor muscles become spastic, not flaccid.
- ④ There is no sensory loss experienced with ALS; the patient remains alert.

68. Comprehension, implementation, prevention/early detection of disease (c)
- ❷ Obesity increases strain on weight bearing joints; reduction of weight minimizes some of the presenting symptoms.
- ① This does not reduce joint strain, but does maintain existing range of motion.
- ③ This will provide comfort but will not reduce strain.
- ④ This does not control strain, but will aid in pain control.

69. Comprehension, assessment, physiological adaptation (b)
- ❶ Tenderness and crepitus are common characteristics of joints involved in osteoarthritis.
- ② Most joints involved in osteoarthritis are on one side of the body. These findings are consistent with rheumatoid arthritis.
- ③ In osteoarthritis, pain is caused by the loss of articular cartilage.
- ④ Rheumatoid arthritis commonly presents with these symptoms.

70. Application, assessment, basic care and comfort (c)
- ❹ As the patient will be staying a short while, this data appears to be the most pertinent, as the nurse will need to ascertain how the patient will ambulate before and after surgery.

① This data would not be particularly relevant at this time.

② Although this is important to note, the nurse will need to assess how the patient will ambulate, as the priority for the short-stay will be on rapid recovery.

③ Although this data is very important, it is not the most pertinent at this time.

71. Application, implementation, physiological adaptation (c)

❹ Concentrated glucose can be absorbed between the buccal mucosa and gum; when patient fully awakens, give a fast-acting carbohydrate by mouth.

① Insulin would further lower the blood glucose reading, and LPN/LVNs are not permitted to administer IV insulin.

② This places the patient in danger for aspiration.

③ This action will most likely result in the patient choking and aspirating.

72. Comprehension, assessment, physiological adaptation (a)

❸ An increase in growth hormone after the epiphyseal plates close leads to acromegaly.

① Prolactin is not associated with acromegaly.

② Cortisol is made by the adrenal cortex and will produce Cushing's syndrome if it is overproduced.

④ An overproduction of thyroid hormone is referred to as hyperthyroidism.

73. Application, implementation, reduction of risk potential (b)

❹ This direction allows the fluid left in the space to consolidate and lessens the possibility of mediastinal shift.

①, ②, ③ These are inappropriate; they increase risk of mediastinal shift when placed on unaffected side.

74. Comprehension, implementation, physiological adaptation (b)

❹ The pulse oximetry machine measures how much of the capillary blood is saturated with oxygen.

① Pulse oximetry does not measure metabolic rate.

② Although most pulse oximetry machines measure the heart rate, that is not the primary purpose of the machine.

③ Only a chest radiograph will be able to show how much fluid is in the lung.

75. Comprehension, implementation, coordinated care (c)

❷ Decreased albumin levels alter the hydrostatic pressure in the liver's portal circulation, forcing fluid into the abdominal cavity.

① Hypertension may contribute to portal hypertension but does not cause ascites.

③ This may cause jaundice but should not cause ascites.

④ Ammonia levels may be elevated but do not cause ascites.

76. Comprehension, implementation, reduction of risk potential (b)

❸ This is standard practice.

① A clean dressing is not a sterile dressing.

② This is not correct, is inappropriate, and is degrading to the physician.

④ This is not a sterile dressing, which is standard practice.

77. Application, implementation, physiological adaptation (b)

❶ A patient with a lobectomy may be turned to either side.

②, ③, ④ These do not allow for full expansion and drainage of all remaining lobes.

78. Comprehension, implementation, basic care and comfort (c)

❸ Bile is needed to emulsify fat. When fat requires bile for emulsification, the gallbladder contracts in an effort to release the bile to be used in this process. A diseased gallbladder that must contract causes a sensation of pain.

① Foods high in fat require bile released by the gallbladder to aid in the emulsification process.

② It is possible that the duct leading from the liver to the gallbladder may become blocked, but it is less likely to involve the pancreas in most acute presentations.

④ Although a portion of this statement is true, this does not explain the mechanism by which pain is produced.

79. Comprehension, assessment, physiological adaptation (b)

❶ Accidental removal of the parathyroid glands can lead to tetany, because the glands secrete a hormone that regulates calcium balance.

② A seizure is possible in tetany but is not one of the initial symptoms.

③ This is not associated with parathyroid removal.

④ Although respiratory compromise is a potential problem with a thyroidectomy, loss of the gag reflex is not associated with parathyroid removal.

80. Application, implementation, prevention/early detection of disease (b)

❸ Elevating the head of the bed will reduce pressure on the cardiac sphincter, reducing the chance of esophageal reflux.

① This suggestion will not reduce bedtime discomfort.

② This will worsen the symptoms; eating is not recommended for 3 hours before bed.

④ This will cause a worsening of symptoms.

81. Application, implementation, reduction in risk potential (b)

❶ This is the appropriate position for the patient undergoing a proctoscopic exam.

② This is not the preferred position for access to the rectum.

③ This will not provide access to the rectum for the procedure.

④ This is not the preferred position for a proctoscopic exam.

82. Comprehension, assessment, prevention and early detection of disease (b)

❹ Alcohol is an irritant that can predispose the patient who is abusing alcohol to cancer.

① Although smoking is a risk factor, it is more a risk for lung cancer.

②, ③ These are not usually risk factors.

83. Application, implementation, prevention/early detection of disease (b)
    ❹ Hypoglycemia can be countered with the ingestion of a rapid-acting sugar.
    ① Running is too strenuous an activity for an individual with diabetes mellitus.
    ② Meals should be spaced no farther than 4 hours apart.
    ③ Medication should be taken first thing in the morning.

84. Application, implementation, prevention/early detection of disease (b)
    ❷ These are the common symptoms of candidiasis.
    ① This is not common in candidiasis, but is common of some systemic infections.
    ③ This is common in genital warts.
    ④ Although a cause for concern, these are not symptoms associated with candidiasis.

85. Application, planning, reduction in risk potential (c)
    ❷ Stress and exertion can overtax the patient and increase the risk of an addisonian crisis.
    ① Although important, planning diversional activities does not take precedence here.
    ③ It is always important for the nurse to provide for a well-balanced diet, but reducing stress is the priority in this plan of care.
    ④ Activity must be planned and moderated for this patient.

86. Application, planning, pharmacological therapies (c)
    ❶ Addison's disease is a failure to produce the needed hormones by the adrenal cortex that help regulate electrolyte balance.
    ② Addison's disease does not affect the white blood cell count, and this goal would cause the patient to be unable to fight off infectious diseases.
    ③ As Addison's disease does not affect the bone marrow, this would not be a goal of therapy.
    ④ The red blood cell count is not affected in Addison's disease and this would not be a goal of therapy.

87. Application, implementation, basic care and comfort (b)
    ❷ Raising the head of the bed may relieve the dyspnea if it is paroxysmal nocturnal dyspnea.
    ① This is helpful but doesn't physically relieve the underlying cause.
    ③ This is not necessary based on information given. Also, suctioning may cause trauma to mucous membranes.
    ④ This intervention would not be appropriate. In addition, some pain medication may depress respirations.

88. Application, implementation, coping and adaptation (b)
    ❹ This may indicate bronchospasm and laryngospasms.
    ① Wheezing is not usual; it may indicate complications.
    ② Wheezing is abnormal; it is not a usual indication that anesthesia is wearing off.
    ③ Return of a gag reflex does not include wheezing.

89. Application, implementation, physiological adaptation (b)
    ❷ Splinting protects the fracture, immobilizes the arm and may prevent worsening of the situation.
    ① Use 911 only in true emergencies.
    ③ Warmth may actually cause an increase in edema and does not immobilize the fracture.
    ④ The extremity should be elevated to prevent edema formation.

90. Application, planning, basic care and comfort (b)
    ❸ If mucus is too thick for the patient to expectorate, aerosol treatments would help.
    ① This is appropriate but may not be as effective or act as quickly as #3.
    ② These actions would relieve the throat irritation but would not assist in making his cough productive.
    ④ This is inappropriate. The high humidity may make breathing more difficult.

91. Application, implementation, reduction of risk potential (b)
    ❹ Coughing when supine may be associated with left-sided heart failure.
    ① Decreased appetite may be caused by a variety of factors.
    ② Respirations should be documented, although easy, regular respirations are normal.
    ③ This may have a variety of causes.

92. Application, implementation, reduction in risk potential (b)
    ❸ This is the only true statement and validates the patient's knowledge deficit while providing information.
    ① The patient did not refuse anything; the patient requires more information.
    ② This may not be true, and it is never a good idea to tell patients what they should do. Provide information so that patients can make an informed choice.
    ④ This response is trite and does not address the problem. The nurse is being judgmental.

93. Knowledge, implementation, reduction of risk potential (a)
    ❹ This is the correct definition.
    ① This is the definition of a bronchoscopy.
    ② This is the definition of an MRI.
    ③ This is the definition of spirometry.

94. Comprehension, implementation, reduction of risk potential (c)
    ❸ It is necessary to assess for a pneumothorax.
    ① Absence of fluid is also possible to note with chest X-ray, but it is not the primary reason for performing one.
    ② This response is inappropriate and unethical relative to the physician.
    ④ This response is true but is stated in a way that would alarm the patient.

95. Application, implementation, reduction of risk potential (a)
    ❷ This is correct based on the use of the contrast medium (dye).
    ①, ③ These are not proper procedures; patient should be NPO.
    ④ This is not necessary; patient's activity has nothing to do with standard protocol for this test under normal circumstances.

96. Comprehension, assessment, reduction of risk potential (b)
    ❶ This is used to determine areas of lung being ventilated, but not perfused, because of an obstruction or clot in the pulmonary circulation.

② This is an inappropriate test for this medical diagnosis (acute myocardial infarction).

③ This is an inappropriate test for this medical diagnosis (pulmonary tumor).

④ This is the definition of a cardiac catheterization.

97. Knowledge, implementation, reduction of risk potential (a)
❹ This is the most common location; it is less likely to puncture the lung.
① This placement is more appropriate for a paracentesis.
②, ③ These indicate improper placements.

98. Application, implementation, basic care and comfort (b)
❷ When flow rate is more than 4L/min, humidification is necessary.
① This is not really responsive to patient's concern.
③ Although true, this response is incomplete in rationale.
④ Humidity does not increase safety factors when oxygen is in use; also, such a statement may be cause for patient concern.

99. Comprehension, planning, reduction in risk potential (b)
❸ Protein is converted to ammonia, and a buildup of ammonia affects brain tissue. Protein should be restricted if ammonia levels rise.
① Soapy enemas assist in the removal of feces but will not prevent hepatic coma from developing.
② Lavages will not prevent the buildup of ammonia levels.
④ Carbohydrates are most easily tolerated by a diseased liver.

100. Application, planning, pharmacological therapies (b)
❸ Regular insulin is fast acting and is used in the acute phase.
① Lente is an intermediate acting insulin that is not used in the acute phase of DKA.
② NPH is an intermediate acting insulin and may be used after the acute phase is passed.
④ This is an oral agent and is not used in the acute phase of DKA.

101. Knowledge, assessment, basic care and comfort (a)
❹ Glucose provides energy for fat and muscle cells.
① Glucose is not used to make protoplasm.
② Protein is used as a repair material.
③ Glucose is a sugar, not a protein.

102. Application, evaluation, prevention/early detection of disease (c)
❷ Infection can cause fluctuations to occur in blood sugar, usually in the form of elevations.
① Stressful situations may precipitate DKA, but an infection is more likely to cause it.
③ Excess insulin would cause hypoglycemia.
④ Insufficient calories in the diet would also cause hypoglycemia.

103. Application, assessment, prevention/early detection of disease (b)
❷ Both of these conditions create regurgitation of blood back through the mitral valve, causing murmurs.
① Angina is not a common assessment finding in valvular disease.
③ Syncope is not normally a finding in these types of valvular disease.

④ Hypertension may be an underlying condition, but it is not specifically associated with either of these diseases.

104. Application, assessment, basic care and comfort (b)
❹ In a patient on bed rest, dependent edema will pool in the sacrum, the lowest point of the patient when lying in bed.
① Because the feet are mostly elevated, edema will not occur in the feet.
② Edema is normally found in the hands of ambulatory patients.
③ Edema is not normally assessed in the knee region.

105. Comprehension, implementation, reduction of risk potential (b)
❸ The funduscopic exam is useful in examining the retina of the eye for changes that are suggestive of those accompanying hypertension.
① A vision screen merely tests visual acuity.
② A tonometer test evaluates pressure within the eye and is useful in monitoring glaucoma.
④ A visual fields exam evaluates peripheral vision and is useful in monitoring glaucoma and in evaluating neurological problems.

106. Application, planning, reduction of risk potential (a)
❸ The incontinence, perspiration, and weight put her at risk for a pressure ulcer.
① This is not appropriate; would also require assistance; shearing forces can cause breakdown.
② She could be positioned on her left side with appropriate support.
④ This is inappropriate and may predispose to complications.

107. Application, assessment, reduction of risk potential (b)
❷ In dark-skinned persons skin under pressure appears darker than surrounding skin and may even take on a purplish hue.
① This may mean she is able to bring up mucus on her own.
③ Complaints of feeling cool may be normal for the patient; age is unknown.
④ Patient may have secondary diagnosis of arthritis; age is unknown; remaining in bed in one position can also contribute to this type of complaint.

108. Application, planning, basic care and comfort (b)
❶ Wound healing is limited by poor protein, vitamin, and caloric intake.
② Exercise is an appropriate action, but not for this patient at this time.
③ An antidepressant order is inappropriate. Nothing indicates that the decreased appetite is caused by depression; nurses do not diagnose.
④ All patients should be given this opportunity; this is not the most appropriate response.

109. Application, implementation, reduction of risk potential (b)
❷ Keeping the head of the bed below 30 degrees will reduce shearing of the skin.
① A turning schedule that is adhered to will be more effective.
③ Incorrect information is being given.
④ This is inappropriately stated; also nerve endings may be compromised and pain may not be present.

110. Comprehension, assessment, pharmacological therapies (a)
- ❸ Eardrops should be warmed to body temperature (no more than 38° C). Vertigo may result from high or low temperatures.
- ① Although eardrops should be slowly instilled and allowed to flow into the canal, the rate most likely did not cause the vertigo.
- ② Occluded canal may cause vertigo. However, his vertigo occurred immediately following administration of the eardrops.
- ④ This is most unlikely, although possible if being given for the first time (not the best response).

111. Application, assessment, prevention/early detection of disease (b)
- ❹ These are common manifestations of hypertension in patients.
- ① Nausea and vomiting are not common symptoms of hypertension.
- ② Increased urination is not a common finding in patients with hypertension.
- ③ These are not common assessment findings for a patient with hypertension.

112. Comprehension, implementation, reduction of risk potential (a)
- ❷ Intermittent catheterization is a part of a bladder retraining program. The objective is to periodically empty the bladder to decrease infections and incontinence.
- ① This response is inappropriate; it doesn't answer the patient's concern.
- ③ This response is inappropriate. The patient may be incontinent between catheterizations.
- ④ This response is inappropriate; it is not a purpose of intermittent catheterization.

113. Knowledge, assessment, physiological adaptation (a)
- ❸ Changes indicating decreased vital capacity or respiratory distress are signs of oxygen toxicity.
- ① This is a sign of digoxin toxicity.
- ② This is a sign of glaucoma.
- ④ This is a sign of alkalosis or electrolyte imbalance.

114. Application, implementation, reduction of risk potential (a)
- ❶ At high end of normal range, failing kidneys cause abnormal buildup of electrolytes such as Na, Cl, K.
- ②, ③, ④ These are normal results.

115. Knowledge, assessment, reduction of risk potential (a)
- ❶ This is a sign of respiratory acidosis.
- ② This is a sign of respiratory alkalosis, metabolic alkalosis.
- ③ This is a sign of tissue hypoxia.
- ④ This is a sign of hypocalcemia.

116. Comprehension, implementation, physiological adaptation (b)
- ❹ The goal of oxygen therapy is to supply the myocardium with additional oxygen, thereby reducing the myocardial oxygen demand and enabling the heart to supply oxygen to the tissues of the body.
- ① Oxygen, in and of itself, will not prevent ventricular fibrillation.
- ② Hypoxia will increase the patient's anxiety and restlessness.
- ③ Oxygen will not prevent cardiogenic shock.

117. Application, implementation, reduction of risk potential (a)
- ❸ These are nonabsorbent, waterproof. Purpose is to protect the ulcer from contamination.
- ① These are absorbent. Purpose is to draw excessive drainage away from ulcer site.
- ② The purpose is to keep skin edges approximated.
- ④ The purpose is to debride or promote drainage.

118. Application, evaluation, reduction of risk potential (a)
- ❸ This may indicate overhydration.
- ① This is normal capillary refill time.
- ② This is normal skin turgor.
- ④ This is the normal color and odor of urine.

119. Application, planning, reduction of risk potential (b)
- ❹ Persons with pulmonary disease are at risk for acidosis, secondary to CO_2 retention.
- ① This does not warrant checking within the next hour.
- ②, ③ There is not enough data to support this assumption.

120. Application, assessment, reduction in risk potential (c)
- ❷ Changes in the circulatory status of the involved extremity indicate a complication.
- ① This is not serious and may be a reaction to the anesthetic.
- ③ This can be handled by the nurse, in most cases, and is not a serious complication of arthroplasty.
- ④ This may not be of any concern, the patient may not have any sputum to produce, and as long as the patient does incentive spirometry, and deep breathing exercises, pulmonary status should be maintained.

121. Application, planning, physiological adaptation (a)
- ❹ These are signs of hyponatremia.
- ① This would be inappropriate to monitor hourly.
- ② This may be appropriate for continued assessment of the patient.
- ③ This is inappropriate without communicating with RN or physician.

122. Application, implementation, basic care and comfort (b)
- ❹ This maintains cleanliness. Preventive skin care is important in maintaining the integrity of the skin and stoma.
- ① Massaging may injure the delicate stoma and is unnecessary unless ordered by the physician.
- ② Oils may be irritating to the skin and stoma; it promotes fungal infection.
- ③ The lotion will provide a medium for fungal growth and may irritate the stoma.

123. Knowledge, evaluation, pharmacological therapies (b)
- ❶ Ditropan acts by exerting a direct antispasmodic effect on smooth muscle such as the bladder.
- ② Cholinergic drugs are helpful with atonic bladder.
- ③ Propantheline bromide is used for complaints of urinary frequency and urgency.
- ④ Trimethoprim sulfamethoxazole is an antiinfective.

124. Application, implementation, reduction of risk potential (a)
- ❹ This ensures a continuous flow of urine in case specimens are needed. It removes bacteria that may be introduced during the procedure.
- ① Bowel prep is required if X-rays are taken. Enemas until clear may be unsafe depending on the number/amount administered.

② This is unnecessary for this procedure.

③ This is inappropriate; see #1 for correct response.

125. Comprehension, implementation, physiological adaptation (a)

❸ The catheter produces the sensation of fullness. Attempting to strain to pass urine around the catheter causes the bladder muscles to contract, resulting in a painful bladder spasm.

① This is not an independent nursing action and may add to patient discomfort.

② This is an unsafe practice and may cause fluid backflow and introduce bacteria into the bladder.

④ This is inappropriate; elevation of the scrotum will not decrease bladder spasms.

126. Comprehension, assessment, physiological adaptation (a)

❶ These are the early symptoms of prostatitis.

② This is related and may indicate a UTI. General.

③, ④ This is a routine part of any general health history.

127. Comprehension, implementation, pharmacological therapies (b)

❶ This keeps the eyes (cornea) from drying out.

② These dilate eyes; do not lubricate.

③ This does not lubricate eyes.

④ This increases risk of corneal abrasion and eye problems.

128. Application, implementation, pharmacological therapies (b)

❷ This drug potentiates muscle weakness because of effect on myoneural junction.

① This drug blocks the action of cholinesterase at the myoneural junction and allows acetylcholine to act. It is therapeutic.

③ Corticosteroids are sometimes used as an adjunct therapy. It is therapeutic.

④ Mestinon blocks the action of cholinesterase at the myoneural junction and allows acetylcholine to act. It is therapeutic.

129. Application, planning, basic care and comfort (b)

❹ This is an alkaline ash diet.

①, ②, ③ These are appropriate as an acid ash diet.

130. Application, implementation, physiological adaptation (a)

❸ The patient is displaying signs of hypovolemia. Initial measures would be those for shock. Turning on side helps prevent aspiration.

① It is important to monitor vital signs; application of a cool cloth is a later measure.

② Sips of water are inappropriate if patient is going into shock.

④ Decreasing the room temperature is not relative to situation; turning on side helps to prevent aspiration.

131. Application, assessment, basic care and comfort (b)

❷ Abduction moves a body part away from the midline.

① Flexion increases an angle at a joint.

③ Adduction is moving a body part toward the midline.

④ Pronation rotates a part to face downward.

132. Application, planning, basic care and comfort (b)

❸ The ventrogluteal is a deep muscle located in the upper, outer quadrant of the hip. It has few superficial blood vessels and makes a good injection site for someone who has muscle atrophy.

① The deltoid is not a good choice because of the patient's muscle atrophy.

② Intramuscular injections are not given in the abdomen.

④ The gluteus maximus is not a good choice because of the muscle atrophy.

133. Application, assessment, reduction in risk potential (b)

❶ An overproduction of cortisol from the adrenal medulla is associated with Cushing's syndrome.

② Overproduction of this hormone leads to acromegaly or gigantism.

③ Elevation of these levels indicates hyperthyroidism.

④ Elevation in epinephrine levels does not indicate Cushing's syndrome.

134. Application, implementation, basic care and comfort (b)

❹ Additional stress placed on the tissues by movement may disrupt the healing tissue. Splinting lessens the chance for this to occur.

① This is true, but the question is specific to ambulation.

② This is too sweeping of a statement. Although there is more pain involved from movement with an abdominal incision, not all patients are hesitant to do so.

③ The binder would be a good choice for the patient if it was applied correctly.

135. Application, implementation, coping and adaptation (b)

❹ This is an open-ended question that seeks to explore the patient's feelings. It is always best to allow the patient to express his or her views.

① This does not address the patient's fears.

② This is defensive and will not help the patient cope.

③ This statement appears to be patronizing. It is best to ascertain what the patient's questions are first.

136. Comprehension, assessment, physiological adaptation (a)

❸ These are low blood sugar (hypoglycemic) symptoms.

①, ② These are not associated with hypoglycemia.

④ These are symptoms of ketoacidosis.

137. Knowledge, assessment, basic care and comfort (b)

❸ This blood type has no A or B antigens and can donate blood to individuals who are type A, B, or O, provided the Rh factor is also compatible.

① Patients with blood type A can receive blood from individuals with A or O blood, if the Rh factors are compatible.

② Patients with Type B blood can receive blood from donors who are type O or B, if the Rh factor is compatible.

④ Patients with Type AB blood must receive blood that is Type AB or O.

138. Application, implementation, physiological adaptation (b)

❹ Because of the neuropathy that can occur in patients with diabetes, they are more sensitive to the cold and could get frostbite more easily.

① This is an abrasion, and if cared for properly should not become infected.

② There are not substantial data given to warrant the need for an X-ray at this time.

③ Rebound swelling should not occur if the time of the cold application is no longer than 20 to 30 minutes.

139. Application, implementation, basic care and comfort (b)
    ❹ This is the most appropriate and least intrusive. Visiting allows the nurse to assess the patient, provides the patient with distraction, and promotes her self-esteem. Repositioning would relieve strain.
    ①, ③ These are inappropriate. The older adult has a greater sensitivity to heat. CVA victims who have some neurosensory impairment may not be able to determine when complications of heat/cold applications occur.
    ② Giving this medication the way the order is written would violate the principles of medication administration.

140. Comprehension, evaluation, physiological adaptation (b)
    ❷ Severe or increased pain in a wound may indicate that an infection or hematoma may be developing.
    ① This is not likely after 6 days.
    ③ This is unlikely; a 4 × 4 is not used as a compression or pressure dressing.
    ④ Inspection of site is necessary; however, a soiled dressing is not always associated with pain.

141. Application, implementation, reduction of risk potential (b)
    ❸ Skin of older adults is fragile and may not tolerate adhesive tape. Frequent tape applications should be avoided.
    ① Although this is true, #3 explains the physiological rationale for use of Montgomery straps, which is given priority over cost.
    ② This is an inappropriate response; increase in infection would not be caused by the method used to secure the dressing.
    ④ The frequency of dressing changes is based on physician orders and/or the amount of drainage. The straps secure the dressing in place.

142. Application, implementation, basic care and comfort (a)
    ❹ This provides countertraction and will minimize trauma of tissues. This should decrease patient discomfort.
    ① This should be done; however, this was not the principle asked for.
    ② Soaking is not necessary. Moistening may be indicated if the dressing adheres to the site or resistance is felt during removal.
    ③ Clean gloves are appropriate for removing dressing. Bringing the edges toward her would expose any drainage present.

143. Knowledge, assessment, reduction of risk potential (a)
    ❷ This is true. In dark-skinned persons, pressure areas appear darker. With blanching, these areas appear gray.
    ① This is descriptive in light-skinned persons.
    ③ This is a sign of pressure, not blanching.
    ④ This may be a sign of pressure.

144. Application, assessment, physiological adaptation (a)
    ❷ All are signs of hyperkalemia.
    ① These are vague, generalized signs and symptoms.
    ③ These are signs of fluid imbalance.
    ④ These are signs of fluid deficit.

145. Application, assessment, reduction in risk potential (b)
    ❶ Rapid administration of blood containing citrate predisposes the patient to hypocalcemia.

② There is no indication that the patient has an existing seizure disorder, and receiving chemotherapy or blood should not cause a patient to have a seizure.
    ③ A carpopedal spasm is unrelated to metastatic carcinoma.
    ④ Adverse signs of chemotherapy include nausea, vomiting, hair loss, and myelosuppression.

146. Comprehension, implementation, pharmacological therapies (a)
    ❷ The feedings do contain water, protein, carbohydrates, fats, electrolytes, vitamins, and trace elements. The subclavian vein or another large vein is used because of the high osmolarity of the nutrients.
    ① Septicemia is a possible complication.
    ③ Nutrients enter the circulatory system.
    ④ This response is inappropriate. Persons may take food orally while receiving TPN.

147. Application, planning, reduction in risk potential (c)
    ❶ The nurse should expect to record the amount of drainage removed (usually 1000 to 1500 cc) and the color and consistency of the fluid.
    ② High-Fowler's is the recommended position.
    ③ A sterile, pressure dressing is applied to prevent leakage.
    ④ The puncture site is prepared aseptically, usually by the physician.

148. Application, assessment, physiological adaptation (c)
    ❷ Damaged parenchymal cells are unable to metabolize bilirubin, which give the stool its normal color; bilirubin in the circulation causes jaundice, pruritus, and dark urine.
    ① Stools are clay colored because of the liver's inability to metabolize bilirubin.
    ③ Clay-colored stools are common in advanced liver disease, urine is dark in color.
    ④ Urine is not blood-tinged, but dark in color with liver dysfunction.

149. Application, implementation, reduction of risk potential (a)
    ❸ This is the appropriate setting for adults.
    ① This is the appropriate setting for infants.
    ② This is the appropriate setting for children.
    ④ This is inappropriate, unsafe; too much pressure is exerted on mucous membranes.

150. Application, implementation, reduction of risk potential (c)
    ❶ Encourages use of the arm and shoulder on the affected side. Movement of the affected side may increase confidence and decrease apprehension. It encourages joint mobility.
    ② This is inappropriate; it discourages normal ADLs and ROM and may increase apprehension.
    ③ This is inappropriate; a Vaseline occlusive dressing should be in place.
    ④ Raising side rails may make him feel more secure or may be a type of restraint.

151. Application, evaluation, reduction of risk potential (a)
    ❸ This would stop the tidaling.
    ① A complete assessment of the patient and the equipment should be performed first.
    ② This is inappropriate; it would not help pinpoint the reason tidaling has ceased.

④ This is inappropriate to do at insertion site. A Vaseline occlusive dressing is at this location. Reinforcing all connecting sites may be helpful if a leak was present.

152. Knowledge, planning, safety and infection control (a)
❶ This maintains healthy oral mucous membranes and decreases the risk of organisms infecting the nasopharynx.
② This may be unrealistic.
③ The increased cost of using disposables is a factor. Proper disposal of used Kleenex would need to be taught.
④ This results in increased cost to patient. It is not proven to be effective and may be a dangerous practice.

153. Application, evaluation, reduction of risk potential (a)
❹ This would indicate that secretions have not accumulated.
① This would indicate an infection and/or dehydration.
② This is inappropriate for this nursing diagnosis.
③ This would give the opportunity to assess the effort of breathing.

154. Knowledge, evaluation, basic care and comfort (a)
❶ Low-Fowler's position provides for better drainage of secretions.
② High-Fowler's position causes more postnasal drip. It is not as comfortable because of frequent swallowing.
③, ④ Secretions may pool. Patent airway may be occluded by this position.

155. Comprehension, planning, basic care and comfort (a)
❹ This would help liquefy secretions.
① Monitoring would give one factor of the patients' hydration status.
② This does not relate to the nursing diagnosis.
③ Humidity would be too high, adding to the effort of breathing. Sometimes increasing room humidity can aid in liquefying mucus that is thick and difficult to expectorate.

156. Application, planning, reduction of risk potential (a)
❹ Placement below her chest allows gravity drainage and prevents fluid backup.
① This is inappropriate; it may interfere with gravity drainage or cause fluid backup, depending on the height of the bed frame.
② This is inappropriate and is unsafe at this level.
③ The towel would not add to or maintain a patent safe drainage system.

157. Comprehension, implementation, physiological adaptation (a)
❸ Persons with pharyngitis caused by streptococci may develop the complication of scarlet fever.
① This is inappropriate. Nothing is ordered until the proper testing is completed. Reporting is necessary to obtain proper testing.
② Penicillin or antibiotics are the treatment of choice for streptococcal pharyngitis. Antibiotics should not be started until the specimen for C&S has been obtained.
④ This is unusual, unless the rash is infected because of scratching.

158. Application, implementation, reduction of risk potential (a)
❷ Lifting heavier items puts unnecessary stress on the healing site.
① The patient may sit on these chairs. He or she should scoot to edge of seat and push up, using legs and arms together to rise up.
③ The patient may shower/bathe. The site may be covered with a piece of plastic wrap.
④ This is an unnecessary restriction.

159. Knowledge, planning, basic care and comfort (b)
❷ Cool temperatures cause vasoconstriction, and a comfortable room humidity prevents skin dryness.
① This would decrease the likelihood of skin excoriation.
③ True that pruritus may be a result of a drug reaction; however, this would not immediately add to the patient's comfort.
④ Administering medications that may not be needed is inappropriate.

160. Comprehension, assessment, physiological adaptation (b)
❶ Because of damage to the nerve, the nurse would expect hoarseness of the voice.
② This may indicate pulmonary edema.
③ This may indicate hemorrhage.
④ This sign indicates tetany and hypocalcemia.

161. Application, assessment, physiological adaptation (b)
❹ Hypocalcemia, which causes tetany, results when the parathyroid glands are removed. The patient will experience facial twitching and carpopedal spasms.
① These are not indicative of tetany.
② These symptoms may signal renal problems.
③ These may be signs of a neurological problem.

162. Application, planning, coping and adaptation (b)
❶ A calm environment is important; these patients are usually in a hyperactive state.
② Visitors may need to be limited to avoid overtaxing the patient's energies.
③ A supportive environment is necessary, but do not overstimulate the patient.
④ A private room ensures better control over the environment.

163. Application, assessment, basic care and comfort (b)
❸ The chest X-ray can reveal an enlarged heart and help augment other diagnostic testing to confirm the diagnosis of heart failure.
① The nurse can give a simple explanation of the test without the physician explaining.
② The nurse is not answering the patient's question; the nurse is capable of giving a short explanation of the test.
④ A chest X-ray does not outline vessels in a way that would confirm the degree or extent of any heart damage. A coronary angiography could do this.

164. Application, assessment, prevention/early detection of disease (b)
❹ Muscle weakness and personality changes herald the possibility of neurological problems.
① Chest pain on exertion is a symptom of angina; this patient does not exhibit this.
② The patient may have no symptoms at all, or symptoms of fatigue and headache.
③ The presenting symptoms indicate a potential neurological complication, not a cardiac one.

165. Comprehension, assessment, reduction in risk potential (b)
- ❸ Following this procedure there may be a loss of sufficient intrinsic factor.
- ① Diabetes mellitus is a pancreatic problem resulting from insufficient amounts of insulin.
- ② Reflux refers to the backward flow of gastric contents through an incompetent sphincter, allowing juices to flow into the esophagus. This is not a complication of a gastrectomy.
- ④ *H. pylori* may be found in the gastric mucosa and may cause peptic ulcers. The incidence of *H. pylori* does not increase after a gastrectomy.

166. Comprehension, planning, prevention/early detection of disease (b)
- ❶ Protection of the blood supply is a sound measure to prevent the transmission of hepatitis B, C and HIV.
- ② One cannot get a blood-borne disease by donating blood.
- ③ This may reduce the risk of ingestion of some pathogens, but not the hepatitis B virus.
- ④ Shellfish are associated with contraction of hepatitis A.

167. Application, planning, physiological adaptation (b)
- ❷ Contact sports that could result in blunt blows to the abdomen should be discouraged.
- ① This noncontact sport poses a reduced risk of injury.
- ③ Although strenuous, this sport poses little risk of injury to the patient's stoma.
- ④ If the patient feels comfortable swimming with an ileostomy, it should not be discouraged.

168. Application, assessment, prevention/early detection of disease (b)
- ❹ These are common assessment findings in peritonitis.
- ① This symptom is common in several conditions, but not peritonitis.
- ② Reduced urine output may occur as a late symptom if the infection is not controlled.
- ③ Frequent stool or diarrhea is not a common assessment finding.

169. Application, planning, prevention/early detection of disease (b)
- ❷ Increased urination, increased thirst, and increased hunger are the cardinal symptoms of diabetes mellitus.
- ① These are symptoms of hypoglycemia.
- ③ These are not the cardinal symptoms of diabetes mellitus but are indicative of hypertension.
- ④ These symptoms are not indicative of diabetes mellitus.

170. Application, planning, physiological adaptation (c)
- ❹ The tube is a triple-lumen tube with an esophageal balloon to control bleeding of varices. One lumen is for lavage and another is used for suction.
- ① Platelets do not need to be replaced. Refrigerated blood lacks prothrombin and coagulation factors needed for clotting.
- ② Iced saline solution is used. Gastric lavage would wash out the stomach, not control bleeding in the esophagus.
- ③ Vasodilators will not control bleeding. Antibiotics and antacids may be used after the acute phase.

171. Application, planning, prevention/early detection of disease (b)
- ❷ Intact skin is the body's first line of defense. Infections that will be difficult to heal will develop if the skin is not intact.
- ① Soap will further compound the dryness associated with stasis dermatitis, but the nurse's main goal is to keep the skin intact.
- ③ Medications are not the treatment of choice for this condition, because it is caused by decreased circulation.
- ④ Ointments/medications are not the treatment of choice; the nurse's main goal to maintain the skin's integrity.

172. Application, implementation, basic care and comfort (b)
- ❶ This may cause infection. The area is usually kept dry.
- ② Activity does not need to be restricted.
- ③ This is appropriate treatment; it maintains patient comfort.
- ④ This is appropriate treatment; it allows more air circulation.

173. Application, planning, safety and infection control (a)
- ❷ Clean technique may be used for allergic reaction.
- ① Sterile technique required if an infection or ulceration is present.
- ③ This is inappropriate. No pressure should be exerted on the eyeball.
- ④ No solution should ever be warmed in a microwave. It is unpredictable. Temperature of compresses should not exceed 49° C (120° F).

174. Knowledge, planning, safety and infection control (a)
- ❷ Gloves should be worn.
- ① Eye pads are contraindicated in general eye infections because they enhance bacterial growth.
- ③ Ointment should be placed in the conjunctiva.
- ④ All patients should have their own tubes of ointment to prevent cross-infection.

175. Knowledge, planning, reduction of risk potential (a)
- ❶ This position prevents pressure on the suture line of the operated eye.
- ② Restricting fluids is inappropriate.
- ③ The patient should avoid showers and shampooing, because soap may irritate the eye.
- ④ TV is okay. Reading is to be avoided. Back-and-forth eye motion may loosen stitches.

176. Comprehension, planning, pharmacological therapies (a)
- ❷ This is the physiological action of the pharmacologic therapy.
- ① This is true of any medication.
- ③ This is true, but it is not the appropriate rationale.
- ④ This may occur after multiple consecutive missed doses.

177. Comprehension, implementation, physiological adaptation (a)
- ❹ This is the only true statement.
- ① This is not directly related to glaucoma.
- ② Blindness is not always a result if glaucoma is diagnosed and treated.
- ③ This is not directly related to glaucoma.

178. Comprehension, implementation, physiological adaptation (b)
- ❶ This is true.

② Bright lights are usually not harmful.
③ Darkness is not necessary.
④ This is not based on a physiological reason.

179. Knowledge, implementation, basic care and comfort (b)
  ① This is a safety precaution.
  ② This may be given if nausea and/or vomiting were present.
  ③ Bed rest is only for the preoperative period and 3 to 5 days postoperatively.
  ④ Retinal detachment produces anxiety and fear but usually not pain.

180. Application, implementation, reduction of risk potential (b)
  ❶ This prevents excessive pressure.
  ② Excessive pressure from nose blowing can force infected secretions up the eustachian tube into the middle ear.
  ③ Keeping mouth open is not necessary. The patient should blow with the nostrils open.
  ④ Excessive pressure from nose blowing can force infected secretions up the eustachian tube into the middle ear.

181. Application, implementation, pharmacological therapies (b)
  ❹ Some diuretics such as Lasix are ototoxic and can cause tinnitus and dizziness.
  ① This is most unlikely; the tinnitus should not affect her ability to drive.
  ② This would not alleviate the patient's concern and is an untrue statement.
  ③ The tinnitus is caused by the ototoxicity of the diuretic.

182. Application, planning, basic care and comfort (b)
  ❹ This is a comfort measure to reduce irritation and promote healing.
  ① Sitz baths are more soothing to the rectum.
  ② Occlusive dressings are not normally used; rectal packing and loose dressings to collect drainage may be used.
  ③ Gas formation is not a common problem with this procedure.

183. Application, assessment, prevention/early detection of disease (b)
  ❹ The involved leg may be shorter because of the pull of the muscles nearest the fracture site, and the leg rotates outward.
  ① Pronation is a term associated with the upper extremities; the leg will be externally rotated.
  ② Supination is a term associated with the upper extremities; the leg will be externally rotated.
  ③ The affected leg is normally shorter than the other and is externally rotated.

184. Comprehension, planning, prevention/early detection of disease (b)
  ❸ An overproduction of cortisone is associated with the development of increased blood sugar, or hyperglycemia.
  ① Hypokalemia may occur as a result of the Cushing's syndrome.
  ② Hypocalcemia is not associated with Cushing's syndrome.

④ An underproduction of insulin is associated with pancreatic dysfunction.

185. Comprehension, assessment, prevention/early detection of disease (b)
  ❷ Hypovolemia may affect kidney perfusion, and it would be prudent of the nurse to monitor the intake and output for the patient.
  ① Pedal pulses can be affected by conditions other than hypovolemia and is not of primary importance in this assessment.
  ③ Although important in any assessment, it is not significant for a patient in hypovolemia.
  ④ As the patient is normally dehydrated, jugular vein distention will not occur.

186. Comprehension, assessment, reduction in risk potential (b)
  ❸ Chemotherapy can cause bone marrow depression. A lowering of the white blood cell count can place the patient at risk for infections.
  ① Thalassemia is not associated with lymphoma treated by chemotherapy.
  ② The CBC can not directly indicate a disease in remission.
  ④ Platelet counts usually decrease rather than increase with chemotherapy.

187. Comprehension, planning, basic care and comfort (b)
  ❹ Diet should supply calories, protein, and carbohydrates to compensate for the increased metabolic demands imposed by the disease.
  ① Restriction of purine is not necessary and there is not enough calories in this diet.
  ② This would provide insufficient calories; it will not meet the metabolic demands of the body.
  ③ Restricting sodium is not necessary.

188. Application, assessment, prevention/early detection of disease (b)
  ❷ These are the classic symptoms of hyperthyroidism.
  ① These symptoms are typical of hypothyroidism.
  ③ These are not indicative of thyroid disease.
  ④ These symptoms are caused by a slowed metabolic rate and are seen in hypothyroidism.

189. Application, planning, basic care and comfort (b)
  ❶ Many diuretics cause excretion of both sodium and potassium; it is important to maintain adequate potassium levels for proper heart function.
  ② This may potentiate a fluid retention problem.
  ③ These foods would not be restricted because the patient is on a diuretic.
  ④ Caffeine is a natural diuretic and is not normally restricted in patients taking diuretics.

190. Comprehension, planning, pharmacological therapies (b)
  ❹ This medication is a diuretic intended to promote fluid loss in an effort to decrease blood pressure in some patients.
  ① This is a cardiotonic and is normally given to individuals who have heart failure, arrhythmias, or atrial fibrillation.
  ② This is an antiinflammatory.
  ③ This is a histamine blocker that suppresses gastric acid secretion.

191. Application, implementation, safety and infection control (a)
   ❷ This maintains an intact drainage system. It is less likely that urine specimen will become contaminated.
   ① This disrupts the patency of the system and increases likelihood of contamination and a urinary tract infection.
   ③ Urine collecting in the drainage bag is likely to have organisms present, thereby giving inaccurate test results.
   ④ These are unnecessary actions and increase risk to patient of acquiring trauma and/or infection.

192. Comprehension, implementation, coping and adaptation (a)
   ❸ This is an emotional change that is common after a CVA. Emotional lability may or may not be appropriate to the situation.
   ① This is common but normal.
   ② This is inappropriate and encourages negative behavior modification technique. The patient has emotional lability.
   ④ This is inappropriate. The patient is not acting this way on purpose.

193. Application, implementation, reduction of risk potential (a)
   ❷ Communication takes longer when speech is impaired.
   ① This is inappropriate and may be a safety hazard.
   ③ Gestures may be appropriate and supplement the intended message. It would be inappropriate if patient is hallucinating or misinterprets.
   ④ This is inappropriate and may add to miscommunication.

194. Comprehension, assessment, reduction of risk potential (a)
   ❹ Dysphagia means difficulty swallowing. He may need to double-swallow between bites.
   ① This is an inappropriate, unnecessary restriction.
   ② This is not necessary. There is no indication that patient is hearing impaired.
   ③ This is a good practice for any person who has had a CVA. However, it is not specific to this question.

195. Comprehension, implementation, basic care and comfort (a)
   ❷ Lubrication would allow easier insertion.
   ① This is a sterile technique, but not the underlying principle.
   ③ This is a result. It is not the underlying principle.
   ④ This may be a result, but it is not the underlying principle.

196. Comprehension, implementation, reduction of risk potential (a)
   ❸ This is true. It also allows rest for the patient and minimizes tissue trauma.
   ① This is an inappropriate principle; action will not maintain patency unless done continuously.
   ② This is an inappropriate principle; action will not prevent contamination of the catheter.
   ④ This is an inappropriate principle; action will not prevent improper tube placement.

197. Knowledge, planning, physiological adaptation (a)
   ❶ This is true. Weakened pelvic muscles may also be a cause.

② This is an inappropriate assumption; this is called "residual" and is not usually a factor in stress inconvenience.
③ This is an inappropriate assumption; muscles and nerves are usually involved, not nerves alone.
④ This is an inappropriate assumption; this may be true but other symptoms would be evident, such as back pain.

198. Comprehension, evaluation, basic care and comfort (a)
   ❹ This question seeks more data and demonstrates attentive listening. Beets, blackberries, rhubarb, and some medications may turn the urine red or orange.
   ① Milk increase is not necessary. Liquids should normally be around 2000 cc/day. This response gives a quick fix.
   ② This response gives false reassurance. This is belittling the patient's concern.
   ③ This response does show the nurse is listening. The nurse is seeking more data. However, response #4 is individualized and therefore a better choice.

199. Comprehension, knowledge, physiological adaptation (a)
   ❷ Injuries above C5 cause quadriplegia.
   ① Emotions remain intact. However, grief and mourning reactions and depression frequently occur.
   ③ Desire remains. However, it may be affected by emotional reactions to the trauma and its effects.
   ④ Speaking ability remains intact.

200. Comprehension, assessment, physiological adaptation (b)
   ❹ These are early signs reflecting heart's attempt to compensate through tachycardia. Yawning is the body's way to take deep breaths to increase oxygen to brain.
   ① These are signs of prolonged or severe oxygen deprivation.
   ② Wheezing usually is not present. Bradycardia and confusion are later signs.
   ③ All are later signs of severe hypoxemia.

201. Comprehension, evaluation, pharmacological therapies (b)
   ❸ Nitroglycerin have a vasodilating effect and are often the cause of headaches, at least in the initial period of therapy.
   ① Tylenol normally alleviates headache discomfort.
   ② Lanoxin is a cardiotonic and does not normally cause headache.
   ④ Potassium chloride is used to counter the side effect of hypokalemia and does not cause headaches.

202. Application, implementation, reduction in risk potential (b)
   ❸ The Holter monitor will record a tracing of the heart during various activities and is compared with activities that the patient is documenting as well.
   ① A glucometer evaluates capillary blood sugar levels.
   ② Urines are used to evaluate various conditions, but not heart activity during exertion.
   ④ This study evaluates blood flow through a carotid artery or extremity.

203. Comprehension, assessment, prevention/early detection of disease (a)
   ❹ Genetic factors that predispose a person to hypertension cannot be controlled by the patient.
   ① Obesity can be controlled by diet and exercise program.

② Smoking can be controlled by smoking cessation.

③ Individuals can choose to start an exercise program.

204. Application, assessment, prevention/early detection of disease (b)

❸ These are the classic symptoms of thrombophlebitis. Additional assessment data may include red streaking along the vein path.

① These are symptoms of a neurological impairment.

② These symptoms may indicate an arterial problem.

④ An arterial occlusion may cause these symptoms.

205. Application, assessment, physiological adaptation (b)

❸ As the heart fails, circulating blood backs up into the pulmonary tree; a sign of congestion is crackles in the lung bases.

① Although fluid does build up in pneumonia, given the patient's history, the crackles most likely signify the beginning of heart failure.

② Dysrhythmias are not assessed by listening to lung sound. A heart monitor, change in vital signs, or patient symptoms will alert the nurse to this complication.

④ This does not normally manifest itself as crackles in the lungs, increased complaints of chest pain or changes in vital signs would alert the nurse to an extension of the MI.

206. Application, implementation, reduction of risk potential (a)

❶ The nurse should stand on the affected side and support with gait belt. The gait belt provides stability and provides greater control in assisting patient without putting undue pressure on patient's body and/or nurse.

② This is inappropriate and does not provide patient with a base of support.

③ This is not a safe practice; the patient may hesitate or tip backward.

④ This is inappropriate. A patient with right-sided weakness requires the nurse to stand on the right side. Reaching over to hold the patient's right hand may change patient's center of gravity and tip her forward. In addition, these are awkward body mechanics for the nurse.

207. Comprehension, planning, psychosocial adaptation (a)

❹ The patient's anxiety and concerns need to be addressed first. This allows her to express any fears and questions. Teaching will be heard once patient's concerns are answered.

① The nurse does not know if this is true. This is an assumption.

② This may be true. However, it is an assumption until patient is given an opportunity to express her concerns.

③ This is an inappropriate assumption.

208. Comprehension, planning, basic care and comfort (b)

❶ Safety should come first. In this patient's case, use Maslow's hierarchy of needs.

② Safety should be first priority.

③ Answer #1 is a better choice. The situation did not indicate pain was present. Assessment of respiratory function would be more appropriate and more individualized.

④ Safety should be first priority.

209. Knowledge, assessment, pharmacological therapies (a)

❸ Toxic levels (lab value of theophylline 20 μg/ml) are accompanied by these signs. The patient may also have palpitations or develop seizures.

①, ②, ④ These are not typical side effects of theophylline/bronchodilators.

210. Knowledge, assessment, physiological adaptation (a)

❸ Characteristic barrel-shaped chest, loss of elasticity, and narrowed bronchioles increase work effort to move air. The patient compensates by using accessory muscles.

① Coughs with copious amount of mucopurulent sputum are characteristic.

② Elevated body temperature is not common.

④ This is not usually present.

211. Application, evaluation, reduction of risk potential (b)

❹ Hearing aids should not be worn during an ear infection. Leaving the hearing aid out allows for drainage and observation of the site and prevents complications.

① This would only distort the sound more. It is unsafe.

② This may damage the ear mold.

③ Hearing aids should not be worn during an ear infection.

212. Knowledge, implementation, basic care and comfort (a)

❷ The patient should receive 1000 cc/12 hr, or 83.383 cc/hr.

①, ③, ④ These are incorrect math calculations.

213. Comprehension, evaluation, physiological adaptation (b)

❶ Persons with a pulmonary embolism experience pain related to ischemia caused by obstruction of small pulmonary arterial branches, process in lung, described as pleuritic chest pain.

② This relates to activity intolerance or interest in doing own self-care. It may be an indication of lessened anxiety.

③ Appetite, weight, nutritional status are not usual problems for patients with a pulmonary embolism.

④ This is related to an ineffective airway clearance problem.

214. Comprehension, evaluation, basic care and comfort (a)

❸ Being able to do own ADLs indicates activity tolerance is increased.

① Anxiety is most likely related to being unable to breathe.

② This is related to a knowledge deficit diagnosis.

④ This is related to the physiological effects.

215. Comprehension, assessment, reduction of risk potential (b)

❷ This is the correct description.

① This describes Level II = Generalized response.

③ This describes Level VI = Confused-appropriate.

④ This describes Level IV = Confused-agitated.

216. Application, assessment, pharmacological therapies (b)

❷ Bleeding is a serious side effect of anticoagulant therapy. Nursing measures focus on monitoring for signs of active bleeding.

① This is a common side effect of any medication. Hematemesis would be of serious concern.

③ This is not a common side effect of this class of medications and is not suggestive of bleeding.

④ This is a common side effect of many medications.

217. Comprehension, assessment, prevention/early detection of disease (b)
❶ Neck pain, decreased neck mobility caused by pain, and upper extremity motor/sensory changes are common symptoms.
② This may be a symptom of lumbar involvement.
③ This may also be a symptom of lumbar involvement.
④ Muscle atrophy of this group is not a finding when the cervical region is involved.

218. Application, planning, physiological adaptation (b)
❻ This reduces risk of constipation and straining, which may put a strain on damaged myocardium.
① This is not a standard of care for a patient having an MI.
② Prolonged bed rest is no longer advocated for patients with myocardial infarction.
③ This is no longer a standard of care.

219. Comprehension, assessment, prevention/early detection of disease (b)
❷ These are the classic signs of cardiogenic shock.
① Fever and bounding pulse are not normally seen in patients with cardiogenic shock.
③ High blood pressure is not a normal symptom in cardiogenic shock.
④ Hot, dry, skin is not normally seen in patients with cardiogenic shock.

220. Comprehension, planning, safety and infection control (a)
❷ OSHA (Occupational Safety and Health Administration) says that unprotected exposure to noise levels of 90 dB (decibels) over an 8-hour day is considered excessive and must be avoided. Ear plugs/protectors can reduce noise reaching the middle ear by 10 dB to 30 dB.
① Does not address the need to reduce the number of decibels of the original noise.
③ This is a possible action. However, it may be unrealistic for all patients to move.
④ This is inappropriate. It does not decrease number of decibels reaching the middle ear.

221. Application, assessment, reduction in risk potential (b)
❸ Diaphoresis is one of the first symptoms of hypoglycemia. Hypoglycemia would result when taking insulin without eating, or from a sudden increase in activity, or body demands such as illness, surgery, or stress.
① Polydipsia is a symptom of hyperglycemia.
② This is a late sign of both hyperglycemia and hypoglycemia. The nurse needs to assess for early signs in order to intervene.
④ This is a symptom of hyperglycemia.

222. Comprehension, evaluation, physiological adaptation (b)
❷ This indicates that sputum has been expectorated from the lungs.
① This relates to decreased appetite and altered nutrition.
③ This demonstrates effectiveness of therapy.
④ This relates to a knowledge deficit nursing diagnosis.

223. Application, implementation, reduction of risk potential (a)
❶ To prevent falling and to decrease vertigo sensation, person has to be still and avoid all head movements that aggravate the spinning sensation.

② This would be appropriate only if a PRN had been ordered.
③ Normal hydration is 2000 cc/day. At times a diuretic may be prescribed to help decrease fluid volume of endolymph.
④ This may increase sensation of vertigo. Bright, glaring lights should be avoided.

224. Comprehension, planning, physiological adaptation (a)
❽ Presbycusis is the term used to describe hearing loss associated with aging.
① This is inappropriate; hearing loss does not usually affect physical comfort.
② This is possible if unaware of environmental sounds. However, it is not a common cause.
③ This is inappropriate; hearing loss does not usually affect family roles.

225. Comprehension, evaluation, physiological adaptation (b)
❸ Widening pulse pressure is a sign of increased ICP.
①, ②, ④ These are not signs of widening pulse pressure.

226. Knowledge, planning, basic care and comfort (b)
❶ Chewing and daily ear hygiene aid in the removal of cerumen.
② This may be necessary. However, subjects patient to a procedure that could be prevented through health-promoting habits.
③ This allows for hydration, but it is not directly related to cerumen buildup.
④ This may damage the hearing aid.

227. Comprehension, assessment, reduction of risk potential (a)
❷ Some patients experience a spinal headache after removal of CSF.
① Capillary refill would assess oxygenation of tissues. It should not be directly related to this procedure.
③ This is inappropriate. Bladder control is affected by many factors and should not be directly affected by this practice.
④ This is inappropriate. Blood pressure is affected by many factors and should not be directly affected by this procedure.

228. Knowledge, evaluation, prevention/early detection of disease (a)
❶ This allows for maximum straightening of the auditory canal.
②, ③, ④ This may occlude auditory canal.

229. Application, assessment, prevention/early detection of disease (a)
❶ This may indicate a problem in inner ear.
② It is important to frequently watch others' faces to lip-read.
③ This may be true if position changes were to lean forward to hear better.
④ This behavior may result from a variety of factors that are not hearing related.

230. Application, implementation, reduction of risk potential (a)
❸ Airway, breathing, and circulation are the first priority. Rapid respirations that are shallow and irregular need immediate action.
① The nurse needs to know patient's previous temperature.

② This may indicate many things. The nurse needs further data. It is not a priority.

④ This may indicate therapy is effective. The nurse needs further data. It is not a priority.

231. Application, assessment, physiological adaptation (b)
❷ Angulation, deformities, shortening of a limb are suggestive of a break in bone continuity.
① Edema is present with both sprains and fractures.
③ Both types of injuries may evidence tenderness.
④ Contused soft tissue structures are tender, thus limiting mobility as well.

232. Application, planning, reduction of risk potential (b)
❹ Traction is commonly used to reduce femoral fractures.
① Buck's traction is not used to treat neck sprains.
② Patients with spinal fractures are normally placed on Stryker frames.
③ Shoulder dislocations are treated with immobilization devices.

233. Application, assessment, reduction in risk potential (b)
❸ Russell's traction uses a sling that may slide up under the knee and cause pressure, compromising circulation.
① There is no cast in this type of traction.
② Compartment syndrome normally develops in cast situations, where there is an encircling, or constricting device.
④ A boot device is not common in this type of traction.

234. Application, planning, physiological adaptation (b)
❶ Delayed wound healing is common in the elderly because of nutritional problems.
② This intervention is appropriate regardless of the patient's age.
③ This is an appropriate intervention no matter what the patient's age.
④ Inspection of the dressings is appropriate no matter what the patient's age.

235. Application, planning, reduction in risk potential (c)
❶ Focusing specifically on rehabilitation and the elements involved and rationale should expedite recovery, by gaining the patient's cooperation.
② This is common of normal preoperative teaching.
③ This information would be given to any individual before surgery.
④ This is common information for any individual before surgery.

236. Application, assessment, reduction in risk potential (b)
❸ When pain is severe, evaluate the neurological and circulatory status first; initial presentation of complications may be that of severe pain.
① Further assessment is needed before giving any pain medication.
② This may be done after the patient is assessed. It is imperative that the assessment be done as soon as possible.
④ Leg rotation is not usually a standard measure.

237. Comprehension, implementation, reduction of risk potential (a)
❸ Hydration and lying flat for 4 to 6 hours helps those individuals who may develop a spinal headache. This response addresses her concerns and gives a plan of action.

① This is not a proven fact. Some individuals will develop a headache.
② Staying prone versus supine does not give any additional benefit. It may increase patient's apprehension, because she may be fearful of moving. This is not a comfortable position to maintain.
④ This may belittle patient's concerns.

238. Comprehension, planning, basic care and comfort (b)
❶ It is easier on the patient to eat small, frequent meals. A large meal is physiologically and emotionally overwhelming to a person with decreased appetite. COPD patients lose weight because of decreased appetite and work of breathing.
② This does not relate to nursing diagnosis.
③ This does help with hydration status and to keep secretions moist.
④ This is unrealistic. As dyspnea progresses, patients are unable to sleep well because of the conscious effort to breathe. Pacing activities would decrease fatigue.

239. Application, assessment, pharmacological therapies (b)
❷ This may also may cause purpura, petechiae.
① The usual adverse skin reaction is an erythematous rash.
③ The adverse skin reaction is rash or urticaria.
④ The adverse skin reaction is urticaria.

240. Knowledge, assessment, physiological adaptation (a)
❶ This answer is accurate. Other behaviors include sleepiness, very short attention span, able to respond verbally. Patient fends off painful stimuli with purposeful movement.
② This is descriptive of deep coma state.
③, ④ These answers are descriptive of stuporous state.

241. Comprehension, implementation, pharmacological therapies (a)
❸ These are also known as hyperosmolar drugs. Mannitol (Osmitrol) is an example. These agents draw water from the edematous brain.
① These should be used carefully; they may mask LOC or cause respiratory depression.
② These may be ordered if nausea is present.
④ These may be ordered if open wound is caused by trauma.

242. Knowledge, assessment, prevention/early detection of disease (a)
❷ This is recommended as an annual test for all men age 50 and older.
① This is a blood test used as a monitoring tool to evaluate a cancer patient's response to treatment or for recurrence of the disease.
③ This is a screening test for BPH or cancer of prostate. It is not a blood test. It is an exam recommended for all men over the age of 40.
④ This is one of the diagnostic tests for HIV.

243. Application, implementation, reduction of risk potential (a)
❸ These will not increase systemic blood pressure because they are not resistive.
①, ② These are unsafe; they cause sudden increase in blood pressure and intracranial pressure.
④ This is unsafe and may cause flexion of hips and/or neck. Both of these positions may cause sudden increase in intracranial pressure.

244. Comprehension, implementation, reduction of risk potential (a)
    ❷ Pantopaque is a heavy dye and the physician strives to remove all the dye to prevent irritation of the meninges. Lying flat may help to lessen chance of headache.
    ① This position is unsafe. Besides headache, must assess for strength and sensation of lower extremities first.
    ③, ④ These positions are inappropriate. Any remaining dye may rise.

245. Comprehension, evaluation, coping and adaptation (a)
    ❹ Discovery of triggering factors demonstrates understanding of disease process and preventative health habit.
    ① This is not directly related. However, it may relieve stress, which is frequently a trigger of headaches.
    ② There is no proof that sunlight triggers these types of headaches.
    ③ Acetylsalicylic acid (aspirin) is seldom effective for classic migraine. Taking it as a preventive may not be a healthful habit.

246. Knowledge, assessment, prevention/early detection of disease (a)
    ❸ The ache may be in the groin. Other signs are a lump or enlargement of a testicle, heaviness or sudden collection of fluid in the scrotum, and/or enlargement or tenderness of the breasts.
    ① This describes phimosis.
    ②, ④ These are not warning signs of testicular cancer.

247. Comprehension, assessment, physiological adaptation (c)
    ❹ Right ventricle problems cause a pooling and backup of blood entering the heart from the systemic circulation. The dyspnea is caused by pressure from the ascites on the lungs. Failure of one of the ventricles normally results in failure of the opposite ventricle.
    ① Patients who have mitral valve disease normally have murmurs. Only in advanced disease do ventricular problems develop.
    ② Patients who have aortic valve problems have murmurs. Only in advanced cases do ventricular problems develop.
    ③ Left ventricular failure would manifest itself as pulmonary edema, dyspnea, and crackles in the lungs.

248. Application, assessment, reduction in risk potential (b)
    ❶ Principal function of white blood cells is to fight infection, which is signaled by an elevation of WBCs. Infection in a patient with diabetes can cause blood sugar fluctuations.
    ② The RBC indices are not as important as the WBC count in this circumstance.
    ③ The hemoglobin and hematocrit are important indicators in evaluating anemia; however, they are not as important in this situation.
    ④ This component of the blood count is not as useful as the WBCs in this situation.

249. Application, assessment, reduction in risk potential (c)
    ❸ A hot spot is usually a sign of inflammation under the cast.
    ① Swelling causes tightness of the cast and affects the neurocirculatory status.

② Tightness of a cast would manifest itself in changes in the neurocirculatory status of the extremity.
④ An object or foreign body beneath the cast, if large enough, may initially be evidenced by changes in neurocirculatory status.

250. Application, implementation, pharmacological therapies (b)
    ❹ This gives the body a chance to adjust the circulation to the effects of gravity.
    ① This will not prevent hypotension.
    ② Hose will not prevent hypotension.
    ③ Limiting dietary sodium is used in the treatment of hypertension but will not prevent hypotension.

251. Comprehension, assessment, prevention/early detection of disease (b)
    ❹ Anginal pain is caused by myocardial ischemia, which is insufficient blood and oxygen to the heart muscle. The pain may be precipitated or exacerbated by exertion.
    ① There is not enough information provided to assume that the patient had a myocardial infarction.
    ② Angina is a cardiac problem, not a cerebral problem.
    ③ An incompetent valve does not normally cause this kind of chest pain.

252. Application, implementation, reduction of risk potential (a)
    ❸ This position promotes venous return.
    ①, ② These may increase intracranial pressure.
    ④ This position causes flexion of the hips and perhaps the neck.

253. Application, implementation, reduction of risk potential (b)
    ❸ Clot may dislodge itself; bright red or darker color may indicate hemorrhage.
    ① This would cause painful bladder spasms.
    ② This may increase the patient's anxiety. The coughing may also increase the patient's discomfort.
    ④ This may increase the patient's discomfort. He is already at risk for fluid and electrolyte imbalance because of absorption of the irrigation fluid.

254. Comprehension, implementation, reduction of risk potential (a)
    ❶ This aids in absorption of dye. Metrizamide dye is water-soluble and does not need to be removed.
    ② This is not usually necessary.
    ③ Common side effects of this dye include nausea, vomiting, seizures with the peak time of risk 4 to 8 hours postprocedure.
    ④ Phenothiazines, tricyclic antidepressants, CNS stimulants, or amphetamines should not be taken 24 to 48 hours preprocedure or immediately postprocedure. These drugs lower seizure threshold.

255. Application, implementation, pharmacological therapies (a)
    ❶ Persons taking this anticonvulsant are especially prone to developing gingival hyperplasia.
    ② This is inappropriate and is not relative to the situation given; see #4.
    ③ This is inappropriate and is not a patient responsibility.

④ Adequate rest and diet are important. Answer #1 is individualized to the situation and is the better choice.

256. Application, planning, reduction of risk potential (a)
❶ Valsalva maneuver is avoided, because it will cause increased thoracic pressure, which indirectly causes increased intracranial pressure.
② Fluids are usually restricted until edema is resolved.
③ This may ease discomfort if patient complains of headache and/or photosensitivity.
④ This may be unsafe. Sensory perceptual alterations may be present. Ambulation may not be ordered until patient is alert, oriented, and has decreased cerebral edema. Certain classifications of pain medications may cause respiratory depression.

257. Application, planning, reduction of risk potential (a)
❶ The patient is at high risk for decubitus ulcer. Sensory loss prevents perception of pain and pressure, the warning signs of tissue injury. If able to, encourage patient involvement.
② This is inappropriate; adequate calcium intake is essential for all individuals.
③ This is inappropriate and is not relative to situation.
④ This is not individualized to persons with sensory/motor loss.

258. Application, planning, basic care and comfort (c)
❹ This has no known effect on urine acidity.
①, ② These cause an alkaline urine.
③ Sulfa drugs require an alkaline urine for maximum drug absorption.

259. Application, evaluation, reduction of risk potential (a)
❸ The diet is high in carbohydrates and restricted in sodium, potassium, phosphorus, and protein.
①, ②, ④ These don't indicate a change in dietary habits.

260. Application, implementation, basic care and comfort (b)
❹ Blood that drained from the legs while in the lithotomy position will flow back into vessels of the feet and legs as the person stands. Dizziness and fainting can occur from the sudden change in distribution.
① Although bleeding, perforation of bladder, and sepsis are complications of this procedure, the effect on VS would not be immediately evident.
② This is not usually necessary.
③ This is inappropriate and is not relevant to the situation.

261. Application, planning, reduction in risk potential (c)
❷ Hydronephrosis can occur rapidly if obstruction occurs.
① Stents are not irrigated.
③ This may be ordered but is not directly related to this situation.
④ The stents are not near the rectum. Contamination with stool is unlikely.

262. Application, evaluation, pharmacological therapies (a)
❶ This is adjunctive treatment, both agents decrease extrapyramidal symptoms.
② The medications mentioned are not antidepressants.
③ VS not affected with Parkinson's; propulsive shuffling gait is a sign of muscular rigidity and loss of postural reflexes.
④ These are not symptoms of Parkinson's.

263. Application, implementation, reduction in risk potential (b)
❹ The patient may have a weakened immune system and should avoid the risk of infection.
① HIV-positive patients can develop AIDS, but there is no fail-safe way to prevent it.
② A specific pneumonia is commonly seen in AIDS, but prevention goes beyond this one problem.
③ Preventing infection is of primary concern over preventing hypotension.

264. Comprehension, planning, pharmacological therapies (b)
❹ Oral agents are useful in treating diabetes when some beta cell function still exists.
① Obesity is not a measurement for beta cell function.
② Most agents are cleared by the liver, but this fact is unrelated to the need for functioning beta cells.
③ Type I diabetes usually is associated with no beta cell function.

265. Application, assessment, prevention/early detection of disease (b)
❷ Infection increases metabolism and increases the demand for insulin.
① This may affect glucose levels but is not a primary cause.
③ This would cause hypoglycemia.
④ This would also cause hypoglycemia

266. Application, planning, pharmacological therapies (b)
❸ Regular insulin is rapid acting and is given during the acute phase of DKA
① This is an intermediate acting insulin and may be given after the acute phase of DKA is over.
② This is also an intermediate acting insulin.
④ This is an extended long acting insulin and is too difficult to control to be used in the treatment of DKA.

267. Application, implementation, pharmacological therapies (b)
❷ This would reduce gastric irritation.
① There is nothing in antiinflammatories that would prevent anyone from driving.
③ Normally, CNS effects are not common when taking an antiinflammatory.
④ This would cause a large amount of gastric irritation.

268. Application, assessment, prevention/early detection of disease (b)
❹ Disorder tends to progress, and involvement of other systems is common with advancement of the disorder.
① This is characteristic of osteoarthritis.
② The disease tends to be chronic in nature.
③ This does not describe rheumatoid arthritis.

269. Knowledge, planning, pharmacological therapies (b)
❸ These drugs reduce the inflammatory process.
① These are not normally used as a first-line drug in the treatment of rheumatoid arthritis.
② These are not used as first-line drugs in the treatment of rheumatoid arthritis.
④ These are not the drug of choice for the treatment of rheumatoid arthritis.

270. Application, implementation, basic care and comfort (a)
    ❹ The dressing is easily soaked with urine through the drain. Urine is irritating to the skin.
    ① No dressing is present. It would be appropriate if patient had a perineal resection.
    ② This is inappropriate; vital signs would be done following usual procedure unless otherwise ordered.
    ③ This is inappropriate. Most patients having a suprapubic prostatectomy also have a CBI for 24 to 48 hours. If no Foley catheter in place, the nurse would need physician's order.

271. Knowledge, assessment, basic care and comfort (a)
    ❶ Awakening at night to void is most common. Pain on urination is sign of cystitis that most men find disturbing.
    ② Hematuria may result from blood vessels that have been overstretched. Groin pain is not present in most men.
    ③ These may result if UTI develops because of stasis of urine.
    ④ These may develop. However, they are not common signs.

272. Comprehension, implementation, pharmacological therapies (a)
    ❶ These decrease tone and involuntary movements and helps relieve anxiety and tension.
    ② These are inappropriate; vasodilators will not decrease spasticity.
    ③ These are inappropriate; narcotic analgesics are not given for spasticity.
    ④ These are inappropriate; NSAIDs will not decrease tone.

273. Application, implementation, reduction of risk potential (a)
    ❸ Taking the BP in left arm may cause compression and/or occlude the fistula. Any compression, tight clothing, or carrying objects with arm bent is to be avoided.
    ① It is unnecessary to do so; patients are discharged with this in place.
    ② This is inappropriate and is not procedure.
    ④ Fluids may be restricted. Some patients may have urine output. Hourly monitoring is usually not appropriate.

274. Application, planning, reduction of risk potential (b)
    ❶ Straining may initiate bleeding.
    ②, ③, ④ These are inappropriate for the expected outcome.

275. Application, assessment, reduction in risk potential (b)
    ❷ These symptoms are indicative of pulmonary edema, a complication of MI caused by heart failure.
    ① These symptoms do not support a diagnosis of emphysema.
    ③ These symptoms do not support a diagnosis of pulmonary embolism.
    ④ Chronic obstructive pulmonary disease does not have these symptoms.

276. Application, implementation, reduction of risk potential (b)
    ❷ Elevating the foot will reduce the swelling of the sprained ankle.

① The foot will have increased swelling because of the effects of gravity.
③ Exercise will increase swelling by increasing blood flow to the area.
④ A warm bath will promote vasodilation, increasing the swelling in the area.

277. Application, implantation, pharmacological therapies (b)
    ❹ The antiinflammatory properties of aspirin decreases joint inflammation and pain.
    ① The primary purpose of aspirin therapy is to decrease joint inflammation. We do not know the dose of the aspirin or the agenda of the physician.
    ② Aspirin does not relax skeletal muscles.
    ③ Aspirin is given to reduce inflammation in joints.

278. Comprehension, assessment, physiological adaptation (b)
    ❶ The signs/symptoms of fat embolism include shortness of breath and restlessness as a result of hypoxia caused by occlusion of pulmonary blood vessels.
    ② Difficulty swallowing and aspiration pneumonia are not symptoms of fat embolism.
    ③ These are symptoms of cholecystitis.
    ④ These symptoms may indicate paralytic ileus.

279. Comprehension, implementation, reduction in risk potential (a)
    ❸ By using the palms of the hands, the nurse has less of a chance for placing indentations in the cast, which could compromise circulatory status when the plaster dries.
    ① The patient will not be able to hold the extremity for a prolonged period of time.
    ② The pillowcase will stick to the cast, causing excess pressure that will mold the cast.
    ④ Not only is this is uncomfortable for the patient but also you will not be able to support the extremity adequately.

280. Application, planning, reduction in risk potential (c)
    ❷ Liver is high in purines, which increase uric acid levels and would exacerbate the patient's condition.
    ① There are no purines in these foods.
    ③ These foods would not exacerbate the patient's arthritis.
    ④ Veal and garlic bread do not have a high purine content.

281. Comprehension, assessment, reduction in risk potential (b)
    ❶ Osteomyelitis most often requires extensive long-term antibiotic therapy.
    ② This activity could have introduced pathogenic bacteria near the bone.
    ③ In the acute phase, mobility should be minimized to decrease the spread of the infection.
    ④ Pain on movement is common in patients with osteomyelitis.

282. Comprehension, assessment, physiological adaptation (c)
    ❸ Crossing of the legs may result in displacement of the new femoral head.
    ① There is no restriction on plantar flexion and should be done to increase circulation to the legs.
    ② Low chairs would cause a greater than 90-degree hip flexion; need elevated toilet seat and chairs.
    ④ Physical therapy, with limited weight bearing and ambulation, begins soon after surgery.

283. Knowledge, assessment, reduction in risk potential (a)
  ❸ The presence of an elevated ESR and rheumatoid factor would indicate rheumatoid arthritis.
  ① Although the WBCs are slightly elevated, the patient should not have an elevated hemoglobin.
  ② Uric acid is elevated in patients with gout.
  ④ Although the rheumatoid factor is present, the LE cells are present in patient with systemic lupus erythematosus.

284. Comprehension, assessment, reduction in risk potential (b)
  ❸ A patient who has developed a thrombosis will exhibit calf pain and swelling of the affected extremity.
  ① This funding is common in a patient with a pulmonary emboli.
  ② This is an assessment finding in heart failure or hypervolemia.
  ④ This may indicate loss of skin integrity or a pin tract infection.

285. Application, evaluation, reduction in risk potential (b)
  ❹ This is the correct rationale behind positioning.
  ① The prone position will not alleviate phantom limb pain.
  ② Although important, this is not the primary reason for the positioning.
  ③ Most patients do not feel that the prone position is the most comfortable. This is not the reason for the positioning.

286. Application, implementation, physiological adaptation (c)
  ❸ Because of the patient's surgery, there is a lack of HCL acid secretion and a lack of intrinsic factor, the patient will not be able to absorb vitamin B_{12}. A lack of vitamin B_{12} causes pernicious anemia.
  ① Although technically correct, this question does not adequately explain the rationale to the patient.
  ② A lack of folic acid does not cause pernicious anemia.
  ④ Untrue, a lack of iron does not cause pernicious anemia.

287. Application, planning, coordinated care (c)
  ❸ The tympanic mode would pose the least chance for injury and bleeding for the patient.
  ① Oral temperatures should not be taken on unconscious adults because of the chance for injury to the mucous membranes.
  ② A rectal temperature may damage the rectal mucosa and cause bleeding.
  ④ Although a safe method, axillary temperatures are less accurate than tympanic.

288. Comprehension, implementation, basic care and comfort (b)
  ❷ This statement provides the best explanation for the patient's symptom.
  ① This is not a true statement.
  ③ This is most likely not true, and it doesn't answer the patient's question.
  ④ This is a true statement but does not answer the patient's question. It assumes that the patient was exercising.

289. Comprehension, evaluation, reduction in risk potential (b)
  ❹ A low platelet count, thrombocytopenia, would cause bleeding tendencies.
  ① A low WBC count might cause inability to fight infection.
  ② A high WBC count would indicate an infectious process.
  ③ An elevated platelet count would cause a high clot situation.

290. Comprehension, implementation, basic care and comfort (c)
  ❸ Exercise increases the oxygen demands of the body, which the failing heart is not able to accommodate.
  ① Bronchi dilate with exercise.
  ② This may be true, exercise must be started gradually, but this statement does not answer the patient's questions.
  ④ The blood vessels of the heart and lungs dilate, increasing blood flow; this does not cause shortness of breath.

291. Application, assessment, reduction in risk potential (b)
  ❸ Monitoring for arrhythmias, shortness of breath (which could indicate a pulmonary embolism) and bleeding at the insertion/access site are the most important assessments at this time.
  ① Leg exercise is discouraged for the first 6 to 8 hours after the procedure.
  ② Early ambulation is discouraged for the first 6 to 8 hours after the procedure.
  ④ The extremity that is accessed should not be exercised in the immediate period following a cardiac catheterization

292. Application, planning, basic care and comfort (b)
  ❶ Corned beef and canned broth have high levels of sodium; eating them each day would not be beneficial.
  ② Both shredded wheat and fruit are low in sodium and consuming them each day should not have an undesirable effect.
  ③ Broccoli and chicken are relatively low in salt and having this lunch once a week should not compromise the patient.
  ④ Although french fries do contain a small amount of salt, consuming this meal three times a week should not adversely effect the patient.

293. Comprehension, assessment, physiological adaptation (c)
  ❸ With left-sided heart failure, blood becomes backed up in the lungs causing crackles or fluid in the lungs.
  ① Nausea is not normally associated with heart failure.
  ② An extra heart sound may be heard (S3), but it is not the sound of a murmur.
  ④ Right ventricular heart failure would result in peripheral edema.

294. Application, assessment, safety and infection control (c)
  ❸ Rheumatic fever and subsequent heart disease is the prominent cause of valvular insufficiency.
  ① An appendectomy should not have any bearing on the patient's present diagnosis.
  ② Although significant for heart disease in general, the history of rheumatic fever is more significant.
  ④ Although significant because of the possible introduction of bacteria into the heart, the history of rheumatic fever is more significant.

295. Application, evaluation, basic care and comfort (b)
    ❷ A fracture would temporarily restrict mobility in the leg, increasing venous stasis and the chance of a blood clot.
    ① Atrial fibrillation may cause clots to form inside the heart.
    ③ Narrow angle glaucoma should not have any effect on the development of blood clots.
    ④ Although small clots eventually effect blood vessels, the fracture is more likely to be significant.

296. Application, implementation, reduction in risk potential (c)
    ❹ The nurse should first check to see that the patient's gag reflex has returned.
    ① The patient will must likely return to their pretest diet, but a gag reflex must be intact first.
    ② There are no time restrictions on this test; a gag reflex must be intact.
    ③ You would do this after checking for an intact gag reflex.

297. Application, planning, safe effective coordinated care (b)
    ❸ Chicken salad is a protein food and would be restricted in someone with elevated ammonia levels.
    ① Pretzels would not be restricted for a person with this diagnosis.
    ② Although cheese does contain some protein, chicken salad would more likely be restricted.
    ④ A bowl of ice cream is mostly fat and carbohydrates and would not be restricted.

298. Comprehension, assessment, physiological adaptation (b)
    ❹ Patients with appendicitis frequently complain of rebound tenderness of the abdomen upon palpation.
    ① Hematemesis is a symptom of perforated ulcers.
    ② Sharp back pain may be a symptom of aortic dissection or pancreatitis.
    ③ Abdominal distention is common with intestinal obstruction or ileus.

299. Application, assessment, basic care and comfort (b)
    ❷ This highly fatty meal may precipitate a gallbladder attack.
    ① Physical activity does not normally prescription gallbladder pain.
    ③ Taking acetaminophen does not normally precipitate pain in this area.
    ④ Although alcohol may cause gastritis, it does not normally cause pain in the gallbladder region.

300. Application, planning, basic care and comfort (b)
    ❸ Abdominal girth alerts the nurse to an accumulation of fluid in the abdomen.
    ① Fluids are sometimes restricted in advanced liver disease.
    ② Low-glucose diets are sometimes indicated in pancreatic disease.
    ④ A high-protein diet would be contraindicated in a person with advanced liver disease.

301. Comprehension, implementation, coping and adaptation (a)
    ❷ Hepatitis A is transmitted by ingestion of contaminated food or liquids.
    ① Hepatitis A is not transmitted by direct contact.
    ③ Hepatitis A is not transmitted by blood or blood products.
    ④ Hepatitis A is not transmitted in this manner.

302. Application, planning, pharmacological therapies (b)
    ❸ Pancreatic enzymes are taken with meals.
    ① The enzymes will not be able to aid digestion if taken between meals.
    ② The enzymes need to be taken when eating any carbohydrates, proteins or fats.
    ④ This would not allow proper digestion to take place.

303. Comprehension, assessment, reduction in risk potential (c)
    ❸ Any increased abdominal pressure will place stress on the surgical incision.
    ① This may be true but would not be the primary reason for notifying the surgeon.
    ② The patient should not have an increased chance for peritonitis because of a respiratory problem.
    ④ Again, this may be true, but it is not the primary reason for notifying the surgeon.

304. Application, evaluation, reduction of risk potential (b)
    ❹ Assess the patency of the tube by checking with an air bolus.
    ① This may be contraindicated and is premature; assess patency first.
    ② This requires a physician order; ascertain whether the tube is patent first.
    ③ Assess patency of tube before notifying the physician.

305. Comprehension, evaluation, reduction in risk potential (b)
    ❹ Stocking shelves would require bending and lifting, which would allow increased abdominal pressure and worsen the patient's symptoms.
    ① Driving should not aggravate the condition.
    ② This activity would not need to be restricted unless there was a lot of bending and lifting involved.
    ③ Typing should not increase abdominal pressure.

306. Application, assessment, pharmacological therapies (b)
    ❶ The need for thyroid replacement therapy would be needed lifelong with medical follow-up.
    ② This is true and may indicate an over dosage of thyroid replacement drugs.
    ③ This establishes an adequate level of the drug in the bloodstream.
    ④ This may indicate hyperthyroidism, which can be caused by the thyroid replacement therapy.

307. Comprehension, implementation, physiological adaption (b)
    ❹ The patient should be placed in low or semi-Fowler's position to decrease the strain on sutures.
    ① Supine would edema of the neck, compromising the patient's airway.
    ② There is no benefit to placing the patient in left lateral Sims'. It will not benefit the patient.
    ③ Trendelenberg's would compromise the airway and place undue strain on the suture line.

308. Application, implementation, basic care and comfort (b)
    ❷ Patients who had adrenalectomies must stay stress free, as they no longer have the ability to respond readily to these situations.
    ① Adrenalectomies do not normally necessitate an accurate intake/output record.
    ③ This is indicated in a person who has Conn's syndrome.
    ④ This is advised for patients who have diabetes insipidus.

309. Comprehension, assessment, basic care and comfort (b)
   ❹ Individuals with diabetes insipidus have an increased intake of fluids coupled with a dilute urine.
   ① A bounding pulse and low urine output are signs of a hypervolemic state.
   ② Individuals who are hypovolemic have low blood pressure; tachycardia is a significant finding for dehydration.
   ③ Individuals with diabetes insipidus have an increased urine output and a low urine specific gravity.

310. Comprehension, evaluation, pharmacological therapies (b)
   ❸ The abrupt withdrawal of steroids can cause an addisonian crisis, an inability to respond to stressful situations.
   ① The withdrawal of insulin in a patient with diabetes mellitus can cause hyperglycemia.
   ② Cardizem is an antiarrythmic/antianginal and will not cause an Addisonian crisis when withdrawn.
   ④ Diltiazem is a cardiotonic; abrupt withdrawal may precipitate heart failure.

311. Comprehension, planning, reduction in risk potential (b)
   ❶ Wearing a medic alert tag will ensure that others will respond appropriately outside the hospital setting.
   ② Although this is advisable, without the medic alert tag, no one would know what to do with the glucose.
   ③ This practice is not advisable and will not assist personnel without a medic alert tag.
   ④ Although this is a good idea, it will not ensure proper care in all locations.

312. Comprehension, assessment, coping and adaptation (a)
   ❷ Patients with hyperpituitarism have structural alterations to their body, which can cause problems with self esteem and body image.
   ① The problems that stem from excess pituitary hormone does not normally cause an alteration in comfort.
   ③ Alteration in fluid and electrolytes is more common with Addison's disease.
   ④ This diagnosis more common in hyperthyroidism.

313. Comprehension, assessment, basic care and comfort (b)
   ❷ Ketones cause metabolic acidosis in DKA.
   ① Both are treated with insulin administration.
   ③ HHNK is found primarily in patients who are non-insulin dependent.
   ④ Serum ketones and glucose are elevated in DKA.

314. Application, assessment, physiological adaptation (b)
   ❸ Swelling in the neck region is of priority as it could compromise the respiratory status.
   ① This is to be expected in the immediate post-op period.
   ② Although a concern, respiratory compromise is of top priority.
   ④ A small amount of bleeding is to be expected and should not be of great concern; further monitoring is indicated.

315. Comprehension, planning, reduction in risk potential (b)
   ❹ Cheese and crackers provide enough complex carbohydrates to sustain the person through the activity.
   ① This provides a rapid form of glucose that would not sustain the person.

② This rapidly acting form of glucose is best taken during a hypoglycemic episode.
   ③ A can of soda, sweetened, would not sustain the person through the activity.

316. Comprehension, planning, reduction in risk potential (b)
   ❷ Patients who have had a conization normally have vaginal packing that needs to be maintained. The nurse should also anticipate monitoring for bleeding.
   ① The patient should not used tampons until instructed to do so by her physician.
   ③ This may disrupt the site and could encourage bleeding.
   ④ Patients should not douche until instructed to do so by their physician.

317. Comprehension, assessment, prevention/early detection of disease (b)
   ❸ Mammograms are recommended yearly for individuals over the age of 40.
   ① Gynecological exams should be done on a yearly basis.
   ② Hepatitis B vaccine is indicated for this individual, because she works in a high-risk occupation.
   ④ TB tests should be done on a yearly basis and the patient's is up to date.

318. Comprehension, implementation, prevention/early detection of disease (b)
   ❹ Breasts should be palpated in a variety of positions to ensure that all areas are assessed.
   ① Breast self-examinations should be conducted 7 days after onset of menstruation.
   ② This could be done, but breasts need to be palpated while lying and standing also.
   ③ The pads of the fingers should be used to feel for lumps.

319. Comprehension, planning, basic care and comfort (b)
   ❷ Drinking warm beverages will help relax the uterine muscles and decrease the pain involved with uterine spasm.
   ① This will cause additional cramping and pain.
   ③ It is recommended that females do not exert themselves during their period.
   ④ Antiinflammatory medication is more effective, with less side effects, than narcotic analgesics.

320. Comprehension, assessment, reduction in risk potential (b)
   ❸ Patients with rectovaginal fistulas will have leakage of fecal matter and flatus from the vagina. This condition causes extreme anxiety in the patient.
   ① This occurs in a ureterovaginal, vesicovaginal, or urethrovaginal fistula.
   ② This is common with hemorrhoids.
   ④ These are common findings in a patient that has *Candida albicans* infection.

321. Comprehension, assessment, prevention/early detection of disease (b)
   ❷ Females rarely have any early symptoms of gonorrhea. The patient should be tested as her partner is infected.
   ① This is not true, gonorrhea does not always cause symptoms in females.
   ③ The patient should be tested now.
   ④ The patient should be tested before giving antibiotics; she may not be infected.

322. Comprehension, implementation, basic care and comfort (b)
❷ Voiding will increase the patient's comfort during the procedure and will keep the patient from voiding during the exam.
① This will impede the exam.
③ Patients can't be menstruating during the time of the exam; visualization and culture is difficult.
④ The patient may need you for support during the exam and may feel abandoned.

323. Comprehension, implementation, reduction in risk potential (c)
❶ Because of the nature of the surgery and the proximity to the urethra, an indwelling catheter is placed during the surgery and will remain for a few days.
② Because of the complications of immobility, patients are ambulated early after surgery, even those surgeries involving internal organs.
③ The patient will most likely resume a normal diet after the bowel sounds have returned.
④ Unless the patient has a preexisting condition, physical therapy would not necessarily be a part of her postsurgical care.

324. Application, assessment, reduction in risk potential (b)
❹ It is generally recommended that family and visitors spend as little time in the direct proximity to the patient as possible. The amount of time visitors stay is limited.
① This is a true statement. It prevents straining of stool, which could dislodge the implant.
② These are the preferred positions, because there is less risk of the implant dislodging.
③ Nausea and vomiting generally accompany radiation therapy.

325. Comprehension, implementation, basic care and comfort (b)
❶ Pizza is high in sodium and would aggravate the symptoms of PMS.
② Mineral water should not aggravate the condition. Beverages with caffeine would worsen the symptoms.
③ Pasta and sauce should not aggravate the condition, unless there is excessive amounts of salt in the sauce.
④ Raw fruits and vegetables are a healthy snack and should not aggravate PMS.

326. Comprehension, assessment, reduction of risk potential (b)
❶ Hypoventilation reduces oxygen to the alveoli and reduces carbon dioxide elimination. The retained CO_2 then combines with H_2O to form an excess of carbonic acid (H_2CO_3), decreasing the blood pH. As a result, concentration of hydrogen ions in body fluids, which directly reflects acidity, increases.
② The lungs excrete carbon dioxide and water. The rate of excretion of CO_2 is controlled by the respiratory center in the medulla of the brain. If increased amounts of CO_2 or hydrogens are present, the respiratory center stimulates an increased rate and depth of breathing.

③, ④ The lungs excrete carbon dioxide and water, which are byproducts of cellular metabolism.

327. Application, assessment, reduction of risk potential, (b)
❷ IgE is the antibody most often associated. Many persons with asthma have an allergic component to their disease.
① INR is a calculated measure as part of a coagulation profile (blood clotting).
③ HCV test done to look for hepatitis C virus and antibody level.
④ CEA is a measure that may be increased with various cancers such as cancer of the colon, liver, and pancreas. CEA levels may also be increased in persons who are chronic cigarette smokers and in persons who have inflammatory bowel disorders.

328. Comprehension, planning, reduction of risk potential (b)
❷ Persons are usually no longer infectious after 2 to 3 weeks of therapy.
①, ③ These are incorrect timeframes. Cell-mediated immunity to the mycobacteria, which develops 3 to 6 weeks later, usually contains the infection and arrests the disease.
④ If these were true, all persons with TB disease would need to remain isolated.

329. Application, implementation, basic care and comfort (b)
❸ This is proper technique. Corticosteroid inhalers should be used last because they require gargling after use to prevent oral candidiasis.
① This may help; it depends on the side effects he is experiencing. Sitting may calm the patient, reduce a sense of panic, and may maximize chest expansion.
② He should be using as prescribed. A few to five minutes is generally recommended between medications.
④ If he is concerned, he needs to call the clinic and make an appointment. He should not stop these medications on his own.

330. Application, assessment, reduction of risk potential (c)
❸ It takes two to three months after exposure to *Mycobacterium tuberculosis* for an infected person to develop skin sensitivity to PPD.
①, ② This would be too soon.
④ It is not recommended to wait this long. This would cause needless anxiety.

331. Comprehension, implementation, coordinated care (a)
❶ The reason for coming as perceived by the patient is defined as the chief complaint. The physician first looks to this part of the admission sheet on which to base the priorities of treatment and care.
② This section refers to environmental, spiritual, cultural aspects, and family dynamics.
③ The past medical history may be important. The reason for seeking treatment today warrants attention. Frequently, the accuracy of this section is not always accurate, depending on how reliable the memory of the person supplying the information.
④ The review of systems is a thorough body system approach of assessment and data gathering. The physician or nurse practitioner fills out this section.

332. Comprehension, implementation, reduction of risk potential (a)
❷ This bacillus is transmitted in the droplet nuclei formed when the person with active TB coughs, sings, talks, laughs, or sneezes.
①, ③, ④ It is highly unlikely to inspire the droplet in these situations. Prolonged contact is necessary.

333. Comprehension, implementation, reduction of risk potential (b)
❹ This allows for time to recover and rest.
①, ②, ③ These are more appropriate if the nursing diagnosis stated a respiratory problem.

334. Application, implementation, reduction of risk potential (b)
❸ Caffeine, carbonated and citrus beverages, as well as alcohol, have been shown to irritate the bladder mucosa.
① Fluids need to be encouraged to flush out irritants and prevent urinary stasis.
② He should urinate every 2 to 3 hours or at the first urge to urinate to flush the urinary tract.
④ He needs to continue to take the Bactrim as prescribed, even if urination and symptoms improve.

335. Comprehension, implementation, coordinated care (b)
❸ Vital signs are objective data.
① Data stated by the patient is subjective, such as the purpose for the clinic visit.
②, ④ These are incorrect and nonexistent.

336. Application, assessment, reduction of risk potential (b)
❹ These are symptoms consistent with chronic bronchitis.
①, ② Although these are forms of COPD, these symptoms may not be present.
③ These symptoms may be present in this disease process, but it is not a form of COPD.

337. Application, assessment, physiological adaptation (b)
④ Gradual loss of peripheral vision is characteristic with this type of glaucoma.
① These are characteristic with retinal detachment.
② Double vision indicates difficulty with both eyes focusing together on an object.
③ Nausea, vomiting, headache, and eye pain or redness are associated with acute closed angle glaucoma.

338. Application, implementation, basic care and comfort (a)
❶ This is unsafe and could cause damage to the ear drum. This would also cause discomfort. It is best if the otoscope is held in a superior position.
②, ③, ④ These are safe and appropriate techniques for an otoscopic exam.

339. Application, planning, reduction of risk potential (b)
❶ An indwelling catheter may be in place for up to 24 hours related to possible edema of the urethra and to decrease the possibility of infection and discomfort. A three-way Foley may be used if bladder irrigation is desired.
②, ④ These statements increase anxiety for the patient and are not usually true in these procedures.
③ These procedures are usually done under local anesthesia.

340. Application, assessment, reduction of risk potential (c)
❶ Fever, chills, nausea, vomiting, flank pain, bloody urine, are all signs of an upper UTI.
②, ③, ④ These complaints are prevalent in lower UTI.

341. Application, assessment, reduction of risk potential (c)
❶ Nephrotic syndrome is a group of symptoms associated with increased glomerular permeability. The primary symptoms are proteinuria, hypoalbuminuria, and edema. Loss of protein leads to the third tissue spacing of fluids as well as vitamin D deficiency. Remember albumin is protein.
②, ③, ④ These are not identified as major factors in the pathophysiology of this syndrome.

342. Knowledge, implementation, pharmacological therapies (b)
❹ The course of therapy is usually longer for upper UTI; expect a 10-14 day course.
①, ②, ③ These are possible courses of antimicrobial therapy, especially with lower UTIs.

343. Application, assessment, reduction of risk potential (b)
❶ In men with chlamydia, urethritis, conjunctivitis, arthritis, and mucocutaneous lesions (Reiter's syndrome) are the common symptoms.
② This is present in syphilis.
③ This is usually not present in sexually transmitted diseases.
④ This is a manifestation of genital warts.

344. Application, assessment, reduction of risk potential (b)
❹ This is correct. The creatinine clearance increases as renal function diminishes.
①, ②, ③ These may be indications of renal function, anemia, or infection, but not GFR.

345. Application, assessment, reduction of risk potential (b)
❸ Painful bladder spasms may indicate trying to void around an obstruction such as blood clots.
① Bowel sounds must be assessed with any surgical patient. However, this data would not relate the cause in this situation.
② An atonic bladder is usually due to a disturbance of innervation or to chronic obstruction. A three-way catheter is in place. Checking for possible obstruction with a catheter is the first priority.
④ Temperature must be assessed with any surgical patient. However, this data would not relate the cause in this situation.

346. Application, implementation, reduction of risk potential (b)
❹ Sexual arousal causes vasodilation and increases discomfort.
① Of the four most common forms of prostatitis, nonbacterial prostatitis may occur after a viral illness or it may be associated with other sexually transmitted diseases, particularly in the young adult. This patient is started on antibiotics, which implies that this is an acute or chronic bacterial prostatitis. A condom will protect the partner from infection.
② Constipation and bearing down to pass a hard stool increase patient discomfort. Stool softeners are often prescribed to provide relief from painful symptoms.
③ Antibiotics should be taken for the full prescribed time.

347. Comprehension, assessment, prevention/early detection of disease (b)
❶ These are the key factors. General nutritional state, age, and any chronic disease state coexisting could influence the rate of wound healing.
②, ③, ④ Skill of closure, mental awareness, type of suture are not key factors.

348. Comprehension, implementation, coordinated care (a)
❹ Purulent drainage indicates that an infection of the wound may be present. This needs to be communicated to the physician if this is a new development.
①, ②, ③ These are expected types of drainage based on the age of the incision. In general, drainage is expected to change from sanguineous (red to serosanguineous [pink]) to serous (straw colored) to clear during a period of hours to days.

349. Application, implementation, reduction of risk potential (b)
❸ This position and the soft textured foods decrease the risk of aspiration
① Suction equipment should be available, however, positioning and the type of foods provided will help the patient more with the actual swallowing.
② Hyperextending the neck serves to increase the possibility of aspiration.
④ It is not necessary to puree or only supply a diet of bland foods. The goal is to provide as normal a diet as possible.

350. Comprehension, assessment, reduction of risk potential (c)
❶ The manifestations of this increased stimulation state are hypertension, blurred vision, headache, sweating, flushed skin, and bradycardia.
②, ③, ④ These are mainly opposite of the increased stimulation manifestations.

351. Application, implementation, reduction of risk potential (a)
❷ Level of consciousness is defined by both the content of consciousness and the arousal level. Confusion is defined as having the described behaviors as well as agitation and irritability. Disorientation to time occurs first, followed by place and place.
① "Difficult" is a value judgment
③ Lethargy is reflective of a patient who is unable to be aroused spontaneously but requires some external stimuli such as touch, voice, etc. Confusion may also be present.
④ Stupor indicates a patient in a deep sleep or unresponsive. Arousal only occurs with vigorous and continuous stimulation.

352. Comprehension, assessment, reduction of risk potential (b)
❷ Although any stimulation can cause this phenomenon to result, the most common are a full bladder, full bowel, wrinkled sheets, etc.
①, ③, ④ Skin stimulation may be a stimulus and needs to be done gently as when taking vital signs. Visitors may unknowingly cause a draft, which may stimulate this reaction.

353. Comprehension, planing, physiological adaptation (b)
❸ Hypovolemic shock may occur as a result of intravascular volume depletion, as fluid moves into the intracellular spaces. Observing and planning for shock is critical. This is a priority. The greatest initial threat to a patient with a major burn is hypovolemic shock.
① Monitoring urine output would better indicate kidney status.
② Skin care and comfort are important
④ A too-rapid IV would increase intravascular volume.

354. Application, assessment, pharmacological therapies (b)
❷ These are common side effects of this classification; they are also common side effects of the methylxanthine derivatives. Other side effects include palpitations, changes in blood pressure, tachycardia, headache, and muscle tremors.
① These are not identified as common side effects for any of the classifications of medications used to treat asthma.
③ These may be associated with large doses of chlorambucil, a drug used in the treatment of neoplastic diseases.
④ These are associated with the antiinflammatory agents that may be given for asthma.

355. Application, implementation, reduction of risk potential (a)
❸ Most policies recommend assessing the site within 48 to 72 hours (2 to 3 days).
①, ②, ④ These are not the recommended times. Inaccurate assessments may result.

356. Application, planning, reduction of risk potential (b)
❶ Retained secretions would indicate her difficulty in removing, because of an ineffective cough. Adventitious breath sounds may also be present.
② This is a symptom of altered tissue perfusion.
③, ④ These complaints by the patient reflect an activity intolerance.

357. Application, implementation, pharmacological therapies (c)
❹ This value may indicate nephrotoxicity. Many antibiotics, such as vancomycin, are nephrotoxic. Normal finding is 0.5 to 1.5 mg/dl. Creatinine indicates impairs kidney function.
①, ②, ③ These are all within normal lab findings.

358. Application, assessment, pharmacological therapies (b)
❶ Hepatitis, with the risk increasing with the age of the patient, needs to be assessed for. Hepatic enzymes are measured before and during therapy.
②, ③, ④ These symptoms have not been noted with active TB.

359. Application, planning, physiological adaptation (b)
❸ Pulse oximetry monitors the actual oxygen content in the blood. A reading of 90% or greater from 79% would indicate that the patient's body is tolerating the activity and better able to meet body requirements.
① Cyanosis indicates poor oxygenation to the tissue.
②, ④ These are later signs indicating activity tolerance. A better indication would be that these rates return to baseline within 1 to 5 minutes.

360. Application, planning, reduction of risk potential (b)
❸ Postural drainage of the lower and middle lobes requires lying in a head-down position that patients in respiratory distress or dyspneic may not be able to tolerate.
① This should be done immediately preceding the CPT.
② The procedures of CPT should be performed at least 1 hour before and 3 hours after meals.
④ There is not need to wait a full hour after CPT to take vital signs.

361. Application, assessment, reduction of risk potential (a)
❹ Cataracts lead to progressive blurring of vision.
① Floaters are characteristics of a retinal detachment.
②, ③ Eye pain or eye dryness is not characteristic of cataracts.

362. Application, implementation, basic care and comfort (b)
❸ The IV and PO intake equals 875 cc.
①, ②, ④ The intake equals the IV and PO. There is a separate area to record the bladder irrigating fluid amount.

363. Application, planning, basic care and comfort (b)
❶ Diminished caliber and/or force of urinary stream and a feeling of incomplete bladder emptying are common complaints.
②, ④ These are more common with UTIs.
③ This is unrelated to the situation.

364. Knowledge, implementation, reduction of risk potential (a)
❷ These patients should avoid douching or using feminine sprays or perfumed feminine hygiene products.
① Voiding is recommended after sexual intercourse.
③ Showers are recommended.
④ Citrus juices are irritating to the bladder. Eight 8-ounce glasses of water and noncaffeine, noncarbonated beverages are recommended.

365. Application, assessment, pharmacological therapies (b)
❶ Calcium channel blockers may affect the ability of the bladder or sphincter to contract or relax normally.
② Anticoagulants may cause hematuria.
③ NSAIDs usually do not affect bladder control.
④ Antiemetics have not been shown to affect bladder or sphincter control.

366. Application, implementation, reduction of risk potential (b)
❶ It has been found that resisting the urge to void for longer than 1 hour can result in a UTI. The distended bladder shortens the urethra.
② Voiding after sexual intercourse is recommended.
③, ④ These actions are not recommended.

367. Comprehension, assessment, reduction of risk potential (b)
❶ Because vitamin D cannot be converted to its biologically active form, which is needed for calcium reabsorption, hypocalcemia may develop.
② WBCs are usually decreased.
③, ④ Both creatinine and BUN increase due to excessive amounts of nitrogenous wastes accumulating in the blood.

368. Application, implementation, pharmacological therapies (a)
❶ Fluid intake is especially important, at least eight 8-ounce glasses a day. Encouraging fluid decreases the potential of the adverse effect of crystal formation
②, ④ These are indirect effects.
③ This is important and best achieved by giving the drug as scheduled.

369. Application, planning, reduction of risk potential (b)
❸ This also involves postoperative suprapubic catheter. The prostate is approached through a low midline abdominal incision that cuts the bladder to the anterior aspect of the prostate.
① This is an incision between the scrotum and rectum.
② This is an abdominal incision without incision of bladder.
④ This is done with a cystourethroscopy.

370. Comprehension, assessment, reduction of risk potential (b)
❸ The body attempts to compensate by increasing respirations and blowing off carbon dioxide.
①, ②, ④ Decreasing respirations may cause retention of CO_2. The kidneys act later than the respiratory system.

371. Comprehension, assessment, reduction of risk potential (b)
❹ The higher the number rating on this scale, which ranges from 0 to 15, the better the prognosis and the likelihood of optimum cerebral functioning.
①, ②, ③ These states would be most likely have rating lower than 13.

372. Comprehension, planning, physiological adaptation (b)
❹ A disruption of the transmembrane potential at the cellular level causes a sodium-potassium pump impairment, resulting in intracellular swelling.
① If the immunoglobulins were decreased, this would affect the immune status not third tissue spacing.
② The cardiac output would be decreased.
③ The hypermetabolic state increases the oxygen consumption.

373. Comprehension, assessment, basic care and comfort (b)
❸ This is the deficit that frequently occurs in right-sided damage and one very distressful for the patient.
①, ②, ④ These are deficits with left-sided brain damage.

374. Comprehension, assessment, physiological adaptation (b)
❷ Some drugs are known to lower the seizure threshold. Other secondary causes of seizures are cerebral ischemia such as in a CVA, or with fevers.
①, ③, ④ These states have not been identified as potential risk factors for seizures.

375. Application, implementation, physiological adaptation (b)
❹ With lower motor neuron pathways disruption in the myoneural junction and muscles occurs. This results in flaccidity. Muscle weakness may also be noted.
①, ② Upper motor neuron lesions lead to spasticity and hypertonia.
③ Hypertrophy, the enlargement of muscle mass, usually occurs from overuse.

376. Application, evaluation, pharmacological therapies (c)
❸ This accurately describes the therapeutic actions for using this thiazide diuretic.
① This agent is thought to stabilize cell membrane and improve autoregulation and blood flow. That is why you may see this agent ordered.
② Phenytoin (Dilantin) is believed to prevent the formation of cerebral edema and control ICP.
④ Mannitol (Osmitrol) withdraws fluid from normal tissue but may increase edema if the blood barrier is damaged.

377. Knowledge, assessment, physiological adaptation (a)
❹ This type of deep partial thickness may involve all layers of the dermis.
① This best describes a superficial partial thickness (first-degree) burn.
② Intact blister formation is indicative of superficial partial thickness burn.
③ This indicates a full-thickness burn.

378. Application, implementation, pharmacological therapies (b)
❶ The reason stated is correct. Also remind him to shake the inhalers before using and to hold his breath for 10 seconds after inhaling the medications.
②, ③, ④ All these statements give incorrect rationale and information. Ventolin is a beta-adrenergic agonist that stimulates beta-adrenergic receptors, producing bronchodilation. Atrovent is an anticholinergic that acts by blocking acetylcholine, resulting in bronchodilation.

379. Application, implementation, reduction of risk potential (a)
❹ This finding is present in both of these forms of COPD.
① This is a finding with emphysema.
②, ③ These usually are present with chronic bronchitis.

380. Comprehension, implementation, reduction of risk potential (a)
❷ This describes the person who is at greatest risk.
①, ③, ④ The spread is by the airborne route. It is very unlikely that the bacillus lives very long outside the host or that a casual contact is a high-risk situation.

381. Application, implementation, reduction of risk potential (b)
❶ Drainage trickling down the posterior pharynx may be indicated by frequent swallowing, belching, hematemesis. The nurse should use a flashlight when assessing the back of the throat.
②, ④ These are very late signs for bleeding from this type of surgery.
③ This would be expected from this type of surgery.

382. Application, implementation, pharmacological therapies (b)
❶ Individuals metabolize xanthines at different rates. Dosage is determined by monitoring response, tolerance, pulmonary function, and serum theophylline levels. Serum theophylline concentrations should range between 10 to 20 mcg/ml; toxicity has been reported with levels above 20 mcg/ml.

②, ③, ④ These levels may be considered toxic. The patient needs to be assessed for theophylline toxicity.

383. Application, planning, reduction of risk potential (c)
❸ A patient with COPD requires additional calories because of the increased work of breathing.
① The meals should be small and offered six times a day, yet the patient needs calories to meet body requirements.
② Fluids should be taken between meals to prevent excess stomach distention but plain water would be better than juice due to the GERD.
④ A diet that is high in carbohydrates should be avoided in patients retaining CO_2.

384. Application, assessment, basic care and comfort (b)
④ Labored breathing is a cardinal symptom.
①, ③ These may also be accompanying complaints, but are not a cardinal symptom.
② Skin turgor does not relate to a respiratory dysfunction.

385. Comprehension, assessment, reduction of risk potential (c)
❶ CO_2 is trapped in the alveoli. This is the basic problem in emphysema. Respiratory acidosis occurs when the lungs can't exhale CO_2 adequately. As a result, the $PaCO_2$ and carbonic acid increase and pH decreases.
② Hyperventilation causes the rapid blowing off of CO_2.
③, ④ These are potential effects of emphysema, not the basic cause of acidosis.

386. Comprehension, implementation, safety and infection control (b)
❸ Hand washing for at least 20 seconds is still found to be the best means of preventing disease transmission.
①, ② These should only be used when medically indicated.
④ Hand washing is part of standard precautions. Potential for exposure to blood and body fluids determine the need for protective equipment.

387. Application, assessment, basic care and comfort (b)
❸ Characteristically vertigo or the sensation of spinning is a chief complaint with Ménière's.
① Hearing loss would be gradual.
②, ④ Ear pain is usually not described, however, a feeling of fullness or headache may be an accompanying complaint.

388. Application, implementation, physiological adaptation (b)
❶ Persons with cataracts need to be encouraged to avoid sunlight and wear sunglasses to decrease glare and the shattering of light.
② Surgical procedures are also available if the patient chooses. The "cataract" glasses are not commonly used today.
③ Eye pain is not associated with cataracts.
④ Persons with cataracts usually have poor night vision. Driving at night is not encouraged.

389. Comprehension, implementation, basic care and comfort (a)
❷ Beverages that irritate the bladder are citrus, alcohol, coffee, tea, colas, and carbonated drinks.

①, ③, ④ These have not been identified as irritating to the bladder.

390. Comprehension, implementation, pharmacological therapies (b)
❷ Serial measurements of peak flow rate provide objective data of the therapeutics of drug response.
①, ④ This may be an indirect result.
③ Blood test monitoring should be done while on bronchodilator therapy.

391. Application, assessment, reduction of risk potential (b)
❶ These are indicative of decreased tissue oxygenation.
②, ③, ④ These are all normal assessment data.

392. Application, assessment, pharmacological therapies (b)
❸ Diuretics increase the quantity and alter the characteristics of the urine.
① Calcium channel blockers may affect the ability of the bladder or sphincter to contract or relax normally.
② Anticoagulants may cause hematuria.
④ Antihistamines may affect the ability of the bladder or sphincter to contract or relax normally.

393. Application, implementation, reduction of risk potential (b)
❶ Ambulation helps to promote passing the stone, as does encouraging fluids.
②, ③ These measures are contraindicated in the patient with urinary tract stones.
④ There is no need to restrict protein.

394. Knowledge, assessment, basic care and comfort (a)
❸ Upper UTIs affect the ureters and kidneys.
① This is cystitis, a lower UTI.
② A UTI ascends up the urethra. This is urethritis, a lower tract urinary infection.
④ UTIs may spread through the bloodstream.

395. Comprehension, implementation, reduction of risk potential (b)
❸ Voiding this often in addition to having adequate fluid intake has been shown to reduce the possibility of urinary stasis and reinfection.
① This is true for those patients who need bladder training such as with incontinence.
② Reflex incontinence is seen in neurogenic disorders. It is the loss of urine because of detrusor hyperreflexia and/or involuntary urethral relaxation in the absence of the desire to void.
④ This is dribbling of urine by reason of the inability of the bladder to empty itself. The cause for this problem should be determined. It is true that this problem may lead to urinary tract infections.

396. Application, implementation, reduction of risk potential (c)
❶ The orange juice is a simple source of carbohydrate, which would increase his glucose level quickly. Remember that the normal glucose level needs to be between 75 to 110 mg/dl.

② This is unsafe. This action would increase his potential for insulin shock.
③ There is no need to call the physician immediately; however, the physician should be made aware of action taken and the patient's response.
④ This action may be appropriate, but it is not the first action.

397. Application, implementation, physiological adaptation (b)
❸ This is the most life threatening.
① This is a normal urine output.
② Hypothermia may result because of fluid evaporation from open wounds.
④ Patient comfort is important. Pain medication may be necessary prior to dressing changes.

398. Comprehension, planning, reduction of risk potential (b)
❶ Fever increases the body's energy expenditures and profuse perspiration causes fluid loss, resulting in the body's increased need for fluids. If fluids are not replaced, dehydration will occur.
②, ③, ④ The opposite occurs due to fluid loss. Respirations increase with fever.

399. Application, assessment, reduction of risk potential (b)
❹ Hypocalcemia may occur in patients with chronic renal failure because the kidneys become unable to excrete phosphorus. Serum phosphorus levels increase and calcium level decrease.
① There is no direct relationship between vitamin C intake and calcium.
② Potassium is the electrolyte most directly affected with diuretic medications.
③ Hyperparathyroidism results in hypercalcemia and bone demineralization.

400. Application, implementation, reduction of risk potential (b)
❹ ICP is the pressure produced by the brain tissue, CSF and blood volume within the skull. Allowing the patient to rest between nursing activities helps to keep the ICP within 5-15 mm Hg. Doing too many activities may increase metabolic demands that would alter the balance of the three components which determine ICP and the brain's inherent compensatory capability.
①, ② Coughing and suctioning as also laying flat, bearing down or Valsalva maneuver may cause ICP to rise.
③ It is necessary to avoid neck and hip flexion. Maintaining the patient's neck, hips, and knees in alignment to promote venous flow. High-Fowler's causes flexion. A semi-Fowler's position improves cerebral perfusion and allows for gravity to drain fluid from the brain.

CHAPTER 6

Mental Health Nursing

The licensed practical/vocational nurse (LP/VN) requires a knowledge of mental health nursing principles in a variety of practice settings. Basic mental health concepts are useful in understanding the response to diseases and dysfunctions of both physical and social systems. Each person responds to disease and disorder in accordance with his or her own basic personality traits, past experiences, intelligence, and innate coping mechanisms. These concepts are explored and studied in mental health nursing.

HOLISM

A. Definition: This concept of health holds that illness results from a complex interaction between the mind and body and the environment

B. Approaches to treatment: multifaceted approaches are used to treat disturbances, rather than simply relying on treatment aimed at specific symptoms; we are no longer content to treat the illness; we are learning to treat the whole person. Approaches include the following dimensions:
  1. Physical
  2. Emotional
  3. Intellectual
  4. Sociocultural
  5. Spiritual

MENTAL HEALTH CONTINUUM

A. Mental health and mental illness are seen as opposite poles on a continuum

B. The precise point at which an individual is deemed mentally ill is determined not only by the specific behavior exhibited but also by the context in which the behavior is seen

C. Some behaviors considered deviant in one setting are considered normal in another setting

D. Variations are based on the culture, the time or era, the specific personal characteristics of the individual, and many other variables

E. Behaviors of the mentally ill are exaggerations of normal human behaviors

MENTAL HEALTH

A. Definition: an individual's ability to manage life's problems and to derive satisfaction from living throughout various life stages

B. Persons may experience times of greater or lesser satisfaction with life, and at times of lesser satisfaction may seek the assistance of a therapist

C. No clear set of characteristics specific to mental health can be identified
  1. All behavior is considered meaningful and may be interpreted as the individual's effort to adapt or cope with the environment
  2. At times some adaptations fail; others are continued long after the need for them has passed; still others may be directed to an undesired end

MENTAL ILLNESS

A. Definition: a pattern of behavior that is disturbing to the individual or the community in which the individual resides. Behaviors may interfere with daily activities, impair judgment, or alter reality. A mental illness is a disturbance of a person's ability to cope effectively, which results in maladaptive behaviors and impaired functioning
  1. The person who is mentally ill acts in ways that seem unrelated to current reality
  2. Relationships with family and friends are disturbed
  3. The person's ability to work and to contribute to his or her own welfare may be impaired
  4. The person often experiences subjective discomfort
  5. The person may exhibit symptoms such as delusions, hallucinations, paranoia, passive-aggressive behavior, or compulsions

B. Historical perspective of mental illness
  1. Early history
    a. Mentally ill persons were thought to be possessed by supernatural forces/evil spirits
    b. Mentally ill persons were ostracized from society or mistreated in other ways
    c. Mentally ill persons were regarded as messengers of the gods or as divinely possessed
    d. Attitudes did not change significantly until the modern era
  2. Classical era (Greco-Roman)
    a. Certain attitudes changed toward mental illness
    b. Early scientific interest led to various descriptive or classification systems
    c. The idea of divine possession was rejected in favor of the Humoral Theory of Disease
    d. Humors were thought to be basic internal fluids capable of controlling behavior
    e. The terms *melancholia* and *hysteria* are derived from these ancient beliefs
  3. The Middle Ages
    a. Return to the idea of divine possession and spiritual explanations of mental illness
    b. The mentally ill person was often mistreated by incarceration
  4. Modern era: numerous reforms were instituted (Box 6-1)
  5. Later modern developments include
    a. Discovery of phenothiazines (the major tranquilizers)
    b. Community mental health: 1960s; still in use today; aim is to provide care of mentally ill persons in their own communities rather than in large institutions: a primary goal of the community mental health concept is to return patients to their homes as quickly as possible and to foster the development of support systems in the community
    c. Patients released from large hospitals: late 1970s; large numbers of mentally ill persons were released into communities where they often did not receive treatment either because they did not seek it out or because adequate types of services were not available; this process is called *deinstitutionalization;* some believe that there is an increase of "street people" as a result of the process
    d. Community mental health centers
    e. Mental health costs were decreased in the United States because of the development and use of psychotropic medications

THE NURSING ROLE

A. The nursing process
  1. Assessment: the licensed practical nurse gathers subjective and objective data through observation, interview, and examination. Data obtained through:
    a. Health history
    b. Mental status exam
      (1) General appearance
      (2) Affect and mood
      (3) Intellect and sensorium
      (4) Thought processes
      (5) Insight

Box 6-1   Historic Highlights

Eighteenth Century

Phillipe Pinel (1745-1826, France): freed mentally ill persons from chains

Benjamin Rush (1745-1813, United States): founded Pennsylvania Hospital; the father of American psychiatry

Nineteenth Century

Florence Nightingale (1860, England): founder of modern nursing

Dorothea Dix (1802-1887, United States): promoted legislation to establish mental hospitals

Linda Richards (1873, United States): first psychiatric nurse

Daniel Tuke (1827-1895, England): founded York Retreat based on Quaker principles

Twentieth Century

Clifford Beers (1876-1943, United States): wrote the book, *The Mind That Found Itself,* generating public concern for the treatment of mentally ill persons

Adolf Meyer (1866-1950, United States): Director of the Johns Hopkins Clinic; founder of the mental hygiene movement

Emil Kraepelin (1856-1926, Germany): classified mental disorders

Eugene Bleuler (1857-1939, Switzerland): coined the word *schizophrenia* and classified it into types

Sigmund Freud (1856-1939, Austria): developed psychoanalytic theory; revolutionized psychiatry

Carl Jung (1875-1961, Switzerland): developed a personality theory that included the concepts of introversion and extroversion

Karen Horney (1885-1952, United States): theorized that culture had a great influence on mental illness

Box 6-2   Psychiatric–Mental Health Nursing's Phenomena of Concern

Actual or potential mental health problems of clients pertaining to the following:

- The maintenance of optimal health and well-being and the prevention of psychobiological illness
- Self-care limitations or impaired functioning related to mental and emotional distress
- Deficits in the functioning of significant biological, emotional, and cognitive systems
- Emotional stress or crisis components of illness, pain, and disability
- Self-concept changes, developmental issues, and life process changes
- Problems related to emotions such as anxiety, anger, sadness, loneliness, and grief
- Physical symptoms that occur along with altered psychological functioning
- Alterations in thinking, perceiving, symbolizing, communicating, and decision making
- Difficulties in relating to others
- Behaviors and mental states that indicate the patient is a danger to self or others or has a severe disability
- Interpersonal, systemic, sociocultural, spiritual, or environmental circumstances or events that affect the mental and emotional well-being of the individual, family, or community
- Symptom management, side effects/toxicities associated with psychopharmacological intervention and other aspects of the treatment regimen

From American Nurses' Association: *A statement on psychiatric mental health clinical nursing practice and standards of psychiatric mental health clinical nursing practice,* Washington, DC, 1994, The Association.

---

   c. Results of psychological testing
      (1) Intelligence testing
      (2) Personality testing
   d. Self assessment; e.g., stress scale; decision-making trees
   e. Physical examination
2. Diagnosis: nurses diagnose and treat human responses to illness; the nursing diagnosis is formulated by the registered professional nurse; the licensed practical nurse contributes to this phase of the nursing process through collection of objective and subjective data; potential nursing diagnoses identify the problem and the etiology of the problem; actual nursing diagnoses identify the problem, etiology, and signs and symptoms; the NANDA listing is used; sample actual and potential nursing diagnoses used in mental health nursing include the following:
   a. Anxiety (panic) related to family rejection; manifested by chest discomfort, palpitations, dizziness, diaphoresis, and trembling
   b. Impaired social interaction related to negative role modeling; manifested by verbalized and observed discomfort in social situations
   c. High risk for violence: self-directed; related to history of suicide attempts.
   d. High risk for trauma; related to muscular incoordination

   The psychiatric-mental health areas of concern for formulating nursing diagnoses appear in Box 6-2
3. Planning: the plan of care is based on the nursing diagnosis; specific nursing interventions are devised to attain specifically stated goals; when possible, goals should be developed jointly with the patient and cooperation enlisted; goals may be short term or long term; all goals should be prioritized, emphasizing reduction or elimination of the identified problem; goals usually include the anticipated length of time for accomplishment and the standard for judging whether the goal has been met
4. Implementation: the planned nursing actions that assist the patient to achieve the identified goal e.g., health teaching, activities of daily living, other prescribed treatments, and medications; this is an ongoing phase, and reactions to treatment are observed and documented so that the care plan may be modified periodically as goals are met
5. Evaluation: outcome achievement is identified as well as the factors that affected the goal being met, partially

met, or not met; this is followed by deciding whether to continue, modify, or terminate the plan; following evaluation of goal achievement the entire nursing process and care plan are reviewed, modified, or updated to reflect new nursing diagnoses

B. Principles of mental health nursing
1. Understand your inner needs, thoughts, and feelings and be aware of how these affect patients
2. Be aware of your own resources and limitations so as to function effectively in mental health nursing
3. Respect the patient as a person; take time to listen to what is said
4. Be aware of the patient's dignity; show patience and understanding
5. Be nonjudgmental and nonthreatening; patients must be accepted as they are to establish a trusting relationship
6. Be honest
7. Reassure patients by being available and allaying fears
8. Explain routine, rules, and regulations when appropriate
9. Maintain a calm, hopeful attitude
10. Encourage reality testing and avoid entering into patient's unrealistic thinking
11. Emphasize strengths that the patient displays by acknowledging healthy behavior; offer warm understanding but do not encourage overdependency or intimacy
12. Remember that all staff members are role models and are often viewed as authority figures by patients
13. Help reduce anxiety by making as few demands as possible on patients
14. Explain what is happening to the patient in simple, understandable language
15. Remain objective but do not display aloofness or distance; maintain your awareness of the patient's humanity and dignity
16. Maintain a nurse/patient relationship that is always realistic and professional
17. Remember that there is a reason for all behavior
18. Note that behavior is changed through emotional experience rather than through rational means
19. Allow patients to exercise all of their basic human rights
20. Use the least restrictive method(s) of controlling behavior, such as communication
21. Respect the confidentiality of the patient

C. Communications in mental health nursing
1. Communication: a complex activity consisting of a series of events, each interdependent on the other, which results in a negotiated understanding between two or more people in a given situation
   a. Communication is not merely the exchange of information
   b. Each message (input) generates an extremely complex reaction that eventually leads to a selective response (output), which in turn becomes a new input for the communicators
2. Modes of communication
   a. The most apparent form is verbal (written or spoken language); spoken is the more important in mental health nursing
   b. Spoken communication is always accompanied by at least one of the following additional communication forms
      (1) Paralanguage: voice quality, tones, grunts, and other nonword vocalizations
      (2) Kinesis: facial expression, gestures, and eye and body movements
      (3) Proxemics: the spatial relationship between persons
      (4) Touch and messages to other sensory organs: aromas and cultural artifacts (jewelry, clothing, hairstyle)
   c. Effective communications are
      (1) Efficient: messages are simple, clear, and timed correctly
      (2) Appropriate: relevant to the situation
      (3) Flexible: open to alteration based on perceived response
      (4) Receptive: allow feedback (checking and correcting by either or both parties)
3. Therapeutic communication (Box 6-3)
4. Blocks to communication (Table 6-1)

D. Nurse-patient relationship
1. One-to-one relationship between a nurse and a patient
2. Patient centered
3. Goal directed
4. Not for mutual satisfaction
5. Focus is on modification of patient behavior, increasing patient's self-worth, and developing patient's coping strategies
6. Therapeutic, not social, relationship
7. Phases
   a. Preorientation: data collection about the patient; self-analysis of attitudes, biases, and perceptions by the nurse
   b. Orientation: 2 to 10 sessions; become acquainted; establish trust and rapport; establish parameters of the relationship; contract discussions; identify patient problems; build on patient's strengths
   c. Working: begins when the patient demonstrates responsibility to uphold terms of the contract; establish priorities and goals with patient; help patient achieve behavior change (e.g., discussion, role playing); focus on the present; reinforce the contract terms as necessary
   d. Termination: begins during orientation phase; purpose is to conclude the relationship; focus on patient growth, help patient with expression of feelings about relationship closure

E. Applications of mental health nursing
1. Community mental health center
2. Partial hospitalization setting: day or night hospitals
3. Mental health clinic
4. Liaison: use of mental health workers in general hospital setting
5. Alcohol and drug-abuse facilities and clinics
6. Inpatient units
7. Crisis intervention
8. Health maintenance organizations

Box 6-3   Therapeutic Communication Techniques

Listening

Definition: An active process of receiving information and examining reaction to the messages received

Example: Maintaining eye contact and receptive nonverbal communication

Therapeutic value: Nonverbally communicates to the patient the nurse's interest and acceptance

Broad Openings

Definition: Encouraging the patient to select topics for discussion

Example: "What are you thinking about?"

Therapeutic value: Indicates acceptance by the nurse and the value of the patient's initiative

Restating

Definition: Repeating the main thought the patient expressed

Example: "You say that your mother left you when you were 5 years old."

Therapeutic value: Indicates that the nurse is listening and validates, reinforces, or calls attention to something important that has been said

Clarification

Definition: Attempting to put into words vague ideas or unclear thoughts of the patient to enhance the nurse's understanding or asking the patient to explain what he means

Example: "I'm not sure what you mean. Could you tell me about that again?"

Therapeutic value: Helps to clarify feelings, ideas, and perceptions of the patient and provide an explicit correlation between them and the patient's actions

Reflection

Definition: Directing back the patient's ideas, feelings, questions, and content

Example: "You're feeling tense and anxious and it's related to a conversation you had with your husband last night?"

Therapeutic value: Validates the nurse's understanding of what the patient is saying and signifies empathy, interest, and respect for the patient

Humor

Definition: The discharge of energy through the comic enjoyment of the imperfect

Example: "That gives a whole new meaning to the word *nervous,*" said with shared kidding between the nurse and patient

Therapeutic value: Can promote insight by making conscious repressed material, resolving paradoxes, tempering aggression, and revealing new options, and is a socially acceptable form of sublimation

Informing

Definition: The skill of information giving

Example: "I think you need to know more about how your medication works."

Therapeutic value: Helpful in health teaching or patient education about relevant aspects of patient's well-being and self-care

Focusing

Definition: Questions or statements that help the patient expand on a topic of importance

Example: "I think that we should talk more about your relationship with your father."

Therapeutic value: Allows the patient to discuss central issues and keeps the communication process goal-directed

Sharing Perceptions

Definition: Asking the patient to verify the nurse's understanding of what the patient is thinking or feeling

Example: "You're smiling but I sense that you are really very angry with me."

Therapeutic value: Conveys the nurse's understanding to the patient and has the potential for clearing up confusing communication

Theme Identification

Definition: Underlying issues or problems experienced by the patient that emerge repeatedly during the course of the nurse-patient relationship

Example: "I've noticed that in all of the relationships that you have described, you've been hurt or rejected by the man. Do you think this is an underlying issue?"

Therapeutic value: Allows the nurse to best promote the patient's exploration and understanding of important problems

Silence

Definition: Lack of verbal communication for a therapeutic reason

Example: Sitting with a patient and nonverbally communicating interest and involvement

Therapeutic value: Allows the patient time to think and gain insights, slows the pace of the interaction and encourages the patient to initiate conversation, while conveying the nurse's support, understanding, and acceptance

Suggesting

Definition: Presentation of alternative ideas for the patient's consideration relative to problem solving

Example: "Have you thought about responding to your boss in a different way when he raises that issue with you? For example, you could ask him if a specific problem has occurred."

Therapeutic value: Increases the patient's perceived options or choices

Modified from Stuart GW, Laraia MT: *Principles and practice of psychiatric nursing,* ed 6, St Louis, 1998, Mosby.

TABLE 6-1   Ineffective Responses That Hinder Therapeutic Communication

Response	Discussion	Nontherapeutic Response	Therapeutic Response
Offering False Reassurance	The nurse, in an effort to be supportive and to make the patient's pain disappear, offers reassuring clichés. This response is not based on fact. It brushes aside the patient's feelings and closes off communication. Often, it is due to the nurse's inability to listen to the patient's negative emotions. No one can predict the outcome of a situation.	"Don't worry, everything will be OK." "Things will be better soon; you'll see."	"I know you have a lot going on right now. Let's make a list and begin to discuss them one at a time. Working toward solutions will assist you to get through this."
Not Listening	The nurse is preoccupied with other work that needs to be done, is distracted by noise in the area, is thinking about personal problems.	"I'm sorry, what did you say?" "Could you start again? I was listening to the other nurse."	"That is interesting. Please elaborate." "I really hear what you are saying . . . it must be difficult."
Offering Approval	It is most important how a patient feels about what he or she said or did. The patient ultimately must approve of his or her own actions.	"That's good." "I agree—I think you should have told him."	"What do you think about what you said to him?" "How do you feel about it?"
Minimizing Problem	The nurse may use this when it is difficult to hear the enormity of a particular problem. This is used in an effort to try to make the patient feel better. It cuts off communication.	"That's nothing compared to that other client's problem." "Everyone feels that way at times, it's not a big deal."	"That is a very difficult problem for you." "That sounds pretty important for you to deal with."
Offering Advice	This response undermines patients' ability to solve their own problems. It serves to render them dependent and helpless. If the solution provided by the nurse does not work, the patient may blame the outcome on the nurse. Patients do not take responsibility for developing outcomes. The nurse maintains control and at the same time devalues the patient.	"I think you should . . ." "In my opinion, it would be wise to . . ." "Why don't you do . . ." "The best solution is . . ."	"What do *you* think you should do?" "There can be several alternatives—let's talk about some. However, the final decision must be yours. I will listen to your problem and help you see it clearly. We can develop a pros and cons list, which may assist you in solving the problem."
Giving Literal Responses	The nurse feeds into a patient's delusions of hallucinations, denies patient the opportunity to see reality. This does not provide a healthy response toward growth.	P: "That TV is talking to me." N: "What is it saying to you?" P: "There is nuclear power coming through the air ducts." N: "I'll turn off the A/C for a while."	"The TV is on for everyone." "There is cool air blowing from the vents. It is the A/C system."
Changing the Subject	The nurse changes the topic at a crucial time because the discussion is too uncomfortable. It negates what the patient seems interested in discussing. Communication will remain superficial.	P: "My mother always puts me down." N: "That's interesting, but let's talk about . . ."	"Tell me about that."

Belittling	The nurse puts down patient's expressed feelings to avoid having to deal with painful feelings.	P: "I don't want to live anymore now that my child is gone." N: "Anyone would be sad, but that's no reason to want to die."	"The death must be very difficult for you. Tell me a little more about how you are feeling."
Disagreeing	The nurse criticizes the patient who is seeking support.	"I definitely do not agree with your view." "I really don't believe that."	"Let's talk about the way you see that." "It seems hard to believe. Please explain further."
Judging	The nurse's responses are filled with his or her own values and judgments. This demonstrates a lack of acceptance of the patient's differences. It will provide a barrier to further disclosures.	"You are not married. Do you think having this baby will solve your problems?" "This is certainly not the Christian thing to do." "You are thinking about divorce when you have three children?"	"What will having this baby provide for you?" "What do you think about what you are attempting to do?" "Let's discuss this option," or "Let's discuss other options."
Excessive Probing	Serves to control the nature of the patient's responses. The nurse asks many questions of patients before they are ready to provide the information. This is self-protective to the nurse by avoiding the anxiety of uncomfortable silences. The patient feels overwhelmed and may withdraw.	"Why do you do this?" "What do you think was the real cause?" "Do you always feel this way?" "Why do you think that way?"	"Tell me how this is upsetting you." "Tell me what you believe to be the cause." "Tell me how you feel when that happens." "Explain your thinking on this if you can."
Challenging	This stems from the nurse's belief that if patients are challenged regarding their unrealistic beliefs, they will be coerced into seeing reality. The patient may feel threatened when challenged, holding onto the beliefs more strongly.	"You are not the Queen of England." "If your leg is missing, then how can you walk this hall?"	"You sound like you want to be important." "It seems to you like you are missing a leg. Tell me more about that."
Superficial Comments	The nurse gives simple or meaningless responses to patients. It suggests a lack of understanding regarding the patient as an individual. The interactions remain superficial, maintaining distance between nurse and patient. Nothing of significance is communicated.	"Great day, huh!" "You should be feeling good; you are being discharged today." "Keep the faith; your doctor should be coming anytime now."	"What kind of day are you having?" "How are you feeling about leaving the hospital today?" "You look worried. Your doctor called and said he would be here within the hour."
Defending	The nurse may believe she or he must defend herself or himself, the staff, or the hospital. The nurse may not take the time to listen to the patient's concerns. Efforts need to be made to explore the patient's thoughts and feelings.	"Your doctor is a good doctor. He would never say that." "We have a very experienced staff here. They would not ever do that."	"What has you so upset about your doctor?" "Tell me what happened on the evening shift."

Continued

From Fortinash KM, Holoday-Worret PA: *Psychiatric-mental health nursing*, ed 2, St Louis, 1999, Mosby.

TABLE 6-1 Ineffective Responses That Hinder Therapeutic Communication—cont'd

Response	Discussion	Nontherapeutic Response	Therapeutic Response
Self-focusing	The nurse focuses attention away from the patient by thinking about sharing his or her own thoughts, feelings, problems. The focus is taken away from the patient who is seeking help. The nurse is more interested in what to say next instead of actively listening to the patient.	"That may have happened to you last year, but it happened to me twice this month, which hurt me a great deal and . . ." "Excuse me but could you say that again? I have a response to make, but I want to be sure of what you said."	"Tell me about your incident and how it might relate to your sadness now." "If I heard you accurately, you said . . ."
Criticism of Others	The nurse puts down others.	P: "The staff members on the day shift let me smoke two cigarettes." N: "The day shift is always breaking the rules. On this shift, we follow the one cigarette policy." P: "My daughter is hateful to me." N: "She must be just awful to live with."	"The policy is one cigarette, which we must follow." "It sounds like you are having a rough time now with your daughter."
Premature Interpretation	The nurse does not wait until the patient fully expresses thoughts and feelings related to a particular problem. This rushes the patient and disregards his or her input. The nurse may miss what the patient wants to explain.	"I think this is what you really mean." "You may think that way consciously, but your unconscious believes . . ."	"What do you think this means?" "So you think . . ."

From Fortinash KM, Holoday-Worret PA: *Psychiatric-mental health nursing*, ed 2, St Louis, 1999, Mosby.

PERSONALITY DEVELOPMENT

A. Definition: a consistent set of behaviors peculiar to a specific individual; the sum of thoughts, feelings, physical characteristics, and sociocultural biases on which all behavior is built
B. Heredity
   1. Personality is influenced by inherited characteristics, both physical and psychological
   2. Controversy exists over the extent of genetic influence on specific human behaviors
C. Environment
   1. The environment is a strong determining factor in the individual's development
   2. Environment includes the intrauterine environment as well as all the external factors that influence the individual after birth
D. Physical basis: personality develops normally if the necessary physical basis is present
   1. The brain is the major organ of thought and is necessary to development of personality
   2. Other influential factors include a normally functioning endocrine system, which strongly influences behavior
E. Major theorists (Table 6-2)
F. Elements of personality (Freud)
   1. Levels of consciousness
      a. The unconscious: always outside the awareness of the individual; influences actions in ways the individual may not understand; thought to include dreams
      b. The preconscious: usually outside awareness; available to conscious mind in special circumstances such as under hypnosis or during therapy
      c. The conscious: ordinary awareness
   2. Structures: some theorists refer to personality structures
      a. Freud: ego, id, superego
      b. Berne: child, adult, parent
   3. Functions: each structure is thought to perform specific functions (Freud)
      a. Id/child: basic, innate psychic energy; emotional
      b. Ego/adult: mediates between person's perception and objective reality; always rational
      c. Superego/parent: incorporates societal values; judgmental and critical
G. Development levels: various theorists describe levels of development
   1. Freud: oral, anal, phallic, latency, genital
   2. Erikson: basic trust vs. mistrust; autonomy vs. shame and doubt; initiative vs. guilt; industry vs. inferiority; identity vs. role diffusion; intimacy vs. isolation; generativity vs. stagnation; ego integrity vs. despair
H. Development of the self-concept
   1. Development through experience with other people, e.g., parents, siblings, relatives, peers, teachers, and other adults
      a. Feelings of adequacy or inadequacy
      b. Feelings of acceptance or rejection
      c. Opportunities for identification
      d. Expectations of values, goals, and behaviors
   2. Self-concept consists of
      a. Body image: one's perception of one's body
      b. Self-ideal: one's idea of what is "good" behavior
      c. Self-esteem: personal judgment of one's own worth

   d. Role: one's perception of how one fits into the society
   e. Identity: the combination of all of the above into a unified whole

Stress

Hans Selye (1956) defined stress as "wear and tear on the body." All people are continuously exposed to varieties of stress: physical, chemical, psychological, and emotional. Almost any situation, pleasant or unpleasant, that requires change leads to some level of stress. Stress produces a clearly identifiable response called the general adaptation syndrome. It is associated with concomitant physical and chemical changes that commonly occur in the body.

EGO DEFENSE MECHANISMS

Ego defense mechanisms are basic psychological tools that individuals use at various times to manage life's crises. They may also be referred to as ego defenses, defense mechanisms, or protective mechanisms. As such, they defend the ego or self from untoward anxiety, help resolve conflicts, and return the individual to a point of psychological homeostasis or comfort. They are usually outside conscious awareness and are not considered pathological in and of themselves. They should not be removed or challenged until the individual is ready and has adequate strength to tolerate the stressful situation. Common defenses are listed in Table 6-3.

MENTAL DISTURBANCES AND RESOURCES
Anxiety

A. Definition: a state of alertness or apprehension, tension or uneasiness; a major component of all mental disturbances. Anxiety is an internal state experienced by the individual when there is a perceived threat to the physical body or to the psychological integrity of the person; it interferes with concentration, focusing attention on the perceived threat; in its mild form anxiety serves to alert the person to danger and to prepare the body to react to danger; in its severe form it is debilitating and may immobilize the person and interfere with activities; anxiety is usually described in degrees or levels
B. Process: coping behaviors
   1. Adaptive coping: the problem creating the anxiety is resolved
   2. Palliative coping: the problem creating the anxiety is not resolved but rather temporarily reduced; the problem returns at a later date
   3. Maladaptive coping: energy is channeled toward reducing the anxiety and no effort is made to solve the problem
   4. Dysfunctional coping: the problem is not solved and the anxiety not reduced
C. Levels
   1. Mild (+1)
   2. Moderate (+2)
   3. Severe (+3)
   4. Panic (+4)
D. Assessment (Table 6-4)
E. Interventions
   1. Remain with the highly anxious patient; leaving the patient alone increases anxiety

Text continued on p. 368

TABLE 6-2 A Comparison of the Development Stages Postulated by Freud, Sullivan, Erikson, and Piaget

Freud	Sullivan	Erikson	Piaget

I. Oral stage (0-18 mo)
a. The mouth is a source of satisfaction
b. Two phases
  1. Passive
    Only interests are satisfying hunger and *sucking*
    Completely helpless, *security* is the greatest need
    Narcissistic and egocentric, operates on *pleasure principle*
    Omnipotent feelings are prevalent
  2. Active
    Biting is a mode of pleasure
    Continuous experimentation and associations
    Sensory discriminations
    Differentiation between mental images and reality
    Differentiation of others and discovery of self
	I. Infancy (0-18 mo)
	a. The mouth is a source of satisfaction
	b. Mouth—takes in (sucking), cuts off (biting), and pushes out (spitting) objects introduced by others
	c. Crying, babbling, and cooing are modes of communication used by the infant to call attention of adults to self
	d. *Satisfaction response (pleasure principle).* Infant's biological needs are met and a mutual feeling of comfort and fulfillment is experienced by mother and infant (mother gives and infant takes)
	e. *Empathic observation.* Capacity to perceive feelings of others as his or her own immediate feelings in the situation
	f. *Autistic invention.* State of symbolic activity in which the infant feels he or she is master of all he or she surveys
	g. Experimentation, exploration, and manipulation are methods used to acquaint self with environment
		I. Oral-sensory stage (0-12 mo)
		a. The mouth is a source of satisfaction and a means of dealing with anxiety-producing situations
		b. Focus is on the development of the basic attitudes of *trust vs. mistrust*
		c. Attitudes are formed through mother's reaction to infant needs
			I. Sensorimotor stage (0-12 mo)
			a. Emphasis is on preverbal intellectual development
			b. Learns relationships with external objects
			c. Focus is on physical development with gradual increase in ability to think and use language

II. Anal stage (1½-3 yr) a. Primary activity is on learning muscular control association with urination and defecation *(toilet training period)* b. Exhibits more self-control; walks, talks, dresses, and undresses c. *Negativism*—assertion of independence d. Introduction of *reality principle,* ego development e. Superego begins to develop f. Engages in parallel play	II. Childhood (1½-6 yr) a. Begins with the capacity for communicating through speech and ends with a beginning need for association with peers b. Uses language as a tool to communicate wishes and needs c. Anus is power tool used to give or withhold a part of self to control significant people in his environment d. Emergence and integration of *self-concept* and *reflected appraisal of significant persons*	II. Anal-muscular stage (1-3 yr) a. Learns the extent to which the *environment* can be influenced by direct manipulation b. Focuses on the development of the basic attitudes of *autonomy vs. shame and doubt* c. Exerts self-control and willpower	II. Preoperational stage (2-7 yr) a. Learns to use symbols and language b. Learns to imitate and play c. Displays egocentricity d. Engages in *animistic thinking*—endowment of objects with power and ability

e. Awareness that postponing or delaying gratification of won wishes may bring satisfaction
f. Begins to find limits in experimentation, exploration, and manipulation
g. More aggressive
h. Uses parallel play and curiosity to explore environment
i. Uses exhibitionism and masturbatory activity to become acquainted with self and others
j. Demonstrates a beginning ability to think abstractly

III. Phallic stage (3-6 yr)
a. *Libidinal energy focus on the genitals*
b. Learns *sexual identity*
c. *Superego becomes internalized*
d. Sibling rivalry and manipulation of parents occurs
e. Intellectual and motor facilities are refined
f. Increased socialization and *associative play*

IV. Latency (6-12 yr)
a. *Quiet stage in which sexual development lies dormant, emotional tension eases*
b. *Normal homosexual phase*
   For boys, gangs
   For girls, cliques
c. Increased intellectual capacity
d. Starts school
e. Identifies with teachers and peers
f. Weakening of home ties
g. Recognizes authority figures outside home, age of *hero worship*

III. Genital-locomotor stage (3-6 yr)
a. Learns the extent to which being *assertive* will influence the environment
b. Focus is on the development of the *basic attitudes of initiative vs. guilt*
c. Explores the world with senses, thoughts, and imagination
d. Activities demonstrate direction and purpose
e. Engages in first real social contacts through *cooperative play*
f. Develops conscience

IV. Latency (6-12 yr)
a. Learns to use energy to create, develop, and manipulate
b. Focus is on the development of basic attitudes of *industry vs. inferiority*
c. Able to initiate and complete tasks
d. Understands rules and regulations
e. Displays competence and productivity

III. Juvenile stage (6-9 yr)
a. Learns to form satisfactory relationship with peers
b. *Peer norms* prevail over family norms
c. Engages in *competition*, experimentation, exploration, and manipulation
d. Able to cooperate and compromise
e. Demonstrates capacity to love
f. Distinguishes fantasy from reality
g. Exerts internal control over behavior

III. Concrete operations stage (7-11 yr)
a. Deals with visible concrete objects and relationships
b. Increased intellectual and conceptual development—uses logic and reasoning
c. More socialized and rule conscious

Continued

Modified from Kreigh H, Perko J: *Psychiatric and mental health nursing: commitment to care and concern*. Reston, 1979, Reston Publishing.

TABLE 6-2   A Comparison of the Development Stages Postulated by Freud, Sullivan, Erikson, and Piaget—cont'd

Freud	Sullivan	Erikson	Piaget
V. Genital stage (12 yr–early adulthood) a. Appearance of secondary sex characteristics, reawakening of sex drives b. Increased concern over physical appearance c. Striving toward independence d. Development of sexual maturity e. Identity crisis f. Identification of love object of opposite sex g. Intellectual maturity h. Plans future	IV. Preadolescence (9-12 yr) a. Learns to relate to a friend of the same sex—*chum relationship* b. Concerned with group success and derives satisfaction from group accomplishment c. Shows signs of *rebellion*—restlessness, hostility, irritability d. Assumes less responsibility for own actions e. Moves from egocentricity to a more full social state f. Uses experimentation, exploration, manipulation g. Seeks *consensual validation* from peers V. Early adolescence (12-14 yr) a. Experiences physiological changes b. Uses rebellion to gain independence c. Fantasizes, overidentifies with heroes d. Discovers and begins relationships with opposite sex e. Demonstrates heightened levels of anxiety in most interpersonal relationships VI. Late adolescence (14-21 yr) a. Establishes an enduring intimate relationship with one member of the opposite sex b. Self-concept becomes stabilized c. Attains physical maturity d. Develops ability to use logic and abstract concepts	V. Puberty and adolescence (12-18 yr) a. Demonstrates an ability to integrate life experiences b. Focuses on the development of the basic attitudes of *identity vs. role diffusion* c. Seeks partner of the opposite sex d. Begins to establish identity and place in society VI. Young adulthood (18-35 yr) a. Primarily concerned with developing an intimate relationship with another adult b. Focus is on the development of the basic attitudes of *intimacy and solidarity vs. isolation*	IV. Formal operations stage (11-15 yr) a. Develops true abstract thought b. Formulates hypothesis and applies logical tests c. Experiences conceptual independence

VII. Adulthood (21 yr and older)
   a. Assumes responsibility relevant to station in life
   b. Maintains balance and involvement between self, family, and community
   c. Further develops creativity
   d. Reaffirms values in life

VII. Adulthood (35-65 yr)
   a. Primarily concerned with establishing and maintaining a family
   b. Focus is on the development of the basic attitudes of *generativity vs. stagnation*
   c. Displays a marked degree of creativity
   d. Adjusts to circumstances of middle age
   e. Reevaluates life's accomplishments and goals

VIII. Maturity (older than 65 yr)
   a. Accepts lifestyle as meaningful and fulfilling
   b. Focuses on the development of basic attitudes of *ego integrity vs. despair*
   c. Remains optimistic and continues to grow
   d. Adjusts to limitations
   e. Adjusts to retirement
   f. Adjusts to reorganized family patterns
   g. Adjusts to losses
   h. Accepts death with serenity

Modified from Kreigh H, Perko J: *Psychiatric and mental health nursing: commitment to care and concern,* Reston, 1979, Reston Publishing.

TABLE 6-3   Ego Defense Mechanisms

Defense Mechanism	Example	Defense Mechanism	Example
Compensation: Process by which a person makes up for a perceived deficiency by strongly emphasizing a feature that he or she regards as an asset	A businessman perceives his small physical stature negatively. He tries to overcome this by being aggressive, forceful, and controlling in business dealings.	**Projection:** Attributing one's thoughts or impulses to another person. Through this process one can attribute intolerable wishes, emotional feelings, or motivations to another person	A young woman who denies she has sexual feelings about a coworker accuses him without basis of being a "flirt" and says he is trying to seduce her.
Denial: Avoidance of disagreeable realities by ignoring or refusing to recognize them; probably simplest and most primitive of all defense mechanisms	Mrs. P has just been told that her breast biopsy indicates a malignancy. When her husband visits her that evening, she tells him that no one has discussed the laboratory results with her.	**Rationalization:** Offering a socially acceptable or apparently logical explanation to justify or make acceptable otherwise unacceptable impulses, feelings, behaviors, and motives	John fails an examination and complains that the lectures were not well organized or clearly presented.
Displacement: Shift of emotion from a person or object to another usually neutral or less dangerous person or object	A 4-year-old boy is angry because he has just been punished by his mother for drawing on his bedroom walls. He begins to play "war" with his soldier toys and has them battle and fight with each other.	**Reaction formation:** Development of conscious attitudes and behavior patterns that are opposite to what one really feels or would like to do	A married woman who feels attracted to one of her husband's friends treats him rudely.
Dissociation: The separation of any group of mental or behavioral processes from the rest of the person's consciousness or identity	A man is brought to the emergency room by the police and is unable to explain who he is and where he lives or works.	**Regression:** Retreat in face of stress to behavior characteristic of any earlier level of development	Four-year-old Nicole, who has been toilet trained for more than a year, begins to wet her pants again when her new baby brother is brought home from the hospital.
Identification: Process by which a person tries to become like someone he or she admires by taking on thoughts, mannerisms, or tastes of that individual	Sally, 15 years old, has her hair styled similarly to her young English teacher whom she admires.	**Repression:** Involuntary exclusion of a painful or conflictual thought, impulse, or memory from awareness. It is the primary ego defense, and other mechanisms tend to reinforce it	Mr. R does not recall hitting his wife when she was pregnant.
Intellectualization: Excessive reasoning or logic is used to avoid experiencing disturbing feelings	A woman avoids dealing with her anxiety in shopping malls by explaining that she is saving the frivolous waste of time and money by not going into them.	**Splitting:** Viewing people and situations as either all good or all bad. Failure to integrate the positive and negative qualities of oneself	A friend tells you that you are the most wonderful person in the world one day, and how much she hates you the next day.
Introjection: Intense type of identification in which a person incorporates qualities or values of another person or group into his own ego structure. It is one of the earliest mechanisms of the child; important in formation of conscience	Eight-year-old Jimmy tells his 3-year-old sister, "Don't scribble in your book of nursery rhymes. Just look at the pretty pictures," thus expressing his parents' values to his little sister.	**Sublimation:** Acceptance of a socially approved substitute goal for a drive whose normal channel of expression is blocked	Ed has an impulsive and physically aggressive nature. He tries out for the football team and becomes a star tackle.
		Suppression: A process often listed as a defense mechanism but really a conscious counterpart of repression. It is intentional exclusion of material from consciousness. At times, it may lead to subsequent repression	A young man at work finds he is thinking so much about his date that evening that it is interfering with his work. He decides to put it out of his mind until he leaves the office for the day.
Isolation: Splitting off of emotional components of a thought, which may be temporary or long term	A second-year medical student dissects a cadaver for her anatomy course without being disturbed by thoughts of death.	**Undoing:** Act or communication that partially negates a previous one; primitive defense mechanism	Larry makes a passionate declaration of love to Sue on a date. On their next meeting he treats her formally and distantly.

From Stuart GW, Laraia MT: *Principles and practice of psychiatric nursing,* ed 6, St Louis, 1998, Mosby.

TABLE 6-4   Levels of Anxiety

Severity of Anxiety	Physical	Intellectual	Social and Emotional

Minimal (near 0)	Basal levels of
	  Blood pressure
	  Pulse
	  Respiration rate
	  O$_2$ consumption
	  Pupillary constriction
	  Muscles relaxed
		Cognitive activity minimal
		Disregard for external environmental stimuli; no attempt to actively process information
		Focus typically on single, nonthreatening mental image
		States of altered consciousness
			No social interaction
			No attempt to deal with environmental stimuli
			Minimal emotional activity
			Feelings of indifference, invulnerability, and contentment prevail

Mild (+1)	Low-level sympathetic arousal Moderate to low skeletal muscle tension Body relaxed Voice calm, well-modulated	Perceptual field open; able to shift focus of attention readily Passively aware of external environment Self-referent thoughts positive; low concern for unexpected or negative outcomes	Behavior primarily automatic; habitual patterns and well-learned skills Positive feeling of security, confidence, and satisfaction dominate Solitary activities

Moderate (+2)	Sympathetic nervous system activation
	  ↑ Blood pressure
	  ↑ Pulse rate
	  ↑ Respiratory rate
	  Pupillary dilation
	  Sweat glands stimulated
	  Peripheral vascular constriction
	Increased muscular tension
	Heightened performance of well-learned skills
	Rate of speech increased, pitch heightened
	Increased alertness
		Narrowing of perception; attentional focus on specific internal or external stimuli
		Conscious effort in processing of information; optimal level for learning
		Self-referent thoughts ± mixed; some concern about personal ability or available resources necessary to solve problems; probability of positive outcomes increasingly uncertain
			Increased skill in learning and refining of skills; analyzing problematic situations; integrating cognitive and motor domains
			Feelings of challenge; drive to resolve problems or dilemmas
			Mixed sense of confidence/optimism with fear, lowered self-esteem, and potential inadequacy

Severe (+3)	Fight-flight response
	Stimulation of adrenal medulla
	  ↑ Catecholamines, accelerated heart rate, palpitations
	  ↑ Blood glucose
	  ↓ Blood flow to digestive system
	  ↑ Blood flow to skeletal muscles
	Muscles extremely tense
	Hyperventilation
	Physical actions increasingly agitated, pacing, wringing of hands, fidgeting, trembling
	May experience loss of appetite, nausea, "cold sweats"
	Rapid, high-pitched speech
	Facial expression: poor eye contact, fleeting eye movements
		Perceptual capacity restricted; exclusive attention to singular stimuli (internal or external) or multifocal, fragmented processing of stimuli
		Problem solving inefficient, difficult
		Some threatening stimuli disregarded, minimized, denied
		Disorientation in terms of time and place
		Expected likelihood of negative consequences or outcomes high; estimates of personal self-efficacy low
			Flight behavior may be manifested by withdrawal, denial, depression, somatization
			Feelings of increasing threat, need to respond to situation are heightened
			Dissociating tendency; feelings are denied

From Keltner NL et al: *Psychiatric nursing: a psychotherapeutic management approach,* St Louis, 1991, Mosby.

Continued

TABLE 6-4   Levels of Anxiety—cont'd

Severity of Anxiety	Physical	Intellectual	Social and Emotional
Panic (+4)	Continued physiological arousal Actions disorganized, directionless; unable to execute simple motor tasks; fumbling, gross motor agitation, flailing May strike out verbally or physically; may attempt to withdraw from situation Eventual depletion of sympathetic neurotransmitters Blood redistributed throughout body Hypotension May feel dizzy, faint, or exhausted Appears pale, drawn, weary Facial expression: aghast, grimacing, eyes fixed Voice louder, higher pitched	Perception severely restricted, may be impervious to external stimuli Thoughts are random, distorted, disconnected, logical processing impaired Unable to solve problems; limited tolerance for processing novel stimuli (verbal, auditory, or visual) Preoccupied with thoughts of highly probable negative outcomes; conclusions may be drawn, negative consequences seen as inevitable	Emotionally drained, overwhelmed Reliance on earlier, more "primitive" coping behaviors: crying, shouting, curling up, rocking, freezing Feelings of impotence, helplessness, agony and desperation dominate; may be experienced as horror, dread, defenselessness; may be converted to anger, rage

From Keltner NL et al: *Psychiatric nursing: a psychotherapeutic management approach,* St Louis, 1991, Mosby.

2. Reduce environmental stimuli or move the patient to a quiet area; the patient's ability to handle stimuli is compromised
3. Remain in control and calm; the patient fears losing control and needs to feel secure
4. Communicate with clear, simple, short sentences because the patient's ability to deal with complex, abstract statements is compromised
5. Use of prn medications may be necessary to decrease patients anxiety to a manageable level (e.g., lorazepam [Ativan] or alprazolam [Xanax])
6. Encourage use of relaxation techniques
7. When appropriate, assist patient with recognizing early signs of anxiety and effective ways to prevent its escalation
8. Provide opportunities for discussion of the relationship of thoughts and verbalizations to anxiety
9. Implement seclusion and/or restraints if patient is a danger to self and/or others

Phobias

A. Definition: irrational, continual fear of an activity, situation, object, or event
B. Types
1. Agoraphobia (literal meaning, "fear of the marketplace") without panic attacks; fear of being away from a safe environment or person
2. Social phobia: irrational fear of exposure to the scrutiny of others
3. Simple phobia: a disabling fear of some specific object or situation, such as the fear of animals or of being in a high place

C. Assessment data
1. Panic anxiety
2. Anticipatory anxiety
3. Recognition of phobia as irrational
4. Uses defense mechanisms of displacement and repression
5. Avoidance behaviors
6. Interference with demands of daily activities
D. Interventions
1. Acceptance of patient and his or her fears
2. Encourage involvement in activities that do not increase anxiety
3. Help patient recognize that his or her behavior is an attempt to cope with anxiety
4. Use a calm, nonauthoritative approach
5. Reassure patient that he or she will not be made to confront the phobia in treatment until ready to do so
6. Systematic desensitization

Obsessive Compulsive Disorder (OCD)

A. Definition: obsessive thoughts (troublesome, persistent thoughts) and compulsions (ritualistic behaviors) that are repetitive
B. Assessment data
1. Compulsive, ritualistic behavior
2. Obsessive thoughts
3. Alterations in normal functioning
4. Fear of loss of control
5. Feelings of guilt
6. Suicidal thoughts/feelings
7. Rumination (persistent meditation on thoughts)
8. Insight impairment

9. Feelings of worthlessness
10. Decreased self-esteem
C. Interventions
1. Allow patient time to perform rituals
2. Ensure basic daily needs are met
3. Redirect rumination positively
4. Do not, initially, call attention to or interfere with the compulsive act
5. Demonstrate concern for and interest in the patient
6. Encourage verbalization of concerns and feelings
7. As anxiety decreases and patient feels comfortable talking with staff, encourage the patient to talk about his or her behavior and thoughts
8. Encourage patient to try to reduce the frequency of compulsive behavior
9. Some people respond to antidepressant medication

Posttraumatic Stress Disorder

Characteristic symptoms after a psychologically traumatic event include numbness of responses, frequently reliving the event, dreams, depression, and anxiety

Perception

A. Definition: awareness acquired through the five senses
B. Alterations: thought to be pathologies resulting from anxiety
1. Illusion: misinterpretation of a sensory input
2. Hallucination: a sensation without an external stimulus; may be
   a. Auditory: hearing nonexistent voices or sounds
   b. Olfactory: smelling nonexistent odors or aromas
   c. Visual: seeing nonexistent things, people, or animals
   d. Tactile: feeling somatic sensations
   e. Gustatory: experiencing flavors or tastes
3. Delusion: a false belief, not based in fact, that cannot be changed by reasoning
   a. Delusions of grandeur: feelings of greatness
   b. Delusions of persecution: feelings of being mistreated
   c. Delusions of sin or guilt: feelings of deserving punishment
   d. Somatic delusions: feelings about the body or part of the body
   e. Ideas of reference: feeling that certain events or words have special meaning for self

Thought Disorders

Schizophrenia is considered the psychiatric manifestation of thought disorder; this group of illnesses represents the largest number of mentally ill persons.
A. Types of schizophrenia
1. Disorganized: includes frequent incoherence, nonsystematized delusions, and inappropriate affect
2. Catatonic: includes stupor, negativity, rigidity, excitement, and posturing
3. Paranoid: includes persecutory delusions, grandiosity, delusional jealousy, and hallucinations
4. Undifferentiated: does not fit criteria of other categories or combines them
5. Residual: presence of residual symptoms (e.g., marked social isolation, inappropriate affect, odd beliefs) without delusions, hallucinations, or gross disorganization

B. Assessment data
1. Delusions of being controlled
2. Somatic delusions (grandiosity, religious, or nihilistic)
3. Persecutory delusions accompanied by hallucinations
4. Auditory hallucinations of a running commentary on behavior or thought
5. Auditory hallucination on several occasions with content of more than one word
6. Incoherence, looseness of association, illogical thinking with a deterioration in function
7. Continuation of symptoms for 6 months or more, occurring before 45 years of age
C. Interventions
1. Establish trust
2. Do not enter into patient's delusions; maintain your own view of reality without demeaning the patient's view of reality
3. Do not argue about hallucinations; the patient views them as real
4. Offer reassurance: most patients are experiencing pain from their symptoms
5. Touch only with permission; the thought-disordered patient may have a distorted sense of his or her own person
6. If you are afraid, be aware that the patient will sense this: be sure you have sufficient backup for your own safety and comfort
7. Maintain patient safety

Affective Disorders

Disturbances in feeling or affective disorders are classified as either depressive disorders or bipolar disorders.

DEPRESSIVE DISORDERS

A. Major depression is the predominant mental illness in the United States and Canada with ranges from 7% to 12% in the male population and 26% to 30% in the female population
B. Assessment data
1. Irritation
2. Loss of interest in some or all usual activities
3. Change in appetite: usually decreased
4. Changes in weight: usually loss in weight
5. Sleep disturbances: usually insomnia, but may be increased hours of sleep per day
6. Withdrawal from family and friends
7. Hopelessness and helplessness may become profound and may lead to delusions or fantasies of "ending it all"
8. If left in this pattern, the patient eventually could justify how nonexistence may solve the problems
9. The patient may start to dwell on death, and to devise a plan of self-destruction
10. Self-destruction becomes the goal; this is suicidal ideation
C. See suicide prevention and suicide intervention

BIPOLAR DISORDERS

A. Category used when one or more manic episodes are noted whether or not a depressive episode is/has been experienced
B. Mania characterized by unstable mood, pressured speech, and increased motor activity

C. Intervention
1. Demonstrate sincere interest
2. Accept patient's feelings; anger may be directed to the nearest safe object: often the nurse
3. Allow patient to express feelings; for example, crying in a dignified environment
4. Encourage only the expression of feelings that you feel capable of handling; for example, do not encourage ventilation of feelings and then go on your lunch hour
5. If patient is overactive, limit setting or reduction of stimuli may be necessary
6. Avoid power struggles: use force only if necessary to protect patient or others in the environment

Eating Disorders

A. Obesity/compulsive overeating: consuming greater than required number of calories, which results in weight gain; not burning as many calories as consumed; usually considered obese when weight is 20% greater than is recommended for one's height
B. Anorexia nervosa: an eating disorder characterized by refusal to maintain a minimally normal body weight; most often seen in adolescent females (may occur with bulimia or separately)
C. Bulimia: an eating disorder characterized by episodes of binging and then purging; person may not appear overweight or underweight; with nonpurging bulimia the person uses laxatives, diuretics, fasting, or exercise to control his or her weight; bulimia leads to other symptoms such as menstrual irregularities, gastric dilation, aspiration pneumonia, dental caries (caused by frequent vomiting), and esophagitis

Personality Disorders

A. Paranoid personality: characterized by suspicion, rigidity, secretiveness, oversensitivity and alertness, distortions of reality, and the use of projection as a major defense mechanism
B. Borderline personality: at times moderately neurotic and at other times, overtly psychotic; extremely difficult to treat and often unstable after numerous treatment attempts
1. Assessment data
   a. Combined anger and depression
   b. Anhedonia (inability to experience pleasure)
   c. Social isolation
   d. Poor impulse control
   e. Dependency
   f. Substance abuse
   g. Sexual promiscuity
2. Interventions
   a. Be honest with patients
   b. These patients are often manipulative and attention seeking
   c. They tend to view people or situations as all good or all bad
   d. Patients need to begin developing meaningful relationships in which they can begin to trust
   e. Consistency is important; patients may split the staff to play one staff member against another
C. Codependency: meeting goals successfully by relying on another person for the answers; characteristics of the codependent person include
1. Partners are dependent on each other to make a whole relationship

2. One of the partners in this relationship assumes a passive role
3. One or both may have low self-esteem
4. One or both may have low self-image
5. One or both may have an addictive disorder (alcohol, drugs, etc.)
6. They tend to be manipulative—there is a constant conflict either between them or within the family
7. They tend to operate in a series of delusions
8. Because of delusions, they tend to promote their version of any story as the absolute truth
9. They exhibit poor boundaries in relationships
10. They are somewhat to totally insensitive to others' emotions and feelings
11. If the codependency exists within family boundaries, it is highly likely that a dysfunctional family unit will emerge and the children will become a part of the codependency
12. Codependency may be intergenerational and therefore cyclical
13. The treatment of codependent persons is designed by identifying the underlying emotions that are fostering the codependency
D. Substance abuse disorders: a pattern of pathological use of substances that entails such things as need for daily use, loss of control, efforts to control use, overdoses, impairment of social functioning, family disruptions, legal problems, and so on; abuse is distinguished from dependency by tolerance of the substance (increasing use requires increasing doses to achieve the same effect) and the presence or absence of a withdrawal syndrome
1. Alcoholism
   a. Abuse is distinguished from recreational use by such features as daily drinking, frequent need for the chemical, blackouts, social impairment, and decreased ability to function, such as job loss, driving while intoxicated, arrests, and so forth
   b. Acute alcohol ingestion may result in a condition formerly known as delirium tremens (DTs), now known as acute alcohol withdrawal syndrome; key features are hallucinations, extreme agitation, and disorientation; treatment includes anxiolytics (benzodiazepines), anticonvulsants, and hydration
   c. Long-term use may lead to peripheral neuropathy, Wernicke's syndrome (confusion, ataxia, and abnormal eye movements), or Korsakoff's syndrome (alcoholic amnesia syndrome), which is manifested by memory loss and confabulation; these effects are largely caused by deficiency of thiamine and may be partially reversed by the provision of thiamine; usually Korsakoff's syndrome is irreversible but may be arrested by thiamine replacement therapy and cessation of alcohol abuse
2. Barbiturate and sedative abuse (barbiturates, minor tranquilizers such as diazepam, benzodiazepines, etc.)
   a. Cross tolerant with alcohol
   b. May be used by "street addicts" when unable to obtain opiates
   c. Second most abused substance after alcohol in the United States
   d. Legally obtained drugs are often used by middle-class women who overuse tranquilizers
   e. Intoxication similar to alcohol

f. There is a withdrawal syndrome similar to alcohol withdrawal
3. Opiates (heroin, morphine, etc.)
    a. Includes street addicts using IV heroin as well as "medical addicts" using various prescribed substances such as codeine
    b. IV drug users are at a high risk for AIDS
    c. Intoxication: pupil constriction, poor attention span, apathy, slurred speech, euphoria, and psychomotor retardation
    d. There is a physical withdrawal syndrome
4. Cocaine
    a. Stimulant
    b. Increasing use among the middle class
    c. Considered a social drug, many believe that it is not addictive
    d. May be snorted or smoked as a "free-base" or as crack
    e. Intoxication: poor judgment, poor impulse control, feeling of confidence, euphoria, talkative, rapid speech, pacing, elevated heart rate and blood pressure, dilated pupils, nausea, and sweating
    f. May lead to hallucinations with prolonged use; severe depression occurs after the substance use is stopped, leading to strong psychological craving
    g. There does not appear to be a true withdrawal syndrome
5. Amphetamines
    a. Abuse may begin in an effort to control weight
    b. May be used IV by street addicts for a "rush"; may be combined with other drugs such as heroin or barbiturates
    c. Intoxication: elevated heart rate and blood pressure, dilated pupils, chills, perspiration, nausea, and vomiting
6. Hallucinogens (LSD, mescaline, etc.)
    a. Used much less than in the early 1970s
    b. Use leads to altered perceptions and hallucinations; distorted perception of colors; illusions and delusions; unpredictable effects
    c. Intoxication: perceptual changes; dilated pupils; increased pulse, sweating, anxiety, tremors; feelings of paranoia; and poor judgment
7. Cannabis (marijuana, hashish, etc.)
    a. Widely used by various groups, usually smoked or eaten
    b. Intoxication: increased pulse rate, bloodshot eyes, increased appetite, dry mouth, distorted perception of time, euphoria, and apathy
    c. May precipitate panic attacks
8. Substance abuse interventions
    a. Severe denial is a common defense mechanism
    b. Keep the patient focused on the purpose of treatment
    c. Manipulation may be used to obtain a substance for abuse
    d. The nurse must remain nonjudgmental
    e. These patients may require repeated attempts at treatment before they can conquer their addiction
    f. Adequate diet, rest, and vitamin supplements are helpful
    g. Long-term success is often achieved through a lifelong affiliation with abstinence programs such as

Alcoholics Anonymous (AA) and Narcotics Anonymous (NA)
    h. Alcoholism is usually treated in several steps, the first being detoxification. In detoxification, the alcoholic is withdrawn from the chemical through the use of a cross-tolerant substance, usually a benzodiazepine, which is administered for 3 to 5 days in decreasing doses. Frequently, alcoholics are referred to Alcoholics Anonymous
        (1) Detoxification should occur in a controlled (monitored) setting because detoxification may become life threatening
        (2) After the acute detoxification period of 3 to 5 days, intense counseling occurs
        (3) The patient may find it beneficial to continue in a peer group setting on a regular full- or part-time schedule
        (4) In some cases, additional treatment may be suggested in the form of halfway houses, which may offer up to 6 months to 1 year of treatment
    i. Other forms of substance abuse are treated similarly, with combinations of detoxification, if needed, and supportive long-term treatment settings; opiate abusers may also be treated with methadone maintenance in attempts to prevent heroin use and allow the addict to return to more socially acceptable behavior patterns

Physically Based Mental Disorders

A. Organic brain syndrome may result from vascular disorders of the brain, brain infections, trauma, altered metabolism, poisoning, endocrine disorders, and deficiencies
    1. Global involvement: confusion, delirium, and dementia
    2. Selective involvement: may be limited to portions of the personality (e.g., amnesia, hallucinations, and psychosomatic disorders)
    3. Functional impairment: has the features of psychosis (e.g. paranoia, depression, and mania)
    4. Special needs of the older adult: special consideration is given to the role of declining physical attributes
        a. There may be prejudices regarding the elderly
        b. Most older adults are not senile
        c. Apparent senile type behavior may be the result of depression or other forms of illness (i.e. alcoholism)
        d. The reaction to drugs of all types may be idiosyncratic among the elderly
        e. Special techniques
            (1) Life review
            (2) Group work aimed at socialization such as remotivation
            (3) Touch: many elderly are deprived of touch in the usual manner because of relational losses
        f. See Chapter 9
B. Mental retardation: subaverage intelligence; there are numerous causes including inherited defects in metabolism, genetic defects, birth injuries, and developmental anomalies
    1. Mental retardation: classified as follows with interventions geared accordingly
        a. Profoundly retarded: needs total nursing care in early stages; later may develop rudimentary ability to care for self; always requires some care
        b. Severely retarded: may be able to care for self in protected environment; requires monitoring

c. Moderately retarded: usually capable of self-care but requires supervision when under stress

d. Mildly retarded: usually self-supporting; may require support of family or others when under stress

2. Special needs of children and adolescents: there are many similarities and some differences in the therapeutics for children and adolescents

a. Services in hospitals are usually short and aimed at assessment and evaluation

b. Most ongoing treatment is on an outpatient basis

c. Treatment is action oriented, using such modalities as play therapy

d. There are many issues of trust vs. mistrust

e. There are issues of self-image, limit testing, and developmentally specific concerns

f. Treatment is selected based on the child's mental age, not his or her physical age

C. Other somatic manifestations of mental disturbance: several conditions have defined or suggested psychological bases

1. Ulcers
2. Bowel disorders
3. Cardiovascular disorders
4. Asthma
5. Allergies
6. Eating disorders: anorexia, bulimia
7. Headache
8. Certain endocrine disorders

DEATH AND DYING

Nursing intervention is aimed at ensuring the transition of the patient through each of the stages listed below. It is important to be aware of your own attitude about death and to ensure that you are meeting the patient's needs and not your own. Being nonjudgmental and allowing the expression of emotions by the patient are essential. Patient defenses are necessary in accepting his or her own death and should not be challenged. Elisabeth Kübler-Ross describes dying as a process that proceeds through the following stages

A. Shock and denial: the patient cannot actually accept or believe that he or she is going to die; may repress information, seek to escape the truth by seeking other opinions, and be unable to hear the real message

B. Anger and rage: the patient becomes angry with the terrible truth of impending death; may be hypercritical of others, demanding, and resentful. Health care workers often bear the brunt of a patient's rage as they represent cure for others but not for him or her

C. Bargaining: acceptance has begun, and the patient begins to bargain for more time or for some specific request; during this stage, wills may be finalized and legacies of various kinds bestowed. If possible, requests should be granted, because they bring comfort to the dying person

D. Depression: after acceptance of the inevitable has begun, the person feels sad and alone. He or she may speak little and cry often. Quiet acceptance is often the most helpful kind of intervention in this stage

E. Acceptance: once this occurs, the person is often seen as tranquil and at peace with himself. Again, the patient may speak little, because most of what he or she has to say to others has been said; although still sad, the patient has made his or her peace with death and has accepted the inevitable. This phase may last for months or longer

GRIEVING

George Engel (1964) defined grieving as a process of sequential steps similar to those in the dying process

A. Shock and disbelief: the person refuses to accept the loss, may feel stunned or numbed; similar to the first stage of dying

B. Developing awareness: the person may experience varying degrees of physical symptoms such as nausea, vomiting, and loss of appetite. Crying is common, anger may be felt and expressed toward the lost person for the act of desertion. Anger may be self-directed and recriminations made

C. Restitution (resolution): acceptance occurs and is aided by the culturally approved modes of grieving such as funerals and wearing black

D. The process of grieving may take more than 1 year; all stages must be experienced for grief to be successfully completed. If grieving is not successful, it may lead to one of the following

1. Delayed reaction: a later reaction to the loss; delay is caused by repressing reality; it may result in more painful experiences than the normal immediate reaction

2. Distorted reactions: may include the development of symptoms similar to the lost person's: medical illnesses, social isolation, agitated depression, increased use of alcohol or other drugs

CRISIS INTERVENTION

Generally, there are common components in all crisis situations. With this knowledge, strategies are developed to assist people through a crisis and minimize its detrimental effects.

A. Crisis: an event that disturbs the equilibrium of the individual or family

B. The disturbance leads to development of certain symptoms, most notably, anxiety and depression

C. These feelings continue until a need is felt to reduce or alleviate them

D. If the person or family has adequate coping mechanisms, the problem will be resolved and balance restored

E. Without coping mechanisms, anxiety and depression increase to intolerable levels

F. Interventions are aimed at providing short-term therapy to increase coping behaviors

G. Most crises are resolved within 6 to 8 weeks

H. Intervention entails

1. A thorough assessment of the situation

2. Planned strategies that do not attempt to rearrange a person's life

3. Strategies that increase intellectual understanding, explore current feelings, offer coping mechanisms, and support existing ties and helpful relationships

CRISIS OF RAPE OR INCEST

Assisting survivors of these violent acts requires substantial time. This intervention begins when the victim calls for help in any form or seeks treatment. There are two possible phases to this violence. One is the acute or immediate phase wherein the victim exhibits fear, confusion, disorganization, and restlessness. The second phase is a long-term process of reorganization and usually begins weeks after the attack.

A. Early relevant feelings include

1. Physical pain
2. Anger

3. Fear of reattack
4. Outrage at the perpetrator
5. Total violation of (emotional) space
6. Fear of involvement with anyone of the same sex as the perpetrator
7. Emotional drain
8. Helplessness
9. Fear of pregnancy
B. If these immediate feelings are not externalized and dealt with, the result may be permanent psychological damage including but not limited to the following psychosexual dysfunctions
   1. Sexual arousal disorders
   2. Sexual deviations (several varieties)
   3. Sexual aversions
   4. Delusions of violent sexual behavior, which could be incorporated in the patient's lifestyle
C. Interventions include
   1. Assess the victim's safety: Are you in a safe place?; Is there help for you?
   2. Listen: accept what is said
   3. Respond as appropriate
   4. Refer patient to appropriate agency

SUICIDE PREVENTION

Suicide ranks as a leading cause of death in the United States. There are specific indicators that assist in assessing suicidal risk.
A. Risk factors include
   1. Age and sex: more women attempt suicide; more men are successful
   2. Men over 35 are at higher risk; most suicides occur in men between the ages of 35 and 50 years
   3. Anxiety and depression: many potential suicide victims report increasing anxiety and depression; most significant is a recent change in these feelings
   4. Past coping pattern: not working in the current situation
   5. Past suicide attempt is always considered a high-risk factor
   6. Alcohol or drug abuse: many suicides are committed by alcoholics
   7. Concrete plan: if there is a plan, considerations are
      a. Is it set in a current time frame?
      b. Is it lethal?
      c. Does the potential victim have the necessary resources to carry out the plan?
   8. Significant others: often a suicide is committed to communicate with others
B. Interventions include
   1. Focus on clear and present danger
   2. Reduce present hazards
   3. Give clear directions for victim to follow
   4. Assign to constant monitoring in a hospital
   5. Mobilize significant others when possible
   6. Mobilize past coping mechanisms
   7. Assign concrete specific tasks
   8. Explore positive alternatives to suicide
   9. Teach problem-solving techniques

SUICIDE INTERVENTION

Intervention becomes critical at the point of suicidal ideation. If intervention does not occur, suicide is highly likely. The patient may be having underlying feelings of hopelessness, help-lessness, and impending doom. Frequently the patient will verbalize the need to "end it all."
A. Always ask
   1. Do I understand that you want to hurt yourself? (confirming suicide ideation)
   2. Do you have a plan or how will you hurt yourself? Will you share your plan with me? (suicidal gesturing may be evident)
   3. If the specific plan calls for using an enabling device or instrument: May I have the _____ that is included in the plan? (specify item: knife, razor, rope, etc.)
B. Ordinarily a loud cry for help can be heard before the suicide occurs if others are perceptive enough to hear it
   NOTE: Severely depressed patients are so physically impaired that they rarely have the energy to commit suicide. As the depression begins to lift, the potential to commit suicide increases, that is, especially if they have communicated that need to "end it all."

TREATMENT MODALITIES
Psychotherapy

A. Individual psychotherapy: one-to-one relationship between a therapist (physician, psychologist, social worker, nurse clinician) and a patient; sessions of 45 to 50 minutes are usually held weekly or more often; the aim is to improve the functioning of the person; it is most effective with the neuroses and in patients who have good verbal skills and high intelligence
B. Family group therapy: a family is seen as a group by a therapist, based on the premise that disturbance arises as a function of family interactions and that treatment must be aimed at the family as a whole
C. Group therapy: treatment provided to a group of persons related by age, symptom, or other commonality; treatment occurs on a weekly or biweekly basis and may include more than one therapist
D. Behavior modification: techniques based on conditioning; undesired behaviors are ignored and desired behaviors are rewarded

Milieu Therapy

Milieu therapy is the use of a controlled environment to influence the treatment of a patient
A. Interactions between patient and staff, as well as interpatient relationships, are used as a basis for treatment
B. Therapeutic communications: behavior modeling and some behavior modification techniques are often used

Therapeutic Community

Therapeutic community (Maxwell Jones, 1968) is a method of establishing a milieu for treatment wherein all members, staff as well as patients, have assigned responsibilities in the community and defined roles. The reasoning is that this type of democratic environment prepares the patient for release into the larger community.

Electroconvulsive Therapy

Use of electroconvulsive therapy (shock therapy, ECT) has recently increased for patients with severe depression who have not responded to other therapies. It is the application of an electrical current through the brain, resulting in a grand mal seizure. Some patients suffer a short-term memory loss as a result of the treatment. The treatments are given by a physician under general anesthesia; the treatment can be given on an outpatient or inpatient basis. Some patients with severe depression can control further episodes with regular periodic treatments.

Psychopharmacological Therapy

Psychopharmacological agents are used in the treatment of mental health disorders. NOTE: When administering medication to the mental health patient, remember to use a tongue blade to examine the interior of the mouth if you suspect the patient is "cheeking" the medication.
A. Anti-extrapyramidal symptoms (anti-EPS): EPS is unusual muscle movement that involves the fine muscles of the body; these symptoms are acute and tonic dystonic reactions to the antipsychotic medication
   1. Frequently EPS appears in the tongue or in the muscles of the upper chest, neck, and shoulders
   2. Anti-EPS medications used to reverse the muscular effects of the antipsychotics are diphenhydramine hydrochloride (Benadryl) and benztropine mesylate (Cogentin)
B. See Chapter 3 for greater detail regarding drugs that are commonly used to treat mental illness

Adjunctive Therapies

A. Occupational therapy: the use of vocational tasks to allow patients to express various underlying feelings
B. Recreational therapy: the use of recreational activities to allow patients to express feelings
C. Art therapy: the use of the plastic and graphic arts to express feeling
D. Other therapies may include vocational counseling, bibliotherapy (writing or reading), and dance therapy

ETHICAL CONSIDERATIONS IN PATIENT CARE

A. In most places, patients may sue institutions under habeas corpus proceedings for their release from treatment
B. Laws guarantee rights to patients
C. Nurses and other staff members may be sued for assault and battery for forcing treatments on patients
D. Wrongful death suits have been brought in circumstances in which a patient has died
E. There is a narrow line between treatment and abuse
F. Local laws vary in different parts of the country, and nurses should be aware of local statutes
G. Confidentiality is essential in mental health nursing
H. Communications between a patient and a nurse may be considered "privileged," whereas most medical records are open to subpoena
I. Documents should contain only factual material not conjecture
J. If a patient threatens bodily harm to others, such information is no longer considered privileged and is required to be reported to the authorities

K. Oppressive mental institutions may infringe on a patient's rights, and nurses should be aware of their responsibilities in such situations

PATIENT'S RIGHTS MOVEMENT

A. Although patients in psychiatric settings are ill, they retain their civil rights and are often specifically protected under special sections of the law
B. In most places, "commitment" removes only the patient's right to leave the hospital or terminate treatment
C. Recent legal decisions indicate that patients may expect treatment and may not simply be detained in hospitals where there is no active treatment available
D. In recent years, patient and former-patient groups have formed and demanded access to records of treatment rationales

CARE AND TREATMENT OF PATIENTS

Basic needs: the basic needs of patients in psychiatric settings are similar to those of other patients; usually, psychiatric patients do not have the accompanying impairments of the physically ill patient
A. Most patients are ambulatory
B. The nurse's role is to guide, encourage, and teach by example
C. Patients may be socially deteriorated and require assistance in activities of daily living such as how to arrange time to complete their own care
D. Reward such as praise is helpful in guiding patients in these activities

SUGGESTED READINGS

American Psychiatric Association: *Diagnostic and statistical manual of mental disorders,* ed 4, Washington, DC, The Association.

Carson VB, Arnold EN: *Mental health nursing: the nurse-patient journey,* Philadelphia, 1996, WB Saunders.

Fontaine KL, Fletcher JS: *Mental health nursing,* ed 4, Upper Saddle River, 1999, Prentice Hall Health.

Fortinash KM, Holoday-Worret PA: *Psychiatric mental health nursing,* ed 2, St Louis, 1999, Mosby.

Haber J, Krainovich-Miller B, McMahon AL: *Comprehensive psychiatric nursing,* ed 5, St Louis, 1997, Mosby.

Keltner NI, Schwecke LH, Bostrom CE: *Psychiatric nursing,* ed 3, St Louis, 1999, Mosby.

Morrison M: *Foundations of mental health nursing,* St Louis, 1997, Mosby.

Rawlins RP, Williams SR, Beck CK: *Mental health-psychiatric nursing,* ed 3, St Louis, 1993, Mosby.

Stuart GW, Laraia MT: *Principles and practice of psychiatric nursing,* ed 6, St Louis, 1998, Mosby.

Townsend M: *Psychiatric mental health nursing,* Philadelphia, 1999, FA Davis Co.

Varcarolis EM: *Foundations of psychiatric-mental health nursing,* ed 3, Philadelphia, 1998, WB Saunders.

REVIEW QUESTIONS

1. The nurse is assigned to work with a depressed patient and wants to make sure that her initial contact does what?
   ① Addresses the root of depression
   ② Keeps communication open
   ❸ Establishes trust
   ④ Raises the patient's spirits

2. A patient who has just been admitted for polysubstance abuse is demanding to leave. Which of the following is the *best* nursing action?
   ① Ask the patient why he or she wants to leave so soon
   ② Inform the patient that no one is allowed to leave once he or she is admitted
   ③ Take the patient to the seclusion room
   ❹ Respond, "I would like you to tell me how you feel. Can you do that?"

3. A nurse is caring for a patient with major depression. When planning activities, the nurse knows that the patient needs:
   ① Frequent changes in activities
   ② Constant redirection into numerous activities
   ③ Behavior modification that restructures feelings
   ❹ Well-defined, structured interactions at the beginning of treatment

4. According to Erikson, the developmental task of the infant is:
   ❶ Trust
   ② Initiative
   ③ Identity
   ④ Integrity

5. A newly admitted patient has not bathed in 4 weeks and is extremely disheveled. To help her with her ADLs (activities of daily living) it is appropriate for the nurse to:
   ① Insist that she bathe before she may have recreational privileges
   ❷ State in a manner-of-fact way that she is expected to bathe each morning at 8 AM, stay with her, and assist her with this task
   ③ Postpone her bath until her symptoms subside, as it is not the major concern now
   ④ Tell her she will be excluded from social groups because she is untidy

6. On the day before finals a student has sweaty palms and "butterflies" in the stomach. The anxiety level is most probably:
   ① Panic level
   ② Free floating
   ❸ Apprehension level
   ④ Alertness level

7. Personality is the result of:
   ❶ Heredity and environment
   ② Temperament and heredity
   ③ Environment and nurturing
   ④ Nurturing and heredity

8. In working with young adults, the nurse recognizes a common developmental task to be:
   ① Achieving economic security
   ❷ Establishing an intimate relationship
   ③ Clarifying values
   ④ Adjusting to decreased health

9. A patient approaches the nurse and says, "I am omnipotent. Some day soon I'm going to take over this unit, you'll see." The appropriate nursing intervention should be to:
   ① Call a code
   ② Tell the patient that no one is omnipotent and to calm down
   ❸ Redirect the patient
   ④ Ask the patient why he thinks he is omnipotent

10. An abnormal excessive fear of a specific situation or object is called a(n):
    ❶ Phobia
    ② Obsession
    ③ Compulsion
    ④ Psychosis

11. Suicide is most likely to occur:
    ① On admission
    ② On discharge
    ③ As the depression deepens
    ❹ As the depression lifts

12. On admission to the psychiatric unit the patient reports, "Sometimes I feel like killing myself but I wouldn't do that." The first response of the nurse should be to:
    ① Determine how severe the risk of suicide is
    ② Ask the patient why he is considering suicide
    ❸ Provide a safe environment for the patient
    ④ Teach the patient alternative coping skills

13. Daydreaming about a super hero is common among:
    ① Toddlers
    ❷ Preschoolers
    ③ School-age children
    ④ Adolescents

14. To help a patient cope with death, the nurse must first:
    ❶ Know how she feels about death
    ② Know how the patient feels about dying
    ③ Know how the family feels about the patient's illness
    ④ Know the meaning of death

15. A short-term expected outcome (goal) for a manic patient is that the patient will gain 3 pounds in 1 week. At the end of the week the patient has gained 2 pounds. The nurse should record which of the following outcomes?
    ① Goal met
    ② Goal will be met in 3 more days
    ③ Goal not met
    ❹ Goal partially met

16. The patient is being admitted to the psychiatric unit. He is extremely agitated and pacing the floor. Which of the following nursing interventions would have priority at this time?
    ❶ Place the patient in a quiet area away from other patients
    ② Encourage the patient to participate in a group activity
    ③ Set firm limits on the patient's behavior
    ④ Orient the patient to his room and the nursing unit

17. The nurse was told in report that she is to observe a particular patient for extrapyramidal side effects, which includes:
    ① Dry mouth and anorexia
    ② GI upset and constipation
    ③ Heart palpitations
    ❹ Muscle rigidity and tremors

18. A nurse working in a hospice overhears one of the patients talking with the physician, begging to be kept alive just 1 more year. The nurse recognizes this as what stage of the grief process?
    ① Denial
    ● Bargaining
    ③ Depression
    ④ Acceptance

19. During the termination phase of the nurse/patient relationship the patient abruptly gets up and leaves. The *most* appropriate nursing action should be to:
    ① Go after the patient and bring him back
    ● Remain at the interaction site until the end of the contracted time
    ③ Resume her regularly scheduled activities
    ④ Speak with the head nurse about assigning another nurse to the patient

20. In caring for the mental health patient the nurse applies Maslow's hierarchy of needs to the development of his care plan. Which level of needs would have the highest priority?
    ● Physiological
    ② Loving and belonging
    ③ Self-esteem
    ④ Self-actualization

21. A nurse is attempting to communicate with a patient. The patient says, "My car is red, your hair is short, my socks are gold, DeWayne, Jewish, my wife's cooking is awful, she burns." This is called:
    ① Word salad
    ② Ambivalence
    ③ Confabulation
    ● Flight of ideas

22. The charge nurse in a long-term care facility finds one of her elderly patients in a confused state this morning. To help with the patient's orientation, the nurse should:
    ● Mark the patient's room with his name
    ● Repeatedly explain to the patient he is in a nursing home
    ③ Involve the patient in group therapy
    ④ Move the patient to a room near the nurses' station

23. The patient was admitted 3 days ago for depression and attempted suicide. Her depression seems to have lifted. The practical nurse knows this means her risk for suicide:
    ① Is less than when she was severely depressed
    ● Is more than when she was severely depressed
    ③ Is gone
    ● Needs to be reevaluated

24. A patient is admitted to a psychiatric unit following an unsuccessful suicide attempt. He repeatedly tells the nurse, "I want to die, please help me die." The *most* appropriate nursing response is:
    ① "Don't worry, you're safe here."
    ② "Relax, nobody's going to kill you."
    ③ "Why do you want to die?"
    ● "You must be feeling very sad right now."

25. The nurse is caring for a patient returning to his room following electroconvulsive therapy (ECT). What behavior should the nurse expect him to exhibit?
    ① The patient complains to the nurse that someone is poisoning his food
    ② The patient goes to the game room to play pool

● The patient is unable to recall the date
④ The patient prepares to go on a field trip

26. A nurse is caring for a college student who is diagnosed with anorexia. The patient is 5′ 8″ and now weighs 105 pounds. Her desired weight is 90 pounds. Because the patient must be weighed, the nurse should know that she may:
    ① Have to be weighed three times a day
    ● Layer her clothes and hide things in her pockets
    ③ Refuse to let you weigh her regularly
    ④ Deny that she has a weight problem

27. Patients who abuse alcohol may become tremulous and have hallucinations when they stop drinking. This is called:
    ① Tolerance
    ② Abstinence
    ● Withdrawal
    ④ Dementia

28. A 14-year-old girl is admitted to the psychiatric unit after superficially cutting her wrist. She has a history of prostitution and minor drug abuse. An appropriate nursing goal for this patient is to:
    ① Show her that her life of prostitution is immoral
    ● Eliminate self-destructive manipulative behavior
    ③ Get her to settle down with a husband
    ④ Convince her to have a tubal ligation to avoid pregnancy

29. The patient tells the nurse to leave her alone; she says, "I'm no good to anyone. Why don't you attend to someone else?" Which response by the nurse would be the most therapeutic?
    ● "I will stay with you for 15 minutes."
    ② "I am responsible for you, so I will stay with you."
    ③ "You are a good person."
    ④ "Why do you say you are no good to anyone?"

30. A hospitalized schizophrenic patient who experiences auditory hallucinations is placed on clozapine (Clozaril) by his physician. The nurse knows the medication is effective when the patient reports that:
    ● He no longer hears voices
    ● The voices aren't as loud
    ③ He is too drowsy to concentrate on the voices
    ④ He does not disturb the other patients any more

31. A patient is admitted to a psychiatric unit. After completing the nursing history and assessment, the nurse determines that a tour of the unit and explanation of the unit rules and regulations is appropriate. The nurse's rationale for this intervention is to:
    ● Reduce the patient's anxiety
    ② Demonstrate that interaction with others is required
    ③ Assure that patient rights aren't violated
    ④ Make sure all the other patients know who the new patient is

32. When the nurse gathered admission data on a patient, it was determined that the patient is on the health end of the mental health/mental illness continuum. Which of the following statements best supports these findings?
    ① The patient is in an abusive marriage
    ② The patient describes her life as boring
    ● The patient is satisfied with her life
    ④ The patient is being checked for terminal disease

33. The nurse is talking with a suicidal patient. Which of the following should the nurse ask first?
    ① "Why do you want to kill yourself?"
    ❷ "Do you have a plan?"
    ③ "What does your family think?"
    ④ "Have you looked at all your options?"

34. The nurse is caring for a patient with obsessive compulsive disorder. Which of the following behaviors would alert the nurse that the patient is under an increased level of stress?
    ① Aggressive behavior
    ② Increased inability to communicate
    ③ Becoming withdrawn from reality
    ❹ An increase in ritualistic behavior

35. The nurse is giving a patient instructions regarding his prescribed MAO inhibitor. Which of the following statements demonstrates the patient understands his instructions?
    ❶ "I need to avoid red wine and hard cheeses."
    ② "I will drink at least eight glasses of water each day."
    ③ "I will avoid fruits and green vegetables."
    ④ "I will avoid milk and fruit juices."

36. A nurse is caring for a mentally ill patient who is convinced that his wife is trying to kill him. There is no evidence to support this belief. The nurse recognizes the patient is suffering from:
    ❶ Delusions
    ② Hallucinations
    ③ Illusions
    ④ Compensation

37. A nurse is caring for a patient with bulimia; the patient tells the nurse she has been bulimic for the past 5 years. In assessing the patient, the nurse hears about the following complaints:
    ① GI upset
    ❷ Toothache
    ③ Diarrhea
    ❹ Sore throat

38. A patient tells the nurse that there are electrodes in her head that are making her arms and legs burn. Which of the following responses is *most* therapeutic?
    ① "That's silly, your legs are okay."
    ② "Does the fire travel from one leg to the other?"
    ③ "If your legs were burning, I would see it."
    ❹ "I understand you feel the fire. How can you stop it?"

39. Paranoid thinking is characterized by feelings of:
    ① Anger and aggression
    ❷ Suspicion and jealousy
    ③ Self-pity and self-centeredness
    ④ Simultaneous hero worship and hero hating

40. The nurse is caring for a patient who is undergoing electroconvulsive therapy (ECT). In planning his care, what should the nurse expect?
    ① The patient will be incontinent
    ② The patient will be at risk for suicide
    ③ The patient will cry and be depressed
    ❹ The patient will be confused and experience a temporary loss of recent memories

41. A nursing diagnosis in psychiatric nursing is:
    ❶ A behavior or problem related to its probable cause
    ② Not used, because nurses do not diagnose
    ③ Based on the medical condition of the patient
    ④ Useful only in general hospital settings

42. A nurse has just received a lab report on patient with a bipolar disorder. The patient's lithium level is 1.9 mEq/L. What should the nurse do first?
    ① Administer the next dose of Lithium
    ❷ Hold the Lithium and call the physician
    ③ Double the Lithium dose
    ④ Hold the Lithium and administer Xanax

43. A patient was admitted with chronic depression that has not responded to antidepressant medications. The doctor has ordered electroconvulsive therapy (ECT) treatments. The patient has signed the permission slip and is asking the nurse what to expect following the treatment. The best answer for the nurse is:
    ① "ECT changes your chemical messengers."
    ② "ECT will change your subconscious thoughts."
    ③ "ECT will cause you to have seizure activity."
    ❹ "The ECT will assist in alleviating your depression."

44. A patient with a personality disorder is brought to the outpatient clinic by her mother, who states her daughter is out of control. The nurse should begin to foster trust by:
    ❶ Telling her you are available regardless of her behavior
    ❷ Telling her you care about her but may not always approve of her behavior
    ③ Avoiding the establishment of trust because the relationship will eventually be terminated
    ④ Letting her know she can call you day or night

45. A patient approaches the nurse and says, "With all my troubles I feel worthless. I would like to end all this misery. Everyone would be better off if I were gone." The nurse's most appropriate response to this statement would be:
    ① "Tell me more."
    ❷ "Are you thinking of killing yourself?"
    ③ "I can see that you are very upset."
    ④ "I have to take blood pressures right now, then we can talk."

46. A nurse is preparing a patient for discharge. Because the patient is on an MAO inhibitor, the nurse will emphasize which of the following instructions?
    ❶ "Avoid aged cheeses."
    ② "Take the medicine with food."
    ③ "Take the medicine at bedtime."
    ④ "Limit caffeine intake."

47. A nurse is assigned to a patient scheduled for electroconvulsive therapy (ECT) in the morning. The patient tells the nurse she is fearful and cannot go through with the treatment as scheduled. The best response from the nurse would be:
    ① "You will be all right."
    ❷ "Tell me how you feel."
    ③ "Do you wish to stay depressed?"
    ④ "ECT is safe for most people."

48. A 42-year-old patient was admitted to the unit for alcohol rehabilitation. The patient tells the nurse he often cannot remember what he does while he is drinking. The nurse asks him additional questions and determines he is suffering from:
    ① Psychosis
    ❷ Blackouts
    ③ Denial
    ④ Alcoholism

49. A patient tells the nurse that the television is cursing her and that there are electrodes in her head that make her arms and legs burn. The idea of the television cursing the patient is an example of:
  ① Persecutory delusion
  ② Visual hallucination
  ③ Incoherence
  ④ Flight of ideas

50. The medication most frequently given to the bipolar (manic depressive) patient is:
  ① Chlorpromazine (Thorazine)
  ② Perphenazine (Trilafon)
  ③ Imipramine (Tofranil)
  ④ Lithium (Lithane)

51. Nurses working on the admissions unit of a psychiatric facility frequently care for aggressive patients. The best nursing intervention in most cases when caring for an aggressive patient is to:
  ① Apply restraints until the patient calms down
  ② Take away privileges if behavior is inappropriate
  ③ Schedule activities with limited stimuli
  ④ Plan a variety of activities to keep the patient occupied

52. A patient is in the clinic waiting room awaiting results of the biopsy of his prostate gland. He is laughing and cracking jokes. The nurse should:
  ① Ask the patient to be quiet
  ② Recognize the patient is manifesting anxiety
  ③ Ignore the patient's behavior
  ④ Overlook the patient's different behavior

53. A nurse is caring for a patient diagnosed with agoraphobia. The nurse understands this means:
  ① Fear of being alone
  ② Fear of physical pain
  ③ Aggressive behavior
  ④ Obsessive-compulsive behavior

54. The nurse is caring for a patient with bipolar disorder who is currently in the manic phase and is trying to get the patient involved in diversional activity. Which of the following would be the most appropriate activity?
  ① Bridge
  ② Jigsaw puzzle
  ③ Ping-pong
  ④ Exercise class

55. A patient rushes up to the nurse and says, "They're after me. They want to torture me and kill me." Which of the following is the most appropriate response?
  ① "Tell me who they are."
  ② "There's no one here except you and me."
  ③ "I need to go look for myself."
  ④ "You are safe here. Can you tell me more?"

56. The nurse is caring for a patient experiencing extrapyramidal side effects from antipsychotic medications. All of the following medications are ordered. Which one should the nurse administer for the side effects?
  ① Furosemide (Lasix)
  ② Benztropine mesylate (Cogentin)
  ③ Prochloperazine (Compazine)
  ④ Acetaminophen (Tylenol)

57. The nurse is caring for an adolescent diagnosed with depression and is establishing rapport with the patient. The nurse understands that the patient's depression may be exhibited by:
  ① Violence
  ② Isolation
  ③ Aggression
  ④ Regression

58. A newly admitted adolescent on the unit has taken on the mannerisms and hair style of a popular singing star. The nurse recognizes this as an example of:
  ① Identification
  ② Compensation
  ③ Conversion
  ④ Displacement

59. During a group therapy session, a patient asks the nurse what the difference is between a psychosis and neurosis. The most appropriate response by the nurse to this question is:
  ① "Psychotics can't think; neurotics can think."
  ② "Psychotics are always depressed; neurotics are not depressed."
  ③ "Psychotics have disorganized thinking; neurotics' thoughts are organized."
  ④ "Psychotics are always in touch with reality; neurotics are not in touch with reality."

60. A patient complains of trouble with control of her or his tongue. Also, the neck muscles are beginning to tighten and the patient is having difficulty keeping her or his head in an upright position. The nurse's *first* response should be:
  ① Check the medication administration record
  ② Call the physician
  ③ Draw blood per standing order
  ④ Fill out an incident report

61. A 46-year-old patient is admitted to the hospital's psychiatric unit because of an increasingly depressed mood. After a few weeks of treatment the nurse observes that the patient has started putting on large amounts of makeup, has become seductive with male patients, and stays up very late pacing the floor. The nurse might conclude that the patient:
  ① Was initially diagnosed incorrectly
  ② May be having a manic episode as part of her illness
  ③ Is showing signs of recovery
  ④ May be having side effects of the medication

62. The nurse is admitting a patient who is delusional and knows a priority nursing measure should be to:
  ① Encourage the patient to talk about the delusions
  ② Explain the delusion to the patient
  ③ Place the patient in seclusion
  ④ Explain to the patient that he is wrong, the delusion is not real

63. A nurse who is doing discharge teaching for a patient on antidepressant therapy should tell the patient he could expect to feel better in what length of time?
  ① 2-3 days
  ② 5-7 days
  ③ 2-4 weeks
  ④ 4-6 weeks

64. Extreme mood swings ranging from deep depression to high activity levels is most often seen in:
   ① Paranoid disorders
   ❷ Bipolar disorders
   ③ Schizophrenia
   ④ Eating disorders

65. A nurse is caring for a patient taking haloperidol (Haldol). What is a common side effect the nurse may see?
   ❶ Sedation
   ② Weight loss
   ③ Dry mouth
   ④ Anxiety

66. The nurse is completing discharge instructions for a patient being discharged on Antabuse to help avoid using alcohol. Which of the following statements should the nurse include in the teaching?
   ① "You will need bi-weekly blood work to determine blood levels of the medication."
   ② "The Antabuse can cause you to be sensitive to the sunlight."
   ③ "This drug causes sedation, do not operate heavy equipment."
   ❹ "The Antabuse can stay in your system as long as 14 days after you stop taking the medication."

67. If a nurse were to select a single identifying characteristic of the obsessive-compulsive patient, it would be:
   ① Seclusiveness
   ② Aggression
   ❸ Orderliness
   ④ Instant gratification

68. A teenager admits to the nurse that he is smoking marijuana on a fairly regular basis. The nurse would know that marijuana is considered a(n):
   ① Highly addictive substance
   ② Amphetamine
   ③ Hallucinogen
   ❹ Cannabinol

69. A nurse is caring for a patient experiencing manic behavior who is too distracted to eat. The most appropriate nursing intervention should be to:
   ① Plan mealtime as a social event
   ② Plan for meals that include the patient's favorite foods
   ❸ Offer finger foods that the patient can eat on the go
   ④ Provide a calm mealtime

70. A patient is hearing voices that are telling him to do harmful things to himself. Which of the following nursing diagnoses should be included on this patient's care plan?
   ❶ Potential for violence
   ② Self-care deficit
   ❸ Sensory perception alteration
   ④ Impaired communication

71. A patient tells the nurse that he is depressed over the recent death of a parent. Which response is the best communication intervention for this patient?
   ① Say nothing
   ② "Wouldn't you rather talk about something else?"
   ❸ "I have some time. Would you like to tell me more about your feelings?"
   ④ "I don't have time for sad people."

72. The nurse is gathering data on a team of patients and notes that one patient has been committed for care. The nurse understands "commitment" to mean:
   ❶ The patient is at risk for harming himself or others
   ❷ The patient will be here indefinitely
   ③ The patient has lost all his rights
   ④ The patient was placed here by the criminal justice system

73. The nurse is preparing the patient for discharge. Which statement by the patient diagnosed with anxiety would indicate he understands his diagnosis?
   ① "Wine with my meals may help me cope better with my anxiety."
   ❷ "I understand that anxiety sometimes will help me perform better."
   ③ "As long as I take my anti-anxiety medication I can continue to work 16-18 hours per day."
   ④ "I understand my life will be great from now on."

74. A nurse enters a patient's room and stands just inside the door. The patient is obviously agitated and is escalating to the point that physical harm may occur. What would be the nurse's most appropriate action?
   ① Take the patient to the seclusion room
   ❷ Talk to the patient and try to identify why he or she is so agitated
   ③ Go to the nurses' station and report the patient's behavior
   ④ Call the physician

75. A nurse working on an inpatient psychiatric unit is also responsible for operating a 24-hour emergency phone line. During the nurse's shift there have been four potential suicide calls. To which of the following calls should the nurse give the greatest priority?
   ① A teenager who is thinking of cutting his wrist
   ② A young adult who agreed to come to the emergency room
   ❸ A young male with a new gun
   ④ A young female who is talking of overdosing on pills

76. The dominant feeling that the patient with major depression is *most* likely to display is:
   ① Agitation
   ② Ambivalence
   ③ Anxiety
   ❹ Hopelessness

77. The nurse is interacting with a patient with obsessive compulsive disorder. What statement by the patient may validate that certain activities help her to deal with her anxiety?
   ❶ "I worry about dirt and germs and I clean a lot."
   ② "I worry about the health of my aging parents."
   ③ "I have a stupid problem, don't I?"
   ④ "I am willing to take medication if necessary."

78. A patient on a psychiatric unit makes all the following comments. Which comment suggests the patient may be suffering from mania?
   ① "I get messages from my dead mother."
   ② "Leave me alone while I'm playing solitaire."
   ❸ "I don't need to sleep."
   ④ "My health is very important to me."

79. In assessing suicidal risk, which of the following is a high-risk factor?
    ① Long psychotherapeutic treatment
    ❷ A concrete plan that is relatively lethal
    ③ Past attempts, because these usually mean the person is now able to cope better with stresses
    ④ Deviance in the person's background

80. A student approaches the school nurse. She is crying and states that her best friend hates her. According to Maslow, the student is expressing a need for:
    ❶ Love and belonging
    ② Self-actualization
    ③ Self-esteem
    ④ Security

81. A depressed patient takes fluoxetine hydrochloride (Prozac). The patient and family should be instructed that:
    ① Dosages are given every 12 hours
    ❷ It may take 1-4 weeks to see improvement in mood
    ③ Anxiety and nervousness should decrease
    ④ Suicidal tendencies may increase

82. The physician slams the chart down and leaves in a huff shortly after meeting with a young patient to discuss her terminal diagnosis. This is an example of which defense mechanism?
    ① Rationalization
    ② Undoing
    ❸ Displacement
    ❹ Compensation

83. A woman brings her father in to the clinic because he has been lost and could not remember his address. Which of the following questions should the nurse ask first to identify a possible cause of the problem?
    ❶ "What medications are you taking?"
    ② "When did you move to this address?"
    ③ "Have you had trouble sleeping lately?"
    ④ "Are you eating balanced meals daily?"

84. Which of the following statements about suicide is *most* correct?
    ① Suicide is 100% preventable
    ② Suicide is only inherited
    ③ Suicide occurs without any prior warning
    ❹ Suicide lethality increases in proportion to the details of the plan

85. Which of the following statements is most true about the difference between a delusion and a hallucination?
    ❶ Delusions are false beliefs; hallucinations are projections
    ② Delusions are systems; hallucinations are beliefs
    ③ Delusions are always true; hallucinations are always false
    ④ Delusions are based on fact; hallucinations are based on belief

86. The nurse is caring for an elderly patient diagnosed with dementia. The nurse tells the patient to "brush her teeth." The patient doesn't seem to comprehend the instructions. What should the nurse do next?
    ❶ Show the patient the toothbrush
    ② Brush the patient's teeth
    ③ Tell the patient again
    ④ Try again later in the day

87. The drug that cannot be given if the patient has consumed alcohol within the past 24 hours is:
    ① Chlorpromazine (Thorazine)
    ② Loxapine succinate (Loxitane)
    ❸ Disulfiram (Antabuse)
    ④ Trifluoperazine (Stelazine)

88. The nurse is caring for female patient in the emergency room. The patient complains of heart palpitations and weakness. No physical cause has been identified for her complaints. What should the nurse do when the patient is having an attack?
    ❶ Acknowledge her discomfort and remain with her
    ② Remind her that all her test were negative
    ③ Encourage the patient to explain the severity of her symptoms to her physician
    ④ Explain anxiety and panic attacks

89. To foster feelings that bolster a patient's self-esteem, it is important that the nurse:
    ① Constantly criticize the patient's behavior
    ❷ Accept and give positive reinforcement for appropriate behavior
    ③ Enforce behavior modification, including ignoring all previous unacceptable behavior
    ④ Remain very strict with unacceptable behavior and structure precise expectations for the patient

90. Which of the following would be the most therapeutic response for the nurse to make to a patient who complains of feeling "blue"?
    ① "You have been so successful."
    ② "Don't be blue, put this out of your mind."
    ③ "Don't let your feelings get the best of you."
    ❹ "Is there something in particular that is worrying you?"

91. The chief defense mechanism used by the alcoholic (addict) is:
    ❶ Denial
    ② Compensation
    ③ Reaction formation
    ④ Sublimation

92. In a crisis the aim of intervention is to:
    ① Rearrange life elements of the people involved
    ② Provide treatment for as long as possible
    ❸ Offer support and explore alternatives
    ④ Avoid old ties because these led up to the crisis

93. The nurse is explaining a diagnostic test to the patient. The patient is very anxious about the test. What should the nurse do to reduce the patient's anxiety?
    ❶ Explain the details of the procedure to the patient
    ② Explain the treatment the test provides
    ③ Explain the patient's NPO status
    ④ Assure the patient that the test is very accurate in identifying health problems

94. A 46-year-old woman is admitted to the hospital's psychiatric unit because of an increasingly depressed mood. She is unable to care for her house, and her husband reports she stays up late at night, has difficulty getting up in the morning, and complains of abdominal pain, which she states is punishment for her sins. The patient's symptoms are characteristic of:
    ① Alcoholic psychosis
    ❷ Affective disorder

③ Schizophrenia

④ Bipolar illness

95. The nurse is caring for a patient recently diagnosed with breast cancer. While discussing the new diagnosis with her, the patient tells the nurse, "You must have me confused with someone else, I have polycystic disease." What defense mechanism is the patient using?

① Repression

● Denial

③ Fantasy

④ Rationalization

96. A patient on suicide precautions reports a recent change in mood. The nurse knows:

● This is a high-risk factor

② The crisis has probably passed

③ The patient may be manic-depressive

● The patient is responding to the added attention of the precautions

97. A promiscuous drug-dependent adolescent is admitted to a psychiatric hospital after superficially cutting her wrist. Her attempted suicide is an example of:

● Poor impulse control

② Regressive behavior

③ Manipulation

④ Depression

98. The nurse just got a call from the emergency room that a patient diagnosed with AIDS is coming to her unit. Which of the following actions should the nurse take first?

① Prepare the patient's room for isolation

● Confront her own feelings about the diagnosis of AIDS

③ Orient the patient to his room

④ Explain unit policies to the patient

99. The nurse is making morning rounds. Upon entering the room of a patient who had a mastectomy for breast cancer, the nurse notes that the room is dark, the curtains are closed, and the lights are off. What objective data would the nurse include in the nurse's notes?

① "Post-op depression noted"

② "Seems to be depressed"

③ "Grieving loss of breast"

● "Sitting in dark room"

100. A severely depressed patient tells the nurse, "There is no reason for me to continue living." Which of the following responses by the nurse would be the most appropriate?

● "Are you thinking about suicide?"

② "There are a lot of people worse off than you."

③ "What would your family do?"

④ "You have a lot to live for."

ANSWERS AND RATIONALES

1. Comprehension, planning, psychosocial adaptation (b)
   ❸ Trust is essential when working with a depressed patient.
   ① This is an ongoing process.
   ② This is not the first priority.
   ④ This is an ongoing process.

2. Comprehension, assessment, psychosocial adaptation (c)
   ❹ Always go for the underlying feeling.
   ① This is a good second-choice answer.
   ② This statement is not true; this is imprisonment.
   ③ This is viewed as punitive for asking a question and has no foundation in fact for such an action.

3. Comprehension, planning, psychosocial adaptation (b)
   ❹ The depressed patient may become overwhelmed if too much is offered too soon; the patient should be engaged in structured, goal-directed activities.
   ① This could lead to withdrawal or seclusive behavior.
   ② This is overwhelming to the patient at the beginning of treatment.
   ③ Feelings cannot be restructured, but they can be dealt with if the patient will allow.

4. Knowledge, assessment, growth and development (a)
   ❶ Trust is seen as the developmental task between birth and 18 months.
   ② This is the developmental task of a preschooler.
   ③ This is the developmental task of an adolescent.
   ④ This is the developmental task in the elderly.

5. Comprehension, implementation, basic care and comfort (b)
   ❷ This gives a clear message, helps organize patient.
   ① This may lead to a power struggle.
   ③ This is not true; she should be encouraged to begin routine self-care as soon as possible.
   ④ Moralizing does not help patient.

6. Comprehension, assessment, coping and adaptation (b)
   ❸ The patient's anxiety is at the apprehension level; anxiety is related to a concrete future event.
   ① Panic includes loss of control.
   ② Free-floating has no specific object or event.
   ④ Alertness level is less severe, only vague symptoms.

7. Knowledge, assessment, growth and development (a)
   ❶ The two factors most associated with personality development are heredity and environment.
   ② Heredity is associated with personality development, but temperament is not.
   ③ Environment is correct, but nurturing is not.
   ④ Heredity is correct, but nurturing is not.

8. Application, assessment, growth and development (a)
   ❶ This is seen in middle adult years.
   ② This is seen in intimacy vs. isolation.
   ③ This is seen in adolescence.
   ④ This is seen in old age.

9. Application, implementation, psychosocial adaptation (c)
   ❸ Of the options given, this is the most appropriate; after very briefly acknowledging the patient's feelings (e.g., "This subject seems troubling for you"), the nurse should distract him from his delusion of grandeur and engage in a less threatening activity or topic.
   ① Measures to reduce the patient's anxiety should be employed at the first sign of discomfort or anxiety.

② Never challenge the patient's delusional system; that may force the patient to defend it.
④ Reinforces the delusion and further distances the patient from reality.

10. Knowledge, assessment, psychosocial adaptation (a)
    ❶ A phobia is an abnormally excessive fear.
    ② Obsession is a recurring thought.
    ③ Compulsion is the urge to engage in a behavior.
    ④ Psychosis is a major mental illness.

11. Comprehension, assessment, coping and adaptation (b)
    ❹ Most authorities agree that as depression lifts the patient is at greatest risk of committing suicide.
    ① The attention of the patient being admitted is diverted and focused on the admission, and he or she is not likely to commit suicide during the admission process.
    ② Discharge will *not* occur if the patient is actively suicidal.
    ③ As the depression deepens, it is less and less likely that suicide will occur, because the patient is experiencing decreasing physical functioning.

12. Comprehension, evaluation, psychosocial adaptation (a)
    ❸ Patient safety is always the number one priority.
    ① This is not the number one priority at this time.
    ② This is not the number one priority at this time.
    ④ This is not a priority at this time.

13. Knowledge, assessment, growth and development (a)
    ❷ Fantasy is common in the preschool-age child.
    ① Daydreaming is not as established at this age.
    ③ They are involved in sports and school activities.
    ④ More mature relationships.

14. Knowledge, assessment, coping and adaptation (a)
    ❶ You must first be in touch with your feelings.
    ② This would be the second most important thing.
    ③ You should also consider this.
    ④ This is not a priority.

15. Comprehension, evaluation, physiological adaptation (a)
    ❹ 3-pound goal was not met but the patient did gain 2 pounds, which is partial goal achievement.
    ① The 3-pound goal was not met.
    ② The goal isn't changed when it's not met; the nursing process is cyclic and has to be reentered.
    ③ The goal was partially met; to not meet the goal, the patient would have to have gained no weight.

16. Application, implementation, coping and adaptation (b)
    ❶ The patient needs to be removed from added stimuli so that he can better cope.
    ② He does not need additional stimuli at this time.
    ③ The client cannot control his anxiety.
    ④ The client does not need additional stimuli at this time.

17. Knowledge, evaluation, pharmacological therapies (a)
    ❹ These are common extrapyramidal side effects.
    ① These are not extrapyramidal side effects.
    ② These are not extrapyramidal side effects.
    ③ These are not extrapyramidal side effects.

18. Knowledge, evaluation, coping and adaptation (a)
    ❷ The patient is bargaining for another year of life.
    ① This is the "No, not me" stage.
    ③ A depressed individual would be found in a darkened room and most likely not be talking to his physician.
    ④ "I'm dying . . ." or any other similar statement indicates acceptance.

19. Application, implementation, coping and adaptation (c)
    ❷ Being dependable is necessary for the patient to trust and feel secure; contracted time with the patient is for that patient only; terminating a session early is a patient response for which the nurse should understand and be prepared.
    ① This is inappropriate; the patient has to assume responsibility for his behavior.
    ③ Contracted time with the patient is time for that patient only; the nurse should remain for the duration of the contracted time.
    ④ This is inappropriate; the focus is always the patient, not the nurse.

20. Comprehension, assessment, basic care and comfort (a)
    ❶ Physiological needs of food, shelter, and clothing are the number one priority.
    ② Loving and belonging are the third-level needs.
    ③ Self-esteem is the fourth-level need.
    ④ Self-actualization is the fifth-level need.

21. Comprehension, assessment, coping and adaptation (a)
    ❹ By definition, the ideas are flying by; hence flight of ideas.
    ① Word salad is a mixture of *just* words.
    ② Ambivalence is "I hate you, I love you"—opposite feelings within the same thought.
    ③ Confabulation is filling in a memory lapse with untrue statements.

22. Application, implementation, psychosocial adaptation (b)
    ❶ This helps with orientation.
    ② This does not help his memory.
    ③ This will probably make him more confused—too much stimuli.
    ④ This will confuse him more.

23. Comprehension, evaluation, psychosocial adaptation (b)
    ❹ Patients who are less depressed have more energy to commit suicide.
    ① The opposite is true.
    ② The opposite is true.
    ③ Patients may not verbalize suicide plans.

24. Application, implementation, psychosocial (b)
    ❹ It is appropriate to recognize the patient's feelings and encourage him to verbalize those feelings.
    ①, ②, ③ These are nontherapeutic. Patient's feelings are not addressed.

25. Application, evaluation, physiological adaptation (b)
    ❸ Amnesia is common following ECT.
    ① Paranoid behavior is not seen with ECT.
    ② The patient will probably be sedated.
    ④ The patient is more likely to be sedated.

26. Application, evaluation, coping and adaptation (b)
    ❷ Patients with anorexia may try to mask their weight loss.
    ① Daily weight is all that is needed.
    ③ This is not a common problem.
    ④ She may not see the problem as you see it.

27. Knowledge, assessment, physiological adaptation (a)
    ❸ Symptoms occur on stopping the drug.
    ① Tolerance means increasing doses to achieve effects.
    ② To abstain is not to drink.
    ④ Dementia is unrelated.

28. Comprehension, planning, physiological adaptation (b)
    ❷ This is clearly a goal that is attainable and appropriate.
    ①, ③, ④ These are unrealistic.

29. Comprehension, planning, psychosocial adaptation (b)
    ❶ This is the best response; it helps develop trust.
    ② This is not a good reason to stay. In this response the nurse, rather than the patient, is the focus; this does not foster trust.
    ③ This is false reassurance.
    ④ This puts client on defensive.

30. Comprehension, evaluation, psychosocial adaptation (c)
    ❷ When the antipsychotic is effective, patients report a decrease in the frequency and/or volume of the voices they hear.
    ① The voices do not disappear.
    ③ Drowsiness is an undesirable side effect; the patient should be assessed and findings reported to the physician and documented.
    ④ The nurse needs to clarify what the patient means by this and validate the patient's behavior.

31. Knowledge, implementation, coping and adaptation (b)
    ❶ The unfamiliar is anxiety provoking; a tour and review of expectations will assist with reducing the patient's anxiety.
    ② Patients are free to interact with others but are never required to do so.
    ③ Patients receive a copy of the Patient Bill of Rights on admission, and either a written copy of the unit rules and regulations or a verbal explanation of them; this builds trust and security.
    ④ This is not the purpose; the patient will be introduced to the group at the first community meeting.

32. Comprehension, assessment, psychosocial adaptation (a)
    ❸ This is a healthy response.
    ① This is unhealthy.
    ② This moves toward the illness end of the continuum.
    ④ This moves toward the illness end of the continuum.

33. Application, assessment, psychosocial adaptation (b)
    ❷ This tells you how serious the threat is.
    ① This is not the number one priority.
    ③ Family support is important, but it is not the number one priority.
    ④ This is not a priority; this comes later.

34. Application, evaluation, psychosocial adaptation (b)
    ❹ Obsessive compulsive behavior is characterized by ritualistic acts; under stress, the ritualistic behavior increases.
    ① Aggressive behavior is not necessarily seen in OCD.
    ② Communication may not be altered.
    ③ Individuals with OCD do not usually withdraw from reality and are aware of ritualistic acts.

35. Comprehension, evaluation, pharmacological therapies (b)
    ❶ This can cause hypertensive crisis.
    ②, ③, ④ These are not related to MAO use.

36. Knowledge, assessment, psychosocial adaptation (b)
    ❶ A delusion is a false fixed idea.
    ② A hallucination is a sensory experience.
    ③ An illusion is a misrepresentation.
    ④ Compensation is a defense mechanism.

37. Application, assessment, coping and adaptation (b)
    ❷ Erosion of tooth enamel is common.
    ①, ③, ④ These complaints are not as common as toothache.

38. Comprehension, implementation, psychosocial adaptation (c)
    ④ This response accepts reality of her experience and suggests self-control.
    ① This response denies reality of her experience.
    ② This response enters into the delusion.
    ③ This response denies reality of her experience.

39. Comprehension, assessment, psychosocial adaptation (b)
    ❷ Suspicion and jealousy are the predominant thoughts of the paranoid patient.
    ① Paranoid patients are so preoccupied with suspicion and jealousy that these are not substantial possibilities.
    ③ Self-pity and self-centeredness are more closely associated with the depressed patient, who is trying to blame self or relieve feelings of guilt.
    ④ This is the definition of ambivalence.

40. Application, planning, psychosocial adaptation (b)
    ④ Temporary amnesia is expected following ETC.
    ① This is not an expected outcome following ECT.
    ② ECT clients are not usually suicidal.
    ③ ECT treats depression.

41. Comprehension, planning, coping and adaptation (b)
    ❶ Nurses diagnose and treat human responses to illness, behaviors, or problems related to their probable causes.
    ② Nurses diagnose responses and not disease entities.
    ③ The medical diagnosis may or may not be related to the nursing diagnosis.
    ④ Nursing diagnosis is useful in many diverse settings.

42. Application, implementation, pharmacological therapies (b)
    ❷ This is a toxic level, so the dose should be held and the physician notified.
    ①, ③ The level is already toxic.
    ④ Xanax is an anti-anxiety medication and will not substitute for Lithium.

43. Knowledge, evaluation, psychosocial adaptation (b)
    ④ This is the desired effect of the treatment.
    ① This is the effect of antidepressant medications.
    ② ECT may cause amnesia of the previous few days, but it will not last.
    ③ This occurs during the treatment.

44. Comprehension, implementation, coping and adaptation (b)
    ❷ This is a realistic, feasible approach.
    ① Blanket approval is unrealistic.
    ③ She should begin to learn to tolerate separation.
    ④ This is unrealistic; leads to mistrust.

45. Comprehension, planning, safety and infection control (b)
    ❷ Identify the plan, then intervene.
    ① "Tell me more" may not identify the plan.
    ③ Although this is true, it does not address the plan.
    ④ This response is incorrect; if anyone approaches you with statements like the ones in this question, find out if they have a plan.

46. Application, implementation, pharmacological therapies (b)
    ❶ This can cause hypertensive crisis.
    ② The medicine can be taken on an empty stomach.
    ③ It is taken in the morning or may be multiple doses.
    ④ This is not necessary.

47. Comprehension, evaluation, coping and adaptation (b)
    ❷ This lets the patient vent her fears.
    ①, ④ This response offers false assurance.
    ③ This is an inappropriate and nontherapeutic remark.

48. Comprehension, evaluation, psychosocial adaptation (b)
    ❷ A blackout is the inability to remember what was done under the influence of alcohol.
    ① Psychosis would include short-term and long-term memory loss.
    ③ Denial is a part of the grieving process.
    ④ He may be alcoholic, but this does not explain the memory loss.

49. Comprehension, assessment, coping and adaptation (c)
    ❶ In a persecutory delusion, the television actually does not curse the patient; she feels persecuted by it.
    ② This is not a visual hallucination.
    ③ This is not incoherent, but structured thought.
    ④ This is not flight of ideas.

50. Comprehension, implementation, psychosocial adaptation (c)
    ④ Lithium is the medication of choice in the treatment of bipolar disorders.
    ① Chlorpromazine (Thorazine) is an antipsychotic; it is not used in bipolar disorder.
    ② Perphenazine (Trilafon) is an antipsychotic-neuroleptic.
    ③ Imipramine (Tofranil) is an antidepressant of the tricyclic group.

51. Comprehension, implementation, coping and adaptation (b)
    ❸ Excessive stimuli can agitate the patient.
    ① Restraints would be a last resort.
    ② Behavior modification may not be appropriate on an admissions unit.
    ④ This would be providing too much stimuli.

52. Application, implementation, psychosocial adaptation (b)
    ❷ This behavior can be anxiety over the unknown biopsy results.
    ① This would be insulting to the patient.
    ③ The nurse needs to acknowledge the behavior.
    ④ The nurse needs to address the behavior.

53. Knowledge, evaluation, coping and adaptation (a)
    ❶ Agoraphobia is fear of being alone.
    ② This is not agoraphobia.
    ③ This is not a symptom.
    ④ This is not seen in agoraphobia.

54. Comprehension, planning, psychosocial adaptation (b)
    ④ Exercise will help the patient burn calories and use energy.
    ①, ② These require the patient to be still and concentrate.
    ③ This is not as good a choice, may be too focused.

55. Comprehension, assessment, coping and adaptation (b)
    ④ Assurance and willingness to listen are keys to good therapeutic relationships.

① You should not acknowledge that you have knowledge and want to know more about "them"; avoid "buying into" the delusion or hallucination.
② Avoid denial of what the patient is seeing or doing. Remember to be nonjudgmental and nonthreatening.
③ See rationale for #1.

56. Comprehension, evaluation, pharmacological therapies (b)
❷ This is the drug of choice.
① This is a diuretic.
③ This is used as a sedative, for nausea.
④ Acetaminophen is an analgesic.

57. Comprehension, assessment, psychosocial adaptation (b)
❶ Adolescents with depression frequently act out.
② Seen in older adult clients that are depressed.
③, ④ These are not seen as part of depression.

58. Application, evaluation, coping and adaptation (b)
❶ Identification is taking on the characteristics of another.
② Compensation is making up for feelings of inferiority.
③ Conversion is channeling anxiety into bodily signs and symptoms.
④ Displacement is redirecting energies into another person or object.

59. Knowledge, implementation, psychosocial adaptation (a)
❸ Of the choices here, this is the most correct one.
① This is not true. Psychotics can think; it is disorganized.
② Psychotics are rarely depressed; mostly they cannot operate in reality.
④ These statements are reversed—the psychotic isn't in reality; the neurotic is in reality, but reality may be distorted.

60. Comprehension, assessment, pharmacological therapies (c)
❶ This is the correct answer; the patient may be experiencing the beginning effect called EPS (extrapyramidal symptoms). These symptoms are associated with the administration of antipsychotic medications. Incidentally, there will probably be an anti-EPS medication ordered to reverse the EPS effects.
②, ③ These are not appropriate as a *first* response.
④ This should not be a first response but may be required at some point in the event.

61. Comprehension, assessment, psychosocial adaptation (a)
❷ The behavioral changes indicate mania.
① This may not be true; diagnosis was accurate for the presenting symptoms.
③ This is not true; change too rapid and extreme.
④ This is unrelated.

62. Comprehension, implementation, psychosocial adaptation (b)
❶ This helps identify the content of the delusion.
② You cannot use logic to explain delusions.
③ Do not leave the patient alone.
④ Do not imply the patient is wrong.

63. Application, evaluation, pharmacological therapies (a)
❸ Patients usually show improvement in 2-4 weeks.
①, ② This is not long enough to see the desired effect.
④ It should not take this long to see improvement.

64. Knowledge, assessment, psychosocial adaptation (a)
❷ Mood swings are the characteristics of bipolar disorder; manic (elation) and depression are two phases.
① Paranoid disorders generally do not involve mood swings at all.
③ Schizophrenia is characterized by disorganized thinking.
④ Persons with eating disorders do not suffer from mood swings.

65. Knowledge, evaluation, pharmacological therapies (a)
❶ Sedation is a common side effect of Haldol.
② Weight gain is more common.
③ Dry mouth is not a common side effect.
④ Agitation is seen with overdose.

66. Comprehension, evaluation, pharmacological therapies (b)
❹ This is a true statement.
① Toxic blood levels are not a concern.
② Photosensitivity is not a problem.
③ Sedation is not a side effect.

67. Knowledge, assessment, psychosocial adaptation (a)
❸ Orderliness is the single feature of the obsessive compulsive disorder; usually done in ritual format.
① The obsessive-compulsive patient is so busy thinking and doing, there would be no time for seclusion.
② Aggression is not an obsessive-compulsive characteristic.
④ Instant gratification is related to poor impulse control; the obsessive-compulsive patient has an overwhelming need to perform activities that release the underlying feelings.

68. Knowledge, assessment, psychosocial adaptation (a)
❹ Marijuana is a cannabinol.
① It is not highly addictive; however, a psychological dependency can develop.
② Amphetamine is a class of psychoactive substance that is a cerebral stimulant.
③ Marijuana causes impaired brain function, but it is generally not known to generate hallucinations.

69. Comprehension, planning, basic care and comfort (b)
❸ During the manic phase patients have trouble being still but may eat on the go.
① This will not make the patient comply.
② This will not make the patient able to comply.
④ The patient will still be experiencing difficulty focusing.

70. Comprehension, assessment, psychosocial adaptation (b)
❶ Safety is always a number one priority.
② Ability to perform self-care is unknown.
③ This is a problem but not as much a priority as safety.
④ He is hearing voices, but safety is more important.

71. Application, implementation, psychosocial adaptation (a)
❸ Open-ended question, with ample time to listen, is the best therapeutic technique in this situation.
① You should indicate an interest in what the patient has said; saying nothing is the wrong activity.
② The pressing issue is death of parents; diversion of discussion is not appropriate.
④ This is inappropriate, and it is insulting.

72. Comprehension, assessment, coordinated care (b)
    ❶ Commitment is to protect the patient and others.
    ② Commitment has a time attached.
    ③ Rights are not lost.
    ④ The criminal justice system does not have to be involved.

73. Comprehension, evaluation, coping and adaptation (b)
    ❷ Anxiety is sometimes a healthy response to problems.
    ① Alcohol is not effective in managing anxiety.
    ③ Leisure time is necessary for a healthy lifestyle.
    ④ The patient will still have good and bad days.

74. Comprehension, assessment, psychosocial adaptation (b)
    ❷ Verbal intervention is always the first course of action.
    ① This action may be required later, depending on the ability to verbally deescalate the situation.
    ③ Go for the underlying feeling *first*.
    ④ Do not do this until it is necessary.

75. Comprehension, assessment, coping and adaptation (a)
    ❸ A gun would be a very serious weapon.
    ① The patient is thinking of it, no exact plan or weapon.
    ② She is seeking help.
    ④ The patient doesn't necessarily have pills.

76. Knowledge, assessment, psychosocial adaptation (b)
    ❹ This is a key indicator of depression.
    ①, ② This is not consistent with depression.
    ③ This is the most distant feeling from depression.

77. Comprehension, assessment, psychosocial adaptation (b)
    ❶ Compulsive behavior helps her cope with the anxiety.
    ② This is normal, not an obsession.
    ③, ④ These don't address specific activities.

78. Comprehension, assessment, psychosocial adaptation (a)
    ❸ This is common among patients with mania.
    ① This behavior is not seen in manic patients.
    ② The patient probably would not be still to play cards.
    ④ This attitude is not associated with mania.

79. Knowledge, assessment, psychosocial adaptation (b)
    ❷ Concrete, lethal plan is a very high-risk factor.
    ① Treatment duration is usually unrelated.
    ③ Past attempt is high risk but not for reason stated.
    ④ This is unrelated.

80. Application, evaluation, psychosocial adaptation (b)
    ❶ Love and belonging were addressed in the student's statement.
    ② This is the level many never reach.
    ③ This is the level next to self-actualization.
    ④ Security refers to a safe environment.

81. Application, implementation, pharmacological therapies (b)
    ❷ This is a true statement.
    ① Prozac is given in the morning and again at noon if more than one dose is required.
    ③ Anxiety and nervousness are side effects.
    ④ They should decrease.

82. Comprehension, evaluation, coping and adaptation (a)
    ❸ The physician is frustrated over the diagnosis and was not able to express this with the patient.
    ① No explanation was given.
    ② Nothing was undone.
    ④ He did not try to make up for a deficiency.

83. Comprehension, assessment, safety and infection control (b)
    ❶ This is the first priority question.

    ②, ③, ④ These questions ask for information that is not important at this time.

84. Comprehension, assessment, psychosocial adaptation (c)
    ❹ The more details contained in the plan of self-destruction, the more likely it is to occur.
    ① Suicide is not 100% preventable; many previous accidental deaths have proven to be suicides; surviving suicide is increasingly difficult as the instances of attempts increase.
    ② This is not a true statement.
    ③ Most suicides occur after ample warnings have been offered.

85. Knowledge, assessment, psychosocial adaptation (a)
    ❶ These are exact definitions of the respective terms.
    ② See rationale for #1.
    ③ Delusions are always false, as are hallucinations.
    ④ See rationale for #3.

86. Comprehension, implementation, basic care and comfort (b)
    ❶ This may jog the patient's memory.
    ② The patient needs to remain as independent as possible.
    ③ This will not make her understand any better.
    ④ She needs her teeth brushed now.

87. Comprehension, assessment, pharmacological therapies (a)
    ❸ Disulfiram (Antabuse) causes violent nausea and vomiting if taken within 24 hours of consuming alcohol.
    ① This is a major antipsychotic.
    ②, ④ These are antipsychotics.

88. Application, assessment, physiological adaptation (b)
    ❶ This is the best answer, these symptoms are real to her.
    ② This does not improve her feelings.
    ③ This will not decrease her symptoms.
    ④ This will not make her feel any better.

89. Comprehension, implementation, psychosocial adaptation (b)
    ❷ This is most therapeutic.
    ① This will have a negative effect.
    ③ Previous unacceptable behavior should be challenged and integrated into current behavioral activities.
    ④ This is not therapeutic.

90. Application, evaluation, psychosocial adaptation (b)
    ❹ You need additional information to help you plan for your patient.
    ① This doesn't help the current situation.
    ② This is false reassurance.
    ③ This doesn't help solve the situation.

91. Comprehension, assessment, psychosocial adaptation (a)
    ❶ Denial is the chief defense mechanism in that the addict can always find a reason to drink.
    ② The addiction is the weakness and has an underlying cause that is uncompensated.
    ③ Underlying feelings of guilt, sadness, etc. are relieved by the addiction, but these feelings return once the drug wears off; the addiction isn't the expression of an opposite attitude; it is relief from the underlying feelings.
    ④ Sublimation does not fit in the discussion of addiction.

92. Knowledge, implementation, psychosocial adaptation (a)
    ❸ Often a new observer is helpful in sorting out complexities and offering useful solutions.
    ① This is not a goal.
    ② Treatment is always time limited.
    ④ Old ties are often strengthened.

93. Application, implementation, reduction of risk potential (b)
    ❶ The more the patient knows, the less anxious he should be.
    ② The test is not treatment.
    ③ This will not decrease anxiety.
    ④ Do not offer false assurance.

94. Comprehension, assessment, psychosocial adaptation (b)
    ❷ Affective disorder is characterized by depressed mood, low energy, and somatic delusions.
    ①, ③ These are not indicated in situation.
    ④ This is unknown from data given; may or may not be true.

95. Application, assessment, psychosocial adaptation (b)
    ❷ Denial is common when diagnosed with a potentially fatal disease.
    ① Repression is a response to painful experience.
    ③ Fantasy is unacceptable behavior.
    ④ Rationalization is using a "good" reason to explain behavior.

96. Comprehension, assessment, coping and adaptation (c)
    ❶ This is high risk: mood change may signal behavior change.

② The nurse should not assume crisis has passed.
③ This is a medical diagnosis, not a nursing assessment.
④ This is not necessarily true.

97. Comprehension, assessment, reduction of risk potential (a)
    ❶ Poor impulse control; superficial wrist-cutting is impulsive behavior.
    ② Regressive is not correct; situation does not indicate earlier, more comfortable behavior.
    ③ May be manipulative, but situation does not indicate this.
    ④ Probably not depressive; situation does not include this.

98. Comprehension, implementation, coping and adaptation (b)
    ❷ You have to deal with your own feelings first.
    ① Universal precautions are all that is required.
    ③ This is not a first priority.
    ④ This is not the first thing to do.

99. Comprehension, evaluation, coping and adaptation (a)
    ❹ This reports what the nurse observed.
    ① The nurse is diagnosing with this written statement.
    ②, ③ The nurse is placing judgment with this written statement.

100. Comprehension, evaluation, psychosocial adaptation (b)
    ❶ This will get the information you need.
    ②, ③, ④ These are nontherapeutic.

CHAPTER 7

Maternity Nursing

The aim of obstetrics is to offer health services to the childbearing mother, her baby, and her family that will ensure a normal pregnancy and a safe prenatal and postnatal experience. This chapter reviews components of the nursing process. Each topic presents pertinent information helpful in planning the nursing assessment and in analyzing the nursing need of the family. Nursing management is outlined giving options for selecting appropriate plans for action. The evaluation of whether outcomes and goals of maternity nursing have been met completes the nursing process. The information presented in this review will assist the nurse in understanding how to:

- Plan, implement, and evaluate the nursing process as it relates to the maternity patient, her baby, and her family.
- Integrate selected theoretic information into the nursing process to effectively meet the basic aims of maternity nursing.

EVOLUTION OF MODERN OBSTETRICS

A. Early influences
1. Middle Ages and early Christianity: pain of childbirth believed to be a means of expiation for sins
2. Judaism: contributed to public health through its kosher dietary laws and to hygiene through its ritual of circumcision
3. Renaissance: Leonardo da Vinci (Italy, 1452-1519): contributed to understanding human anatomy through his anatomic drawings

B. Western European influence
1. Ambroise Paré (France, 1510-1590): started trend of doctors replacing midwives
2. Peter Chamberlen (England and Holland, 1560-1631): introduced forceps, paving the way for mechanical devices to assist in difficult deliveries
3. William Smellie (England, 1697-1763): published book on midwifery in 1752 and wrote rules for the use of forceps during a delivery
4. William Hunter (England, 1718-1783): described placental anatomy
5. Jean Louis Baudelocque (France, 1746-1810): described positions, presentations, and pelvic measurements
6. Ignaz Philipp Semmelweiss (Austria, 1818-1865): a pioneer in obstetric asepsis, Semmelweis found that handwashing before attending mothers greatly reduced the incidence of puerperal (child-bed) fever
7. Louis Pasteur (France, 1822-1895): discovered *Streptococcus* as the causative organism in puerperal fever (1860)

C. Contributors in the United States
1. Anne Hutchinson (1634): midwife who delivered many babies of early settlers
2. William Shippen: established first lying-in hospital and midwifery school in the United States in 1762
3. Oliver Wendell Holmes (1809-1894): stressed cleanliness and hand washing before caring for new mothers
4. Margaret Sanger Research Bureau (1923): first organization to address question of contraception and planned parenthood

D. United States legislation affecting mothers and children
1. 1921: Sheppard Towner Act: promoted health and welfare for mothers and children
2. 1936: Social Security benefits begun; later to include entitlement benefits for mothers and their dependent children
3. 1943: Emergency Maternal and Infant Care Act to assist families of soldiers during World War II
4. 1973: Supreme Court legalizes abortion
5. 1974: WIC: federally funded nutritional program providing supplementary food to eligible pregnant, lactating, or postpartum women, their infants, and children under 5 years of age
6. 1995-1996: several states enacted legislation to lengthen a postpartum stay to 48 hours for a vaginal delivery and 96 hours for a cesarean birth. Early discharge would be voluntary

DEFINITIONS COMMONLY USED IN OBSTETRICS
Statistics

Birth Rates
number of live births per 1000 population
Fetal Death (Stillborn)
fetus of 20 weeks or more gestational age who dies in utero prior to birth
Infant Mortality Rate
number of deaths before the first birthday per 1000 live births
Maternal Mortality Rate
number of mothers dying in or because of childbearing per 100,000 live births
Neonatal Death
death within first 4 weeks of life
Neonatal Death Care
number of deaths within the first 4 weeks of life per 1000 live births

Abbreviations (Limited Listing)

ABC
alternative birthing center
ARM
artificial rupture of membranes
BOW
bag of waters; amniotic sac
CPD
cephalopelvic disproportion
CS
cesarean section
DIC
disseminated intravascular coagulation
EDC
estimated date of confinement; due date for birth
EDD
estimated date of delivery
FHR
fetal heart rate
FHT
fetal heart tone
G
gravida; number of pregnancies
GTPAL
gravida, term, premature, abortions, living children; identification of pregnancy status
HCG
human chorionic gonadotropin
HELLP
hemolysis, elevated liver enzymes, low platelet count; extention of pathology related to severe preeclampsia
HIV
human immunodeficiency virus
LDRP
labor/delivery/recovery/postpartum; all phases of maternal and child care occur in the same room with the same staff member
LGA
large for gestational age
LMP
last menstrual period
P
para; number of viable births

PIH
pregnancy-induced hypertension
PROM
premature rupture of membranes
Q
quadrant; one of four equal parts into which the abdomen is divided to designate position of fetus in uterus
RhoGAM
antibody against Rh factor given early prenatally or within 72 hours postpartum to mother
SGA
small for gestational age
TORCHES
a group of intrauterine infections including toxoplasmosis, rubella, cytomegalovirus, herpes, and syphilis; these are commonly associated with high infant mortality

Common Obstetric Terminology

Apgar Score
method of evaluating infant immediately after delivery; usually at 1 minute and at 5 minutes
Advanced Maternal Age (Elderly Primapara)
pregnant woman over 35 years of age giving birth to her first child
Braxton-Hicks Contractions
painless uterine contractions felt throughout pregnancy, becoming stronger and more noticeable during second and third trimester
Caput
head; cephalic portion of infant
Cyesis
pregnancy
Dystocia
long, painful labor and delivery
Gestation
developmental time of embryo, fetus, in utero
Grand Multipara
more than five children
High Risk
pregnant woman with preexisting problems that could jeopardize the pregnancy, the fetus, or herself; under 18 years of age or over 35 years of age with no prenatal care (any one or more of these conditions)
Lightening
moving of the fetus and uterus downward into the pelvic cavity during the last 2 weeks before EDC (usually just before labor in multiparas)
Low Birth Weight
weight less than 2500 grams because of the baby being preterm (premature) or because of intrauterine growth retardation.
Low Risk
pregnant woman with normal history, between ages 18 and 34, with no medical, psychological, or other preexisting problems, and under good prenatal care
Meconium
first bowel movement of the newborn—thick, tarlike, greenish-black substance
Multigravida
pregnant more than one time
Multipara
given birth to more than one child

Postmature Infant
one born after 42 weeks' gestation
Premature Infant
one born anytime before 37 weeks' gestation
Primigravida
pregnant for the first time
Primipara
giving birth to first child
Pseudocyesis
false pregnancy
Quickening
first movements of the fetus felt by the mother (16 to 18 weeks' gestation)
Secundines
afterbirth of placenta and membranes
Term Infant
one born between 38 and 42 weeks' gestation
Vernix Caseosa
cheesy material covering the fetus and newborn that acts as a protection to the skin
Viable
capable of developing, growing, and sustaining life such as a normal human fetus at 24 weeks' gestation
Vis a Tergo
external pressure on the fundus to assist in the delivery of the infant

TRENDS

A. Cost containment: rising health care costs are a national concern; increased home care, shortened stays, and increased emphasis on prenatal care are interventions to help control cost and maintain quality; regionalization of services for high-risk childbearing families and managed care are newer methods to attempt to control costs

B. Prenatal care: emphasis must be placed on improving access to prenatal care; particularly for low-income women. Prenatal care can avoid many conditions that can be prevented with adequate monitoring during pregnancy

C. Early discharge: may be discharged home within 12 to 24 hours (uncomplicated labor and delivery) and 3 to 4 days or less for a cesarean. These shortened stays are an attempt to control health care costs. These shortened stays are creating an increased need for prenatal education materials and follow-up phone numbers to reinforce education

D. Early discharges: these have caused an increased demand for home care and other community services. This home follow-up is especially important for adolescents or other families with psychosocial complications. Nurse entrepreneurs have helped to bridge this gap for many families

E. High-technology care: technological developments including fetal surgery have often outpaced society's ability to determine ethical implications of their use

F. Changing demographics: women are waiting longer in life to have their first babies. Nurses need to be familiar with effects of pregnancy on older women

G. Teen pregnancy: nurses need to identify and implement strategies to decrease incidence of adolescent pregnancy

H. Changing cultures: nurses need to be sensitive to different cultures' ideas and health practices

I. Prepared childbirth experience: mother and father (or alternate) jointly attend childbirth education classes to prepare for the child and for the childbearing and childbirth experience

J. Alternative birth settings
1. Birthing centers outside of hospital; ABC (alternative birth centers)
2. Individual's home
3. Use of the birthing chair instead of traditional table
4. Birthing room: labor, delivery, and postpartum hospital stay incorporated into one cheerful, homelike room set up with necessary labor and delivery equipment

K. Variety of positions used to assist labor and delivery (squat, side position, etc.)

L. Showering during first or second stage of labor

M. Inclusion of father or alternate: support person stays in labor and delivery area for both vaginal and cesarean section deliveries

N. Rooming in: allows newborn in room with mother for the day; fathers allowed unlimited visiting time

O. Sibling visits: designated hours that children may visit and see baby

P. Use of midwives: many hospitals and birthing centers throughout the United States now have nurse-midwives as the primary care person conducting prenatal, labor, delivery, and follow-up care

Q. Cesarean sections: more frequent now because of sophisticated fetal monitoring; controversial because of high numbers of sections in recent years

R. Breast-feeding: accepted and encouraged; societies such as La Leche League and popularity of "natural" foods encourage breast-feeding

S. Genetic counseling: increasingly accurate, safe amniocentesis and advances in genetics encourage counselors to advise couples with genetic problems

T. In vitro method of fertilization to assist pregnancy/fetal development: usually chosen by couples with fertility problems after exploring various methods, including fertility drugs and other insemination practices

U. Students are advised to review the U.S. Department of Health and Human Services: *Healthy People 2000: national health promotion and disease prevention objectives,* http://odphp.Osophs.dhhs.gov/pubs/hp2000/

PROCEDURES TO DETERMINE MATERNAL/FETAL PROBLEMS

A. Alpha fetoprotein (AFP) test
1. Screening procedure, not diagnostic
2. Serum from maternal blood sample is tested; best results if sample is taken at 16 to 18 weeks' gestation; identifies unrecognized high-risk pregnancies
3. Elevated levels of maternal serum indicate 5% to 10% open neural tube defect (spina bifida) in developing fetus
4. Recommend two samples of test followed by ultrasound and amniocentesis to confirm findings; genetic counseling availability if confirmed
5. Other causes of elevated AFP levels: multiple gestation, missed abortions, other abnormalities

B. Amniocentesis: invasive procedure during which a needle is inserted through abdomen and uterus to withdraw amniotic fluid; usually done after 14th week
1. Used for determination of sex, defects in fetus (e.g., Down syndrome); fetal status (Rh isoimmunal problem, fetal maturity, other tests as listed below)
2. Lecithin/sphingomyelin ratio (L/S ratio): used to determine fetal lung maturity by testing surfactant by 35th week of pregnancy; lecithin level two times greater than sphingomyelin level indicates that lungs are mature
3. Creatinine level: used to test fetal muscle mass and fetal renal function; 0.2 mg/100 ml amniotic fluid at 36 weeks is normal level; large amount may also indicate large fetus, such as fetus of diabetic mother
4. Bilirubin level: used for determination of fetal liver maturity; should decrease as term progresses; 450 μm is optimal density
5. Cytological testing: determines percentage of lipid globules present in amniotic fluid, indicates fetal age

C. Chorionic villi test
1. Permits first-trimester testing for biochemical and chromosomal defects; invasive and high-risk procedure during which a plastic catheter is inserted vaginally into the uterus; ultrasound guides catheter to chorionic frondosum
2. Can be done 9 to 11 weeks after LMP
3. Done earlier than amniocentesis; recent evidence shows that test may increase risk of babies born with missing toes and fingers or shortened digits

D. Fetoscopy: invasive procedure using transabdominal insertion of metal cannula into abdomen; visualization of fetus and placenta for developing abnormalities and to obtain fetal skin or blood samples
1. High-risk procedure; complications include spontaneous abortion and premature labor
2. Has limited usage, only if defect cannot be detected otherwise

E. Umbilical cord technique: evaluates condition of fetus
1. Superior technique because fetal blood can be analyzed as early as 18th week of gestation
2. Can evaluate blood count, liver function, blood gases, acid-base status
3. Invasive procedure; limited use because of risk of injury to fetus

F. Estriol level study: 24-hour urinalysis of urine from mother; determines estriol level to ascertain fetal well being and placental functioning
1. Done at third trimester (32 weeks)
2. 12 mg in 24 hours is good; below 12 mg indicates that infant is in jeopardy (related to decreased placental functioning)
3. Decreasing estriol levels can be used in combination with other diagnostic tests to indicate a compromised placenta or fetus

G. Heterozygote testing (mother's blood): done to detect clinically normal carriers of mutant genes
1. Tay-Sachs disease: common fatal genetic disease affecting children of Ashkenazi Jews (Eastern Europe)
2. Sickle cell anemia: common disorder among black Americans of African descent; 1 in 10 African-Americans is a carrier

3. Cooley's anemia (beta thalassemia): genetic disorder frequent among Mediterranean ethnic groups: Italians, Sicilians, Greeks, Turks, Middle Eastern Arabs, Asian Indians, Pakistanis

H. Contraction stress test: late trimester test to measure placental insufficiency and measure fetal reaction to uterine contractions (potential fetal compromise);
   1. Usually done after estimated date of confinement (EDC) has passed
   2. Invasive procedure during which IV oxytocin is administered, baseline recorded on monitor; takes 20 minutes to 1 hour
   3. Breast stimulation techniques are done in some health care settings in place of oxytocin infusion during a contraction stress test
   4. Results: late decelerations during contraction for at least three contractions indicate a positive test; no decelerations during three successive contractions within 10 minutes indicate a negative test; occasionally inconsistent decelerations indicate suspicious conditions

I. Nonstress test (NST): assesses and evaluates fetal heart tone (FHT) response to uterine movement or increased fetal activity

J. Ultrasound procedure: use of high-frequency sound waves to determine fetal size, estimate amniotic fluid volume, neural tube defects, limb abnormalities, evaluation of fetal presentation, diagnosis of breech presentation, etc.
   1. Usually a second-trimester procedure
   2. Risks still under investigation
   3. Acoustic sound waves can be used to help stimulate an inactive fetus during a nonstress test

K. Biophysical profile: using ultrasound and a nonstress test, this profile evaluates five fetal variables: breathing movements, body movements, muscular tone, qualitative amniotic fluid volume, and heart rate

L. Doppler flow studies: use ultrasound techniques to evaluate blood flow studies in deep-lying vessels; these are particularly useful in managing high-risk pregnancies

M. Fetal movement: Noninvasive method of determining fetal well being; if patterns deviate from normal pattern it may be an indication for further studies

ANATOMY AND PHYSIOLOGY OF REPRODUCTION
Obstetric Pelvis

A. Types (Fig. 7-1)
   1. Gynecoid: "true" female pelvis
   2. Anthropoid: narrow from side to side
   3. Android: male pelvis
   4. Platypoid: flat pelvis narrow from front to back
   Types 3 and 4 are not adequate for vaginal delivery

B. Components
   1. Ilium: flat or lateral, flaring part of pelvis or hip; iliac crest is top part of ilium
   2. Ischium: inferior dorsal or lower part of hip bone; the ischial spines, sharp projections of the ischium, are important in obstetrics because they are landmarks to measure progress of presenting part of fetus
   3. Sacrum: triangular bone between the two hip bones; flat part of the lower back (spine)

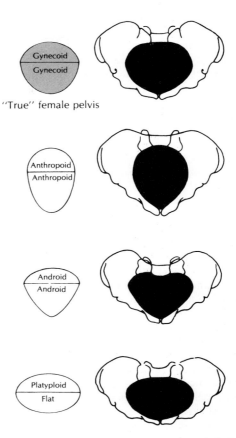

PURE TYPES

"True" female pelvis

Figure 7-1 Female pelvis: pure types. (From Bobak IM, Jensen MD: *Essentials of maternity nursing,* ed 2, St Louis, 1987, Mosby.)

   4. Coccyx: two to five rudimentary vertebrate that are fused and attached to lower part of sacrum (tailbone)

C. Measurements
   1. Diagonal conjugate: measured through vagina from lower border of symphysis pubis to promontory of sacrum (12.5 to 13 cm)
   2. Conjugate vera (true conjugate): measured from upper margin of symphysis pubis to promontory of sacrum by x-ray examination or sonogram (11 cm)
   3. Transverse diameter: distance between inner surfaces of the tuberosities of ischium (13 to 13.5 cm)
   4. Obstetric conjugate: measured by x-ray examination or sonogram or by subtracting 1.5 to 2 cm from diagonal conjugate (9.5 to 11.5 cm)

Fertilization and Implantation

A. Definitions
   1. Fertilization: occurs when the sperm and ovum join, usually at the distal third of the fallopian tube within 12 to 48 hours after intercourse
   2. Zygote: product of the union of a sperm and ovum
   3. Implantation: occurs when zygote burrows into the endometrium of the uterus, approximately 7 days after fertilization
   4. Nidation: completion of implantation

B. Processes
   1. Mitosis: rapid cell division
   2. Blastoderm: first division of the zygote
   3. Morula: ball-like structure of the blastoderm; sometimes referred to as mulberry-like
   4. Blastocyst: as morula enters uterus
   5. Trophoblast: as blastocyst implants in the uterus, the wall becomes the trophoblast
   6. Chorionic villi: trophoblasts develop villi that become fetal portion of the placenta
   7. Decidua: endometrium undergoes a change when pregnancy occurs
   8. Decidua vera: that portion of the decidua that becomes the lining of the uterus except for around implantation site
   9. Decidua basalis: where implantation occurs and where chorionic villi become frondosum or the beginning of the placental formation
   10. Decidua capsularis: covers blastocyst and fuses to form fetal membranes
   11. Amnion: inner membrane, which comes from the zygote and blends with the cord
   12. Chorion: outer membrane, which comes from the zygote and blends with the fetal portion of the placenta

Development of Human Organism

A. Ovum stage: preembryonic stage from conception until the primary villi appear (first 14 days)
B. Embryo: end of ovum stage to 8 weeks from LMP; period of rapid cellular development: disruption will cause developmental abnormality
C. Fetus: from end of embryonic stage (8 weeks) to term
D. Placenta: membrane weighing about 450 g (1 lb); develops cotyledons that act as areas for nourishing fetus; maternal surface is beefy and red; fetal surface is shiny and gray
E. Amnionic cavity: fills with fluid (1000 ml) that is replaced every 3 hours; shelters fetus

Sex Determination

A. Normal sperm: carries 22 autosomes and 1 sex chromosome (either an X or a Y chromosome)
B. Normal ovum: carries 22 autosomes and 1 sex chromosome (always an X chromosome)
C. Combined number of chromosomes: 44 autosomes and 2 sex chromosomes (at conception)
D. Genetic component of sperm determines sex of child (Box 7-1)
E. Chromosome carries genes plus DNA and proteins
F. Genes: factors in chromosomes carrying hereditary characteristics

PHYSIOLOGY OF FETUS

A. Membranes and amniotic fluid
   1. Protect from blows and bumps mother may experience
   2. Maintain even heat to fetus
   3. Act as an excretory system
   4. Supply oral fluid for fetus
   5. Allow free movement of fetus
B. Placenta
   1. Transport organ: passes nutrients from mother to fetus and relays excretory material from fetus to mother
   2. Formation completed by 3 months

Box 7-1   Sex Determination

Sperm supplies 22 autosomes and an X sex chromosome
Ovum supplies 22 autosomes and an X sex chromosome
Result: 44 autosomes and an XX = female
Sperm supplies 22 autosomes and a Y sex chromosome
Ovum supplies 22 autosomes and an X sex chromosome
Result: 44 autosomes and an XY = male

---

   3. Functions: kidney, lungs, stomach, and intestines
   4. Requirement: adequate oxygen from mother to function well
C. Monthly development
   1. Embryonic stage (1st to 8th week)
      a. Beginning: pulsating heart, spinal canal formation: no eyes or ears; buds for arms and legs
      b. By end: little over 1 inch (2.5 cm) long; eyelids fused; distinct divisions of arms, legs; cord formed; tail disappears
   2. Fetal stage (9th week to term)
      a. Between 20 and 24 weeks is considered the legal threshold for viability, the age at which the fetus is capable of surviving outside of the uterus
      b. The embryo or fetus is most vulnerable to damaging effects of tetragenic agents during the first trimester; tetracycline, caffeine, and many over-the-counter drugs are examples of drugs that are tetragenic
      c. 3 months: 3 inches (7.5 cm) long; weighs 1 oz (28 g); fully formed arms, legs, fingers; distinguishable sex organs
      d. 4 months: development of muscles, movement; mother feels quickening; 6 to 7 inches (15 to 17.5 cm) long; weighs 4 oz (112 g); lanugo over body; head large
      e. 5 months: 10 to 12 inches (25 to 30 cm) long; weighs ½ to 1 lb (225 to 450 g); internal organs maturing; lungs immature; FHT heard on examination; eyes fused; rarely survives more than several hours
      f. 6 months: 11 to 14 inches (27.5 to 35 cm) long; weighs 1 to 1½ lb (450 to 675 g); wrinkled "old man" appearance; vernix caseosa covers body; eyelids separated; eyelashes and fingernails formed
      g. 7 months: begins to store fat and minerals; 16 inches (40 cm) long; may survive with excellent care
      h. 8 months: beginning of month weighs 2 to 3 lb (900 to 1350 g); by end of month, 4 to 5 lb (1800 to 2250 g); continues to develop; loses wrinkled appearance
      i. 9 months: 19 inches (47.5 cm) long; weighs 7 lb (3200 g) (girl) 7½ lb (3400 g) (boy); more fat under skin; vernix caseosa; has stored vitamins, minerals, and antibodies; fully developed
D. Fetal circulation
   1. Special structures
      a. Ductus venosus: passes through liver; connects umbilical vein to inferior vena cava; closes at birth

b. Ductus arteriosus: shunts blood from pulmonary artery to descending aorta; closes almost immediately after birth

c. Foramen ovale: valve opening that allows blood to flow from right atrium to left atrium; functionally closes at birth; all three fetal structures listed above allow blood to bypass the fetal lungs and liver

d. Umbilical arteries (2): transport blood from the hypogastric artery to the placenta; functionally closes at birth

e. Umbilical vein (1): transports oxygenated blood from placenta to ductus venosus and liver, then to the inferior vena cava (IVC); closes at birth

2. Fetal circulation (Fig. 7-2)

a. Oxygenated blood from placenta goes through umbilical vein, bypassing portal system of the liver by way of the ductus venosus

b. From the ductus venosus blood goes to the ascending vena cava (inferior) to the heart, right auricle

c. From the right auricle through the foramen ovale

d. To the left auricle, then to the left ventricle

e. Leaves the heart through the aorta to the arms and head

f. The blood then returns to the heart, passing through the descending vena cava (superior)

g. To the right auricle, then to the right ventricle

h. Blood leaves the heart through the pulmonary arteries, bypassing the lungs

i. Blood goes through the ductus arteriosus to the aorta and down to the trunk and lower extremities

j. It then goes through the hypogastric arteries to the umbilical arteries on to the placenta, carrying carbon dioxide and waste materials

NORMAL ANTEPARTUM (PRENATAL)
Physiological Changes During Pregnancy

A. Reproductive system

1. External changes

a. Perineum: increased vasculature; enlarges

b. Labia majora: change especially in parous woman; separate and stretch

c. Anal and vulvar varices: caused by increased pelvic congestion

2. Internal changes

a. Uterus: enlarges to accommodate growing fetus; walls thicken first trimester; *Hegar's* sign (soft, lower lip of uterus)

b. Cervix: *Goodell's* sign (thickens, softens) 6 weeks from LMP because of vascular changes

c. Vagina: *Chadwick's* sign (bluish violet color); mucosal changes about 8 weeks from LMP; estrogen activity may cause thick vaginal discharge

B. Other body system changes

1. Breasts

a. Increased size, tingling sensations, heavy

b. Increased pigmentation, darkened areolae

c. Montgomery's tubercles on areolae

2. Cardiovascular changes

a. Slight enlargement of heart resulting from increased blood volume

b. Increased circulation (47%)

c. Cardiac output increased 30% first and second trimester, then levels off until term; during labor and delivery increases; and about 13% above normal during postpartum period

3. Hematologic changes

a. Increased RBC count; decreased hemoglobin level

b. Increased tendency for blood to coagulate during pregnancy

c. Coagulation factors return to normal during postpartum, increasing likelihood of thromboembolism

4. Respiratory/pulmonary changes: enlarging uterus presses on diaphragm, causing difficulty breathing

5. Skin: increased pigmentation

a. Linea nigra: darkening line from below breast bone (sternum) down midline of abdomen to symphysis pubis

b. Chloasma gravidarum (mask of pregnancy): dark, frecklelike pigmentation over nose and cheeks; disappears after delivery

c. Stria gravidarum: stretching of skin with silvery to reddish, bluish stretch marks on breasts, abdomen, thighs, never disappears completely; lotion, cocoa butter lubricants may help

6. Urinary system changes

a. Traces of sugar in urine resulting from activity of lactiferous ducts

b. Even though glucosuria is common in pregnancy, all women should be screened for diabetes

c. Transitory albumin: may be indication of pending pregnancy-induced hypertension

d. Cystitis: frequent because ureters lose some compliance or elasticity

7. Endocrine system

a. Variable production of insulin during pregnancy

b. Mother's cells become more insulin resistant

c. Thyroid gland increases in size, resulting in increased basal metabolic rate (BMR)

8. Digestive system

a. Morning sickness: nausea and vomiting common during first trimester

b. Increased appetite after first trimester

c. Indigestion (heartburn): caused by increasing upward pressure of enlarging uterus or by relaxin hormone, which slows metabolism and keeps food in stomach longer in pregnant women

d. Constipation: caused by changes in organ positions; pressure of growing uterus on sigmoid colon

9. Musculoskeletal system

a. Normal lumbar curve becomes more pronounced as weight of pelvic contents tilts the pelvis forward

b. Extra weight may lead to backache experienced in late pregnancy

10. Weight gain: total weight gain varies from 25 to 30 lb (12 to 13.5 kg) (Table 7-1)

Duration of Pregnancy

A. Length in terms of time

1. 9 calendar months

2. 10 lunar months

3. 280 days (266 days from time of ovulation)

4. 40 weeks

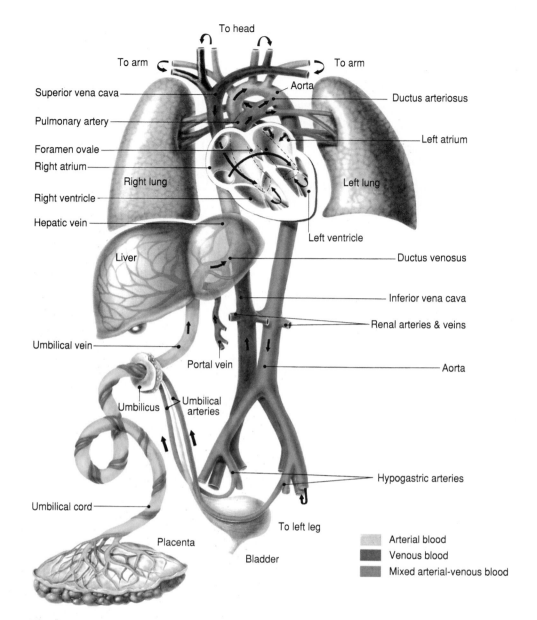

Figure 7-2   *Fetal circulation. Before birth.* Arterialized blood from the placenta flows into the fetus through the umbilical vein and passes rapidly through the liver into the inferior vena cava; it flows through the foramen ovale into the left atrium, soon to appear in the aorta and arteries of the head. A portion bypasses the liver through the ductus venosus. Venous blood from the lower extremities and head passes predominantly into the right atrium, the right ventricle, and then into the descending pulmonary artery and ductus arteriosus. Thus the foramen ovale and the ductus arteriosus act as bypass channels, allowing a large part of the combined cardiac output to return to the placenta without flowing through the lungs. Approximately 55% of the combined ventricular output flows to the placenta; 35% perfuses body tissues; and the remaining 10% flows through the lungs. *After birth.* The foramen ovale closes, the ductus arteriosus closes and becomes a ligament, the ductus venosus closes and becomes a ligament, and the umbilical vein and arteries close and become ligaments. (Used with permission of Ross Products Division, Abbott Laboratories, Columbus, Ohio.)

B. Nägele's rule: to calculate EDC count back 3 months from the month of the LMP and add 7 days to the first day of LMP

EXAMPLE: first day of LMP was July 17

$$\begin{array}{ll} 7 \;\;(\text{July}) & 17 \\ \underline{-3 \;\; \text{months}} & \underline{+7} \\ 4\text{th month} & 24 = \text{EDC April 24} \end{array}$$

Signs and Symptoms of Pregnancy

A. Presumptive signs (subjective: mother usually notices)
  1. Missed menstrual period
  2. Breast changes; nipples tingle, fuller, darker areola in about 6 weeks
  3. Frequency of urination in about 6 weeks
  4. Morning sickness: nausea and vomiting in 4 to 6 weeks

TABLE 7-1 Distribution of Weight Gain During Pregnancy

Distribution	Pounds	Grams
Fetus	7½	3400
Placenta	1	450
Amniotic fluid	2	900
Uterus	2½	1125
Increased blood volume	3-4	1350-1800
Breasts	2-3	900-1350
Mother's gain (fat, tissue, etc.)	4-8	1800-3600
Total weight gain	21-28 lb	9.5-12.7 kg

5. Skin changes: chloasma, linea nigra, striae (some authors call this "probable" sign)
B. Probable signs (objective examiner usually notices)
  1. Uterus: enlarges; shape changes at 12 to 16 weeks; Hegar's sign: 8 weeks
  2. Cervix: Goodell's sign
  3. Vagina: Chadwick's sign
  4. Implantation site: softens, enlarges (von Fernwald's sign) 6 to 7 weeks
  5. Laboratory tests:
    a. Immunological: widely used today; faster, 90% accurate; beta subunit of Hcg can be used even before missed period
    b. Commercially sold pregnancy test: an HAI in-home test, results in 4 minutes; should be confirmed by a physician
  6. Braxton-Hicks contractions
  7. Ballottement
C. Positive signs (by examiner)
  1. Palpate: can feel fetal parts
  2. Hearing: fetal heart tone
    a. Electronic Doptone scope (audible at 8 to 11 weeks)
    b. Sonogram (can ascertain at 12 weeks)
    c. Auscultation (17 to 24 weeks) with fetoscope (headscope) or Leff stethoscope
  3. Ultrasonographic (echographic) evidence of pregnancy visualized on screen
  4. Fetal movement palpable after 20 weeks

Prenatal Care

A. Importance
  1. Regular assessment and monitoring detect early signs and symptoms disrupting normal, healthy pregnancy
  2. Early evaluation of problem permits development of an appropriate plan of action based on findings
B. Visits and examinations
  1. Initial visits: establish diagnosis of pregnancy
  2. Lab work drawn during prenatal visits
    a. Alpha fetoprotein (AFP): AFP measurements in maternal serum are used for early diagnosis of fetal neural tube defects, such as spina bifida and anencephaly
    b. Estriol: estriol levels are done as part of a "triple marker test"; in the presence of a fetus with Down's syndrome, the AFP levels and estriol levels are low and the Hcg levels are low; these tests in combination with maternal age are used to calculate the risk

c. Human placental lactogen (HPL): a placental hormone that may be deficient in certain abnormalities of pregnancy
3. Complete medical history
  a. General personal health, habits, diseases, and medical or surgical problems
  b. History of communicable diseases, especially scarlet fever, measles, rubella, streptococcal infections, kidney conditions that might adversely affect pregnancy, and sexually transmitted diseases
  c. Psychosocial history: assess substance use or abuse (including alcohol, tobacco, illegal prescription or over-the-counter drugs), social support, physical abuse, stress, employment, physical activity, cultural influences, and sibling adjustment; siblings of the baby should be provided with explanations of pregnancy appropriate for the child's age
  d. Previous pregnancies, miscarriages, abortions, blood transfusions, gynecological problems
  e. Family health status: diabetes, tuberculosis, heart disease, cancer, epilepsy, allergies, mental problems
4. Complete examination to include
  a. Routine laboratory tests
    (1) Matching blood type and Rh factor
    (2) Antibody screen (rubella, sickle cell) if appropriate
    (3) Hemoglobin and hematocrit
    (4) Venereal Disease Research Laboratory (VDRL) test (for syphilis)
    (5) Herpes 1 and 2 tests
    (6) HIV testing for the AIDS virus
    (7) Hepatitis A and B tests
    (8) Pap smear
    (9) PPD test used for tuberculosis
  b. Physical examination to include
    (1) Pelvic examination and measurements
    (2) Abdominal palpation
    (3) Examination of breasts, nipples
    (4) Vital signs: blood pressure, weight, temperature, respirations
    (5) Urinalysis for sugar and albumin
    (6) Smears (Papanicolaou's test) for cytology, gonorrhea, chlamydia
5. Usual schedule for prenatal visits
  a. Every month for 28 weeks
  b. Every 2 weeks thereafter to 36th week
  c. Every week from 37th week to term
  d. Adjusted to individual needs
6. Usual routine for prenatal visits:
  a. Urinalysis each visit for sugar, acetone, albumin
  b. Capillary blood testing on a glucose oxidase strip for gestational diabetes mellitus (GDM); followed by plasma glucose testing at 12 weeks' gestation on all high-risk pregnancies
  c. Check vital signs (especially blood pressure)
  d. Check weight gain every visit
    (1) First trimester: 3 to 4 lb (1.5 to 2 kg) total
    (2) Second trimester: 1 lb (0.5 kg) per week; 12 to 14 lb (6 to 7 kg) total
    (3) Third trimester: 1 lb (0.5 kg) per week; 8 to 10 lb (4 to 5 kg) total
  e. Measure height of fundus to evaluate growth of fetus (Fig. 7-3)

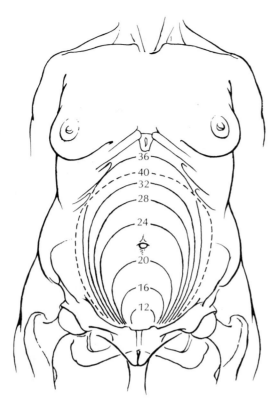

Figure 7-3 Height of fundus by weeks of normal gestation with a single fetus. Dotted line indicates height after lightening. (Modified from Barkauskas V et al: *Health and physical assessment*, ed 2, St Louis, 1998, Mosby.)

    f. Listen to FHT and FHR by Doptone or auscultation
    g. Ask about fetal activity, attitude of family; answer mother's questions, fears
    h. Recommend childbirth education classes
C. Promotion of positive health
  1. Nutritional counseling
    a. Fetus receives all nourishment from mother
    b. Teenage pregnant mother requires extensive counseling (nutritional pattern poor); focus on positive effect of good nutrition on teenager as well as on fetus
    c. Salt restrictions may be advised in presence of edema, retention of fluids, sudden change in blood pressure
    d. Direct relationship between maternal nutrition and mental development of the child
    e. Megavitamins should be avoided during pregnancy; they can be dangerous for the developing fetus
    f. Long-term users of oral contraceptives may have depleted the body's reserves of vitamin B_6 and folate
    g. High folic acid intake may disguise vitamin B_{12} deficiency (pernicious anemia), which can lead to neurological damage; folic acid intake should not exceed 400 μg/day.
    h. Energy needs during pregnancy increases little (300 kcal/day) compared with the increased need for nutrients
  2. Nutritional needs during pregnancy
    a. See Table 7-2
    b. See Food Pyramid in Chapter 4

3. General health teaching
    a. Daily baths for cleanliness; showers during last 6 weeks for safety's sake
    b. Moderate exercise, especially walking
    c. Douching only on advice of physician
    d. Sexual intercourse permissible as long as it is not uncomfortable, cervix is closed and membranes are intact
    e. Good support bra
    f. Unrestrictive comfortable clothing, hose
    g. Good mental attitude; discuss ambivalent feelings
    h. Smoking: nicotine retards growth of fetus, constricts blood vessels in mother, decreases placental function, and may cause premature labor; growing evidence shows that secondary smoking has damaging effects on the mother, fetus, children, and spouses; research has shown a relationship between mothers who smoke excessively and the incidence of pneumonia and bronchitis in babies at 6 to 9 months of age
    i. Alcohol: research has yet to determine minimum safe amounts of alcohol (if any) that can be consumed in pregnancy
    j. Caffeine: caffeine has been shown to cause tetragenic effects in animals; pregnant women should be counseled to avoid foods containing caffeine (found in coffee, tea, chocolate, colas, and some analgesics); newer evidence indicates a higher incidence of Sudden Infant Death Syndrome (SIDS) in infants of mothers who consumed significant amounts of caffeine during pregnancy
    k. Drugs: may pass placental barrier and affect fetus; greatest danger is during first trimester, but effects may not be evident for years after birth; new evidence shows that crack or cocaine may cause significant complications for mother and newborn; pregnant women should be counseled to avoid over-the-counter or prescription medications without the advice of a physician; pregnant women should be counseled about their regular use of vitamins and warned against taking megadoses
4. Childbirth and parent education classes
    a. Dick-Read method ("childbirth without fear") (1944): philosophy of relaxation coupled with abdominal and chest breathing and education
    b. Lamaze method, American Society for Prophylaxis in Obstetrics [ASPO]; psychoprophylactic method [PPM]) 1960: combines breathing techniques with preparation for childbirth by training mother to anticipate various stages of labor and meet each stage with practiced relaxation and breathing methods; coach to support mother and direct her if necessary.
    c. Bradley method, 1965: husband-coached childbirth, emphasizing quiet, darkened atmosphere, no stress
5. Teaching danger signs (those that must be reported to physician immediately)
    a. Persistent, severe vomiting beyond first trimester
    b. Epigastric or abdominal pain
    c. Edema: face, fingers; especially in the morning
    d. Visual disturbances: blurring, double vision, spots
    e. Frequent or continuous headaches
    f. Bleeding or "leakage of fluid" from vagina
    g. Absence of fetal movements (after quickening)

TABLE 7-2   Nutritional Needs During Pregnancy

Nutrient	Nonpregnant Woman (19-22 yr)	Pregnant Woman	Usage	Food Source
Protein	44 g	74-100 g; needs twice as much	Growth of fetus Placental growth During labor and delivery During lactation	Milk, cheese, eggs, meat, grains, legumes, nuts
Major minerals Calcium	800 mg	1200 mg; needs one and a half times as much	Fetal skeleton Fetal tooth buds Calcium metabolism in mother	Milk, cheese, whole grains, leafy vegetables, egg yolk
Phosphorus	800 mg	1200 mg; needs one and a half times as much		Milk, cheese, lean meats
Iron (Fe)	18 mg	30-60 mg supplement; needs almost two to three times as much	Increased maternal blood volume Fetus stores iron in third trimester	Liver, meats, eggs, leafy vegetables, nuts, legumes, whole wheat
Vitamin C (not stored in body so pregnant mother should take at least 1 serving per day)	60 mg	80 mg	Tissue formation Increased iron absorption	Citrus fruits, berries, melon, tomatoes, green peppers, green leafy vegetables, broccoli
Vitamin D	5-10 μg*; 200-400 IU†	10-15 μg; 400-600 IU; needs almost twice as much	Tooth buds Mineralize bone tissue Aid absorption of calcium and phosphorus	Fortified milk Fortified margarine
Folic acid	180 μg	400 μg	Increase red blood cell formation; prevention of macrocytic and megaloblastic anemia and neural tube defects	Green leafy vegetables, oranges, broccoli, asparagus and liver

*μg = microgram.
†IU = international units.

h. Chills and fever (signs of infection)
i. Rapid weight gain (signs of possible preeclampsia)

Normal Discomforts of Pregnancy
Table 7-3

ABNORMAL ANTEPARTUM
Hypertensive States
A. Definition: a group of conditions that occur during pregnancy usually after 20 weeks' gestation: symptoms can range from high blood pressure (BP) to headaches, blurred vision, and convulsions with ensuing coma
  1. Frequent in high-risk mothers
  2. Greater likelihood during first pregnancies
  3. Incidence: 5% to 7% of all pregnancies
B. Types
  1. Pregnancy-induced hypertension (PIH): increase of blood pressure to or above 140/90 mm Hg
    a. Increased BP only symptom
    b. Disappears within 10 days following delivery

  2. Preeclampsia: an acute hypertensive condition resulting in elevated BP (increased systolic BP 30 mm Hg or increased BP 15 mm Hg over baseline) and proteinuria; edema may also be present
    a. Mild preeclampsia:
      (1) BP 140/90
      (2) Proteinuria 1+
      (3) Rapid weight gain
    b. Moderate-to-severe preeclampsia:
      (1) Hospitalize stat
      (2) BP 160/110
      (3) Albumin 2+ to 4+
      (4) Persistent, severe headaches with visual disturbances
      (5) Epigastric pain (late sign)
      (6) Hyperactive deep tendon reflexes (DTR) clonus: an abnormal pattern of neuromuscular activity, characterized by rapidly alternating involuntary contraction and relaxation of skeletal muscle

TABLE 7-3   Normal Discomforts of Pregnancy

Discomfort	Probable Cause	Relief Measures
First Trimester		
Breasts: painful	Hypertrophy of glandular tissue Increased blood flow to area Hormonal effects	Firm, supportive bra; even a nursing bra
Urinary frequency	Pressure on bladder from expanding uterus reduces bladder capacity; increased vascular content	Pads if necessary
Yawning (tired, sleepy)	Whether result of relaxin hormone is questionable; possibly caused by sudden chemical changes in body	Frequent rest periods Balanced diet to prevent anemia

Nausea/vomiting	Hormonal changes
	Ambivalent feelings regarding pregnancy
		Small, frequent meals
		Limited fluids
		  Dry crackers with tea
		  Avoid greasy fried foods

Second Trimester		
Heartburn (acid taste in mouth)	Relaxin hormone effect Enlarging uterus displaces stomach upward	Avoid fatty foods Antacids: Milk of Magnesia, Gelusil, Maalox, Amphojel
Pigmentation	Hormonal	Reassure mother that it is temporary and will disappear after delivery
Leg cramps	Calcium-phosphorus imbalance	Position relief Calf stretching Calcium supplements, milk
Constipation	Hormonal: slowing down of peristaltic movements Compression of colon by uterus and baby	Adequate fluids, fruits, foods with roughage Exercises Stool softener but no mineral oil
Third Trimester		
Urinary incontinence	Lightening/dropping of fetus into pelvic cavity pushes presenting part on bladder	Pelvic floor exercise (Kegel): tighten perineal muscles, relax, then repeat
Hemorrhoids	Pressure from fetal presenting part Increased vascular activity	Knee-chest (elevate hips): Kegel exercises Comfort measures: frequent rest periods; sitting in warm tub; supporting legs with pillows
Low back pain	Increased pressure Fatigue Poor weight distribution	Pelvic exercises Pushing, stretching Comfort massaging Good posture
Insomnia	Increased fetal movements Muscular cramping Frequency Dyspnea	Adequate rest periods Warm milk at bedtime Relaxing shower Support with pillows Deep breathing
Varicosities (leg, vulva)	Hereditary disposition Pelvis vasocongestion Pull of gravity Pressure of uterus Forcing stool (constipation)	Support stockings Changing position frequently Abdominal support Keeping legs uncrossed
Edema (legs, feet)	Immobility (staying in one position for a prolonged time)	Periodic resting Moving around Support stockings Elevating legs Plenty of fluids (to serve as a diuretic)
Dyspnea (shortness of breath)	Pressure on diaphragm from expanding uterus	Sitting erect Deep breathing Putting arms above head Keeping weight down
Leaking of colostrum	Increased blood supply Prominent nipples	Support bra Pads if necessary (keep clean and dry)
Supine hypotension syndrome (feel faint)	Pressure on ascending vena cava by uterus	Lying on left side with legs flexed or semi-sitting position
Vaginal discharge	Hormonal	No douching Keep area clean, dry (perineal care)

3. Eclampsia
   a. Definition: most severe form of the hypertensive states, characterized by hypertensive crisis, shock, followed by grand mal seizure and possibly coma
   b. Signs and symptoms
      (1) Alarming weight gain
      (2) Scanty urine (less than 30 ml/hour)
      (3) Proteinuria 4+, red blood cells (RBCs) in urine
      (4) BP 200/100 or higher
      (5) Edema of retina; can cause blindness
      (6) Severe epigastric pain
      (7) Hyperactive deep tendon reflexes
      (8) Convulsions: tonic and clonic

NOTE: May start labor prematurely; infant may be severely compromised and die

1. HELLP (hemolysis, elevated liver enzymes, and low platelets) syndrome: a severe form of PIH that involves multiple organ damage. The exact cause is unknown. HELLP syndrome is thought to arise as a result of changes occurring with preeclampsia. Arteriolar vasospasm, endothelial damage, and platelet aggregation lead to decreased tissue perfusion and organ damage

C. Treatment and nursing management
   1. According to classification and severity of symptoms; varies from home care precautions to absolute bed rest in a hospital with patient lying on left side
   2. Reduce stimuli
   3. Convulsion precautions
   4. Selective antihypertensive and diuretic therapy may be ordered (e.g., hydralazine [Apresoline] hydrochloride, furosemide [Lasix], magnesium sulfate, mannitol labetelol); nurse should know effects and untoward symptoms
   5. Monitor edema, BP, FHT, levels of consciousness, deep tendon reflexes, impending labor signs

Hyperemesis Gravidarum

A. Definition: pernicious vomiting of pregnancy lasting into second trimester
B. Signs and symptoms
   1. Excessive nausea and vomiting
   2. Considerable weight loss
   3. Severe dehydration
   4. Depletion of essential electrolytes (sodium and potassium)
   5. Vitamin, glucose, and protein deficiencies
   6. Ketone bodies in urine: 1+ protein
   7. Elevated hemoglobin level, RBC count, and hematocrit
C. Treatment and nursing management: untreated will lead to death of mother, fetus, or both
   1. Hospitalize in well-ventilated, private, pleasant environment
   2. Restrict visitors
   3. Nothing by mouth (NPO) first 48 hours
   4. Record intake and output (I & O)
   5. If vomiting occurs, antiemetic medications may be administered
   6. Intravenous (IV) fluids to replace losses in nutrition
   7. Gradual serving of attractive, small portions of food on china dishes, starting with dry toast and tea
   8. Nonjudgmental nursing attitudes
   9. Refer for psychotherapy when appropriate

Hemorrhagic Conditions

A. Abortion (early pregnancy bleeding)
   1. Definition: the expulsion of uterine contents before viability of the fetus for medical reasons or spontaneously
   2. Types
      a. Induced abortion
         (1) Termination of pregnancy (therapeutic): legal aborting of the fetus for medical or psychological reasons by a licensed physician under controlled, aseptic conditions
         (2) Criminal: an abortion performed under illegal, unsafe conditions
      b. Spontaneous abortion
         (1) Definition: an abortion that occurs naturally (usually in the first trimester)
         (2) Possible causes: hormonal deficiencies, abnormalities of the fetus, incompetent cervix, abnormalities of the reproductive organs, emotional shock, physical injury, acute infections, growths, and so on
   3. Terminology of abortions
      a. Habitual abortion: three or more consecutive spontaneous abortions for unknown reasons
      b. Threatened abortion: minimal signs and symptoms of abortion such as bleeding and cramping but with no loss of uterine contents
      c. Imminent abortion: considerable blood loss, severe contractions, urge to push that without treatment will result in loss of uterine contents
      d. Inevitable abortion: bleeding, contractions, rupture of membranes, and cervical dilatation in which the uterine contents will be lost, so treatment will concentrate on the mother
      e. Incomplete abortion: part(s) of uterine contents retained, necessitating administration of oxytocins to accelerate expulsion of remaining contents, or dilatation and curettage (D&C; a minor surgical intervention) to prevent prolonged bleeding
      f. Complete abortion: entire uterine contents are expelled
   4. Signs and symptoms of abortion
      a. Vaginal bleeding: scant to profuse
      b. Abdominal cramping: slight to severe
      c. Contractions: intermittent, steady, mild, or severe
   5. Treatment and nursing management
      a. Prompt and immediate bed rest
      b. Hospitalization when appropriate
      c. Prevention of blood loss and shock
      d. Replacement blood treatment if necessary
      e. Checking vital signs and temperature for 24 hours
      f. Endocrine therapy when appropriate
      g. Surgical intervention when appropriate: Shirodkar operation (purse-string suturing) for known incompetent cervix
      h. Psychotherapy when appropriate
         (1) Prepare for grieving process
         (2) Provide assistance for burial regulations
         (3) Let mother vent feelings of love, loss, guilt
         (4) Quiet, supportive, compassionate nursing care
B. Ectopic pregnancy (early pregnancy bleeding)
   1. Definition: an extrauterine pregnancy in which the products of conception are implanted outside the uter-

ine cavity; 90% occur in the fallopian tube (right tube more frequent); other sites include the abdomen or the ovary

2. Signs and symptoms
   a. Abnormal or missed menstrual period
   b. Slight uterine bleeding or spotting
   c. Possible mass on affected side; pain, tenderness, rigid abdomen
   d. If tube ruptures, may be little bleeding externally, but massive internal hemorrhaging with accompanying severe shock
   e. A diagnosis via transvaginal ultrasound is possible before tube rupture; if diagnosed before rupture, a laparoscopy is done to remove portion of the tube; goal is to remove ectopic pregnancy and preserve reproductive function; may also treat with methotrexate

3. Treatment and nursing management
   a. Hospitalization stat
   b. Treat shock (warm, quiet, replacement therapy—IV fluids, oxygen, etc.)
   c. Crossmatch and other blood work: transfusion readiness
   d. Support mother, who will be extremely frightened
   e. Prepare for stat surgery if appropriate
   f. Arrange for baptism of fetus when appropriate
   g. Postsurgical care with IV fluids, medications, other appropriate treatments (RhoGAM if necessary)
   h. Provide emotional support to mother and family; get assistance of clergy when requested

C. Gestational trophoblastic neoplasm (formerly known as hydatidiform mole)
1. Definition: rare degeneration of chorionic villi into a benign neoplasm in which the villi fill with clear viscous fluid and form grapelike clusters; the neoplasm fills the decidua and expands the uterus to larger than normal for gestational age
2. Signs and symptoms
   a. Enlarging uterus, greater than for normal gestation
   b. Missed period; spotting to profuse bleeding
   c. Several shiny, tapioca-like "grape clusters" escape through vaginal tract
   d. Nausea and vomiting
   e. Signs of pregnancy-induced hypertension (PIH); usually before 20 weeks' gestation
   f. No FHT
   g. Ultrasound reveals no fetal structures
   h. Laboratory findings: human chorionic gonadotropin (HCG) titers up to 1 to 2 million (normally 350,000 to 400,000 at 8 weeks)
3. Treatment and nursing management
   a. Termination as soon as diagnosis confirmed
   b. Blood transfusion if indicated
   c. Assistance in grieving process of mother and family
   d. Follow-up very important
      (1) Contraceptive advice (no oral since that will distort HCG titers)
      (2) HCG titers for at least 6 months

D. Placenta previa (third-trimester bleeding)
1. Definition: abnormal implantation of a normal placenta for unknown reasons, usually in the lower segment of the uterus; condition usually occurs in multiparas, and incidence appears to increase with age; may also be caused by fibroids
2. Types (Fig. 7-4)
   a. Partial (incomplete): incomplete coverage of the uterine os
   b. Complete (total): entire uterine os completely covered
   c. Marginal (low lying): located in lower uterine segment but away from the os
3. Signs and symptoms
   a. Painless uterine bleeding: may be intermittent or occur in gushes; scanty to severe; bright red
   b. Third-trimester occurrence
4. Treatment and nursing management
   a. Diagnosis confirmed by ultrasound or x-ray examination
   b. Avoidance of vaginal examinations
   c. Hospitalization stat

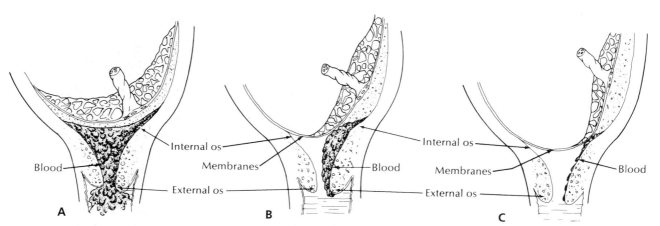

Figure 7-4 Types of placenta previa after onset of labor. **A,** Complete, or total. **B,** Incomplete, or partial. **C,** Marginal, or low-lying. (From Lowdermilk DL, Perry SE, Bobak IM: *Maternity nursing,* ed 5, St Louis, 1999, Mosby.)

d. Quiet environment; fetus uncompromised; station high
e. Fowler's position (head at 30-degree angle)
f. Tocolytic therapy with use of magnesium sulfate to manage uterine irritability under certain circumstances
g. Have double set-up ready so that if vaginal examination is imperative, emergency cesarean section equipment is available and blood is ready for transfusion
h. Foley catheter if condition is severe; shock care
i. Count pads to determine amount, color, duration of bleeding
j. Monitor vital signs, especially blood pressure
k. Monitor FHT and FHR
l. IV fluids
m. Support patient and family; keep them informed

E. Abruptio placentae (third-trimester bleeding)
1. Definition: premature separation of a normally implanted placenta before the birth of the fetus
2. Causes
   a. Trauma
   b. Chronic maternal disease
   c. Grand multipara
   d. Unknown
3. Types (Fig. 7-5)
   a. Complete: separation of the placenta from the uterine wall before birth of the fetus
   b. Partial: separation of a portion of the placenta from the wall of the uterus before the birth of the fetus
4. Signs and symptoms
   a. Severe abdominal pain; sometimes called "exquisite" or unrelenting
   b. Patient is distressed, depressed, and exhibits signs of shock
   c. Painful bleeding: moderate to severe; internal or external; dark red, not clotted; amount varies
   d. Abdomen tense, boardlike; nurse unable to feel contractions; uterus irritable
   e. Hypovolemic shock can result in renal failure
   f. Sudden change in heartbeat or bradycardia, or absence of FHT

5. Treatment and nursing management
   a. Depends on stage and intensity of condition; for reasons not clearly understood, partial abruptio placentae may seal off bleeding spontaneously, and labor will proceed normally
   b. Check coagulation profile: fibrinogen/fibrin, platelets
   c. Prevent hypovolemic shock and fetal hypoxia
   d. Crossmatch, type, readiness for transfusions
   e. Monitor contractions, FHT, and vital signs
   f. Slight or moderate bleeding may indicate artificial rupture of membranes (ARM or AROM) to hasten delivery or seal off bleeding
   g. Severe bleeding (dark red) may indicate immediate cesarean section
   h. Support mother and family
   i. Continued bleeding after delivery may necessitate hysterectomy

F. Disseminated intravascular coagulation (DIC)
1. Cause
   a. Unknown
   b. Coincidental with abruptio placentae, postabortal infection, amniotic fluid emboli, placenta previa, and uterine atony
2. Pathology: not clearly understood; massive clotting, depletion of coagulant factor
3. Signs and symptoms: excessive bleeding at placental site, incisional site, nose, mouth, gums
4. Treatment and nursing management
   a. Halt or reverse DIC
   b. Eliminate cause
   c. Delivery stat
   d. Blood replacement
   e. IV fibrinogen/heparin

Medical and Infectious Conditions

A. Chickenpox (varicella)
1. Causative agent: herpesvirus; varicella zoster virus (VZV)
2. Effect on mother
   a. May manifest itself as herpes zoster (shingles)
   b. May be fatal if severe
   c. May cause abortion

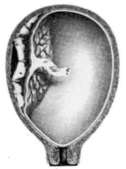
Partial separation
(Concealed hemorrhage)

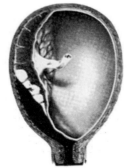
Partial separation
(Apparent hemorrhage)

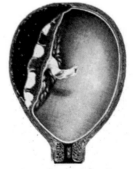
Complete separation
(Concealed hemorrhage)

Figure 7-5   Abruptio placentae. Premature separation of normally implanted placenta. (From Lowdermilk DL, Perry SE, Bobak IM: *Maternity nursing,* ed 5, St Louis, 1999, Mosby.)

3. Effect on fetus
   a. May cause defects of skin, bones, hydrocephalus if contracted during first trimester
   b. Fetal death

B. German measles (rubella or 3-day measles)
   1. Causative agent: virus
   2. Effect on mother
      a. Rash, fever, photophobia
      b. Possible abortion
   3. Effect on fetus if infected during first trimester
      a. Rubella syndrome: heart defects, blindness, deafness, mental retardation
      b. Delayed effect on brain (15 to 20 years of age)

C. Genital herpes
   1. Causative agent: herpes simplex virus 2
   2. Effect on mother
      a. Vaginal discharge
      b. Genital blisters, ulcers
      c. Fever
      d. Painful inguinal lymph nodes
   3. Effect on fetus
      a. Abortion or premature birth
      b. Neonatal infections
      c. Survivors may have CNS symptoms

D. Group B *streptococcus*
   1. Causative agent: *Streptococcus* bacterium found in the lower genital tract or rectum of 10% to 30% of all healthy pregnant women
   2. Effect on mother
      a. Asymptomatic carriers
      b. Increased risk of abnormal vaginal discharge, UTIs, endocarditis
   3. Effect on fetus
      a. Pneumonia and sepsis, which can result in death in 12 to 24 hours
      b. Blindness, deafness, and mental retardation
   4. Treatment
      a. Prenatal screening: if cultures are positive, the drug of choice is penicillin G
      b. High-risk women should be offered prophylactic antibiotics in labor

E. Hepatitis A
   1. Causative agent: virus
   2. Effect on mother
      a. Abortion
      b. Liver failure
   3. Effect on fetus
      a. First-trimester infection: fetal anomalies
      b. Premature birth
      c. Neonatal hepatitis

F. Hepatitis B (serum hepatitis)
   1. Causative agent: virus (HBV); contact with blood and through sexual intercourse
   2. Effect on mother
      a. May be asymptomatic
      b. Low-grade fever, fatigue, joint pain, nausea, and vomiting
      c. Liver and spleen enlargement, cirrhosis
      d. Vaccine available for high-risk women and health care workers
   3. Effect on fetus
      a. Avoid exposure of newborn to blood of mother
      b. Preterm at birth
      c. May be asymptomatic at birth
      d. May exhibit signs of acute hepatitis
      e. Possible carrier
      f. Infants born to women who have hepatitis B should receive appropriate vaccinations

G. Influenza
   1. Causative agent: virus
   2. Effect on mother
      a. Pneumonia
      b. Abortion
      c. Premature labor
   3. Effect on fetus
      a. Abortion or premature birth
      b. Fetal death
   4. Vaccine for pregnant women available; live viral vaccine can infect fetus

H. Gonorrhea (clap)
   1. Causative agent: *Neisseria gonorrhoeae* bacterium
   2. Effect on mother
      a. Vaginal discharge
      b. Cervical tenderness
      c. Dysuria
      d. Affects ovaries, tubes, causing sterility
   3. Effect on fetus
      a. Ophthalmia neonatorum
      b. Conjunctivitis
      c. Mild-to-severe infections

I. Syphilis (lues)
   1. Causative agent: *Treponema pallidum* bacterium
   2. Effect on mother (if untreated)
      a. Primary chancre
      b. Secondary skin rash
      c. Latent or tertiary CNS problems
   3. Effect on fetus
      a. Rhagades of the corners of mouth and anus
      b. Snuffles
      c. Maceration of palms of hands and soles of feet
      d. Congenital syphilis (symptoms appearing later in life)
      e. Death (stillborn)

J. Cytomegalovirus (CMV)
   1. Causative agent: cytomegalovirus of the herpes group, transmitted by close bodily and sexual contact
   2. May be transmitted by asymptomatic woman to fetus causing fetal damage, retardation, or fetal death
   3. The infant may acquire the virus by exposure to cervical mucus during vaginal birth
   4. No satisfactory treatment for maternal or neonatal CMV

K. Chlamydia
   1. Causative agent: bacterial microorganism *Chlamydia trachomatis* (CT)—transmitted by close bodily and sexual contact
   2. May initiate pelvic inflammatory disease (PID) leading to ectopic pregnancy and infertility
   3. Some evidence suggests relationship between CT and premature rupture of membranes, preterm labor and delivery, low birth weight, increased perinatal mortality, and late onset endometritis
   4. Treated with extended erythromycin
   5. Transmission from infected birth canal may result in conjunctivitis and/or pneumonia

L. Cardiac disease
   1. Classification
      a. Class I: no limitation of activity
      b. Class II: slight limitation of activity
      c. Class III: considerable limitation of even ordinary activity
      d. Class IV: symptoms of cardiac insufficiency even at rest
   2. Treatment and nursing management
      a. Close medical and nursing supervision
      b. Watch for signs and symptoms of fatigue, dyspnea, coughing, palpitations, tachycardia
      c. Promote rest
      d. Hospitalize at end of second trimester
      e. Breast-feeding contraindicated
      f. Contraceptive education
      g. Nutrition: offer foods high in iron and protein; avoid raw, deep green vegetables because vitamin K counteracts effects of heparin
      h. Prevent infections: report first signs of exposure
      i. Teach comfortable positions: pillows, support, left side
      j. During labor and delivery: epidural or caudal anesthesia (blocks) block to minimize discomfort on bearing down
      k. Watch for cardiac decompensation (pulse rate over 100 beats/min; respirations, 25+)
      l. Vaginal delivery preferred
         (1) Episiotomy, low forceps
         (2) Oxygen to decrease pulmonary edema
         (3) Medication to regulate heart rate
         (4) Diuretic to reduce fluid retention
      m. Postpartal care
         (1) Hospitalization longer than normal to stabilize cardiac output
         (2) Application of abdominal binder (because of rapid change in intraabdominal pressure)
         (3) Bed rest with progressive bathroom privileges dependent on progress
         (4) Prevent overdistention of bladder
         (5) Encourage bonding; nurse should hold baby at eye level to allow mother to touch and talk to baby
         (6) Inform mother and family of progress
M. Diabetes mellitus
   1. Definition: inborn error in the transportation and metabolism of carbohydrates
   2. Classification: see Table 7-4

   3. Effects of diabetes on pregnancy
      a. Difficult to control because of changing patterns of fetal growth and development and maternal demands
      b. Fluctuating insulin requirements
      c. Tendency to develop acidosis (diabetic coma) from lack of insulin
      d. Increased tendency to infection (urinary tract, vaginal tract), preeclampsia, and polyhydramnios
      e. Increased incidence of premature labor
      f. Macrosomia (oversized baby)
      g. Possibility of dystocia
      h. Increased danger of placental deterioration causing hypoxia in fetus
      i. Tendency to abruptio placentae
   4. Changing insulin requirements during pregnancy
      a. First trimester: insulin requirement decreased
      b. Second trimester: insulin requirement increased
      c. Third trimester: careful regulation (blood sugar); evaluation of placenta, oxytocin challenge test (CST)
      d. Intranatal: labor depletes glycogen
      e. Postpartum: insulin reaction resulting from sudden drop in need
      f. Watch for hypoglycemia, shock, infection, bleeding
      g. No need for insulin 24 to 48 hours after delivery
      h. Hospitalized until insulin balance restored
   5. Early recognition of insulin reaction and diabetic coma
   6. Treatment and nursing management
      a. Weekly prenatal visits
      b. Regulation of insulin dosage and dietary management
      c. Mother taught to test blood three or four times a day
      d. Testing for placental adequacy: CST (stress test) measures fetal response to uterine contractions; late deceleration indicates problem
      e. Teach good nutrition
      f. Help allay fears and anxieties
N. Addiction and pregnancy
   1. Drug addition
      a. Effect on mother
         (1) Abortion
         (2) Premature birth
         (3) Stillbirth
      b. Effect on neonate: see section on abnormal newborn

TABLE 7-4 Classifications of Diabetes

Classification	Characteristics	Treatment During Pregnancy
Type 1: Insulin-dependent diabetes mellitus (IDDM)	Usually juvenile onset; prone to ketosis	Diet control and insulin
Type 2: Non–insulin-dependent diabetes mellitus (NIDDM)	Usually adult onset; ketosis resistant; may require insulin for hyperglycemia during stress; requires insulin during pregnancy	Diet control and insulin
Other: Gestational diabetes mellitus (GDM)	Develops during pregnancy	Diet control alone or insulin

2. Alcohol and pregnancy
   a. Effect on mother
      (1) Poor nutritional habits
      (2) Poor hygiene
      (3) Physical, psychosocial deterioration
   b. Effect on neonate: see section on abnormal newborn
3. Treatment and nursing management
   a. Supervised withdrawal
   b. Substitute therapy

Acquired Immunodeficiency Syndrome (AIDS)

Pregnant women whose partners were drug users sharing common needles, high-risk category men (bisexual or homosexual), or men who were infected with the disease have been known to become infected. Transmission of the HIV virus to the unborn fetus has now been confirmed.

A. Confirmed avenues of transmission
   1. Anal/vaginal intercourse
   2. Drug addicts sharing needles of infected users
   3. Contaminated blood transfusions
   4. Transmission to the fetus or neonate can occur transplacentally or by exposure to blood and vaginal secretions at delivery and or by exposure to maternal secretion such as breast milk
   5. Cesarean section does not appear to totally prevent the transmission of the virus
B. Treatment and nursing management
   1. Pregnant HIV-infected women should receive pneumovax, influenza, and hepatitis vaccines and should be screened for sexually transmitted diseases
   2. HIV testing is voluntary and must be accompanied by informed consent and counseling; results are confidential
   3. Immune status needs to be monitored; if immune status falls physicians may elect to administer azidothymidine (AZT) to delay onset of illness
   4. HIV-positive women need counseling to practice safe sex to decrease risk of repeatedly exposing fetus
   5. Infants need to be followed and tested for a minimum of 2 years to determine if they have the disease
C. Centers for Disease Control and Prevention (CDC) guidelines for preventing transmission of the AIDS virus
   1. Wear gloves when in contact with body fluids, mucous membranes, and nonintact skin; wear gloves when performing venipuncture or when handling items soiled with blood or body fluids
   2. Change gloves after caring for each patient; wash hands and most of your exposed surfaces with soap and water
   3. Wear masks, gown, and apron (if available); protect mucous membranes of your mouth, nose, and eyes
   4. Prevent injuries from needles, sharp instruments, toys, and other products; be alert when handling, cleaning, and disposing of instruments
   5. Avoid needle pricks; all sharp items that have been used should be placed in puncture-resistant containers; do not recap needles
   6. To minimize need for emergency mouth-to-mouth resuscitation, keep resuscitation bags, mouthpieces, and ventilation devices in easily located areas
   7. Refrain from direct patient care and do not handle patient care equipment if you have open lesions, weeping dermatitis, and so forth

8. Pregnant nurses should be especially careful, as an HIV infection could place the fetus at risk
D. Minimum precautions for invasive procedures
   1. Wear gloves, surgical masks, and protective eyewear for all invasive procedures
      a. Prevent skin and mucous membrane contact with blood and other body fluids by using appropriate barrier precautions
      b. Wear protective eyewear or face shields, gowns, or aprons for procedures resulting in splashing to protect from blood or other body fluids
   2. Wear gloves and gowns when handling placenta or the infant until blood and amniotic fluid have been removed from the infant's skin and during postdelivery care of the umbilical cord
   3. Put on new gloves as soon as patient safety permits should you tear a glove or be injured by a needle-stick or other injury; always check gloves for holes

Tuberculosis

Tuberculosis is an increasingly prevalent health problem throughout the world; its resurgence in the United States is attributed to homelessness, drug abuse, poverty, and human immunodeficiency virus (HIV); rates are particularly high among minorities and recent immigrants to the United States.

A. Confirmed avenues of transmission
   1. Airborne: coughs or sneezes of a person with infectious tuberculosis
   2. Shared air: persons in close air contact for a prolonged period of time
B. Treatment and nursing management
   1. Preventive therapy postponed until after delivery
   2. A pregnant woman with active disease needs immediate treatment of 2 to 3 antituberculosis drugs
   3. Breast-feeding is permitted; however, infant still needs to undergo prophylactic treatment

Asthma

A. Definition: chronic lung disease in which airways are overly responsive to stimuli such as allergens, pollutants, exercise, and cold air
   1. Asthma occurs in approximately 1% of all pregnant women
   2. The incidence of preeclampsia is higher in asthmatic patients
B. Signs and symptoms: cough, wheezing, dyspnea, and chest tightness
C. Treatment and nursing management:
   1. Pulmonary function tests to monitor lung function
   2. NSTs to monitor fetal well being
   3. Avoiding allergens
   4. Pharmacological therapies
   5. Breast-feeding to provide some neonatal protection against respiratory allergens

Premature Labor

A. Definition: labor occurring before 37 to 38 weeks' gestation
B. Effect on family (focus on psychosocial problems)
   1. Mother not ready for delivery: apprehensive and frightened; may feel guilty
   2. Family plus professional staff: restrained, quiet, anticipating complications

C. Effect on fetus: see Preterm (Premature) Infant under Abnormal Newborn, pp. 419-420
D. Treatment and nursing management
  1. Usually premature rupture of membranes precedes premature labor; test fluid with nitrazine paper: if alkaline, positive for amniotic fluid
  2. If membranes intact and cervix undilated, halt labor if possible; magnesium sulfate and terbutaline are frequently used to halt premature labor
  3. Bed rest stat
  4. Monitor maternal pulse and blood pressure
  5. Know untoward effects of medications
  6. Prevent infection
  7. Offer constant emotional support to mother and family: inform, reassure, encourage mother and family

NORMAL INTRAPARTUM (LABOR AND DELIVERY)

A. Fetal head (passenger)
  1. Two parietal bones: one each side of head
  2. Two temporal bones: one each side of head near temple
  3. Two frontal bones: one each side of forehead
  4. One occipital bone: lower back of head
  5. Sutures: membranous spaces between bones
    a. Sagittal suture: separates parietal bones and extends longitudinally back to front
    b. Frontal suture: between two frontal bones and is continuation of the sagittal suture
    c. Coronal suture: like a crown, separates frontal and parietal bones
    d. Lambdoidal suture: separates occipital bone from two parietal bones
  6. Fontanels: formed by intersection of sutures; allow head bones to override and accommodate to birth passage
    a. Anterior fontanel: membranous, diamond-shaped space (bregma) formed by intersection of sagittal, frontal, and coronal sutures; called "soft spot"; closes within 12 to 18 months
    b. Posterior fontanel: small, membraneous triangle-shaped space between occipital bone and two parietal bones; closes within 6 to 8 weeks
  7. Principal measurements of the fetal head
B. Presentations, positions, station
  1. Presentation
    a. Definition: refers to that part of the passenger (fetus) that enters the passage (true pelvis, uterine os, vaginal canal) first
    b. Types of presentations
      (1) Cephalic: head, vertex, occiput (93%)
      (2) Breech: buttocks, sacrum, leg(s), foot (feet) (3%)
      (3) Shoulder: scapula (3%)
  2. Lie (Fig. 7-6)
    a. Definition: refers to the relationship between the long axis of the passenger and the long axis of the mother
    b. Types
      (1) Longitudinal (99%)
      (2) Transverse (sideways)
  3. Position (Fig. 7-7)
    a. Definition: the way in which the presenting part of the fetus lies in relation to the four quadrants of the

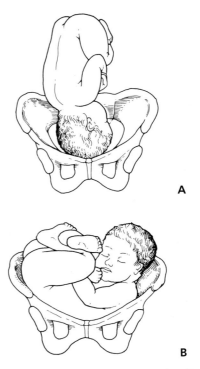

Figure 7-6 **A,** Longitudinal lie. **B,** Transverse lie. (From Phillips CR: *Family-centered maternity and newborn care: a basic text,* ed 4, St Louis, 1996, Mosby.)

mother's pelvis and to her back (posterior) and her front (anterior)
    b. To determine position, fetal "reference points" are used, and they are
      (1) Occiput (back of fetal head): O
      (2) Chin (mentum): M
      (3) Brow (bregma): B
      (4) Buttocks (sacrum): S
      (5) Shoulder (scapula): Sc
      (6) Transversus
    c. Types of position with occiput presentations: LOA, LOT, LOP, ROA, ROT, ROP (see Fig. 7-7)
  4. Attitude
    a. Definition: relationship of the various fetal parts to one another, or the relationship of the fetal extremities to its body (trunk)
    b. Normal attitude: flexed; fetal head on sternum, arms folded against chest; knees bent, pressing abdomen; legs flexed so toes touch arm
  5. Station
    a. Definition: degree to which presenting part is located in the true pelvis; points of reference are the ischial spines, which are designated as *0* (zero)
    b. Levels
      (1) Minus: as in -1, -2, -3 station, means that presenting part is above the ischial spines
      (2) Plus: as in $+1$, $+2$, $+3$ station, means that the presenting part is below the ischial spines
      (3) -5 = floating; $+5$ = presenting part on perineum; or -3 to -5 = floating; $+3$ to $+5$ = presenting part on perineum; check with agency for the numbers used

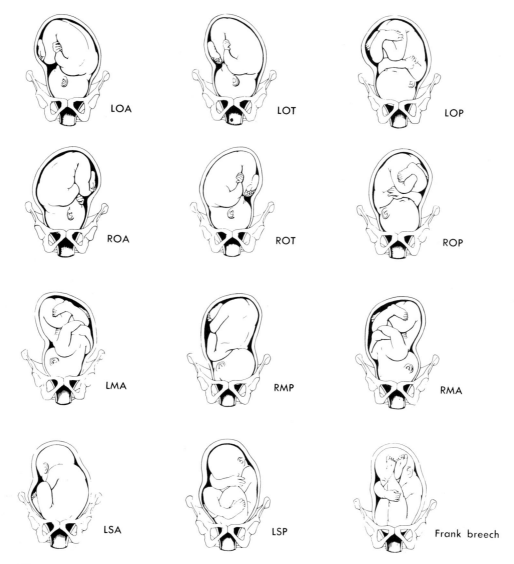

Figure 7-7 Categories of presentations. (Used with permission of Ross Products Division, Abbott Laboratories, Columbus, Ohio.)

C. Mechanisms and stages of labor: labor cannot progress without power
 1. Definition: the steps or maneuvers the fetus must undertake to accommodate to the passage and be delivered
 2. Process (mechanisms) (Fig. 7-8)
   a. Engagement: passage of the passenger into the pelvic inlet
   b. Descent: continuous slow progress of the fetus through the pelvis and the birth canal
   c. Flexion: head slowly adapts to birth canal by flexing chin
   d. Internal rotation: fetal head turns in corkscrew maneuver so the long diameter of the head is parallel to the longest diameter of the pelvic outlet
   e. Extension: the back of the fetal head goes under the pubic arch; the spine of the fetus extends to adapt itself to the curvature of the birth canal, and the head is delivered
   f. Restitution: as the head emerges, it rotates back 45 degrees to the position it was before internal rotation, which helps the shoulders accommodate to the outlet
   g. External rotation: the shoulders drop down and turn to the anteroposterior (AP) position, and the head slowly turns so both head and shoulders are aligned
   h. Expulsion: the posterior (underneath) shoulder is delivered by lateral flexion (upward motion); then the anterior upper shoulder will slide out (downward motion) from under the pubic arch, and the body is easily expelled
 3. Stages of labor
   a. First stage: begins with the first true labor contraction; ends with complete dilatation and effacement of the cervix
   b. Second stage (expulsion): from complete effacement and dilatation to expulsion of the infant

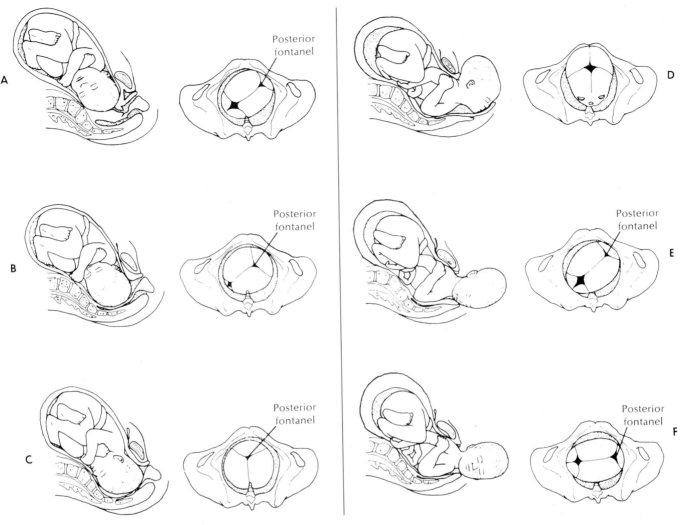

Figure 7-8 Mechanism of labor in left occipitoanterior (LOA) presentation. **A,** Engagement and descent. **B,** Flexion. **C,** Internal rotation to OA. **D,** Extension. **E,** Restitution, **F,** External rotation.

c. Third stage (placental): from delivery of the infant to delivery of the placenta and membranes (5 to 20 minutes)

d. Fourth stage: from delivery of the secundines and repair of the perineum to 1 hour thereafter

D. Fetal evaluation during labor and delivery and immediately after
1. During labor
   a. Fetal monitoring devices
      (1) Phonotransducer: amplification of fetal heart activity
      (2) Doppler transducer: ultrasonic device
   b. Special stethoscopes for monitoring FHT
      (1) Headscope (fetoscope): stethoscope on a head device; FHT conducted through monitor's frontal bone
      (2) Leff stethoscope: stethoscope with large, heavy conductor
      (3) External fetal monitor (EFM): applied to abdomen; FHT monitored electronically

   c. Direct fetal monitoring: an electrocardiogram (ECG) fetal scalp electrode (FSE) is placed directly to the fetal head
2. Evaluation immediately after delivery
   a. Establishment of patent airway
   b. Apgar scoring (Fig. 7-9): system of evaluating newborn response 1 minute after birth and 5 minutes after birth
   c. Observation for any visible anomalies

E. Nursing assessment
1. Premonitory (impending) signs and symptoms of labor
   a. Lightening: descent of fetus down pelvic cavity
   b. Braxton-Hicks contractions: painless contractions more frequent, regular
   c. Breathing easier; heartburn disappears; hungry
   d. Weight loss (decrease in water retention)
   e. Frequency (pressure on bladder by presenting part)
   f. Bloody show (slight pinkish discharge with or without discharge of mucous plug)

APGAR SCORING CHART

Sign	0	1	2
HEART RATE	Absent	Slow (below 100)	Over 100
RESPIRATORY EFFORT	Absent	Weak cry, hypoventilation	Good strong cry
MUSCLE TONE	Limp	Some flexion of extremities	Well flexed
REFLEX RESPONSE 1. Response to catheter in nostril (tested after oro-pharynx is clear)	No response	Grimace	Cough or sneeze
2. Tangential foot slap	No response	Grimace	Cry and withdrawal of foot
COLOR	Blue, pale	Body pink, extremities blue	Completely pink

Figure 7-9   The Apgar scoring chart. (From Phillips CR: *Family-centered maternity and newborn care: a basic text,* ed 4, St Louis, 1996, Mosby.)

g. Bag of waters (BOW) ruptures spontaneously without prior contractions
2. Differences between true and false labor
  a. False labor
    (1) Contractions irregular
    (2) No progress in interval or duration of contractions
    (3) Some abdominal discomfort
    (4) No bloody show
    (5) Relief by walking
    (6) No cervical change
    (7) Discomfort mostly in front (lower abdomen)
  b. True labor
    (1) Contractions regular and progressive
    (2) Not relieved by walking
    (3) Cervical changes
    (4) Progressive discomfort starting in back, going around lower abdomen, indentable fundus
3. Spontaneous rupture of membranes
  a. Note time, amount, and color of fluid; note fetal heart tones
  b. Prevent infection (hand washing, good hygienic practice)
  c. Observe for prolapsed cord (notify physician immediately)
  d. If leakage minimal, spontaneous resealing may occur
  e. If close to EDC, contractions may begin, usually within 4 to 16 hours
F. Nursing intervention
1. Nursing management during first stage of labor
  a. Admit patient to labor room
  b. Establish rapport; ask pertinent questions regarding labor; observe reaction to labor process
  c. Offer bedpan frequently (keep bladder empty)
  d. Usually an IV is started to keep a vein open (KVO) (get equipment, solutions)
  e. Monitor contractions, FHR
    (1) Hook up to fetal monitoring device

    (2) Check every 30 to 60 minutes (depending on progress)
    (3) Frequency, duration, and intensity of uterine contractions are assessed to help determine the progress of labor
    (4) When there are ominous FHR patterns (e.g., late decelerations, lack of variability), the nurse must document interventions and subsequent fetal response
  f. Keep mother, father informed on status and progress
    (1) Effacement, dilatation, station
    (2) Encourage father to follow monitor readout
    (3) Encourage father to use comfort measures for mother
2. Nursing management during second stage of labor
  a. Uterine muscles bring about effacement and dilatation; abdominal muscles bring fetus down after dilatation and effacement are complete, and levator ani muscles assist in pushing and expelling fetus
  b. All monitoring equipment removed from mother
    (1) Explain procedures
    (2) Clean perineal area according to hospital policy
    (3) Computers are frequently used to monitor fetal heart rates. Electronic fetal monitoring and/or a fetoscope are also used; inform physician on rate, strength, position
    (4) Check blood pressure every 15 minutes as necessary
    (5) Prepare necessary equipment for delivery readiness and for reception of baby
    (6) Instruct mother to push with contractions when indicated
    (7) When infant delivered completely, note time
    (8) Establish patent airway
    (9) Encourage mother and father to see, touch, and speak to infant
    (10) Carefully place prophylactic drops in each eye

(11) Follow proper identification routine
(12) Transfer infant into warm crib for further evaluation and care
3. Nursing management during third stage (placental)
   a. Be sure cord blood specimen is taken
   b. Placenta delivered within 5 to 20 minutes from expulsion of infant
   c. Note time and which side of placenta delivered
      (1) Maternal side, raw and meaty: Duncan delivery
      (2) Fetal side, shiny and neat: Schultze delivery
   d. Administer oxytocin immediately following delivery of placenta to contract uterus and prevent hemorrhage
   e. Check blood pressure every 15 minutes
   f. Check fundus for firmness; soft, boggy indicates possible hemorrhaging
   g. Check and clean perineal area; apply sanitary napkin
   h. Mother may experience knees shaking, teeth chattering
      (1) Sudden changes in abdominal pressure plus hormonal changes trigger these symptoms
      (2) Place several warm blankets over mother
      (3) Reassure mother and family that it is a normal physiological phenomenon
   i. Transfer mother to recovery area (if not in birthing room)
4. Nursing management during fourth stage of delivery
   a. Critical hour after delivery; watch for complications, especially hemorrhaging
   b. Perform fundal check every 5 minutes; massage gently if necessary
   c. Check blood pressure and vital signs every 10 to 15 minutes until stable
   d. After about 1 hour, when vital signs are stable
      (1) Offer warm drink, toast, or even meal tray if mother wishes and physician approves
      (2) Offer bedpan frequently to prevent bladder distention, which will impede involution; if unable to void, catheterization is usually a standing order
      (3) Give sponge bath to refresh and clean body
      (4) Teach perineal care with peribottle
      (5) Transfer to postpartum room
      (6) Advise mother to request help the first time she wishes to use the bathroom
5. Commonly used medications during labor and delivery: prepared childbirth has greatly diminished use of analgesics and anesthetics during labor and delivery; patients who experience dystocia may need some medication for relief from exhaustion, fright, or prolonged pain
   a. Amnesic
   b. Tranquilizer
   c. Analgesic
   d. Regional anesthesia
      (1) Paracervical block: anesthetizes cervical area
      (2) Pudendal block: peripheral nerve block; may also block urge to push for 30 minutes
      (3) Caudal block (spinal): used during first and second stages; continuous or one dosage
      (4) Saddle block: third, fourth, or fifth lumbar interspace; anesthetizes saddle area (inner groin, perineal area)
      (5) Epidural: also administered into lumbar interspace; uses less anesthetic than caudal; blocks urge to push
      (6) Spinal block: most commonly used for cesarean birth
   e. Nursing management
      (1) Encourage urination, force fluids
      (2) Observe for postspinal headache; treatment includes bed rest, ibuprofen, intravenous caffeine; the definitive treatment is a blood patch
   f. General anesthesia: rare

ABNORMAL INTRAPARTUM
Dystocia
A. Definition: prolonged, difficult, painful labor or delivery involving any one or more problems with the three *P*s: passage, power, and passenger
B. Problems with passage
   1. Inadequate pelvis
   2. Soft-tissue deviation: a full bladder is the most common cause
C. Problems with the power (uterine contractions)
   1. Primary uterine inertia: inefficient contractions from the beginning
   2. Secondary uterine inertia: well-established labor with good contractions at first; then progress suddenly or gradually slows and stops altogether
   3. Hypotonic contractions (atonic uterus); most common; no progress in effacement or dilatation
   4. Hypertonic uterine contractions
      a. Intense, titanic
      b. No interval between contractions
   5. Dystonic contractions
      a. Painful
      b. Ineffective
      c. Asymmetrical (contractions in different segments of the uterus)
D. Problems with passenger (fetus)
   1. Excessive size
   2. Fetal anomaly
   3. Fetal malposition or malpresentation
      a. Occiput posterior (most common)
      b. Breech
      c. Transverse
      d. Face
      e. Soldier (military) presentation
   4. Cephalopelvic disproportion (CPD)
      a. Accommodation impossible
      b. May note unusual contour of uterus or abdomen
E. Complications
   1. Premature rupture of membranes
   2. Predisposition to infection
   3. Trauma
   4. Hemorrhage
   5. Prolapse of cord
   6. Hypoxia of fetus
   7. Severe molding of fetal head: danger of intracranial hemorrhage
   8. Extreme backache (posterior positions)

9. Flowering of anus early because of pressure of occiput on lower sacral region, with subsequent residual of hemorrhoids
10. Extreme fatigue

F. Treatment and nursing management
1. Electronic monitoring of fetus and mother
2. Frequent confirmation of cervical progress
3. Sterile techniques during vaginal examination
4. Check status of BOW
5. Check vital signs
6. Observe condition of mother
   a. Need for pain relief
   b. Sometimes after a medicated sleep or rest dystocia disappears
7. Support physical and psychological needs
8. Watch for dehydration
9. Spontaneous rotation toward end of transition may occur in occiput posteriors

Supine Hypotensive Syndrome

A. Definition: condition caused by compression of vena cava by heavy uterus for a prolonged period; caused by mother's staying in one position for a long time
B. Signs and symptoms
1. Pallor
2. Light-headedness
3. Dizziness
4. Slight nausea
C. Treatment and nursing management: turn patient on left side to relieve pressure; advise frequent turning and changing of position

Ruptured Uterus

A. Causes
1. Tetanic, pauseless or continuous contractions
   a. Possible cause: unmonitored pitocin infusion
   b. Unknown
2. Stretching of uterine walls by extensive, rapid growth of hydatidiform mole
3. Attempted vaginal birth after cesarean (VBAC) and uterine scar ruptures during labor
4. Cephalo pelvic disproportion (CPD)
5. Forceps delivery
B. Treatment and nursing management
1. Prepare for emergency cesarean section
2. Monitor for signs of hypovolemic shock and fetal distress
3. Prepare for all anticipatory nursing responsibilities, surgical or medical

Prolapsed Cord

A. Definition: displacement of the cord below the presenting part and into the vaginal passage before delivery of fetus
B. Causes
1. Spontaneous rupture of the membranes before engagement
2. Breech presentations
3. Prematurity
4. Polyhydramnios
5. Abnormal presentations
C. Signs and symptoms
1. Cord may be seen, felt, or palpated
2. Fetal heart pattern abnormal (baseline bradycardia with decelerations)

D. Treatment and nursing management
1. Do not compress cord; do not try to reposition it
2. Sterile saline compress to keep cord moist and protected from infection
3. Place mother in knee-chest position or in Trendelenburg's position so that presenting part is pushed away from cord by gravity
4. Preparation for cesarean section, blood crossmatch, IV fluids, and so on
5. Check FHR or use continuous electronic fetal monitor (EFM)
6. Support frightened mother and family
7. If not a standing order obtain an order for the mother to receive oxygen by mask

Multiple Pregnancies

A. Definition: simultaneous gestation; twins, triplets, quadruplets, quintuplets, sextuplets, septuplets
B. Signs and symptoms
1. History of multiple gestation (female lineage)
2. Hearing two FHTs, each with own rate
3. Disclosure of multiple limbs, heads, by palpation
4. Larger than normal gestation uterus
5. Weight gain increased more than in normal gestation
6. Striae gravidarum more noticeable early on
7. Confirmation by sonogram
8. X-ray may be done, but only in the third trimester
C. Types (Fig. 7-10)
1. Single-ovum twins (monozygotic, identical)
   a. Union of one sperm with one ovum
   b. During mitosis divides into two embryos
   c. One placenta, two amniotic sacs
   d. Same sex
   e. Heredity a factor
2. Fraternal twins (dizygotic, unidentical)
   a. Union of two sperm with two separate ova
   b. Two amniotic sacs
   c. Separate or fused placenta
   d. Same or different sex
   e. Do not look identical
   f. Age of mother a factor; older women tend to release more than one ovum
3. Formation of triplets and so on is varied
D. Treatment and nursing management
1. Prenatal care
   a. Visits increased
   b. Observe for signs and symptoms of preeclampsia
   c. Premature labor common
   d. Backaches common: support girdle, longer rest periods
   e. Varicosities common
   f. Watch for complications resulting from position, presentation, lie of fetuses
   g. Size of fetuses may cause problems
   h. Be alert for possible cesarean section
2. Intrapartal care
   a. Be prepared for premature labor and premature babies
   b. High-risk second stage
3. Third and fourth stages
   a. Possibility of hemorrhage because of oversized uterus
   b. Blood loss greater than for single births

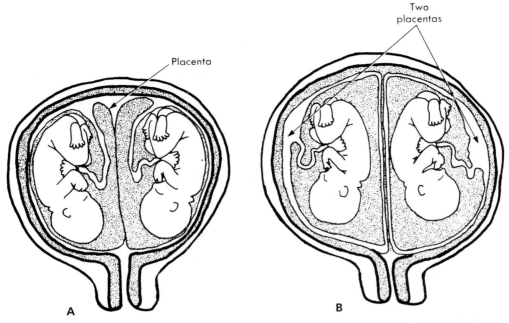

Figure 7-10   Multiple pregnancy. **A,** Identical (monozygotic) twins: two sacs, one placenta. **B,** Fraternal (dizygotic) twins: two sacs, two placentas. (From Phillips CR: *Family-centered maternity and newborn care: a basic text,* ed 4, St Louis, 1996, Mosby.)

c. Oxytocin not administered to mother until all babies delivered

d. Risk of infection greater than in normal single births

e. Perinatal mortality greater than in single deliveries

Induction of Labor

A. Definition: the use of medication (oxytocin) to stimulate contractions before spontaneous onset

B. Indications
1. Overdue fetus (over 42 weeks' gestation)
2. Fetal death
3. Prolonged rupture of membranes (over 24 hours) if uterine contractions have not begun
4. Premature rupture of membranes
5. Diabetic mother
6. Severe preeclampsia (exercise extreme caution)
7. Steeply rising Rh titer

C. Contraindications
1. Cephalopelvic disproportion (CPD)
2. Fetal distress
3. Previous cesarean section
4. Multiple births
5. Heart conditions
6. Prematurity
7. Unengaged presenting part
8. Placenta previa
9. Abnormal fetal position (breech or transverse lie)
10. Active genital herpes

D. Treatment and nursing management
1. Monitor contractions carefully with external fetal monitor
2. If there are no intervals between contractions, stop medication drip and call physician immediately
3. Monitor FHR and report any changes stat

4. Check blood pressure: gradual elevation warrants immediate discontinuation of medication and prompt notification of doctor
5. Keep family and mother informed of progress and procedure
6. Monitor vital signs, I&O
7. The physician or nurse midwife will assess for cervical dilation as needed and observe for the resting tone of the uterus before increasing the pitocin dose

Augmentation of Labor

A. Definition: the use of medication to enhance existing contractions

B. Uses
1. Uterine inertia: primary or secondary
2. Atonic or hypotonic uterine contractions (may be enhanced by a boost of oxytocin)

Operative Obstetrics

A. Episiotomy
1. Definition: surgical incision of the perineum during delivery to enlarge the vaginal outlet
2. Types (Fig. 7-11)
3. Indications
   a. To avoid tearing
   b. To shorten second stage of labor
   c. Fetus or mother is in jeopardy
4. Treatment and nursing management
   a. Comfort measures (promote healing); sitz bath and ice pack first 12 hours
   b. Encourage Kegel exercises—lessen pain and promote healing
   c. Apply witch hazel pads to perineal area (decrease swelling, promote healing)

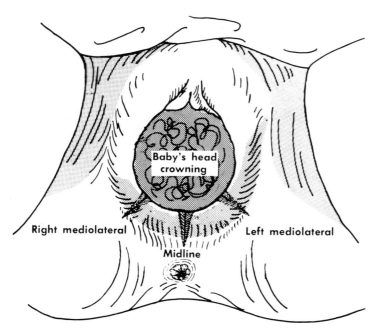

Right mediolateral　　　Left mediolateral

Baby's head crowning

Midline

Figure 7-11 Three types of episiotomies. (From Hamilton PM: *Basic maternity nursing,* ed 6, St Louis, 1988, Mosby.)

B. Forceps deliveries
 1. Definition: an operative procedure using various instruments to deliver the presenting part
 2. Indications for use
   a. To shorten second stage
   b. Assist in descent of presenting part when there has been poor progress or fetal distress
   c. Maternal exhaustion
   d. When rotation (of head) is necessary, e.g., left occiput posterior (LOP) to occiput anterior (OA)
   e. To save fetus in jeopardy
 3. Requirements for application
   a. No cephalopelvic disproportion
   b. Presenting part engaged and below ischial spines
   c. Full dilatation and effacement
   d. Ruptured membranes
   e. Empty bladder
   f. FHR checked before and after application
 4. Complications
   a. Lacerations and tears
   b. Hemorrhage
   c. Rupture of uterus
   d. Facial marks or facial paralysis of fetus
   e. Intracranial hemorrhage or brain damage to fetus
C. Vacuum extraction
 1. Definition: a soft, flexible cup placed over the fetal head as a machine exerts suction; allows practitioner to turn or pull the fetal head to assist delivery; an alternative to the use of forceps
 2. Problems for the fetus can be observed at the attachment site, including caput succedaneum or cephalhematoma
D. Cesarean section
 1. Definition: an operative procedure to deliver the fetus through a surgical incision made through the abdominal and uterine walls

 2. Indications
   a. Cephalopelvic disproportion
   b. Fetal distress
   c. Prematurity
   d. Dystocia
   e. Prolapsed cord
   f. Oversized infant (macrosomia)
   g. Positions and presentations undeliverable through the vagina
   h. Some hypertensive states, placenta previa, abruptio placentae, prolapsed cord abnormalities
   i. Maternal exhaustion
 3. Types
   a. Elective
     (1) Anticipated difficulties: for example, inadequate pelvis or vaginal deliveries inadvisable because mother has AIDS or herpes
     (2) Previous cesarean sections (selective)
   b. Emergency
     (1) Sudden fetal distress (e.g., rupture of the uterus)
     (2) Accident
     (3) Breech presentation
 4. Treatment and nursing management
   a. Routine surgical preoperative and postoperative care plus normal postpartum care
   b. Promote involution
   c. Perineal care
   d. Lochia; color amount same as for vaginal delivery
   e. Support mother and family; allay fears
   f. Watch for signs and symptoms of infection (chills, fever)
 5. Vaginal birth after cesarean (VBAC): vaginal delivery after a cesarean section may be encouraged; depends on reason for cesarean section

NORMAL POSTPARTUM

A. Definition: period from end of fourth stage of labor to 6 weeks after day of delivery
B. Immediate care following delivery
 1. Continue checking of vital signs
 2. Encourage urination
   a. Full bladder impedes involution
   b. Full bladder may cause excessive bleeding
 3. Offer food: if policy permits, offer food and drink to mother after vital signs are stable
 4. Care of fundus
   a. Check for firmness
   b. Lochia checked for color, amount, and presence of clots
 5. Provide perineal care and care of breasts
 6. Check incision (episiotomy or abdominal)
 7. General hygiene: shower may be permissible to clean, refresh mother after vital signs are stable (policies vary)
 8. Encourage putting infant to breast for feeding and bonding
C. Physiological changes during puerperium
 1. Reproductive organs
   a. Uterus: involution (return of uterus to normal size and function)
     (1) Walls of uterus return to normal in 3 to 4 weeks
     (2) Menstruation may return in 3 to 4 weeks
     (3) Nursing mothers: menstruation may be delayed several months

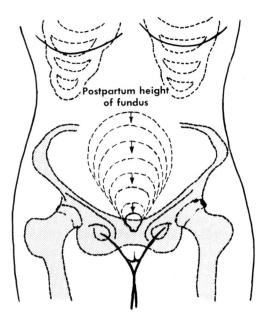

Figure 7-12 Involution. Height of fundus as it descends to prepregnant levels postpartum. (From Hamilton PM: *Basic maternity nursing*, ed 6, St Louis, 1988, Mosby.)

 (4) Fundus involutes 1 finger-width every day if umbilicus is used as point of reference (Fig. 7-12)
 b. Vagina
  (1) Returns to normal within 3 to 6 weeks after delivery, depending on type of delivery, length of labor, lacerations, healing process, and so on
  (2) Cesarean sections: vaginal recovery rapid
 c. Perineal area
  (1) Should be intact and clean
  (2) Complete healing should take 5 to 7 days
2. Return to normal of body system and functions
 a. Hormonal recovery begins immediately
 b. Lochia: vaginal discharge coming from decidual lining of uterus after delivery
  (1) Lochia rubra: dark red to bright red; occasional clots; flow lasts 2 to 3 days
  (2) Lochia serosa: pale pink to brownish lochia; lighter flow, dependent on ambulation; lasts 2 to 5 days
  (3) Lochia alba: yellowish, creamy discharge consisting of leukocytes and dead cells; lasts 5 to 10 days
  (4) Prolonged or recurring bleeding may indicate a medical problem
 c. Vascular system
  (1) Average loss of blood at delivery: 250 to 400 ml
  (2) Blood loss of 500 ml or more considered hemorrhage
 d. Urinary tract
  (1) Perineal soreness may temporarily reduce voiding reflexes
  (2) Marked diuresis 8 to 12 hours postpartum
D. Treatment and nursing management during postpartum
 1. Objectives for daily care
  a. Assist in normal process of involution; examples include assessing the fundus and promoting urination

  b. Assist in preventing infection; examples include proper hand washing and promoting proper breast-feeding technique
  c. Promote infant bonding with mother and family; examples include sibling visits when appropriate and encouraging partner to participate in care
 2. Nursing techniques for postpartum care
  a. Vital signs: watch for symptoms of hypovolemic shock and hemorrhage (fainting); stay with mother who is out of bed (OOB) for the first time since delivery
  b. Check breasts
   (1) Should be soft until milk comes in
   (2) Daily cleansing in shower
   (3) Daily breast examination to note any complications; nodules may be felt second or third day as milk production begins; teach breast self-examination; report any abnormalities
  c. Engorgement
   (1) Nursing usually prevents this; breast pump; nipple shield
   (2) Nonnursing mother
    (a) Cold compresses or ice bag on breasts
    (b) Supportive bra
    (c) Follow steps a and b only if requested
  d. Infections
   (1) Redness, warmth, pain, elevated temperature ≥100.4° F after 24 hr
   (2) May require minor surgical intervention to release drainage
  e. Check fundus
   (1) Height and firmness for proper involution
   (2) Relaxed fundus may indicate problem (hemorrhage or infection)
  f. Check lochia: color, amount, odor
  g. Check perineal area: healing and cleanliness
  h. Check legs: pain, tenderness, swelling (thrombi); check for Homans' sign
  i. Check urination: overdistention (subinvolution)
  j. Bowels: keep open (encourage fluids with balanced diet): administer stool softener (e.g., docusate sodium sulfosuccinate [Colace])
  k. Afterpains: involution
  l. Postpartum blues (baby blues): possible hormonal transitory depression; usually noted after discharge
 3. Teaching: important component of postpartum nursing management
  a. Personal hygiene
  b. Weight loss
   (1) Immediately after delivery, 7- to 10-lb weight loss
   (2) Total weight loss of pregnancy may take 6 weeks to 6 months or more to achieve
  c. PKU tests: requirement by law to test for inborn error of metabolism involving proteins and amino acids
  d. Discuss with mother and father
   (1) Importance of bonding
   (2) Readiness for parenthood
  e. Postpartum exercises
  f. Review methods of holding, bubbling, or burping baby

ABNORMAL POSTPARTUM
Postpartum Infection

A. Definition: any infection in the reproductive organs during labor, delivery, or up to 1 month postpartum
B. Signs and symptoms
  1. Chills, fever, localized back pain (kidney involvement)
  2. Malaise
  3. Lower abdominal tenderness, lower back pains
  4. Foul-smelling lochia (retained placental infection)
  5. Fundal height changes abnormal
C. Treatment and nursing management in general
  1. Administration of appropriate antibiotics on time and as directed
  2. Comfort measures appropriate to discomfort
  3. Check vital signs q4h
D. Specific infections
  1. Urinary tract infection (cystitis, pyelitis)
    a. Cause: trauma (stretching or tearing) or by an organism
    b. Signs and symptoms
      (1) 3 days postpartum
      (2) Low back pain
      (3) Localized pain (pyelitis)
      (4) Chills, high fever, apprehension
      (5) Frequency and burning urination (cystitis)
      (6) Discomfort
    c. Treatment and nursing management
      (1) Bed rest until symptoms subside (1 day)
      (2) Drugs (antibiotics)
      (3) Force fluids
      (4) Careful hand washing by mother and nursing staff
  2. Mastitis
    a. Definition: inflammation of the glands in the breast(s); if untreated could lead to abscess complications
    b. Cause
      (1) *Staphylococcus* infection
      (2) Stasis of milk (usually occurs 2 to 4 weeks postpartum)
      (3) Bruising of breast tissue
      (4) Open cuts in nipple or areola
    c. Signs and symptoms
      (1) High fever (103° F; 39.5° C)
      (2) Chills
      (3) Red, tender, painful, hard
    d. Treatment and nursing management
      (1) Support bra
      (2) Antibiotic therapy
      (3) Check incision for drainage
      (4) Heat to area
      (5) Increase fluid intake
      (6) Reassurance of mother
      (7) Continue breast-feeding if permitted by health care provider
  3. Thrombophlebitis
    a. Definition: a clot (thrombus) formed in response to an inflammation of the vessel wall
    b. Signs and symptoms
      (1) Local tenderness: femoral vein
      (2) 1 to 2 weeks postpartum
      (3) Swelling, chills, fever

    c. Treatment and nursing management
      (1) Administration of anticoagulant
      (2) Bed rest
      (3) Antibiotic therapy
      (4) Elevation of legs
      (5) Warm, wet compresses every 15 to 30 minutes
      (6) Never massage

Postpartum Hemorrhage

A. Definition: any loss of 500 ml or more of blood during first 24 hours following delivery
B. Types
  1. Early postpartal hemorrhage resulting from uterine atony (1 to 3 days)
  2. Late postpartal hemorrhage resulting from subinvolution (inability of the uterus to involute or return to its prepregnant state) or placental infection
C. Causes
  1. Uterine atony
  2. Retained placental fragments
  3. Overdistention of the uterus
  4. Grand multiparity
  5. Lacerations
  6. Trauma of the uterus due to forceps delivery
  7. Inversion of the uterus (an abnormal condition where the uterus is turned inside out)
D. Signs and symptoms
  1. Visible blood loss
  2. Shocklike symptoms: pale, clammy, hypotensive, apprehensive
E. Treatment and nursing management
  1. NPO, warm covers, oxygen as ordered
  2. IV fluids (ordered meds—examples include Pitocin and Methergine)
  3. Replacement transfusion if ordered
  4. Massage boggy uterus until firm
  5. Offer assurance and support to family and mother
  6. Medical management of cause (repair of laceration, possible D&C)

Hematomas

A. Definition: local accumulation of blood caused by injury to a blood vessel from the following:
  1. Undue pressure of heavy gravid uterus
  2. Bearing down inappropriately
  3. Long second stage
  4. Primigravida's prolonged pushing
B. Signs and symptoms
  1. Severe pain in perineal area
  2. Visible vaginal hematoma
  3. Vulvular hematoma
  4. Large blood-filled sac visible
C. Treatment and nursing management
  1. Ice to area for 24 hours (for a small hematoma)
  2. Antibiotics if ordered, analgesics if ordered
  3. Incision or ligation if necessary, vaginal packing and retention catheter
  4. Comfort measures similar to episiotomy care, that is, sitz bath

Subinvolution

A. Definition: inability of the uterus to return to its normal size after delivery; failure to involute; diagnosed 4 to 6 weeks postpartum
B. Causes
   1. Retention of placental pieces
   2. Infection (endometrium)
C. Signs and symptoms
   1. Involution process abnormal
   2. Boggy uterus (not firm); foul odor
   3. Lochia remains rubra for 2 weeks or longer
D. Treatment and nursing management
   1. Surgical intervention (D&C) (for retained placenta)
   2. Support and reassurance to mother and family
   3. Administration of medications to facilitate involution and cure infection

NORMAL NEWBORN

A. Immediate care following delivery
   1. Maintain patent airway
   2. Apply cord clamp, check for bleeding, follow procedure for daily cord care
   3. Maintain warmth
      a. Wrap in prewarmed receiving blankets or
      b. Place in preheated crib
   4. Preventive care
      a. Instill prophylactic eye drops in each eye as required by law to treat *Chlamydia trachomatis* and to prevent opthalmia neonatorum
      b. Commonly used prophylactic drugs: erythromycin, penicillin ointments/drops; silver nitrate frequently used in the past is no longer as commonly seen
      c. Administer intramuscular (IM) injection of vitamin K to reduce likelihood of hemorrhagic disease of the newborn
      d. Hepatitis B vaccination is recommended for all neonates regardless of HbsAg status (first dose within 12 hours of birth, second 1 month of age, third 6 months of age)
   5. Identification procedures
      a. Complete identification bands as required
      b. Record footprints of baby and pointer fingerprint of mother
   6. Apgar scoring
   7. Initial observation of newborn
      a. Is the primary responsibility of physician/pediatrician
      b. Nurse should wear gloves when handling newborn during immediate care and until initial bath; regulations differ for daily routines
      c. Nurse also makes quick observation, checking for visible anomalies such as cleft lip, cleft palate, extra digits, spinal column, limbs, skin, head
      d. Reflexes that nurse may check include Moro, sucking, rooting, blinking, grasping
   8. Encourage bonding
      a. After initial delivery room care, wipe off excess blood and debris from baby; wrap securely in clean, warm receiving blanket and let parents hold baby
      b. Allow time for mother and father to look at touch, and hold infant; allow time to initiate breastfeeding if mother desires

B. Normal physiology of newborn
   1. Vital signs
      a. Temperature
         (1) Axillary: 97.7° F to 98.6° F (36.5° C to 37° C)
         (2) Rectal: 97.7° F to 99° F (36.5° C to 37.3° C)
         (3) Rectal temperatures taken only on initial reading, or if temperature elevated, to avoid damage to the large intestine
      b. Pulse rate: 120 to 160 beats/min
         (1) Apical pulse rate
         (2) Irregular in rate and cadence (normal)
      c. Respirations: abdominal and irregular, 30 to 60 per minute
   2. Measurements
      a. Weight
         (1) Girls 7 lb (3100 g)
         (2) Boys 7½ lb (3300 g)
         (3) 5.5 to 9 lb (3000 to 4500 g) considered normal
         (4) 5% to 10% weight loss in first 2 to 3 days
         (5) Regains birth weight in 5 to 7 days
      b. Length: 18 to 22 inches (45 to 55 cm) long
      c. Head circumference: 13 to 14 inches (33 to 35 cm)
      d. Chest circumference: 12 to 13 inches (30 to 33 cm)
   3. Skin
      a. Milia: small, white sebaceous glands visible about nose, forehead, chin
      b. "Stork bites": telangiectasis or capillary hemangiomas
      c. Red nevi: discoloration, circumscribed, blanch on touch, prominent during crying, disappear in 6 months to a year
      d. Mongolian spots: bluish, bruiselike spots on buttocks, back, shoulders; disappear by toddler or preschool age and found in babies of Hispanic, black, Slavic, or Asian background
      e. Erythema toxicum neonatorum (newborn rash): appears as scratches and pimples; may be nosocomial infection
      f. Nevi vasculosus (strawberry mark): bright red or dark capillary hemangiomas with raised, rough surfaces; usually disappear by school age
      g. Nevi flammeus (port-wine stain): reddish purple raised capillary hemangiomas; do not blanch on pressure and may not disappear
      h. Lanugo: soft, downy hair on top of skin on ears, forehead, neck, shoulders; disappears in weeks
      i. Vernix caseosa: cheeselike protective material coating fetus, especially under arms, beneath knees, and in folds of thighs and groin
      j. Acrocyanosis: are bluish for several hours after delivery (hands and feet)
      k. Physiological jaundice: caused when excessive amounts of hemoglobin needed for intrauterine life decrease to extrauterine levels; the immature liver cannot process the bilirubin fast enough, and jaundice results
         (1) 50% of normal newborns and 80% of premature newborns have some level of jaundice
         (2) Treatment includes bilirubin test, increased formula, possible phototherapy

4. Elimination
   a. Urine: 3 to 4 times a day for first few days; usually urinates after every feeding
   b. Bowel movement: 5 to 6 times a day for first week
      (1) Meconium: expelled within 2 to 12 hours; black, tarry, thick unformed stool
      (2) Transient stool: blackish or greenish stool expelled after first few feedings
   c. Breast-fed stool: yellow, odorless, slightly runny
   d. Bottle-fed stool: formed, brownish yellow, distinct odor
   e. Each infant establishes own pattern of stool movement
5. Hyperestrogenism and its effect on the newborn
   a. Swelling of the breasts in male or female infant because of hormones from mother; the ensuing discharge is called "witch's milk"
   b. Swelling of the male scrotum: large, with rugae; disappears within days
   c. Pseudomenses with female
6. Reproductive organs of the male newborn
   a. Cryptorchidism: testes have not descended into scrotum; often present in premature infants
   b. Occasionally testes are in inguinal sac at birth but will descend within hours or more; if undescended after 1 month, pediatrician should evaluate
   c. The foreskin should not be retracted until at least 3 years of age if newborn is circumcised
7. Circulatory system: pulmonary circulation established within minutes of birth
8. Digestive system: immature at birth but can metabolize nutrients except fats
9. Visual capabilities: immature coordination and muscle control
10. Hearing capabilities: acute hearing within 2 minutes of birth
11. Taste perception: can distinguish sweet and sour in 1 to 3 days
12. Smelling perception: can distinguish smell of mother at 5 days
13. Sleep patterns
    a. Unstable for 6 to 8 hours after birth
    b. Has regular and irregular sleep cycles
14. Newborn reflexes
    a. Sucking, rooting, swallowing, extrusion reflexes
    b. Tonic neck (fencing) should disappear in 3 to 4 months
    c. Grasping (palmar) and plantar lessens in 3 to 4 months
    d. Moro's (startle) disappears in 2 months
    e. Stepping disappears in 3 to 4 weeks
    f. Babinski's (plantar): absence indicates CNS damage
    g. Blinking, sneezing
15. Immunity in the newborn
    a. Has 3-month supply (passive immunity) from mother if baby is term
    b. Begins own synthesis (active immunity) by 3 months of age
C. Daily observation and nursing care
   1. Newborn nursery care and observation
      a. Constant, careful observation
      b. Place infant in warmer until vital signs are stable

c. Check temperature; follow agency policy (rectal, axilla, etc.)
   (1) Infant is placed under warmer to prevent cold stress
   (2) Heat production normal in 2 to 3 days
   (3) Newborn loses heat through convection, conduction, radiation, and evaporation
d. Check respirations
e. Place infant on right side to promote expansion of lungs and drain excess mucus
f. Observe for signs and symptoms of respiratory distress syndrome (RDS)
g. Cord
   (1) Removal of cord clamp within 8 to 24 hours
   (2) Daily application of antigermicidal agent to prevent infections
h. Check eyes and ears for abnormal drainage
2. Daily nursery routine
   a. Daily weight and vital signs, especially temperature
   b. Observation and recording condition of skin, cord, eyes, elimination
   c. Daily care and changing of crib linen
      (1) Daily cord care
      (2) General observation
   d. During feeding routine observe infant-mother bonding
3. Teaching mothers care of newborn: mothers' classes should incorporate the care, handling, and dressing of the newborn in addition to procedures and demonstrations in sponge baths, tub baths, and cord care
4. Daily bath routine
   a. Purpose
      (1) Cleansing
      (2) Exercise time
      (3) Play, social time with parents (bonding time)
   b. Prepare environment: select safe, convenient, warm area
   c. Select and prepare equipment
      (1) Utensils for sponge bath
      (2) Necessary articles for procedure
      (3) Clean clothing
   d. Sponge baths: recommended for babies with cord intact
   e. Tub baths: recommended for babies whose cord has fallen off—10 to 14 days after birth
5. Cord care
   a. Wipe base of cord with alcohol or designated antiseptic every time diapers are changed and during bath time
   b. After cord falls off
      (1) Wipe with alcohol as instructed after daily bath routine for first day or two
      (2) If drainage persists, cleanse with alcohol and notify pediatrician
6. Diaper rash
   a. Change diapers frequently
   b. Wash area with warm tap water
   c. May apply A and D Ointment as a preventative and protective measure
   d. Expose to air if possible
      (1) Lay infant on abdomen and expose buttocks to air

(2) Apply Desitin or Balmex if A and D Ointment does not help
7. Circumcision
   a. Definition: the surgical cutting and removal of foreskin; usually done 1 to 3 days after birth
   b. Treatment and nursing management
      (1) Observe for bleeding, edema
      (2) Treatment may include petroleum jelly (Vaseline) for 3 days depending on the type of instrument used for circumcision
      (3) Check and record first voiding after procedure
      (4) Complications: rare
8. Facts about feeding the newborn
   a. Newborn metabolic rate twice that of adult
   b. Carbohydrates needed for brain growth and as source of energy
   c. Protein needed for building tissue; inadequacy results in infection, slow growth, flabby muscles
   d. Fat difficult to digest and metabolize but needed to maintain integrity of skin
   e. Iron: continuous supply needed for growth and development; storage from mother depleted in 4 to 6 months
   f. At birth can take 1 to 2 oz (30 to 60 ml) per feeding
   g. By 1 to 2 weeks, can nurse 4 oz (120 ml) per feeding
   h. Gradual increase to 6 to 8 oz (180 to 240 ml) per feeding in 1 month
9. Facts about breast milk
   a. Less protein than cow's milk; easier to digest
   b. More lactose than cow's milk, which facilitates metabolism and is good for bones
   c. Lactoferrin decreases dangers to infection
   d. Sucking stimulates posterior pituitary of mother to trigger let-down reflex, which allows milk to flow
10. Guidelines for breast-feeding
   a. A general rule of thumb is to nurse until breasts are soft once milk is established
   b. To ensure a good supply of breast milk, the mother should
      (1) Have adequate rest
      (2) Drink sufficient fluids
      (3) Eat a balanced, nutritious diet
      (4) Maintain psychological equilibrium (maternal-infant bonding)
11. The length of time for breast-feeding varies considerably from infant to infant and is normally 10 to 30 minutes. Limiting the time of nursing on each breast is no longer considered effective in preventing sore nipples. It is more important to use correct technique and empty the breasts completely
12. Contraindications to breast-feeding
   a. Mother with AIDS
   b. Baby with galactosemia/PKU

ABNORMAL NEWBORN
The Preterm (Premature) Infant

A. Definition: a baby born before 37 weeks' gestation and weighing less than 5½ lb (2500 g)
B. Infants may be small for gestational age (SGA) because they are preterm or from genetic or intrauterine causes
C. Statistics
   1. Of all live births 7% are premature
   2. Incidence of prematurity increases to 10% in some minority populations
   3. Prematurity is leading cause of death in infants in the United States
D. Cause
   1. Young, adolescent mothers
   2. Elderly primigravidas
   3. Multiple births
   4. Poor prenatal care
   5. Congenital anomalies
   6. Diseases or conditions that compromise fetus
      a. Pregnancy-induced hypertension
      b. Diabetes
      c. Heart disease
      d. Nutritional deficits
      e. Preterm labor
      f. Drug or alcohol addictions
      g. Smoking
      h. Placental insufficiency
E. Characteristics of a premature infant
   1. Central nervous system
      a. Poor muscle tone
      b. Poor reflexes
      c. Limp
      d. Assumes froglike position
      e. Weak, feeble cry
      f. Unstable heating mechanism: temperature fluctuates from 94° F to 96° F (34° C to 36° C)
      g. Poor sucking reflexes
      h. Weak gagging and sucking reflexes
   2. Respiratory system
      a. Insufficient surfactant
      b. Immature lungs, rib cage, muscles
      c. Prone to respiratory distress syndrome (RDS)
      d. Poor oxygenation
   3. Digestive system: immature gastric system; decreased ability to convert protein and fat to energy, able to digest simple sugars
   4. Integumentary system
      a. Harlequin pattern observed (a temporary flushing of the skin on the lower side of the body with pallor on the upward side); commonly seen in normal infants and disappears as the child matures
      b. Veins and capillaries visible
      c. Lanugo prominent
      d. Vernix prominent
      e. Decreased subcutaneous fat, thinner skin
      f. Skin tight, shiny, taut
   5. Circulatory system
      a. Fragile capillaries
      b. Susceptible to hemorrhages (intracranial)
   6. Renal system
      a. Inability to urinate properly
      b. Easily dehydrated (decreased concentrated urine leading to fluid retention)
      c. Fragile electrolyte balance (metabolic acidosis, Na bicarbonate decreased, and decreased excretion of drugs)
   7. Immune system
      a. Too young to have obtained any immunity from mother
      b. Vulnerable to infection

8. Endocrine system: a common complication is hypoglycemia
9. Head
   a. Fontanels large
   b. Suture lines prominent
   c. Old looking
F. Treatment and nursing management
   1. Maintain patent airway
   2. Frequently monitor blood gases to determine oxygen need
   3. Maintain body temperature by placing in heater
   4. Conserve energy: basic care only
   5. Provide adequate nutrition
      a. Nasogastric feedings
      b. Special soft nipples
      c. Parenteral fluids
   6. Prevent infection
      a. Prevent skin breakdown: change positions
      b. Keep dry and clean
   7. Length of hospitalization: usually until a weight of 5½ lb (2500 g) is reached
   8. Mothering stimulation taught and practiced
      a. Encourage parents to stroke, cuddle, talk
      b. Feed, diaper infants
      c. Play soft music
      d. Encourage tapping on Isolette and talking
   9. Listen to concerns of mothers and fathers

Post-Term Infant

A. Definition: over 42 weeks' gestation
B. Cause: unknown
C. Characteristics of postmature infant
   1. Old looking
   2. No vernix; no lanugo
   3. Color: yellow-green or meconium stained
   4. Desquamation of hands (palms) and feet (soles)
   5. May have respiratory problems
D. Nursing management
   1. Observe for hypoglycemia
   2. Observe for RDS
   3. Look for birth injuries
   4. Symptomatic nursing care

Neonatal Respiratory Distress Syndrome

A. Definition
   1. A series of symptoms signifying respiratory distress
   2. Synonyms: RDS, hyaline membrane disease (HMD)
B. Statistics
   1. Common in premature babies
   2. Leading cause of death in infants in the United States
C. Causes
   1. Lack or loss of surfactant in lungs
   2. Immaturity
   3. Hypoxia
   4. Hypothermia
D. Signs and symptoms
   1. Appears within minutes to hours after birth
   2. Grunting, rib retraction, nasal flaring (RDS symptoms)
   3. Inadequate oxygen: 60 or more respirations per minute
E. Diagnosis: x-ray examination shows collapsed portions of lungs; arterial blood gases reveal hypoxia

F. Treatment and nursing management
   1. Transfer to intensive care unit and Isolette care
   2. Initiate oxygen therapy: 60%; hood is best
      a. Intermittent positive-pressure breathing (IPPB)
      b. Continuous positive airway pressure (CPAP)
      c. Positive end-expiratory pressure (PEEP)
      d. Surfactant replacement
      e. Monitor blood gases
   3. Endotracheal tube if necessary
   4. IV hydration and nutrition and antibiotic therapy
   5. Elevate head of bed slightly
G. Complication
   1. Retinopathy of prematurity (ROP)
   2. Causes
      a. High arterial oxygen levels
      b. Retinal vascular immaturity

Birth Injuries

A. Normal deviations of the head
   1. Caput succedaneum (Fig. 7-13)
      a. Definition: edema (swelling) of soft tissues of scalp
      b. Cause: continuous pressure of the fetal head on cervix
      c. Signs and symptoms
         (1) Crosses suture lines
         (2) Appears at birth
         (3) Disappears in 3 to 4 days
      d. Treatment: none
   2. Cephalhematoma (see Fig. 7-13)
      a. Definition: blood between the periosteum and bone
      b. Cause: pressure during delivery (forceps; prolonged labor)
      c. Signs and symptoms
         (1) Never crosses suture lines
         (2) Appears several hours to several days after birth
         (3) Disappears within 3 to 6 weeks
      d. Treatment: none
   3. Molding (Fig. 7-14)
      a. Definition: changes in the shape of the head
      b. Cause: accommodation of fetal bones to birth canal during labor and delivery
      c. Signs and symptoms: visual
      d. Treatment: disappears without treatment in 3 days
   4. Soft tissue injuries (subcutaneous fat necrosis)
      a. Definition: pressure necrosis
      b. Signs and symptoms: purplish, movable mass
      c. Treatment: resolves spontaneously
B. Subconjunctival hemorrhage (scleral or retinal)
   1. Definition: rupture of small capillaries in eye
   2. Cause: increased intracranial pressure of birth
   3. Signs and symptoms: small, red pin dots in white of sclera, or hemorrhaging in retina
   4. Treatment: resolves without treatment in 5 days
C. Ecchymosis, petechiae, edema
   1. Definition: blood within tissues; does not blanch with pressure
   2. Cause: forceps, manipulation, pressure
   3. Signs and symptoms: visual in affected areas
   4. Treatment: resolves without treatment in 2 days
D. Skeletal injuries
   1. Skull fracture: rare, and unless blood vessels are involved, heals without treatment

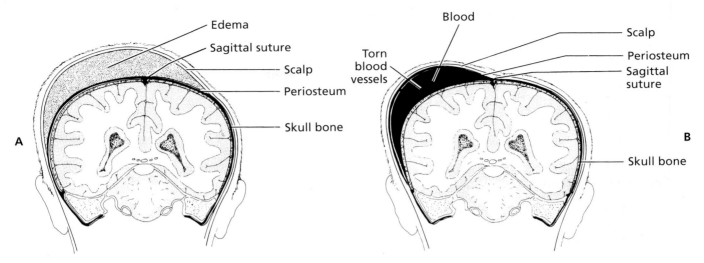

Figure 7-13 Differences between caput succedaneum and cephalhematoma. **A,** Caput succedaneum: edema of scalp noted at birth; crosses suture line. **B,** Cephalhematoma: bleeding between periosteum and skull bone appearing within first 2 days; does not cross suture lines.

2. Fracture of the clavicle: most common fracture; usually caused by shoulder impaction; dystocia
    a. Treatment: handle infant with care
    b. Prognosis: good
3. Fracture of the humerus or femur: rare
    a. Cause: dystocia and difficult delivery
    b. Treatment
        (1) Immobilize
        (2) Heals rapidly
    c. Complications: rare
E. Neurological injuries
    1. Brachial paralysis of upper arm: Erb-Duchenne paralysis (Erb's palsy)
        a. Definition: traumatic injury to the upper brachial plexus, with damage to one or more cervical nerve roots
        b. Cause
            (1) Difficult labor
            (2) Shoulder impaction; dystocia
            (3) Malposition of forceps
        c. Treatment: immobilize with brace or splint
        d. Nursing management
            (1) Skin care as necessary
            (2) Gentle range-of-motion exercises after healing
    2. Brachial paralysis of lower arm: Klumpke's
        a. Definition: nerves of hand and wrist crushed or severed
        b. Treatment
            (1) Pad wrist and fingers
            (2) Corrective surgery
            (3) Gentle massage after surgery
            (4) Range-of-motion exercises when appropriate
        c. Prognosis: good
    3. Facial paralysis
        a. Definition: crushed or severed nerves of face that cause grimacing and distortion, especially when crying; asymmetric paralysis
        b. Cause: misapplication of forceps
        c. Treatment: condition transitory; reassure parents

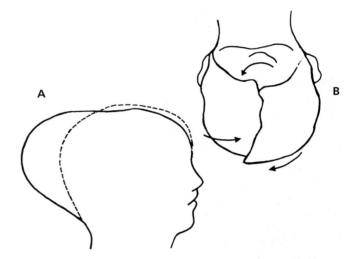

Figure 7-14 **A,** Various types of molding. **B,** Bones overlapping during molding. (From Hamilton PM: *Basic maternity nursing,* ed 6, St Louis, 1988, Mosby.)

F. Central nervous system injuries
    1. Definition: injuries causing intracranial hemorrhaging
    2. Cause
        a. Prematurity
        b. Large full-term babies
        c. Dystocia
        d. Hypoxia
        e. Hypovolemia
    3. Types
        a. In brain itself
        b. Subdural hematoma
    4. Signs and symptoms
        a. Suture line separation
        b. Bulging anterior-fontanel
        c. High-pitched cry
        d. Abnormal respirations
        e. Cyanosis

f. Irritability or lethargy
g. Twitching; convulsions
5. Treatment and nursing management
a. Head higher than hips
b. Warmth
c. Oxygen
d. IV therapy
e. Minimal handling
f. Surgical aspiration (if appropriate)
g. Measurement of head size weekly
h. Convulsion precautions

Infections of the Newborn

A. Causes
1. Dystocia
2. Premature rupture of the membranes of 24 hours or more (sepsis neonatorum)
3. Clinical amnionitis
4. Maternal infection (toxoplasmosis, syphilis, rubella)
5. Nosocomial infection (hospital-based infection; usually staph)
6. *Monilia* or yeast infection in mother's vagina
B. Signs and symptoms
1. Appears within first 48 hours
2. Vague symptoms
3. Lethargy, irritability, lack of appetite
4. Low-grade temperature
5. Diarrhea
6. Jaundice
C. Treatment and nursing management
1. Take cultures of blood, urine, throat
2. Administer antibiotic therapy
3. Keep warm
4. Administer oxygen therapy if necessary
5. Isolate if appropriate
6. Weigh daily
7. Watch for signs of jaundice
8. Keep parents informed of progress

Congenital Malformations

A. Perinatal signs
1. Polyhydramnios: excessive amniotic fluid; may occur with other congenital anomalies
2. Oligohydramnios: scant amniotic fluid; indicates urinary tract anomalies and renal disturbances
B. Postnatal congenital malformations
1. Choanal atresia (gastrointestinal anomaly)
a. Definition: blockage between the nose and throat; can be unilateral or bilateral
b. Signs and symptoms
(1) Cyanotic at rest
(2) Color improves when crying
(3) Snorts when feeding
c. Treatment and nursing management
(1) Physician may pierce obstruction with a probe if it is only a membrane
(2) Minor surgical repair if bone involved; prognosis excellent
(3) Feeding problems; positioning important
(4) Gavage feeding may be necessary
(5) Watch closely for aspiration
2. Esophageal atresia: refer to Chapter 8

3. Congenital laryngeal stridor
a. Definition: abnormal condition around larynx that causes noisy respiration, especially a crowing sound on inspiration
b. Cause:
(1) Flabby epiglottis
(2) Extraglotteal structures
(3) Relaxation of laryngeal wall
(4) Absence of tracheal rings
(5) Deformity of vocal cords
c. Signs and symptoms
(1) Noisy respirations on inspiration
(2) Most noticeable when crying
(3) Mild-to-severe intercostal or supraclavicular retractions
(4) Cyanosis
(5) Dyspnea
d. Treatment and nursing management
(1) Depends on cause
(2) Mild stridor may subside in 6 to 18 months
(3) Mother taught to position baby upright for feeding
(4) Feed slowly, pausing to let infant catch his or her breath
(5) Use small nipple
(6) Watch for aspiration of feedings
(7) Prevent respiratory complications
(8) Keep infant warm, dry, away from drafts
(9) Oxygen in readiness
(10) Tracheotomy preparedness
e. Prognosis: good
4. Cleft lip and cleft palate
a. Definition: bilateral or unilateral fissure or opening on the palate or the upper lips resulting from failure of the bony and soft tissue structures to unite
b. Cause: developmental failure during the embryonic stage because of heredity, age, or a variety of other factors such as radiation or viral infections
c. Signs and symptoms
(1) Visual on lips
(2) Palate more difficult to notice sometimes
(3) Occurs more frequently in males
(4) Difficulty feeding
(5) Choking
(6) Drooling
(7) Milk may drain through nostrils
d. Treatment
(1) Cleft lips may have butterfly adhesive taping as initial treatment; may be helpful in feeding so milk does not continually drain through fissure
(2) Cleft lip may be surgically repaired at 1 to 2 weeks of age, or at 12 lb (5.5 kg)
(3) Cleft palate; first repair usually by 18 months
e. Nursing management
(1) Feeding precautions
(a) Use soft duck nipple, medicine dropper with rubber tip
(b) Place nipple away from cleft side
(c) Feed slowly
(d) Bubble frequently
(e) Rinse mouth after feedings

(f) Watch for aspiration, respiratory distress, gastrointestinal disturbances

(2) Mouth care: prevent cracks, fissures on lips

(3) Postoperative care for cleft lip

    (a) Place infant on side

    (b) Mouth care important because of Logan bar applied to prevent stretching of sutures

    (c) Prevent crying

    (d) Check swelling (tongue, nose, mouth)

    (e) Watch for hemorrhage

    (f) Apply elbow restraints

    (g) Prevent crust formation

    (h) Feed on opposite side of surgery

    (i) Use rubber-tipped dropper (3 weeks)

5. Diaphragmatic hernia

  a. Definition: herniation of abdominal viscera into the thoracic cavity as a result of incomplete development during embryonic stage, ranging from minimal to complete herniation

  b. Signs and symptoms

    (1) Constant respiratory distress

    (2) Bowels distended

    (3) Bowel sounds heard in chest

    (4) Asymmetrical chest contour

  c. Treatment and nursing management

    (1) Early recognition and prompt surgery

    (2) Usual preoperative and postoperative management

  d. Prognosis guarded, depending on severity

6. Omphalocele: see Chapter 8

7. Imperforate anus: see Chapter 8

C. Congenital anomalies of central nervous system

1. Spina bifida occulta

  a. Definition: defect in vertebral column without protrusion of spinal cord and meninges; this is one of three types of spina bifida, which is a malformation of the spine, most common in the lumbosacral region, in which the posterior portion of the vertebrae fails to close

  b. Signs and symptoms

    (1) Dimple in lower lumbosacral skin

    (2) Hair over area sometimes

    (3) X-ray film confirmation

  c. Treatment and nursing management: no treatment necessary unless neurologic symptoms occur

2. Meningocele (another form of spina bifida)

  a. Definition: defect in spinal cord with protrusion of meninges through an opening in spinal canal; paralysis is present

  b. Surgical correction

3. Myelomeningocele

  a. Definition: both spinal cord and meninges protrude through defective bony rings in spinal cord; possible paralysis below sac

  b. Signs and symptoms

    (1) Visual signs

    (2) Observe for change in intracranial pressure

    (3) Check head measurements for hydrocephalus

    (4) Report signs and symptoms of CNS involvement

  c. Preoperative management

    (1) Flat on abdomen with sterile gauze, petroleum jelly (Vaseline), Telfa pad, normal saline

    (2) No diapers

    (3) Keep clean

    (4) Use care to prevent sac from breaking

    (5) Prevent infection: sterile technique

    (6) Prevent deformity

    (7) Prevent injury

  d. Postoperative management

    (1) Vital signs

    (2) Symptoms of shock

    (3) Oxygen readiness

    (4) Head measurements

    (5) Cast care if necessary; sometimes casts applied to legs

    (6) Importance of good nutrition

    (7) Orthopedic and urological habilitation

    (8) Encourage normal use of functions

    (9) Minimize disabilities

    (10) Paralysis (if present) may not be alleviated, but further damage could be prevented; aim of surgery is to give infant opportunity for optimal growth and development

    (11) "Crede" bladder to keep it empty and free from infection

4. Hydrocephalus: refer to Chapter 8

5. Congenital dislocation of the hip: refer to Chapter 8

6. Talipes equinovarus (clubfoot): refer to Chapter 8

7. Phocomelia

  a. Definition: developmental congenital anomaly in which only stubs or parts of arms and legs are present; degree of severity varies

  b. Cause: interference with embryonic development of long bones; is rare and seen as a result of the drug thalidomide taken during early pregnancy to relieve nausea

  c. Treatment and nursing management

    (1) Psychosocial problems for family and infant

    (2) Body surface limited, so heating mechanism overheats rest of body, causing diaphoresis

    (3) Personal hygiene; frequent baths

    (4) Special education imperative

8. Polydactyly

  a. Definition: supernumerary fingers or toes

  b. Cause: possibly hereditary

  c. Treatment and nursing management

    (1) Usually no bone or nerve involvement

    (2) Tie digit with silk suture in newborn nursery; it falls off

    (3) Surgical intervention necessary with bone involvement; X-ray done first to assure no bone or ligaments present

9. Hypospadias: refer to Chapter 8

10. Epispadias: refer to Chapter 8

Hemolytic Disease of Newborn

A. Pathological jaundice

1. Cause: Rh factor incompatibility; occurs only when mother is Rh negative and fetus is Rh positive

2. Pathophysiology: the Rh-negative mother is exposed to and develops antibodies against the Rh antigen (sensiti-

zation); sensitization to Rh-positive blood can be caused by exposure to the antigen during amniocentesis or if there is a transplacental bleed during a miscarriage or abortion; the most common time for sensitization to occur is birth
3. Signs and symptoms
    a. Jaundice
    b. Anemia
    c. Enlarged liver and spleen
    d. Generalized edema
    e. If untreated, "yellow bodies" will travel to brain, causing brain damage, heart failure, kernicterus, and death
4. Treatment and nursing management
    a. Blood types of mother and father important for anticipatory guidance
    b. Usually first babies do not present a problem
    c. If baby's bilirubin is above 10 or 12 mg/dl, phototherapy may be applied to reduce jaundice; exchange transfusions may be necessary
    d. After birth of Rh-positive baby, an unsensitized Rh-negative mother is given RhoGAM, a specific gamma globulin that will prevent the production of Rh antibodies; this must be given within 72 hours after delivery; the effect is the assurance that subsequent pregnancies will not be harmful to the baby
    e. Rh-antibody titers can be monitored throughout pregnancy (prenatal)
    f. Amniocentesis will reveal, by indirect Coombs' test, if mother has antibodies circulating in the maternal plasma or serum
B. Erythroblastosis fetalis (hydrops)
    1. Definition: most severe form of fetal hemolysis
    2. Rarely seen since the development of Rhogam
    3. Signs and symptoms include anemia, congestive heart failure, and ascites
C. ABO incompatibility
    1. Definition: an incompatibility of blood groups A and B because of the presence of antigens developed and passed on to the fetus by a type O mother
    2. Signs and symptoms
        a. Jaundice: mild, occurring during first day or two
        b. Slight enlargement of liver and spleen
    3. Treatment and nursing management
        a. Phototherapy
        b. If bilirubin is above 20 mg/dl, an exchange transfusion with group O and appropriate Rh type
        c. Observe for progressive lethargy
        d. Level of jaundice (visual and laboratory)
        e. Observe color of urine
        f. Observe for edema
        g. Observe for convulsions
        h. Symptomatic nursing care

Down's Syndrome (Trisomy 21)
Refer to Chapter 8

Drug Addiction in Newborns
A. Definition: secondary addiction, caused by drugs being ingested or injected by mother-addict; drugs cross placental barrier and create a drug-dependent newborn (immature liver unable to excrete drug rapidly during fetal life)

B. Signs and symptoms
    1. Low birth weight
    2. Premature
    3. Immature
    4. Withdrawal symptoms within 48 to 72 hours; watch for
        a. Sneezing
        b. Respiratory distress
        c. Excessive sweating
        d. Feeding problems
        e. Frantic sucking of fists
        f. High-pitched cry
        g. Irritable, hyperactive, tremors
        h. Fever
        i. Diarrhea
C. Treatment and nursing management
    1. Prevent infection
    2. Promote good nutrition
    3. Keep quiet (quiet, darkened environment)
    4. Offer loving, soothing, cuddling care
    5. Give medications on time
    6. Monitor vital signs
    7. Keep warm
    8. Protect from injury because child is hyperactive
    9. Good skin care because of excessive sweating and diarrhea
    10. Adequate fluids (prevent dehydration)
    11. Encourage mother to assist in care
        a. Teach holding, diapering, talking, bathing
        b. Encourage visits

Infants of Diabetic Mothers
A. Complications
    1. Delivery date may be recommended before EDC or about 36 to 37 weeks' gestation to prevent:
        a. Oversized baby (macrosomia)
        b. High-risk infant (diabetic babies have high rate of infant mortality)
    2. Neonatal hypoglycemia common
    3. RDS complications
    4. Hyperbilirubinemia (severe jaundice)
    5. Intracranial hemorrhage (birth trauma, LGA)
    6. Congestive heart failure
    7. Congenital anomalies in 5% of infants
    8. Hypocalcemia
B. Signs and symptoms
    1. Lethargic
    2. Plump, puffy face
    3. Long and heavy
    4. Respiratory problems evident
    5. Enlarged heart, liver, and spleen
    6. Symptoms of hypoglycemia
    7. Symptoms of hypocalcemia (tremors)
C. Treatment and nursing management
    1. Medical management difficult because of rapid, changing growth patterns, nutritional demands, illness
    2. Parents must be taught techniques for blood glucose monitoring
    3. Short-acting insulin best (easier to control)
    4. Treat hypoglycemia and hypocalcemia
    5. Oral feedings when tolerated and blood sugar levels stable

Cretinism (Congenital Hypothyroidism)
Refer to Chapter 8

FAMILY PLANNING
A. Trends
1. Smaller families (except for the poor and disadvantaged)
2. Delayed parenthood by choice
   a. Career women
   b. Desire for higher education
   c. Alternate living arrangements
3. Single parents
   a. High divorce rate
   b. Expanding role of father as single parent because custody of children, traditionally awarded to mother, is now being awarded to fathers
   c. Lessening barriers for adoption by single men and women
   d. Cultural and ethnic acceptance of unmarried mothers
   e. Opportunities to continue education for pregnant teenager without pressure of forced marriage
B. Communes: labor and delivery in communal community homes
C. Early sexual encounters (teenage pregnancies)
1. Need for referrals to family planning centers for guidance and counseling
   a. Teach use of condoms (controversial)
   b. Practice abstinence
2. Problems originating from early sexual encounters
D. Surrogate mothers
1. In vitro transplantation of embryo in the uterus of a woman who agrees to have a full-term pregnancy for another woman
2. Moral and legal implications

Possible Influential Factors
A. Sex education: incorporation of sex education in public and parochial schools at an early age
B. Freedom of choice
1. Availability of over-the-counter pregnancy tests
2. Availability of over-the-counter contraceptives
3. Abortions mandated as legal by the United States Supreme Court, 1977
C. Postponement of family: using available contraceptive devices
D. Economic factor: high cost of medical care forces young people to consider waiting until affluent enough to "afford" a family

Common Methods of Birth Control (Contraception)
A. Natural
1. Rhythm (calendar) method
   a. Based on the principle that ovulation occurs during midcycle of a menstrual period; that is, in a 28-day cycle, ovulation would occur on the 14th day
   b. Accordingly the most fertile days are considered to be 3 to 4 days before and 3 to 4 days after ovulation
2. Basal metabolism method: daily monitoring of early morning temperature for a period of several months and entering it on a graph (Fig. 7-15) will establish an ovulation time; "safe" and "fertile" times can be determined, and mother advised on use of this method

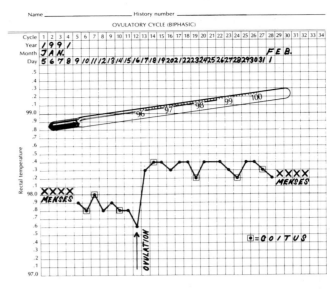

Figure 7-15 Basal temperature record shows drop and sharp rise at time of ovulation. (From Lowdermilk DL, Perry SE, Bobak IM: *Maternity nursing,* ed 5, St Louis, 1999, Mosby.)

B. Coitus interruptus
1. Penis is withdrawn from vagina just before ejaculation
2. Least effective of all methods
C. Condom (sheath, snakeskin, rubbers): thin rubber or plastic sheath that fits over penis and acts as barrier, preventing sperm from entering the vagina
D. Diaphragm: mechanical barrier placed at mouth of cervix; used with contraceptive cream or jelly to be effective; may engage in intercourse immediately after placement; should be left in place for 6 hours after intercourse; spermicide must be added each time intercourse occurs
E. Chemical agents: foam, creams, jelly, vaginal suppositories, and sponges form a chemical barrier in the vagina and render the area unsafe for sperm
F. Intrauterine devices (IUD)
1. Devices come in various shapes made of memory plastic inserted in the uterine cavity immediately following the woman's menstrual cycle
2. Mode of action unclear; thought to interfere with implantation by creating peristaltic waves
3. Disadvantages
   a. Excessive bleeding during menstrual cycle
   b. Extremely controversial; Dalkon Shield taken off the market because of permanent sterility and multiple gynecological problems
   c. Possible contamination from IUD string hanging in vaginal orifice
4. Advantage: once IUD inserted, only periodic checking (usually monthly) to confirm it is still intact
G. Oral contraceptive (birth control pill)
1. Most widely used
2. Considered 90% or more effective
3. Prevents anterior pituitary from releasing follicle stimulating hormone (FSH); artificially raises estrogen and progesterone levels and prevents ovulation
4. Stimulates endometrium, creating hostile environment for sperm

5. Minor side effects, lasting a few weeks to months: nausea, weight gain, full breasts
6. Major side effects: thrombophlebitis, hypertension, embolism, cardiovascular disturbances

H. Cervical cap
1. A small rubber cap fitted over the cervix to prevent sperm from entering the cervical canal
2. More comfortable than the diaphragm
3. May be left safely on the cervix for longer periods of time and remain effective

I. Female condom
1. A sheath secured by two rings that cover the cervix and vulva; coated with a spermicide preparation
2. Protects against both pregnancy and disease
3. May cause a decrease in sensation during intercourse

J. Operative sterilization
1. Vasectomy
   a. Removal of a portion of both vasa deferentia; prevents the transport of sperm into the seminal fluid
   b. Temporary birth control should be used for 2 to 3 months until a semen analysis determines that no viable sperm are present
   c. Reversal may be possible using microsurgery
2. Tubal ligation (bilateral partial salpingectomy)
   a. Fallopian tubes are clipped, cut, or cauterized
   b. Sexual activity can resume whenever woman is comfortable enough
   c. Reversal is possible; however, the probability of regaining fertility is seriously decreased

RESOURCES

Healthy People 2010
Office of Disease Prevention and Health Promotion
Hubert H. Humphrey Building, Room 738G
200 Independence Avenue, SW.
Washington, DC 20201
Fax (202) 205-9478

American Academy of Pediatrics
141 Northwest Point Boulevard
P.O. Box 927
Elk Grove Village, IL 60009-0927
(708) 228-5005

American College of Obstetrics and Gynecology
409 12th Street SW
Washington, DC 20024
(202) 863-2518

Health Resources and Services Administration
Maternal and Child Health Bureau
Parklawn Building, Room 18A-05
5600 Fishers Lane
Rockville, MD 20857
(301) 443-2170

March of Dimes Birth Defects Foundation
1275 Mamaroneck Avenue
White Plains, NY 10605
(914) 428-7100

National Center for Education and Maternal and Child Health
2000 15th Street North, Suite 701
Arlington, VA 22201
(703) 524-7802

National Perinatal Information Center
1 State Street, Suite 102
Providence, RI 02908-5035

SUGGESTED READINGS

Anderson B, Shapiro P: *Basic maternal and newborn nursing,* ed 6, Albany, 1995, Delmar Publishers.
Eschleman M: *Introductory nutrition and nutrition therapy,* ed 3, St Louis, 1996, Mosby.
McKenry LM, Salerno E: *Pharmacology in nursing,* ed 20, St Louis, 1998, Mosby.
Novak JC, Broom BL: *Ingalls and Salerno's Maternal and child health nursing,* ed 9, St Louis, 1999, Mosby.
Phillips CR: *Family-centered maternity and newborn care,* ed 4, St Louis, 1996, Mosby.
Wold GH: *Contemporary maternity nursing,* St Louis, 1997, Mosby.

REVIEW QUESTIONS

1. A pioneer who helped decrease puerperal infection is:
   ① William Smellie
   ② Ignaz Semmelweiss
   ③ Louis Pasteur
   ④ Peter Chamberlain

2. An additional method of determining the estimated date of delivery (EDD) aside from Naegle's rule is:
   ① Rupture of the membranes
   ② Audible fetal heart tones
   ③ Lightening
   ④ Quickening

3. A couple planning their first pregnancy asks the nurse about the accuracy of home pregnancy tests. The nurse replies that, "Home pregnancy tests are widely used today." However, it is most important that prospective parents:
   ① Wait at least 3 weeks after the first missed period
   ② Wait at least 9 days after the first missed period
   ③ Make certain that the blood is correctly placed on the stick
   ④ Use a sterile urine specimen to complete the test

4. A patient who is a mother of a 5-year-old son and is now pregnant again should be classified as:
   ① Gravida I Para I
   ② Gravida II Para II
   ③ Gravida II Para I
   ④ Gravida II Para 0

5. One of the earliest presumptive signs of pregnancy is:
   ① Hegar's sign
   ② Missed menstrual period
   ③ Linea nigra
   ④ Braxton-Hicks contractions

6. A couple is thrilled to hear their baby's heart rate with a Doppler. The gestation of the couple's pregnancy at this time is most likely:
   ① 4 weeks
   ② 10 weeks
   ③ 18 weeks
   ④ 24 weeks

7. To confirm a patient's pregnancy the nurse should give which of the following instructions regarding the required urine specimen:
   ① Give a voided specimen during her first visit
   ② Instruct her on how to give a sterile specimen in the office
   ③ Tell her to withhold fluid intake during the night and bring in the first voided specimen in the morning
   ④ A catheterized specimen will be required

8. Which female hormone is said to "hold" the pregnancy:
   ① Estrogen
   ② Luteinizing hormone
   ③ Progesterone
   ④ Human gonadotropic hormone

9. A prenatal patient asks when she should stop working. The most appropriate response for the nurse is:
   ① "Around the start of the eighth month."
   ② "Everyone is different; it is up to you."
   ③ "What do you do for a living?"
   ④ "Two weeks before your EDC."

10. Which of the following statements in a prenatal class would indicate to the nurse that a family is beginning to accept the newborn into their world?
    ① A father states, "Everyone is going to have to pitch in and help."
    ② An 8-year-old sibling states, "I can help mommy with the new baby."
    ③ A mother states, "I cannot wait to go back to school."
    ④ A 3-year-old asks, "Am I going to have to share my toys?"

11. A patient is interested in having a vaginal birth after cesarean (VBAC). One factor in her obstetrical history that would help the physician/midwife evaluate whether this would be an option is:
    ① The first cesarean was because of hypertension
    ② The patient has a history of substance abuse
    ③ The first cesarean was caused by a breech presentation
    ④ The mother is a gestational diabetic

12. The communicable (childhood) disease most likely to affect pregnancy, with harmful effects to the fetus is:
    ① Chickenpox
    ② Rubella
    ③ Varicella
    ④ Rubeola

13. A nurse is teaching a prepared childbirth class. She is asked which method is the best way? The most appropriate reply is:
    ① "The Dick Reed method is my favorite."
    ② "Any combination that works best for you."
    ③ "Strict adherence to any method is what is important."
    ④ "The Hegar method is the one that is currently favored."

14. During a prenatal class, a father asks, "When does the embryo becomes a fetus?" The nurse explains:
    ① "The term *embryo* is used for the first 3 weeks."
    ② "The term *embryo* is used for the first 8 weeks of pregnancy."
    ③ "The embryo becomes a fetus after the first week."
    ④ "The embryo becomes a fetus when the fetal heart is heard."

15. The nurse is teaching a class on fetal development. She explains that the product of conception is called a blastocyst:
    ① After the first division of the zygote
    ② When it is in the fallopian tube
    ③ After 3 weeks
    ④ As the morula enters the uterus

16. Implantation of the zygote occurs:
    ① Approximately 3 weeks after fertilization
    ② Approximately 7 days after fertilization
    ③ When the sperm and ovum join
    ④ Within 12 to 48 hours after intercourse

17. Fetal circulation is different from circulation following birth because:
    ① Blood leaves the heart through the pulmonary arteries bypassing the lungs
    ② Blood leaves the heart through the pulmonary veins
    ③ The chambers are not fully developed until after birth
    ④ Blood goes through the ductus arteriosus to the lungs

18. A student nurse asks, "How is the baby's sex determined?" The nursing instructor responds:
    ① X chromosome from the ovum
    ② A random number of chromosomes
    ③ Y or X chromosome from the sperm
    ④ Genes that are carried by DNA and protein

19. The basal metabolic rate of a prenatal patient generally increases. An explanation of this would be:
    ① Hormone production is increased
    ② The thyroid gland increases in size
    ③ Cardiac output and rate increases
    ④ The baby causes a need for excess energy

20. Which of the following statements by a teenage mom would most indicate to the nurse that the patient is accepting her new role?
    ① "My mom is taking care of the baby so that I can stay in school."
    ② "The baby is going to cause many changes in my schedule."
    ③ "She is so cute, I just love her so much."
    ④ "My friends have all promised to help."

21. A couple asks why it is so important to the fetus for both of them to stop smoking. The nurse responds:
    ① "Smoking and secondhand smoke causes decreased oxygenation to the fetus."
    ② "Pregnant women who smoke or who are around smoke tend to have larger babies."
    ③ "Pregnant women who smoke tend to have babies who are diabetic."
    ④ "Pregnant women who smoke tend to have babies with cardiac anomalies."

22. A couple of Eastern European–Jewish heritage is referred for genetic counseling. Which of the following conditions would be of most concern to this couple?
    ① Sickle-cell anemia
    ② Tay-Sachs disease
    ③ Thalassemia
    ④ Cystic fibrosis

23. A mother in her first trimester confides to the nurse she is worried she will not be a good mother. She is disappointed that she will not be able to go back to school as she had planned. The nurse should:
    ① Reassure the mother that her feelings of ambivalence are normal in the first trimester
    ② Tell her she has to let everyone in the family help her
    ③ Instruct her that she made the baby and she has to take responsibility for it
    ④ Assure her that as the pregnancy progresses, her feelings will become more positive

24. The patient who is 28 weeks pregnant is having a routine prenatal visit. A trace of albumin is discovered in her urine. The nurse is concerned because this may be an indication of:
    ① Pregnancy-induced hypertension
    ② Cystitis
    ③ Diabetes
    ④ Heart disease

25. A nurse is teaching a class on childbirth during a prenatal clinic. She is asked by a patient what is meant by stretch marks. She explains that stretch marks are called striae gravidarum and look like:
    ① A darkening line from below the breast bone to the symphysis pubis

② A dark freckle-like pigmentation over nose and cheeks
③ A stretching of skin with silvery to reddish-bluish stretch marks on breasts and abdomen
④ A darkening and increased size of areolar tissue of the breast

26. A nurse is teaching a bath class to a group of new parents. Which of the following instructions would be correct concerning cord care?
    ① "The baby can take a tub bath when the cord falls off."
    ② "Wipe around the base of the cord every day with alcohol until the cord falls off."
    ③ "Place antibiotic ointment around the base of the cord."
    ④ "There really is nothing special that needs to be done with the cord."

27. A nurse is asked by her neighbor if it is safe for her to have her baby delivered by a midwife. The first question that should be asked by the nurse is:
    ① "Is a physician available if complications develop?"
    ② "What is your medical and obstetrical history?"
    ③ "Have you asked your physician?"
    ④ "What training has the midwife received?"

28. A patient asks the health care provider why is it necessary to take so many measurements of her pelvis. The best response would be:
    ① "You are below average in height and weight. We want to be certain there is room for the baby to come out."
    ② "You are above average in height and weight. We want to make certain there is room for the baby to come out."
    ③ "We have to make certain that you have a platyploid pelvis."
    ④ "We make an estimate of the size of your pelvis to be certain that the opening is wide enough for an average size baby."

29. A patient in her sixth month of pregnancy is complaining of difficulties with insomnia. The intervention that the nurse might suggest includes:
    ① Keeping legs uncrossed
    ② Elevate hips
    ③ Warm milk at bedtime
    ④ Balanced diet

30. A patient in a prenatal class asks about whether Kegel exercises are beneficial in pregnancy. The most appropriate response by the nurse would be:
    ① "Absolutely not!! They are dangerous to your heart."
    ② "They help some people, but the benefit is minimal."
    ③ "Yes, they can help to tighten the pelvic floor muscles."
    ④ "Yes, these exercises will help with leg cramps."

31. A couple asks the nurse, "When during the pregnancy do we have to stop having sex?" The nurse responds:
    ① "By the eighth month, it becomes dangerous for the fetus."
    ② "It is safe as long as the patient douches each time."
    ③ "Sexual intercourse is okay if the cervix is closed."
    ④ "Generally by the third trimester it is not advisable."

32. A patient is curious to know when the fetal heart begins to function. The nurse tells her it is usually:
    ① By the third or fourth week after LMP
    ② Within 6 weeks after implantation

③ By the first trimester
④ By the time the placenta is formed

33. A prenatal patient is complaining of low back pains. A nurse might suggest:
① Sitz baths
② Heating pads to her back
③ Pelvic rocking or pelvic tilting exercises
④ Visits to the chiropractor

34. A primigravida in the sixth month of pregnancy is complaining of indigestion. The nurse explains that this is caused by:
① A growing uterus pushing on the diaphragm
② Eating small frequent meals increases gastric acid secretion
③ An increasing basal metabolic rate leading to increased appetite
④ Increased nausea and vomiting, common in this trimester

35. A prenatal patient is experiencing leg cramps. A nursing intervention should include:
① Advising hot compresses bid
② Instructing her to elevate her legs at least 15 minutes 3 times daily
③ Informing her of the cause (excessive phosphorus) and encouraging her to drink milk
④ Advising her to chew Tums for calcium

36. A patient is 36 weeks pregnant and in danger of becoming eclamptic. Delivery is induced. She delivers a 5 lb 8 oz (2500 g) boy after just 6 hours of labor. She must continue to be watched for impending eclampsia for how long?
① 1 hour
② 2 hours
③ 24 hours
④ 72 hours

37. Orders for a patient, recently admitted to the unit, include notifying the physician immediately of any changes in status, no vaginal or rectal examinations, fetal monitoring, pad count, oxygen if necessary, and laboratory work (type and cross match, Hgb, Hct). These orders would alert the nurse to prepare for which of the following?
① Pending abortion
② Ectopic pregnancy
③ Third-trimester bleeding
④ Missed abortion

38. Estriol testing is a urine test taken at certain intervals to determine:
① Fetal age
② Lung surfactant of the fetus
③ Uterine nomenclature
④ Placental functioning

39. A patient is a chain-smoker. The prenatal nurse has taught her the effect of nicotine and hazards of passive smoking. She does not drink, but the nurse has taught her that fetal alcohol syndrome is a major concern today. In addressing the abuse of tobacco, the nurse would stress that it:
① Is a dirty, nasty habit that yellows your teeth, can cause lung cancer, and can offend nonsmokers
② Is becoming socially unacceptable and has widespread negative effects on children as well as grown-ups
③ May cause adverse physiological effects on the fetus
④ Retards fetal growth, constricts blood vessels in the mother, decreases placental function, and may cause premature labor

40. A patient has learned that the placenta is an all-purpose organ that nourishes the fetus, excretes waste materials, and acts as a respiratory organ. She is curious about the role of the umbilical cord. The best explanation should be:
① The cord is the staff of life and is surrounded by Wharton's jelly for protection of its contents
② It contains two veins and an artery that carry the vital life-sustaining products to the fetus
③ The umbilical cord contains the umbilical vein, which supplies oxygen and nutrients to the fetus while two arteries carry away the waste products
④ The oxygen flows from the umbilical vein to the liver through a fetal structure called the ductus venosus; then the arteries go through another fetal structure called the ductus arteriosus into the aorta and eventually back to the umbilical arteries

41. Which of the following statements is correct relative to differences between a stress and a nonstress test?
① A nonstress test is done by abdominal palpation by the physician
② A nonstress test is done early in pregnancy to determine sex of the infant
③ A stress test is usually done late in pregnancy to measure fetal response to uterine contractions
④ A stress test is done after the mother has been given orange juice to drink

42. Mothers are routinely screened during their first prenatal examination for a variety of conditions. One of the most important tests is the alpha-fetoprotein (AFP) test, which:
① Determines fetal maturity
② Detects a neural tube defect such as spina bifida
③ Detects Tay-Sachs disease
④ Detects respiratory distress syndrome (RDS)

43. As a rule, the nurse should schedule the high-risk pregnant mother to be screened for gestational diabetes mellitus (GDM) at:
① 12 weeks' gestation
② 20 to 24 weeks' gestation
③ 32 weeks' gestation
④ 40 weeks' gestation

44. The nurse should explain to the patient that the CST test is an invasive test because medication is given in the veins and it:
① Is uncomfortable for a short while
② Is not painful at all
③ Will take a few minutes to complete
④ Is a routine procedure for all pregnant women

45. Prenatal care is considered the primary means of circumventing complications during pregnancy. Which complication would you consider as most affected by good prenatal care?
① Placenta previa
② Hyperemesis gravidarum
③ Pregnancy-induced hypertension (PIH)
④ Abortion

46. The symptom that is often considered a warning sign of an impending convulsion in the eclamptic mother is:
① Headache
② Severe epigastric pain
③ Scotoma
④ Puffy face

47. A patient in her second pregnancy has occasional traces of albumin in her urine specimen. What should the nurse's assessment of these findings be?
① She is eating a diet high in carbohydrates
② She is showing an indicator of pregnancy-induced hypertension
③ This is probably the result of absorption of lactose from the breasts
④ Because she is a multipara there is more absorption of lactose from the breasts

48. A patient is diagnosed with abruptio placenta. The physician orders fibrinogen levels every 15 minutes. The patient's husband is frightened and asks the nurse why the physician has to withdraw so much blood. The nurse's best response should be:
① "You may ask the physician yourself."
② "Would you like me to inquire for you?"
③ "This test determines the status of the clotting factor."
④ "The physician is determining whether to give her a transfusion or whether to operate."

49. During a nutritional assessment a nurse is concerned when the patient makes which of the following statements?
① "I love vegetables, especially broccoli."
② "Some days I am so busy I eat fast food."
③ "I take a lot of different vitamins."
④ "I hate milk, but I guess I need it for the baby."

50. During a class on fetal development the nurse is asked, "What is the major function of the placenta?" The most appropriate response would be:
① "It passes medications from mother to fetus."
② "It allows the fetus to develop more rapidly."
③ "Nutrients are passed from mother to fetus."
④ "It functions as the kidney and the stomach of the fetus."

51. Which of the following would not be a routine assessment at 10 weeks' gestation?
① Goodell's sign is felt by the examiner
② Complaints of nausea and vomiting
③ Feelings of quickening by the mother
④ Increased feelings of tingling in the breast

52. A nurse is teaching a parent's class. She is asked, "When is it appropriate to give my baby a tub bath?" Which of the following statements by the nurse is the most appropriate response?
① "A sponge bath or a tub bath is fine at any time, as long as you hold him carefully and support his head."
② "A tub bath is fine at any time after the cord falls off, usually in 3 to 5 days."
③ "A tub bath is fine any time after the cord falls off in 10 to 14 days."
④ "A tub bath is fine as soon as he can maintain a sitting position."

53. A nurse is caring for a 26-year-old primigravida. She is 24 weeks' gestation. She has been admitted for observation because of premature labor contractions. The patient states, "I feel a rush of fluid between my legs." Which of the following actions should the nurse perform first?
① Perform a nonstress test to determine viability of infant

② Perform a nitrazine test for ferning.
③ Check fetal heart tones
④ Prepare patient for a vaginal exam

54. A primigravida who is 30 weeks' gestation is admitted to the maternity unit after having been involved in an automobile accident. She is complaining of dull pain in her lower abdomen. Which of the following assessments would be of the most concern to the nurse?
① A fetal heart rate of 140 to 160
② Complaints of irregular contractions relieved by walking
③ Regular contractions occurring at intervals unrelieved by walking
④ Complaints of shortness of breath

55. A prenatal patient who has had diabetes for 2 years is admitted to a maternity unit for hyperglycemia. She is 9 weeks pregnant and she admits to the nurse that she does not always take her diabetes medications. Which of the following would most likely be ordered for this patient?
① Oral hypoglycemics
② Regular insulin to cover elevated blood sugars
③ Oral antibiotics to protect against infection
④ NPH and regular insulin

56. A newly arrived immigrant woman is being seen by the health care provider for the first time. It is determined that she is pregnant with her first child. The health care provider is concerned, however, because she is also complaining of fever, weight loss, night sweats, and a persistent cough. A diagnosis of active TB is made. The most appropriate course of action for this patient at this time should be:
① Begin a drug treatment regimen according to drug susceptibility and patient's response to treatment
② Do nothing until the pregnancy is over because of the risk of injury to the fetus
③ Start with a mild drug and monitor the pregnancy carefully for any signs of complications
④ Monitor the pregnancy carefully and begin treatment in the third trimester after the major fetal structures are complete

57. The patient is 4 weeks pregnant. She is gravida II para I. Her 3-year-old child was born with spina bifida. In addition to regular vitamin supplements, the health care provider prescribes an additional supplement. The nurse should know that this supplement would most likely be:
① Vitamin K
② Thiamine
③ Vitamin E
④ Folic acid

58. A prenatal patient is diagnosed with group B *Streptococcus* infection. The treatment should be:
① Obtain cultures to identify the organism responsible
② Treat with a course of penicillin
③ Wait until labor and then treat with antibiotic
④ Educate the patient on how to prevent future infection

59. Because of her past history of diabetes a patient is classified as a high-risk pregnancy. The health care provider knows that her prenatal visits will be scheduled approximately as follows:
① 2 times a month for the first 28 weeks
② Every 2 weeks after the thirty-eighth week

③ Every week from the thirty-sixth week and after

④ Scheduled on a week-to-week basis

60. A patient in her twentieth week is admitted with hyperemesis gravidarum. The priority nursing intervention should be:

① Providing diversion to decrease pain

② Monitoring accurate intake and output

③ Weighing the patient daily

④ Providing attractive nourishing meals

61. A woman is admitted with a diagnosis of gestational trophoblastic neoplasm. The nursing priority for this patient would be:

① Explanation of the importance of birth control

② Monitoring intravenous fluids

③ Monitoring the need for blood transfusion

④ Referral for counseling to deal with grief

62. A patient who is 30 weeks pregnant is concerned because her hemoglobin level is 11.5g/dl. The nurse explains:

① "This is a concern and needs to be followed closely by the physician."

② "Double the dose of iron for the first trimester."

③ "Circulation increases so it may appear to be decreased but it is actually diluted."

④ "Have your blood work rechecked in a week to see if it continues to drop."

63. A statement that would indicate to the nurse that a teenage mother understands the importance of birth control would be:

① "My boyfriend promises he will use condoms all of the time."

② "I am going to get a shot of Depo-Provera before I leave this hospital."

③ "I am not going to have sex again until I am married."

④ "I am going to have to remember to take a pill every day."

64. A couple is planning to use condoms and spermicide as a method of birth control. Which of the following statements should most concern the nurse?

① "My husband has a history of allergy to latex."

② "Sometimes I have to remember to buy the condoms."

③ "I trust my boyfriend, I know he will remember."

④ "If condoms don't work, I will get a shot of Depo-Provera."

65. Which newborn condition is not considered normal?

① Milia

② Mongolian spots

③ Erb-Duchenne palsy

④ Cephalhematoma

66. A new mother is concerned and asks the nurse why her baby has acne. The first response by the nurse would be:

① "These are called milia and they are caused by hormones transferred at birth."

② "They generally disappear after birth."

③ "If they do not disappear you can take the baby to a dermatologist."

④ "The doctor might want to start her on antibiotics to stop the infection."

67. If a patient is truly overdue, her newborn is at risk for:

① Polydactyly and jaundice

② Desquaminated palms of hands and soles of feet

③ Lanugo and small amounts of ear cartilage

④ Mongolian spots and milia

68. Which of the following should be of most concern to the nurse caring for a newborn?

① A newborn who has not voided in 24 hours

② A newborn whose hands and feet are slightly cyanotic

③ A newborn who passes greenish tarry stool

④ A newborn who seems to sleep all the time

69. At a 2-week newborn exam, which of the following assessments would be of most concern to the nurse?

① The Babinski reflex is present

② A cephalhematoma is present

③ Small red pin dot present in white of sclera

④ The infant is waking up twice a night

70. A staff nurse is concerned that the father of the baby is very quiet and does not seem to want to participate in the baby's care. The first priority in this case should be:

① Make a special effort to cuddle and care for the baby to set an example for the parents

② Insist that the father sit and hold the baby

③ Identify the cultural norms of the couple

④ Refer the couple to Social Services for counseling sessions

71. During a newborn class the mother asks when the "soft spots" on her baby's head will close. The nurse replies:

① "The one on the top will close in 12 to 18 months. The posterior will close in 6 to 8 weeks."

② "The posterior will close in 12 to 18 months and the anterior in 6 to 8 weeks."

③ "The anterior fontanel will close in 4 to 6 weeks and the posterior in 1 year."

④ "You don't have to worry about those spots. They will close."

72. A new mother asks why her baby's breasts are so swollen. The nurse replies:

① "You don't have to do anything; the swelling will disappear."

② "The doctor is aware and he will speak with you about it."

③ "It is normal due to exposure to your hormones during pregnancy."

④ "It is called 'witch's milk' and some babies produce it."

73. Which of the following statements by a new mom would indicate she understands the steps necessary for circumcision care?

① "I need to check and record every time my baby urinates."

② "I need to place petroleum gauze on the penis every time the baby urinates for 3 days."

③ "A small amount of bleeding is normal."

④ "I have to keep the penis exposed to air as much as possible."

74. A new father is concerned because his baby is under a warmer. The nurse explains:

① "This is a normal procedure until his temperature is stable."

② "We are a bit concerned but we are watching his vital signs carefully."

③ "His heat production will be normal in 2 to 3 days."

④ "A newborn loses heat easily."

75. New parents ask why antibiotic ointment is placed in the baby's eyes. The most appropriate response by the nurse is:
① "It is administered to prevent gonorrhea from being transmitted."
② "It is state law."
③ "It is administered to prevent infection."
④ "It prevents blindness caused by infection."

76. The nurse takes an axillary temperature on a 6-hour-old newborn. The most appropriate action for a reading of 96° F should be:
① Place the newborn under the warmer until temperature stabilizes at 97.6° F to 99° F
② Double wrap the infant and place a hat on his head
③ Recheck the temperature in an hour
④ Do nothing; this is a normal reading

77. Which of the following evaluations would be indicative of an infant with respiratory distress syndrome?
① Grunting, rib retraction, and nasal flaring
② Retrolental fibroplasia
③ Breathing with abdominal muscles
④ Breathing irregularly at 38 breaths/minute

78. Signs and symptoms that may indicate a diaphragmatic hernia to the nurse include:
① Bowel sounds heard in chest
② Difficulty feeding
③ Dimple in lower lumbosacral skin
④ Respiratory difficulty

79. Phototherapy may be indicated for a 1-day-old infant
① Born to a drug-addicted mother
② Whose bilirubin is elevated above 12 mg/dl
③ With congestive heart failure
④ Born to a diabetic mother

80. Which of the following assessments would indicate a premature infant?
① Mongolian spots
② Paralysis of lower extremities
③ "Frog-like" position
④ Positive Babinski sign

81. New parents are concerned because the baby's head looks like a "conehead." The best response for the nurse is:
① "Don't worry; it is normal."
② "The odd shape will disappear in a few weeks."
③ "The doctor is aware and will monitor the condition."
④ "It is from the birth process and will disappear in a few days."

82. The parents of a newborn insist on seeing and holding their newborn immediately after birth. The most appropriate action for the nurse is:
① Allow them a quick glance and then place the baby in the warmer
② Wrap the baby in blankets to be certain it is warm and then allow the parents to hold the baby
③ Place the antibiotic ointment in the baby's eyes and then allow the parents to hold the baby
④ Explain to the parents that the baby has to stay in the warmer until the temperature stabilizes

83. Newborn parents are concerned because their baby's eyes seem to be crossed at times. The most appropriate response for the nurse at this time should be:
① "This is normal. Newborns eyes often seem uncoordinated for the first few days."
② "We have called the eye doctor in on consult."

③ "This is often caused by the ointment that we put in their eyes at birth."
④ "New parents worry about everything."

84. Newborn parents are absolutely delighted that their baby is able to grasp their fingers. The most appropriate response for the nurse is:
① "This is a normal reflex and it is fun to be involved with."
② "Your baby is very special. Enjoy him."
③ "It will disappear in 3 to 4 months."
④ "This reflex occurs in only about 50% of all newborns."

85. Which of the following evaluations would indicate increased intracranial pressure?
① Ruptured small capillaries in eye
② Bulging anterior fontanel
③ Edema under the scalp
④ Difficulty feeding

86. Cocaine is addictive to newborns because of:
① The inability of the newborn's immature liver to excrete the drug rapidly
② The mother's long-term use of drugs before conception
③ The mother's ingestion of several different drugs is doubly addictive to the newborn
④ The mother's impaired uterine growth, resulting in the newborn having respiratory distress syndrome (RDS) after birth

87. There are identical twins and fraternal twins. How would you distinguish the kind of twins a patient has if she delivered a boy and a girl?
① Monozygotic or single-ovum twins: union of one sperm and one ovum, divides during mitosis into two embryos; one placenta, two amniotic sacs; heredity is a factor
② Dizygotic twins: union of two sperms with two ovas; two amniotic sacs; separate or fused placenta; same or different sex
③ They look exactly alike even though they are of a different sex; blood tests will reveal if they are identical or fraternal
④ DNA will identify the type of twins they are

88. A home health care provider is assessing a newborn who is 36 hours old and was discharged home from the hospital 12 hours ago. Which of the following should be of concern to the nurse?
① The infant produces a greenish, tarry stool
② A positive Babinski reflex is elicited
③ The infant's elbows are fully flexed when lying in a supine position
④ A respiratory rate greater than 70 breaths per minute is counted

89. What Apgar score would be given to a newborn who exhibited the following?
Heart rate—below 100 beats/min
Respiratory effort—weak cry
Muscle tone—some flexion
Reflex response—cough or sneeze
Color—body pink; extremities blue
① 4
② 6
③ 7
④ 8

90. A newborn is diagnosed with pathological jaundice. His sclera is yellow, his bilirubin index is 17, and he is not nursing well. If the newborn's index continues to rise, the nurse should:
   ① Tell the mother the baby will probably need an exchange transfusion and plan a teaching module of pros and cons
   ② Prepare unit for possible exchange transfusion procedure; obtain supplies, review procedure, wait for physician's orders
   ③ Place the baby under phototherapy light for longer periods of time; offer water every 2 hours until jaundice begins to fade
   ④ Suggest that the family all be tested for proper blood type

91. Why does a fetal position of left occiput posterior (LOP) create dystocia and severe back pain?
   ① The baby's face is descending, facing toward the spine
   ② The fetus is descending with its occipital bone against the mother's spine
   ③ The left shoulder is against the mother's spine
   ④ The presenting part is pressing against the symphysis pubis

92. After a precipitous delivery in the emergency room, the responsibilities of the emergency room nurse should include:
   ① Performing an admission assessment and bath
   ② Following hospital protocol for nonsterile births
   ③ Placing a baby in an isolette for observation
   ④ Administering vitamin K to prevent hemorrhage

93. A gravida II para I goes into labor at 24 weeks and gives birth prematurely. Physically the infant's appearance would most closely resemble which of the following descriptions?
   ① 12 inches long, 1½ pounds, covered with vernix caseosa
   ② 19 inches, 7 pounds, small amount of vernix
   ③ 7 inches, 6 ounces, lanugo covered
   ④ 10 inches, 1 pound, covered with vernix

94. Which of the following situations would most likely indicate to the physician the need to augment labor?
   ① Maternal heart condition
   ② Unengaged presenting part
   ③ Primary uterine inertia
   ④ Previous cesarean section

95. A physician has determined that it is necessary to do a forceps delivery. One of the assessments that may have lead to this decision is:
   ① An extended stage two of labor and maternal exhaustion
   ② The existence of cephalopelvic disproportion
   ③ Full dilation and effacement
   ④ Presenting part engaged and below the ischial spines

96. During a vaginal examination the health care provider states that the fetus is engaged. The nurse explains to the patient that this means:
   ① The fetus is at the ischial spines
   ② The fetus is floating high in the perineum
   ③ The presenting part is crowning
   ④ The infant has passed into the pelvic inlet

97. The health care provider is evaluating whether the second stage of labor has begun. The nurse knows that this would be when:
   ① The woman feels the urge to push
   ② The fetus is at +1 station
   ③ The cervix is fully dilated at 10 cm
   ④ The placenta is delivered

98. A woman is admitted with a history of cardiac disease. Which of these special nursing interventions should be indicated in the course of labor?
   ① Use of epidural anesthesia
   ② Checking carefully for signs of cardiac decompensation
   ③ Encourage voiding at regular intervals
   ④ Monitoring the fetal monitor carefully for any abnormalities

99. After the birth of an infant, the physician examines the umbilical cord carefully. The nurse understands that he is checking for the normal pattern, which is:
   ① 2 arteries and 1 vein
   ② 2 veins and 1 artery
   ③ 1 vein and 1 artery
   ④ 2 veins and 2 arteries

100. A patient in labor is experiencing dystocia. One possible cause for this is:
   ① The cervix is just about to reach full dilation
   ② The mother is experiencing extreme fatigue
   ③ Excessive size of the fetus
   ④ Prolapsed cord

101. The fetal monitoring strip should be evaluated and documented on a regular basis. Which of the following monitor patterns should be considered ominous?
   ① Fetal heart rate accelerations
   ② Early decelerations
   ③ Late decelerations
   ④ Isolated variable decelerations

102. The nurse is very careful to evaluate the fundus of the uterus every 15 minutes during the fourth stage of labor. A fundus that indicates a normal finding would be:
   ① Soft to touch, but firms up when massaged
   ② Firm and at the umbilicus
   ③ Firm and deviated to the right
   ④ Soft and deviated to the left

103. While caring for a patient in labor, the nurse observes the umbilical cord protruding from the vagina. After calling the health care provider, the priority nursing intervention would be:
   ① Attempting to reposition the cord in the vagina
   ② Sterile saline compresses to keep cord moist and protected from infection
   ③ Place a pillow under the hips
   ④ Check the fetal heart rate every 5 minutes

104. A doctor has just ruptured the patient's membranes. The primary responsibility of the attending nurse is to:
   ① Clean up after the procedure
   ② Note the time of the procedure, color, odor of fluid and fetal heart tones
   ③ Chart the physician's name and the procedure done, sign her name in full
   ④ Hold patient's hand, reassure her, change the bed

105. The greatest comfort a nurse can give a patient in labor is to assure her that:
    ① Her progress is normal
    ② She will not be left alone
    ③ Her physician is in the building
    ④ She will be able to hold the baby after delivery

106. The labor-room nurse should encourage a patient to void because a full bladder:
    ① During labor may cause postpartum hemorrhage
    ② May cause a rupture of the bladder during descent of the head
    ③ May cause cystitis
    ④ May slow the progress of labor

107. To relieve supine hypotensive syndrome in a patient, the nurse should:
    ① Massage her leg
    ② Instruct her to breathe deeply
    ③ Turn her on left side
    ④ Advise her to walk slowly and carefully

108. Nursing management during the first stage of labor includes which of the following?
    ① Admit patient to labor room, establish rapport, monitor FHT, keep patient and significant others apprised of progress
    ② Monitor FHT, monitor blood pressure (BP) q 15 min, give pushing instructions, maintain patent airway for newborn, follow proper identification routine
    ③ Be sure cord blood specimen is obtained, observe time and delivery of placenta, check perineal area, check fundus, administer oxytocin IV after placenta is delivered; check BP and fundus q 5 min
    ④ Watch for hemorrhaging, check fundus q 15 min, monitor BP q 15 min, offer warm food and fluid, offer bedpan for urination, teach perineal care, transfer patient to postpartum room when condition is stable

109. After the placenta is delivered and episiotomy suturing is completed, the nurse notices that the patient has begun to shiver. What should the nurse suspect as the probable cause of the shivering?
    ① The sudden emptying of the uterine contents, plus the return of the body chemistry and hormones to the prepregnant state, causes a certain shock to the system
    ② Loss of blood, length of labor, and a certain tiredness cause the lowering of the body temperature; the warm blankets will help
    ③ Pitocin is given after the delivery of the placenta and may cause the body to respond by shivering
    ④ The shiver is a normal reaction, because she has been swallowing ice chips and only covered with a thin sheet

110. A couple arrive at the emergency room visibly upset and frightened. She has been in labor for 3 hours and suddenly had a sudden sharp pain that made her gasp for breath. The nurse notices that she is diaphoretic, ashen, cold, and clammy. The nurse also assesses her abdomen to be rigid and boardlike. Judging from the symptoms described, the most likely complication for the nurse to suspect would be:
    ① Low marginal placenta previa
    ② Appendicitis
    ③ Premature separation of the placenta
    ④ Rupture of the uterus

111. A patient is admitted to the maternity care department. The mother-to-be has been having contractions intermittently at 10- to 20-minute intervals for the past 12 hours. The contractions are relieved by ambulation. Her EDC is 2 weeks away. The physician examines her and finds her to be 0 centimeters dilated and just slightly effaced. The nurse should know that these contractions are most likely:
    ① True labor and will progress rapidly
    ② True labor and will progress differently for every woman
    ③ False labor, as they are relieved by activity
    ④ False labor that most likely will change to true labor in 24 hours

112. After a particularly stormy labor, posterior presentation, severe back pains, nausea, and vomiting during transition and difficulty pushing, the patient delivered a 9 lb 14 oz baby boy. The placenta was not yet delivered when suddenly the patient started to hemorrhage profusely from the vaginal orifice. Within minutes the nurse sees blood trickling from the patient's nose and mouth. What can the nurse do to help in alleviating this condition, which the physician has labeled as disseminated intravascular coagulation (DIC)?
    ① Call the laboratory for blood replacement (fresh whole blood) and assist the physician to deliver the placenta as quickly as possible
    ② Prepare for possible blood transfusions, monitor vital signs, and prepare for heparin administration
    ③ Apply fundal pressure to help deliver the placenta stat
    ④ Hold patient's hand and reassure her; use extra blankets to prevent shock

113. A patient is admitted to the emergency department in active labor. She delivers a baby girl spontaneously after one contraction. The nurse is still alone with the patient; her first responsibility is to:
    ① Ascertain whether the fundus is likely to hemorrhage
    ② Establish an airway for the baby by milking the trachea and maintaining the head lower than the body
    ③ Quickly tie and cut the umbilical cord
    ④ Look for the uterus to rise, watch the perineum for a trickle of blood, and deliver the placenta

114. A patient in labor is admitted to the maternity department. The physician's diagnosis is abruptio placenta. Her partner asks why she is so pale and weak when there is no significant bleeding. The nurse's explanation should be:
    ① "The bleeding is all internal; perhaps you should line up some blood donors."
    ② "In this condition, shock is out of proportion to the blood loss, but we are watching her closely and will not leave her bedside."
    ③ "It is a good sign that you cannot see much bleeding."
    ④ "As you can see, we are doing everything to treat the shock. She should be coming out of it soon."

115. As the nurse watches the monitor during an CST procedure on a patient, she notes at least 3 late decelerations during at least 3 contractions. What should the nurse do?
    ① This indicates a positive test; call the midwife or physician immediately
    ② This is not a positive test; wait until the pattern changed

③ Stop the oxytocin (Pitocin) and administer nasal oxygen

④ Prepare her for immediate delivery

116. A patient is uncertain whether or not she wishes to breastfeed her newborn. Which of these statements should the nurse make to assist the patient in making a choice?
① "Breastfeeding is the absolute best!!! There is nothing healthier for the baby."
② "Ask your mother. She will help you decide what is best."
③ "Let's discuss your questions and concerns about breast-feeding."
④ "Whatever choice you make, the important thing is that the baby gets enough to eat."

117. A patient delivered a macrosomic infant, which means the infant is:
① Small for gestational age (SGA)
② Large, weighing more than 4000 g
③ Covered with newborn milia, which will disappear without treatment
④ Definitely diabetic and will be insulin dependent

118. Magnesium sulfate is used for preeclampsia and should not be given if:
① BP is elevated
② DTRs are absent
③ DTRs are brisk
④ Albumin is 3$^+$

119. A nurse on a postpartum unit has just completed a parents' class for six couples. Which of the following statements should indicate to the nurse that at least one of the partners has understood bath safety as a major concept of the class?
① "This is a lot of work; my partner is going to have to be very organized."
② "Having a schedule everyday is extremely important, so that we can keep our life organized."
③ "My wife is breastfeeding, so this is something that I can do to help."
④ "Staying with the baby and maintaining safety precautions is a top priority."

120. A patient whose last menstrual period began on May 18 should have an estimated date of confinement (EDC) of:
① February 9
② February 11
③ February 18
④ February 25

121. Postpartum teaching of a gestational diabetic should include which of the following?
① Her elevated blood glucose levels should disappear in about 6 weeks
② She must be careful because she may become insulin dependent
③ She should try not to gain over 25 lb
④ She should have her glucose level checked for 5 years

122. A patient admitted with abruptio placenta delivers a healthy baby girl via cesarean. After the delivery the physician examines the placenta very thoroughly. Why?
① The placenta will reveal a tear where any separation might have occurred
② The placenta will clearly show calcified areas that caused the problem
③ A placenta that is heavier than normal may indicate additional abnormalities
④ The location of the tear in the placenta will affect the course of treatment

123. After reviewing prenatal care with a patient the nurse should instruct the patient to notify the physician immediately if she experiences:
① Abdominal pain, bright red bleeding, chills, and fever
② Blood-streaked mucus, Braxton-Hicks contractions
③ Constipation, urgency, hemorrhoids
④ Quickening, varicosities, and discomfort

124. The patient is a primipara. She has passed her due date by 2 weeks. She is apprehensive and does not know why she was instructed to come in for a nonstress test. She appears confused and bewildered. How can the nurse help her?
① To ease her distress the nurse could engage her in trivial conversation regarding the weather, current styles, and so forth
② Explain that she will be placed on a monitor for 20 minutes to an hour to see if her baby responds to her drinking juice or to gentle external pressure by the nurse on her abdomen. The procedure is called a nonstress test
③ Tell the patient she may have to have a nonstress test at a later date but that it is invasive
④ Tell the patient that many people are often past due, and she probably miscalculated her dates

125. The physician arrives after a precipitous delivery. He examines the baby, then examines the mother. He has her wheeled into a delivery room, where he delivers the secundines intact. He reexamines the mother internally, orders oxytocin (pitocin) IV and starts an IV with a piggyback of an antibiotic. Because the patient had a precipitous delivery, a nursing responsibility should be to:
① Watch for infiltration of the IV and observe for antibiotic reaction
② Watch for excessive bleeding or signs of hemorrhage
③ Anticipate the patient's legs shaking and chills
④ Watch for sudden elevation of temperature as a forerunner of an infection or infectious process

126. The patient who is in her third trimester of pregnancy suddenly notices that she is bleeding. At first the bleeding was scanty but has become heavier. She reports she has no pain. A nurse should suspect:
① Abruptio placentae
② Placenta previa
③ Ruptured uterus
④ Vasa previa

127. In looking over a patient's chart a nurse sees that her hemoglobin is 9.5 g/dl. The patient is 32 weeks' gestation. What does this mean to the nurse?
① That the patient is anemic and needs treatment stat
② That this is probably resulting from increased blood volume of pregnancy
③ That this must be her baseline
④ That Z-track iron should be administered to this patient

128. A patient is admitted to the labor and delivery room with a diagnosis of abruptio placenta. The nurse caring for the patient should expect to prepare equipment for a:
① Cesarean section
② Natural vaginal delivery
③ Double set up
④ Precipitate delivery

129. A patient who is 38 weeks pregnant is admitted to the maternity ward complaining of headaches and "blind spots" for about a week. She complained of upper abdominal pain in the AM. Emergency services brought her to the hospital immediately.

Admitting record:
BP 140/112
Albumin 4+
FHT 140 strong
Cervix effaced, dilated 3 cm
Presenting part; station 0
Membranes intact

The admitting nurse, knowing the situation, would place her in:
① A semiprivate room with plenty of sunlight and air
② A semiprivate room, darkened and quiet; restricted visitors
③ A single, darkened room; no visitors, close to nurses' station
④ Single room, plenty of sunlight; no visitors, away from the nurses' station

130. A patient who is 2 months pregnant asks the nurse if it is all right to exercise during pregnancy. The nurse's most appropriate answer should be:
① "It depends on your previous exercise patterns."
② "Absolutely. It will help you and your baby to feel better."
③ "Do not do any exercise that will jar the baby, such as horseback riding or skydiving."
④ "Make certain that you let your physician know if you experience any pain or discomfort."

131. A patient delivered her first baby, a boy, several hours ago. She has been admitted to her postpartum room in stable condition and is euphoric over her successful implementation of the Lamaze techniques. The nurse finds her uterus firm, slightly above the umbilicus. She has saturated one pad with lochia rubra. Her episiotomy appears clean, but her labia and perineal area are swollen and slightly ecchymotic. The nurse's first priority in nursing care should be to:
① Apply an ice glove to the perineal area
② Massage her uterus so it will go down below the umbilicus
③ Administer a tranquilizer because she is so euphoric
④ Watch for hemorrhage because her lochia is so red

132. A 38-year-old primigravida is scheduled to undergo an amniocentesis. She and her significant other are very apprehensive and ask the nurse to reinforce the explanation that the physician has already given to them. The nurse should explain:
① "It is not my place to explain procedures after the physician has already done so."
② "It is a procedure where a small amount of amniotic fluid is withdrawn from the uterus via a needle inserted in the mother's abdomen."

③ "Would you like me to ask the physician to explain the procedure to you again?"
④ "Don't worry! It is a very short procedure and the risks are minimal."

133. A home care nurse is interviewing and assessing a mother who gave birth 10 days ago. Which of the following items should be reported to the physician?
① A fundus that is not palpable
② Reports by the mother of problems with constipation
③ Reports by the mother of periods when she just cannot stop crying
④ Reports of the mother of dark red lochia with small clots

134. A patient appears to be an impending eclamptic. She has complained of visual disturbance and severe epigastric pain. The nurse should observe her closely for signs of:
① Seizure
② Elevated BP
③ Lowered BP
④ Labor

135. Magnesium sulfate in 100 ml D5W is due to run out in 1 hour. The administration set has 15 gtt/ml. How many drops per minute would you run the IV?
① 15 gtt/min
② 18 gtt/min
③ 25 gtt/min
④ 100 gtt/min

136. Which of the following mothers would receive Rhogam within 72 hours after giving birth?
① An Rh-negative mother giving birth to an Rh-negative child
② An Rh-positive mother giving birth to an Rh-positive child
③ An Rh-negative mother who did not receive Rhogam after a previous miscarriage of a negative fetus
④ An Rh-negative mother giving birth to her first Rh-positive child

137. Which of the following statements is most indicative to the nurse that the mother understands the proper technique for breast-feeding?
① "10 minutes on each side is generally adequate."
② "A strict time schedule is not necessary as long as the baby receives adequate nutrition."
③ "Sometimes the baby has trouble latching on."
④ "The football hold feels the most comfortable for me."

138. A patient is a 2-day postoperative cesarean birth. She is of Asian heritage. Her bowel sounds are positive, so she is advanced to a clear liquid diet. She is refusing to drink any clear liquids except for hot water, hot tea, and a special broth that her mother brings her from home. Which of the following interventions is appropriate for the nurse at this time?
① Insist that the patient consult a dietician for additional clear liquids
② Set the patient up and assist as needed with the clear liquids she will drink
③ Speak with the family about encouraging the patient to drink more of a variety of clear liquids
④ Explain to the patient that hospital clear liquids are healthier

139. For the past 3 days a day-5 postop cesarean patient has been experiencing frequent episodes of diarrhea. She is extremely weak and diaphoretic. She is breast-feeding and bonding well with the baby. For infection control purposes, which of the following interventions would be most appropriate?
    ① Have the patient placed on strict respiratory isolation
    ② Discontinue breast-feeding and have the baby remain in the nursery
    ③ Have the baby remain in the room with the mother and have one nurse care for both
    ④ Contact the physician for blood, sputum, and stool cultures

140. The nurse evaluates when it is appropriate to let a patient out of bed after epidural anesthesia. The most appropriate time should be:
    ① As soon as the catheter is removed from the epidural space
    ② When full sensation has returned to the patient's legs
    ③ When the baby is born and she feels up to it
    ④ After her first meal

141. Although rare, a spinal headache is often treated conservatively. If conservative treatment is not adequate, which of the following interventions may be attempted?
    ① Epidural anesthesia
    ② Transcutaneous electrical nerve stimulation
    ③ A blood patch
    ④ Antibiotics

142. Which finding in a 10-day postpartum patient would indicate that involution is proceeding at a normal rate?
    ① The uterus is firm, midline, and three fingers below the umbilicus
    ② The uterus is firm, deviated to the right, and three fingers below the umbilicus
    ③ The uterus is no longer palpable in the abdominal cavity
    ④ The uterus is firm and at the umbilicus

143. Nursing care for a patient who has a cesarean birth includes all of the following except:
    ① Assessing amount and color of vaginal discharge
    ② Encouraging coughing and deep breathing
    ③ Assessing the episiotomy for intactness
    ④ Checking the color and characteristics of urinary output

144. The nurse will be certain that the patient understands pericare when she:
    ① Verbalizes the proper method
    ② Demonstrates the proper method
    ③ Attends a class for new mothers
    ④ Exhibits no signs and symptoms of infection

145. A mother who is 2 weeks postpartum asks, "How can I be certain that my baby is receiving enough nourishment?" The most appropriate reply by the nurse would be:
    ① "When he falls asleep after nursing, he is satisfied."
    ② "If he nurses at least 10 minutes on each side, he is satisfied."
    ③ "If he urinates 6 to 8 times a day, he is adequately nourished."
    ④ "If he gains weight on a regular basis, he is fine."

146. A new mother asks why it is so important for her to breast-feed her infant. The most appropriate response by the nurse should be:
    ① "Breast-feeding helps your uterus to contract more rapidly."
    ② "The newborn will receive excellent vitamins and minerals."
    ③ "Breast milk provides increased immunity to the newborn."
    ④ "Breast milk is easier for the newborn to digest."

147. Which of the following assessments would be of most concern to the nurse? The patient is a 2-day postpartum mother.
    ① A firm fundus two fingers below the umbilicus
    ② Frequency and burning on urination
    ③ Breasts that are firm and engorged
    ④ Lochia rubra with small clots

148. A patient who is 2 weeks postpartum is admitted to the emergency room. Which of the following evaluations would be indicative of late postpartum hemorrhage?
    ① Boggy uterus, shocklike symptoms
    ② Elevated respirations, back pain
    ③ Intermittent abdominal cramping, elevated blood pressure
    ④ Foul-smelling vaginal drainage, uterus hard to the touch

149. During evaluation of a midline episiotomy, the nurse suspects that the patient may have a hematoma. Which assessment by the nurse might lead to this conclusion?
    ① The patient had a prolonged second stage
    ② The patient is complaining of severe perineal pain
    ③ A blood-filled sac is visible in the vaginal area
    ④ The episiotomy is swollen and slightly reddened

150. A patient is admitted to your med-surg unit after delivering a full-term infant who was stillborn. The husband says to the nurse, "I will see my baby and take care of the arrangements. I don't want anyone to say anything to my wife about what happened." The most appropriate action of the nurse should be to:
    ① Reassure the husband that his wishes will be respected
    ② Explain to the husband that no one will initiate the specific topic with his wife but they will not stop her from talking about it
    ③ Encourage the husband to talk with his wife so that they can support each other through the grieving process
    ④ Explain politely to the husband that his wife is the patient and it is your responsibility to encourage communication in every way possible

ANSWERS AND RATIONALES

1. Knowledge, implementation, safety and infection control (a)
   ❷ Discovered the importance of hand washing.
   ① He published a book on midwifery.
   ③ He discovered *Streptococcus.*
   ④ He introduced the use of forceps in obstetrics.
2. Comprehension, assessment, growth and development (b)
   ❹ Quickening is the first movements of the fetus felt by the mother; this normally occurs at approximately 16 weeks.
   ① If this occurs prematurely in a pregnancy, it is an emergency situation.
   ② This occurs at about 10 weeks but is not used as an indicator for EDD.
   ③ This occurs during the last 2 weeks (earlier for multigravidas) and is not a reliable indicator.
3. Comprehension, assessment, growth and development (b)
   ❷ Most tests are accurate at this time.
   ① It will be accurate; it is not generally necessary to wait that long.
   ③ Urine is used for home pregnancy tests.
   ④ A sterile specimen is not needed.
4. Comprehension, assessment, growth and development (a)
   ❸ The patient has been pregnant twice and has one child.
   ① This means pregnant once, one child.
   ② This means pregnant twice, two children.
   ④ This means twice pregnant, no children.
5. Knowledge, assessment, growth and development (a)
   ❷ This is the first sign that will usually cause a woman to seek medical attention.
   ① This is a probable sign at about the sixth week.
   ③ There is debate about whether this is presumptive or probable; it occurs late in first trimester.
   ④ This is a probable sign.
6. Comprehension, assessment, growth and development (a)
   ❷ This is the correct time.
   ① This is too early.
   ③, ④ At this point the heart rate should be audible with a fetoscope.
7. Knowledge, implementation, growth and development (a)
   ❸ These are the correct instructions.
   ① This is acceptable for a routine urinalysis.
   ② Pregnancy tests do not require a sterile specimen.
   ④ This is untrue.
8. Knowledge, assessment, growth and development (a)
   ❸ This is the correct answer. Without this, the embryo and fetus could not survive; this hormone changes the walls of the endometrium to prepare to accept a fertilized ovum.
   ① Estrogen stimulates endometrium to thicken; a "preparation" hormone to thicken uterine lining.
   ② Luteinizing hormone controls ovarian function.

④ This is secreted by the fertilized ovum and helps the corpus luteum to produce progesterone for the first trimester; this hormone affects pregnancy testing, and without it there would be no positive test results.
9. Application, planning, growth and development (b)
   ❸ Further information is required; how long a woman works depends on the degree and type of activities required by her job.
   ① This is not necessarily true.
   ② This is true, but more information is required to give advice.
   ④ This is not necessarily true.
10. Application, evaluation, coping and adaptation (b)
    ❷ An 8-year-old is capable of helping with the baby under supervision.
    ① The fact that it is said does not mean it will be reality.
    ③ This is also normal; however, circumstances may or may not allow it in the immediate future.
    ④ 3-year-olds do not like to share toys or their mom and dad.
11. Application, evaluation, physiological adaptation (c)
    ❸ The first cesarean was caused by a breech; chances are not likely that this would be repeated.
    ① PIH is an ongoing condition and is likely to be present in the second pregnancy.
    ② This would not preclude a VBAC.
    ④ This would probably preclude a VBAC because these moms tend to have larger babies and are classified as high risk.
12. Knowledge, assessment, prevention and early detection of disease (a)
    ❷ German measles have a devastating effect on fetal growth: physical abnormalities, mental retardation, hearing impairment or deafness, blindness.
    ① Chickenpox may have a more severe action on the mother, but will not cause fetal physiological defects or problems.
    ③ This is a synonym for chickenpox.
    ④ This is regular measles; it does not affect the unborn.
13. Comprehension, implementation, basic care and comfort (a)
    ❷ Being educated and knowing different techniques available is the priority.
    ① This method is one of many available.
    ③ It is not necessary to adhere to one method.
    ④ This is a fictitious method; it is a presumptive sign of pregnancy.
14. Application, planning, growth and development (b)
    ❷ This is the correct length of time.
    ① The first 2 weeks are the ovum stage.
    ③ This is too soon.
    ④ This occurs 8 to 11 weeks with a Doppler.
15. Application, planning, growth and development (b)
    ❹ This is the correct definition.
    ① This is too soon; at this stage it is called a blastoderm.
    ② This is too soon; this is called a morula.
    ③ This is too late; at this point it is an embryo.
16. Knowledge, planning, growth and development (a)
    ❷ This is the correct answer.
    ① This is too long.
    ③ This is called fertilization.
    ④ This is the incorrect definition.

17. Knowledge, planning, growth and development (b)
❶ This is the correct path.
② There are differences.
③ The chambers are developed before birth.
④ Blood goes to the aorta.

18. Knowledge, planning, growth and development (a)
❸ This is the correct answer.
① The ovum carries two X chromosomes.
② This is not true.
④ This is true; it does not answer the question.

19. Knowledge, planning, growth and development (b)
❷ Increased thyroid hormones cause an increase in BMR.
① This is true but is not specific enough.
③ This is true; however, it does not respond to the question.
④ Increased caloric energy is needed, but this is not the cause for the increased BMR.

20. Application, evaluation, coping and adaptation (b)
❷ This shows more reality in her planning.
① This is fine, but the baby is still her responsibility.
③, ④ This is fine; however, it does not show the acceptance of responsibility.

21. Application, planning, prevention and early detection of disease (a)
❶ Smoking causes vasoconstriction and decreased oxygenation.
② Women who smoke actually tend to have smaller babies.
③, ④ There is no documented connection.

22. Knowledge, planning, growth and development (a)
❷ An inherited neurodegenerative disease of lipid metabolism.
① This is an anemia more common in African-Americans.
③ This is an anemia common in people from the Mediterranean area.
④ This is more common in Caucasians, a disorder of fat metabolism.

23. Application, planning, coping and adaptation (b)
❶ In the first trimester the mother generally thinks more about herself and how the pregnancy will affect her life.
② This is fine, but it does not answer her concerns.
③ This is judgmental and does not offer therapeutic communication.
④ This is what is hoped for; however, it is not guaranteed.

24. Comprehension, assessment, prevention and early detection of disease
❶ Albumin is a protein; protein in the urine is a possible sign of PIH.
② Frequency or burning would be a sign of cystitis.
③ Glucose is the urine would be a sign of diabetes.
④ This is not an indication of heart disease.

25. Knowledge, assessment, growth and development (a)
❸ This is the correct definition.
① This is the linea nigra.
② This is cholasma, sometimes called "the mask of pregnancy."
④ This is a normal change in pregnancy.

26. Application, implementation, growth and development (b)
❷ This is recommended as a preventive measure.
① This is true; however, it does not answer the question.
③ This may be ordered if there is evidence of infection.
④ This is not a factual statement.

27. Application, assessment, coordinated care (b)
❷ Women who may be classified as high risk should not generally be attended by a midwife.
①, ③ These are fine questions that can be asked later.
④ Midwives are required to attend colleges and receive advanced degrees, although questions about experience would be in order.

28. Application, assessment, prevention and early detection of disease (a)
❹ This answers the question in the least alarming way with accurate information.
①, ② Size of the woman has nothing to do with pelvic measurements.
③ This is not the "true" type of the female pelvis.

29. Application, implementation, basic care and comfort (a)
❸ This helps to relieve muscle cramping.
① This promotes circulation and helps to prevent thrombophlebitis.
② This relieves urinary incontinence.
④ This prevents anemia.

30. Application, implementation, basic care and comfort (b)
❸ This is the correct use of Kegel exercises.
① They are not dangerous to the heart.
② This is not a correct statement.
④ ROM exercises will help with leg cramps.

31. Application, planning, basic care and comfort (b)
❸ This is a factual statement.
① This is incorrect information.
② Pregnant women should not douche unless ordered by a physician.
④ This is not a factual statement.

32. Knowledge, assessment, growth and development (b)
❶ The heart begins beating during embryonic period.
② This is incorrect.
③ This is the third month; heart and cardiovascular system would have been working long before.
④ Placenta begins to form shortly after implantation and continues to form for 16 to 20 weeks into gestation, so this answer is wrong.

33. Application, implementation, basic care and comfort (b)
❸ This is the best answer.
① These relieve perineal discomfort.
② These provide temporary relief at best.
④ This is improper advice.

34. Application, planning, basic care and comfort (b)
❶ The growing uterus leaves less space for the stomach and therefore food will sometimes remain there longer.
② This does not cause heartburn; it is sometimes recommended to decrease symptoms.
③ This does not cause heartburn.
④ These symptoms are not common in this trimester and if they are present may be an indication of hyperemesis gravidarum.

35. Application, implementation, basic care and comfort (b)
    ❸ This is correct information and advice; decreased use of carbonated beverage will also assist in decreasing phosphorus.
    ① This does not alleviate leg cramps.
    ② This is for relief from the discomfort of varicose veins.
    ④ This is not incorrect but not best answer.

36. Comprehension, implementation, physiological adaptation (c)
    ❹ Within 72 hours, danger of seizure passes.
    ①, ② Danger of seizure lasts longer; normal recovery may be 1 to 2 hours or more.
    ③ Danger of seizure lasts longer than 24 hours.

37. Knowledge, planning, physiological adaptation (c)
    ❸ Third-trimester bleeding conditions, particularly because physician orders include no vaginal/rectal examinations.
    ① The bleeding, pain, or contractions would not be as acute.
    ② The pregnancy in itself would not necessitate these nursing measures unless the mother had symptoms.
    ④ This is fetal death without expulsion of products of conception; symptoms include slight bleeding, brownish discharge, no cramping; treatment is D&C.

38. Comprehension, planning, prevention and early detection of disease (b)
    ❹ Usually estriol levels are tested for placental functioning in the third trimester; a level of 12 mg is good, but below 12 mg in 24 hours may place the fetus in jeopardy.
    ① Fetal age is determined by uterine height, calculation of EDC.
    ② Amniocentesis procedure may reveal surfactant lecithin/sphingomyelin ratio and help determine lung maturity.
    ③ Human gonadotropin hormonal levels in the urine are tested early on in pregnancy, but the words *uterine nomenclature* are not related to the question.

39. Application, planning, psychosocial adaptation (b)
    ❹ This is the correct answer.
    ① This is all true, but not a good answer to a pregnant mother.
    ② This is also true but is not the best answer.
    ③ This is too vague; it is not the best answer.

40. Knowledge, planning, growth and development (a)
    ❸ This is the correct and direct answer to the patient's question.
    ① This is a correct statement but is irrelevant to the question.
    ② This is incorrect information.
    ④ This is wrong; this is a partial explanation of fetal circulation.

41. Comprehension, planning, growth and development (a)
    ❸ This is the correct answer.
    ① This is ballottement or locating of fetal parts; it is not a part of a nonstress test.
    ② Sex of an infant may be seen on a screen during a sonogram, but not by a fetal monitoring device, which only measures fetal heart tones—strength of contractions and fetal movements through the FHT response.

④ This is wrong; the mother is given orange juice for a nonstress test; for the stress test she is given oxytocin intravenously.

42. Comprehension, planning, prevention and early detection of disease (a)
    ❷ This is the correct answer; elevated levels of AFP indicate up to 5% to 10% of a neural defect, but must be followed by two consecutive AFP tests, ultrasound readings, and an amniocentesis.
    ① Fetal maturity is tested by an L/S ratio that determines lung maturity by measuring the ratio of the two components of surfactant (lecithin and sphingomyelin); an amniocentesis done after the 35th week of pregnancy should show an increase in the amount of lecithin and a decrease in sphingomyelin.
    ③ Genetic work-up, including family history and a series of blood tests, can evaluate risk of disease in offspring.
    ④ Respiratory distress syndrome is most likely to occur in low–birth-weight babies, premature babies, or babies known to be at risk for immature lung development following delivery.

43. Comprehension, planning, physiological adaptation (a)
    ❶ This is the correct answer; the sooner the mother is seen and evaluated, the better.
    ② If the opportunity to see the high-risk mother was not before this time (20 to 24 weeks' gestation), by all means see her. It is never too late.
    ③ Although scheduled evaluation should be even before, it is never too late to schedule continuing evaluations.
    ④ Evaluation scheduling should have been started as early as possible and continue at appropriate times throughout pregnancy.

44. Comprehension, planning, prevention and early detection of disease (c)
    ❶ This provides reassurance and explanation.
    ② Levels of perception of pain differ, so do not promise there will be "no pain."
    ③ This test takes from 20 minutes to over an hour.
    ④ This is untrue; most women will never need this test.

45. Comprehension, assessment, prevention and early detection of disease (b)
    ❸ This is the correct answer; early, frequent, and continual testing of urine and blood pressure would signal early signs that could be addressed rapidly and appropriately.
    ① This is usually a third-trimester complication and would not be considered a preventable condition.
    ② This is not exactly preventable but can be helped by easing discomfort, teaching, and advising on care.
    ④ Abortions—spontaneous ones might have some early signs and symptoms that alert pending conditions, but this is not the best answer.

46. Knowledge, assessment, physiological adaptation (b)
    ❷ This is the significant symptom of an impending convulsion.
    ① This is a sign of change in blood pressure, preeclampsia.
    ③ Eye changes would not be noticed by the mother.
    ④ This is not necessarily a sign of impending convulsions; rather of fluid retention.

47. Comprehension, assessment, prevention and early detection of disease (a)
   ❷ This is an indicator of possible pregnancy-induced hypertension
   ① Albumin is a protein; it may indicate kidney damage.
   ③, ④ Albumin is not an indicator of either of these conditions.

48. Application, planning, coping and adaptation (c)
   ❸ The nurse is explaining procedure and giving reassurance.
   ① This response is rude, curt, and did not answer the question.
   ② The physician was in the room, but he asked the nurse.
   ④ This answer creates unnecessary anxiety with no explanation.

49. Application, assessment, basic care and comfort (b)
   ❸ Megadoses of vitamins can be teratogenic.
   ① This is OK as long as the diet is balanced.
   ② This is OK as long as healthy choices can be made.
   ④ Alternatives can be offered for milk.

50. Application, planning, growth and development (a)
   ❸ This answers the question most accurately.
   ① Certain medications are passed to the fetus; however, this is not a function.
   ② This is not true.
   ④ This is not true.

51. Knowledge, assessment, growth and development (a)
   ❸ Fetal movement is normally felt at about 16 weeks.
   ① The cervix thickens and softens; this is normally felt by 6 weeks.
   ② This is normal during the first trimester.
   ④ This is normal.

52. Application, planning, growth and development (a)
   ❸ This is correct and the cord generally does fall off in between 10 to 14 days.
   ① Babies should always be held carefully with the head supported.
   ② This is partially correct, but the cord does not fall off in 3 to 5 days.
   ④ This is not a requirement for a tub bath.

53. Comprehension, assessment, prevention and early detection of disease (b)
   ❸ The physician or nurse midwife will want to know the status of the fetus. This is an emergency situation and the health care provider must be notified to prepare for a possible premature delivery.
   ① Test is not indicated at this point; it may have been done prior to this.
   ② This would be done second.
   ④ This is not indicated and could be dangerous at this time.

54. Application, assessment, prevention and early detection of disease (b)
   ❸ This is one sign of true labor.
   ① This is a normal range for a fetal heart rate.
   ② Contractions relieved by walking are Braxton-Hicks contractions.
   ④ This is normal in the beginning of the third trimester, caused by a growing baby putting pressure on the diaphragm.

55. Comprehension, planning, prevention and early detection of disease (b)
   ❹ A combination of types of insulin with different durations allows for a steadier therapeutic level of insulin in the body.
   ① Oral hypoglycemics are contraindicated during pregnancy, because their effect on the fetus is uncertain.
   ② Regular insulin is short acting and therefore would not act on a long-term basis.
   ③ There is no mention of infection in the question.

56. Application, implementation, physiological adaptation (b)
   ❶ A pregnant woman with active disease needs effective treatment to protect herself and her unborn fetus.
   ② Preventive therapy can be postponed until after pregnancy; the risks of doing nothing in active disease are too great.
   ③ Treatment for active disease includes a minimum of two to three drugs.
   ④ Risk to the mother and fetus is too great to wait until the third trimester.

57. Application, implementation, basic care and comfort (b)
   ❹ Folic acid has been shown to be a benefit in preventing neurological conditions.
   ① This is given to newborns to prevent hemorrhaging.
   ② A B-complex vitamin involved in carbohydrate metabolism.
   ③ This is useful in preventing certain forms of anemia in newborns.

58. Comprehension, implementation, physiological adaptation (b)
   ❷ Treatment prior to birth of the infant is preferred; it decreases the chance of the infant's exposure to the organism.
   ① This has already been done.
   ③ This is an option for high-risk women; however, treatment should not wait if a diagnosis has been made.
   ④ This is also important; treatment takes priority.

59. Comprehension, planning, physiological adaptation (b)
   ❹ It will be necessary to evaluate each pregnancy individually.
   ① This would be possible but not guaranteed.
   ② There are only approximately 40 weeks in a pregnancy.
   ③ A high-risk pregnancy would generally start weekly visits sooner.

60. Application, implementation, basic care and comfort (b)
   ❷ Monitoring intravenous and urinary output is the priority.
   ① Patients need quiet; there is not usually pain.
   ③ A baseline is important, but this is not a priority.
   ④ Small meals may be provided after the intestinal tract has had the opportunity to rest.

61. Application, implementation, physiological adaptation (c)
   ❸ Patients with this diagnosis frequently lose a great deal of blood.
   ① This is important and should be handled when the patient is physically stable.
   ② This should be done with all patients.
   ④ This is absolutely appropriate and can be dealt with after the patient is stable.

62. Application, evaluation, physiological adaptation (b)
    ❸ A slight drop in HgB is not unusual; solid particles seem less in an increased cardiac output.
    ① This statement causes undue anxiety; the physician is always responsible for monitoring bloodwork.
    ②, ④ These are not indicated and not within the scope of nursing practice.

63. Application, evaluation, growth and development (b)
    ❷ This is the best method that does not require any further effort for 3 months.
    ① This is a fine statement, but it puts the responsibility on someone else to follow through.
    ③ This is also fine; however, it may be easier said than done.
    ④ It is not a good sign if remembering to take a pill is seen as a burden.

64. Application, evaluation, prevention and early detection of disease (a)
    ❶ Many condoms are made of latex and could pose a problem for the couple.
    ② This will work only as long as somebody remembers.
    ③ This is fine, as long as he does remember.
    ④ This is good as long as she realizes before she gets pregnant.

65. Comprehension, evaluation, growth and development (a)
    ❸ Birth injury occurs when the upper arm has been injured in such a way that the nerves of the brachial plexus are severed or injured, resulting in a paralysis.
    ① These are small, white sebacious glands found in the chin, forehead, nose, cheek, and upper lip.
    ② These are dark pigmented areas on the lower back and buttock.
    ④ This is normal cranial deviation resulting from normal vaginal delivery; these conditions occur as the caput descends through the birth canal.

66. Application, evaluation, growth and development (b)
    ❶ This is factual.
    ② This is true; however, it does not totally answer the question.
    ③ This is an unnecessary action.
    ④ Infection is not a cause.

67. Knowledge, planning, growth and development (a)
    ❷ Post-term infants' skin is very dry and cracked in appearance.
    ① These are genetic anomalies not caused by an overdue date.
    ③ These are characteristics of preterm infants.
    ④ These are normal.

68. Comprehension, assessment, prevention and early detection of disease (b)
    ❶ This is a priority and should be reported to the physician.
    ② This is normal.
    ③ This is normal and called meconium.
    ④ It is not unusual for newborns to sleep many hours.

69. Comprehension, assessment, growth and development (b)
    ❸ This should resolve in 5 days.
    ① This plantar reflex is normal for a year.
    ② This should disappear in 3 to 4 weeks.
    ④ This is normal; sleep patterns vary widely.

70. Application, assessment, coordinated care (b)
    ❸ This may be the way that they were brought up in their culture. The father may be very proud of the infant and shows it privately.
    ① This is fine but further information needs to be gathered first.
    ② This is not appropriate.
    ④ This is very premature until a great deal of further information is gathered.

71. Application, implementation, growth and development (b)
    ❶ This is factual information.
    ② This is the opposite.
    ③ This is not true.
    ④ She did not say she was worried, and this does not completely answer the question.

72. Application, implementation, growth and development (b)
    ❸ This provides accurate information without inducing undue anxiety.
    ① This is true but does not answer the question.
    ② This is not necessary.
    ④ This is also true; however, it does not answer the question.

73. Application, implementation, growth and development (b)
    ❷ This is a generally recommended procedure in most cases, depending on the type of method used.
    ① It is generally necessary to record only the first voiding after the procedure.
    ③ This is true; however, it does not answer the question.
    ④ This is false and may actually increase the child's discomfort.

74. Application, implementation, basic care and comfort (b)
    ❶ This is the correct information.
    ② There is no need for concern, causes undue anxiety.
    ③, ④ These are true; however, they do not answer the question.

75. Application, evaluation, prevention and early detection of disease (a)
    ❸ This is factual without causing undue alarm.
    ① This is true, but it may be insulting.
    ② This is true; however, it does not answer the question.
    ④ This causes undue alarm.

76. Application, implementation, physiological adaptation (b)
    ❶ Cold stress is dangerous for infants; this is the appropriate action.
    ② This can be done after the infant has spent time in the warmer.
    ③ This should also be done after the first two interventions are completed.
    ④ This is incorrect.

77. Application, evaluation, physiological adaptation (b)
    ❶ These are signs of respiratory distress.
    ② This is a possible complication of RDS.
    ③, ④ These are normal characteristics of an infant.

78. Knowledge, evaluation, physiological adaptation (b)
    ❶ These are indicative of diaphragmatic hernia.
    ② This is indicative of a cleft lip or palate
    ③ This is an indication of spina bifida.
    ④ This is not a sign; it may occur if patient chokes while feeding.

79. Comprehension, evaluation, physiological adaptation (b)
    ❷ This is a treatment for an elevated bilirubin caused by Rh or ABO incompatibility.
    ① These infants are extremely irritable and should be placed in a quiet, darkened place.
    ③, ④ This is not an indicated therapy for these conditions.

80. Comprehension, evaluation, growth and development (b)
    ❸ This is a neurological symptom.
    ① These are normal, particularly with darker-skinned infants.
    ② This is called Klumpkes' syndrome, indicative of neurological injury.
    ④ This is normal.

81. Application, evaluation, growth and development (b)
    ❹ This statement gives an explanation and reassurance.
    ① This is true but does not provide information or reassurance.
    ② This is too long, provides incorrect information.
    ③ The doctor is aware; there is no need for monitoring.

82. Application, implementation, coping and adaptation (b)
    ❷ The first hour after birth the baby is very alert and it is an important time to bond; studies have shown that the baby will stay warm in his parent's arms.
    ① This is not sufficient.
    ③ The baby's eyes will be blurry, which may be a hindrance to bonding.
    ④ This is not true.

83. Application, evaluation, growth and development (b)
    ❶ This is correct, reassuring information.
    ② This is not necessary and alarming.
    ③ This is incorrect information.
    ④ This is a demeaning statement.

84. Application, evaluation, growth and development (a)
    ❶ This is factual information and promotes bonding.
    ② This is true for all parents but does not provide information.
    ③ This is true but can be said at a later time.
    ④ This is incorrect information.

85. Application, evaluation, physiological adaptation (c)
    ❷ This is a sign of fluid buildup.
    ① This is normal and resolves without treatment in approximately 5 days, caused by increased intracranial pressure during the birth process.
    ③ This is normal; cephalhematoma disappears without treatment in 3 to 4 days.
    ④ This is a sign of a cleft palate.

86. Comprehension, evaluation, psychosocial adaptation (c)
    ❶ This is the correct answer. Because all newborns have an immature liver, putting a drug into the system jeopardizes the infant.
    ② Prolonged use of a drug by the mother just before conception does not necessarily cause newborn addiction unless the mother continues the habit from conception throughout pregnancy to term.
    ③ This answer in itself is not correct; usage must be continued during pregnancy.
    ④ Drugs may affect uterine growth because the addictive mother seldom has good nutritional habits, but if carried through term, the infant does not necessarily have RDS.

87. Knowledge, assessment, growth and development (b)
    ❷ Because the patient delivered a boy and a girl, they must be fraternal or unidentical; if they had been the same sex, the placenta and sacs would have to be identified.
    ① Monozygotic twins are always the same sex.
    ③ Blood tests are not the *best* answer; a nurse should know the status by identifying the placenta and sacs.
    ④ DNA tests are not the *best* answer; a nurse should know the status by identifying the placenta and sacs.

88. Application, assessment, prevention and early detection of disease (b)
    ❹ This may be a sign of illness.
    ① This is meconium, which is normal stool for about 48 hours.
    ② This is normal for a newborn; in older children and adults it may indicate possible CNS abnormality.
    ③ This is normal for full-term infants.

89. Comprehension, assessment, prevention and early detection of disease (a)
    ❷ This is the correct answer; the Apgar score is 6 (see Fig. 7-9 on p. 410).
    Heart rate = 1
    Respiratory effort = 1
    Muscle tone = 1
    Reflex response = 2
    Color = 1
    ①, ③, ④ These are incorrect.

90. Application, planning, physiological adaptation (a)
    ❷ This is the best response; preparation is started, so if the procedure is ordered, time is not lost.
    ① Responsibility is not assumed until order is given by physician.
    ③ Unless there is a standing order, this would not be appropriate.
    ④ Alarming family without proper teaching or preparation is inadvisable.

91. Knowledge, assessment, growth and development (b)
    ❷ This is the correct answer. The LOP position means the bony back of the head presses against the spine, causing lower back pain because it presents bone against bone. The head must turn until the face is against the spine; this may happen spontaneously or by artificial means (maneuvers by the physician). It is usually a slow and painful process of descent.
    ① This is a more normal descent and does not present itself to dystocia and pain.
    ③ This is almost an impossible vaginal delivery position or lie; most certainly a cesarean section elective.
    ④ This does not describe a presentation.

92. Comprehension, planning, prevention and early detection of disease (b)
    ❷ Normally hospitals have protocols in place that include additional observations for signs of infection.
    ① The maternity nurse can perform this after the baby's temperature has stabilized.
    ③ The baby and the mother are normally not separated and transferred to the maternity department as quickly as possible.
    ④ This can be completed by the maternity nurse at a later point in time.

93. Comprehension, assessment, growth and development (b)
   ❶ This is appropriate for an infant at 24 weeks.
   ② This is appropriate for a full-term infant.
   ③ This is appropriate at 16 weeks.
   ④ This is appropriate at 20 weeks.
94. Knowledge, evaluation, prevention and early detection of disease (b)
   ❸ This is an indication for induction; it is the failure of the uterus to contract effectively from the start.
   ①, ②, ④ These are all contraindications for induction.
95. Comprehension, evaluation, physiological adaptation (b)
   ❶ These are two indications for a forceps delivery.
   ② This is a contraindication; it is an indication for a cesarean.
   ③, ④ These are two of the requirements for application of forceps.
96. Application, implementation, growth and development (b)
   ❹ This is the definition for engagement.
   ① This would be 0 station.
   ② This means that the baby is high in the pelvis.
   ③ This would mean that the presenting part is visible to the health care provider.
97. Knowledge, evaluation, growth and development (a)
   ❸ Stage 2 is from full dilation of the cervix until birth of the fetus.
   ① Pushing before full dilation can be dangerous to the fetus and exhausting to the mother.
   ② This is still too high.
   ④ This is stage 3.
98. Comprehension, implementation, physiological adaptation (c)
   ❷ The heart may be under stress if the rate is above 100.
   ① The use of epidural anesthesia is normal.
   ③ This should be done with all women; a full bladder may impede labor.
   ④ This should be done with all women.
99. Comprehension, evaluation, prevention and early detection of disease (b)
   ❶ This is the normal pattern.
   ②, ③, ④ Any deviations may be indicative of fetal anomalies.
100. Knowledge, evaluation, physiological adaptation (a)
   ❸ This is a problem with the passenger (fetus), which is one of many causes of dystocia.
   ① This is normal as labor progresses.
   ②, ④ These are complications, not causes.
101. Application, evaluation, growth and development (c)
   ❸ A pattern of decelerations late in the contraction may indicate utero-placental insufficiency.
   ① Accelerations typically occur in response to fetal movement, uterine contractions, or maternal abdominal contractions.
   ② This deceleration is generally benign and is a result of fetal head is pressing on the perineum.
   ④ If these are repetitive and worsen as labor progresses, they may be indicative of cord compression.
102. Comprehension, evaluation, growth and development (a)
   ❷ This is a normal finding at the first stage of labor.
   ① It should not be soft; the patient may need Pitocin in her intravenous infusion.

   ③ It should be midline; deviation may mean a full bladder.
   ④ Soft may be an indication of uterine atony and is a cause for hemorrhage.
103. Assessment, implementation, physiological adaptation (c)
   ❸ This would take pressure off fetal head by lifting it off the cord.
   ① Further damage can be caused by trying to reposition cord.
   ② This can be done second.
   ④ This of course should be done and preparations should be made for a cesarean birth.
104. Application, evaluation, basic care and comfort (a)
   ❷ This is correct, a responsible nursing procedure.
   ① This is done as part of the routine responsibility, but #2 is specific to procedure accomplished.
   ③ This is incomplete recording.
   ④ This is part of the routine nursing care and not specific to this question.
105. Knowledge, implementation, basic care and comfort (a)
   ❷ Fear is a major threat to women in labor.
   ① Whatever progress is made, the fear of facing labor alone is worse.
   ③ This statement is of no help if the physician is not beside her.
   ④ It is during labor she needs support.
106. Comprehension, implementation, basic care and comfort (a)
   ❹ As the fetal presenting part descends down the birth canal, a full bladder will create an impediment to descent.
   ①, ②, ③ These are possible but unlikely.
107. Knowledge, implementation, physiological adaptation (b)
   ❸ This is correct, simply relieving pressure by changing positions.
   ① The symptoms are pallor, light-headedness, dizziness, and slight nausea—rubbing the legs does not correct the syndrome.
   ② This is incorrect. It is caused by the heavy uterus exerting pressure on the aorta and hampering good circulation; Determine the cause and effect first, then plan the intervention.
   ④ Know cause and effect; Because the patient is dizzy, the nurse would not recommend walking.
108. Comprehension, planning, growth and development (a)
   ❶ This is the correct answer.
   ② These are nursing responsibilities for the second stage of labor.
   ③ These are major nursing interventions for the third stage of labor.
   ④ These are nursing care measures for the fourth stage of labor, or 1 hour after delivery, usually in the recovery room.
109. Knowledge, planning, physiological adaptation (b)
   ❶ This is the correct answer.
   ② This does not explain the physiological dynamics.
   ③ Pitocin is an oxytocic acting on the uterus.
   ④ This does not explain the physiological dynamics of immediate postpartum phenomenon.
110. Comprehension, assessment, physiological adaptation (a)
   ❸ Symptoms are indicative of abruptio placentae.
   ① This would give rise to painless bleeding.

② Onset is gradual, accompanied by nausea, possibly vomiting, and gradual shock; abdomen is tender but not boardlike.

④ This would not cause a rigid, boardlike abdomen.

111. Knowledge, assessment, growth and development (a)
   ❸ False labor is generally relieved by activity.
   ① True labor will have a regular interval between contractions and progress is shown in effacement and dilation of cervix.
   ② True labor does progress differently; however, this is not true labor.
   ④ There is no way to determine when true labor will occur after an episode of false labor.

112. Comprehension, planning, physiological adaptation (b)
   ❷ Interpreting what is happening to the patient, the best assistance would be to prepare for medical interventions and anticipate what nursing actions to implement.
   ① The nurse will anticipate this, but will have the necessary equipment ready.
   ③ The nurse would not intervene unless requested to do so by the physician.
   ④ With massive bleeding, the patient is probably in shock and needs nursing and medical intervention stat.

113. Comprehension, implementation, growth and development (b)
   ❷ First priority is to establish patent airway so that baby can breathe, cry, and fill her lungs with oxygen.
   ① This is not first priority.
   ③ Umbilical cord can be left attached; there is no danger in delaying the cutting of the cord while tasks with a higher priority are performed.
   ④ The delivery of the placenta may take anywhere from 5 to 20 minutes, because it must separate from the walls of the uterus; therefore this is not top priority.

114. Comprehension, implementation, physiological adaptation (a)
   ❷ This explanation attempts to teach, reassure, and describe condition.
   ① This is an alarming, senseless, and incorrect response; insensitive as well.
   ③ This is an inappropriate, incorrect answer.
   ④ This does not reassure or answer the partner's concern.

115. Comprehension, implementation, prevention and early detection of disease (b)
   ❶ This analysis and plan of action is correct.
   ② It is a positive test for trouble, and waiting for the pattern to change may compromise the fetus.
   ③ The nurse may proceed to this together with the head nurse.
   ④ There is nothing in this situation that indicates an imminent delivery.

116. Application, implementation, coping and adaptation (b)
   ❸ This is factual information; allows communication to be open.
   ① This is factual information; however, it does not allow patient to express concerns.
   ② Mothers may have definite feelings, which may or may not be backed up with facts.
   ④ Breast-feeding has advantages for mother and baby.

117. Knowledge, evaluation, growth and development (b)
   ❷ This is the correct answer by definition, usually born of mothers with diabetes.
   ① *Macro* is large; *micro* is small.
   ③ Milia are small white visible papules on the face of the newborn and have nothing to do with infant size.
   ④ Large babies are screened and tested for diabetes, but this does not necessarily mean that they are or will become insulin-dependent diabetics.

118. Comprehension, evaluation, physiological adaptation (b)
   ❷ DTRs are absent; respiratory effort may quickly be impaired.
   ① BP is not affected by the drug; as a result of CNS depression, BP will decrease.
   ③ It is being given to decrease the DTRs.
   ④ Proteinuria ($+1$ to $+2$) is a classic sign of preeclampsia; proteinuria ($3+$) is extremely high, which may indicate use of medication in a closely monitored setting.

119. Application, evaluation, growth and development (a)
   ❹ Never leaving the baby alone is essential to prevent injuries.
   ① Organization is important; both partners are capable of providing the newborn with a bath.
   ② A schedule is not needed; infants can be bathed any time day or night. Infants do not necessarily need a bath every day, but their face and perineal area have to be washed every day.
   ③ This is true; however, it is not the most important thing that is ascertained from a class.

120. Comprehension, planning, growth and development (a)
   ❹ According to Nägele's formula this is correct.
   ①, ②, ③ These are wrong according to Nägele's formula.

121. Knowledge, planning, growth and development (b)
   ❶ This is the correct answer: most patients with pregnancy-induced diabetes or gestational diabetes mellitus (GDM) will return to normal by the 6-week checkup with the obstetrician.
   ② This is not a good statement for health teaching; this is a scare tactic and not accurate. Some studies indicate that women who have successive large babies, and gain considerable weight, or are grossly overweight-before and after pregnancy, may experience some problems, but good follow-up teaching with emphasis on weight and nutritional care should help in maintaining sugar-free urine, etc.
   ③ There is no indication that a blanket number ensures against diabetes; there is considerable evidence to support the claim that excess weight is detrimental to health.
   ④ This is not necessary; see rationale for #1.

122. Comprehension, assessment, prevention and early detection of disease (b)
   ❶ This is a true statement; physician and nurse should check to determine location of tear.
   ② Calcification indicates age, not a tear.
   ③, ④ These statements are not true; the postpartum treatment is the same regardless of the location of the tear or the weight of the placenta; there is no research that indicates the weight of the placenta is of any significance.

123. Comprehension, planning, prevention and early detection of disease (a)
    ❶ These are reportable signs and symptoms that should be taught to the patient.
    ② These are usual signs and symptoms and are normal.
    ③ These are nonemergency signs and symptoms, which can be addressed during regular visits.
    ④ These are later signs and symptoms; nonemergency.

124. Comprehension, assessment, coping and adaptation (b)
    ❷ Explain procedure. Nonstress tests are done to see how the uterus is adapting to the fetal environment.
    ① She wants to know what is going to happen to her, nothing else.
    ③ This is an unnecessary anxiety-causing statement, irrelevant at this time.
    ④ This is not a comforting statement; implies stupidity.

125. Comprehension, assessment, physiological adaptation (b)
    ❷ The suddenness of precipitous delivery always predisposes the patient to possible hemorrhage.
    ① This is not top priority; usual checking of IV and administration of any drug.
    ③ Many women experience this after delivery.
    ④ Precipitous delivery does not of itself cause massive infection.

126. Knowledge, assessment, physiological adaptation (c)
    ❷ This is the correct answer; signs and symptoms are bright red clots first, then light, painless bleeding.
    ① In abruptio placentae, there is pain, and there may or may not be bleeding; if there is bleeding, it is dark red and usually not clotted.
    ③ Bleeding would be bright red in variable amounts with pain.
    ④ The patient would experience painless vaginal bleeding with bloody amniotic fluid.

127. Comprehension, assessment, physiological adaptation (b)
    ❷ This is the correct statement and correct answer.
    ① The nurse would consider doing follow-up tests to determine precise findings, and the physician would consider what medical treatment is needed.
    ③ This is a false assumption.
    ④ It is not a part of the nursing process to make this kind of determination.

128. Comprehension, implementation, physiological adaptation (b)
    ❸ In abruptio placentae this is standard practice.
    ① If bleeding subsides or stops, vaginal delivery is preferable.
    ② Should bleeding continue, a vaginal delivery places both mother and fetus in jeopardy.
    ④ This is unlikely; emergency delivery tray items are limited.

129. Comprehension, implementation, physiological adaptation (a)
    ❸ Prevent convulsions; be able to respond stat.
    ① A severely eclamptic mother should not be in a semiprivate room, and certainly not in a sunny room with visitors.
    ② The room must be quiet with absolutely no visitors.
    ④ Bright sunshine will aggravate the central nervous system, and being far from the nurses' station will hamper emergency nursing care.

130. Application, implementation, basic care and comfort (b)
    ❶ Exercise is generally safe in pregnancy if the woman has exercised previously; otherwise it may be necessary to begin slowly.
    ②, ③ These are true, however; they do not completely answer the question.
    ④ A physician should be consulted before starting exercise. A patient should not wait until pain is experienced.

131. Application, implementation, basic care and comfort (a)
    ❶ This will reduce perineal swelling and edema.
    ② This is the normal location of the fundus a few hours after delivery.
    ③ Natural reaction is to be happy over an apparently successful birthing experience.
    ④ One pad saturated with red lochia several hours after delivery is normal and not a sign of hemorrhage.

132. Application, implementation, prevention and early detection of disease (a)
    ❷ This statement gives correct information without raising unnecessary alarm.
    ① It is within the scope of nursing practice to reinforce explanations of diagnostic procedures.
    ③ This is not what they asked the nurse; if they want information from the physician they should be encouraged to ask the physician themselves.
    ④ This does not answer the question and raises unnecessary alarm.

133. Application, implementation, physiological adaptation (b)
    ❹ Return of lochia rubra after its initial cessation may be indicative of uterine subinvolution or hemorrhage.
    ① At 10 days postpartum the fundus has returned to its position as a pelvic organ and is no longer palpable.
    ② Mothers commonly experience constipation; simple interventions can be suggested.
    ③ Postpartum blues occur most commonly during the third to tenth day postpartum.

134. Knowledge, implementation, physiological adaptation (b)
    ❶ When the patient becomes eclamptic, she has a seizure.
    ②, ③ BP should be watched but is an indication of preeclampsia.
    ④ The nurse should watch all pregnant patients for labor; this does not cause eclamptic conditions.

135. Knowledge, implementation, prevention and early detection of disease (b)
    ❸ 100 ml in 1 hr
    $\times$ 15 gtt ml
    1500 gtt in 1 hr
    1500 gtt divided by 60 min = 25 gtt/min
    ①, ②, ④ These are incorrect calculations.

136. Comprehension, implementation, prevention and early detection of disease (b)
    ❹ Rhogam prevents the development of antibodies when given either prenatally or within 72 hours of delivery.
    ①, ② These are compatible.
    ③ A negative blood type would not have caused the development of antibodies.

137. Application, evaluation, basic care and comfort (b)
❷ A time limit on each breast is no longer considered needed to prevent complications.
① A strict schedule is no longer considered necessary.
③ This is an indication of the need for further teaching.
④ This is fine; however, it does not indicate understanding.

138. Comprehension, planning, basic care and comfort (b)
❷ In many cultures drinking hot liquids after childbirth is important to restore the balance of nature.
① A clear liquid diet is fairly self-explanatory; a dietician can basically offer the same items as the nurse.
③ The patient is able to decide what she will drink or not drink according to her likes and desires.
④ This is not true and is judgmental.

139. Comprehension, implementation, safety and infection control (b)
❸ Bonding and breast-feeding can continue with minimal exposure to other patients and staff.
① Standard precautions and gown and gloves for direct care are appropriate.
② If the baby is breast-feeding well, there is no reason to discontinue; there is also no reason to expose other babies in the nursery to potential infection.
④ Diagnosis is important, but precautions can start before that.

140. Comprehension, evaluation, physiological adaptation (b)
❷ In addition, she has to be able to support herself.
① It takes time for sensation to return after the catheter is removed.
③ Further assessments need to be made other than these.
④ It is helpful for the patient to eat something, but it is not the only criteria.

141. Knowledge, planning, physiological adaptation (b)
❸ This procedure attempts to form a small clot to stop the leaking fluid.
① This is done prior to childbirth and involves invading the epidural space.
② This is done for chronic pain.
④ Infection is not a cause.

142. Application, evaluation, growth and development (a)
❸ This would indicate a healthy involution.
① This would be normal for the 2 to 3 days after birth.
② If the uterus is deviated to the right, the bladder needs to be emptied.
④ This is healthy immediately after birth.

143. Application, evaluation, reduction of risk potential (a)
❸ With a cesarean section there is no episiotomy.
①, ②, ④ These are required nursing interventions for this patient.

144. Application, evaluation, reduction of risk potential (a)
❷ Actual demonstration is the best way to be sure that a skill is understood.
① This is fine, but demonstration is better.
③ Attendance is no proof of understanding.
④ The goal is for no one to exhibit signs and symptoms of infection.

145. Application, evaluation, basic care and comfort (b)
❸ This evaluation is the most accurate way of ensuring that the baby is receiving adequate nourishment and is not becoming dehydrated.
① Many babies will fall asleep part way through a feeding and need to be stimulated to feed a little longer.
② Time is no longer considered relevant for nourishment or to prevent complications.
④ This is a measurement, but not on a short-term basis.

146. Application, planning, prevention and early detection of disease (b)
❸ This is accurate and provides incentive.
① While this is true and may provide additional incentive for the mother to breast-feed, it is not the most important reason for breast-feeding.
② This is factual; however, formula-fed infants receive required nutrients as well.
④ This is true and may provide additional incentive for the mother to breast-feed; however, most women will not choose to breast-feed for this reason alone.

147. Cognitive, assessment, growth and development (a)
❷ This may be indicative of urinary infection.
①, ③, ④ These are normal at this time.

148. Application, evaluation, physiological adaptation (c)
❶ These are classic signs of postpartum infection.
②, ③, ④ These are not typical signs; need further evaluation to determine cause.

149. Application, evaluation, physiological adaptation (b)
❷ This needs to be evaluated; complaints of severe perineal pain is abnormal.
① This is a risk factor, not an assessment.
③ Hematomas may or may not be visible.
④ This is more indicative of infection.

150. Application, implementation, coping and adaptation (b)
❸ This answer allows for communication that will encourage the couple to deal with their pain as a family unit and allows for more effective coping with grief.
① The patient is an adult who cannot have her rights for appropriate standards of care taken away from her.
② Nurses should implement therapeutic methods of communication as an appropriate standard of care.
④ Patients exist as part of a family unit; family members' needs should be considered.

CHAPTER 8

Pediatric Nursing

Pediatric nursing includes the care of both well and sick children and covers both preventive health care and restorative nursing care. This chapter is divided into the following age groups: infancy, toddlerhood, preschool, school age, and adolescence. The areas covered include normal growth and development, psychosocial development, health promotion, and health problems specific to each age group. Other topics discussed include the battered child syndrome, hospitalization and the child, and nursing care of the hospitalized child. The information provided in this chapter presents both the physical and psychological aspects of care necessary in providing pediatric nursing care.

ASSESSMENT OF CHILD AND FAMILY

A. Functions and structure of family
   1. The functions and structure of the family are vital to the normal growth and development of the child
   2. Three primary functions of the family
      a. Providing physical care such as food, clothing, shelter, safety, prevention of illness, and care during illness
      b. Education and training: language, values, morals, and formal education
      c. Protecting psychological and emotional health
B. Physical assessment of child
   1. Performing a health history, including the child's past history as well as current complaints or problems, is done by the nurse, physician, or nurse practitioner
   2. Assessment of child's physical growth and development level is done by the physician or nurse practitioner
C. Concepts of child development (Table 8-1)
   1. Freud's theory of development is based on the child's psychosexual development
   2. Erikson's theory of development is based on psychosocial development as a series of developmental tasks
   3. Piaget's theory of development is based on intellectual (cognitive) development: how the child learns and develops his or her intelligence

INFANCY (AGES 4 WEEKS TO 1 YEAR)
NORMAL GROWTH AND DEVELOPMENT
Physical Development*

A. 1 month
   1. Physical
      a. Weight: gains about 150 to 210g (5 to 7 oz) weekly during the first 6 months of life
      b. Height: gains about 2.5 cm (1 inch) a month for the first 6 months of life
   2. Motor
      a. May lift the head temporarily, but generally the head must be supported
      b. Holds the head parallel with the body when placed prone

---

*From Saxton DF, Nugent PM, Pelikan PK: *Mosby's comprehensive review of nursing*, ed 16, St Louis, 1999, Mosby.

      c. Can turn the head from side to side when prone or supine
      d. Asymmetrical posture dominates, such as tonic neck reflex
      e. Primitive reflexes still present and strong (grasp, Moro, tonic neck)
   3. Sensory
      a. Follows a light to midline
      b. Eye movements coordinated most of the time
      c. Visual acuity 20/100 to 20/50
      d. Quiet when hears a voice
   4. Socialization and vocalization
      a. Smiles indiscriminately
      b. Makes small throaty sounds
      c. Watches parent's face when he or she talks to infant
B. 2 to 3 months
   1. Physical: posterior fontanel closed
   2. Motor
      a. Holds the head erect for a short time and can raise chest supported on the forearms
      b. Can carry hand or an object to the mouth at will
      c. Reaches for attractive objects but misjudges distances
      d. Grasp, tonic neck, and Moro reflexes are fading
      e. Can sit when the back is supported; knees will be flexed and back rounded
      f. Step or dance reflex disappears
      g. Plays with fingers and hands
   3. Sensory
      a. Follows a light to the periphery
      b. Has binocular coordination (vertical and horizontal vision)
      c. Locates sounds by turning head in direction of the sound
   4. Socialization and vocalization
      a. Smiles in response to a person or object
      b. Coos and gurgles; shows pleasure in making sounds
      c. Stops crying when parent enters the room
C. 4 to 5 months
   1. Physical: drools because salivary glands are functioning, but the child does not have sufficient coordination to swallow saliva
   2. Motor
      a. Balances the head well in a sitting position
      b. Sits with little support; holds the back straight when pulled to a sitting position
      c. Symmetrical body position predominates

TABLE 8-1 Concepts of Child Development

Age	Developmental Stage	Freud's Theory	Erikson's Theory	Piaget's Theory
4 wk-1 yr	Infancy	Oral stage	Trust vs. mistrust	Sensorimotor phase
1-3 yr	Toddlerhood	Anal stage	Autonomy vs. shame and doubt	Preoperational phase
3-5 yr	Preschool age	Oedipal stage Latency stage	Initiative vs. guilt	Preoperational phase continued
6-12 yr	School age	Latency stage continued Genital stage	Industry vs. inferiority	Concrete operational phase Formal operational phase
13-18 yr	Adolescence	Genital stage continued	Identity vs. identify confusion	Formal operational phase continued

    d. Can sustain a portion of own weight when held in a standing position

    e. Reaches for and grasps an object with the whole hand

    f. Can roll over from back to side

    g. Lifts the head and shoulders at a 90-degree angle when prone

    h. Primitive reflexes (e.g., grasp, tonic neck, and Moro) have disappeared

  3. Sensory

    a. Recognizes familiar objects and people

    b. Beginning eye-hand coordination

  4. Socialization and vocalization

    a. Laughs aloud

    b. Definitely enjoys social interaction with people

    c. Vocalizes displeasure when an object is taken away

D. 6 to 7 months

  1. Physical

    a. Weight: gains about 90 to 150 g (3 to 5 oz) weekly during second 6 months of life; weight doubles by 6 months

    b. Height: gains about 1.25 cm (½ inch) a month

    c. Teething may begin with eruption of two lower central incisors, followed by upper incisors (Fig. 8-1)

  2. Motor

    a. Can turn over equally well from stomach or back

    b. Sits fairly well unsupported, especially if placed in a forward-leaning position

    c. Hitches or moves backward when in a sitting position

    d. Can transfer a toy from one hand to the other

    e. Can approach toy and grasp it with one hand

    f. Plays with feet and puts them in mouth

    g. When lying down, lifts head as if trying to sit up

    h. Transfers everything from hand to mouth

  3. Sensory

    a. Has taste preferences; will spit out disliked foods

    b. Responds to own name

  4. Socialization and vocalization

    a. Begins to differentiate between strange and familiar faces and shows "stranger anxiety"

    b. Makes polysyllabic vowel sounds (baba, dada)

    c. Plays peekaboo

    d. Responds to word no

E. 8 to 9 months

  1. Motor

    a. Sits steadily alone

    b. Has good hand-to-mouth coordination

    c. Developing pincer grasp, with preference for use of one hand over the other

    d. Crawls and then creeps (creeping is more advanced because the abdomen is supported off the floor)

    e. Can raise self to a sitting position but may require help to pull self to feet

  2. Sensory

    a. Depth perception is beginning to develop

    b. Displays interest in small objects

  3. Socialization and vocalization

    a. Shows anxiety with strangers by turning or pushing away and crying

    b. Definite social attachment is evident: stretches out arms to loved ones

    c. Is voluntarily separating self from mother by desire to act on own

    d. Reacts to adult anger: cries when scolded

    e. Dislikes dressing, diaper change

    f. No true words as yet, but comprehends words such as bye-bye, no-no

F. 10 to 12 months

  1. Physical

    a. Has tripled birth weight by 1 year

    b. Upper and lower lateral incisors usually have erupted for total of 6 to 8 teeth

    c. Head and chest circumferences are equal

    d. Lumbar curve develops; lordosis evident when walking

  2. Motor

    a. Stands alone for short times

    b. Walks with help; moves around by holding onto furniture

    c. Can sit down from a standing position without help

    d. Can eat from a spoon and drink from a cup but needs help; prefers using fingers

    e. Can play pat-a-cake

    f. Can hold a crayon to make a mark on paper

    g. Helps in dressing, such as putting arm through sleeve

  3. Sensory

    a. Visual acuity 20/50+

    b. Amblyopia may develop with lack of binocularity

    c. Discriminates simple geometric forms

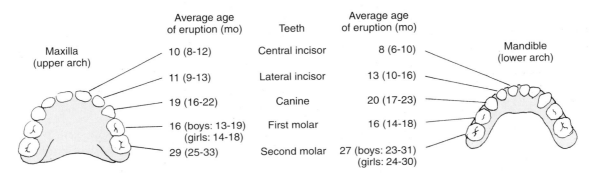

Figure 8-1. Sequence of eruption of primary teeth. Range represents ±1 standard deviation or 67% of subjects studied. (Data from McDonald RE, Avery DR: *Dentistry for the child and adolescent*, ed 6, St Louis, 1994, Mosby.)

4. Socialization and vocalization
   a. Shows emotions such as jealousy, affection, anger
   b. Enjoys familiar surroundings and will explore away from mother
   c. Fearful in strange situation or with strangers; clings to mother
   d. May develop habit of "security" blanket
   e. Can say 3-5 words besides *Dadda* or *Mama*
   f. Understands simple verbal requests, such as "Give it to me"
   g. Knows own name

Psychosocial Development

A. Infants are in Erikson's stage of "trust vs. mistrust." Infants will develop a sense of trust or mistrust depending on how their needs are met by their parents (or other caregivers)
B. As infants grow older, they slowly realize that they are separate from their environment and that they influence their environment with their actions
C. Infants' early activities are mostly reflexes: crying, sucking, kicking, and so on. As the months progress, they learn to move in certain ways, follow with their eyes, and smile in response to a smile and soft words

HEALTH PROMOTION

A. Immunizations should be given on schedule; Fig. 8-2
B. Nutrition appropriate to the age and needs of the infant should be provided
   1. Human milk is the most desirable complete diet for the first 6 months of life
   2. Introduction of strained foods may begin at 6 months of age, starting with strained fruits
   3. Solid foods should be introduced slowly, in small amounts, and one at a time, to determine the infant's likes and dislikes; this also helps detect possible allergies to certain foods. Allow 4 to 7 days between introduction of each new food
   4. Weaning from breast or bottle to a cup can begin between 5 and 6 months of age, although the infant cannot be weaned completely until between 12 and 24 months of age
C. Safety and accident prevention includes a safe home environment, safe toys, use of car seats, and close attention to the infant who is crawling or walking

HEALTH PROBLEMS
Nutritional Disorders
FAILURE TO THRIVE (FTT)

A. Definition: a state of inadequate growth resulting from inability to obtain and/or use calories; leads to malnutrition
B. Symptoms: below normal weight and height (below 5th percentile for age), listlessness, poor feeding habits, unresponsive to holding and attention, voluntary regurgitation, prolonged periods of sleep
C. Diagnosis
   1. Based on symptoms and a continued deviation from an established growth curve
   2. Three general categories of FTT
      a. Organic: result of a physical cause such as congenital defects of gastrointestinal (GI) system or heart
      b. Nonorganic: unrelated to a disease; usually caused by psychosocial factors

c. Idiopathic: unexplained cause; may be grouped with nonorganic FTT
D. Treatment/nursing interventions (directed at correcting the malnutrition)
   1. Correction of organic causes, if possible
   2. Development of a structured routine
   3. Sensory stimulation
   4. Adequate food for weight gain; this may include nasogastric feedings as well as bottle feedings during early treatment
   5. Tender loving care; holding and cuddling, talking to the infant
   6. Teaching and encouraging the mother and father regarding feeding, infant care, and parenting skills
   7. Family counseling when needed

COLIC

A. Definition: paroxysmal abdominal pain or cramping that is manifested by crying and drawing the legs up to the abdomen; colic is most commonly seen in infants under the age of 3 months
B. Symptoms: episodes of loud crying accompanied by abdominal cramping; despite obvious indications of pain, the infant usually tolerates feedings well and gains weight
C. Diagnosis: based on symptoms reported by parents/caregivers
D. Treatment/nursing interventions
   1. If child is bottle-fed, investigation of possibility of cow's milk allergy; substitution of another formula (such as casein hydrosolate [Nutramigen]) may be tried
   2. Comfort measures that can be used by the parents/caregivers:
      a. Place infant prone over a covered hot-water bottle or covered heating pad (ensure that hot water bottle is warm, not hot)
      b. Massage infant's abdomen
      c. Change infant's position frequently
      d. Provide smaller, frequent feedings; burp infant during and after feedings, and place infant in an upright seat after feeding
      e. Introduce pacifier for added sucking
   3. Pharmacological agents such as sedatives, antispasmodics, antihistamines, and antiflatulents are sometimes recommended

Respiratory Disorders
UPPER RESPIRATORY INFECTIONS (URIs)

A. Definition: viral or bacterial infection affecting the upper respiratory tract; nasopharyngitis or the "common cold" is particularly common in children of all ages
B. Symptoms: fever, sore throat, sneezing, nasal congestion, occasional cough, irritability, anorexia
C. Diagnosis: based on the symptoms
D. Treatment/nursing interventions
   1. Bed rest until free of fever
   2. Encourage oral fluids
   3. Antipyretics for fever (acetaminophen, ibuprofen; not aspirin)
   4. Nose drops to relieve nasal congestion
   5. Oral decongestants as ordered
   6. Adequate nutrition for age; high-calorie fluids and soft foods are better tolerated by infants and young children

Recommended Childhood Immunization Schedule
United States, January - December 2000

Vaccines[1] are listed under routinely recommended ages. ⬚Bars⬚ indicate range of recommended ages for immunization. Any dose not given at the recommended age should be given as a "catch-up" immunization at any subsequent visit when indicated and feasible. ⬭Ovals⬭ indicate vaccines to be given if previously recommended doses were missed or given earlier than the recommended minimum age.

Age ▶ Vaccine ▼	Birth	1 mo	2 mos	4 mos	6 mos	12 mos	15 mos	18 mos	24 mos	4-6 yrs	11-12 yrs	14-16 yrs
Hepatitis B[2]	Hep B											
			Hep B			Hep B					(Hep B)	
Diphtheria, Tetanus, Pertussis[3]			DTaP	DTaP	DTaP		DTaP[3]			DTaP	Td	
H. influenzae type b[4]			Hib	Hib	Hib	Hib						
Polio[5]			IPV	IPV		IPV[5]				IPV[5]		
Measles, Mumps, Rubella[6]						MMR				MMR[6]	(MMR[6])	
Varicella[7]						Var					(Var[7])	
Hepatitis A[8]										Hep A[8]-in selected areas		

Approved by the Advisory Committee on Immunization Practices (ACIP), the American Academy of Pediatrics (AAP), and the American Academy of Family Physicians (AAFP).

On October 22, 1999, the Advisory Committee on Immunization Practices (ACIP) recommended that Rotashield (RRV-TV), the only US-licensed rotavirus vaccine, no longer be used in the United States (MMWR Morb Mortal Wkly Rep. Nov 5, 1999;48(43):1007). Parents should be reassured that their children who received rotavirus vaccine before July are not at increased risk for intussusception now.

1. This schedule indicated the recommended ages for routine administration of currently licensed childhood vaccines as of 11/1/99. Additional vaccines may be licensed and recommended during the year. Licensed combination vaccines may be used whenever any components of the combination are indicated and its other components are not contraindicated. Providers should consult the manufacturers' package inserts for detailed recommendations.

2. **Infants born to HBsAg-negative mothers** should receive the 1st dose of hepatitis B (Hep B) vaccine by age 2 months. The 2nd dose should be at least 1 month after the 1st dose. The 3rd dose should be administered at least 4 months after the 1st dose and at least 2 months after the 2nd dose, but not before 6 months of age for infants. **Infants born to HBsAg-positive mothers** should receive hepatitis B vaccine and 0.5 mL hepatitis B immune globulin (HBIG) within 12 hours of birth at separate sites. The 2nd dose is recommended at 1 month of age and the 3rd dose at 6 months of age. **Infants born to mothers whose HBsAg status is unknown** should receive hepatitis B vaccine within 12 hours of birth. Maternal blood should be drawn at the time of delivery to determine the mother's HBsAg status; if the HBsAg test is positive, the infant should receive HBIG as soon as possible (no later than 1 week of age). **All children and adolescents (through 18 years of age)** who have not been immunized against hepatitis B may begin the series during any visit. Special efforts should be made to immunize children who were born in or whose parents were born in areas of the world with moderate or high endemicity of hepatitis B virus infection.

3. The 4th dose of DTaP (diphtheria and tetanus toxoids and acellular pertussis vaccine) may be administered as early as 12 months of age, provided 6 months have elapsed since the 3rd dose and the child is unlikely to return at age 15 to 18 months. Td (tetanus and diphtheria toxoids) is recommended at 11 to 12 years of age if at least 5 years have elapsed since the last dose of DTP, DTaP, or DT. Subsequent routine Td boosters are recommended every 10 years.

4. Three *Haemophilus influenzae* type b (Hib) conjugate vaccines are licensed for infant use. If PRP-OMP (PedvaxHIB or ComVax [Merck]) is administered at 2 and 4 months of age, a dose at 6 months is not required. Because clinical studies in infants have demonstrated that using some combination products may induce a lower immune response to the Hib vaccine component, DTaP/Hib combination products should not be used for primary immunization in infants at 2, 4, or 6 months of age unless FDA-approved for these ages.

5. To eliminate the risk of vaccine-associated paralytic polio (VAPP), an all-IPV schedule is now recommended for routine childhood polio vaccination in the United States. All children should receive four doses of IPV at 2 months, 4 months, 6 to 18 months, and 4 to 6 years. OPV (if available) may be used only for the following special circumstances:
   1. Mass vaccination campaigns to control outbreaks of paralytic polio.
   2. Unvaccinated children who will be traveling in <4 weeks to areas where polio is endemic or epidemic.
   3. Children of parents who do not accept the recommended number of vaccine injections. These children may receive OPV only for the third or fourth dose or both; in this situation, health care professionals should administer OPV only after discussing the risk for VAPP with parents or caregivers.
   4. During the transition to an all-IPV schedule, recommendations for the use of remaining OPV supplies in physicians' offices and clinics have been issued by the American Academy of Pediatrics (see *Pediatrics*, December 1999).

6. The 2nd dose of measles, mumps, and rubella (MMR) vaccine is recommended routinely at 4 to 6 years of age but may be administered during any visit, provided at least 4 weeks have elapsed since receipt of the 1st dose and that both doses are administered beginning at or after 12 months of age. Those who have not previously received the second dose should complete the schedule by the 11- to 12-year-old visit.

7. Varicella (Var) vaccine is recommended at any visit on or after the first birthday for susceptible children, i.e., those who lack a reliable history of chickenpox (as judged by a health care professional) and who have not been immunized. Susceptible persons 13 years of age or older should receive 2 doses, given at least 4 weeks apart.

8. Hepatitis A (Hep A) is shaded to indicate its recommended use in selected states and/or regions; consult your local public health authority. (Also see *MMWR Morb Mortal Wkly Rep.* Oct 01, 1999;48(RR-12); 1-37).

Immunization Protects Children
Regular checkups at your pediatrician's office or local health clinic are an important way to keep children healthy.

By making sure that your child gets immunized on time, you can provide the best available defense against many dangerous childhood diseases. Immunizations protect children against: hepatitis B, polio, measles, mumps, rubella (German measles), pertussis (whooping cough), diphtheria, tetanus (lockjaw), *Haemophilus influenzae* type b, and chickenpox. All of these immunizations need to be given before children are 2 years old in order for them to be protected during their most vulnerable period. Are your child's immunizations up-to-date?

The chart at the top of this fact sheet includes immunization recommendations from the American Academy of Pediatrics. Remember to keep track of your child's immunizations—it's the only way you can be sure your child is up-to-date. Also, check with your pediatrician or health clinic at each visit to find out if your child needs any booster shots or if any new vaccines have been recommended since this schedule was prepared.

If you don't have a pediatrician, call your local health department. Public health clinics usually have supplies of vaccine and may give shots for free.

American Academy of Pediatrics

The information contained in this publication should not be used as a substitute for the medical care and advice of your pediatrician. There may be variations in treatment that your pediatrician may recommend based on individual facts and circumstances.

Figure 8-2. Recommended childhood immunization schedule, approved January 2000. Updated on an annual basis.

7. Cool air humidifier for moistened air (to assist in decreasing congestion)

ACUTE OTITIS MEDIA

A. Definition: middle ear infection; frequently caused by nasopharyngeal infections that travel through the infant's shortened, widened eustachian tubes
B. Symptoms: fever, irritability, restlessness, pulling or rubbing of the ears, loss of appetite; otoscopy reveals a bright red, bulging tympanic membrane
C. Diagnosis: based on the symptoms and history of recent URI
D. Treatment/nursing interventions
    1. Antibiotics as ordered for bacterial infections (usually oral and/or ear drops)
    2. Antipyretics for fever
    3. Analgesics/antipyretics for discomfort (acetaminophen, ibuprofen)
    4. Encourage oral fluids
    5. Promote rest and quiet environment
    6. Myringotomy and insertion of polyethylene tubes by the physician, to allow for drainage of fluid
    7. Observe for drainage; keep ears clean

LOWER RESPIRATORY INFECTIONS
RESPIRATORY SYNCYTIAL VIRUS (RSV)/ BRONCHIOLITIS

A. Definition
    1. Bronchiolitis is an acute viral infection that occurs primarily in winter and spring, and is most common in infants and children up to 2 years of age; it causes the bronchioles to become plugged with mucus, and the bronchiole mucosa to swell; the mucus traps the air in the lungs, making it difficult for the infant to expel the air
    2. RSV is related to the parainfluenza virus; it is responsible for at least 50% of the diagnosed cases of bronchiolitis; the peak incidence for RSV infection is 2 to 5 months of age; it is transmitted predominantly through direct contact with respiratory secretions; RSV has been known to survive for hours on countertops, gloves, and cloth, and for half an hour on skin
B. Symptoms
    1. Usually begins with an upper respiratory infection; symptoms include rhinorrhea, coughing, sneezing, pharyngitis, wheezing, and intermittent fever
    2. With progression of the disease, there is increased coughing and wheezing, air hunger, tachypnea, retractions, and cyanosis
    3. Symptoms of severe illness include tachypnea of more than 70 breaths per minute, listlessness, poor air exchange, apneic spells, O_2 saturation less than 95%
C. Diagnosis
    1. Based on clinical symptoms
    2. RSV can be identified by various tests done on nasal/nasopharyngeal secretions to detect RSV antigen
D. Treatment/nursing interventions
    1. Humidified oxygen inhalation (to relieve dyspnea and hypoxia)
    2. Elevate head of crib
    3. Monitor vital signs and oxygen saturation (via pulse oximeter)

4. Adequate fluid intake, including IV fluids as needed for hydration
5. Allow infant to rest as much as possible
6. Medical therapy for bronchiolitis has not proved to be effective; however, Ribavirin, an antiviral agent, may be used specifically for RSV infection
    a. Ribavirin is administered by nebulization via an oxygen hood, tent, or mask for 12 to 20 hours per day, for 1-7 days
    b. It is most commonly used in children with RSV infection who are at high risk for complications caused by other conditions, including chronic lung conditions, immunodeficiency, and certain neurologic diseases (such as severe cerebral palsy)

VIRAL PNEUMONIA

A. Definition: inflammation of the lung, characterized by interstitial pneumonitis with inflammation of the mucosa and walls of bronchi and bronchioles
B. Symptoms: fever, cough, rapid respiratory rate, listlessness
C. Diagnosis: based on the symptoms and results of chest x-ray films
D. Treatment/nursing interventions
    1. Elevate the head of the crib
    2. Croup tent for humidified oxygen inhalation
    3. Chest physiotherapy and postural drainage
    4. Antibiotics as ordered (for bacterial pneumonia)
    5. Antipyretics for fever
    6. Monitor vital signs frequently
    7. Encourage clear fluids by mouth
    8. Allow infant to rest to prevent dyspnea

Gastrointestinal Disorders
INFECTIOUS GASTROENTERITIS

A. Definition: diarrhea and vomiting that may be caused by viral or bacterial infections
B. Symptoms: frequent, loose stools, irritability, vomiting, abdominal distention, dehydration, sunken fontanel, poor skin turgor, weak, rapid pulse
C. Diagnosis: based on the symptoms; specific bacterial cause can be isolated in a stool culture (most commonly *Escherichia coli* or rotavirus in the infant)
D. Treatment/nursing interventions
    1. Oral rehydration therapy (with commercially prepared solutions such as Pedialyte); amount is based on infant's weight, and percentage of dehydration
    2. IV fluids with electrolytes as ordered, if oral rehydration therapy is not effective, or if dehydration is severe
    3. Return to normal diet (including formula, cow's milk, and age-appropriate solids) should be started as soon as they are tolerated; the "BRAT" diet (bananas, rice cereal, applesauce, tea/toast) is contraindicated for the infant with acute diarrhea because it has little nutritional value
    4. Note amount, color, and consistency of stools and emesis
    5. Keep accurate intake and output record (if necessary, weigh diapers to measure urine output)
    6. Maintain proper isolation technique (enteric precautions)
    7. Provide good skin care to buttocks and perineum after each diaper change; cleanse well; leave area open to air when possible; apply ointments as ordered
    8. Provide time for stimulation, holding, and cuddling

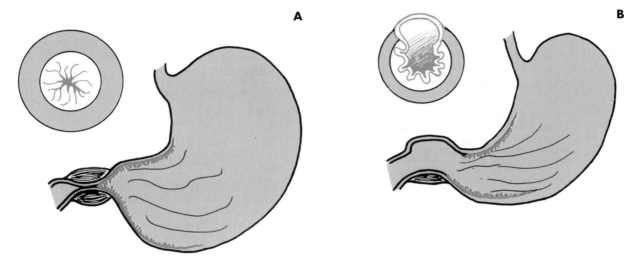

Figure 8-3. Hypertrophic pyloric stenosis. **A,** Enlarged muscular tumor nearly obliterates pyloric channel. **B,** Longitudinal surgical division of muscle down to submucosa establishes adequate passageway. (From Wong DL et al: *Whaley and Wong's Nursing care of infants and children,* ed 6, St Louis, 1999, Mosby.)

HYPERTROPHIC PYLORIC STENOSIS

A. Definition: hypertrophy of the pyloric muscle fibers and narrowing of the pylorus, which is at distal end of the stomach (Fig. 8-3)
B. Symptoms: usually appear between 3 and 8 weeks of age; projectile vomiting of formula and mucus, irritability, weight loss, and dehydration; the physician can often palpate the olive-size pyloric mass in the abdomen
C. Diagnosis: based on the symptoms, physical examination, and, if necessary, upper gastrointestinal radiographic or ultrasound studies
D. Treatment/nursing interventions
   1. Preoperative
      a. IV fluids with electrolytes as ordered
      b. NPO unless ordered to feed
      c. Nasogastric (NG) tube is often inserted to remove excess stomach contents immediately before surgery (pyloromyotomy)
   2. Postoperative
      a. Position the infant on right side or abdomen or in infant seat to prevent aspiration
      b. NPO; first feeding begins about 4 to 6 hours after surgery (glucose water); amounts are increased slowly, to administer small frequent feedings as ordered, formula is started 24 hours postoperatively if clear fluids are retained
      c. General postoperative nursing care

Nervous System Disorders

FEBRILE SEIZURES

A. Definition: seizures caused by high fever (102° F to 105° F; 38.8° C to 40.5° C); most often seen between 6 months and 3 years of age
B. Symptoms: seizures characterized by stiffening of the body, with jerking movements of the extremities and face, ending with a lapse of consciousness
C. Diagnosis: based on evidence of seizure activity preceded by high fever
   1. Simple febrile seizures are brief and generalized
   2. Complex febrile seizures are prolonged and may have focal features
D. Treatment/nursing interventions
   1. Anticonvulsant (phenobarbital) and antianxiety (diazepam) medications to control the seizures; antipyretics (acetaminophen) to control fever (see Chapter 3)
   2. Padded side rails
   3. Airway and suction equipment at bedside
   4. During seizure, do not restrain the infant; turn his or her head to the side to allow saliva to drain out of the mouth; *do not* try to insert a seizure stick or airway in the infant's mouth during a seizure; observe the seizure and protect the infant from harm
   5. Documentation: note the kinds of movements, behavior before the seizure (if known), duration of the seizure, skin color and vital signs during and after the seizure, and medications given during the seizure, including the infant/toddler's reaction to the medications
   6. Parent teaching should include care of the infant during a seizure

MENINGITIS

A. Definition: infection of the spinal meninges and fluid; caused by several bacteria and viruses
B. Symptoms: elevated temperature, irritability, poor feeding, high-pitched cry, nuchal rigidity, seizures, bulging fontanel
C. Diagnosis: based on the symptoms and the presence of cloudy spinal fluid when lumbar puncture is performed (increased WBC count; decreased glucose level and increased protein level in the spinal fluid) (Fig. 8-4)
D. Treatment/nursing interventions
   1. Isolation from other children (for bacterial meningitis)

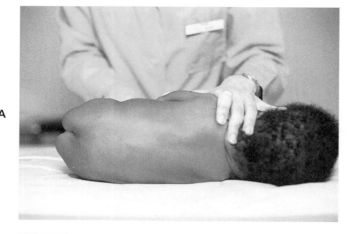

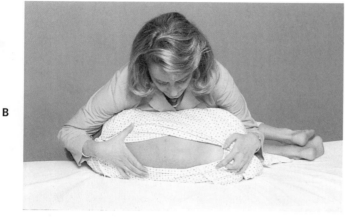

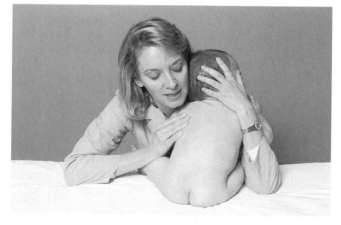

Figure 8-4. **A,** Modified side-lying position for lumbar puncture. **B,** Older child in side-lying position. **C,** Infant sitting position allows for flexion of lumbar spine. (From Wong DL et al: *Whaley and Wong's Nursing care of infants and children,* ed 6, St Louis, 1999, Mosby.)

2. IV antibiotics as ordered
3. Monitor vital signs, neurologic status, and level of consciousness frequently
4. IV fluids as ordered
5. Diet: infant may be NPO at first, until liquids can be tolerated
6. Antipyretics to reduce elevated temperature

7. Handle the infant as little as possible when the infant is irritable and uncomfortable; keep room quiet
8. Seizure precautions (padded side rails)
9. IV Dexamethasone (for *Haemophilus influenzae* type B meningitis)

Integumentary Disorders
INFANTILE ECZEMA
A. Definition: atopic dermatitis caused by an allergic reaction to some irritant; usually begins between 2 and 6 months of age and undergoes spontaneous remission around age 3
B. Symptoms: reddened, raised rash starting on cheeks and spreading to arms and legs; itching, oozing of vesicles
C. Diagnosis: based on the story and symptoms; the cause of the eczema (the allergen) must also be determined to control further episodes
D. Treatment/nursing interventions
  1. Good skin care; keep affected areas clean
  2. Tub baths with tepid water, baking soda, and corn starch to relieve the itching
  3. Keep skin well hydrated; various lubricants or moisturizing lotions may be ordered
  4. Antihistamines and topical steroids as ordered to control itching
  5. "Mittens" to prevent scratching
  6. Elbow restraints to prevent scratching (only if necessary)
  7. Provide for sensory stimulation, holding, and cuddling at frequent intervals

IMPETIGO
A. Definition: infection of the skin caused by *Streptococcus* or *Staphylococcus* bacteria; occurs in nurseries when strict handwashing technique is not followed (impetigo neonatorum); also occurs in preschool and school-age children
B. Symptoms: reddened, vesicular lesions (pustules)
C. Diagnosis: based on the symptoms; specific bacterial cause can be determined by culture of the draining lesions
D. Treatment/nursing interventions
  1. Isolation of infant (child)
  2. Strict handwashing technique by all persons coming in contact with the infant
  3. Warm saline compresses to lesions, followed by a gentle cleansing and topical antibiotic ointment
  4. Systemic antibiotics and corticosteroids may be ordered for infants/children with widespread lesions

Congenital Defects and Hereditary Disorders
GASTROINTESTINAL SYSTEM
HIRSCHSPRUNG'S DISEASE
A. Definition: distention of a portion of the lower colon caused by a congenital lack of nerve cells in the wall of the colon just below the distended section (Fig. 8-5)
B. Symptoms: constipation (including a lack of meconium stool in the newborn in the first 24 hours), abdominal distention, bile-stained mucus and emesis, inadequate weight gain
C. Diagnosis: based on the symptoms, results of barium enema, rectal biopsy, and/or anorectal manometry

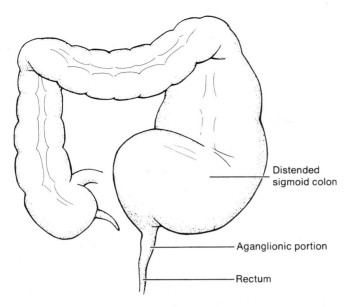

Figure 8-5. Hirschsprung's disease. (From Wong DL et al: *Whaley and Wong's Nursing care of infants and children,* ed 6, St Louis, 1999, Mosby.)

Labels: Distended sigmoid colon; Aganglionic portion; Rectum

D. Treatment/nursing interventions: based on the type of surgery done (bowel resection, sometimes with temporary colostomy); surgery done in two or three stages
  1. Preoperative
     a. Observation of stools: color, amount, and consistency
     b. IV fluids and electrolytes as ordered
  2. Postoperative
     a. NG tube to low-suction or gravity drainage
     b. General postoperative care
     c. Routine colostomy care as necessary (prn)
     d. Vital signs as ordered; axillary temperatures should be taken
     e. IV fluids as ordered
     f. NPO; resume diet as ordered
     g. Record intake and output (I&O) every shift
     h. Observe stools and record amount and characteristics
     i. Observe for rectal bleeding and abdominal distention
     j. Parent teaching and support

OMPHALOCELE

A. Definition: the abdominal organs protrude through an abnormal opening in the abdominal wall and form a sac lying on the abdomen
B. Diagnosis: based on symptoms and physical examination
C. Treatment/nursing interventions
  1. Preoperative
     a. Keep the omphalocele covered with sterile gauze, moistened with normal saline and a plastic drape until surgery can be performed
     b. Maintain sterile technique as much as possible in caring for the omphalocele

  2. Postoperative
     a. Surgery: the organs are returned to the abdominal cavity, and the abdominal wall is closed
     b. General postoperative care, including mechanical ventilation for several days
     c. Parenteral nutrition for several days
     d. Observe stools and record amount and characteristics

IMPERFORATE ANUS

A. Definition: the rectal pouch ends blindly at a distance above the anus; sometimes there is no anal opening; there are various forms of this defect
B. Symptoms: no stools in the first 24 hours after birth; rectal thermometer cannot be inserted properly
C. Diagnosis: made by digital rectal examination, intestinal x-ray examination, and endoscopy
D. Treatment/nursing interventions
  1. Surgical procedure to reconnect the ends of the rectum and form an anal opening
  2. General postoperative nursing care

ESOPHAGEAL ATRESIA

A. Definition: the upper end of the esophagus ends in a blind pouch; the lower end may also end in a blind pouch or may be connected to the trachea by fistula defect (tracheoesophageal fistula) (Fig. 8-6)
B. Symptoms: excessive salivation and drooling, coughing and choking during feedings, regurgitation of all feedings
C. Diagnosis: based on symptoms as well as passage of an NG tube or catheter down the esophagus to test for patency; exact anomaly is determined by x-ray studies
D. Treatment/nursing interventions
  1. NPO with administration of IV fluids as ordered
  2. Suctioning of nose and mouth as needed
  3. Insertion of an NG tube to drain mucus and fluid from the blind pouch
  4. Antibiotic therapy as ordered (for probable aspiration pneumonia)
  5. Surgical repair to correct the defects and reconnect the ends of the esophagus

INTUSSUSCEPTION

A. Definition; telescoping of one portion of the bowel into a distal portion; the most common site is at the ileocecal valve; usually occurs between 3 and 12 months of age
B. Symptoms: appear suddenly; pallor; sharp colicky pain causes infant to draw up legs and cry out (this occurs every 5 to 10 minutes); vomiting; stools with blood and mucus ("red currant jelly" stools); signs of shock
C. Diagnosis: based on symptoms; definitive diagnosis can be made radiographically with barium enema
D. Treatment/nursing interventions: this is an emergency that requires immediate treatment. The initial treatment of choice is hydrostatic reduction by barium enema; if this is not effective, surgery is necessary
  1. Preoperative
     a. Careful observation and recording of vital signs frequently
     b. IV fluids with electrolytes as ordered
     c. NPO

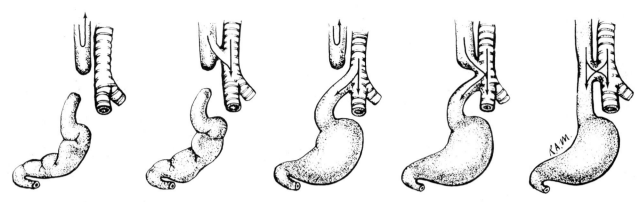

Figure 8-6.   The five most common types of esophageal atresia and tracheoesophageal fistula. (From Wong DL et al: *Whaley and Wong's Nursing care of infants and children,* ed 6, St Louis, 1999, Mosby.)

    d. NG tube to remove gastric contents
    e. Emotional support for parents; explain all procedures; answer questions
    f. Observe for passage of abnormal brown stool (indicates the intussusception has reduced itself); report to physician immediately
  2. Postoperative
    a. General postoperative care
    b. IV fluids as ordered; NPO
    c. Record intake and output
    d. Auscultate for return of bowel sounds
    e. Observe all stools and record
    f. Resume feedings slowly as ordered

NERVOUS SYSTEM

HYDROCEPHALUS

A. Definition: disorder caused by an obstruction of cerebrospinal fluid drainage or by impaired absorption of CSF fluid in the subarachnoid space; characterized by an excess of cerebrospinal fluid (CSF) within the cranial cavity, which causes an enlarged head and potential brain damage or retardation; it occurs in association with several other anomalies
B. Symptoms: bulging of the anterior fontanel, enlargement of the head, irritability, lethargy, opisthotonos, "setting-sun" sign (sclera can be seen above the iris because of increased intracranial pressure); lower extremity spasticity
C. Diagnosis: based on the symptoms, frequent measurements of head circumference, computerized tomography (CT), and magnetic resonance imaging (MRI)
D. Treatment/nursing interventions
  1. Surgical repair is necessary to relieve the obstruction or to shunt the CSF from the ventricles of the brain into the abdomen (ventriculoperitoneal shunt) (Fig. 8-7)
  2. Postoperative care includes frequent position changes to prevent pressure on the head, care of the shunt, general postoperative care, and observation for complications (infection, shunt malfunction, return of increased ICP)
  3. Measure head circumference daily

DOWN'S SYNDROME

A. Definition: an abnormality caused by extra chromosome 21 (trisomy 21). Children with Down's syndrome are born

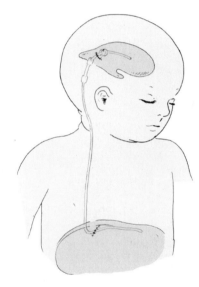

Figure 8-7.   Ventriculoperitoneal shunt. Catheter is threaded beneath the skin. (From Wong DL et al: *Whaley and Wong's Nursing care of infants and children,* ed 6, St Louis, 1999, Mosby.)

to women of all ages. The risk is higher in women over age 35, but infants with Down's syndrome are born to women under age 35 although the risk is much lower. Today, with the availability of prenatal diagnosis, fewer infants with trisomy 21 are born to older women.
B. Symptoms: hypotonia; small, low-set ears; slanted eyes; protruding tongue; small, flattened nose; short, broad neck; single transverse palmar (simian) crease; dry, cracked skin; congenital heart defects; and mental retardation
C. Diagnosis: based on the physical defects; chromosomal studies are done to determine specific defects
D. Treatment/nursing interventions
  1. Emotional support for parents; they expected a "normal" infant without defects
  2. Assist family in preventing physical problems (respiratory, integumentary, nutrition)
  3. Promote the child's developmental progress, and help parents to set realistic goals for the child

4. Encourage activity and intellectual stimulation for the child through early intervention programs and school
5. Genetic counseling for the parents

GENITOURINARY SYSTEM
EPISPADIAS AND HYPOSPADIAS
A. Definition: congenital conditions in male infants where urethra ends on the under side (hypospadias) or the top side (epispadias) of the penis, rather than at the end
B. Symptoms: obvious physical defects evident on physical examination; abnormal stream of urine
C. Diagnosis: based on physical examination
D. Treatment/nursing interventions
    1. The surgery to extend the urethra to the end of the penis is usually done in several stages when the child is 6 to 18 months of age. Infant should not be circumcised, because foreskin may be needed for later surgery
    2. Postoperative care includes inspection of the operative site for bleeding, catheter care, and emotional support for the child and parents, as well as general postoperative care

CRYPTORCHIDISM
A. Definition: failure of one or both testes to descend into the scrotal sac; sterility may result if not treated
B. Symptoms: testes not palpable in the scrotal sac on physical examination
C. Diagnosis: based on symptoms
D. Treatment/nursing interventions
    1. The testes often descend by 1 year of age
    2. Hormonal therapy (human chorionic gonadotropin [HCG]) may be used at an early age to promote descent of the testes into the scrotum
    3. Surgical intervention (orchiopexy) is usually necessary to bring the testes down the inguinal canal and into the scrotum; routine postoperative care

WILMS' TUMOR
A. Definition: tumor (nephroblastoma) in the kidney region
B. Symptoms: sometimes not symptomatic, discovered on routine exam; there may be occasional hematuria and elevated blood pressure; swelling or mass in the abdomen
C. Diagnosis: the tumor is often palpable through the abdominal wall; it occurs most often in children under 2 years of age and is usually found by the caregiver before the child reaches the age of 3
D. Treatment/nursing interventions
    1. Surgery to remove the tumor is performed within 48 hours of diagnosis; routine postoperative care is given
    2. Radiation therapy is given postoperatively as ordered
    3. Chemotherapy as ordered (see Chapter 3)
    4. Emotional support/education for parents
E. Prognosis is good with early diagnosis and treatment for children under 2 years of age

MUSCULOSKELETAL SYSTEM
CONGENITAL CLUBFOOT (TALIPES EQUINOVARUS)
A. Definition: defect in which the entire foot is inverted, heel is drawn up, and front of the foot is adducted; can affect one or both feet (Fig. 8-8)
B. Symptoms: obvious physical defect evident on physical examination

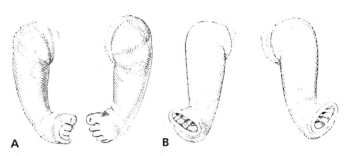

Figure 8-8. Feet casted for correction of bilateral congenital talipes equinovarus. **A,** Before correction. **B,** Undergoing correction in plaster casts. (From Brashear HR Jr, Raney RB: *Shands' handbook of orthopaedic surgery,* ed 10, St Louis, 1986, Mosby.)

C. Diagnosis: based on the presence of the physical defect on examination
D. Treatment/nursing interventions
    1. The deformity is usually repaired in stages; the type of treatment depends on the severity of the defect
    2. Various methods of treatment include manipulation and serial casting, splints, and surgery when necessary to repair the deformities; nursing care depends on method chosen

DEVELOPMENTAL DYSPLASIA OF THE HIP (DDH)
A. Definition: DDH describes a group of disorders related to abnormal development of the hip, in which there is a shallow acetabulum, subluxation, or dislocation; DDH may result from laxity of the supporting capsule or an abnormality of the acetabulum
B. Symptoms: limited hip abduction, apparent shortening of femur, asymmetry of gluteal and thigh folds (Fig. 8-9)
C. Diagnosis: symptoms found on physical examination by the physician/nurse practitioner
D. Treatment/nursing interventions
    1. Treatment is started as soon as the defect is diagnosed; the hip is manipulated into proper position and an abduction device (Pavlik harness, Fig. 8-10) or hip spica cast is applied; Bryant's traction, modified Bryant's traction, or modified Buck's extension may also be used
    2. Nursing care includes parent teaching regarding application of the harness and cast care

CARDIOVASCULAR SYSTEM
CONGENITAL HEART DEFECTS (CYANOTIC AND ACYANOTIC)
A. Atrial septal defect (ASD): abnormal opening in the septum between the two atria, or a patent foramen ovale, that causes left-to-right shunting of the blood (acyanotic)
B. Ventricular septal defect (VSD): abnormal opening in the septum between the two ventricles that causes left-to-right shunting of the blood (acyanotic)
C. Patent ductus arteriosus (PDA): the ductus arteriosus remains open after birth instead of closing off as normal, causing an overload of the left heart and a slight murmur (acyanotic)
D. Coarctation of the aorta: constriction of the aortic arch, causing hypertension in the upper body and hypotension in the lower body (acyanotic)

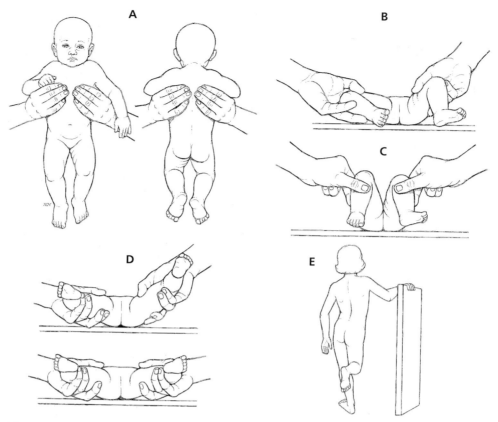

Figure 8-9.   Signs of developmental dysplasia of the hip. **A,** Asymmetry of gluteal and thigh folds. **B,** Limited hip abduction, as seen in flexion. **C,** Apparent shortening of the femur, as indicated by the level of the knees in flexion. **D,** Ortolani click (if infant is under 4 weeks of age). **E,** Positive Trendelenburg sign or gait (if child is weight bearing). (From Wong DL et al: *Whaley and Wong's Nursing care of infants and children,* ed 6, St Louis, 1999, Mosby.)

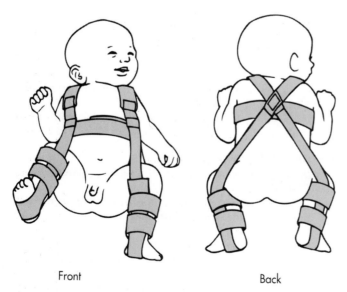

Front   Back

Figure 8-10.   Child in Pavlik harness. (From Ball JW: *Mosby's pediatric patient teaching guides,* St Louis, 1998, Mosby.)

E. Tetralogy of Fallot: consists of four congenital defects: pulmonary stenosis, ventricular septal defect, overriding of the aorta, and right ventricular hypertrophy (cyanotic)
F. Classic symptoms of congenital heart defects: dyspnea, difficulty with feeding, clubbing of fingers, cyanosis (in certain defects), heart murmurs, rapid pulse, recurrent respiratory infections, edema
G. Diagnosis: based on the symptoms, electrocardiograms, echocardiograms, cardiac catheterizations, and chest x-ray films
H. Treatment/nursing interventions
  1. Most defects must be corrected by surgical intervention, often in stages; some symptoms can be treated with medications as ordered
  2. Nursing care measures depend on the type of treatment or surgery; most often, immediate postoperative care is given in intensive care units
  3. Patient/parent teaching should include instructing parents to help the child conserve energy, without being overprotective

SICKLE CELL ANEMIA

A. Definition: autosomal disease occurring mainly in blacks, but also occurs on occasion in whites of Mediterranean descent; causes breakdown of red blood cells carrying an ab-

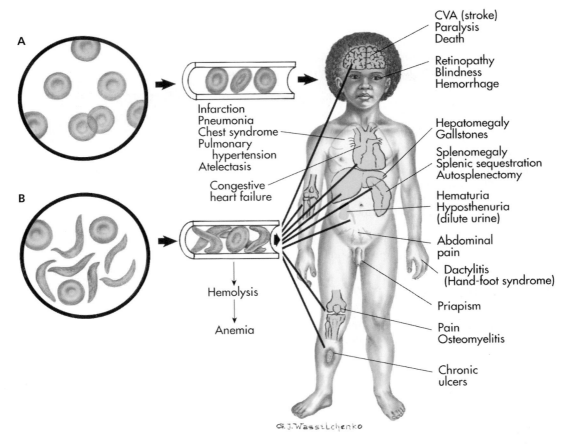

Figure 8-11. Differences between effects of **A,** normal, and **B,** sickled RBCs on circulation with selected consequences in a child. (From Wong DL et al: *Whaley and Wong's Nursing care of infants and children,* ed 6, St Louis, 1999, Mosby.)

normal hemoglobin S, which leads to a severe hemolytic anemia; the disease may not be recognized until the toddler or preschool period

B. Symptoms: appear only in children who inherit the trait from both parents; fatigue, anorexia, decreased hemoglobin; sickle cell crisis may occur, causing severe joint pain, abdominal pain, fever, and firm, distended abdomen (Fig. 8-11)

C. Diagnosis: based on the symptoms, family history of the disease, and specific blood tests including the sickle-cell slide preparation, sickle-turbidity test (Sickledex), and hemoglobin electrophoresis ("Fingerprinting")

D. Treatment/nursing interventions
  1. IV fluids and fluids by mouth (PO) as ordered
  2. Oxygen therapy, especially during sickle cell crisis
  3. Bed rest
  4. Electrolyte replacement
  5. Analgesics for pain as ordered
  6. Blood transfusions as ordered (packed red blood cells)
  7. Antibiotic therapy as needed
  8. Genetic counseling for parents
  9. Proper nutrition, as tolerated
  10. Avoid exposure to people with colds and infections

ENDOCRINE SYSTEM
HYPOPITUITARISM (DWARFISM)

A. Definition; growth retardation resulting from deficiency of the growth hormone (GH)

B. Symptoms: short stature, well-nourished appearance, delayed physical development

C. Diagnosis: based on the family history, child's growth patterns, physical examination, x-ray studies, and endocrine studies

D. Treatment/nursing interventions
  1. Replacement of the growth hormone by subcutaneous injections
  2. Early diagnosis and treatment help to prevent many physical and emotional problems that occur later in childhood
  3. Provide emotional support for the child and parents during diagnostic procedures and early stages of treatment (even after growth hormone therapy is started, growth will be slower than normal)

CONGENITAL HYPOTHYROIDISM (CRETINISM)

A. Definition: lack of thyroid function resulting from a failure of the embryonic development of the thyroid gland

B. Symptoms: usually do not appear until 6 to 12 weeks of age in bottle-fed infants and after weaning in breast-fed infants; include feeding problems, inactivity, anemia, thick, dry, mottled skin, bradycardia, relaxation of the abdominal muscles, and delayed development of the nervous system, which leads to mental retardation

C. Diagnosis: based on the symptoms and tests of thyroid function, such as initial measurement of the newborn's T_4 (thyroxin) and thyroid stimulating hormone (TSH) level

D. Treatment/nursing interventions
   1. Early diagnosis and treatment are essential in preventing retardation and other severe physiological symptoms
   2. Treatment is indefinite replacement therapy of the thyroid hormone
   3. Parent teaching concerning administration of the thyroid hormone, including signs and symptoms of thyroid overdose

Sudden Infant Death Syndrome (SIDS)

A. Definition: sudden death of an infant under 1 year of age that remains unexplained after a complete postmortem examination, including an investigation of the death scene and a review of the infant's clinical history; the leading cause of death in children between 1 and 12 months of age; the peak age for SIDS is 2 to 4 months; 95% of cases occur by the age of 6 months

B. Research: Numerous theories have been proposed regarding the cause of SIDS, but the exact cause is unknown; many researchers believe that it may be related to a brainstem abnormality in the regulation of cardiorespiratory control; other studies have demonstrated that infants sleeping in the prone position are at an increased risk for SIDS; because of these findings, the American Academy of Pediatrics recommends that healthy infants up to 6 months of age sleep on their side or back

C. Emotional support for the parents
   1. Parents always feel guilty and must be reassured that SIDS is not their fault
   2. Encourage them to allow an autopsy to try to determine a specific cause of death; this helps to allay their guilt and feelings that they could have prevented it
   3. Allow parents to spend some time with the child to say goodbye
   4. Refer the parents to the SIDS Foundation for counseling and support
   5. After the parents return home from the hospital, emotional support should continue to be provided for them by qualified healthcare professionals

TODDLERHOOD (AGES 1 TO 3)
NORMAL GROWTH AND DEVELOPMENT
Physical Development

A. Toddlerhood shows a decrease in the rate of growth but an increase in the rate of development

B. Toddlers gain approximately 4 to 6 lb (1.8 to 2.7 kg) each year, and add 3 inches (7.5 cm) in height per year

C. They have learned, and continue to learn, to walk between 1 and 2 years of age

D. Visual acuity of 20/20 is achieved during the toddler years

E. Toddlers continue to learn to talk, learning new words and phrases; their favorite word is "no!"

Psychosocial Development

A. Behavior in the toddler is characterized by several things
   1. Negativism: toddlers say "no!" to almost everything; this is part of their becoming an individual person separate from their parents
   2. Ritualism: developing and following certain patterns of behavior to develop their own security
   3. Temper tantrums: toddlers like to do everything for themselves; when they can't, they are frustrated, and this frustration leads to temper tantrums; tantrums should be ignored as much as possible, and the child should be dealt with after the "storm" is over

B. Toddlers are in Erikson's stage of "autonomy vs. shame and doubt"; they need to develop a sense of autonomy and self-control; to do this, toddlers must be able to make some choices as well as learn to function within the limits set for them

C. Discipline and limit setting must be consistent to be effective; it is also important to remember to criticize the behavior, not the child

D. Toilet training is an important part of the socialization process in toddlers; they should be praised when they use the "potty chair" or toilet properly, rather than being punished for not using it; toilet training should only begin when the toddler is physically capable of controlling bowel and bladder (18 to 24 months)

HEALTH PROMOTION

A. Nutrition needs change because of change in growth rate; toddlers need less food, and their appetites decrease (18 months of age)
   1. Teach parents that the decrease in food intake is normal
   2. The child is more autonomous now; should be allowed to feed himself or herself as much as possible; "finger foods" are ideal
   3. Snacks should be nutritious; cheese, fruits, and crackers are good choices
   4. Desserts should not be used as rewards; this gets the toddler into a habit of expecting something sweet whenever doing something good

B. Prevention of accidents is a major responsibility with toddlers; keep dangerous items (sharp objects, medications, cleaning supplies) out of their reach; toddlers should not be left unattended near a bathtub, swimming pool, whirlpool bath, or hot objects, such as pans on the stove or open flames

C. Teaching the toddler good oral hygiene habits is necessary to prevent early tooth decay and problems with gums
   1. Brushing the teeth should begin between 12 and 18 months of age
   2. Dental checkups with the dental hygienist or dentist should begin at about 1 year of age
   3. Proper nutrition helps prevent a large amount of early dental caries

HEALTH PROBLEMS
Respiratory Disorders
EPIGLOTTITIS

A. Definition: one of the croup syndromes; a severely inflamed epiglottis; begins abruptly and progresses rapidly into severe respiratory distress; usually caused by *Haemophilus influenzae* bacteria

B. Symptoms: fever, sore throat, difficulty swallowing; child insists on sitting up, leaning forward with chin thrust out, mouth open, and tongue protruding; drooling is common

C. Diagnosis: based on the symptoms and visualization of enlarged reddened epiglottis on careful throat examination and enlarged epiglottis on lateral neck x-ray examination

D. Treatment/nursing interventions
   1. Do *not* examine throat unless immediate intubation can be performed if necessary
   2. Keep child as quiet as possible; allow child to sit up in bed or on lap of parent
   3. Keep emergency tracheostomy tray (and intubation tray) with patient at all times
   4. Administer IV fluids and antibiotics as ordered
   5. Monitor child closely

CYSTIC FIBROSIS

A. Definition: an autosomal recessive hereditary disease affecting the exocrine glands; the lungs, pancreas, liver and small intestine produce abnormal mucus secretions and become obstructed

B. Symptoms
   1. In newborns: meconium ileus, bile-stained emesis, distended abdomen, no stools, and salty "taste" to the skin resulting from increased sodium in the perspiration
   2. In infants and children: harsh, dry cough, frequent bronchial infections, malnutrition, distended abdomen, barrel chest, clubbed fingers, and bulky, greasy, foul-smelling stools (steatorrhea)

C. Diagnosis: based on family history, a history of FTT, the symptoms, lung changes revealed by chest x-ray films, an elevated sweat chloride level (increased sodium in the perspiration), and stool analysis for fat and enzymes

D. Treatment/nursing interventions
   1. Pancreatic enzymes are given as ordered with food to improve digestion of fats and proteins
   2. High-carbohydrate, high-protein, and low-fat diet
   3. Increased amounts of salt and water-soluble vitamins
   4. Inhalation therapy: nebulizer treatments of bronchodilators (see Chapter 3) and recombinant human deoxyribonuclease (Dnase) to decrease the viscosity of the mucus
   5. Postural drainage and chest physiotherapy to help in expectoration of mucus
   6. Physical exercise to stimulate mucus secretion
   7. Antibiotics for all pulmonary infections
   8. Parent teaching regarding diet, medications, and inhalation therapy for proper home care after discharge

   9. Referral to the Cystic Fibrosis Foundation for financial or emotional support
   10. Genetic counseling for parents

Cardiovascular Disorder: Kawasaki Disease (Mucocutaneous Lymph Node Syndrome)

A. Definition: an acute inflammation of the vascular system; cause unknown; it is most common in children under age 5, with peak incidence seen in the toddler age group; diagnosed in every racial group, but is most common in Japanese children; most cases diagnosed in late winter and early spring; with proper treatment, 25% of children develop cardiac complications, including damage to the cardiac blood vessels and the heart muscle itself

B. Symptoms/diagnosis: child must exhibit five of the following six criteria, including fever: fever for 5 or more days; bilateral conjunctival inflammation; changes in the oral mucus membranes, including dryness and erythema; changes in the extremities, such as erythema and peeling of the palms and soles, and peripheral edema; cervical lymphadenopathy; and polymorphous rash

C. Treatment/nursing interventions
   1. High dose IV immune globulin (IVIG) to decrease the fever and incidence of coronary artery damage
   2. Salicylate therapy to control fever and symptoms of inflammation
   3. Intake and output, daily weight (to assess for signs of CHF)
   4. Mouth care
   5. Careful observation of the IV site
   6. Quiet environment and proper rest
   7. Emotional support for the child and family
   8. Long-term follow-up should include monitoring of heart disease risk factors (BP, cholesterol levels) and promotion of a heart-healthy lifestyle (proper nutrition, exercise, and avoidance of smoking)

Gastrointestinal Disorder: Celiac Disease (Gluten Enteropathy)

A. Definition: a defect of metabolism precipitated by the ingestion of wheat or rye gluten, leading to impaired fat absorption; exact cause unknown

B. Symptoms: usually appear between 1 and 5 years of age; chronic diarrhea with bulky, greasy, foul-smelling stools; malnutrition; anorexia; unhappy disposition; retardation of growth; distended abdomen; and muscle wasting especially of extremities and buttocks

C. Diagnosis: laboratory tests including stool analysis for fecal fat; blood studies for anemia, hypoproteinemia, and serum iron; definitive diagnosis is based on these tests, the symptoms, and a jejunal biopsy to demonstrate changes in the jejunal mucosa

D. Treatment/nursing interventions
   1. Gluten-free, low-fat diet; rice cereal for infants
   2. Parent teaching regarding diet and specific foods to avoid
   3. The child should be protected from respiratory infections, which may lead to exacerbations of the disease known as celiac crisis (characterized by severe vomiting and diarrhea, dehydration, and acidosis)

Neurosensory Disorders

EYE DISORDERS

STRABISMUS

A. Definition: failure of the eyes to direct and focus on the same object at the same time
B. Symptoms: deviation of one eye to the center (esotropia) or to the other corner (exotropia)
C. Diagnosis: based on the symptoms
D. Treatment/nursing unaffected interventions
 1. Patching of unaffected eye to increase visual stimulation of weaker eye
 2. Glasses and exercise to help improve vision
 3. Surgery to correct the muscle defects is often necessary when conservative treatment is ineffective
 4. Preoperative and postoperative nursing care as indicated

AMBLYOPIA ("LAZY EYE")

A. Definition: reduced visual acuity in one eye, usually caused by strabismus; the eyes are unable to focus and work together, and blindness may occur in the weaker eye if there is no treatment
B. Symptoms: blurred vision, double vision, development of a "blind spot"
C. Diagnosis: based on results of Snellen's eye test and the symptoms
D. Treatment/nursing interventions: patching of the unaffected eye so that the child is forced to use and focus the weaker eye; the best time for treatment is during early childhood

CEREBRAL PALSY

A. Definition: a group of nonprogressive disorders caused by a malfunction of the motor centers of the brain; oxygen deprivation (anoxia) damages the brain's motor centers prenatally, during or immediately after delivery, or during childhood after an accident or disease
B. Symptoms: abnormal muscle tone and coordination, delays in development, hearing and vision impairment, seizures, and, in some cases, mental retardation
C. Diagnosis: based on the mother's prenatal history, birth history, history of an accident or disease, presence of delays in growth and development, and abnormal neurological examination (Table 8-2)
D. Types of cerebral palsy
 1. Spastic: hypertonicity with poor control of posture, balance, and coordination; impaired motor skills; hypertonicity of muscles and tendon reflexes lead to development of contractures
 2. Dyskinetic: abnormal involuntary movement; athetosis, characterized by slow, writhing movements that involve extremities, trunk, neck, facial muscles, and the tongue
 3. Ataxic: wide-based gait; disintegration of movements of the upper extremities when the child reaches for objects
 4. Mixed type: combination of spasticity and athetosis
E. Treatment/nursing interventions
 1. Treatment and care are supportive to ensure optimal level of development for the child

TABLE 8-2   Cerebral Palsy: Predisposing Factors and Known Causes

Risk Factors	Associated Causes
Prenatal	
Maternal	Metabolic diseases
	Nutritional deficiencies (e.g., anemia)
	Twin or multiple births
	Bleeding
	Toxemia
	Blood incompatibilities
	Exposure to radiation
	Infection (e.g., rubella, toxoplasmosis, cytomegalic inclusion disease)
	Premature labor
Prematurity	Asphyxia leading to cerebral hemorrhage
Genetic factors	Absence of corpus callosum, aqueductal stenosis, cerebellar hypoplasia
Congenital anomalies of the brain	Unknown causes not evident on clinical examination
Perinatal	Anesthesia or analgesia during labor and delivery
	Mechanical trauma during delivery
	Immaturity at birth
	Metabolic disorders (e.g., hyperbilirubinemia, hypoglycemia, amino acid disorders, hyperosmolality)
	Electrolyte disturbances (e.g., hypernatremia, hypoglycemia)
Postnatal	Head trauma
	Infections (e.g., meningitis, encephalitis)
	Cerebrovascular accidents
	Toxicosis
	Environmental toxins (e.g., lead ingestion, methyl mercury ingestion from contaminated fish)

From McCance KL, Huether SE: *Pathophysiology: the biologic basis for disease in adults and children,* ed 3, St Louis, 1999, Mosby.

2. Physical and occupational therapy to help the child learn some control over muscle movements
3. Braces/splints as needed to hold extremities in correct positions of function
4. Use of wheelchairs, walkers, and crutches as needed for ambulation/locomotion
5. Speech therapy/assistance with feeding as needed
6. Treatment for respiratory problems, seizures, contractures as needed
7. Emotional support for the family and child; most often, cerebral palsy children are of normal intelligence and have only physical handicaps
8. Encourage the child to live as normal a life as possible; refer the family to supportive groups such as the Easter Seal Society

Accidents

A. Accidents are the major cause of death in children between 1 and 4 years of age, chiefly because of their ability to walk and move about more freely than during infancy, along with their unawareness of danger within the environment
B. Accident prevention during toddlerhood is a major task requiring the involvement of both parents and other family members; following are several basic suggestions for accident prevention
   1. Supervise play, especially around dangerous areas such as cars, swimming pools, and open flames or hot appliances
   2. Use well-designed, safe car seats or restraints
   3. Turn all handles of pots and pans in toward the stove, away from the child's reach
   4. Cover electrical outlets with protective plastic caps
   5. Do not allow the child to play with the bathtub faucets; do not leave the child unattended in the bathroom
   6. Keep all medications and poisonous substances out of the child's reach (preferably in a locked cabinet)
   7. Know the number and location of the nearest poison control center and hospital
   8. Put up gates at the top and bottom of stairwells
   9. Choose well-made toys appropriate for the child's age, without sharp edges or small removable pieces
   10. Store all guns, dangerous tools, and equipment in a locked cabinet
   11. Teach the toddler about common dangers such as "hot" items, looking "both ways" before crossing the street, and water safety
   12. Provide bicycle helmets for toddlers to wear every time they ride a bike

PRESCHOOL AGE (AGES 3 TO 5)
NORMAL GROWTH AND DEVELOPMENT
Physical Development

A. Growth is slow during the preschool years; children gain approximately 5 lb (2.3 kg) and 2 to 3 inches (5 to 7.5 cm) in height each year
B. Deciduous teeth are being replaced by permanent teeth; there is a definite need for proper dental hygiene and regular dental checkups at this age level and throughout childhood

C. Language development of preschoolers is rapid; 3-year-olds talk to themselves and their toys; 4-year-olds begin to talk and communicate more with other people

Psychosocial Development

A. Preschoolers are in Erikson's stage of "initiative vs. guilt"; at this age level they learn how to interact with other children and adults; they also learn the difference between proper and improper behavior, and the rewards and disciplines associated with each; without proper adult guidance, preschoolers can learn improper behavior and develop a sense of guilt and inferiority rather than a sense of initiative and accomplishment
B. Preschoolers begin to develop their imaginations; they use "magical thinking" and have difficulty distinguishing fantasy from reality
C. Preschoolers become acutely aware of their sexuality, including their roles as boys or girls and their sex organs; parents must work with their children in a positive way to help them develop healthy attitudes toward themselves and their bodies
D. Preschoolers continue to learn through play; they still use parallel play but also begin to use associative play (play with other children) and imitative play (play by imitating the actions of adults or other children)

HEALTH PROMOTION

A. Immunizations started in infancy and toddlerhood should continue according to schedule (see Fig. 8-2)
B. Nutrition should be appropriate to age, keeping in mind that growth is slow during this period; preschoolers should be eating foods from all four basic food groups

HEALTH PROBLEMS
Communicable Diseases

See Appendix G

Respiratory Disorders: Tonsillitis and Adenoiditis

A. Definition: inflammation of the tonsils and adenoids caused by chronic upper respiratory infection
B. Symptoms: sore throat, difficulty in swallowing and breathing ("mouth breathers"), hoarseness, harsh cough
C. Diagnosis: based on the symptoms and the presence of swelling and redness of the tonsils and adenoids on examination
D. Treatment/nursing interventions
   1. Acute infections are treated with antibiotics as ordered, increased oral fluids, and warm saltwater gargles
   2. If chronic infections continue after antibiotic treatment, surgery is often indicated (tonsillectomy and adenoidectomy); however, surgery is less common today than in the past
   3. Postoperative nursing care measures include keeping the child in a prone position with head to the side until fully awake; monitoring vital signs frequently; checking the throat and nares for active bleeding; keeping the suction equipment at the bedside for emergency use; observing the child for frequent swallowing (this may indicate oozing of blood in the nasopharynx or pharynx); analgesic/antipyretic drugs for discomfort; and encouraging cool clear oral fluids after the nausea subsides

(synthetic juices less irritating than natural juices). Warm saltwater gargles may be used beginning 1 week after the surgery

4. Teach the child not to cough, clear the throat, or blow the nose, to help decrease risk of bleeding. Provide written instructions to parents regarding post-op care and possible complications

Genitourinary Disorders

NEPHROTIC SYNDROME

A. Definition: massive proteinuria, hypoalbuminemia, hyperlipemia, and edema; is the most common glomerular injury in children; it can be classified as primary (restricted to glomerular injury) or secondary (when it develops as part of a systemic illness)

B. Symptoms: edema of the face, extremities, and abdomen; proteinuria, hypoalbuminemia, respiratory distress; malnutrition; irritability; increased susceptibility to infection

C. Diagnosis: based on decreased serum protein levels and increased proteinuria, edema, and hypocholesterolemia, and on results of a renal biopsy

D. Treatment/nursing interventions
1. Nephrotic syndrome is a chronic disorder, with remissions and exacerbations, usually lasting 12 to 18 months; treatment measures continue for an extended period
2. Corticosteroids as ordered to reduce the edema
3. Administration of an oral alkylating agent, usually Cytoxan, alternating with prednisone, to reduce the relapse rate and induce long-term remission
4. Frequent urine testing for protein and albumin
5. Recording of intake and output
6. Diuretics as ordered (not always effective)
7. Low-salt diet during exacerbations
8. Antibiotics as ordered during exacerbations
9. Parent teaching for home care regarding medications, diet, and follow-up

ACUTE GLOMERULONEPHRITIS

A. Definition: inflammation of the glomeruli and nephrons of the kidney; it may occur as a primary event, or as a reaction to an infection (most often streptococcal, pneumococcal, or viral)

B. Symptoms: edema of the face and eyes, anorexia, dark-colored ("tea") urine, oliguria, listlessness, irritability, headache, abdominal discomfort, vomiting, slightly elevated blood pressure, proteinuria; if the disease occurs as a result of a systemic infection, the symptoms occur approximately 10 days after the infection

C. Diagnosis: based on the symptoms and a positive recent history of streptococcal or other infection

D. Treatment/nursing interventions
1. Bed rest for 2 to 4 weeks until the symptoms subside
2. Antibiotics as ordered (see Chapter 3)
3. Liquid diet, progressing to a regular, low-salt diet
4. Measurement of intake and output and observation of color of urine
5. Frequent checking and recording of blood pressure
6. Urine testing for protein and specific gravity
7. Daily weights
8. Antihypertensives and diuretics for elevated BP, as ordered

Circulatory Disorders

HEMOPHILIA

A. Definition: an X-linked recessive disorder of metabolism that results in a delayed coagulation of blood; hemophilia is typed according to which clotting factor is affected

B. Symptoms: prolonged bleeding and clotting times; easy bruising and bleeding into tissues and joints; joint pain

C. Diagnosis: based on the symptoms, as well as family health history, and a prolonged clotting time

D. Treatment/nursing interventions
1. Observations for any signs of internal bleeding and shock
2. Transfusions as ordered with the missing clotting factor
3. Frequent laboratory tests, such as partial thromboplastin time (PTT), clotting time, complete blood count (CBC); screening for HIV (from receiving contaminated transfusions or clotting factors)
4. Corticosteroids and nonsteroidal antiinflammatory drugs as ordered
5. Exercise and physical therapy to strengthen muscles around joints
6. Protection of the child from injuries as much as possible
7. Emotional support and counseling for the child and parents
8. Parent teaching regarding follow-up physical examinations, protecting the child from physical harm, the need for immediate care if any injury occurs, and administering the clotting factor to the child
9. Referrals to community resources, such as the National Hemophilia Foundation
10. Genetic counseling for parents

LEUKEMIA

A. Definition: a broad term given to a group of malignant diseases of the bone marrow and lymphatic system; an unrestricted proliferation of immature WBCs in the bloodforming tissues of the body; classified according to its predominant cell type and level of maturity, acute lymphocytic leukemia (ALL) is the most common childhood leukemia

B. Symptoms: the three main consequences of bone marrow dysfunction are anemia, infection, and bleeding; other symptoms include lethargy, pallor, anorexia, fever, pain in the bones and joints; petechiae, easy bruising, and sores in the mouth; decreased RBCs and WBCs

C. Diagnosis: made on the basis of history, symptoms, an elevated WBC count, and presence of immature leukocytes and blast cells in a bone marrow biopsy or aspiration

D. Treatment/nursing interventions
1. Leukemia is a chronic, sometimes fatal disease with remissions and exacerbations; the child and family need a great deal of emotional support from the physician and nursing staff
2. Chemotherapy drugs and corticosteroids as ordered (see Chapter 3)
3. IV fluids and blood transfusions as ordered
4. Administration of pain medications as ordered; joint pain during exacerbations may be severe, especially in

the more advanced stages; higher-than-normal doses are often required

5. Proper skin and mouth care
6. Providing proper nutrition as the child's condition allows
7. Prevention of infections whenever possible; chemotherapy drugs lower the WBC count, which in turn decreases the child's resistance to infection
8. Observation for possible side effects of chemotherapy drugs
9. Bone marrow transplants may be ordered in certain types of leukemia to replace unhealthy bone marrow; an exact "match" is often difficult to find

Musculoskeletal Disorder: Muscular Dystrophy

A. Definition: a group of hereditary muscle diseases (recessive trait) characterized by gradual degeneration of muscle fibers, which is evidenced by muscle wasting and weakness and increasing disability and deformity
B. Symptoms: gradual muscle weakness including difficulty walking, standing up, a "waddle" gait, and mild mental retardation; most symptoms appear in children between 3 and 5 years of age
C. Diagnosis: based on the history of the symptoms, family history, muscle biopsy to determine muscle degeneration, electromyography (EMG), and serum enzyme measurement
D. Treatment/nursing interventions
  1. There is no cure for muscular dystrophy, so treatment is supportive
  2. Encourage the child to be as active and to lead as normal a life as possible
  3. Range-of-motion exercises and physical therapy as ordered to prevent contractures
  4. Use of walkers, crutches, braces, and wheelchairs as needed
  5. Emotional support for the parents and child; this is a progressive disease, and the family requires ongoing support by the health care team
  6. Frequent medical checkups to observe for progressive symptoms such as respiratory distress
  7. Genetic counseling for the parents

SCHOOL AGE (AGES 6 TO 12)
NORMAL GROWTH AND DEVELOPMENT
Physical Development

A. Growth is slow in children between the ages of 6 and 10 years; the child gains 4½ to 6½ lb (2 to 3 kg) and 2 inches (5 cm) per year
B. Bone growth is slow; the cartilage is replaced by bone at the bone epiphyses
C. Middle childhood (ages 6 to 12) is the stage of development when deciduous teeth are shed

Psychosocial Development

A. School-age children are in Erikson's stage of "industry vs. inferiority"; an eagerness to develop new skills and interests, and the processes of cooperating and competing with other children are characteristics of this age that engender a sense of accomplishment rather than a sense of inferiority and poor self-worth
B. Children ages 7 to 10 start to become more influenced by their peer group than by their parents; they develop "best friends" and start to separate into boy and girl groups
C. The most significant skill acquired during the school-age period is the ability to read

HEALTH PROMOTION

A. Communicable disease prevention is accomplished by timely immunizations, proper rest and diet, and frequent medical and dental check-ups
B. Accident prevention remains a major factor at this age level; safety measures should include rules for bicycle and skateboard safety (helmets and pads for safety in competitive sports such as baseball, football, and soccer)
C. Sex education should begin at this age level and should be presented by the parents in simple, honest terms; audiovisual aids such as books and pictures are available to assist parents in presenting the information on the child's level
D. Promotion of a balanced diet continues to be important at this age level; high-calorie, low-nutrition snacks are popular with school-age children but often lead to excess weight gain

HEALTH PROBLEMS
Respiratory Disorders: Allergic Conditions
ASTHMA

A. Definition: an obstructive airway disease caused by spasms of bronchial tubes; results from hypersensitivity of the airways, accompanied by inflammation and edema of the bronchial mucosa and increased production of bronchial mucus; it is often caused by an allergic response to allergens ("triggers") such as pollen, animal fur, food, or irritants, such as tobacco smoke, exercise, cold air, respiratory infections, and changes in the weather; it is the most common chronic disease of childhood
B. Symptoms: irritability; restlessness; tightness in the chest; hacking, nonproductive cough; dyspnea; wheezing
C. Diagnosis: based on the symptoms, physical examination, the child's history, family history, chest x-ray films that rule out other respiratory diseases, and pulmonary function studies
D. Treatment/nursing interventions
  1. Bronchodilator medications as ordered (administered by inhalation, by mouth, or by injection) (see Chapter 3)
  2. Antiinflammatory medications, either corticosteroids (prednisone) or nonsteroidal agents (cromolyn sodium) administered by inhalation, by mouth, or by injection
  3. Chest physiotherapy
  4. IV fluids as ordered
  5. Liquid diet, progressing to a regular diet
  6. Identification and removal of the allergens if possible
  7. Parent and child teaching regarding home care including medications, removal of any potential "triggers," use of peak flow meter to measure peak expiratory flow rate, and follow-up examinations

ALLERGIC RHINITIS (HAY FEVER)

A. Cause: an allergy to some pollen, dust, or animal fur
B. Symptoms: sneezing, runny nose, postnasal drip, and watery, itchy eyes

C. Diagnosis: based on the symptoms and results of allergy testing done to discover specific allergen
D. Treatment/nursing interventions
1. Find and remove the allergen if possible
2. Antihistamines or decongestants as ordered
3. Immunotherapy may be necessary if symptoms cannot be controlled

Gastrointestinal Disorders
APPENDICITIS
A. Definition: inflammation of the appendix, often following an infection elsewhere in the body
B. Symptoms: localized abdominal tenderness in the right lower quadrant (increased on rebound during palpation), abdominal rigidity, decreased bowel sounds, fever, nausea and vomiting, and constipation
C. Diagnosis: based on the symptoms and usually an elevated WBC count
D. Treatment/nursing interventions
1. Removal of the inflamed appendix (appendectomy), preferably before it ruptures and spreads the infection throughout the abdomen, causing peritonitis
2. Routine postoperative care, including monitoring vital signs, frequent observation of the incision or dressing for bleeding, careful recording of intake and output, and administration of IV fluids as ordered
3. Antibiotics may be ordered if there is a possibility of infection (especially with a ruptured appendix)
4. Pain medication as ordered

PINWORMS
A. Definition: worms that affect the intestine; the worms or eggs are swallowed and are spread easily from person to person by the hands, linen, or food
B. Symptoms; itching around the anus, anorexia, and diarrhea
C. Diagnosis: made by the cellophane tape test; the eggs are captured from the anal area during the night or early morning hours by placing a tongue blade covered with cellophane tape at the anal opening; the worms come out of the intestine at night to lay their eggs, and the eggs are picked up on the tape
D. Treatment/nursing interventions
1. Good handwashing technique to prevent spread of the worms and reinfection; keep fingernails short
2. Frequent changes of underwear and linen
3. Medication of choice is mebendazole (see Chapter 3)
4. Examination and treatment of all family members, because pinworms are easily transmitted

Nervous System Disorder: Epilepsy
A. Definition: chronic seizure disorder with recurrent and unprovoked seizures; although there are many causes for seizures, most are idiopathic
B. Symptoms: classification of seizures (Box 8-1)
C. Diagnosis: based on the evidence of seizures; differentiation of the type of seizure by physical examination, neurological assessment, patient history, and changes in the electroencephalogram (EEG) (changes in the brain wave patterns)
D. Treatment/nursing interventions
1. Anticonvulsant medications as ordered (see Chapter 3)
2. Parent and child education regarding medications and

Box 8-1   International Classification of Epileptic Seizures

I. Partial seizures (seizures beginning locally)
  A. Simple partial seizures (with elementary symptoms; consciousness unimpaired)
   • With motor symptoms
   • With somatosensory or special sensory symptoms
   • With autonomic symptoms
   • Compound forms (with psychic symptoms)
  B. Complex partial symptoms (temporal lobe or psychomotor; generally with impaired consciousness)
   • With impairment of consciousness only
   • With cognitive symptoms
   • With affective symptoms
   • With psychosensory symptoms
   • With psychomotor symptoms
   • Compound forms
  C. Partial seizures, secondarily generalized
II. Generalized seizures (bilaterally symmetrical; without local onset; with impairment of consciousness)
   • Tonic-clonic (grand mal) seizures
   • Tonic seizures
   • Clonic seizures
   • Absence (petit mal) seizures
   • Atonic seizures
   • Myoclonic seizures
   • Infantile spasms
   • Akinetic seizures
III. Unilateral seizures (those involving one hemisphere)
IV. Unclassified epileptic seizures (incomplete data)

Modified from Commission on Classification and Terminology of the International League Against Epilepsy: Proposal for revised clinical and electroencephalographic classification of epileptic seizures, *Epilepsia* 22:489-501, 1981.

---

the necessity of taking them as prescribed; safety factors; actions to take if the child has a seizure at home; the importance of follow-up physical examinations and laboratory work (to measure blood levels of anticonvulsants)
3. In children with poorly controlled seizures, a ketogenic diet (either with or without the use of anticonvulsants) has been tried with moderate success in some children; children on this strict diet must be followed closely by a dietitian, neurologist, and pediatrician; the length of time of the diet ranges from 1 to 3 years
4. Community referrals to support groups such as the National Epilepsy Foundation

Musculoskeletal Disorder: Scoliosis
A. Definition: a lateral S-shaped curvature of the spine; it can be congenital or caused by a variety of conditions, but most often has no known cause (idiopathic); most often seen in young girls, and is most noticeable at the time of the preadolescent growth spurt

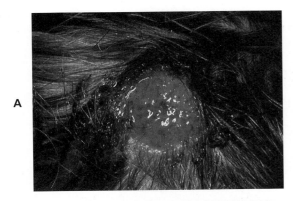

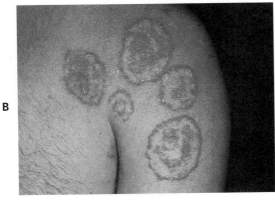

Figure 8-12. **A,** Tinea capitis. **B,** Tinea corporis. Both infections are caused by Microsporum canis, the "kitten" or "puppy" fungus. (From Habif TP: *Clinical dermatology: a color guide to diagnosis and therapy,* ed 3, St Louis, 1996, Mosby.)

B. Symptoms: poor posture; uneven length of legs; asymmetry of shoulder and hip height; pelvic obliquity
C. Diagnosis: based on symptoms, x-ray films, and physical examination
D. Treatment/nursing interventions
1. A brace (Milwaukee brace or Boston brace) or splint is often used along with exercises to prevent an increase in the degree of curvature; this may be the only treatment, or may be used before surgery
2. Spinal fusion may be necessary to correct severe scoliosis; postoperative care as indicated

Integumentary Disorders

RINGWORM
A. Definition: a fungal infection transferred from person to person or from animal to person; it can occur on the scalp (tinea capitis), the body (tinea corporis), and the feet (tinea pedis) (Fig. 8-12)
B. Symptoms: small papules, dry, scaly skin, and itching on the affected part
C. Diagnosis: based on the symptoms
D. Treatment/nursing interventions
1. Washing the affected areas with soap and water and removal of crusts
2. Antifungal ointment to affected areas as ordered
3. Antifungal oral medication as ordered (see Chapter 3)

PEDICULOSIS
A. Definition: infestation by lice of the scalp and hairy areas of the body
B. Symptoms: severe itching in the affected area and appearance of lice on the hair or clothing
C. Diagnosis: based on the symptoms
D. Treatment/nursing interventions
1. Pediculicide shampoo to hair/scalp as ordered; remaining nits are removed with an extra-fine-tooth comb
2. Washing of all linens and clothing in hot water to destroy the nits (small lice) and eggs of the lice
3. Emphasis on importance of follow-up treatment to prevent reinfestation
4. Examination and treatment of other family members (if affected)
5. Report to school, day-care facility

HIVES (URTICARIA)
A. Definition: an allergic reaction on the skin, usually caused by an allergy to food or drugs
B. Symptoms: bright red, raised wheals on the skin and itching of the affected areas
C. Diagnosis: based on the symptoms; allergy testing may be done to determine the specific allergen
D. Treatment/nursing interventions
1. Determination and removal of the allergen
2. Antihistamines as ordered to decrease the swelling and inflammation
3. Cool-water soaks to the affected areas to decrease the itching
4. Local soothing antipruritic lotions to affected areas as ordered
5. Keep the child's nails short to avoid itching and possible infection

Rheumatic Fever
A. Definition: autoimmune reaction to a group A beta hemolytic streptococcal pharyngitis (strep throat); it involves the joints, skin, brain, and heart
B. Symptoms: begin 2 to 6 weeks after the initial streptococcal infection; lethargy, anorexia, muscle and joint pain, fever, polyarthritis, chorea (muscle tremors and emotional upset), and carditis (Fig. 8-13)
C. Diagnosis: based on the symptoms; specific diagnosis based on the Jones criteria (Box 8-2)
D. Treatment/nursing interventions
1. Bed rest to decrease the workload on the heart and help prevent or ease the carditis
2. Feeding meals to the child during strict bed rest
3. Medications as ordered including salicylates for pain, steroids to decrease inflammation o the muscle and connective tissue, and antibiotics to fight infection (penicillin is the drug of choice) (see Chapter 3)
4. Emotional support and nonstressful diversion for the child during bed rest
5. Monitoring of frequent laboratory tests, including the WBC count and the erythrocyte sedimentation rate (ESR) (elevated in inflammatory diseases)
6. Parent and child teaching for home care, including the need for rest, proper nutrition, proper administration of medications, and the need for prophylactic anti-

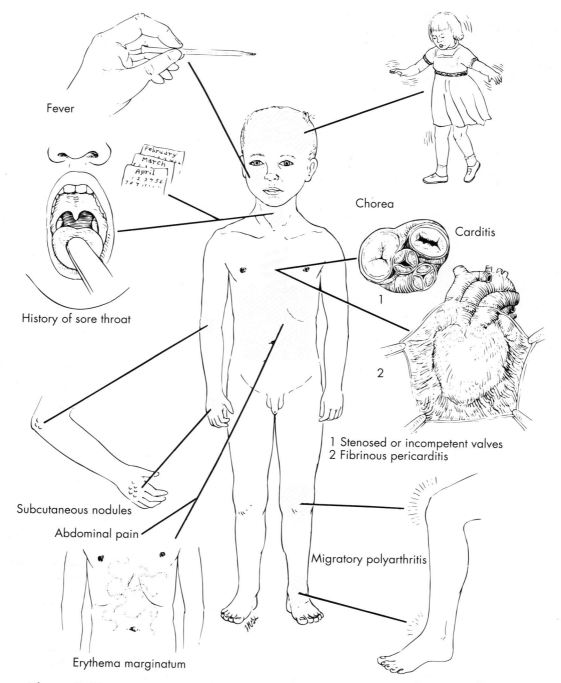

Fever

History of sore throat

Subcutaneous nodules

Abdominal pain

Erythema marginatum

Chorea

Carditis

1 Stenosed or incompetent valves
2 Fibrinous pericarditis

Migratory polyarthritis

Figure 8-13.   Signs and symptoms of rheumatic fever. (From Novak JC, Broom BL: *Ingalls & Salerno's maternal and child health nursing*, ed 9, St Louis, 1999, Mosby.)

biotic therapy before dental work and invasive procedures

Diabetes Mellitus

A. Definition: in Type I diabetes the beta cells of the pancreas stop producing insulin, which is necessary for the metabolism of fats, carbohydrates, and proteins; peak incidence is 10 to 15 years of age

B. Symptoms: rapid onset of symptoms, including easy fatigability, polydipsia (excessive thirst), polyphagia (increased

appetite), polyuria (increased urine output), glycosuria (glucose in the urine), and weight loss

C. Diagnosis: based on the symptoms, blood glucose levels, and the presence of glucose and ketones in the urine

D. Treatment/nursing interventions
   1. Daily insulin administration by subcutaneous injections (usually twice a day), or by a means of a portable insulin pump (see Chapter 3)
   2. American Diabetes Association diet as ordered
   3. Routine blood sugar monitoring; Chemstrips, Accu-

Box 8-2 **Guidelines for the Diagnosis of Initial Attack of Rheumatic Fever (Jones Criteria, 1992 Update)***

Major Manifestations

Carditis
Polyarthritis
Chorea
Erythema marginatum
Subcutaneous nodules

Minor Manifestations

Clinical findings
Previous rheumatic fever or rheumatic heart disease
Arthralgia
Fever
Laboratory findings
Acute phase reactants
Erythrocyte sedimentation rate
C-reactive protein, leukocytosis
Prolonged PR interval

Supporting Evidence of Streptococcal Infection

Increased titer of streptococcal antibodies
ASO (antistreptolysin O)
Other antibodies
Positive throat culture for group A *Streptococcus*
Recent scarlet fever

From Guidelines for the diagnosis of rheumatic fever, *JAMA* 268:2070, 1992. Copyright 1992, American Medical Association.
*The presence of two major criteria or of one major and two minor criteria indicates a high probability of the presence of rheumatic fever. Evidence of a preceding streptococcal infection greatly strengthens the possibility of acute rheumatic fever; its absence should make the diagnosis doubtful (except in Sydenham's chorea or long-standing carditis.)

check, or one-touch glucometers are commonly used for this
4. Routine urine testing for glucose and ketones may be done
5. Child and parent teaching regarding insulin injection technique, diet, exercise, urine testing, blood glucose monitoring, signs of hypoglycemia and hyperglycemia, and need for regular follow-up visits to the pediatrician
6. Support group for parents and child

ADOLESCENCE (AGES 13 TO 19)
NORMAL GROWTH AND DEVELOPMENT
Physical Development

A. During the adolescent period there is a growth spurt. This accelerated growth includes an increase in both height and weight. In girls, this occurs between 10 and 12 years of age; in boys it occurs between 12 and 14 years of age

B. Secondary sex characteristics also develop during early adolescence
1. In girls the pelvis widens, the breasts develop and enlarge, and body hair starts to appear
2. In boys the penis and scrotum enlarge and pubic and facial hair start to appear, puberty in boys officially begins with the first nocturnal emission

Psychological and Emotional Development

A. Adolescence is the time of transition from childhood to adulthood; adolescents are in Erikson's stage of "identity vs. role confusion"; they are in the process of developing a self-image or a sense of identity about who they are and what they want in life; if they do not develop a positive self-image and identity, they may develop a sense of inferiority, or a negative self-image

B. Development of a positive self-image and healthy personality depends a great deal on the adolescents' relationships with their peer group as well as with their family

C. Body image is the major part of adolescents' self-concept; sexuality and sexual feelings are a new part of their body images; physical appearance is important to how they perceive themselves as being accepted by their peer group
1. Boys' responses to puberty include pleasure at becoming a "man" as evidenced by enlargement of the sex organs, being able to shave, and the sexual feelings they begin to have during this stage; because of their strong sex drive, they often masturbate to relieve themselves of strong sexual tension
2. Girls' responses to puberty include a developing awareness of their bodily changes, both internal and external (such as hormonal changes and menstruation); the sex drive in girls is usually not as strong as it is in boys

HEALTH PROMOTION

A. Immunizations and physical examinations should continue according to schedule
B. Counseling and sex education, especially concerning AIDS, venereal disease, and birth control, should be made available to all adolescents
C. Counseling regarding drug and alcohol abuse should be presented and readily available to all adolescents who are in need of it
D. Emotional stress is high during adolescence; psychiatric counseling is necessary for some adolescents to work through their stresses and fears
E. Proper nutrition needs may not be met because of increased snacking, especially on high-calorie, high-fat foods; nutritional counseling may be helpful

HEALTH PROBLEMS
Substance Abuse (Drugs, Alcohol)

A. Definition: abuse of alcohol or mood-altering drugs, usually because of peer pressure or increased tension and stress
B. Signs of abuse: increased school absences, poor academic performance, changes in behavior patterns, wearing dark glasses inside, wearing long-sleeved shirts/blouses every day, and a sloppy, unclean appearance; signs often depend on drug being used

C. Diagnosis: based on the symptoms (signs of abuse)
D. Substances abused
  1. Alcohol
  2. Narcotics
  3. Psychedelic drugs (LSD, marijuana, PCP)
  4. Depressants (barbiturates, methaqualone [Quaalude])
  5. Minor tranquilizers (Valium)
  6. Hallucinogens (marijuana, LSD, PCP)
  7. Analgesics (codeine)
  8. Opiates (heroin, morphine, methadone)
  9. Valium
  10. Organic solvents (e.g., glue, cleaning fluids)
  11. Stimulants (amphetamines ["speed"], cocaine)
  12. Inhalants
E. Treatment/nursing interventions
  1. Prevention of the problem is of course the best treatment
  2. Emergency measures when necessary (such as cardiopulmonary resuscitation [CPR] and gastric lavage)
  3. Psychiatric counseling as needed for the adolescent and family; identify reason(s) for drug abuse
  4. Follow-up health care; group support and counseling as needed for adolescent and family

Suicide

A. Definition: the act of taking one's own life voluntarily
B. Etiology: suicide usually does not occur without warning; the adolescent usually has a history of emotional problems, difficult relationships, and emotional upsets including such things as divorce in the family, death of a family member or friend, or a self-identity crisis
C. Treatment/nursing interventions
  1. Prevention is the best treatment; listen for verbal clues, such as "after tomorrow, it won't matter anymore"; and watch for warning signs, such as giving away favorite possessions
  2. Psychiatric counseling to determine the reasons for the adolescent's actions; this should also include the family members
  3. Follow-up medical care as needed
  4. Emotional support and counseling for the family members, especially during the crisis stages

Anorexia Nervosa and Bulimia

A. Definition (these disorders can occur together or separately)
  1. Anorexia nervosa: an eating disorder characterized by a refusal to maintain a minimally normal body weight; most often seen in adolescent females
  2. Bulimia: an eating disorder characterized by repeated episodes of "binge eating," followed by inappropriate compensatory measures, such as self-induced vomiting; misuse of laxatives, diuretics, or other medications; fasting; or excessive exercise
B. Symptoms
  1. With anorexia nervosa there are three basic psychological disturbances: the inability to correctly perceive body size, the absence of hunger or inability to perceive hunger, and feelings of inadequacy or lack of self-esteem; other symptoms include amenorrhea, constipation, dry skin, low blood pressure, anemia, and lanugo (fine, soft hair) on the back and arms

  2. With bulimia, as the disease increases, the frequency of binges increases; the adolescent loses control over the binge/purge cycle; other symptoms are similar to those seen in anorexia nervosa
C. Diagnosis: based on the symptoms, family history, and psychologic evaluation
D. Treatment/nursing interventions
  1. The adolescent is usually hospitalized to correct the malnutrition and to identify and treat the psychological cause
  2. Behavior modification techniques are often used to assist in changing the adolescent's behavior; for example, privileges or visitors are withdrawn until the adolescent begins to gain weight
  3. Psychological counseling for the adolescent and family members to determine the cause

Crohn's Disease

A. Definition: a chronic, recurrent inflammatory disorder of the intestines; it occurs most often in upper-middle-class men and women, aged 15 to 35 years
B. Symptoms: regional ileitis causing acute low abdominal pain, fever, chronic diarrhea, weight loss, abdominal tenderness and distention, anemia, and failure to grow
C. Diagnosis based on the symptoms, x-ray films of the intestine (barium enema), endoscopy, and mucosal biopsy of the intestines
D. Treatment/nursing interventions
  1. The goal of treatment is to relieve the symptoms and discomfort
  2. Adequate rest and relaxation to alleviate stress
  3. Soft, low-fiber diet
  4. Corticosteroids as ordered to decrease inflammation of the intestines
  5. Sulfasalazine as ordered (as this interferes with the absorption of folic acid, folic acid may be ordered)
  6. Antidiarrheal drugs as ordered
  7. Antispasmodic drugs as ordered to relieve intestinal spasms
  8. Emotional support and psychological counseling as needed to decrease the stress level

Mononucleosis

A. Definition: an acute infectious viral disease causing an increase in mononuclear WBCs and signs of general infection; it is usually thought to be only mildly contagious and is spread by oral contact; the Epstein-Barr virus is the principal cause
B. Symptoms: general malaise, sore throat, fever, enlarged lymph glands, lack of energy, headache, red, flat rash on the body, and tonsillitis
C. Diagnosis: based on the symptoms, an elevated WBC count, and a positive Monospot blood test (which indicates increased agglutinins in the blood count)
D. Treatment/nursing interventions
  1. Antibiotics as ordered
  2. Antipyretics to relieve fever and discomfort
  3. Increased oral fluids; IV fluids may be ordered for severe dehydration
  4. Gargles or lozenges as ordered for sore throat
  5. Adequate rest and sleep

6. Diet as tolerated; if the patient can only tolerate fluids, high-calorie fluids should be provided

7. Patient teaching regarding follow-up care, including the need for adequate rest and sleep

Acne Vulgaris

A. Definition: a disorder of the sebaceous glands; the glands become irritated with the secretion of sebum and the interaction of the sebum with the hormones; the glands become impacted with sebum and form comedones (noninflamed) and papules and pustules (inflamed)

B. Symptoms: the appearance of the comedones, papules, and pustules on the face; they can also appear on other places on the body such as the chest and back

C. Diagnosis: based on the symptoms

D. Treatment/nursing interventions

1. Cleaning the affected areas with soap or soap substitute and water daily

2. A diet low in greasy foods, chocolate, and nuts may help decrease the amount of oil in the skin, avoid other foods that tend to exacerbate the condition

3. Nonprescription topical creams and lotions have limited effectiveness; retinoic acid and benzoyl peroxide, when used together (one in the morning, the other in the evening), are the most effective

4. Encouraging the adolescent to keep stress levels to a minimum when possible may help in keeping acne to a minimum

5. Patient teaching: papules and pustules should not be squeezed; they can become infected and spread

6. Counseling for the adolescent to maintain a positive body image

Acquired Immunodeficiency Syndrome (AIDS)

A. Definition: an immune disorder caused by a retrovirus, the human immunodeficiency virus (HIV)

1. The AIDS virus is known to be transmitted by blood and other body fluids containing blood (semen; saliva) (see Chapter 5, Chapter 7)

2. Three primary modes of transmission of the AIDS virus in children are prenatal exposure to infected mothers, blood transfusion, and engaging in high-risk activities (sexual or IV drug use, specifically with adolescents)

3. As of June 1997, more than 7900 children with AIDS had been reported to the Centers for Disease Control and Prevention (CDC); the majority of children with HIV are less than 7 years of age; the number of adolescents with HIV is increasing rapidly; AIDS is the sixth leading cause of death among children ages 1-4 years, and the seventh leading cause of death in children ages 5-14 years

B. Symptoms: recurrent or chronic infections (because of decreased number of CD-4 T-cells) including meningitis, pneumonia, and urinary tract infections; fever; weight loss; failure to thrive; anemia; hepatosplenomegaly; persistent lymphadenopathy

C. Diagnosis: abnormal laboratory values, including abnormal T-cell ratio, decreased T-lymphocytes and hypergammaglobulinemia; history of possible exposure to AIDS virus; positive HIV test; and history of recurrent infections

D. Treatment/nursing interventions

1. There is no cure for AIDS, so treatment and nursing care measures are supportive and designed to prevent and alleviate opportunistic infections

2. Antiretroviral drugs work to prevent reproduction of new virus particles; varying combinations of these drugs are used to slow progression of the disease (see Chapter 3)

3. Antibiotics/antifungal drugs as ordered (see Chapter 3)

4. IV gamma globulin may be helpful in compensating for the deficiency of B-lymphocytes

5. Adequate nutrition and fluid intake

6. Use of universal precautions when caring for the child in the hospital, clinic, or home

7. Maintenance of an environment as free from infection as possible

8. Immunizations against childhood diseases (as well as the pneumococcal and influenza vaccines) should be given; however, inactivated poliovirus should be given rather than the oral poliovirus

9. Promotion of normal development of the child

10. Education and emotional support for the child and family

E. Prognosis: poor, especially in children with AIDS who are under 1 year of age

THE BATTERED CHILD SYNDROME

A. Definition: abuse of children by parents or other caregivers; the abuse can be physical, sexual, nutritional, or emotional; can occur at any age

B. Characteristics of battered children

1. They are often from a unplanned pregnancy

2. Many of them were premature, had a low birth weight, or had major birth defects

3. They sometimes resemble a person that the parents disliked

C. Characteristics of abusive parents

1. One parent often has a previous emotional problem

2. The abuse is usually done by one parent; the other parent knows about the abuse but usually does not report it

3. Abusive parents often have very high expectations of their children; if they do not "perform" up to these expectations, they are "punished"

4. Abusive parents are often substance abusers

5. The most common characteristic of abusive parents is that often they were abused themselves as children; however, this is not always true

6. They come from all socioeconomic levels

D. Identifying the battered child

1. The child has many unexplained scars, bruises and injuries; many of these markings are characteristic of abuse (Fig. 8-14)

2. Bone fractures may be seen on x-ray examination at various stages of healing

3. The child exhibits signs of physical neglect: malnourishment or improper or dirty clothing

4. The parents' explanations of the child's injury are inconsistent; one parent's explanation differs from the other's, or it changes from one time to the next

5. The child withdraws when approached by the parents, nurse, or physician

6. The parents' emotional reaction is consistent with the extent of the child's injury

E. Nursing interventions for the battered child and parents
1. Interview the parents calmly regarding the history of the incident; document all information carefully
2. Nursing personnel must control their own feelings and attitudes toward the parents to work effectively with the family
3. Provide physical care for the child as needed
4. Emotional care for the child should include providing a safe environment, explaining all procedures, providing toys and familiar belongings while the child is hospitalized, and physical cuddling and holding when appropriate
5. Referrals should be made to the hospital social worker, the local department of children and family services, the police, and the psychologist as needed

HOSPITALIZATION AND THE CHILD

A. Preparation for hospitalization
1. The rationale for preparing children for hospitalization is based on the theory that fear of the unknown is more severe than fear of the known
2. Preadmission preparation can be done by both parents and professionals (nurses and physicians) honestly at a level the child can understand
3. Hospital admission procedures include the admission history, blood tests, chest x-ray studies when necessary, physical examination, and placement in the child's room and bed; these should be explained to the child during preadmission preparation
4. In preparing the child for any hospital procedure the nurse or parent should include all necessary information regarding the procedure and any necessary preparation; time should be allowed for questions by the child and parents

B. Hospitalization as a crisis
1. Children are more vulnerable to the crisis of illness and hospitalization because stress is a change from their usual state of health and routine, and children have a limited number of coping mechanisms to deal with stressful events
2. Their reactions to stress differ in each developmental age group
   a. Infants and toddlers: their major stress is separation anxiety (fear of being separated from their parents and family)
   b. Preschoolers: their major stresses are separation anxiety and fear of loss of body control and of bodily injury and pain
   c. School-age children: their major stresses are fear of separation (sometimes more from peers than from family), of loss of body control, and of bodily injury, mutilation, pain, and death
   d. Adolescents: their major stresses are fear of separation from their peer group; of loss of body control,

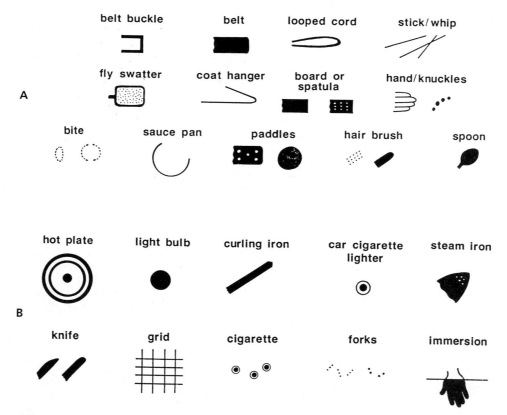

Figure 8-14. Characteristic markings often seen in child abuse. **A,** Marks from objects. **B,** Marks from burns. (From Reece RM, Smith MK, editors: Inflicted injury versus accidental injury, *Pediatr Clin North Am* Aug 1990.)

independence and identity; and of bodily injury and pain, especially concerning sexual changes

3. Nursing measures that can be used to minimize the hospitalized child's fears and stresses
   a. Open visiting for parents and siblings; visiting by peers in the school-age and adolescent groups should be encouraged
   b. Explain procedures or preparation for procedures at the child's age level (medical play)
   c. All the child to have favorite toys and games from home
   d. Nursing personnel should not lie to the child about the parents' visits; the visits should not be used as rewards or as something to be withheld if the child does not cooperate or behave
   e. Allow the child as much physical freedom as his or her condition will allow
   f. Allow the child to participate in decision making as much as possible, especially regarding treatments and procedures; this allows the child some control in the situation
   g. Encourage the parents to visit as much as possible; explain all procedures to them and encourage them to assist in their child's care if they are comfortable in doing so
   h. Instruct the parents not to lie to the child; lying only sets up a sense of mistrust among the child, the parents, and the hospital staff
   i. Administer pain medications as ordered whenever necessary; a child's pain response is affected by developmental level
   j. Expect some regressive behavior during the child's hospital stay; tell the parents that this is normal during stressful periods

C. Use of play during hospitalization
   1. Play in the hospital helps relieve tension and anxiety, lessens the stress of separation and feelings of homesickness, and helps the child to relax and feel more secure
   2. The play activities should be based on the child's age, interests, and limitations
   3. Play can be used for diversion, for recreation, and to play out the child's fears and anxieties over his illness and treatment
   4. Toys can come from home or from the hospital play area; they can even be adapted from hospital "stock" supplies
   5. Play therapy can be used to teach the child about procedures and surgery, as well as to help the child work through fears and anxieties about hospitalization

D. Preparation and teaching for discharge
   1. Preparation for discharge should begin during the admission by setting long-term goals concerning discharge
   2. Discharge planning should include several areas
      a. Parent-child teaching regarding home care procedures and medication regimen
      b. Follow-up care including physician appointments and the importance of keeping them
      c. Referrals to community agencies, public health nurses, and other resources as needed

Nursing Care of the Hospitalized Child

A. Safety factors
   1. Side rails should be kept up at all times when the child is in bed; if the bed is adjustable, it should be kept in the low position
   2. When restraints are used, they should be applied securely to the child; extremities should be checked frequently for impaired circulation caused by tight restraints; appropriate charting should be done
   3. Small toys, game pieces, and other small objects should be kept away from infants and toddlers who may swallow them
   4. Toddlers and young children should not be left unattended in their rooms or hallways; if they are out of bed, they should be observed continuously to avoid accidents and injuries
   5. Medications, needles, and syringes should be kept out of the reach of all children

B. Medication administration
   1. General guidelines in giving medications to children
      a. Approach the child with a cheerful, positive attitude and explain what you are going to do
      b. Be honest when talking to the child; tell the child it is medicine, not "juice" or "candy"
      c. When necessary, use foods or liquids to disguise the taste of bad-tasting medications
      d. Oral syringes or syringes without needles may be used to deliver oral medications to infants and young children
      e. Allow the child some control in the situation; make sure the question you ask the child is appropriate to the child's age level and the situation
      f. Intramuscular (IM) injections are safer and easier to give to a young child if a second person helps restrain the child
      g. Tell the child that it is all right to cry if the shot "hurts"; offer a Band-aid
      h. Teach the child to "say no" to street drugs but that the medicines received in the hospital are okay to take
   2. Safe IM injection technique includes the same steps used for IM injections in adults
      a. In infants the lateral thigh (vastus lateralis muscle) should be used
      b. In toddlers and preschoolers, the ventrogluteal area is the preferred site (lateral thigh can also be used)
      c. In older children and adolescents, other regularly used injection sites may be used (ventrogluteal muscle is the safest; deltoid and dorsogluteal muscles may also be used) (Fig. 8-15)

C. Assisting with treatments and procedures
   1. All tests and procedures should be explained to the child in an honest, simple manner; older children and adolescents should be allowed to ask questions and receive answers
   2. All children should be allowed to say "ouch" or to cry if the procedure is a painful one; rewards are often given after a painful procedure (a reward sticker, toy, or special food treat)
   3. The child may need to be held or restrained in certain positions for procedures; all equipment should be as-

sembled before the procedure is started so that the nurse can stay with the child as much as possible

D. Preoperative teaching
1. Patient teaching in pediatrics should include the child (preschool age and older) and the parents; both should be involved in the teaching and preparation for surgery
2. Use words that the child can understand; audiovisual aids (pictures, dolls, puppets, and bandages) are extremely useful in helping the child understand the procedure or surgery

3. Be honest with the child, especially regarding procedures or treatments that may be uncomfortable or painful
4. Tell the child that he or she will not feel any pain during the surgery because of the "special sleep" of anesthesia and that he or she will wake up after surgery is over in the recovery room
5. Include details specific to the child's surgery such as dressings, tubes, IV fluids, medications, the specific site of the pain or discomfort, and the diet restrictions before and after surgery

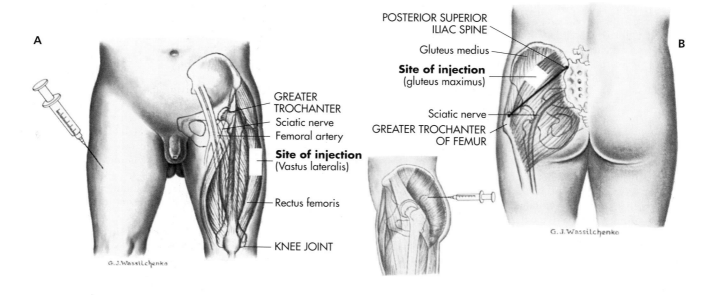

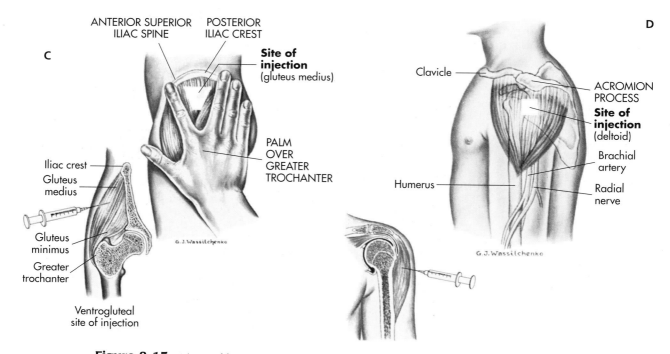

Figure 8-15. Acceptable intramuscular sites in children. **A,** Vastus lateralis. **B,** Dorsogluteal. **C,** Ventrogluteal. **D,** Deltoid. (From Wong DL et al: *Whaley and Wong's Nursing care of infants and children,* ed 6, St Louis, 1999, Mosby.)

E. General postoperative care
  1. Basic postoperative care is similar to nursing care of adult postoperative patients
     a. Frequent vital signs; pulse oximetry, as needed
     b. Observation of the incision or dressings
     c. Level of consciousness
     d. Intake and output, IV fluids, Foley catheter, nasogastric (NG) tube
     e. Administer pain medications as needed (IV, PO, epidurals; IM may be used, but should be avoided)
  2. Allow the child's parents to assist in the child's care if they desire to do so
  3. Explain all postoperative procedures before doing them
F. Care of the child in a cast
  1. The cast should be handled lightly with open palms while it is still damp to avoid indentations
  2. Observe and record the condition of the skin at the edges of the cast for color, warmth, irritation, sensation, and edema
  3. Check the color of the nail beds below the cast; check the pulse in the area below the cast if it is in an accessible area (radial or pedal pulse)
  4. Teach the child not to put anything inside the cast or to "scratch" the skin beneath the cast

  5. Check the cast for drainage or discoloration; any drainage should be marked, timed, dated, and documented
  6. Protect the cast from water, urine, and stool
  7. "Petal" the edges of the cast before the patient goes home (if cast is damp, teach parents the proper way to do it)
  8. Before discharge, talk to the parents regarding a safe method for restraining the child with a cast while in the car; infants and children in long leg and hip spica casts will need adapted car seats/safety belts
G. Care of the child in traction
  1. Types of traction
     a. Skeletal: uses pins, wires, and tongs
     b. Skin; uses tapes, plastic, and bandages attached to the skin
     c. Bryant's/modified Bryant's: a type of skin traction; it is most commonly used in infants and toddlers for treatment of a fractured femur and congenital hip dislocation (Fig. 8-16)
  2. Nursing care measures for the child in traction
     a. Explain the traction apparatus to the child; allow the child to participate in his or her care as much as possible

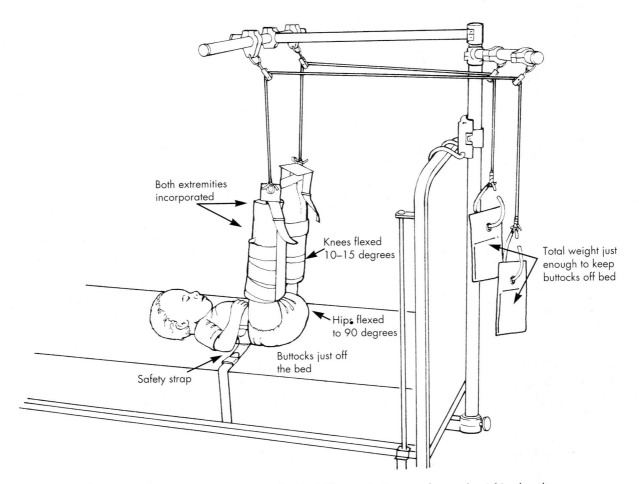

Both extremities incorporated

Knees flexed 10–15 degrees

Total weight just enough to keep buttocks off bed

Hips flexed to 90 degrees

Buttocks just off the bed

Safety strap

Figure 8-16. Bryant's traction is used with children under 3 years of age and weighing less than 35 lb (15.9 kg) who have developmental dysplasia of the hip (DDH). (From Folcik MA, Carina-Garcia G, Birmingham JJ: *Traction: assessment and management,* St Louis, 1994, Mosby.)

b. Maintain traction alignment; be sure that all ropes are in the center tracks of the pulleys and that the weights are hanging freely

c. Provide proper skin care; observe for reddened, irritated areas at the edges of the tape and elastic bandages, as well as at other pressure sites

d. Observe skeletal pin sites for bleeding, inflammation, and signs of infection; provide pin-site care as ordered

e. Observe affected extremity for skin color, nail bed color, and changes in sensation and mobility

f. Administer pain medications as ordered and keep the child as comfortable as possible

g. Provide range-of-motion exercises to the unaffected body parts to help prevent contractures and muscle atrophy

h. Provide toys and activities appropriate to the child's age level and limited mobility

SUGGESTED READINGS

Ball JW: *Mosby's pediatric patient teaching guides,* St Louis, 1998, Mosby.

Jackson PL, Vessey JA: *Primary care of the child with a chronic condition,* ed 2, St Louis, 1996, Mosby.

McCance KL, Huether SE: *Pathophysiology: the biologic basis for disease in adults and children,* ed 3, St Louis, 1999, Mosby.

Miller S, Fiorvanti J: *Pediatric medications: a handbook for nurses,* St Louis, 1997, Mosby.

Novak JC, Broom BL: *Ingalls & Selerno's maternal and child health nursing,* ed 9, St Louis, 1999, Mosby.

Opperman CS, Cassandra KA: *Contemporary pediatric nursing,* St Louis, 1998, Mosby.

Wong DL et al: *Whaley & Wong's nursing care of infants and children,* ed 6, St Louis, 1999, Mosby.

Wong DL: *Clinical manual of pediatric nursing,* ed 4, St Louis, 1996, Mosby.

REVIEW QUESTIONS

1. A Wilms' tumor is an adenosarcoma found in the:
   ① Brain
   ② Small intestine
   ③ Colon
   ④ Kidney

2. Infancy is that period from:
   ① Birth to 6 weeks of age
   ② Birth to 1 year of age
   ③ 4 weeks to 1 year of age
   ④ 4 weeks to 2 years of age

3. The nurse's neighbor, age 7 years, has developed a red, raised rash on her face, neck, and trunk. She also has a temperature of 101.4° F (38.5° C) and whitish spots on the back of her throat. From these symptoms, the nurse knows that the child has:
   ① Chickenpox
   ② Measles (rubeola)
   ③ Mumps
   ④ German measles (rubella)

4. The patient, age 4, was admitted with a diagnosis of possible epiglottitis. If the nurse suspects the patient has epiglottitis, the nurse should:
   ① Check her throat carefully with a flashlight
   ② Increase her oral intake
   ③ Direct warm steam toward the patient
   ④ Have emergency tracheostomy equipment immediately available

5. The patient, age 3, has an order for sulfisoxazole (Gantrisin) 750 mg po q AM. On hand, the nurse has sulfisoxazole 0.5 g/5 ml. The nurse should give the patient:
   ① 2 ml
   ② 4 ml
   ③ 1½ tsp
   ④ 2 tsp

6. Adolescence begins when:
   ① The growth rate increases rapidly
   ② The child develops a positive self-image
   ③ Secondary sex characteristics appear
   ④ The child starts to be attracted to the opposite sex

7. Hospitalized teenagers have the most difficulty with:
   ① Dependence vs. independence
   ② Trust vs. autonomy
   ③ Reality vs. fantasy
   ④ Initiative vs. guilt

8. According to Erikson's theory of psychosocial development, preschoolers are in the stage of:
   ① Trust vs. mistrust
   ② Industry vs. inferiority
   ③ Autonomy vs. shame and doubt
   ④ Initiative vs. guilt

9. The best way for the pediatric nurse to establish a good working relationship with parents is to:
   ① Avoid contact whenever possible
   ② Answer their questions honestly
   ③ Refer all questions to the physician
   ④ Keep them out of their child's room as much as possible

10. Rheumatic fever is caused by:
    ① A fungus
    ② Staphylococcus bacteria
    ③ A virus
    ④ Streptococcus bacteria

11. Which of the following pathophysiological mechanisms is responsible for respiratory alterations seen in children with cystic fibrosis?
    ① Decreased ciliary action causing stasis of mucus in lungs
    ② Edema of the epiglottis causing upper airway occlusion
    ③ Excessive production of thick mucus leading to airway obstruction
    ④ Laryngeal stricture leading to bronchospasm

12. The child with cystic fibrosis takes pancreatic enzymes with each meal. The purpose of this therapy is to facilitate:
    ① Absorption of vitamins A, C, and K
    ② Increased carbohydrate metabolism for growth
    ③ Digestions and absorption of fats and proteins
    ④ Sodium excretion and electrolyte balance

13. In caring for a child with Down's syndrome, the nurse should be aware that a frequent accompanying defect is:
    ① Congenital heart disease
    ② Congenital hip dysplasia
    ③ Central auditory imperception
    ④ Pyloric stenosis

14. The safest place to give an infant in intramuscular (IM) injection is the:
    ① Deltoid muscle
    ② Vastus lateralis muscle
    ③ Ventrogluteal muscle
    ④ Dorsogluteal muscle

15. Celiac disease is characterized by disturbance in the absorption of:
    ① Proteins
    ② Carbohydrates
    ③ Vitamins
    ④ Fats

16. Symptoms of celiac disease include which of the following?
    ① Constipation, anorexia, and malnutrition
    ② Malnutrition, distended abdomen, constant appetite for sweets
    ③ Distended abdomen, constipation, anorexia
    ④ Bulky, greasy stools, distended abdomen, and malnutrition

17. The best, most reliable method of assessing for pinworms in a child is by:
    ① The history, symptoms, and a stool culture
    ② A blood culture
    ③ Capturing the eggs from the anal edge on cellophane tape
    ④ Sending a stool culture to the laboratory

18. A 2-year-old patient is diagnosed with leukemia. The most common signs and symptoms of leukemia related to bone marrow involvement are:
    ① Headache, papilledema, and irritability
    ② Muscle wasting, weight loss, and fatigue
    ③ Decreased intracranial pressure, psychosis, and confusion
    ④ Anemia, infection, and bleeding

19. The lateral S-shaped curvature of the spine that most often occurs in school-age girls is:
    ① Scoliosis
    ② Nephrosis
    ③ Lordosis
    ④ Kyphosis

20. The most notable symptoms the nurse would observe in a 13-month-old with meningitis would be:
    ① Weak or absent cry, coma
    ② Bulging fontanel, irritability
    ③ Absent reflexes, rigid digits
    ④ Dilated and fixed pupils

21. A 2-year-old female patient has a complex febrile seizure in her crib while the nurse is caring for her. What is the most important nursing activity at this time?
    ① Place a seizure stick between her jaws
    ② Prepare the suction equipment
    ③ Observe the seizure and protect her from harm
    ④ Restrain her to prevent injury

22. A male patient, age 18 months, is admitted to the hospital for a bilateral myringotomy because of frequent occurrences of otitis media. Otitis media occurs more frequently in young children than in older children because of the different position and shape of the young child's:
    ① Esophagus
    ② Tympanic membranes
    ③ External ear canals
    ④ Eustachian tubes

23. Which of the following is responsible for airway narrowing characteristic of an asthma episode?
    ① Laryngeal edema, dehydration, and anxiety
    ② Bronchospasm, edema, and increased accumulation of mucus
    ③ Increased negative pleural pressure, laryngospasm, and mucus plugging
    ④ Carbon dioxide retention, pharyngeal hyperemia, and alveolar collapse

24. The nurse is caring for a child who weighs 25 lb. The usual dose for ampicillin for children is 100 mg/kg/day. Which of the following would be an appropriate order for this child?
    ① Ampicillin 25 mg q4h
    ② Ampicillin 250 mg qid
    ③ Ampicillin 100 mg q6h
    ④ Ampicillin 100 mg qid

25. Bulimia is an eating disorder characterized by:
    ① Anorexia with severe weight loss
    ② Binge eating followed by induced vomiting
    ③ Sudden weight gain
    ④ Chronic diarrhea

26. The childhood disease that exhibits symptoms of lethargy, muscle pain, polyarthritis, and chorea and is diagnosed by using the Jones criteria is:
    ① Infectious mononucleosis
    ② Muscular dystrophy
    ③ Cystic fibrosis
    ④ Rheumatic fever

27. A 3-month-old infant is admitted to the pediatric unit for treatment of bronchiolitis. Oxygen therapy is ordered for the infant primarily to:
    ① Reduce fever
    ② Allay anxiety and restlessness
    ③ Liquefy secretions
    ④ Relieve dyspnea and hypoxemia

28. Fluids by mouth are initially contraindicated for an infant with bronchiolitis because of feeding difficulty caused by:
    ① Tachypnea
    ② Bradycardia
    ③ Irritability
    ④ Fever

29. The stage of development where parallel play takes place is:
    ① Infancy
    ② Toddler
    ③ Preschool age
    ④ School age

30. The disorder characterized by a malfunction of the motor centers of the brain (because of lack of oxygen to the brain) is:
    ① Down's syndrome
    ② Scoliosis
    ③ Osteomyelitis
    ④ Cerebral palsy

31. Which of the following statements about pain in children is true?
    ① A child's behavioral response to pain is affected by his or her age and developmental stage
    ② Recovery from a painful experience occurs at a faster rate in children than in adults
    ③ Narcotic use in children is dangerous because of the increased risk of addiction and respiratory depression
    ④ Immaturity of the nervous system in young children provides them with increased thresholds for pain

32. The first immunizations an infant receives at 2 months of age are:
    ① DPT only
    ② PPD, OPV, first hepatitis B vaccines
    ③ DTP, OPV, MMR
    ④ DTP, OPV, Hib, second hepatitis B vaccine

33. The leading cause of death in children between 1 year and 14 years of age is:
    ① Meningitis
    ② Leukemia
    ③ Accidents
    ④ AIDS

34. A disorder caused by an obstruction of cerebrospinal fluid drainage is:
    ① Opisthotonos
    ② Wilms' tumor
    ③ Hydrocephalus
    ④ Meningitis

35. Characteristics of an infant diagnosed as failure to thrive (FTT) include:
    ① Sociable smile at 2 months
    ② Weight below 25th percentile
    ③ Distrust of human contact
    ④ No interest in toys

36. In caring for a child in a full leg cast, which of the following findings should the nurse report to the physician immediately?
    ① The cast is still damp after 4 hours
    ② The child's pedal pulse is 80

③ The child complains of pain in his leg

④ The child is unable to move his toes

37. Of the following, the most important criterion on which to base the decision to report suspected child abuse is:
① Inappropriate parental concern for the degree of injury
② Absence of the parents for questioning about the child's injuries
③ A complaint other than the one associated with the signs of abuse
④ Incompatibility between the history given and the injury observed

38. By the end of the school-age years, a child should have developed a sense of:
① Initiative, purpose
② Industry, competence
③ Identity, role
④ Intimacy, fidelity

39. Your patient is 2 years old. Her favorite word is "No!" She is in Erikson's developmental stage of:
① Trust vs. mistrust
② Initiative vs. guilt
③ Autonomy vs. shame and doubt
④ Industry vs. inferiority

40. A 5-week-old infant is brought to the pediatrician's office with symptoms of irritability, weight loss, and projectile vomiting. On physical examination the infant appears dehydrated. From these symptoms you know that the infant probably has:
① Hirschsprung's disease
② Pyloric stenosis
③ Esophageal atresia
④ Intussusception

41. A 12-month-old female with sickle cell anemia is admitted in sickle cell crisis. Her symptoms might include:
① Fever, seizures, coma
② Abdominal pain, swollen painful joints
③ Polycythemia, tachycardia
④ Severe itching, vomiting

42. A female patient, 18 months of age, has developmental dysplasia of her right hip and will be hospitalized for surgery and application of a hip spica cast. Which of the following measures will be necessary in caring for her?
① Avoid giving her pain medication as much as possible, to prevent constipation
② Limit fluids, so she will be less likely to get the cast wet when she voids
③ Tell the parents that they can take her home in the car propped up on pillows, with her legs down
④ Assess sensation, circulation, and motion of her feet and toes

43. Many researchers believe that SIDS may be related to a brainstem abnormality in the regulation of cardiorespiratory control. Other recent studies have demonstrated that there is an increased risk of SIDS in infants who:
① Breast feed rather than bottle feed
② Sleep in the prone position
③ Are more than 10 months of age
④ Use a pacifier while they sleep

44. The treatment of a child with nephrotic syndrome includes administration of corticosteroids to:
① Decrease the amount of proteinuria
② Increase the amount of albumin in the blood
③ Help control hypertension
④ Reduce edema of the face, extremities, and abdomen

45. A ketogenic diet is sometimes used in the treatment of:
① Epilepsy
② Crohn's disease
③ Bulimia
④ Acute glomerulonephritis

46. A child with asthma would most likely present with which of the following symptoms?
① Laryngitis, sore throat, and productive cough
② Fever, rhinorrhea, and coarse breath sounds
③ Tightness in the chest, nonproductive cough, and wheezing
④ Rapid respiratory rate, difficulty swallowing, and fever

47. The two main types of medication used to treat asthma are:
① Antiinflammatory agents and immunosuppressants
② Bronchodilators and antiinflammatory agents
③ Antibiotics and bronchodilators
④ Decongestants and antihistamines

48. The hepatitis B vaccine series should begin at what age?
① Newborn
② 2 months
③ 6 months
④ 12 months

49. A female patient, age 2 months, presents at the pediatrician's office with a 2-week history of paroxysmal abdominal cramping. Her mother states that she is very fussy and cries as if she is in pain. She is tolerating her normal amounts of formula well and has gained weight since her last visit. These signs and symptoms indicate that she most likely has:
① An intussusception
② Colic
③ A pyloric stenosis
④ Hirschsprung's disease

50. A 5-month-old infant with chronic lung disease is admitted with a severe case of RSV. Treatment for this child will include:
① Cromolyn (Intal) nebulizer treatments and IV fluids
② Ribavirin (Virazole) and humidified oxygen
③ Antibiotics and IV fluids
④ Prednisone (LiquiPred) and oxygen

51. Which of the following statements about RSV/bronchiolitis is true?
① It occurs primarily in fall and winter
② Peak incidence for RSV infection is 6 to 18 months of age
③ RSV can survive for hours on gloves, countertops, and skin
④ It causes the bronchioles to plug with mucus, trapping air in the lungs

52. At the time of delivery, an infant is born with its abdominal organs, covered by a sac, protruding through an abnormal opening in the umbilical ring. This condition is known as:
① Intussusception
② Diaphragmatic hernia
③ Omphalocele
④ Gastroschisis

53. The preoperative injection order reads: "Meperidine (Demerol) 35 mg and Atropine 0.1 mg IM." The meperidine is supplied at 50 mg/ml, and the atropine at 0.2 mg/ml. What volume of meperidine and the volume of atropine should the nurse give?
    ① Meperidine 0.35 ml and atropine 0.5 ml
    ② Meperidine 0.6 ml and atropine 0.4 ml
    ③ Meperidine 0.7 ml and atropine 0.5 ml
    ④ Meperidine 0.85 ml and atropine 0.1 ml

54. The nurse is about to give an oral medication to an uncooperative 2-year-old toddler. Which of the following actions would be the best way to give the child the medication?
    ① Get an order to change the medication to an injectable form
    ② Sedate the child
    ③ Allow a parent to assist
    ④ Use wrist and ankle restraints

55. The nurse has an order to administer ampicillin 425 mg IVPB. Ampicillin is supplied as 1 g/4 ml. What volume of ampicillin should the nurse draw from the vial?
    ① 0.9 ml
    ② 1.25 ml
    ③ 1.7 ml
    ④ 1.9 ml

56. A patient has an order for an IV of D5.45 NS to be infused at 80 ml/hr. If the IV tubing delivers 10 gtt/ml, at what rate should the nurse infuse the IV fluid?
    ① 8 gtt/min
    ② 13 gtt/min
    ③ 16 gtt/min
    ④ 21 gtt/min

57. The treatment of choice for children with infectious gastroenteritis is:
    ① Oral rehydration therapy
    ② IV fluids and antibiotics
    ③ The "BRAT" diet
    ④ Low fiber diet and skim milk

58. The symptoms of croup are caused by:
    ① A bacterial infection of the larynx
    ② Inflammation of the trachea and esophagus
    ③ Spasms of the larynx
    ④ Inflammation of the lungs

59. The foul-smelling, frothy stools seen in children with cystic fibrosis result from the presence of large amounts of:
    ① Proteins and enzymes
    ② Carbohydrates
    ③ Sodium and glucose
    ④ Undigested fats

60. The organ of the digestive system most commonly involved in cystic fibrosis is the:
    ① Pancreas
    ② Small intestine
    ③ Esophagus
    ④ Liver

61. Discharge planning and preparation for home care of the hospitalized child should begin:
    ① On the day of the discharge
    ② As soon as the discharge order is written
    ③ During the admission, by setting long-term goals
    ④ Only if the child will need home care and treatment

62. Down's syndrome is:
    ① A chromosomal abnormality
    ② Caused by a bacterial infection
    ③ Caused by a viral infection
    ④ A result of a lack of oxygen to the brain at birth

63. Which of the following foods is contraindicated in the diet of the child with celiac disease?
    ① Wheat and rye breads
    ② Lean meats
    ③ Strawberries
    ④ Green beans

64. The most common method of treatment for an infant with a fractured femur is:
    ① Surgery and placement of a pin to set the fracture
    ② Putting the child in skeletal traction
    ③ Immediate setting and casting of the fractured leg
    ④ Putting the child in Bryant's or modified Bryant's traction

65. Sickle cell disease is caused by:
    ① A virus
    ② An abnormal hereditary trait
    ③ *Streptococcus* bacteria
    ④ A mismatched blood transfusion

66. A fungal infection of the skin that can occur on the scalp, body, and feet is:
    ① Ringworm
    ② Pediculosis
    ③ Herpes type II
    ④ Urticaria

67. The total number of deciduous teeth is:
    ① 18
    ② 20
    ③ 22
    ④ 24

68. The pediatrician ordered aspirin gr. v PO. On hand the nurse has aspirin 300 mg tablets. The nurse should give:
    ① ½ tablet
    ② 1 tablet
    ③ 1½ tablets
    ④ 2 tablets

69. A 4-year-old boy is admitted with a diagnosis of nephrotic syndrome. Treatment for this child will include:
    ① High-Fowler's position
    ② Regular diet
    ③ Diuretics as ordered
    ④ Sodium and potassium supplements

70. Nursing care for the child with eczema includes:
    ① Keeping the child in the same position
    ② Keeping the child fully clothed
    ③ Keeping the skin clean and dry
    ④ Warm, moist dressings to relieve the itching

71. An 18-year-old is seen in the clinic and is diagnosed with anorexia nervosa. Her symptoms would most likely include:
    ① Dysmenorrhea
    ② Periods of hyperactivity
    ③ Tachycardia
    ④ Diarrhea

72. The nurse needs to instill ear drops into a 2-year-old's left ear. The correct way to position her ear for administration of the ear drops is to:
    ① Pull the outer ear up and toward the back of the head

② Pull the outer ear down and toward the back of the head
③ Pull the ear lobe down and toward the chin
④ Pull the ear lobe up and toward the nose

73. Treatment of the preschooler with Kawasaki disease (KD) includes the administration of high-dose IV immune globulin (IVIG). This is used to:
① Treat the infection causing the Kawasaki disease
② Relax the child and allow the child to get the appropriate rest they need
③ Maintain proper hydration and blood pressure levels
④ Decrease the fever and incidence of coronary artery damage

74. The nurse completes her nursing assessment of a normal 18-month-old boy and begins to document her findings. An expected characteristic of a normal 18-month-old child is:
① Moving slowly and carefully
② "Getting into everything"
③ Playing quietly and cooperatively with other children
④ Preferring toys that can be played while sitting still

75. A 2-week-old infant has been admitted to the hospital with a diagnosis of possible hydrocephalus. Which assessment would be most important for the nurse to make?
① Daily weight
② Frequent neurovascular checks
③ Specific gravity on all urine output
④ Daily head circumference measurement

76. A mother of an otherwise healthy 18-month-old tells the nurse that the child has had two diarrhea stools. When she asks what fluids and foods she can safely give the child, the nurse tells her to:
① Keep the child NPO until 24 hours after the diarrhea stops
② Continue to offer normal diet items, but substitute foods the child especially likes
③ Encourage fluids (diluted juice, soda, Pedialyte) and offer small crackers
④ Offer constipating foods, such as cheese, with each meal, and decrease fluid intake

77. The nurse is assigned to care for a male 3-year-old on the pediatric unit that has a Wilms' tumor. Which nursing intervention is appropriate?
① Encourage the child to choose his own activities, but tell him he must accept responsibility for his own safety
② Avoid manipulation or pressure on the child's abdomen that could increase the possibility of metastasis
③ Palpate the tumor each shift to determine any change in size or configuration
④ At regular intervals, position the child appropriately and perform postural drainage techniques

78. The nurse is admitting a child with a diagnosis of trisomy 21. Another term for this genetic problem is:
① Hurler syndrome
② Cri du chat syndrome
③ Turner's syndrome
④ Down's syndrome

79. The nurse is caring for a child in acute respiratory distress from bronchitis. One appropriate nursing intervention is to provide a cool moist environment, because it:
① Relieves symptoms immediately
② Prevents drug toxicity by liquid dispersion in the lungs
③ Promotes adequate hydration and fever reduction
④ Reduces inflammation and keeps secretions thin

80. A teenage girl at the pediatrician's office has been diagnosed with infectious mononucleosis. When her mother asks how her daughter could have gotten the disease, the nurse explains to her that it is caused by:
① Kissing
② Poor health habits
③ A virus
④ Bacteria

81. When talking to a mother of a 6-month-old girl that has just been diagnosed as having an intussusception, she asks what intussusception means. The nurse's best response is:
① "A hole has developed between two parts of her intestine, the duodenum, and the ileum."
② "The lower segment of her bowel has no anal opening."
③ "One portion of her intestine has telescoped into another portion of the intestine."
④ "A portion of her bowel has twisted around itself, causing a blockage."

82. A preschooler visiting the pediatrician is diagnosed with eczema. His father asks what could be causing the disease, and the nurse tells him that a likely cause is:
① A metabolic disorder
② An allergic disorder
③ An infectious disorder
④ A nutritional disorder

83. At what age would an infant be expected to triple his birth weight?
① 6 months
② 9 months
③ 12 months
④ 18 months

84. Which child is most likely to develop osteomyelitis?
① A child that has experienced a traumatic birth experience
② A child that inherited the gene for osteomyelitis
③ A child that had trauma to a long bone in an extremity
④ A child that experienced protein loss as a result of inadequate calcium intake

85. Which organism is the major cause of osteomyelitis?
① Beta-hemolytic *Streptococcus*
② *Haemophilus influenzae*
③ *Escherichia coli*
④ *Staphylococcus aureus*

86. The desired clinical outcome for a child experiencing respiratory distress from epiglottitis is:
① Child remains asleep for 8 hours a night
② Child is in no pain or discomfort
③ Airway remains patent
④ Oral mucus membranes remain moist and pink

87. A 6-year-old child with a 3-year history of celiac disease comes into the clinic for a check-up. If the child and his family have been in compliance with the necessary diet regimen, the nurse should expect to see:
① Slow, steady weight loss
② Increase in appetite
③ Hemoglobin level above 12.0
④ Decrease in steatorrhea

88. Hirschsprung's disease is caused by:
   ① A congenital absence of the ganglion nerve cells in the lower colon
   ② An infectious organism, that causes inflammation and swelling in the lower bowel
   ③ An autoimmune reaction causing damage to the muscles of the large intestine
   ④ Damage to the bowel resulting from an allergic reaction to cow's milk

89. An 8-year-old girl is admitted to the unit complaining of localized abdominal tenderness, rigidity, and a fever. She has rebound abdominal tenderness, and decreased bowel sounds. These are characteristic signs of:
   ① Meckel's diverticulum
   ② Acute appendicitis
   ③ Rheumatic fever
   ④ Ulcerative colitis

90. During a physical assessment of a young infant, the nurse palpates his suture lines and fontanels. The nurse should expect the anterior fontanel of a normal child to be completely closed at:
   ① 3 to 4 months of age
   ② 6 months of age
   ③ 9 to 17 months of age
   ④ 18 to 24 months of age

91. In a 6-month-old infant who is teething, which teeth would the nurse expect to erupt first?
   ① Two lower lateral incisors
   ② Two lower central incisors
   ③ Four first molars
   ④ Four upper molars

92. During the physical assessment of a child with glomerulonephritis, the nurse's priorities should be:
   ① Color, motion, and sensation of lower extremities
   ② Severity of abdominal pain, bowel sounds
   ③ Blood pressure, observation for dependent edema
   ④ Neurological checks, level of consciousness

93. The posterior fontanel of an infant is expected to be closed:
   ① At the time of birth
   ② Within hours after birth
   ③ By the end of the first month of life
   ④ By the age of 2 to 3 months

94. During the initial assessment of an 8-year-old boy who has nephrotic syndrome, the nurse should expect to see:
   ① Absence of tears
   ② Increased urine output
   ③ Flushed skin
   ④ Scrotal edema

95. What is the legal responsibility of a nurse regarding the reporting of suspected child abuse or neglect?
   ① None; nurses can be sued if they report suspected child abuse or neglect
   ② Nurses must report abuse and neglect to the child's pediatrician prior to calling a child abuse center
   ③ Only physicians are legally required to report abuse or neglect
   ④ Nurses must report all suspected and confirmed abuse or neglect

96. Prednisone is often used in the treatment of rheumatic fever because it:
   ① Prevents infection
   ② Cures the disease
   ③ Suppresses inflammation
   ④ Takes the place of antibiotic prophylaxis

97. A 3-month-old infant is receiving continuous IV fluids because of dehydration. In providing nursing care for her, the nurse's priority should be to:
   ① Help the infant adjust to restricted activities
   ② Relieve the infant's anxiety
   ③ Promote fluid elimination
   ④ Prevent interference with the IV therapy

98. The theory of child development that is based on psychosocial development as a series of developmental tasks is known as:
   ① Freud's theory
   ② Erikson's theory
   ③ Masterson's theory
   ④ Piaget's theory

99. Piaget's theory of child development is based on:
   ① Intellectual (cognitive) development
   ② Psychosexual development
   ③ Psychosocial development
   ④ Social and physical development

100. Normal physical development characteristics for a 1-month-old infant include:
   ① Closed posterior fontanel
   ② Can raise chest supported on forearms
   ③ Can turn the head from side to side when prone or supine
   ④ Can carry hand or an object to the mouth

101. Primitive newborn reflexes disappear at:
   ① 2 weeks of age
   ② 6 to 8 weeks of age
   ③ 3 months of age
   ④ 5 months of age

102. Teething usually begins at the age of:
   ① 3 to 4 months
   ② 5 months
   ③ 6 to 7 months
   ④ 8 months

103. "Stranger anxiety," fear of strangers demonstrated by pushing away and crying, usually begins at age:
   ① 4 to 5 months
   ② 6 to 7 months
   ③ 8 to 9 months
   ④ 10 to 11 months

104. Erikson's theory of development states that the developmental task of infancy is:
   ① Autonomy
   ② Trust
   ③ Initiative
   ④ Gratification

105. According to the July 1999 revision to the immunization schedule, clinicians were advised to suspend the administration of:
   ① MMR vaccine
   ② Third DTP vaccine
   ③ Varicella vaccine
   ④ Rotavirus vaccine

106. An infant with a congenital heart defect that is not eating or growing normally may also be diagnosed with which type of failure to thrive (FTT)?
   ① Organic FTT

② Systemic FTT
③ Nonorganic FTT
④ Idiopathic FTT

107. When asked to explain the pathophysiology of RSV to an infant's caregiver, the nurse should tell her that RSV is:
① A bacterial infection of the lungs, similar to pneumonia
② A viral infection of the lungs and trachea that causes inflammation
③ An inflammation of the pleural cavity that can be prevented with ribavirin
④ A viral infection that causes the bronchioles to become plugged with mucus

108. Ribavirin, an antiviral agent given in the treatment of RSV, is administered:
① Via slow IV infusion
② Via an oxygen hood or mask
③ Via IM injection
④ Orally; can be given with juice or formula

109. Infectious gastroenteritis in the infant is most often caused by:
① Staphylococcal infection
② *E. coli* infection
③ MRSA infection
④ Rotavirus infection

110. The nurse is providing postoperative care for an infant that has had a pyloromyotomy for pyloric stenosis. The first feeding of glucose water will most likely be given:
① 4 to 6 hours after surgery
② 8 hours after surgery
③ 12 hours after surgery
④ 24 hours after surgery

111. A child with *Haemophilus influenzae* type B meningitis is usually treated with IV fluids, antibiotics, and:
① IV dexamethasone
② IM ribavirin
③ PO Benadryl
④ IV Lasix

112. A newborn with Hirschsprung's disease will often exhibit classic signs and symptoms including:
① Respiratory distress and wheezing
② Pallor, bruising, and low hemoglobin
③ An olive-shaped mass in the abdomen and projectile vomiting
④ Lack of meconium stool and bile-stained emesis

113. Treatment for an infant newly diagnosed with esophageal atresia should include:
① Liquid diet, monitoring of vital signs, accurate I&O
② NPO, IV fluids, suctioning of mouth and nose as needed
③ Oxygen via nasal cannula and bronchodilators
④ Half-strength formula in small, frequent amounts, IV fluids

114. Daily head circumference measurements are important nursing interventions postoperatively for the child with a:
① Wilms' tumor
② Seizure disorder
③ Ventriculoperitoneal shunt
④ Spinal cord injury

115. The failure of one or both testes to descend into the scrotal sac is known as:
① Epispadias
② Hypospadius
③ Cryptorchidism
④ Nephrotic syndrome

116. A drug that is sometimes given to promote the descent of the testes into the scrotum is:
① Dexamethasone
② Human chorionic gonadotropin
③ Growth hormone
④ Recombinant human DNA

117. Tetralogy of Fallot consists of four separate cardiac defects:
① Atrial septal defect, ventricular septal defect, coarctation of the aorta, and PDA
② Ventricular septal defect, pulmonary stenosis, overriding of the aorta, and right ventricular hypertrophy
③ Coarctation of the aorta, pulmonary stenosis, atrial septal defect, right ventricular hypertrophy
④ Ventricular septal defect, left ventricular hypertrophy, PDA, overriding of the aorta

118. Treatment for a child in sickle cell crisis includes:
① IV fluids, oxygen, analgesics for pain
② NPO, NG tube to suction, bed rest
③ Bone marrow transplant, IV fluids, oxygen
④ Analgesics for pain, pancreatic enzymes, bed rest

119. To promote healthy psychosocial development in the toddler, it is important to remember to:
① Attempt to quiet and reason with a toddler during a temper tantrum
② Criticize the child's bad behavior, not the child
③ Help him or her to develop a strong sense of initiative, not a sense of guilt
④ Make every attempt to have them potty trained by age 2 years

120. The condition in which a child's eyes are unable to focus and work together, and there is reduced visual acuity in one eye is called:
① Strabismus
② Esotropia
③ Amblyopia
④ Exotropia

121. Spastic cerebral palsy is characterized by:
① Mental retardation, wide-based gait, flexion contractures, and involuntary movements
② Disintegration of movements of the upper extremities, hypertonicity of the lower extremities
③ Abnormal involuntary movement, athetosis, and slow, writhing movements
④ Hypertonicity of muscles and tendon reflexes, poor coordination, contractures

122. Suggestions to parents to help avoid accidents in children include:
① Allow the preschool-age child to ride his or her bike without a helmet, as long as an adult is nearby
② Keep all medications and poisonous substances in the back of a low cabinet in the kitchen
③ Turn all handles of pots and pans outward so that the child can see them and learn not to touch them
④ Supervise play, especially around dangerous areas such as cars, pools, and open flames

123. The age level in which children begin to learn the difference between proper and improper behavior is part of Erikson's developmental task of "initiative vs. guilt." The age level for this task is:
    ① Toddler
    ② Preschooler
    ③ School-age
    ④ Adolescent

124. A normal part of the development of preschoolers is:
    ① Developing their imagination using "magical thinking"
    ② Developing a sense of trust, depending on how their caregivers treat them
    ③ Developing "best friends" and beginning to be influenced by their peer group
    ④ Developing and following certain regular patterns of behavior

125. Immediate postoperative care of the child after a tonsillectomy includes:
    ① Supine position, with head of bed slightly elevated
    ② Offering the child cold fluids and ice cream when awake
    ③ Placing the child in an oxygen tent with cool mist
    ④ Observing the child for frequent swallowing and active bleeding

126. Diagnosis of nephrotic syndrome in a child is based on:
    ① Symptoms of edema, hyperalbuminemia, and tea-colored urine
    ② Results of renal ultrasound, proteinuria, and increased levels of protein in the blood
    ③ Increased proteinuria, edema, decreased serum protein, and renal biopsy
    ④ Edema of face and abdomen, positive renal MRI, increased serum protein

127. Treatment of nephrotic syndrome includes frequent urine testing for protein and albumin, measurement of intake and output, low salt diet, and several medications including:
    ① Corticosteroids and oral alkylating agents
    ② Diuretics and antibiotics
    ③ Antihypertensives and diuretics
    ④ Antibiotics and corticosteroids

128. An X-linked recessive disorder of metabolism that results in a delayed coagulation of blood is known as:
    ① Sickle cell anemia
    ② Thalassemia major
    ③ Hemophilia
    ④ Leukemia

129. The mother of a school-age child with hemophilia asks the nurse what sport would be safest for her child to participate in during gym: football, basketball, swimming, or archery. An appropriate response by the nurse would be:
    ① Football
    ② Basketball
    ③ Swimming
    ④ Archery

130. In leukemia, the three main consequences of bone marrow dysfunction are:
    ① Anemia, increased blood clotting, infection
    ② Infection, anemia, bleeding

③ Decreased clotting, increased hemoglobin, sickling of the RBCs
④ Prolonged bleeding time, decreased WBCs, increased coagulation

131. Treatment of leukemia includes administration of chemotherapy agents to lower the WBC count. This decrease in WBC count may:
    ① Lower the child's resistance to infection
    ② Cause joint pain and sores in the mouth
    ③ Lead to a decrease in hemoglobin and increased anemia
    ④ Lead to lethargy, petechiae, and bruising

132. A hereditary musculoskeletal disorder that exhibits symptoms of gradual muscle weakness, a "waddle" gait, and difficulty standing and sitting is known as:
    ① Multiple sclerosis
    ② Cerebral palsy
    ③ Developmental dysplasia of the hip
    ④ Muscular dystrophy

133. At which age level is cartilage replaced by bone at the bone epiphyses?
    ① Toddler
    ② Preschool
    ③ School-age
    ④ Adolescent

134. According to the International Classification of Epileptic Seizures, tonic-clonic (grand-mal) seizures are classified as:
    ① Simple partial seizures
    ② Complex partial seizures
    ③ Unilateral seizures
    ④ Generalized seizures

135. Care of the child with pediculosis includes:
    ① Antifungal oral medication and pediculicide shampoo
    ② Corticosteroids and antifungal ointment
    ③ Pediculicide shampoo and removal of eggs with comb
    ④ Antibiotic shampoo and ointment and destruction of linens

136. Which of the following is an important concept to be taught to parents and a school-age child that has recently been diagnosed with insulin-dependent diabetes?
    ① Blood sugar monitoring will be required every 1 to 2 days
    ② Symptoms of hypoglycemia include glycosuria, blood sugar over 120, and dizziness
    ③ Insulin injections will be required, and the child and the parents should be taught how to do injections
    ④ The child's diet will remain the same, as long as the child exercises daily

137. The growth spurt in adolescent boys occurs:
    ① Earlier than girls, at age 10 to 12
    ② Later than girls, at age 14 to 16
    ③ At the same time as girls, at age 10 to 12
    ④ Later than girls, at age 12 to 14

138. An adolescent that exhibits changes in behavior patterns, an increase in school absences, a decrease in academic performance, and starts to spend time with people other than his regular friends, may be showing signs of:
    ① Manic-depression
    ② Bulimia
    ③ Drug abuse
    ④ Schizophrenia

139. Retinoic acid is used in the treatment of:
① Acne vulgaris
② Tinea corporis
③ Pediculosis
④ Ringworm

140. Antiretroviral agents are used to treat a child with AIDS to slow progression of the disease by:
① Killing the bacteria that lead to the development of AIDS
② Working to prevent the reproduction of new virus particles
③ Decreasing inflammation and promoting formation of healthy T-cells
④ Compensating for the deficiency of B-lymphocytes in the body

141. The rationale for preparing children for hospitalization is based on the theory that:
① Children have a right to know what is going to happen to them
② It will then be easier for the parents to leave their child in the hospital overnight
③ Fear of the unknown is more severe than fear of the known
④ If they are well prepared, parents will not have to visit as often

142. Which of the following promotes age-specific care and safety of the child in the hospital?
① Allow a toddler to keep her "Candyland" game in her bed at all times
② Keep one side rail down at night, so the child can get out of bed to go to the bathroom
③ If using a restraint, it should be applied securely, and the extremity's circulation checked frequently
④ Allow the adolescent to keep her medication from home in her bedside table

143. Bryant's traction, used with infants for the treatment of fractured femur, is a type of:
① Skin traction
② Skeletal traction
③ Wire traction
④ Pelvic traction

144. When providing care for a child with an extremity in a new cast, the nurse should:
① Use a hairdryer to circulate the air and speed up the drying time of the cast

② Handle the cast using your fingertips to prevent pressure areas under the cast
③ Turn and/or reposition the child every 2 hours to ensure that the cast dries evenly
④ Keep the casted extremity covered with a sheet or blanket

145. The cancer that is seen most often in children is:
① Lymphoma
② Leukemia
③ Melanoma
④ Osteosarcoma

146. The diagnosis of Hirschsprung's disease is usually confirmed by a:
① Rectal biopsy
② Upper GI series
③ Esophagoscopy
④ Gastroscopy

147. Projectile vomiting in an infant is a classic sign of:
① Intussusception
② Celiac disease
③ Tracheoesophageal fistula
④ Pyloric stenosis

148. Of the following antibiotics, which one is usually ordered for the treatment of acute otitis media?
① Vancomycin
② Amoxicillin
③ Gentamycin
④ Ribavirin

149. An adolescent presents at the pediatrician's office with symptoms of mononucleosis: malaise, sore throat, fever, and lack of energy. Which of the following is another common symptom in the early stages of mononucleosis?
① Acute otitis media
② Red, flat rash on the body
③ Cardiac enlargement
④ Edema in the lower extremities

150. An infant weighing 11 pounds has been ordered to receive morphine sulfate 0.5 mg SQ for postoperative pain. The normal dose of morphine is 0.1 mg/kg. The ordered dose of IV morphine is:
① Too low, based on the weight of the infant
② Too high, based on the weight of the infant
③ Inappropriate; morphine should not be given SQ
④ Correct, based on the weight of the infant

ANSWERS AND RATIONALES

1. Knowledge, assessment, physiological adaptation (b)
   ❹ A Wilms' tumor is found only in the kidney and kidney area.
   ① It is not found in the brain.
   ② It is not found in the small intestine.
   ③ It in not found in the colon.

2. Knowledge, assessment, growth and development through the life span (b)
   ❸ This is the period of life known as infancy.
   ① Birth to 4 weeks is the newborn period; birth to 6 weeks includes newborn and part of infancy.
   ② Birth to 4 weeks is the newborn period and is not considered part of the infancy period.
   ④ After 1 year of age until 3 years of age is considered the toddler period.

3. Comprehension, assessment, physiological adaptation (c)
   ❷ These are symptoms of rubeola.
   ① Symptoms of chickenpox include a clear, vesicular rash, fever, irritability, and pruritus.
   ③ Symptoms of rubella do not include a high fever or white spots at the back of the throat.
   ④ Symptoms of mumps include enlarged parotid glands and fever, with no rash.

4. Application, implementation, reduction of risk potential (a)
   ❹ This equipment may be necessary if the enlarged epiglottis completely obstructs the airway.
   ① Any examination of the throat could lead to laryngospasm.
   ② The child with epiglottitis has difficulty swallowing.
   ③ Warm steam is not a method of treatment in epiglottitis.

5. Application, implementation, pharmacological therapies (b)
   ❸ DD = 750 mg
   DH = 0.5 g (500 mg)
   V = 5 ml

   $$\frac{DD}{DH} = \frac{750 \text{ mg}}{500 \text{ mg}} \times 5 \text{ ml} = 7.5 \text{ ml} = 1\frac{1}{2} \text{ tsp.}$$

   ①, ②, ④ These are not the correct answer.

6. Comprehension, assessment, growth and development through the life span (b)
   ❸ This is when adolescence is considered to begin in each child's life.
   ① This occurs more than once in childhood.
   ② Developing a self-image is part of adolescence, but it may be positive or negative during the teenage years.
   ④ Adolescent boys are often attracted to adolescent girls at an earlier age than the girls are attracted to the boys.

7. Knowledge, assessment, growth and development through the life span (a)
   ❶ Adolescents are at the stage where they are constantly struggling to develop a positive self-image and their own identity and independence.
   ② These are the developmental skills developed during infancy and toddlerhood.
   ③, ④ This occurs during the preschool stage.

8. Knowledge, assessment, growth and development through the life span (a)
   ❹ Preschoolers are at the stage where they are learning how to interact with other people, as well as proper behavior; this helps them develop a sense of initiative and accomplishment.
   ① This is the stage of infants.
   ② This is the stage of school-age children.
   ③ This is the stage of toddlers.

9. Comprehension, implementation, coordinated care (a)
   ❷ The parents will deal best with a nurse who is open and honest with them.
   ① This will put a strain on the relationship between the parents and the nurse.
   ③ The nurse should answer as many questions as possible and refer only questions that she cannot answer to the physician.
   ④ The parents should be involved as much as possible in their child's care recovery, and this should be encouraged by the nurse.

10. Knowledge, assessment, physiological adaptation (b)
    ❹ Rheumatic fever is a chronic disease caused by a streptococcal infection.
    ① It is not caused by a fungus.
    ② It is not caused by *Staphylococcus* bacteria.
    ③ It is not caused by a virus.

11. Comprehension, assessment, physiological adaptation (a)
    ❸ Large amounts of abnormally thick mucus are produced in the lungs, as well as the pancreas and liver.
    ①, ④ These do not occur in cystic fibrosis.
    ② This occurs in epiglottitis.

12. Knowledge, assessment, pharmacological therapies (b)
    ❸ Pancreatic enzymes are given regularly with food to improve the digestions and absorption of proteins and fats in the small intestine.
    ① Pancreatic enzymes do not directly affect vitamin absorption.
    ② Pancreatic enzymes do not affect carbohydrate metabolism.
    ④ Although sodium levels are a problem in the child with cystic fibrosis, pancreatic enzymes do not affect them.

13. Comprehension, assessment, reduction of risk potential (a)
    ❶ Some form of congenital heart defect is often seen in children with Down syndrome.
    ②, ③, ④ These are not frequently seen in children with Down syndrome.

14. Knowledge, implementation, reduction of risk potential (b)
    ❷ This is the best-developed muscle in infants and therefore is the safest for IM injections.
    ① This muscle is not well developed in infants, toddlers, and or young children.
    ③, ④ These muscles are not well developed in infants and toddlers.

15. Knowledge, assessment, physiological adaptation (a)
    ❹ Celiac disease is a basic defect of metabolism, leading to impaired fat absorption.
    ① Celiac disease does not affect absorption of proteins.
    ② Celiac disease does not affect absorption of carbohydrates.
    ③ Celiac disease does not affect absorption of vitamins.

16. Knowledge, assessment, physiological adaptation (b)
    ❹ These are all common symptoms of celiac disease.
    ①, ③ Constipation is not a symptom of celiac disease.
    ② An appetite for sweets in not a symptom of celiac disease.

17. Knowledge, assessment, prevention and early detection of disease (a)
    ❸ The cellophane tape test is used in diagnosing pinworms.
    ① The child's history and symptoms are not enough to definitely diagnose pinworms; a stool culture will not diagnose pinworms.
    ② A blood culture would not be helpful in diagnosing pinworms.
    ④ A stool culture will not diagnose pinworms.

18. Comprehension, assessment, physiological adaptation (b)
    ❹ These symptoms of leukemia result directly from changes in the bone marrow.
    ① These symptoms are caused by leukemic effects on the nervous system that lead to increased intracranial pressure.
    ② These symptoms result from the body's increasing need to meet the metabolic needs of the leukemic cells.
    ③ These are not symptoms of leukemia.

19. Knowledge, assessment, reduction of risk potential (a)
    ❶ Scoliosis of the spine often occurs because of rapid growth; seen most often in girls.
    ② Nephrosis is a disease of the kidneys, causing edema and proteinuria.
    ③ Lordosis is a concave curvature of the spine; called sway-back.
    ④ Kyphosis is a convex curvature of the spine; called hunchback.

20. Comprehension, assessment, physiological adaptation (b)
    ❷ These signs are the most notable, because these symptoms are caused by increased intracranial pressure, a serious complication in meningitis.
    ① The child's cry would be shrill and high-pitched.
    ③, ④ These are not signs seen in meningitis.

21. Application, implementation, safety, and infection control (b)
    ❸ Observing the length and type of seizure is important, as is preventing the child from injuring herself.
    ① This could injure the child's mouth.
    ② Suctioning may be needed, but would not be feasible until the seizure was over.
    ④ Restraints could lead to severe injury.

22. Comprehension, assessment, growth and development through the life span (b)
    ❹ The eustachian tubes are shorter and wider in the young child than in the older child, which allows for easier introduction of bacteria.
    ①, ② The shape and position of these do not affect otitis media.
    ③ The external ear canals are basically the same shape and in the same position in young and older children.

23. Comprehension, assessment, physiological adaptation (b)
    ❷ These changes in the respiratory system lead to narrowing of the child's airway.
    ①, ③, ④ These do not occur in asthma.

24. Application, implementation, pharmacological therapies (b)
    ❷ 25 lb = 11.3 kg
    100 mg × 11.3 kg/day = 1130 mg/day
    $\dfrac{1130 \text{ mg}}{4 \text{ doses}}$ = 282 mg
    Appropriate order = 250 mg qid
    ①, ③, ④ These are not appropriate orders for this child.

25. Knowledge, assessment, physiological adaptation (a)
    ❷ Binge eating followed by induced vomiting is the classic symptom of bulimia.
    ① This is a symptom of anorexia nervosa.
    ③, ④ These are not symptoms of bulimia.

26. Comprehension, assessment, physiological adaptation (a)
    ❹ The Jones criteria are used only to diagnose rheumatic fever.
    ① This is a viral disease diagnosed by the symptoms and the Monospot test.
    ②, ③ These are hereditary diseases.

27. Comprehension, assessment, basic care and comfort (b)
    ❹ The infant with bronchiolitis needs oxygen to relieve his extreme dyspnea and resultant hypoxemia.
    ① Oxygen would not reduce a fever.
    ② This is not the primary reason for oxygen therapy.
    ③ Oxygen would not liquefy secretions.

28. Comprehension, assessment, reduction of risk potential (b)
    ❶ Severe tachypnea seen in bronchiolitis is a contraindication for oral feedings.
    ② Bronchiolitis normally causes tachycardia.
    ③, ④ These are not contraindications for oral fluids.

29. Knowledge, assessment, growth and development through the life span (b)
    ❷ Toddlers use parallel play when playing with other children.
    ① Infants usually play alone or with an adult.
    ③ Preschoolers use associative play.
    ④ School-age children use associative play.

30. Comprehension, assessment, physiological adaptation (b)
    ❹ Cerebral palsy is a disorder that affects the motor centers of the brain; it is usually caused by birth trauma or head trauma.
    ① This is a chromosomal abnormality.
    ② This is an S-shaped curvature of the spine.
    ③ This in an infection of the bone.

31. Comprehension, assessment, physiological adaptation (a)
    ❶ This statement is true.
    ② Recovery from a painful experience does not occur faster in children.
    ③ Narcotics are both safe and often necessary in the management of children's pain.
    ④ Children do not have increased pain thresholds.

32. Knowledge, assessment, prevention and detection of disease (a)
    ❹ These are the immunizations normally given at 2 months of age.
    ① The OPV is also given.
    ② The PPD is not given.
    ③ The MMR vaccine is not given.

33. Comprehension, assessment, growth and development through the life span (b)
    ❸ Accidents of all types are the leading cause of death in this age level.
    ① Meningitis is not always fatal.
    ② Leukemia occurs less often than accidents.
    ④ AIDS occurs less often than accidents.

34. Knowledge, assessment, physiological adaptation (a)
    ❸ Hydrocephalus occurs when there is an obstruction of the cerebrospinal fluid drainage pathways.
    ① Opisthotonos is a sign of creased intracranial pressure.
    ② It does not cause the formation of a Wilms' tumor.
    ④ It does not cause meningitis.

35. Knowledge, assessment, physiological adaptation (b)
    ❸ The infant with FTT is distrustful of people.
    ① This is a characteristic of a healthy infant.
    ② This could be caused by other medical conditions/prematurity.
    ④ The infant with FTT prefers inanimate objects such as toys.

36. Comprehension, implementation, reduction of risk potential (b)
    ❹ This may indicate nerve damage at the fracture site or pressure from a tight cast and should be reported immediately.
    ①, ② These are normal findings.
    ③ This is usually a normal finding; any sudden increase in pain or severe muscle spasms should be reported to the physician.

37. Knowledge, assessment, psychosocial adaptation (b)
    ❹ In cases of child abuse, the history given by the caregiver does not fit with the severity or type of injury.
    ① This may occur with other types of injury as well as child abuse.
    ②, ③ These are not indications of abuse.

38. Knowledge, assessment, growth and development through the life span (a)
    ❷ School-age children are in the stage of industry vs. inferiority.
    ① This is the developmental task in the preschooler.
    ③ This is the developmental task in the adolescent.
    ④ This is the developmental task in the young adult.

39. Knowledge, assessment, growth and development through the life span (b)
    ❸ Toddlers (age 1 to 3 years) are in the stage of autonomy vs. shame and doubt.
    ① Infants are in the stage of trust vs. mistrust.
    ② Preschoolers are in the stage of initiative vs. guilt.
    ④ School-age children are in the stage of industry vs. inferiority.

40. Comprehension, assessment, physiological adaptation (b)
    ❷ These are classic symptoms of an infant with pyloric stenosis.
    ① These are not symptoms of Hirschsprung's disease.
    ③ These are not symptoms of esophageal atresia.
    ④ These are not symptoms of intussusception.

41. Knowledge, assessment, physiological adaptation (a)
    ❷ A child in sickle cell crisis often experiences abdominal pain, swollen, painful joints, and fever.
    ① These do not occur in sickle cell crisis.
    ③ This is not a symptom of sickle cell crisis.
    ④ These are not symptoms of sickle cell crisis.

42. Application, planning, basic care and comfort (b)
    ❹ Assessing sensation, circulation, and motion in affected extremities is necessary for all children in a cast.
    ① Children having pain should be medicated for pain as needed.
    ② Fluids should be encouraged; the cast can be kept dry by careful diapering and padding of the cast.
    ③ The child will need an adapted car seat to take her home safely.

43. Knowledge, evaluation, reduction of risk potential (b)
    ❷ Several studies have demonstrated that infants sleeping prone are at a greater risk for SIDS.
    ① This is not applicable to SIDS.
    ③ The peak age for SIDS is 2 to 4 months.
    ④ This is not applicable to SIDS.

44. Comprehension, planning, pharmacological therapies (b)
    ❹ The antiinflammatory effects of corticosteroids will decrease the edema commonly seen with nephrotic syndrome.
    ① Steroids have no effect on proteinuria.
    ② Steroids have no effect on increased albumin levels.
    ③ Steroids are not antihypertensive drugs.

45. Application, planning, physiological adaptation (b)
    ❶ In epileptic children with poorly controlled seizures, a ketogenic diet is often suggested as a method of treatment.
    ② Children with Crohn's disease are usually on a soft, low-fiber diet.
    ③ Children with bulimia are not placed on a ketogenic diet.
    ④ Children with acute glomerulonephritis are usually on a low-sodium diet.

46. Comprehension, application, physiological adaptation (c)
    ❸ The bronchoconstriction and inflammation of the airways seen in asthma cause these symptoms.
    ① These are symptoms of a cold; a child with asthma has a nonproductive cough.
    ② Asthma does not produce a fever or rhinorrhea.
    ④ These are symptoms of epiglottitis.

47. Comprehension, planning, pharmacological therapies (c)
    ❷ Bronchodilators (to relieve bronchial constriction) and antiinflammatory agents (to relieve inflammation of bronchial mucosa) are most often used together to treat asthma.
    ① Immunosuppressants are not regularly used to treat asthma.
    ③ Antibiotics are not used to treat asthma.
    ④ Decongestants and antihistamines are not effective in relieving the bronchoconstriction and inflammation seen in asthma.

48. Knowledge, planning, prevention and early detection of disease (b)
    ❶ The first hepatitis B vaccine is given to the newborn infant, usually within the first 24-48 hours after delivery.
    ② At 2 months, the infant receives the DTP, OPV, Hib, and the second dose of hepatitis B vaccine.
    ③ At 6 months, the infant receives the DTP, OPV, and the third dose of hepatitis B vaccine.

④ At 12 months, the infant receives the MMR, the varicella zoster vaccine, and the DTP.

49. Comprehension, assessment, physiological adaptation (b)
❷ The infant with colic demonstrates these signs and symptoms.
① Signs and symptoms of intussusception begin suddenly and include vomiting and bloody stools.
③ Signs and symptoms of pyloric stenosis include projectile vomiting and weight loss.
④ Signs and symptoms of Hirschsprung's disease include abdominal distention, vomiting, and inadequate weight gain.

50. Application, planning, pharmacological therapies (c)
❷ Ribavirin (Virazole), an antiviral agent, is used specifically for an RSV infection, especially in children with chronic conditions; humidified oxygen relieves the dyspnea and hypoxia seen with RSV disease.
① Cromolyn (Intal), a nonsteroidal antiinflammatory agent, is used in the treatment of asthma.
③ Antibiotics are not used for RSV infection.
④ Prednisone (LiquiPred) is not used for RSV infection.

51. Knowledge, assessment, physiological adaptation (c)
❹ This is the pathophysiology of RSV bronchiolitis.
① RSV occurs primarily in the winter and spring.
② Peak incidence for RSV infection is 2 to 5 months of age.
③ RSV can survive for hours on many surfaces, but for only half an hour on skin.

52. Knowledge, assessment, physiological adaptation (b)
❸ An omphalocele is a defect in which the abdominal contents protrude through the abdominal wall in an intact sac.
① Intussusception is a telescoping of the bowel and occurs within the abdomen.
② A diaphragmatic hernia is a congenital defect in the diaphragm that allows the abdominal contents to enter the thoracic cavity.
④ Gastroschisis is a herniation of the abdominal contents, not covered by a peritoneal sac, that herniates lateral to the umbilical ring.

53. Application, implementation, pharmacological therapies (c)
❸ Meperidine: DD = 35 mg
DH = 50 mg
V = 1 ml
$$\frac{DD}{DH} = \frac{35 \text{ mg}}{50 \text{ mg}} \times 1 \text{ ml} = 0.7 \text{ ml}$$
Atropine: DD = 0.1 mg
DH = 0.2 mg
V = 1 ml
$$\frac{DD}{DH} = \frac{0.1 \text{ mg}}{0.2 \text{ mg}} \times 1 \text{ ml} = 0.5 \text{ ml}$$
①, ②, ④ These are not the correct doses.

54. Application, planning, safety and infection control (b)
❸ Having a parent assist in procedures such as this often helps to calm the child, making it easier to give the medication.
① Giving a medication orally is much less traumatic and more preferable than giving it via an injection.

② Sedation is used only as a last resort for traumatic procedures, not for administering medications.
④ Restraints should be used only if there is no parent or other nurse to assist.

55. Application, implementation, pharmacological therapies (b)
❸ DD = 425 mg
DH = 1 g (1000 mg)
C = 4 ml
$$\frac{DD}{DH} = \frac{425 \text{ mg}}{1000 \text{ mg}} \times 4 \text{ ml} = 1.7 \text{ ml}$$
①, ②, ④ These are not the correct dose.

56. Knowledge, implementation, pharmacological therapies (b)
❷ This is the correct rate of infusion.
① This rate is too slow.
③, ④ These rates are too fast.

57. Comprehension, planning, physiological adaptation (b)
❶ This is the preferred method of treatment for infectious gastroenteritis.
② IV fluids may be used if oral therapy does not work, but it is not the preferred method.
③, ④ These are incorrect treatments for this disease.

58. Comprehension, analysis, physiological adaptation (c)
❸ Croup is also known as spasmodic laryngitis.
① Croup is usually of viral origin.
② The esophagus is not involved in croup.
④ This would be pneumonia or pneumonitis.

59. Comprehension, analysis, physiological adaptation (a)
❹ Fats are not completely digested in a child with cystic fibrosis because of the lack of the enzyme lipase. These fats are excreted with the stool, making it frothy and foul smelling.
①, ②, ③ These do not cause the abnormal stools.

60. Knowledge, analysis, physiological adaptation (b)
❶ The pancreas is the organ most severely affected in cystic fibrosis.
②, ③ These are not involved in cystic fibrosis.
④ The liver is not directly involved in cystic fibrosis.

61. Application, planning, coordinated care (b)
❸ This is the best time to begin planning for the child's discharge.
①, ② These are much too late to begin discharge planning.
④ All children need to have some form of discharge planning to make the transition from hospital to home go smoothly.

62. Knowledge, analysis, physiological adaptation (a)
❶ Down syndrome is a chromosomal abnormality (trisomy 21).
②, ③ Down syndrome is not caused by an infection.
④ It is not caused by a lack of oxygen at birth.

63. Comprehension, analysis, physiological adaptation (b)
❶ Celiac syndrome is a metabolic defect precipitated by the ingestion of rye or wheat gluten.
②, ③, ④ These are not contraindicated for children with celiac disease.

64. Comprehension, analysis, reduction of risk potential (b)
    ❹ Bryant's/modified Bryant's traction is the usual method of treatment for an infant with a fractured femur.
    ① This is more extensive treatment than is usually needed.
    ② Skeletal traction is not usually used for infants with fractured femurs; often used in older children.
    ③ Traction is usually necessary before casting can be done if the fracture is to heal properly.

65. Knowledge, analysis, physiological adaptation (a)
    ❷ Sickle cell disease is caused by a hereditary trait that occurs primarily among African-Americans.
    ① It is not a viral disease.
    ③ It is not a bacterial disease.
    ④ It is not caused by a mismatched blood transfusion.

66. Comprehension, assessment, physiological adaptation (a)
    ❶ Ringworm is caused by a fungus and can occur on the scalp (tinea capitis), body (tinea corporis), or feet (tinea pedis).
    ❷ This is an infestation of lice.
    ③ This is caused by a virus.
    ④ This is hives, often caused by allergies to foods or animal fur.

67. Knowledge, assessment, growth and development through the life span (b)
    ❷ This is the total number of deciduous (baby) teeth.
    ① This figure is too low.
    ③, ④ These figures are too high.

68. Application, implementation, pharmacological therapies (b)
    ❷ gr. v = 300 mg; one tablet is the correct answer.
    ①, ③, ④ These are not the correct answer.

69. Analysis, implementation, physiological adaptation (b)
    ❸ Use of diuretics is necessary because of the patient's edema.
    ① Semi-Fowler's position in the most comfortable position to facilitate respiration.
    ② The normal diet for a child with nephrotic syndrome is a high-protein diet.
    ④ Sodium and potassium supplements are not usually given; sodium is limited.

70. Application, implementation, physiological adaptation (b)
    ❸ This aids in the prevention of infection.
    ① The child's position should be changed frequently to avoid pressure areas and severe itching.
    ② To reduce itching and subsequent scratching, a minimum amount of clothing is recommended.
    ④ Warm, moist dressings would increase the itching; cool, moist dressings should be used.

71. Comprehension, assessment, physiological adaptation (b)
    ❷ This is a symptom of the condition.
    ① Amenorrhea, not dysmenorrhea, is commonly seen in these patients.
    ③ Bradycardia and hypotension are common, probably because of the state of starvation.
    ④ Constipation, not diarrhea, is a symptom of anorexia nervosa.

72. Application, implementation, pharmacological therapies (b)
    ❷ In a 2-year-old, pulling the outer ear down and back straightens the ear canal so that the drops can be properly instilled.
    ① This is the correct position for children over 3 years of age.
    ③, ④ These are not the correct positions.

73. Application, planning, physiological adaptation (c)
    ❹ IV immune globulin (IVIG) is given to help decrease the fever and to decrease the incidence of coronary artery damage commonly seen as a complication of KD.
    ① The cause of KD is unknown.
    ② IVIG does not promote rest or sleep.
    ③ IVIG does not regulate fluid levels or BP.

74. Knowledge, assessment, growth and development through the life span (b)
    ❷ This is normal behavior for toddlers at this age level.
    ① Toddlers do not move carefully; they tend to run and bump into objects and people.
    ③ Toddlers are noisy; typical play at this age is known as "parallel play," in which the toddler plays next to another toddler, but not with them.
    ④ Toddlers like to move when they play.

75. Application, assessment, physiological adaptation (b)
    ❹ This is the most important assessment to make on a child with hydrocephalus.
    ①, ③ These are not important assessments to make on this child.
    ② Frequent neurological checks may be necessary, not neurovascular checks.

76. Application, implementation, basic care and comfort (b)
    ❸ These are appropriate fluids and food for a child with mild diarrhea.
    ① This could lead to dehydration.
    ②, ④ These are inappropriate choices for a child with diarrhea.

77. Application, planning, reduction of risk potential (b)
    ❷ Palpation of the tumor is to be avoided to decrease the chance of cancer metastasis.
    ① A 3-year-old cannot be held responsible for his or her own safety.
    ③, ④ These are not part of the care of a child with Wilms' tumor.

78. Knowledge, assessment, physiological adaptation (a)
    ❹ This is another name for trisomy 21.
    ①, ②, ③ These are other types of genetic syndromes.

79. Application, planning, physiological adaptation (c)
    ❹ The cool, moist air helps to reduce inflammation in the airway and helps to keep secretions moist.
    ① Symptoms are relieved over a period of time.
    ② The cool, moist air does not prevent drug toxicity.
    ③ The cool, moist air may assist in reducing fever but does not promote hydration.

80. Comprehension, implementation, physiological adaptation (b)
    ❸ The Epstein-Barr virus is the principal cause of mononucleosis.
    ① Kissing is one of the methods that this virus can be passed.

② This is not a cause of mononucleosis.

④ Mononucleosis is a viral, not a bacterial, disease.

81. Comprehension, implementation, physiological adaptation (b)

❸ An intussusception occurs when one part of the intestine telescopes into another part of the intestine.

①, ②, ④ These are not what happens with an intussusception.

82. Comprehension, implementation, physiological adaptation (b)

❷ Eczema (atopic dermatitis) is usually associated with an allergy, along with a family history of the disease.

① Eczema is not a metabolic disorder.

③ Eczema is not an infectious disorder, but a secondary infection may result without proper treatment.

④ Eczema is not a nutritional disorder, but it can be a result of a food allergy.

83. Knowledge, assessment, growth and development through the life span (b)

❸ An infant normally triples his or her birth weight at 12 months of age.

① At 6 months, an infant normally doubles his or her birth weight.

② This is too early of an age to expect tripling of birth weight.

④ By this age, the birth weight of the infant should be more than tripled.

84. Comprehension, assessment, prevention and early detection of disease (c)

❸ Osteomyelitis most often occurs after an injury to a long bone.

①, ④ These do not lead to the development of osteomyelitis.

② There is no gene for osteomyelitis.

85. Knowledge, assessment, prevention and early detection of disease (b)

❹ *Staphylococcus aureus* is the main organism that causes osteomyelitis.

①, ②, ③ These organisms do not normally cause osteomyelitis.

86. Comprehension, evaluation, physiological adaptation (c)

❸ The most important clinical outcome for a child in respiratory distress is that the airway remains patent.

①, ② These are not appropriate clinical outcomes for a child in respiratory distress.

④ Although this is a positive outcome, it is not the most important clinical outcome for a child in respiratory distress.

87. Comprehension, evaluation, physiological adaptation (c)

❹ A child who follows the appropriate diet should have less fat in their stools.

① The goal should be a slow, steady weight gain.

②, ③ These are not related to a child with celiac disease following their diet.

88. Knowledge, assessment, prevention and early detection of disease (b)

❶ Hirschsprung's disease is a congenital anomaly (absence of the ganglion nerve cells) that results in a mechanical obstruction of the colon.

②, ③, ④ These are not the causes of Hirschsprung's disease.

89. Comprehension, assessment, physiological adaptation (b)

❷ These are classic symptoms of acute appendicitis.

①, ②, ④ These are not signs of this disease.

90. Knowledge, assessment, growth and development through the life span (b)

❹ The anterior fontanel begins to close throughout infancy, but is not completely closed until 18-24 months of age.

①, ②, ③ The anterior fontanel is still open at these ages.

91. Knowledge, assessment, growth and development through the life span (b)

❷ The two lower central incisors erupt first, between 6 and 8 months of age.

① These teeth erupt at the age of 12 to 13 months.

③, ④ These teeth erupt at the age of 16 months.

92. Application, assessment, basic care and comfort, (b)

❸ Blood pressure measurement and observation for edema are your assessment priorities when caring for a child with glomerulonephritis.

①, ②, ④ These parts of the assessment are not appropriate for a child with glomerulonephritis.

93. Knowledge, assessment, growth and development through the life span (b)

❹ The posterior fontanel is closed between 2 to 3 months of age.

①, ②, ③ The posterior fontanel remains open at these ages.

94. Comprehension, assessment, physiological adaptation (b)

❹ Scrotal edema, along with edema to the face, extremities, and abdomen are common signs of nephrotic syndrome.

① This is a sign of severe dehydration.

② There is a decreased urinary output in a child with nephrotic syndrome.

③ The skin is very pale in a child with nephrotic syndrome.

95. Application, implementation, psychosocial adaptation (b)

❹ Nurses are considered "mandated reporters" of actual and suspected child abuse and neglect.

① Because nurses are mandated reporters, they are legally bound to report abuse and neglect, regardless of possible legal consequences.

② Nurses are not required to report abuse to a physician prior to calling a child abuse center.

③ Nurses are also required to report abuse.

96. Comprehension, evaluation, pharmacological therapies (c)

❸ Prednisone is given to decrease inflammation.

①, ②, ④ Prednisone is not used for this reason in the treatment for rheumatic fever.

97. Application, planning, reduction of risk potential (b)

❹ In an infant receiving IV therapy, special attention should be paid to maintaining the IV line and infusion of IV fluids.

①, ② These are part of the infant's care but are not a priority.

③ This is not generally a necessary part of the infant's care.

98. Knowledge, assessment, growth and development through the life span (c)
    ❷ This is Erikson's theory of child development.
    ① Freud's theory is based on psychosexual development.
    ③ There is no theory of child development by this name.
    ④ Piaget's theory is based on intellectual (cognitive) development.
99. Comprehension, assessment, growth and development through the life span (c)
    ❶ This is the basis of Piaget's theory of child development.
    ② This is the basis of Freud's theory of child development.
    ③ This is the basis of Erikson's theory of child development.
    ④ This is not a theory of child development.
100. Knowledge, assessment, growth and development through the life span (c)
    ❸ This is a normal characteristic for a healthy 1-month-old infant.
    ①, ②, ④ These are normal characteristics for a healthy 2- to 3-month-old infant.
101. Knowledge, assessment, growth and development through the life span (b)
    ❹ Primitive reflexes (grasp, tonic neck, etc.) disappear between 4 and 5 months of age.
    ①, ② Primitive reflexes remain strong at these ages.
    ③ Primitive reflexes are still present, but fading.
102. Knowledge, assessment, growth and development through the life span (b)
    ❸ Teething normally begins at this age.
    ①, ② These are earlier than the time teething normally begins.
    ④ Infants usually have 4 to 6 teeth by this age.
103. Comprehension, evaluation, growth and development through the life span (c)
    ❸ Infants at this age first begin to consistently demonstrate fear of strangers.
    ①, ② Fear of strangers has not developed at this age.
    ④ The infant continues to be fearful of strangers; demonstration of anxiety begins earlier.
104. Knowledge, assessment, growth and development through the life span (b)
    ❷ Trust is Erikson's developmental task of infancy, and is developed depending on how their needs are met by their parents/caregivers.
    ① This is the developmental task of toddlers.
    ③ This is the developmental task of preschoolers.
    ④ This is not a developmental task.
105. Knowledge, implementation, prevention and early detection of disease (c)
    ❹ The American Academy of Pediatrics advised that all clinicians should suspend the administration of the rotavirus vaccine pending collection of additional information.
    ①, ②, ③ These vaccines should still be given according to schedule; their use was not suspended.
106. Comprehension, evaluation, physiological adaptation (c)
    ❶ Organic FTT occurs as a result of a physical cause, such as congenital heart disease.
    ② This is not a classification of FTT.
    ③ Nonorganic FTT is unrelated to a disease.
    ④ Idiopathic FTT has no explained cause.
107. Comprehension, assessment, physiological adaptation (c)
    ❹ RSV bronchiolitis is a viral infection that causes the bronchioles to swell and become plugged with mucus. The trapped mucus makes it difficult for the infant to expel air.
    ①, ②, ③ These are not the pathophysiology of RSV.
108. Application, implementation, pharmacological therapies (b)
    ❷ Ribavirin is administered by nebulization via an oxygen hood, tent, or mask for 12 to 20 hours per day, for 1 to 7 days.
    ①, ③, ④ These are inappropriate ways to administer ribavirin.
109. Comprehension, assessment, physiological adaptation (b)
    ❹ The most common cause for infectious gastroenteritis in infants is the rotavirus.
    ①, ③ These are not causes for infectious gastroenteritis.
    ② This is a cause for infectious gastroenteritis but is not as common as rotavirus in the infant.
110. Application, planning, basic care and comfort (b)
    ❶ Normally, the first glucose water feeding will be attempted 4 to 6 hours after the surgery.
    ②, ③ These are later than the first feeding is normally given.
    ④ This is when formula is started after surgery.
111. Application, implementation, pharmacological therapies (b)
    ❶ This steroidal medication is usually used for this specific type of meningitis.
    ①, ②, ③ These drugs are not used for the treatment of *Haemophilus influenzae* type B meningitis
112. Knowledge, assessment, physiological adaptation (b)
    ❹ Hirschsprung's disease, caused by a congenital lack of nerve cells in the wall of the colon, will exhibit these symptoms during the first several hours of life.
    ①, ② These are not signs of Hirschsprung's disease.
    ③ These are symptoms of pyloric stenosis.
113. Comprehension, planning, physiological adaptation (c)
    ❷ The infant with esophageal atresia must be kept NPO and on IV fluids until after surgery is completed to correct the defects. Suctioning of excess mucus is often necessary.
    ①, ④ The infant must be NPO.
    ③ This is not the treatment for esophageal atresia.
114. Application, implementation, reduction of risk potential (b)
    ❸ Nursing care of the child after a ventriculoperitoneal shunt should include head circumference measurements to help determine if the shunt is draining cerebrospinal fluid properly.
    ①, ②, ④ These are not necessary postoperative nursing interventions for this disorder.
115. Knowledge, assessment, physiological adaptation (b)
    ❸ This is the term for the condition when one or both of the testes fail to descend into the scrotal sac.
    ① Epispadias is a congenital condition in which the urethra ends on the top side of the penis.
    ② Hypospadias is a congenital condition in which the urethra ends on the bottom side of the penis.
    ④ Nephrotic syndrome is a kidney disorder.

116. Comprehension, implementation, pharmacological therapies (b)
   ❷ This drug (HCG) is sometimes given to young males with cryptorchidism.
   ①, ③ These drugs are not given for cryptorchidism.
   ④ This drug is given in the treatment of cystic fibrosis.

117. Comprehension, assessment, physiological adaptation (c)
   ❷ These are the four separate cardiac defects known as Tetralogy of Fallot.
   ①, ③, ④ These conditions do not make up the condition Tetralogy of Fallot.

118. Comprehension, planning, pharmacological therapies (c)
   ❶ Treatment for sickle cell crisis includes IV fluids, oxygen as needed, bed rest, analgesics for pain, blood transfusions as needed, proper nutrition, oral fluids, antibiotic therapy as needed.
   ② Children in sickle cell crisis need increased fluids, and do not need an NG tube.
   ③ Children with sickle cell disease do not require bone marrow transplants.
   ④ Pancreatic enzymes are used in the treatment of cystic fibrosis.

119. Application, planning, coping and adaptation, (c)
   ❷ Bad behavior should be criticized, and limits set; criticizing the child only leads to development of shame and self-doubt.
   ① Reasoning with a toddler should be attempted after the temper tantrum.
   ③ This is the developmental task of a preschooler.
   ④ Many toddlers are not "ready" to be potty trained at age 2.

120. Knowledge, assessment, physiological adaptation (b)
   ❸ These are the symptoms of amblyopia, or "lazy eye."
   ① Strabismus is a condition in which the eyes fail to direct and focus on the same object at the same time.
   ②, ④ These are types of strabismus.

121. Comprehension, assessment, physiological adaptation (c)
   ❹ These are characteristic signs of the spastic type of cerebral palsy.
   ①, ② This is the mixed type of cerebral palsy.
   ③ These are signs of ataxic cerebral palsy.

122. Application, planning, prevention and early detection of disease (a)
   ❹ This type of advice will help prevent childhood accidents.
   ① All children of all ages should wear bicycle helmets every time they ride a bike.
   ② Medications and poisonous substances should be placed in a high, locked cabinet.
   ③ Handles of pots and pans should be turned inward, away from the reach of children.

123. Comprehension, assessment, growth and development through the life span (b)
   ❷ Preschooler (3 to 5 years of age) is the age level of children developing this task.
   ① The developmental task of toddlers is "autonomy vs. shame and doubt."
   ③ The developmental task of school-age children is "industry vs. inferiority."
   ④ The developmental task of adolescents is "identity vs. role confusion."

124. Comprehension, assessment, growth and development through the life span (b)
   ❶ This is a normal developmental stage in preschoolers.
   ② This is a normal developmental stage in infants.
   ③ This is a normal developmental stage in school-age children.
   ④ This is a normal developmental stage in toddlers.

125. Application, implementation, basic care and comfort (c)
   ❹ Postoperative care for the child after a tonsillectomy includes these nursing interventions.
   ① The child should be kept prone, with the head to the side, until fully awake.
   ② Clear, cool fluids should be given to the child, after the nausea subsides.
   ③ This is not usual postoperative care for a child after tonsillectomy.

126. Knowledge, assessment, physiological adaptation (c)
   ❸ These are signs and symptoms of nephrotic syndrome.
   ① Nephrotic syndrome includes hypoalbuminemia.
   ②, ④ Nephrotic syndrome is diagnosed via renal biopsy; there are decreased levels of protein in the blood.

127. Comprehension, implementation, pharmacological therapies (b)
   ❶ Nephrotic syndrome is treated with corticosteroids to decrease the edema and oral alkylating agents to reduce the relapse rate and induce long-term remission.
   ②, ④ Antibiotics are not used to treat nephrotic syndrome.
   ③ Antihypertensives are not used to treat nephrotic syndrome.

128. Knowledge, assessment, physiological adaptation (b)
   ❸ This clotting disorder is known as hemophilia.
   ①, ②, ④ These are not the definitions for this blood disorder.

129. Application, implementation, prevention and early detection of disease (b)
   ❸ Swimming is the safest of the four sports listed for a child with hemophilia.
   ①, ②, ④ These are not safe sports for a child with hemophilia.

130. Comprehension, assessment, physiological adaptation (c)
   ❷ These are the three main consequences of bone marrow dysfunction seen in leukemia.
   ①, ③, ④ Blood clotting function is not a consequence of bone marrow dysfunction in leukemia.

131. Comprehension, evaluation, reduction of risk potential (b)
   ❶ A decreased WBC count often lowers a child's resistance to infection.
   ②, ④ These symptoms of leukemia are not all caused by a decrease in WBCs.
   ③ This is not caused by a decreased WBC count.

132. Knowledge, assessment, physiological adaptation (b)
   ❹ These are all characteristic signs of muscular dystrophy.
   ①, ②, ③ These are not characteristic signs of this disease.

133. Knowledge, assessment, growth and development through the life span (b)
❸ This is the age where bone growth slows, and cartilage is replace by bone at the epiphyses.
①, ② These ages are too young for cartilage to be replaced.
④ At this age, most of the cartilage has already been replaced by bone at the epiphyses.

134. Comprehension, assessment, physiological adaptation (b)
❹ Generalized seizures are bilaterally symmetrical, and accompanied by impaired consciousness; grand mal seizures are one type of generalized seizure.
①, ②, ③ Grand mal seizures are not classified as this type of seizure because of their characteristics.

135. Application, planning, pharmacological therapies (a)
❸ This is the appropriate treatment for pediculosis.
① Corticosteroids are not used in the treatment of pediculosis.
②, ④ These are not used in the treatment for pediculosis.

136. Application, implementation, coping and adaptation (c)
❸ The child with insulin-dependent diabetes should be taught how to do insulin injections, along with his or her parents (or other caregivers).
① Blood sugar (glucose) monitoring will most likely be required more than once a day.
② Symptoms of hypoglycemia include low blood sugar and a normal glucose in the urine.
④ The child's diet will be different than before the diagnosis; he or she will also be required to exercise, to help maintain a regular blood sugar.

137. Knowledge, assessment, growth and development through the life span (b)
❹ The growth spurt in adolescent boys is later than in girls and usually occurs between 12 and 14 year of age.
①, ②, ③ These are not the time that the growth spurt occurs in adolescent boys.

138. Comprehension, assessment, prevention and early detection of disease (b)
❸ These are typical signs of an adolescent that is abusing drugs/alcohol.
①, ②, ④ These are not all typical signs of this disease.

139. Application, implementation, pharmacological therapies (b)
❶ Retinoic acid is commonly used in combination with benzoyl peroxide in the treatment of acne vulgaris.
②, ④ Tinea corporis and all forms of ringworm are treated with antifungal creams/ointments.
③ Pediculosis is treated with a pediculicide shampoo.

140. Comprehension, planning, pharmacological therapies (c)
❷ This is the action of antiretroviral agents in the treatment of HIV.
①, ③, ④ These are not the actions of antiretroviral agents.

141. Application, implementation, coping and adaptation (b)
❸ This is the rationale for preparing children for hospitalization.
① This is true, but it is not the rationale for preparing children prior to hospitalization.

②, ④ These are not the rationales for preparing children for hospitalization.

142. Application, implementation, safety and infection control (b)
❸ Restraints may be necessary; if used, they should be on securely, and circulation should be checked regularly and documented.
① "Candyland" has small pieces that a toddler could choke on or swallow.
② A child's side rails should always be up when they are in bed.
④ No medications should be left with any age child.

143. Comprehension, implementation, physiological adaptation (b)
❶ Bryant's traction is a type of skin traction.
②, ③ Bryant's traction is not these types of traction.
④ Pelvic traction is another type of skin traction, but it is not the same as Bryant's traction.

144. Application, implementation, reduction of risk potential (b)
❸ For the entire cast to dry, all areas must be allowed to be open to the air.
① Hairdryers should not be used to dry the cast.
② The cast should be handled using open palms, not fingertips, to avoid denting the cast.
④ The cast should remain open to the air in order to dry.

145. Knowledge, assessment, physiological adaptation (b)
❷ Leukemia is the most common cancer seen in children.
①, ③, ④ This type of cancer is seen in children but is not as common as leukemia.

146. Comprehension, implementation, prevention and early detection of disease (b)
❶ This test, along with a barium enema, is used to confirm Hirschsprung's disease.
②, ③, ④ These tests are not used to confirm Hirschsprung's disease.

147. Knowledge, assessment, physiological adaptation (b)
❹ The symptom of projectile vomiting is a classic sign of pyloric stenosis.
①, ②, ③ These are not classic signs of this disease.

148. Application, implementation, pharmacological therapies (c)
❷ Amoxicillin is most commonly ordered for treatment of otitis media.
①, ③ These antibiotics are not usually used in the treatment of otitis media.
④ This is not an antibiotic.

149. Knowledge, assessment, physiological adaptation (b)
❷ A red, flat rash is normally seen on the body of an adolescent with mononucleosis.
①, ③, ④ These are not common symptoms of mononucleosis.

150. Application, intervention, pharmacological therapies (c)
❹ This is the correct dose.
2.2 lb = 1 kg; 11 pounds × 2.2 pounds = 5 kg
DD = 0.1 mg/kg
0.1 mg × 5 kg = 0.5 mg
①, ② These are not the correct dose.
③ Morphine can be given via SQ, IM, IV, and epidural routes.

CHAPTER 9

Nursing Care of the Aging Adult

The percentage of the American population over age 65 is rapidly passing 13% and continues to constitute our fastest-growing age group. As the life expectancy of Americans continues to lengthen, the year 2010 will see the first baby boomers retiring. By the year 2030 we will be challenged to care for an aging adult population that constitutes 22% of the total population. Maintenance of health and wellness, and caring for increasingly older adults will be the emphasis in future years. How we address these future trends will be reflected in history as a measure of our civility.

It is nursing's challenge to meet the care needs of our older adults, who are so vulnerable to the biases of our fast-paced, youth-oriented society. As nurses we have an opportunity to play a significant role in determining whether these will be years of continued growth and development, years of happiness and accomplishment, or years of forced shame, illness, and neglect.

This chapter focuses on aging as a normal process and strives to increase the practitioner's knowledge of and understanding for a stage of life through which we will all pass.

"For age is opportunity no less than youth itself, though in another dress."
—Longfellow

GOVERNMENT RESOURCES FOR THE OLDER ADULT

Income

A. Social Security (Federal Old-Age, Survivors, and Disability Insurance, FOASDI)-first adopted in 1935
   1. Funded by employee and employer payroll taxes
   2. Entitlement determined by United States Social Security Administration; benefits are granted in accordance with:
      a. Age
      b. Lifetime earnings record—retirement age is steadily increasing
      c. Free earnings credits for active military service
      d. Whether required number of work credits have been earned (work credits are measured in quarters)
   3. Specific maximum benefit amount with cost-of-living protection against inflation
   4. Minimum retirement benefits begin at age 62
   5. Railroad workers have a separate retirement system; workers who have less than 10 years of railroad service may transfer earnings to Social Security to be counted toward Social Security benefits
   6. Federal employees are covered under the Civil Service Retirement System, the Federal Employees Retirement System, and the Thrift Savings Plan
   7. Social Security benefits are reduced according to monies earned over a stated maximum annual allowable income
   8. No reduction in Social Security benefits for full-time employees over the age of 70
   9. Payments are indexed according to inflation rate
B. Supplemental Security Income (SSI)—established in 1972.
   1. Funded from general tax revenues
   2. Cash assistance program
   3. Administered by Social Security Administration
   4. Designed to provide for disabled, blind, or aged with limited incomes and resources
   5. Medicaid eligibility in many states is based on SSI eligibility

Health

A. Medicare (Title XVIII of Social Security Act)—established in 1965
   1. Administered by Health Care Finance Administration of U.S. Department of Health and Human Services
   2. Designed to help those over 65 years of age and certain disabled people under 65, who are eligible under Social Security, to meet medical care costs regardless of income, and people of any age with permanent kidney failure
   3. Major insurance companies in each state handle claims (e.g., Travelers Insurance Company in New York)
   4. Pays for only limited time in long-term care
   5. Do not have to be retired to receive benefits
   6. Financed by employer and employee payroll taxes and by self-employment tax monies
   7. Everyone over 65 who is entitled to Social Security benefits receives hospital insurance without paying premium charges
   8. Automatic hospital insurance is provided to disabled persons who have been entitled to Social Security disability benefits for 24 consecutive months
   9. Initial enrollment period begins 3 months before the month individual will become 65 and continues for 4 months after individual turns 65
   10. Annual enrollment periods (January 1 through March 31)
   11. Premiums generally increase if people do not apply when they are eligible
   12. Deductible is applied to each benefit period
   13. Two parts
      a. Part A designed as hospital insurance that has certain exclusions
      b. Part B covers physician services and outpatient services
      c. If subscribing to part A, automatically enrolled in part B unless it is declined
B. Medicaid (Title XIX of Social Security Act)—established in 1965
   1. Purposes
      a. To cover specific expenses not provided for by Medicare
      b. To reduce expenses of those who have exhausted their Medicare benefits
      c. To defray medical expenses of those who cannot afford Medicare premiums
   2. Funded by federal and state contributions
   3. State-operated programs
   4. Funds the majority of long-term care, after Medicare and personal funds are depleted
   5. Other programs
      a. Qualified Medicare Beneficiary (QMB) Program
         (1) Annual income must be below or at the national poverty level—12% of older adults fall below the poverty line
         (2) Functions like Medigap policy
         (3) State Medicaid program helps pay
         (4) Pays Medicare Part B premium
         (5) Pays Medicare Part A premiums for eligible older adults and disabled persons, Medicare deductible, and co-insurance fees
      b. Specified Low-Income Medicare Beneficiary (SLMB)
         (1) Income cannot be more than 20% above the national poverty level
         (2) Must be eligible for Medicare Part A
         (3) State will pay Medicare Part B premiums
         (4) Does not pay Medicare co-insurance or deductibles
C. Private health insurance
   1. Medigap
      a. Medicare Supplement Insurance
      b. Regulated by state and federal law
      c. Ten standard plans
      d. Lifetime maximums are established
      e. Not government sponsored
      f. Policies of choice may be purchased from any insurer doing Medigap business in one's state of residency for a 6-month period from date enrolled in Medicare Part B; and age 65 or older
      g. Plans pay all or most medical co-insurance amounts; some policies pay for Medicare deductibles
   2. Medicare Select
      a. Purchase of Medicare Select Plan is Medigap insurance
      b. Supplements Medicare's benefits
      c. Sold by insurance companies and HMOs

d. Difference between Medicare Select and Medigap is that specific doctors and certain hospitals must be used for nonemergent care to qualify for full benefits

e. Federally approved through 1998 in all states

Housing

A. Department of Housing and Urban Development
   1. Rent Supplement Program: rent-subsidized apartments for older adult, disabled, or low-income families
      a. Utility and rent costs in existing buildings
      b. Renovations of existing units
      c. Building of new units
   2. Provides home improvement loans
   3. Provides mortgage insurance
   4. Age, asset, income eligibility requirements
B. Older adult and handicapped housing (Housing Act of 1959)
   1. Funding to private, nonprofit organizations for renovation or building of units for the older adult and handicapped
   2. Low-interest federal loans for same
C. National Housing Act (Housing and Urban Development Act, 1968): funding to private corporations for construction of low- and middle-income housing
D. National Housing Act of 1952: funding to private, profit, or nonprofit groups for nursing home construction or renovation

Title XX of the Social Security Act

A. Federal monies for social programs that are available and appropriate for the older adult
B. State administered
C. Individual must be eligible for SSI

Food Stamp Program

A. Administered by U.S. Department of Agriculture
B. Must meet income requirements
C. Each state's welfare department determines eligibility
D. Components
   1. Home-delivered meals
   2. Grocery store food purchases

Administration on Aging

A. State, regional, area, and local units: area units responsible for providing program coordination and development expertise
B. Major services
   1. Nutritional programs
      a. On-site meals
      b. Home-delivered meals
   2. Senior centers
      a. Services
      b. Programs
   3. Home care
      a. Homemaker
      b. Home health aide
      c. Home visits
      d. Telephone calls
      e. Chore maintenance
   4. Information and referral
   5. Transportation
      a. Urban Mass Transit Act
      b. Area agencies on aging

LEGISLATION AFFECTING THE OLDER ADULT

1. Social Security—established in 1935 by Theodore Roosevelt. Legislators predict benefits may be depleted by the year 2015
2. Medicare and Medicaid Programs—developed in 1965, programs have been through many reforms
3. Older Americans Act—first initiated in 1987 and revised in 1992; established standards for safeguarding the rights of the older adult
4. The Omnibus Budget Reconciliation Act (OBRA) of 1991—established to improve the lives of those individuals residing in nursing homes; attached stringent guidelines for the use of physical and chemical restraints
5. The Patient Self Determination Act—established in 1991, developed in an effort to allow individuals to control end-of-life care
   a. Living wills—completed while the individual is well, and outlines what the individual may or may not want done if unable to make decisions regarding end-of-life care
   b. Healthcare proxy—the individual designates a person to make end-of-life care decisions for them should they become incapacitated

NURSING ROLES AND THE CARE OF THE OLDER ADULT

1. Care provider—nurses are in the unique position to meet the healthcare needs of the older adult
   a. Nursing's goal in the care of the older adult is assisting the individual to their optimum state of health
   b. Nursing care focuses on prevention of acute and chronic health problems, promotion of a healthy lifestyle, and management of the symptoms of chronic health problems
2. Educator
   a. Nurses educate the older adult concerning health promotion and maintenance of acute and chronic health problems
   b. Nurses increase public awareness of problems affecting the older adult
3. Data collection
   a. Nurses must assess the older adult's need for services
   b. Area agencies on aging are the best resource regarding services for older adults in the community
4. Patient advocate
   a. Nurses act as patient advocates to ensure that the rights of the older adult are preserved in regards to health care practices, treatment modalities, and end-of-life care
   b. The American Nurses Association's Council on Gerontological Nursing has established Nursing Standards of Gerontological Practice
   c. Nurses recognize the older adult as a unique individual, molded by life experience, family, society, religion, and culture (Box 9-1)

THEORIES OF AGING
Sociological Theories

A. Disengagement
   1. Controversial
   2. Mutual withdrawal from social interaction by aged individual and society
   3. Theory describes engagement as active occupation and devotion

Box 9-1   Cultural Considerations

Chinese—achieving old age is a blessing, family is expected to take care of the older adult. Use alternative medicine such as herbs, acupressure, and acupuncture. May be hesitant to seek out services for the older adult.

Japanese—the older adults are viewed with respect, close family bonds are established. Many Japanese men would wed younger wives—higher proportion of widows. May reject modern medicine in favor of traditional practices.

Hispanic—describes individuals from Spain, Cuba, Mexico, and Puerto Rico. View illness as an act of God. Old age is viewed as a positive time. Families avoid long term care and this ethnic group has the lowest rate of institutionalization.

Native American—the older adults are respected as leaders in the community. Illness and health are viewed as good and evil and evil actions are punished by illness. Many elders feel that the questions used by nurses are too probing and inappropriate.

African-Americans—many Afrian-Americans never reach old age, therefore old age is viewed as a goal. There is a low rate of institutionalization among this ethnic group. The older adults look to family members for advice and care before contacting service agencies.

Jewish Americans—although not actually a particular culture, the Jewish religion dictates the customs and practices of these people. Illness typically draws the family together, and this group, who are normally highly educated, do not hesitate to seek out modern medicine as needed.

4. Supports leisure as a form of activity
5. Respects individual-initiated withdrawal
B. Activity
   1. Individual remains active and interacts with society's events
   2. Pursues new interests, friends, and roles to substitute for lost roles
   3. Supports social activity as beneficial
C. Continuity or development
   1. Lifelong personality characteristics and coping strategies continue
   2. Sense of inferiority develops
   3. Supportive network of relationships established
D. Passages: life cycle changes can be identified, predicted, planned for, and managed

Biological Theories

A. Wear-and-tear
   1. Stress and use deplete the body cells of repair ability
   2. Coping mechanisms decline because of decrease in available energy
B. Collagen
   1. Most abundant body protein
   2. Collagen molecules held together by bonds

3. Chemical reactions cause a switching of bonds between collagen molecules, resulting in structural changes characteristic of the aging process
C. Lipofuscin accumulation
   1. Lipofuscins or age pigments are insoluble end products of cell metabolism
   2. Accumulate in the cell, altering the cell's ability to function normally
D. Immunologic responses
   1. Aging is an autoimmune disease process
   2. Cells change, and the body does not recognize its own cells
   3. Autoimmune responses damage the cells, causing cell death
E. Cell death of genetic programming
   1. Cell reproduction is programmed
   2. The programming determines the rate and time a given species ages and dies
F. Free radical
   1. Molecules that have an extra electron are free radicals
   2. Free radicals attach to other molecules, altering function or structure
   3. There are internal and external sources of free radicals
   4. It is believed that the free radicals damage membrane function and structure (vitamins A, C, and E are thought to reduce free radical activity)
G. Mutation and error
   1. Cell division errors occur progressively over time
   2. Mutated cells are altered in their function and effectiveness
   3. Error theory expands mutation theory to include errors in interpretation of cell messages

Psychological Theories

A. Freud: did not recommend psychoanalysis for the aged population (see Chapter 6)
B. Sullivan: see Chapter 6
C. Maslow: see Chapter 2
D. Erikson: see Chapter 6
   1. Eighth stage (65 to 100 years of age) identified as "integrity vs. despair" (Fig. 9-1)
   2. Older adult who views own life as having no meaning ends life's stages in despair; older adult who can review his or her accomplishments and errors derives a sense of integrity
E. Peck
   1. Expanded Erikson's developmental theory of the eighth stage of man
   2. Focuses on alternatives to preoccupation with body changes and illness, thereby achieving life satisfaction (Fig. 9-2)

ROLE CHANGES

A. Types
   1. Crisis
      a. Sudden
      b. Not able to plan for appropriate replacement
      c. Substitute not readily available
      d. Stress producing
   2. Gradual
      a. Develops slowly

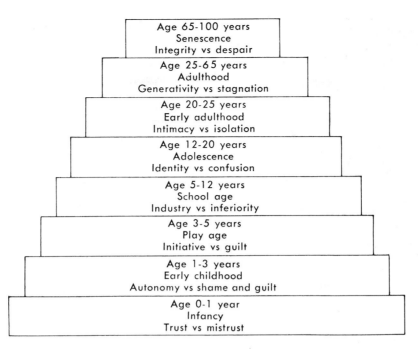

Figure 9-1 Erikson: Eight stages of man. (From Forbes ES, Fitzsimmons VM: *The older adult: a process for wellness,* St. Louis, 1981, Mosby.)

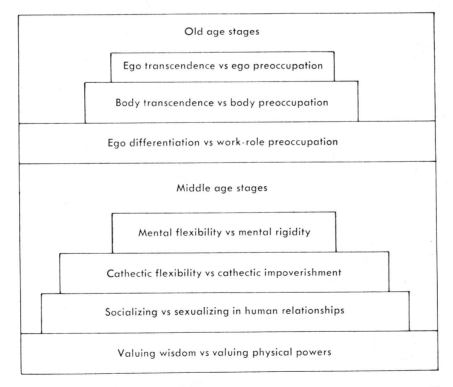

Figure 9-2 Peck: Stages of middle age and old age. (From Forbes ES, Fitzsimmons VM: *The older adult: a process for wellness,* St. Louis, 1981, Mosby.)

b. Time available for preparation, which eases transition
c. Control over whether to develop a substitute
B. Sufficient preparation and adequate support determine adjustment success or failure

C. Role changes that occur to the older adult are predominantly crisis oriented
  1. Forced retirement
  2. Alteration in income
  3. Loss of spouse

4. Illness
5. Friends move away or die
6. Family members relocate, assume new roles, have increasingly less time for relationships
7. Society's assigned role of decreased psychological and physiological functioning
D. Role losses
  1. Work
    a. No longer the breadwinner
    b. Job-related companionship
    c. Usefulness, competence, identity
    d. Income
    e. Sense of purpose
    f. Self-esteem
  2. Family
    a. May no longer be the decision maker
    b. May not be held in the same esteem
    c. Loss of independence; reversal of roles with children
E. Role gains
  1. Grandparenthood or great-grandparenthood
  2. Family support roles assumed
    a. Economic
    b. Child care
    c. Caring role in illness
    d. Care of the home
  3. Community activities
  4. Religious activities
  5. Recreational activities
  6. Clubs, organizations, and associations
  7. Advisory roles
  8. New friends
  9. Adult education
  10. Volunteerism

ALTERATIONS IN LIFESTYLE
Employment
A. Society emphasizes the employed as valuable and the unemployed as useless
B. Increase in the number of older women working
C. Decrease in the number of older men working
D. Part-time employment more common
E. Trend toward early retirement
F. Serial careers emerging in keeping with interest changes
G. More women are joining the workforce at a time when men are winding down their working lives
H. Older worker possesses involuntary limitations
  1. Health problems
  2. Sensory or perceptual alterations, for example, in vision and auditory acuity
  3. Decline in physical strength, endurance, and speed
I. Older workers possess innumerable strengths
  1. Reliability
  2. Dependability
  3. Knowledge
  4. Expertise
  5. Experience

Retirement
A. Mandatory retirement in federal employment eliminated
B. Mandatory retirement age raised to 70 in private employment
C. Changes in the economy leading to forced retirements

D. More people taking advantage of early retirement due to incentives by companies to retire older workers, and replace with younger workers
E. Health problems are primary reason for voluntary retirement
F. Increase in leisure time
G. May create tremendous anxiety for some older adults
H. Some derive an initial feeling of relief, but for most it is a loss that comes at a time of meaningful productivity
I. Adjustment depends on previously established patterns of adjustment, degree of financial security, state of health, and future outlook
J. For most it creates an additional series of losses and problems at a time in life when coping and problem-solving abilities are fragile
K. Job loss
  1. Loss of daily routine
    a. Alters household routine
    b. Alters lifestyle
    c. Creates discouragement, depression, and loneliness
    d. Alters family relationships
    e. Alcohol abuse
  2. Loss of income
    a. Relocation
    b. Daily decision-making determined by economics
    c. Decreases self-esteem
    d. Increases fear and anxiety
    e. Increases insecurity
L. Welcome changes
  1. New friends
  2. New activities
  3. New interests
  4. Renewal of marriage
  5. Seek new and different employment
  6. Find purpose and opportunity
  7. Rest and relaxation

Economic Changes
A. Most older adults live on fixed incomes
B. Of older adult persons, 1 out of 10 lives below the nation's poverty level
C. Independence declines as costs increase and buying power decreases
D. For many Social Security is the sole source of income
E. Many older adults are not receiving the assistance to which they are entitled
  1. Lack of resource knowledge
  2. Inability to find out about resources
    a. Lack of mobility
    b. Health problems
F. Supplemental Social Security: may qualify for in addition to or instead of Social Security benefits
G. Economic penalties: limit on the amount a Social Security beneficiary can earn annually without losing some monthly payments
H. Income tax reforms, for example a once-in-a-lifetime capital gains tax exemption on sale of personal residence for person over 55 years of age
I. Income sources
  1. Public
    a. Social Security (Federal Old-Age, Survivors, and Disability Insurance)
    b. Supplemental Social Security income

2. Private (e.g., pensions and investments)
3. Other (e.g., Railroad Retirement System, Federal Employee's Retirement System, and Civil Service Retirement System)

Health

A. Most older adults have more than one chronic disease
B. Health care needs increase with age
C. Cost of health care is increasing as financial income is either decreasing or fixed
D. Older adults account for one third of the nation's health care costs

Housing

A. Most older adults prefer to remain independent as long as family and friends live nearby
B. Most live with spouse, alone, or with family
C. Large percentage continue to own their own home and prefer this lifestyle
   1. Security
   2. Privacy
   3. Independence
   4. Sense of purpose
   5. Familiarity
   6. Household activities
   7. Pride
   8. Socialization
D. Other housing alternatives
   1. Mobile homes
      a. Convenient
      b. Economical
   2. Retirement communities
      a. Minimum age requirement
      b. Different cost levels, for example, houses, apartments, and condominiums
   3. Foster home
   4. Life care facilities: living, recreational, medical facilities on the premises
   5. Nursing homes—5% of those individuals aged 65-85 live in nursing homes; after the age of 85, 25% live in nursing homes
   6. Assisted living facilities
   7. House sharing
   8. Public housing
   9. Rooming houses
   10. Hotels: SROs (single room occupancy)
E. Special assistance needs of the older adult that enable them to remain in their own homes longer
   1. Transportation
      a. Reliable
      b. Nearby
      c. Inexpensive
      d. Safe
   2. Meals available in the event of illness or disability
   3. Health hotlines: most older adults are institutionalized because of health needs and lack of convenient community health services
   4. Housecleaners
   5. Homemaker services
   6. Social services
   7. Home care services
   8. Neighborhood safety

Recreation

A. Older adults have more time for recreation, but deterring factors exist
   1. Cost
      a. Transportation
      b. Special equipment
      c. Special clothing
      d. Fees for membership and use of facilities
   2. Health problems
   3. Diminished energy level
   4. Lack of incentive
   5. Sensory losses
   6. Lack of environmental aids
   7. Lack of conveniently located facilities, for example, rest rooms
   8. Lack of handicapped facilities
B. Most older adults depend on a family as the major source of activity and interaction
C. Alternatives
   1. Religious activities
   2. Community activities, for example, volunteerism
   3. Day care
   4. Senior citizen centers
   5. Clubs, organizations, and associations
   6. Recreation centers
   7. Adult education
   8. Shopping
   9. Cultural events
   10. Elder hostel

SOCIAL ISOLATION

A. Four classifications (Ebersole and Hess, 1985)
B. Attitudinal: that which is self-imposed and that imposed by society
   1. Self-imposed aloneness, loneliness
   2. Society imposes myths about the aged, perceptions of aging
C. Presentational: set apart or sets one apart
D. Behavioral: exhibits behaviors that are not acceptable to a youth-oriented society, for example, confusion, eccentricity
E. Geographic
   1. Lack of resources to relocate
   2. Psychological safety and security at present location
   3. Fear of being victims of crime
   4. Distance from family and friends who have moved away
F. Rural areas have a higher proportion of older people

Drug Use

A. Largest users of prescription medications are those over the age of 65
B. Tendency to self-medicate
C. Higher frequency of hospital admissions that are drug-related than that for other age groups
D. Self-administration errors are common
E. Slower ingestion of drug into the system as a result of a decline in gastric acid secretion and decreased gastric motility
F. Circulatory alterations affect drug distribution
G. Drug metabolism altered by such factors as a diminished rate of body metabolism
H. Drug excretion time reduced by illness, disease, and the aging process
I. Management
   1. Patient education

2. Medication administration times more compatible with lifestyle
3. Color coding
4. Larger print on labels
5. Easily removable bottle and vial caps
6. Monitoring of drug effectiveness and compatibility
7. Drug holidays
8. Daily/weekly medication containers

Alcohol Abuse

A. High-risk group for alcoholism
   1. Significant number of alcohol abusers are over age 60.
   2. Adult men have a higher incidence of abuse than adult women
   3. Statistics are inaccurate due to protection by family members
B. Tolerance to alcohol decreases with age, as the body systems do not excrete and detoxify as rapidly as those of a younger adult
C. Substitution for unmet psychological needs and untreated physiological problems
D. Cause of accidents, nutritional deficiencies, drug incompatibilities, self-neglect, alterations in self-esteem, psychosocial and physiological health care problems

Elder Abuse

A. Physical (Box 9-2)
   1. Battering
   2. Neglect
   3. Sexual abuse
   4. Confinement or restraint
B. Psychologic: threatened or forced
   1. Relinquishment of assets
   2. Institutionalization
   3. Loss of control over independent functioning
   4. Social isolation
   5. Sensory deprivation
C. Prevention
   1. Acquire knowledge of family abuse and patterns of violence
   2. Identify predisposing factors
   3. Incorporate assessment tools into interviewing and counseling strategies
   4. Increase public awareness and education
   5. Identify actual and potential sources of emergency protection
   6. Acquire knowledge of community resources

THE HEALTHY OLDER ADULT

A. Although older adults are sometimes plagued by chronic health problems, most live in the community
B. Focus of education for the older adult in regards to healthy living include:
   1. Disease Prevention—prevention of acute/chronic health problems
      a. Self maintenance—take responsibility for own health practices
      b. Maintenance of activity—engage in moderate physical activity at least three times/week
      c. Dietary practices—eat a varied diet that includes adequate amounts of carbohydrates, proteins, and fats

---

Box 9-2 Physical Indicators of Actual or Potential Elder Abuse/Neglect

General Appearance

Anxious, fearful, and passive
Poor eye contact
Looks to caregiver for answers
Poor hygiene and inappropriate dress
Underweight or malnourished
Physically handicapped
No glasses, false teeth, or hearing aid despite need

Skin

Contusions, abrasions, burns, and scars in various stages of healing
Decubitus ulcers, urine burns
Rope marks

Abdominal/rectal

Distended
Internal bleeding
Fecal impactions

Musculoskeletal fractures

Evidence of old healed fractures
Current fractures and sprains
Limited range of motion
Contractures

Genital/urinary

Vaginal lacerations, bruises, and infections
Urinary tract infections

Neurologic

Slurred speech
Confusion

From Fortinash KM, Holoday-Worret PA: *Psychiatric-mental health nursing*, ed 2, St Louis, 1999, Mosby.

---

   d. Diagnostic testing—should regularly undergo examinations for the detection and early treatment of disease (mammograms, prostate exams, colorectal screening)
   e. Influenza and pneumonia vaccines as recommended by a physician
   f. Management of stress
   2. Health promotion—maintenance of chronic health problems
      a. Regularly visit physician for examinations
      b. Engage in healthy lifestyle practices
      c. Take prescribed medications

Physiological Alterations (Normal Aging Process) and Selected Disorders (Abnormal)

A. Normal aging changes are gradual and begin in early middle age
B. Specific changes of aging do not alter the older adult's ability to cope on a day-to-day basis

C. Due to specific changes of aging, the older adult has a decreased capacity to "bounce back" from stress or illness

Integumentary System

A. Alterations
   1. Moisture loss, dryness
   2. Epithelial layer thinning; fragility
   3. Shrinkage and rigidity of elastic collagen fibers: sagging and wrinkling
   4. Sweat glands decrease in number, activity, and size: less efficient body cooling system
   5. Subcutaneous fat loss deepening of hollows and more prominent contours
   6. Loss of capillaries and melanocytes: skin sallowness
   7. Skin pigmentation increases: keratoses (scaly, raised areas), senile lentigines (liver spots: brown or yellow spots)
   8. Hair changes in color (gray, white), changes in texture (becomes fine or coarse), and thins (balding)
   9. Appearance of facial hair for women; decrease in facial hair for men
B. Factors contributing to problems of the integumentary system
   1. Peripheral circulation diminishes, causing thick brittle nails
   2. Cardiovascular changes cause decreased healing of wounds
   3. Immune system decreases ability to heal disease
C. Resulting problems
   1. Skin tears
   2. Decubitus ulcers
D. Nursing management of the dependent older adult
   1. Use extra lotions/creams on dry skin
   2. Gentle handling when moving
   3. Extra care when performing venipunctures

Musculoskeletal System

A. Alterations
   1. Loss of lean muscle mass and muscle cells: decreased muscle strength, size, and tone
   2. Loss of elastic fibers in muscle tissue: increased stiffness and decreased flexibility
   3. Thinning of long bones: brittle, porous bones
   4. Thinning of intervertebral disks: height loss and changes in posture
B. Factors contributing to general musculoskeletal problems
   1. Poor nutritional patterns
   2. Endocrine system changes: decreased estrogen and testosterone
   3. Gastrointestinal system changes: decreased absorption of vitamins and minerals
   4. Cardiovascular system changes: poor circulation
   5. Neurological deficits causing safety hazards
   6. Decreased level of activity and periods of prolonged bed rest
   7. Side effects of medications, for example, steroids
C. Resulting problems
   1. Increased susceptibility to fractures
   2. Altered body image
   3. Pain and discomfort
   4. Decreased mobility
   5. Impaired ability to perform activities of daily living (ADLs)

6. Increasing feelings of dependency
7. Calcium deposits in blood vessels and renal structures
8. Weakened muscles affecting other systems
   a. Diaphragm
   b. Bladder
   c. Myocardium
   d. Abdominal wall

D. Nursing management of the dependent older adult
   1. Handle patient gently
   2. Reduce environmental safety hazards
   3. Encourage mobility and exercise
   4. Allow extra time for performing activities
   5. Assist with ADLs and exercises as needed
   6. Provide encouragement and support for accomplishments
   7. Prevent deformities
      a. Proper positioning
      b. Exercises such as range of motion (ROM)
   8. Alleviate pain
      a. Rest periods
      b. Positioning
   9. Encourage liberal fluid intake

Respiratory System

A. Alterations
   1. Structural alterations (scoliosis, kyphosis, osteoporosis): decrease in lung expansion
   2. Alveoli enlarge and thin out: decreased oxygen and carbon dioxide diffusion
   3. Loss of bronchiole elasticity: decreased breathing capacity, increased residual air
   4. Diaphragm becomes fibrotic and weakened; diminished efficiency
   5. Respiratory muscle structure and function decrease: diminished strength for breathing and coughing
   6. Changes in larynx: weaker, higher-pitched voice
   7. Decrease in ciliary function: increased susceptibility to upper respiratory tract infection
B. Factors contributing to respiratory problems
   1. Decreased resistance to infection
   2. Musculoskeletal system changes: weakened muscles and postural changes
   3. Longer history of smoking and exposure to pollutants
   4. Periods of prolonged bed rest
   5. Cardiovascular system changes
   6. Side effects of medications, for example, sedatives and hypnotics
C. Resulting problems
   1. Dyspnea
   2. Chronic cough
   3. Fatigue and debilitation
   4. Cerebral hypoxia
      a. Confusion
      b. Restlessness
      c. Behavioral changes
   5. Decreased activity tolerance
   6. Cardiovascular problems, for example, congestive heart failure
   7. Anorexia
D. Nursing management of the dependent older adult
   1. Assist with ADLs as necessary
   2. Encourage breathing exercises

3. Administer oxygen therapy
4. Change position frequently
5. Encourage liberal fluid intake
6. Discourage smoking
7. Position for maximum comfort and efficiency of respiration, for example, extra pillows, Fowler's position
8. Allow rest periods
9. Assess pulmonary status when assessing behavioral changes

Cardiovascular System

A. Alterations
   1. Decrease in enzymatic stimulation: longer and less forceful contractions
   2. Increase in fat and collagen amounts: decline in cardiac output
   3. Increase in oxygen demands of coronary arteries and brain: decreased peripheral circulation
   4. Loss of elasticity of vessel walls; decrease in contraction and recoiling responses
   5. Reduced or unaltered heart rate at rest
   6. Mild tachycardia on activity
   7. Slow increase in serum cholesterol
B. Factors contributing to problems of the cardiovascular system
   1. Poor nutritional patterns
   2. Anxiety and stress
   3. Decreased activity level
   4. Arteriosclerosis and hypertension
   5. Pulmonary system changes
   6. Side effects of medications
C. Resulting problems
   1. Fatigue and decreased activity tolerance
   2. Increased anxiety
   3. Edema
   4. Hypertension: increased risk of cerebrovascular accident (CVA)
   5. Behavioral changes
   6. Poor circulation to other systems and extremities: delayed healing, decreased efficiency of kidneys
   7. Potential risk for coronary artery disease, heart failure
D. Nursing management of the dependent older adult
   1. Assist with ADLs prn
   2. Encourage moderate activity and exercise
   3. Patient teaching considerations
      a. Confusion
      b. Forgetfulness
      c. Resistance to change
   4. Avoid excess pressure on the skin
      a. Change position frequently
      b. Sheepskin; water mattress
      c. Bed cradle
   5. Assess cardiovascular status when assessing behavioral changes
   6. Avoid tight, constrictive clothing and shoes
   7. Special foot care
      a. Prevent trauma
      b. Prevent infection

Gastrointestinal System

A. Alterations
   1. Muscle atrophy in the tongue, cheeks, mouth
   2. Esophageal wall thinning
   3. Decrease in ptyalin and amylase secretion by salivary gland: alkaline saliva
   4. Decrease in saliva secretion: thicker mucus and dryness
   5. Oral sensitivity loss, loss of taste discrimination
   6. Ill-fitting dentures, periodontal disease, lack of teeth: nutritional deficiencies
   7. Shrinkage of bony structures of mouth
   8. Gastric mucosa shrinks: decline in digestive enzyme secretion leads to delayed digestion
   9. Decrease in lipase secretion: fat intolerance
   10. Decrease in gastric acid: diminished ability to use calcium
   11. Decrease in intrinsic factor: pernicious anemia
   12. Decrease in iron absorption: iron-deficiency anemia
   13. Internal sphincter muscle tone loss: alterations in bowel evacuation
B. Factors contributing to problems of the gastrointestinal system
   1. Decreased level of activity
   2. Dental problems
   3. Poor nutritional patterns
   4. Weakened muscles
   5. Nervous system changes
   6. Overuse of laxative and enemas
   7. Anorexia
   8. Side effects of medications; for example, opiates and steroids
C. Resulting problems
   1. Discomfort
   2. Constipation and impaction
   3. Fecal incontinence
   4. Anorexia
   5. Increased risk of aspiration
D. Nursing management of the dependent older adult
   1. Promote nutritional intake
      a. Consistency of food
      b. Ability to manage utensils
      c. Extra time for feeding (oral and tube)
   2. Provide good oral hygiene
   3. Encourage mobility and exercise
   4. Provide adequate fluid intake
   5. Educate patient regarding constipation and laxative abuse
   6. Check bowel habits regularly
   7. Give prompt assistance to bathroom or with bedpan
   8. Prevent skin and mucosal breakdown
      a. Prompt, thorough cleansing of anal area
      b. Extra gentleness when inserting rectal and feeding tubes

Renal System

A. Alterations
   1. Decrease in kidney size
   2. Decline in renal blood flow
   3. Reduced ability of nephron to filter urine: decreased clearance
   4. Reduced ability of tubule cells to selectively secrete and reabsorb: fluid and electrolyte alterations
   5. Bladder capacity decreases: frequency and urgency
   6. Loss of muscle tone of bladder and uterus
   7. Loss of pelvic muscle tone
   8. Decreased urine concentration ability
   9. Prostate gland enlargement

B. Factors contributing to problems of the renal system
   1. Periods of prolonged bed rest
      a. Increased urinary stasis
      b. Renal calculi formation
   2. Cardiovascular system changes, for example, decreased renal perfusion
   3. Nervous system changes
   4. Decreased fluid intake
   5. Muscle weakness
   6. Social withdrawal and apathy, for example, sensory deprivation
   7. Side effects of medication, for example, diuretics, antiparkinsonian drugs
C. Resulting problems
   1. Hyperglycemia
   2. Behavioral changes, for example, confusion, elevated BUN, electrolyte imbalance
   3. Interference with sleep and recreational patterns
      a. Urinary frequency
      b. Urinary urgency
      c. Nocturia
   4. Increased chance of skin breakdown; for example, incontinence
   5. Feelings of embarrassment, rejection, and withdrawal
D. Nursing management of the dependent older adult
   1. Prevent urinary stasis
      a. Encourage liberal fluid intake
      b. Encourage frequent change of position
      c. Encourage ambulation
   2. Prevent skin breakdown: prompt and thorough cleansing
   3. Bladder retraining
   4. Promptly respond to call for bathroom or bedpan
   5. Leave night light on if patient experiencing nocturia
   6. Assess renal status when assessing behavior changes
   7. Early recognition of urinary tract infection

Neurological System

A. Alterations
   1. Decrease in weight and size of brain
   2. Decline in number of neurons
   3. Diminished nerve conduction speed
      a. Voluntary movement slower
      b. Decreased reaction time
      c. Delayed decisions
   4. Alterations in sleep-wake cycle
      a. Less rapid eye movement (REM) sleep
      b. Less deep sleep: tendency to catnap
      c. Easily awakened
      d. Difficulty falling asleep
      e. Average 5 to 7 hours sleep at night
      f. Need less sleep but require more rest periods
   5. Brain tissue atrophy and meningeal thickening: short-term memory loss
B. Factors contributing to problems of the neurological system
   1. Poor nutrition patterns
   2. Cardiovascular system changes, for example, decreased circulation
   3. Pulmonary system changes, for example, cerebral hypoxia
   4. Sensory deprivation
   5. Side effects of medications, for example, sedatives

C. Resulting problems
   1. Safety hazards
      a. Impaired senses, for example, vision, hearing, pain, and temperature
      b. Forgetfulness and confusion
   2. Anorexia, for example, decreased taste buds
   3. Social isolation and rejection
   4. Impaired ability to perform ADLs
      a. Decreased coordination
      b. Safety hazards
   5. Increased sense of dependency
   6. Incontinence
   7. Altered self-image and declining confidence
   8. Behavioral changes, for example, forgetfulness and confusion
D. Nursing management of the dependent older adult
   1. Provide for safety
   2. Establish means of communication if patient has hearing impairment
   3. Assess all systems when assessing behavioral changes
   4. Maintain sense of independence when possible
   5. Assist with ADLs only when necessary; allow extra time
   6. Encourage socialization
   7. Provide sensory stimulation
   8. Consider forgetfulness and confusion when teaching
      a. Be consistent
      b. Provide repetition when necessary
      c. Be patient
      d. Provide positive reinforcement and encouragement
   9. Assess other symptoms carefully when assessing for infection and trauma: decreased temperature control and pain perception mask these symptoms
   10. Carefully check temperature of bath water and forms of heat therapy to avoid burns: discrepancy in sensation of heat and cold
   11. Maximize use of environmental aids

Endocrine System

A. Alterations
   1. Decline in growth hormone secretion
   2. Estrogen secretion diminishes
   3. Uterus becomes smaller
   4. Fallopian tubes decrease in size and motility
   5. Vagina loses elasticity
   6. Vulva and external genitalia shrink with loss of subcutaneous fat
   7. Vaginal secretions diminish
   8. Response to sexual stimulation takes longer
   9. Elasticity of breast tissue is reduced
   10. Testosterone secretion decreases
   11. Testes become smaller and less firm
   12. Sperm production is slowed
   13. Erection takes longer to achieve and subsides more rapidly
   14. Development of new drug, Viagra, treats erectile dysfunction in some men
   15. Ejaculation is shorter and less forceful
   16. Time between erection and orgasm lengthens
   17. Basal metabolism rate is decreased
   18. Glucose metabolism diminishes
   19. Pancreatic secretions decrease

B. Factors contributing to problems of the endocrine system Related changes in other body systems
C. Resulting problems
   1. Adult-onset diabetes mellitus
   2. Musculoskeletal system changes
   3. Hypothyroidism
   4. Sexual dysfunction
D. Nursing management of diabetes mellitus: special considerations
   1. Poor vision
   2. Lack of coordination
   3. Poor nutritional patterns
   4. Forgetfulness and confusion
   5. Resistance to change
   6. Masking of symptoms by physiological changes of aging and disease
   7. Decreased activity level
   8. Stress and anxiety
   9. Increased susceptibility to complications

Autoimmune System

A. Alterations
   1. Diminished immunoglobulin production
   2. Weakened antibody response
   3. Atypical signs and symptoms frequently a response to infection, for example, subnormal temperature, behavior changes, and decreased pain sensation
B. Factors contributing to problems in the autoimmune system
   1. Weakened antibody response
   2. Reduced immunoglobulin production
      a. Thymus gland wasting
      b. Reticuloendothelial system alterations
C. Resulting problems
   1. Self-destructive autoaggressive phenomenon
   2. Increased susceptibility to infection
   3. Increased susceptibility to disease
   4. Misdiagnosis
D. Nursing management of the dependent older adult
   1. Be careful in observation and assessment
   2. Be aware that atypical symptoms of infection are common among the older adult; for example, with otitis media, difficulty in hearing is too often dismissed as a typical aging problem
   3. Use early nursing intervention
   4. Educate regarding available vaccines

Sense Organs

A. Vision
   1. Alterations
      a. Pupil size diminishes: loss of responsiveness to light
      b. Decline in peripheral vision
      c. Accommodation ability decreases, causing presbyopia (farsightedness)
      d. Decrease in tear production
      e. Decrease in lens transparency and elasticity
      f. Decline in ability to focus quickly
      g. Decline in color discrimination
      h. Difficulty in adjusting to dark-light changes
      i. Altered depth perception
   2. Selected Disorders
      a. Cataracts
      b. Glaucoma
      c. Senile macular degeneration
B. Auditory alterations
   1. Progressive loss of hearing, starting with high-frequency tones
      a. Presbycusis (loss of sound perception)
      b. Otosclerosis (bone cell overgrowth)
      c. Cerumen accumulation
   2. Eardrum thickens and becomes more opaque
C. Taste bud alterations
   1. Number of taste buds decline
   2. Taste sensation declines
D. Olfactory alterations
   1. Olfactory nerve fibers decrease
   2. Sense of smell diminishes
E. Tactile alterations
   1. Sense of touch dulled
   2. Pain threshold higher
   3. Sense of vibration diminished
   4. Heat/cold discrimination declines
F. Vestibular/kinesthetic alterations
   1. Diminished proprioception
   2. Decrease in coordination
   3. Decline in equilibrium

SPECIAL CONSIDERATIONS
Nutrition

A. Diet
   1. Nutrition needs same as those of other adults
   2. Decreased need for calories
   3. Adequate protein to prevent muscle wasting and weakness
   4. Adequate fats for padding, insulation, and energy; low saturated fat intake recommended by physician
   5. Adequate carbohydrates from unprocessed foods for energy: older adults have a tendency to buy high-carbohydrate, empty-calorie foods because they:
      a. Are less costly
      b. Are filling
      c. Are easy to chew
      d. Require minimal preparation
   6. Ethnic, cultural, and lifestyle preferences should be encouraged for identity reinforcement and appetite stimulation
   7. Fluid intake should be 1500 to 2000 ml per day: tendency is to reduce intake because of urinary frequency, urgency, and incontinence
   8. Vitamin supplements to prevent deficiencies: women should continue with increased intake of calcium supplements.
   9. Lactose deficiency common: calcium can be obtained from other sources, for example, spinach, asparagus, broccoli, and sardines
   10. Fiber, roughage, bulk to aid elimination
   11. Consistency and preparation in accordance with chewing, swallowing, and digestive abilities
   12. Small, frequent meals are easier to digest and conserve energy
   13. Attention to cholesterol and fat intakes
   14. Awareness of food-drug and food-food interactions
B. Unhurried atmosphere to increase appetite and incentive to eat

C. Caution against food fads and megavitamin therapy
D. Assess facilities for appropriateness
  1. Storage
  2. Cooking
  3. Refrigeration
E. Financial assistance and planning
F. Transportation to and from grocery store
G. Assistance with packages because of weakness and physical disabilities
H. Mealtime socialization
I. Assistance for the confused, forgetful, and ill
J. Encourage regular meals; older adults have a tendency to skip meals
K. Education classes on purchasing healthful foods on limited income
L. Factors that increase risk of nutritional problems in the older adult (Box 9-3)

Hygiene

A. Skin
  1. Water temperature 100° to 105° F (37.7° to 40.5° C)
  2. Daily baths not necessary
  3. Oil-base or emollient lotion
  4. Alcohol and dusting powder not appropriate because they dry out the skin (dusting powder can be inhaled)
  5. Avoid friction
  6. Avoid pressure
  7. Neutral-reaction or oil-based soap
  8. Susceptible to bruising and skin tears

Box 9-3   Factors That Increase Risk of Nutritional Problems in the Older Adult

Physiological Factors

Decreased secretion of enzymes; indigestion, gastric reflux common
Decreased absorption of nutrients and minerals
Reduced mobility of stomach; slowing of peristalsis
Restricted intake of nutrients caused by problems with teeth and dentures (e.g., ill-fitting dentures, periodontal disease, missing teeth)
Decrease in production of saliva
Reduced sensitivity to sweet and salty flavors
Low activity level
Disease-related symptoms that can reduce appetite, energy, or ability to ingest food
Side effects of medications

Psychosocial Factors

Limited finances that prohibit purchase of proper food
Lack of knowledge regarding nutritional needs, nutritional value of foods
Inability to shop, store foods, or cook (e.g., lack of transportation, no kitchen facilities, dementia)
Personal preferences that violate principles of good nutritional intake
Loneliness or eating alone
Mood disturbances (e.g., depression, anxiety)

From Eliopoulos C: *Manual of gerontologic nursing*, ed 2, St Louis, 1999, Mosby.

B. Nose: blunt-end scissors to trim nasal hairs that extend beyond nares
C. Oral hygiene
  1. Dentures
    a. Take out at night and reinsert the next morning to prevent tissue swelling unless contraindicated by dentist
    b. Frequent cleaning
    c. Proper storage
    d. If patient is institutionalized, make sure dentures are labeled
  2. Soft nylon toothbrush, electric toothbrush, or adaptive toothbrush
  3. Mouthwash (optional)
  4. Lanolin to lips
  5. Encourage semiannual dental visits
  6. Frequent mouth inspection for food accumulation, injury, disease, and infection (tendency to pocket food can lead to infection)
D. Ears
  1. Clean with warm, soapy water and dry with towel
  2. Do not use cotton swabs because they force cerumen back against the tympanum
  3. Trim ear hair growth in men
  4. Hearing aids
    a. Wash mold and receiver with mild soap and warm water
    b. Check cannula for patency, and clean and dry with pipe cleaner
    c. Remove batteries when aid is not in use
    d. Store batteries in refrigerator to retain freshness
    e. Turn aid to off position when inserting in patient's ear
    f. Turn aid on to adjust volume
    g. Store aid in its original box away from cold, heat, and sunlight
    h. Components, styles, nursing care (Box 9-4)
E. Eyes
  1. Decreased tear production may necessitate use of artificial tears
  2. Eyeglass care
    a. More frequent cleaning of eyeglasses required
    b. Use warm water to clean eyeglasses
    c. Store only in eyeglass case
    d. If patient is institutionalized, make sure glasses are labeled
F. Nails
  1. Daily care
  2. Use moisturizer on nails and cuticles
  3. Encourage circulation with buffing of nails
  4. File with emery board (cutting makes them more brittle and risks injury)
G. Hair
  1. Use mild shampoo that is not irritating to the eyes
  2. Remove facial hair from women with tweezers or waxing
  3. Use of a shaving brush is recommended for men
  4. Moisturizers are beneficial for men's facial hair
H. Feet
  1. Give daily care (washing, inspection, skin care)
  2. Inspect between and under toes for abrasions, cracking, lacerations, and scaling

---

Box 9-4   Hearing Aids

Components

Microphone: converts sounds into electric energy
Amplifier: increases energy
Receiver: converts energy back into sound waves
Volume control
On/off switch

Styles

Behind the ear: limited amplification
In the ear: entire unit worn in the ear; limited amplification
Eyeglass attached: unit built in the frame of the eyeglass; limited amplification
Body aided: amplifier housed in a case worn on body; offers most amplification of all

Nursing Care

Encourage client to obtain hearing aid from a reputable dealer after a full audiometric examination has been done
Ensure that batteries are functioning before the aid is applied; it is recommended that batteries be changed weekly
Identify common hearing aid problems:
- Whistling sound: bad connection between earpiece and amplifier; excessively high volume
- Insufficient amplification: volume set too low; weak or dead battery; blockage from cerumen; disconnected tubing or wiring
- Periodic loss of amplification: loose connection; poor battery contact; dirt in switch; cracked case

Recognize that adjustment to a hearing aid is difficult and may take time, and reassure the client that this is not unusual.

Adapted from Eliopoulos C: *Manual of gerontologic nursing,* ed 2, St Louis, 1999, Mosby.

---

3. Clip toenails straight across
4. Pumice stone should be used to remove dry, hard skin
5. Discourage use of irritants
6. Avoid elastic-top socks or knee-high stockings
7. Emphasize the danger of roll garters
8. Recommend properly fitting shoes with low, broad, rubber heels for safety, comfort, and fatigue reduction

Safety

A. Susceptibility to accidents increased by
 1. Decline in sensory acuity
 2. Decreased ability to interpret environment
 3. Increased reflex time
 4. Postural change sensitivity
 5. Gait disturbances
 6. Muscular weakness
 7. Urinary urgency and frequency
 8. Confusion
 9. Judgment alterations
 10. Forgetfulness
 11. Proprioceptive inadequacies
 12. Improper footwear
 13. Depression
 14. Environmental hazards
 15. Medications that cause drowsiness
B. Accident prevention
 1. Attire
  a. Short or three-quarter–length sleeves as opposed to long, loose-fitting sleeves
  b. Avoid long garments
  c. Velcro closures
 2. Furniture
  a. Proper height
  b. Chairs with arms
 3. Floors
  a. No-slip wax
  b. No scatter rugs or deep-pile carpeting
  c. Avoid clutter
  d. Rubber tips on ambulation aids
 4. Kitchen
  a. Tong reachers instead of footstools, chairs, and step ladders
  b. Temperature-controlled faucets
  c. Electric rather than gas stoves
  d. Stoves with controls on the front
  e. Shelves within comfortable reach
  f. Wall cabinets at comfortable height instead of floor-based cabinets to avoid bending and stooping
  g. Avoid trash accumulation
  h. Easy-grip utensils
 5. Bathroom
  a. Nonskid strips or rubber mats in tub and shower
  b. Temperature-controlled faucets
  c. Good soap containers
  d. Tub and toilet handrails
  e. Bathtub seats
  f. Shower chairs
  g. High toilet seats
  h. Colored toilet seats
  i. Night light
 6. Bedroom
  a. Bedside commode
  b. Side rails
  c. Night light
  d. Telephone next to bed (amplifier; dial enlarger)
 7. General
  a. Proper lighting
  b. Railings on stairways
  c. Safe electric appliances
  d. No overloading of electric outlets
  e. No frayed wiring or extension cords
  f. Securely taped cords
  g. Emergency telephone numbers readily available at telephone
  h. Smoke detectors
  i. Crime prevention assessment and implementation
  j. Medications
   (1) Separate from those of other household members
   (2) Internal and external medications in different locations
   (3) Large print labels
   (4) Color coded labels

(5) Daily supply containers

(6) Calendar or alarm clock reminders

(7) Discard outdated medications and prescriptions

k. Medical emergency alarm system

8. Mobility aids (Table 9-1)

Vision

A. Bright, diffused light is best

B. Place items on better-vision side

C. Avoid glare

D. Strips on stairs improve depth perception

E. Glasses should be kept clean (the older adult frequently forget or ignore this)

F. Use colors that increase visual acuity, for example, red, orange, and yellow

G. Avoid night driving

H. Use resources and aids for visually handicapped

I. Preserve independence

J. Visual losses increase susceptibility to illusions, disorientation, confusion, and isolation

K. Place objects directly in front of individual with decreased peripheral vision

L. Stimulate other senses

Hearing

A. Older adults usually do poorly on hearing tests because of their cautious responsiveness

B. Reduce distractions

C. Do not fatigue with unnecessary noise and talk

D. Speak in a normal tone of voice; shouting is misinterpreted by those who have normal hearing

E. Observe for signs of developing hearing loss

1. Leaning forward

2. Inappropriate responses

3. Cupping ear when listening

4. Loud speaking voice

5. Requests to repeat what has been said

F. Reduce background noise before speaking, for example, television and radio

G. Hearing deficits increase social isolation, suspiciousness, and fears

H. Speak toward the better ear

I. Be sure to have the person's attention before speaking

J. Use resources and aids for the hearing impaired, for example, television and telephone amplifiers, sound lamps, and alarm clocks that shake the bed

K. Keep hands and objects away from mouth when speaking

Activities of Daily Living

A. Older adults may ignore appearance because of fatigue, unawareness, or lack of incentive

B. Clean clothing is essential for maintaining pride and dignity

C. Choosing what to wear provides a source of control over one's life, fosters independence, and increases self-confidence and self-esteem

D. Lifelong sleeping attire or lack of attire should be encouraged

1. Reinforces individuality

2. Reduces sleep interference

E. Standard clothing sizes no longer fit; loose-fitting, comfortable clothing should be encouraged

F. Front closures are more easily managed

G. Cotton socks absorb perspiration

H. Zippers, Velcro, and large buttons make dressing easier

I. Layering and/or sweat suits provide warmth in cold weather

J. Daily exercise should be encouraged and paced

K. Increase self-awareness with mirrors

L. Use daily living resources and aids

1. Zipper aids

2. Extra-long shoehorns

3. Shoelace tiers, Velcro fasteners

4. Adaptive utensils

M. Functional independence—ability to perform ADLs and instrumental activities of daily living (IADLs). Examples of IADLs include shopping, using the telephone, ability to pay bills, obtaining meals, obtaining transportation.

Sexuality

A. Cultural stereotypes deny freedom of sexual expression for the older adult

B. Lifelong sexual adjustment will determine how the older adult deals with sexual needs

C. Partner availability is made difficult

1. More older adult women than men

2. Social and business roles change

D. Physiological alterations affect self-image and foster non-participation

E. Families of older adult persons tend to discourage sexual relationships because of stereotypes and inheritance threats

F. Sexual focus shifts to companionship

G. Older persons continue to enjoy sexual activity; decrease is primarily a result of declining health or lack of available partner (Box 9-5).

Speech

A. Older adults tend to rely on speech more than action

B. Speak slowly and clearly

C. Allow sufficient time for comprehension and response

D. Speak to and treat the individual as an adult

E. Explanations will reduce fear

F. Recovery of speech is influenced by multiple impairments and dependency

---

Box 9-5   Encouraging Intimacy in the Older Adult

Educate others, including family members, concerning need for intimacy in old age.

If sexual intimacy is not possible, promote expression of intimacy in other ways (hugging, cuddling, spending time together).

Avoid belittling the older person's desire for intimacy.

Provide education for the older adult concerning intimacy, as it is not always comfortable for the older adult to inquire about this subject.

Older adults may need detailed instruction after life-altering events such as myocardial infarction, cerebrovascular accident, or other acute or chronic illness.

TABLE 9-1   Mobility Aids

Aid	Characteristics	Fit	Use
Cane	Assists balance by widening base of support; not intended for weight bearing. Comes in a variety of styles: • Regular (straight): provides minimal assistance with balance • Three- and four-point (quad): broader base of support, more cumbersome	Length should approximate distance between greater trochanter and floor. Elbow should be flexed slightly when cane rests 6 inches from side of foot	Use on unaffected side. Advance when affected limb advances (i.e., if right leg is weak, the cane is held on the left and moved forward as the right leg steps). Hold close to body; do not move forward beyond toes of affected foot. All canes should have suction grips to prevent slippage on floor
Walker	Broader base of support; more stability than a cane. Comes in a variety of styles: • Pickup: assists with weight bearing • Rolling: pushed on wheels rather than lifted; reduces physical strain; often have seats to allow rest after several steps or propulsion from a sitting position	Height equivalent to distance between greater trochanter and floor. Elbows slightly flexed when hands on sides of walker	When weight bearing is allowed, advance walker and step normally. When partial or no weight can be borne on one limb, thrust weight forward, then lift walker and replace all four legs on floor. Always use both hands when transferring from chair or commode; back walker to seat and use arms of chair or commode to assist in standing
Wheelchair	Used when client's disability prohibits other walking aids. Should not be used for convenience or speed of client or staff	Individually prescribed based on height, weight, limb use, arm strength, and self-propulsion capacity	Prepare environment for wheelchair use: widen doorways and toilet stalls; plan a functional furniture layout with no rugs; lower mirrors, telephones, drinking fountains, counters; install ramps. Use special pads and cushions to reduce pressure damage; shift weight and reposition frequently. Lock wheels and remove footrests when transferring to/from chair
Crutches	Frequently difficult for older person to use because of inadequate upper body strength, arthritic hands, and balance problems. Not as stable as other mobility aids	Individually sized. Length should be equivalent to 2 inches below axilla to point on floor 6 inches in front of client. Hand bars placement crucial because hands should bear total weight. Elbow should be flexed, wrist slightly hyperextended. Axillary pressure can cause radial nerve paralysis	Tailor gait to client's needs; consult with physical therapist. Use good posture and pay particular attention to foot position on affected side (walking exclusively on ball of foot or toes can cause footdrop). General rule when climbing stairs: stronger foot goes up first, down last. Upstairs: step up with stronger foot; bring crutches to that step; raise affected foot. Downstairs: crutches to lower step; lower affected foot; follow with stronger foot. Eliminate obstacles: • Waxed floors • Throw rugs • Extension cords • Uneven surfaces • Clutter

From Eliopoulos C: *Manual of gerontologic nursing*, ed 2, St Louis, 1999, Mosby.

Box 9-6   Organic Mental Syndromes

Delirium

A reduced ability to maintain attention to external stimuli and to appropriately shift attention to new external stimuli; disorganized thinking, as manifested by rambling, irrelevant, or incoherent speech; reduced level of consciousness; sensory misperceptions; disturbances of the sleep-wake cycle and level of psychomotor activity; disorientation to time, place, or person; memory impairment

Dementia

Impairment of short- and long-term memory; changes in abstract thinking; impaired judgment

Amnestic Syndrome

Impairment in short- and long-term memory that is attributed to a specific organic factor; immediate memory is not impaired

Organic Delusional Syndrome

Delusions resulting from specific organic factor such as amphetamine use or cerebral lesions of the right hemisphere

Organic Hallucinosis

Hallucinations that are persistent or recurrent and caused by a specific organic factor such as use of hallucinogens that produce visual hallucinations, or alcohol, which induces auditory hallucinations

Organic Mood Syndrome

Persistent depressed, elevated, or expansive mood caused by a specific organic factor such as a toxic effect of substances, including reserpine or methyldopa, an endocrine disorder such as hyperthyroidism, or structural brain disease that results from hemispheric strokes

Organic Anxiety Syndrome

Recurrent panic attacks or generalized anxiety caused by a specific organic factor such as endocrine disorder, use of psychoactive substances, brain tumors in the vicinity of the third ventricle, vitamin B_{12} deficiency, aspirin intolerance, heavy metal intoxication

Organic Personality Syndrome

Persistent personality disturbance caused by a specific organic factor such as structural damage to the brain caused by neoplasms, head trauma, cerebrovascular disease

Intoxication

Maladaptive behavior and a substance-specific syndrome caused by the recent ingestion of a psychoactive substance such as alcohol, cannabis, amphetamine, cocaine

Withdrawal

Development of a substance-specific syndrome that follows the cessation of, or reduction in, intake of a psychoactive substance that the person previously used regularly

Adapted from Haber J et al: *Comprehensive psychiatric nursing,* ed 5, St Louis, 1998, Mosby.

NEUROLOGICAL SYSTEM (SELECTED DISORDERS)
Organic Mental Syndromes (Box 9-6)

A. Onset may be rapid or progressive
B. Cognitive function alterations
   1. Judgment
   2. Memory
   3. Intellect
   4. Orientation
   5. Affect
C. Associated factors (Table 9-2)
D. Cognitive dysfunction dementia

DEMENTIA

A. Alzheimer's disease: progressive, deteriorating, chronic dementia
   1. Types
      a. Senile dementia Alzheimer's type (SDAT): onset over age 65
      b. Presenile dementia: onset between ages 40 and 60
   2. Cerebral pathophysiology
      a. Senile plaques
      b. Neurofibrillary tangles
      c. Neurotransmitter abnormalities
      d. Atrophy
   3. Diagnosis confirmed by above findings on autopsy
   4. Assessment
      a. Personality changes
      b. Memory changes
      c. Behavioral changes
      d. Impaired cognition
      e. Late-stage physical alterations affecting mobility and swallowing
   5. Nursing intervention/management
      a. Support independence with ADL
      b. Provide structured, consistent environment
      c. Facilitate sleep-activity balance
      d. Promote bowel and bladder continence
      e. Provide reality orientation, remotivation, reminiscence
      f. Provide for patient safety:
         (1) At risk for wandering
         (2) Becomes lost easily
         (3) Fails to recognize environmental hazards
      g. Encourage socialization, because withdrawal and social isolation are common
      h. Reduce anxiety-provoking situations
      i. Provide for nutritional needs
      j. Recognized self-concept needs
      k. Encourage verbal communications
      l. Monitor effectiveness of medications, for example, antidepressants
B. Multi-infarct dementia: cognitive impairment caused by cerebrovascular disease
C. Psychoactive substance-induced mental disorders: chemically induced organic disease

TABLE 9-2   Factors Associated with Organic Mental Syndromes and Disorders

Influential Factors	Examples
Volatile agents	Gasoline, aerosols, glues, paint removers, solvents, lacquers, varnishes, dry-cleaning agents, home cleaning products alone or when mixed
Heavy metals	Lead paints, ceramic glazes, moonshine whiskey, mercury, arsenic, manganese
Insecticides	DDT, parathion, malathion, diazine
Brain trauma	Concussion, contusion, hemorrhage, thrombosis, penetrating wounds, blast effects, electrical trauma; exposure to repeated courses of electroconvulsive therapy; oxygen deprivation
Drugs	Alcohol, barbiturates, opioids, cocaine, amphetamines, cannabis, hallucinogens such as lysergic acid diethylamide (LSD) and phencyclidine (PCP)
Infections	Tuberculous and fungal meningitis, viral encephalitis, neurosyphilis (tabes dorsalis), Jakob-Creutzfeldt disease, human immunodeficiency virus (HIV) related disorders (AIDS, ARC)
Neoplasms, tumors	Astrocytoma, medulloblastoma, meningioma
Metabolic and endocrine disorders	Hepatic disease, uremic encephalopathy, porphyria; thyroid, parathyroid, and adrenal dysfunction; Wernicke-Korsakoff syndrome
Nutritional deficiencies	Lack of protein; deficiencies in vitamin C and the B vitamins (folic acid, niacin, pyridoxine, riboflavin, thiamine, B_{12}); fluid and electrolyte imbalance
Seizures	Petit mal, grand mal, focal seizures, psychic seizures
Hypoxia-ischemia	Anoxia related to delayed or prolonged cardiopulmonary resuscitation
Neurological disease (possible genetic influence)	Huntington chorea, multiple sclerosis, Pick's disease, cerebral degeneration, Parkinson's disease
Cerebral changes associated with Alzheimer's disease	Loss of neurons, plaques, neurofibrillary degeneration, tangles, amyloid deposits, loss of dendritic tree, choline acetyl transferase, CAT defects, degeneration of basal forebrain, elevated platelet fluidity, inherited genetic factor

From Haber et al: *Comprehensive psychiatric nursing,* ed 5, St Louis, 1998, Mosby.

PARKINSONIAN SYNDROME
Progressive neurological movement disorder
A. Primary
    1. Parkinson's disease
    2. Paralysis agitans
B. Secondary
    1. Tumors
    2. Drugs
    3. Infection
C. Assessment
    1. Slowness of movement
    2. Waxlike rigidity of extremities
    3. Facial masking
    4. Tremors while at rest; characteristic pill-rolling motion
    5. Muscular weakness
    6. Shuffling gait
    7. Stature alterations
    8. Drooling; swallowing difficulties
    9. Cognitive impairment
    10. Mood swings
D. Nursing intervention/management
    1. Foster independence with ADLs
    2. Maintain physical mobility
    3. Provide adequate nutrition
      a. Keep swallowing difficulties in mind
      b. May require suction; prone to aspiration
      c. Monitor weight weekly
      d. Provide adaptive eating devices
      e. Provide thick liquids
    4. Prevent constipation
    5. Encourage communication
      a. Be attentive: speech is soft and low pitched
      b. Allow time: speech is slow and monotonous

    6. Enhance self-concept
      a. Focus on patient's strengths
      b. Encourage activities that foster success
      c. Give positive feedback
      d. Establish realistic goals
      e. Encourage verbalization of feelings
      f. Maintain intellectual activity stimulation
    7. Monitor effectiveness of medications in controlling tremors and rigidity and alleviating characteristic depression
      a. Tricyclic antidepressants; monoamine oxidase inhibitors (MAOIs)
      b. Antihistamines
      c. Anticholinergics
      d. Levodopa (eliminate Vitamin B_6 from diet)
    8. Provide safety
    9. Decrease stress

PSYCHOLOGICAL CHANGES (NORMAL AGING PROCESS)
Self-Image
A. Physiological alterations
B. Youth-oriented society
C. Retirement
D. Income alterations
E. Role changes
F. Sexual expression alterations

Intelligence
A. Verbal ability and retained information remain unchanged
B. Abstract thinking and performance response decline
C. Performance of activities involving neuromuscular learning decline

D. Attention span shortens
E. Literal approach to problem-solving affects ability
F. Fluid intelligence declines after adolescence
G. Crystallized intelligence continues to increase throughout life
H. Learning capacity continues

Memory

A. Short term: concentration and retention decline
B. Long term: minimal impairment
C. Remote
   1. Remote memory is better than short-term memory
   2. Involved in reminiscence

Motivation

A. Not risk takers
B. Do not actively seek change
C. Possess fear of failure
D. Self-fulfilling prophecies
E. Competitiveness declines
F. Energy levels decline

Attitudes, Beliefs, Interests

A. General attitude realignment
B. Interests either narrow or expand
C. Tend to keep lifelong beliefs amid rapidly changing society

Personality

A. Basically unchanged
B. Some exaggeration of behavioral responses is evident
C. Adaptive capacities are diminished
D. Reduced ability to handle stress

PSYCHOLOGICAL DISORDERS (ABNORMAL)

Depression

A. Reaction to loss of:
   1. Independence
   2. Status
   3. Spouse, relatives, and friends
   4. Possessions
   5. Income
   6. Mobility
B. Medications can cause depression (e.g., digitalis)
C. Physical illness and changes
   1. Lowered self-esteem
   2. Self-concept alterations
   3. Feelings of hopelessness and worthlessness
D. Types
   1. Exogenous
      a. Referred to as neurotic; external, caused by outside events
      b. Common in the older adult
      c. Usually a reaction to losses
   2. Endogenous
      a. Referred to as psychotic; caused by internal events
      b. Characterized by:
         (1) Guilt
         (2) Reduced self-regard
         (3) Early morning awakening
         (4) Slowing of thought, verbalization, and level of activity

TABLE 9-3 Symptoms of Depression as Observed in Cognitive, Affective, and Somatic Changes

Cognitive	Affective	Somatic
Indecisiveness	Fear*	Tearful
Confusion*	Anxiety	Crying spells
Impaired thinking*	Sadness	Agitation*
Poverty of thought	Irritability	Anorexia
Hopelessness/emptiness	Anger*	Weight loss
Suicidal ideation*	Feels distant	Constipation
Guilt	from others*	Palpitations
Inability to concentrate	Depersonalized	Fatigue/
Worry		weakness
Believes self a failure*		Insomnia
Believes self causing harm to others*		Restlessness*
Believes self going crazy*		
Believes self deserving of punishment*		

Data from Morris J, Wolf R, Kerman L: *J Gerontol* 30:209, 1975; Zung W: *Arch Gen Psychiatry* 29:328, 1973.
*Presence of clinically significant depression.

   c. Classifications
      (1) Unipolar: life history of depression
      (2) Bipolar (manic-depressive psychosis)
         (a) Mood swings from depression to euphoria
         (b) More likely to have hallucinations and delusions
E. Symptoms of depression (Table 9-3)
F. Nursing intervention
   1. Encourage self-expression; increase self-esteem
   2. Improve appearance
   3. Provide structure, routine
   4. Assist with maintaining or regaining control
   5. Have kind, understanding attitude
   6. Provide physical care as needed; encourage independence
   7. Provide safety, security
   8. Reduce environmental stimuli and stress
   9. Continuously test reality perception
   10. Ascertain emotional support network
   11. Prevent isolation and avoidance
   12. Realize potential for suicide exists
      a. Suicide is an act that stems from depression
      b. Approximately 25% of suicides occur in persons over age 65
      c. White males over age 75 have the highest rate
      d. Refer to Chapter 6 for suicidal risk assessment, crisis intervention, and nursing interventions

Aggressive Behavior

A. Abnormal anger, rage, or hostility, which if turned inward would lead to depression and if turned outward would lead to aggressiveness
B. Response to
   1. Anxiety
   2. Stress

3. Guilt
4. Insecurity
5. Loss of self-esteem
6. Loss of control of destiny
7. Forced dependency

C. Clinical manifestations
1. Lack of cooperation
2. Irritability
3. Demanding
4. Hostility
5. Demonstration of coping mechanisms characteristically used to decrease stress, for example, rationalization and repression
6. Altered interpersonal relationships
7. Altered reality testing

D. Nursing intervention
1. Reduce stress source and sensory overload
2. Encourage verbalization
3. Set realistic, reachable goals
4. Respond to questions directly and briefly
5. Allow ample time for task completion
6. Meet physical needs as necessary
7. Encourage environmental participation and activity involvement
8. Positively recognize attainments
9. Set limits on activities
10. Anticipate hostile, demanding behavior
11. Allow only the degree of independence that can be successfully handled
12. Avoid responses and action that could lead to guilt, feelings of rejection, bother, or dislike
13. Increase feeling of self-worth
14. Medication
15. Therapy if indicated

REGRESSION

The display of regressive behavior, an ego defense mechanism, is not an uncommon response in the older adult to external stressors; this return to an earlier behavioral stage (e.g., temper tantrums, rocking, or incontinence) requires prevention, early detection, and prompt intervention (remove source of stress and reverse the behavior)

Paranoid Behavior

A. Inappropriate attempt of coping with stress
B. Response to:
1. Physical impairments
2. Sensory deprivation
3. Loss
4. Loneliness
5. Medications
6. Environmental changes
7. Isolation
8. Vision alterations
9. Auditory alterations

C. Clinical manifestations
1. Secretiveness
2. Mistrust
3. Mood disturbances
4. Oversensitivity
5. Insecurity
6. Superiority attitude
7. Alterations in behavior

8. Delusions
9. Withdrawal
10. Fearfulness
11. Aloofness
12. Refusal to take medications, eat, or carry out normal self-care activities

D. Nursing intervention
1. Attempt to allay anxiety
2. Allow patient to refuse treatments
3. Don't argue with patient
4. Try not to take patient's anger personally
5. Administer medication
6. Don't make promises to patient
7. Look for alterations in ADLs as cues to whether the patient's verbalizations are of real concern or are for attention
8. Be aware of events precipitated by environment
9. Use stress-management techniques
10. Patient-predicted events that do not occur should be brought to patient's attention
11. Encourage independence
12. Monitor impact on hygiene and nutrition
13. Encourage socialization

REHABILITATION/MAINTENANCE OF COGNITIVE FUNCTION
Reality Orientation (Table 9-4)

A. A total approach to keeping individuals oriented. Small groups that emphasize time, place, and person; weather; holidays, etc.
B. First used with disoriented, confused older adults at Veterans Administration Hospital in Tuscaloosa, Alabama, in 1965
C. Orientation boards may be used to provide contact with reality
D. Program success depends on total staff commitment and 24-hour implementation
E. Many facilities that care for the older adult have implemented modified programs
F. Program implementation not limited to an institutional setting
G. Components
1. Small groups
2. Formal classroom sessions
   a. 20 to 30 minutes
   b. Morning sessions recommended (older adults are more alert in the morning)
   c. Reality orientation board, calendars, clocks, and other materials used according to instructor plan
   d. Positive verbal feedback emphasized
   e. Confusion never reinforced
H. All personnel who come in contact with patients participating in the program are expected to use reality orientation
1. Address patient by name and title
2. Orient patient to time, place, and person
3. Give positive verbal feedback
4. Do not reinforce confusion

Remotivation

A. Similar to reality orientation
B. Normal behavior reinforced through structured group program

TABLE 9-4 Differences Between Remotivation and Reality Orientation

Reality Orientation	Remotivation
1. Correct position or relation with the existing situation in a community. Maximum use of assets	1. Orientation to reality for community living; present oriented
2. Called reality orientation and classroom reality orientation program	2. Called remotivation
3. Structured	3. Definite structure
4. Refreshments or food may be served for identification	4. Refreshments not served
5. Appreciation of the work of the world. Constantly reminded of who they are, where they are, why they are here, and what is expected of them	5. Appreciation of the work of the group stimulates the desire to return to function in society
6. Classes range from 3 to 5 patients, depending on degree/level of confusion or disorientation from any cause	6. Group size: 5 to 12 patients
7. Meeting ½ hour daily at same time in same place	7. Meeting once to twice weekly for an hour
8. Planned procedures: reality-centered objects	8. Preselected and reality-centered objects
9. Consistence of approach response of resident responsibility of teacher	9. No exploration of feelings
10. Periodic reality orientation test pertaining to residents' level of confusion or disorientation	10. Progress ratings
11. Emphasis on time, place, person orientation	11. Topic: no discussion of religion, politics, or death
12. Use of portion of mind function still intact	12. Untouched areas of the mind
13. Residents greeted by name, thanked for coming, and extended handshake and/or physical contact according to attitude approach in group	13. No physical contact permitted. Acceptance and acknowledgment of everyone's contribution
14. Conducted by trained aides and activity assistants	14. Conducted by trained psychiatric aides

From Barns E, Sack A, Shore H: *The Gerontologist* 13:513, 1973.

C. Stimulating participation and interest in the environment are key components
D. Sessions average 20 to 60 minutes
E. Visual aids used, for example, items that stimulate sensory responses
F. Client behavior recorded
G. Staff support and involvement essential

Reminiscence

A. Small group sessions
B. Based on life-review process
C. Older adults with cognitive dysfunction retain long-term memory and through reminiscence can adapt to the aging process
D. Purposes
   1. Conflict resolution
   2. Sharing of memories
   3. Sense of identity and self-importance achieved
   4. Focus is on a life that has meaning as opposed to a life viewed as a waste of time
   5. Natural for older adult persons to reminisce
      a. Feel comfortable
      b. They're good at it
      c. Reinforces sense of belonging (everyone talks about life's trials and tribulations)
   6. Therapeutic relationship with leader more likely to develop as patients realize their memories are important and valued
   7. Depressed patients find a caring listener and an opportunity to externalize their anger

8. Psychologically disturbed patients receive acceptance, group validation, and a forum for expression: encourage active exploration of past strengths
9. Strive to change outlook on the past rather than establishing new future directions
10. Psychological assessment tool (e.g., insight into past coping mechanisms)
11. Reduces isolation, insecurity, and negative self-esteem
12. Confused patients can be assisted to explore a memory that will stimulate latent thoughts, become more oriented, and improve ability to focus
13. Current circumstances are often reflected through memories
E. If patients have difficulty focusing their thoughts, assist by selecting a specific memory
F. Stimulation of dormant thoughts to the surface decreases disorientation
G. Patients who are reluctant to talk can usually be stimulated with topics of food, movies, or music
H. Program implementation is not limited to institutional settings

Cognitive Training

A. Consists of memory exercises, problem-solving situations, and memory training
B. Leader must be familiar with patient's past leisure time utilization, hobbies, and occupations
C. Individual, small, or large groups
D. Purpose is to maintain mental activity

Relaxation Therapy

A. Promotes sense of physical well-being, reduces stress, releases tension
B. Small groups
C. Involves rhythmic breathing, tension-relaxation exercises, and altered state of consciousness

Bladder Retraining: Urinary Incontinence

A. Causes
  1. Physiological changes
    a. Decline in muscle support of pelvis
    b. Reduction in bladder's capacity to hold urine
    c. Sphincter weakness
  2. Behavioral alterations
    a. Regression
    b. Insecurity
    c. Rebellion
    d. Attention seeking
    e. Dependency
    f. Sensory deprivation
  3. Drugs
  4. Consciousness alterations
  5. Disease
  6. Obstruction
  7. Trauma
  8. Immobility
  9. Bedpans and urinals
  10. Lack of privacy
  11. Lack of time
B. Types
  1. Stress or passive
    a. Bladder outlet weakness
    b. Involuntary
    c. Frequency when sneezing, coughing, laughing, and lifting
  2. Paradoxical or overflow
    a. Uncontrollable contraction waves
    b. Bladder does not empty
    c. Frequency accompanied by retention
    d. At risk for urinary tract infection
  3. Total
    a. Constant dribbling
    b. Storage problem
C. Older adults susceptible to
  1. Urinary tract infections
  2. Urgency
  3. Frequency
D. Patient reactions to incontinence
  1. Insecurity
    a. Social withdrawal
    b. Isolation
    c. Sensory deprivation
    d. Avoidance of previously developed relationships
  2. Depression
    a. Embarrassment
    b. Guilt
    c. Shame
E. Intervention
  1. Pelvic exercises
    a. Bearing down
    b. Push-ups from a chair
  2. Indwelling catheter as a last resort if skin integrity threatened

  3. Condom drainage
  4. Absorbent, waterproof underpants
  5. Keep patient clean and dry
  6. Skin care
  7. Retraining
    a. Assess and record voiding pattern for minimum of 72 hours
      (1) Time
      (2) Place
      (3) Quantity
      (4) Activity
      (5) Patient awareness
      (6) Significant medications
      (7) Character of urine
      (8) Presence or absence of constipation or discharge
      (9) Problems: for example, clothing and ambulation hindrances
    b. Reestablish voiding pattern
      (1) First scheduled voiding of the day should be attempted immediately after awakening in the morning even if bed is wet
      (2) Voiding should be attempted at intervals determined from the assessment period (usually at 1-, 2-, or 3-hour periods; goal is every 4 hours)
      (3) Patient takes one or two 8-oz (240-ml) glasses of fluid 1 hour before attempting to urinate
      (4) No fluids should be taken between 6 PM and 6 AM if no urinating is desired
      (5) Fluid intake should be at least 2000 ml per day
      (6) Alcoholic drinks contraindicated
      (7) Soft drinks, tea, and coffee should be avoided
      (8) All fluid intake should be measured and recorded
      (9) All urine output should be measured and recorded

Bowel Retraining: Fecal Incontinence

A. Causes
  1. Physiological changes
    a. External anal sphincter relaxation
    b. Perineal relaxation
    c. Muscle atony
  2. Behavioral alterations
    a. Regression
    b. Rebellion
    c. Dependency
    d. Sensory deprivation
  3. Central nervous system injury
  4. Obstruction
  5. Impaction
  6. Consciousness alterations
  7. Immobility
  8. Trauma
B. Intervention
  1. Keep patient clean and dry
  2. Absorbent, waterproof underpants
  3. Skin care
  4. Retraining
    a. Bowel retraining is easier than bladder retraining; if patient is incontinent of urine and stool, start bowel retraining program first

b. Use no laxatives
c. Ensure adequate fluid intake (2 L per day)
d. Fluids and solids that promote patient's bowel movements (e.g., bran and orange juice) and roughage should be included in the diet
e. Encourage physical activity
f. Obtain bowel history
g. Procedure
   (1) Establish regular days(s) and time to assist patient to the toilet for evacuation; preferably after a meal
   (2) After 20 minutes if patient has not had a bowel movement, insert a lubricated glycerine suppository
      (a) Do not use directly from refrigerator
      (b) Do not insert into a bolus of stool (ineffective)
      (c) After ascertaining that patient requires the suppository for training, it can be inserted 1 to 2 hours before the scheduled training time and after a meal

   (3) Digital stimulation is recommended after 48 hours if the above procedure is not successful
   (4) Take patient to the bathroom at the scheduled time daily, even if he or she has had a bowel movement between scheduled times

SUGGESTED READINGS

Eliopoulus C: *Manual of gerontologic nursing,* ed 2, St Louis, 1999, Mosby.

Eliopoulus C: *Gerontological nursing,* ed 4, Philadelphia, 1997, Lippincott-Raven.

Feldman RS: *Development across the life span,* Englewood Cliffs, NJ, 1999, Prentice Hall.

Hamdy RC, Edwards J, Turnbull JM: *Alzheimer's disease, a handbook for caregivers,* ed 2, St Louis, 1998, Mosby.

Hogstel MO: *Clinical manual of gerontological nursing,* St Louis, 1992, Mosby.

Hogstel MO: *Geropsychiatric Nursing,* ed 2, St. Louis, 1995, Mosby.

Morice SV: *Geriatric nursing,* Aurora, 1996, Skidmore-Roth Publishing.

Polan E, Taylor DC: *Journey across the life span,* 1998, FA Davis.

REVIEW QUESTIONS

1. An older adult with osteoarthritis is admitted to the hospital for a total knee replacement. Of the following baseline data, which is most important for the nurse to obtain?
   ① Usual sleeping habits
   ② Food likes and dislikes
   ③ Mental health status and history
   ④ Extent of knee flexion and extension

2. A patient with Parkinson's disease has difficulty swallowing. The patient will be able to meet dietary requirements when he can:
   ① Eat solid food
   ② Drink thin liquids
   ③ Eat a meal in 20 minutes
   ④ Swallow without choking

3. Which of the following is included in the preoperative teaching for a 71-year-old patient scheduled for a total knee replacement?
   ① Russell traction
   ② Cast brace application
   ③ Principles of Buck's extension
   ④ Continuous passive motion (CPM) device

4. Routine nursing care following a total knee replacement in an older adult should include which of the following?
   ① Keeping the affected leg in abduction
   ② Elevating the affected knee when out of bed
   ③ Using wedge pillows between the patient's legs
   ④ Keeping the head of the bed elevated up to 45 degrees

5. Which of the following statements is accurate regarding ice application to the affected knee following a total knee replacement?
   ① Reduces edema and bleeding
   ② Reduces the chance of infection
   ③ Increases circulation and movement
   ④ Reduces fluid accumulation in the joint

6. Which of the following measures should be reinforced in the discharge teaching plan for an older adult recovering from a total knee replacement?
   ① Full weight bearing in the affected leg
   ② Non-weight bearing in the affected leg
   ③ Weight bearing only as tolerated by the patient
   ④ Weight bearing only as prescribed by the physician

7. An 89-year-old patient is alert and active. On annual physical examination, she complains of hemorrhoids and annoying constipation. Her physician instructs her to increase her fluid and dietary fiber intake. Which of the following snacks, if selected by the patient, would indicate that she can identify food sources high in fiber?
   ① Cucumber
   ② Apple juice
   ③ Bran cereal
   ④ Small banana

8. A 62-year-old male patient has a diagnosis of hiatal hernia (gastric reflux). Which of the following nursing measures should be included in his plan of care?
   ① Eat three good meals a day
   ② Eat high-protein, high-fat foods
   ③ Lie down for 1 to 2 hours after meals
   ④ Sleep with the head of the bed elevated

9. Which of the following procedures can give a positive diagnosis of Alzheimer's disease?
   ① Neural tissue evaluation on autopsy
   ② Computer tomography scanning (CT)
   ③ Positron emission tomography (PET)
   ④ Serial evaluations of neuropsychologic testing

10. A 67-year-old patient is admitted to a nursing home with a diagnosis of senile dementia Alzheimer's type (SDAT). The nurse observes the resident moving toward the exit door. The nurse meets the resident at the door and volunteers assistance. The resident responds, "You can leave me alone. I'm going home." Which of the following nursing actions is most appropriate?
   ① Go with the resident
   ② Engage him in an activity
   ③ Call the security department
   ④ Physically prevent him from leaving

11. An older adult with Alzheimer's disease is restless and agitated. Which of the following activities is most appropriate for the patient?
   ① Taking a nap
   ② Taking a walk
   ③ Listening to music
   ④ Watching television

12. Which of the following activities is most appropriate for an Alzheimer's patient who is demonstrating increasing difficulty with planning and decision making?
   ① Sorting the laundry
   ② Hoeing in the garden
   ③ Planning the dinner menu
   ④ Writing out the grocery list

13. A patient with Alzheimer's disease demonstrates progressive personality changes. The patient begins to show signs of hostility and combativeness. The nurse should include which of the following in his plan of care?
   ① Use memory aids
   ② Simplify daily activity
   ③ Decrease environmental stimuli
   ④ Secure doors leading from the house

14. When caring for the elderly, the nurse must know that the most common and easily reversed cause of dementia is:
   ① Pick's disease
   ② Drug toxicity
   ③ Parkinson's disease
   ④ Alcoholism

15. An 82-year-old patient has periods of confusion and disorientation as well as difficulty remembering where the bathroom is. Which of the following nursing actions should be most helpful?
   ① Take him to the bathroom every hour
   ② Place a sign saying *"Here it is"* on the door
   ③ Place a picture of a toilet on the bathroom door
   ④ Tell him if he can't find the bathroom he'll have to wear diapers

16. An 89-year-old nursing home resident with a history of poor nutritional intake takes a few mouthfuls of dinner and then gets up and leaves the table. Which of the following nursing approaches is most appropriate?
   ① Apply a vest restraint during meals
   ② Offer five to six small feedings daily

③ Have a staff member feed him his meals

④ Provide him with a variety of finger foods

17. A 79-year-old nursing home resident is confused. Which of the following nursing measures would best reduce his confusion?

① Place a weekly activity calendar in his room

② Speak clearly, calmly, and in short sentences

③ Leave him alone and let him do what he wants

④ Explain the planned daily activities to him each morning

18. The physician orders a restraint chair to be used in accordance with agency policy when a nursing home resident becomes overly agitated and combative. Which of the following statements by the nurse indicates the best understanding of the resident's response to the chair?

① The use of a restraint chair causes decubiti

② The use of a restraint chair fosters incontinence

③ The use of the chair can increase a patient's agitation level

④ All agitated patients should be restrained for their own safety

19. How should the nurse address Mr. Jake Walters, a resident in a long-term care facility? The nurse knows that the resident is sometimes called "Pops" and was the school crossing guard in the nurse's old neighborhood.

① "Hi Jake. I'm your nurse, Karen."

② "Hi there, Mr. Walters, remember me?"

③ "Hi, aren't you Pops, the school crossing guard?"

④ "Mr. Walters. Hello. I'm your nurse for today."

20. A nurse responds to a resident's call bell and finds the patient standing at the bedside in a puddle of urine, with his pajamas soaked. Which of the following is the most appropriate response by the nurse?

① "Not again. You may need to wear Attends from now on."

② "Now look what you've done. Let's go to the bathroom again."

③ "Next time, wait for help before getting out of bed. That's why I'm here."

④ "Let's go to the bathroom where you can wash up and put on clean pajamas."

21. A patient diagnosed with Parkinson's disease is placed on Sinemet 10/100 PO tid by his physician. As he is leaving the doctor's office, he asks the nurse what the drug will do. Which of the following explanations by the nurse is most correct?

① "You'll have to discuss that with the physician."

② "It can decrease your tremors and improve your gait."

③ "It's the carbidopa-levodopa content ratio of the drug."

④ "It's really very complicated and not necessary for you to know."

22. Which of the following assessments of a patient on Sinemet should indicate possible drug toxicity to the nurse?

① Akinesia and drooling

② Muscle stiffness and rigidity

③ Muscle and eyelid twitching

④ Slow movements and handwriting changes

23. A patient with Parkinson's disease has been on Sinemet 10/100 PO tid for 2 weeks. The patient calls the doctor's office and tells the nurse that he has seen no improvement since the Sinemet was started and perhaps another drug should be tried. Which of the following responses by the nurse is most appropriate?

① "What makes you think you're not improving?"

② "I'll let the physician know you want a medication change."

③ "It frequently takes several months to achieve maximum effect."

④ "Why don't you call the doctor tomorrow when he is in the office?"

24. A patient on Sinemet reports to the nurse that he really doesn't want to eat and occasionally vomits when he does eat. To reduce the gastrointestinal side effects of Sinemet and enhance its absorption, which of the following instructions should the nurse give the patient?

① Take the medication after meals

② Take the medication before meals

③ Crush the medication and mix it with his food

④ If any problems, call the physician to lower the dosage

25. Which of the following facts reported by a patient with Parkinson's disease would indicate to the nurse that the patient has a basic understanding of his disease process?

① Autosomal dominant genetic disorder

② Progressive, fatal disease caused by a virus

③ Chronic progressive hereditary disease of the nervous system

④ Progressive damage to neurons that regulate and control movement

26. A 66-year-old skilled nursing facility (SNF) resident has rheumatoid arthritis resulting in severe deformities of both hands. Her medications consist of prednisone (Prednisone) 5 mg PO qd and auranofin (Ridaura) 2 mg PO tid. She refuses her qd dose of prednisone. Which of the following actions should the nurse take?

① Chart the refusal in the nurses' notes and inform the head nurse

② Chart *"refused"* on the medication sheet and report it to the physician

③ Return to the patient in a half hour and offer her the medication again

④ Call the physician and get an order for an injectable adrenocorticosteroid

27. An older nursing home resident has a history of paranoid behavior. When planning care for the patient, which of the following demonstrated behaviors should the staff identify as unusual?

① Verbalized hallucination

② Demonstrated superiority

③ Verbalized oversensitivity

④ Refusal of meals and treatments

28. The nurse brings a 90-year-old hospitalized patient his breakfast tray. The patient says, "Take it away; I don't want it." What is the most appropriate response?

① "I'll tell the dietitian you don't like the food here."

② "I'll call the kitchen and order something else for you."

③ "I'll leave the tray here just in case you change your mind."

④ "I'll throw it out and record that you refused your breakfast."

29. A 73-year-old nursing home resident reports that the staff ignores her needs but takes care of all the other patients. The nurse knows this to be inaccurate and understands that the patient is:
    ① Looking to cause trouble
    ② Experiencing active hallucinations
    ③ Attempting to manipulate the staff
    ④ Demonstrating manifestations of paranoia

30. Which of the following activities would be most therapeutic for a 78-year-old resident with deformities of both hands (related to rheumatoid arthritis) who has a history of paranoid behavior?
    ① Making her own bed daily
    ② Greeting visitors at the front desk
    ③ Participating daily in arts and crafts
    ④ Independently preparing her meal tray

31. An 80-year-old widower lives with his four cats in a two-bedroom, fourth-floor walkup. His children want him to move to a ground floor smaller apartment. He refuses and says he'll stay where he is until he dies. It is important that his children recognize that their father is:
    ① Afraid to move
    ② Becoming paranoid
    ③ Displaying eccentricity
    ④ Feeling secure where he is

32. A 75-year-old man falls in the street and is taken to the hospital by EMS (Emergency Medical Service). He is diagnosed with a mild concussion and a fractured left radius. His two children live nearby and are notified of their father's hospitalization. He tells the nurse that he can't stay in the hospital because he lives alone and has four cats that he needs to take care of. Which of the following actions should the nurse take?
    ① Offer to go to his home once a day to care for the cats
    ② Speak with the patient's children about arranging care for his cats
    ③ Remind the patient that cats are independent and can care for themselves
    ④ Tell the patient that he has too many cats and should give them to the ASPCA

33. A 78-year-old widow is brought to the local emergency room by the police, who found her wandering aimlessly about the street. She is confused, disoriented, and hospitalized for pneumonia. The nurse should recognize that the cause of her confusion and disorientation is:
    ① Infection
    ② Unknown
    ③ Arteriosclerosis
    ④ Organic brain syndrome

34. An elderly man is hospitalized with pneumonia and has a poor nutritional intake. The patient's appetite may improve if:
    ① His food is blenderized
    ② All liquids are served warm
    ③ A roll is served with each meal
    ④ He is served small meals frequently

35. An elderly patient hospitalized with pneumonia asks the time of each staff member who enters his room. The nurse knows that this is characteristic of:
    ① Confusion
    ② Disorientation
    ③ Memory deficit
    ④ Impaired judgment

36. A 70-year-old nursing home resident has not had a bowel movement in 3 days. The nurse identifies the problem as constipation and knows that constipation in the elderly is frequently the result of:
    ① Poor eating habits
    ② Lack of daily exercise
    ③ Too much fiber in the diet
    ④ Usage of medications that cause constipation

37. A 78-year-old nursing home resident's bedside stand is found to be full of packets of sugar, salt, jelly, napkins, and straws, which he has removed from his meal trays. The nurse understands that this behavior indicates:
    ① Increased insecurity
    ② Increased confusion
    ③ Decreased self-esteem
    ④ Increased disorientation

38. The night staff in a nursing home expresses concern about an elderly resident who is awake most of the night. Which of the following would be the most appropriate response by the nurse?
    ① "We'll increase his day activities."
    ② "I'll get a physician's order for a sedative."
    ③ "As people get older, they require less sleep."
    ④ "The elderly require less sleep at night, and more rest periods."

39. An elderly stroke survivor is being followed in the Outpatient Clinic. He is on sodium warfarin (Coumadin) daily. His prothrombin times have been unstable and the physician requests the nurse to review the patient's dietary intake for indications of possible food-drug interactions. The nurse ascertains that the patient eats large quantities of the following foods. Which foods high in vitamin K should he avoid ingesting in large quantities?
    ① Rice and beans
    ② Chicken and rice
    ③ Spaghetti and meatballs
    ④ Broccoli and turnip greens

40. Which of the following patient concerns would result from the age-related change of loss of subcutaneous tissue?
    ① Foot pain
    ② Muscle cramps
    ③ Increased urination at night
    ④ Increased susceptibility to infection

41. Given the normal aging changes in the sensory system, which of the following colors would be most effective when color coding the door to the room of an elderly nursing home resident?
    ① Red
    ② Pink
    ③ Blue
    ④ Green

42. To evaluate the judgment of a patient in the early stages of Alzheimer's disease, the nurse should pay particular attention to the patient's ability to:
    ① Set the dining room table
    ② Cooperate with caregivers
    ③ Manage personal finances
    ④ Navigate in familiar surroundings

43. The nurse should anticipate that a patient with early Alzheimer's disease would have difficulty:
    ① Remembering how to operate an automobile
    ② Remembering she has put a meal in the oven

③ Remembering where she put the house keys the evening before

④ Recalling a telephone conversation right after hanging up the phone

44. An 80-year-old patient with diabetes mellitus is hospitalized and scheduled for a right below-the-knee amputation. On the fifth postoperative day the nurse notices that the residual limb is edematous. The nurse should plan to:
① Elevate the limb on a pillow
② See if the patient has an order for a diuretic
③ Instruct the patient to sit on the edge of the bed and dangle
④ Assure proper application of the Ace bandage to the residual limb

45. A patient's son comes to the nurse's station and remarks that his mother can't remember what she had for breakfast, but can remember every detail of his wedding 30 years ago. The most accurate response from the nurse would be:
① Older adults tend to remember happy events in their lives
② This is a normal manifestation of the mother's disease process
③ This is not unusual; there is long-term memory loss in older adults
④ This is not unusual; there is short-term memory loss in older adults

46. Aging causes respiratory changes that may result in:
① A lower-toned, frailer voice and dyspnea
② A much higher-pitched, stronger, resonant voice
③ Decreased activity tolerance, dyspnea, and fatigue
④ Decreased activity tolerance, orthopnea, and fatigue

47. A nurse instructs a nursing assistant not to fully bathe a resident with extremely dry skin every day. Which of the following is the best reason why older adults do not need to have a complete bath every day?
① Body odor is diminished
② Activity level is decreased
③ Interest in hygiene is diminished
④ Sweat and oil glands are less active

48. Which of the following foods should be suggested to combat constipation in older adults?
① Fruit juices and dairy products
② Meats, cheese, and poultry products
③ Processed carbohydrates and milk products
④ Whole-grain cereals, fresh vegetables, and water

49. Which of the following activities would an individual with presbyopia have the most difficulty completing?
① Walking and gardening
② Needlepoint and knitting
③ Playing bingo and shopping
④ Seeing road signs while driving

50. The nurse suggests to an older adult that she wear some makeup and a pretty robe when she goes to physical therapy. The nurse's suggestion is:
① Inappropriate because it infantilizes her
② Appropriate because it may increase her self-esteem
③ Appropriate because she needs encouragement to bathe
④ Inappropriate because she is unaware of her surroundings

51. A hospitalized older adult is on a regular diet but will not eat because he claims the food has no flavor. The nurse's best course of action is to:
① Explain the complications of poor nutrition
② Teach the patient about adequate calorie intake
③ Ascertain what condiments the patient uses at home
④ Describe that salt is never acceptable for older adults to consume

52. The normal inflammatory response is not always a reliable indicator of disease in the older adult because:
① Aging changes heighten the older adult's pain perception
② Cardiovascular changes heighten the erythema that develops around infection sites
③ Changes in the hypothalamus diminish the ability of the older adult to produce a fever
④ Changes in the hypothalamus grossly elevate temperature changes in the older adult

53. The nurse realizes that the teaching of older adult patients may be more difficult because they:
① Have a pronounced loss of intelligence
② Learn more quickly but have a slower reaction time
③ Respond better to verbal teaching than demonstrative teaching
④ Are susceptible to background noise, making distraction a problem

54. Which of the following is a characteristic of Alzheimer's disease?
① Has a sudden, rapid onset
② Is curable if the cause is found
③ Average age at onset is 35-40 years
④ Is a progressive, neurological disorder of the brain

55. Which of the following hospital rooms would the nurse choose as being the best for a wandering patient with dementia?
① A room by the elevators
② A room by the nurse's station
③ A room with a talkative, chatty roommate
④ A room where the nurse's station must be passed to leave

56. When attempting to teach a patient with dementia, it is important to remember to:
① Speak quickly and repeat several times in succession
② Talk in a very animated, loud voice so the patient can hear you
③ Eliminate background noise by shutting doors and turning off the TV
④ Talk to the patient when she is stress free, such as while watching TV

57. The nurse is caring for a 72-year-old patient who has no known organic disease. The patient often calls the nurse by her daughter's name. The best course of action would be to:
① Tell her that her daughter will be visiting soon
② Go along with it since she is unlikely to re-orient well
③ Tell her the nurse's name and explain what the nurse will be doing for her
④ Tell her that the daughter went home for a rest and will be back soon

58. A nurse begins a reality orientation program for a group of older adults. The nurse is applying a program to emphasize:
① Reinforcement of "normal behavior"
② Orientation to time, place, and person
③ Conflict resolution and sharing of memories
④ Participation and interest in the environment

59. A confused, demented patient should bring personal items along to a long-term care facility. The purpose of doing this is to:
① Increase attention span
② Decrease dementia behaviors
③ Facilitate short-term memory
④ Foster recognition in the environment

60. The nurse is administering medications via a small-bore feeding tube to a 68-year-old individual. Which of the following is the correct sequence of administration?
① Check residual, give med, flush with at least 150 cc of water
② Check tube placement, flush with water, give med, check residual
③ Flush tube with water, check residual, give med, flush with water again
④ Check tube placement, flush with water, give med, flush with water again

61. The charge nurse at a long-term care facility needs to communicate information to the nursing assistants on her shift. Which of the following communication methods would be <u>best</u> to utilize?
① E-mail them on their home computers
② Post a memo in the bathroom for all to read
③ Verbally present the information in a short staff meeting
④ Allow an RN to communicate the information to the nurse's aides

62. A charge nurse has the following tasks to perform at 9 AM; vitals on two residents; medications for four residents; attend an interdisciplinary care team meeting; and documentation for four residents. Which of the previous tasks would be most appropriate to assign to a nursing assistant?
① The documentation
② Administering meds
③ Monitoring vital signs
④ Attending the care planning meeting

63. When assessing the functional status of the older adult, it is important for the nurse to remember that:
① Older adults should be assessed on more than one occasion
② The best setting for a functional assessment is in a hospital setting
③ Older adults will usually verbally tell the nurse they are having difficulty with their ADLs
④ Assistive aids such as walkers/wheelchairs should not be included in the functional assessment

64. A patient states that he has difficulty climbing stairs. Which of the following would be the <u>best</u> way for the nurse to validate this claim?
① Ask a family member if it is true
② Watch the patient as he climbs the stairs
③ Ask for a physical therapy referral for the patient
④ Ask the patient what happens when he climbs the steps

65. In which of the following facilities would the resident most likely receive skilled nursing care?
① Nursing home
② Adult day care
③ Personal care home
④ Senior citizen center

66. A nurse working in a hospital is approached by a nursing assistant who is concerned about a geriatric patient is restless and attempting to get out of bed. The assistant says "If she doesn't quit that, I will have to tie her down." What is the nurse's best response to the comment?
① "I'll have to call and get an order for the restraint."
② "Try to put her in a restraint chair; we'll see if that helps."
③ "Let me take a look at her; maybe she's having trouble and can't tell us."
④ "Why don't you just sit with her? Someone else can finish the water pitchers."

67. Which of the following nursing interventions should be the priority after a fall has occurred?
① Move the patient to a bed or stretcher
② Check the extremities for symmetry and alignment
③ Assess for skin intactness and any bruises or swelling
④ Survey the patient's airway, and any difficulty breathing

68. One day after open reduction internal fixation (ORIF) of the right hip, an 80-year-old patient is exhibiting extremely restless behavior. What is the <u>first</u> nursing action at this time?
① Medicate him for pain
② Ask his wife what is wrong with him
③ Assess his cardiac and respiratory status
④ Call the physician from the nurse's station to see him

69. A nurse is instructing an older adult concerning the Patient Self-Determination Act. Which of the following statements by the nurse accurately describes a healthcare proxy or durable power of attorney?
① The healthcare proxy is able to make financial decisions for the patient
② The state appoints a guardian who is given the power to make healthcare decisions for the patient
③ The patient forms a list of activities that he does not want done if he should become incapacitated
④ The patient appoints an individual who is given power of attorney to make medical decisions for the patient

70. According to the Patient Self-Determination Act, information about advance directives is given to patients when they are:
① Admitted to the hospital
② Involved in a life-threatening crisis
③ Discharged into a home health agency
④ Willing to discuss the issue with the physician

71. An 80-year-old patient asks the nurse what is included in an advance directive. Which of the following statements by the nurse contains accurate information concerning advance directives?
① Guardianships and living wills
② Organ procurement and donation
③ Living wills and healthcare proxy
④ Active and passive acts of euthanasia

72. An LPN is assisting an RN in counseling an older couple concerning finances and long-term care. The couple relate that they thought that medicare would cover nursing homes. The nurse advises the couple that:
① Medicare should cover all of the expenses of long-term care
② Medicare only covers 1 or 2 years of long-term care expenses
③ Social Security will cover the expenses incurred during nursing home stays
④ The majority of the expenses incurred in nursing home care are covered by medicaid

73. According to Erikson's theory of life stages, older adults spend a great deal of the latter part of their life managing the task of:
① Intimacy vs. isolation
② Ego integrity vs. despair
③ Generativity vs. stagnation
④ Identity vs. role confusion

74. A nurse is presenting a seminar on culture to a group of nursing assistants. The nurse relates that the culture most likely to use traditional or alternative therapies before accessing health care is:
① African-Americans
② Jewish Americans
③ Chinese Americans
④ Hispanic Americans

75. Which culture boasts the lowest rate of nursing home utilization?
① Caucasians
② Asian Americans
③ Jewish Americans
④ Hispanic Americans

76. Which of the following provides income for the majority of retired older adult's income?
① Medicare
② Medicaid
③ Social Security
④ Tax-sheltered annuities

77. A nursing assistant that has not worked in long term care for a number of years inquires why restraints aren't used as much as they used to be. The nurse responds that restraints were heavily regulated by the
① Administration on Aging
② Title XX of the Social Security Act
③ The Patient Self-Determination Act
④ Omnibus Budget Reconciliation Act

78. The nurses in a long-term care facility are attending a meeting by a noted gerontologist who is sharing his theories of aging. The gerontologist believes that by consuming the Vitamins A, C, and E, individuals can slow the aging process. The gerontologist most likely adheres to the:
① Free-radical theory of aging
② Collagen-fiber theory of aging
③ Immunologic-response theory of aging
④ Lipofuscin-accumulation theory of aging

79. A patient presents to the emergency department with acute myocardial infarction. A family member states that the patient has been depressed since his retirement 3 months ago. Which of the following may have been a contributing factor to the patient's current health status?
① An inability to "let go" of work problems
② Excitement caused by the prospect of retirement

③ Excess stimulation from new friends and activities
④ Stress over the loss of income and change in daily routine

80. The primary focus in the care of the older adult lies in:
① Prevention of acute illness
② Prevention of chronic illness
③ Health maintenance of acute illnesses
④ Symptom management of chronic illnesses

81. A 76-year-old patient is being discharged 2 days after a cholecystectomy. A family member inquires why he is being discharged so soon after surgery. Which of the following responses by the nurse accurately defines the trend in today's managed healthcare system?
① "Why don't you ask the physician to keep him longer?"
② "Because of insurance we can't keep patients too long after simple surgery."
③ "Home health agencies need the elderly to return home so they can be taken care of at home."
④ "Patients are given a certain period of time to recuperate in the hospital, but most recovery is done at home."

82. An 81-year-old patient presents to the physician's office with a fractured right ankle. A family member states that the individual fell down the stairs. Which of the following additional assessments most strongly suggests elder abuse?
① Anorexia and ill-fitting dentures
② Chronic cough and shortness of breath
③ Confusion and abrasions in various stages of healing
④ Fatigue and extreme pain upon palpation of the right ankle

83. A 69-year-old patient is admitted with an accidental drug overdose. The patient states that she is unable to read how many pills to take because the print on the bottle is too small. The nurse should:
① Call for a psychiatric consult
② Call the patient's pharmacist to request large-print bottles
③ Advise the family that they need to fill pill boxes for the patient
④ Consult a home health nurse to go to the patient's home to give medications

84. An older adult is admitted to the hospital with acute alcohol intoxication. The family member states "He used to be able to drink a few beers a day without any problems." Which of the following is the nurse's best response?
① "Would you like to talk to one of our counselors?"
② "It is time he stopped drinking now that he is older."
③ "He should know that he can't drink like he used to."
④ "Older adults can't metabolize alcohol like young people do."

85. A 77-year-old individual is brought to the emergency department after being found lying in the street by a neighbor who states that his apartment is filthy and there is no food in the cupboards or refrigerator. The patient appears to be intoxicated. Which of the following questions should the nurse ask during her data collection?
① "Do you drink too much?"
② "Do you eat three meals a day?"
③ "How much alcohol did you drink today?"
④ "Do you have any family members living near you?"

86. Individuals who would benefit the least from reality orientation programs are those who are:
    ① In the early stages of Alzheimer's disease
    ② Suffering from medication-induced delirium
    ③ Experiencing confusion related to hospitalization
    ④ In the latter stages of dementia from Parkinson's disease

87. The physician explains to the family of a patient with newly diagnosed Alzheimer's disease that he is to begin taking the drug Cognex as part of his medication regime. Which of the following statements made by the son would indicate understanding of the purpose of the drug?
    ① "He should be cured in about 3 months."
    ② "The progression of Alzheimer's should slow down."
    ③ "The drug should be stopped if we don't see any improvement."
    ④ "I should start to see improvement in my dad's memory in 3 to 4 weeks."

88. Which of the following is a reason that adverse drug reactions occur in the older adult?
    ① Older adults excrete drugs more effectively
    ② Older adults have a higher percentage of muscle tissue
    ③ Older adults have altered drug distribution due to circulatory changes
    ④ Increased gastric motility causes changes in the absorption of drugs

89. Which of the following would be an appropriate nursing intervention when giving an older adult oral medications?
    ① Elevate head of bed 15 degrees
    ② Give fluids before and after medications
    ③ Give all medications at one time to enhance absorption
    ④ Crush the medications and mix them with the patient's food

90. Which of the following eye conditions is the most common reason for blindness in the older adult?
    ① Glaucoma
    ② Cataracts
    ③ Presbyopia
    ④ Macular degeneration

91. A caretaker for an older adult expresses concern that the person frequently goes to the bathroom at night without contacting her. The nurse advises the caretaker that she should:
    ① Buy siderails for his bed
    ② Give him a sedative at night
    ③ Provide a clear path to the bathroom
    ④ Restrain her if she gets up more than once

92. An older patient asks the nurse if the new drug, Viagra, would be something that would help him resume sexual relations with his wife. The most correct response by the nurse would be:
    ① "Viagra allows for a more intimate sexual experience."
    ② "It is best that you put that part of your life behind you."
    ③ "Viagra assists some individuals in achieving an erection."
    ④ "Viagra helps some people become more sexually excited."

93. A nursing assistant asks the nurse why some older residents fail to fill in all the responses to a multiple-choice survey concerning nutrition. The nurse responds that older adults:
    ① Have brain atrophy that affects intelligence

② Do not care about surveys concerning nutrition
③ May be afraid to take the risk of answering "wrong"
④ Probably were unable to see the small circles on the paper

94. An agitated, delusional resident is receiving haloperidol (Haldol) due to extreme acting out behavior. The nurse is concerned because of this drug's side effects. The nurse asks the nursing assistants to alert her if the patient exhibits:
    ① Increased urine output
    ② Jaundice and lethargy
    ③ Confusion and dizziness
    ④ Headache and swollen glands

95. A 92-year-old woman confides in the nurse that she finds another resident attractive. Which of the following is the nurse's best response?
    ① "Aren't you a little old for that?"
    ② "Do you want me to introduce you?"
    ③ "We don't encourage that type of relations here."
    ④ "Maybe we should go to the activities room now."

96. The nurse is instructing a nursing assistant to put in a patient's hearing aid. The nurse instructs the assistant to turn the hearing aid on:
    ① Before placing it in the ear
    ② While inserting it in the ear canal
    ③ Only after the aid is in the ear canal
    ④ When the person decides to turn it on

97. A family member complains that his father, who has a hearing aid, no longer seems able to hear him speak. Which of the following is the best suggestion by the nurse?
    ① "Let's check the batteries on that aid."
    ② "I'll have his physician come in and check him out."
    ③ "Maybe he is just tired and doesn't want to listen now."
    ④ "Let's make him an appointment at the hearing aid clinic."

98. A 78-year-old man is returning home with his daughter. The daughter is concerned that her home is not safe for her father. Which of the following may indicate a possible safety hazard?
    ① Electric stoves
    ② Hardwood floors
    ③ Non-glare lighting
    ④ Elevated toilet seats

99. The nurse is evaluating the best possible mobility aid for a patient with vertigo. Which of the following mobility aids would be the most stable for this patient?
    ① Cane
    ② Walker
    ③ Crutches
    ④ Wheelchair

100. A 79-year-old woman states that she needs respite care for her husband, who has dementia, while she undergoes a diagnostic procedure in an outpatient clinic. To which of the following types of facilities should the nurse refer the couple?
    ① Nursing home
    ② Personal care home
    ③ Local area agency on aging
    ④ Social Security administration

ANSWERS AND RATIONALES

1. Comprehension, assessment, basic care and comfort (b)
   ❹ Pain and limited motion occur as the disease progresses; extent of the knee flexion and extension is essential baseline data to provide a clear understanding of the patient's health status.
   ① Sleep habits are important, but not considered a priority.
   ② Postoperatively, this information will be important; however, it is not a priority at this time.
   ③ The initial baseline data should focus on the disorder leading to the patient's admission.

2. Application, evaluation, basic care and comfort (b)
   ❹ When the patient swallows without choking and takes his time eating, he's safely able to meet dietary requirements.
   ① It is inappropriate to feed a patient who has difficulty swallowing any type of solid food.
   ② Thin liquids are very difficult to swallow for individuals who have dysphagia.
   ③ It may take much longer for this patient to eat, because special precautions must be taken.

3. Application, planning, safety and infection control (b)
   ❹ Continuous passive motion device is used postoperatively to facilitate joint range of motion. Equipment to be used postoperatively should be introduced, demonstrated, and made familiar to the patient preoperatively.
   ① Not appropriate; Russel traction is used for tibia fractures.
   ② Not appropriate; a cast brace enhances fracture healing.
   ③ Not appropriate; skin traction is used for hip injuries before surgery.

4. Application, implementation, physiological adaptation (b)
   ❷ This is routine postop total knee replacement care to control edema and bleeding.
   ① Abduction is used postop for total hip replacement to prevent hip flexion.
   ③ Wedge pillows are used to abduct the leg postoperatively for total hip replacements.
   ④ This is not appropriate for a total knee replacement.

5. Application, assessment, physiological adaptation (b)
   ❶ The cold will cause vasoconstriction, which will control bleeding and edema.
   ② Cold will not reduce the incidence of infection.
   ③ CPM machines will increase circulation and movement.
   ④ Drains should reduce fluid accumulation.

6. Comprehension, planning, reduction of risk potential (b)
   ❹ Weight bearing limits are always determined by the physician and depend on the surgical technique used, the patient's postoperative condition, and type of prosthesis.
   ① Full weight bearing is not normally ordered; this is determined by the physician.
   ② Physicians do not normally order this, but once again, it must be ordered by the physician.
   ③ Patient tolerance is important, but progress must be made in physical therapy, which the physician will order.

7. Comprehension, evaluation, prevention and early detection of disease (b)
   ❸ Bran cereal has a higher fiber content than any of the other sources.
   ① Cucumbers have a low fiber content.
   ② Apple juice contains low fiber content.
   ④ Bananas contain some fiber, but not as much as the bran cereal.

8. Application, planning, basic care and comfort (b)
   ❹ Sleeping with the head of the bed elevated prevents the hernia from shifting with gravity, causing reflux.
   ① Frequent small meals are indicated to reduce symptoms.
   ② High-protein and fatty foods are more difficult to digest and more irritating.
   ③ Patients should sit up for at least 1 hour after eating to prevent gastric reflux.

9. Knowledge, assessment, basic care and comfort (b)
   ❶ Alzheimer's disease is diagnosed by exclusion and confirmed only by autopsy.
   ② CT may support or refute a diagnosis, but it can't confirm.
   ③ PET cannot confirm a positive diagnosis.
   ④ These are used to track progression of cognitive disorders, but they are not diagnostic.

10. Application, implementation, safety and infection control (b)
    ❷ The nurse uses the short-term memory loss to her advantage; this produces little anxiety in the resident.
    ① Accompanying the resident may be appropriate if diversion does not work.
    ③ Show of force will only further agitate the resident.
    ④ Agitation will increase if the resident is confronted.

11. Application, implementation, psychosocial adaptation (c)
    ❷ Agitation is best reduced by an active diversion such as walking.
    ① Although this choice appears calming, it will not calm an agitated patient.
    ③ Listening to music is a passive exercise that will not reduce agitation.
    ④ This passive activity will not reduce restlessness or agitation.

12. Application, planning, psychosocial adaptation (b)
    ❷ Hoeing is a repetitive action that does not require decision-making or planning.
    ① Sorting laundry has some measure of decision making.
    ③ Too much planning is involved in this activity.
    ④ The patient will become frustrated because of inability to plan the grocery list

13. Comprehension, planning, psychosocial adaptation (b)
    ❸ Agitated and hostile individuals should remain in as nonstimulating, calm an environment as possible in order to defuse aggressiveness.
    ① Memory aids will serve to preserve the patient's memory, but this does not address the hostility issue.
    ② This also helps the patient's memory, but it does not decrease hostile tendencies.
    ④ This will preserve the patient's safety.

14. Knowledge, assessment, prevention and early detection of disease (b)
    ❷ Drug toxicity is the only reversible cause of dementia listed.
    ① Pick's disease is a progressive neurological disease that is not reversible.
    ③ Parkinson's disease is progressive and results in dementia, and it is not reversible.
    ④ The effects of alcoholism may be reversed, but not quite as easily as the effects of drug toxicity.

15. Application, implementation, psychosocial adaptation (b)
    ❸ Pictures reduce environmental confusion and are good memory aids for the cognitively impaired.
    ① This promotes dependence and is unrealistic.
    ② This sign may confuse the patient, who may no longer be able to read.
    ④ This response is demeaning and threatening.

16. Application, implementation, basic care and comfort (b)
    ❹ This is the best choice for the resident who does not sit at mealtime; it ensures proper nutritional intake.
    ① Restraints should be used for resident safety only.
    ② Normally, this would be a good choice; however, the resident does not sit at the table.
    ③ This is inappropriate, as it promotes dependence.

17. Application, planning, psychosocial adaptation (b)
    ❷ By using short sentences and speaking clearly, short-term memory is maximized.
    ① This is too much information for the resident to remember.
    ③ This does not support the resident's cognitive function.
    ④ This is too much information given to him at one time.

18. Comprehension, planning, psychosocial adaptation (b)
    ❸ Physically restraining a resident will increase the agitation level of the resident.
    ① The chair itself does not cause decubitus ulcers.
    ② If the resident is toileted by the staff, the chair itself should not foster incontinence.
    ④ This is a sweeping statement that does not demonstrate knowledge of agitated patients.

19. Application, assessment, coordinated care (b)
    ❹ This is the only appropriate response that does not humiliate the resident.
    ① This is too familiar and fails to demonstrate respect.
    ② This response conveys failure if the resident does not remember.
    ③ This does not convey respect or compassion.

20. Application, implementation, psychosocial adaptation (b)
    ❹ This is the only response that conveys dignity and respect for the resident.
    ① This response is humiliating and degrading.
    ② This response demeans the resident.
    ③ Chastising the resident demeans the resident's dignity.

21. Application, implementation, pharmacological therapies (b)
    ❷ This is the only response that answers the patient's question.
    ① This does not acknowledge the patient's question.

③ This response does not answer the patient's question.
④ This is demeaning to the patient.

22. Application, assessment, pharmacological therapies (b)
    ❸ These are toxic effects of Sinemet.
    ①, ② These are symptoms of Parkinson's disease.
    ④ Patients with Parkinson's disease have these changes.

23. Comprehension, implementation, pharmacological therapies (b)
    ❸ This is an accurate response and may allay the patient's concerns.
    ① This is a very threatening statement.
    ② This is not conveying the appropriate information.
    ④ This response does not assist the patient's needs.

24. Application, implementation, pharmacological therapies (b)
    ❷ Administering the drug before meals with enhance absorption and decrease GI irritation.
    ① This will diminish absorption of the drug.
    ③ This is inappropriate; medications should not be mixed with the patient's food.
    ④ There is no indication that this may be necessary; the physician determines this.

25. Comprehension, evaluation, psychosocial adaptation (b)
    ❹ This is the only remark that describes Parkinson's disease.
    ① This describes Huntington's disease.
    ② This describes Creutzfeldt-Jakob disease.
    ③ This describes Huntington's disease.

26. Application, implementation, pharmacological therapies (b)
    ❸ It is not imperative that the individual take the qd medication at exactly 9 AM. She may have mood swings, and may take the medication at a later time.
    ① This may eventually be the correct course of action, but the patient should be offered the medication first.
    ② It is appropriate to do this eventually, but not until the resident has been offered the medication.
    ④ This would be the last course of action and would be done only after repeatedly trying to get the resident to take the oral form.

27. Application, assessment, psychosocial adaptation (b)
    ❶ Hallucinations are not usually characteristic of paranoid behavior in the elderly.
    ② This is an expected characteristic of paranoid behavior.
    ③ Oversensitivity is also a characteristic of paranoia.
    ④ Many paranoid individuals refuse meals and treatments.

28. Application, implementation, basic care and comfort (b)
    ❸ Refusal is not uncommon as the patient is in new and unfamiliar surroundings; he may wish to try the tray later.
    ① This assumes that the patient doesn't like the food, which may not be the case.
    ② The nurse does not know whether the patient likes the food or not.
    ④ This is inappropriate; the nurse should allow sufficient time for the patient to consume the breakfast.

29. Comprehension, evaluation, coping and adaptation (c)
    ❹ These actions are characteristic of paranoia.

① This is judgmental and does not correctly describe the behavior.

② The resident is not displaying hallucinations.

③ Although this may be the outcome of her actions, the resident is displaying paranoid behavior.

30. Application, planning, physiological adaptation (c)
   ❷ This allows the patient to function independently in an area where she can be successful.
   ① This activity would be frustrating because the resident would have difficulty due to her deformities.
   ③ The resident may not be successful in these activities.
   ④ This would cause frustration and failure due to limitations.

31. Comprehension, assessment, growth and development through the life span (b)
   ❹ The patient most likely feels secure, and moving at this time would contribute further to his losses.
   ① The patient may not be afraid to move, but wishes to lessen his losses.
   ② These actions do not indicate paranoid behavior.
   ③ This situation does not indicate eccentric behavior.

32. Application, implementation, coordinated care (b)
   ❷ Informing the family of his concern should be sufficient to activate an appropriate plan of action in this case.
   ① This would establish an inappropriate nurse-patient relationship.
   ③ This is an inappropriate response because it ignores his concern.
   ④ This is an inappropriate response because it suggests he should experience another loss.

33. Comprehension, assessment, basic care and comfort (b)
   ❷ Not enough information is given to arrive at a diagnosis.
   ① This may be the cause; however, further evaluation is necessary.
   ③ There is no indication that this may be the cause of the episode.
   ④ Further testing is required before this diagnosis can be made.

34. Comprehension, planning, basic care and comfort (b)
   ❹ Frequent small meals are easier to digest and not as overwhelming to the patient.
   ① There is no indication for blenderized foods.
   ② There is no reason to believe that warm liquids would increase his appetite.
   ③ Rolls would most likely not stimulate his appetite.

35. Comprehension, assessment, coping and adaptation (b)
   ❷ This situation is presented as an impairment in orientation to time, place, and person.
   ① Manifestation of a physiological problem and may be present; however, the patient is specifically having difficulty with time orientation.
   ③ Although memory deficit may be present, the situation describes time disorientation.
   ④ There is no evidence that impaired judgment is present.

36. Comprehension, assessment, basic care and comfort (b)
   ❶ An absence of sufficient water and fiber in the diet are common causes of constipation.

② Lack of daily exercise may contribute to the problem of constipation, but poor eating habits are more problematic.

③ Too much fiber in the diet does not cause constipation.

④ Some medications may cause constipation, but not all older adults are on these drugs, and there is no indication that this resident takes these drugs.

37. Comprehension, assessment, coping and adaptation (c)
   ❶ Hoarding is a manifestation of insecurity.
   ② The situation does not present any indication of confusion.
   ③ Decreased self-esteem is not related to hoarding behaviors.
   ④ The resident does not appear to be exhibiting problems with disorientation.

38. Comprehension, planning, growth and development through the life span (b)
   ❹ This is a normal aging change.
   ① This would not be compatible with the rest needs of the patient.
   ② A more thorough assessment is needed before medication is given.
   ③ The quality and continuity of sleep patterns change.

39. Application, assessment, pharmacological therapies (c)
   ❹ Broccoli and turnip greens are high in vitamin K.
   ① These are not vitamin K rich foods.
   ② These are important to the diet and not high in vitamin K.
   ③ This is not an especially rich source of vitamin K.

40. Comprehension, assessment, basic care and comfort (c)
   ❶ Loss of fat tissue on the soles of the feet, coupled with the trauma of walking, places the patient at risk for foot problems.
   ② With the decrease in muscle mass, tendons shrink and sclerose.
   ③ Changes in the kidney predispose the patient to nocturia.
   ④ Respiratory system changes alter the body's ability to handle foreign particles and secretions, which increases susceptibility to infection.

41. Application, planning, safety and infection control (b)
   ❶ Because of the yellowing of the lens of the eye, the elderly can see reds, oranges, and yellows best.
   ② This is a lower color tone, which is not seen well by the elderly.
   ③ Blue is difficult for the elderly to differentiate.
   ④ Green is difficult for the elderly to distinguish from other colors.

42. Comprehension, evaluation, psychosocial adaptation (b)
   ❸ Difficulty managing personal finances indicates impaired cognition. Because of poor judgment, the patient may make unwise financial decisions and have difficulty with bill paying and checkbook balancing.
   ① Although the patient may have a decreased ability to do this, it does not demonstrate a cognitive function; it is most likely due to deficits in the sensory and motor system.
   ② Resistance to care is an abnormal behavior pattern, not a cognitive deficit.
   ④ This is a visual-spatial impairment.

43. Comprehension, assessment, psychosocial adaptation (b)
❷ In early Alzheimer's disease, short-term memory, which spans a few minutes or hours, is impaired.
① This is long-term memory, which is usually preserved in early Alzheimer's disease.
③ This is benign forgetfulness, which is usually limited to trivial matters, and tends to occur in all individuals at some time in their lives.
④ This is an example of immediate memory, which is not impaired in early Alzheimer's disease.

44. Application, planning, physiological adaptation (c)
❹ A properly applied Ace wrap will reduce edema and shape the limb in preparation for prosthesis application.
① The stump is elevated for the first 24 hours postoperatively; after that it is not elevated to prevent hip flexion contractures.
② A diuretic is not indicated in this situation.
③ This will not decrease the amount of edema in the stump; it will create further edema.

45. Comprehension, implementation, coordinated care (b)
❹ Older adults generally exhibit short-term memory loss. The ability to remember details from 30 years ago is not unusual.
① This statement is too sweeping to apply to the entire elder population.
② It has not been established that the patient has a cognitive disorder.
③ Usually long-term memory is preserved in older adults.

46. Comprehension, assessment, growth and development through the life span (b)
❸ Changes in the respiratory system can cause decreased tolerance in activity, dyspnea, and fatigue.
① These changes cause a higher-pitched, frailer voice; dyspnea is a common complaint.
② The voice is not stronger or more resonant.
④ Aging changes do cause a decrease in activity tolerance, but do not cause orthopnea.

47. Comprehension, assessment, growth and development through the life span (b)
❹ As individuals age, the action of the sweat and oil glands become less active, so daily bathing is not required.
① Body odor may not diminish, although perspiration does.
② This may not be true of all older adults.
③ This is not a true statement.

48. Comprehension, assessment, prevention and early detection of disease (b)
❹ These foods will increase the amount of bulk and fiber in the diet.
① Although fruit juices do contain some fiber, the dairy products will constipate the individual.
② Meat, cheese, and poultry products will not increase fiber in the diet.
③ Processed carbohydrates and milk products will not combat constipation.

49. Comprehension, evaluation, safety and infection control (b)
❷ Individuals with presbyopia have difficulty with near vision; activities that require near vision such as needlepoint and knitting will be the most difficult for them to complete.

① These activities should not be difficult for individuals with presbyopia.
③ Bingo and shopping require very little near vision and should not pose a problem.
④ Driving requires far vision, and viewing road signs should not be a problem.

50. Comprehension, assessment, psychosocial adaptation (c)
❷ Applying makeup and wearing appealing clothing may increase the patient's self-worth.
① This suggestion, as it is presented, does not appear to demean the individual.
③ There is no indication that the patient has not bathed.
④ As presented, the situation does not involve a patient who is unaware of her surroundings.

51. Comprehension, implementation, basic care and comfort (c)
❸ By inquiring about normal condiment use at home, the nurse will be better able to make suggestions to the older adult patient.
① The individual may already know the complications, and this response does not address the patient's difficulty.
② This is not indicated at this time.
④ This is untrue and it does not address the patient's problem.

52. Knowledge, assessment, growth and development through the life span (b)
❸ The changes in this portion of the brain diminish the ability of older adults to produce a fever in response to an inflammatory agent.
① Aging changes normally increase the older adult's pain threshold.
② Cardiovascular aging changes do not increase erythema.
④ Older adults generally have normal to subnormal temperature readings.

53. Comprehension, planning, growth and development through the life span (b)
❹ Older adults are very susceptible to background noise, and the nurse may have to turn off appliances, shut doors, and eliminate other noise in order for teaching to be done.
① There is no loss of intelligence with normal aging.
② Older adults do not learn more quickly than others, and reaction time is slower.
③ Older adults respond well to verbal instruction combined with demonstrations.

54. Comprehension, evaluation, psychosocial adaptation (b)
❹ Alzheimer's disease is a progressive, neurological disorder of the brain and is not reversible.
① Onset of Alzheimer's disease is insidious and can be diagnosed as depression.
② There is no known cure for Alzheimer's disease.
③ Onset is usually after age 60.

55. Application, planning, psychosocial adaptation (b)
❹ If the patient tries to leave the unit, a nurse may see the patient if the patient must pass the nurse's station in order to leave.
① This provides too much opportunity for elopement and would be too noisy.
② The nurse's station would be too stimulating to patients with dementia.

③ This would provide too much stimulation for the patient.

56. Application, implementation, psychosocial adaptation (b)
  ❸ This will be the best way to get the patient's attention.
  ① Speaking too quickly will confuse the patient.
  ② Talking loudly may agitate the individual.
  ④ Watching the TV would provide too much distraction.

57. Application, implementation, coping and adaptation (b)
  ❸ Since the patient has no known organic disease, she may be confused and would most likely re-orient well to the situation.
  ① This may not be true and gives false reassurance.
  ② There is no indication that this patient will not re-orient to time, place, and person.
  ④ This may not be true, and will give false reassurance to the patient.

58. Knowledge, planning, psychosocial adaptation (b)
  ❷ Reality orientation programs reinforce time, place, and person on a continuous, 24-hour basis.
  ① There is no one definition of "normal behavior." Behavior modification programs attempt to sculpt behavior.
  ③ Reality orientation programs emphasize a continuous reinforcement of time, place, and person.
  ④ Although important, reality orientation programs do not directly emphasize interest in the environment.

59. Comprehension, planning, psychosocial adaptation (b)
  ❹ Surrounding the patient with familiar objects will increase a feeling of recognition in the new facility.
  ① Bringing along familiar objects will not increase the attention span of the individual.
  ② Although the familiar objects will be calming, they will not decrease dementia behaviors.
  ③ The objects would most likely facilitate long-term memory, if they facilitate memory at all.

60. Application, implementation, basic care and comfort (c)
  ❹ This is the proper sequence to administer medications through a small-bore feeding tube.
  ① The tube should be flushed with a small amount of water (unless specified by physician) before and after the medication.
  ② Checking residual after giving the med will result in withdrawing some of the medication from the tube; the nurse will not get a true residual amount.
  ③ Residual amounts should be checked before flushing with water.

61. Comprehension, implementation, coordinated care (b)
  ❸ It is best to communicate information verbally, in person, during a short meeting.
  ① This is impersonal; instructions need to be given verbally.
  ② This is also impersonal and does not signify effective communication techniques.
  ④ The information will be more effective if given by the charge nurse for those nurse's aides.

62. Application, planning, coordinated care (b)
  ❸ Monitoring vital signs is within the nursing assistant's scope of practice.
  ① Documentation should be done by the individual who cared for the residents, presumably the nurse.

② Administering medications is not within the scope of the nursing assistant.
  ④ The nurse should provide the input concerning the resident's care.

63. Application, assessment, growth and development through the life span (b)
  ❶ Older adults have both good and bad days and should be assessed on more than one occasion to gather the most correct data.
  ② The best setting for a functional assessment is in the patient's own environment.
  ③ Older adults have difficulty relating any problems with activities of daily living.
  ④ Any assistive aids that are used on a day-to-day basis should be included in the functional assessment.

64. Application, assessment, basic care and comfort (b)
  ❷ The best way to assess for this patient problem is to actually watch the patient perform the activity.
  ① Although helpful, this will not provide as much information as watching the patient perform the activity.
  ③ This is an assessment that the nurse is capable of making.
  ④ This is descriptive, but it still does not provide as much information as watching him perform the task.

65. Knowledge, evaluation, coordinated care (b)
  ❶ This is the only choice where skilled nursing care is performed.
  ② Adult day care provides a structured environment for individuals for less than a 24-hour basis.
  ③ Personal care homes assist residents in the activities of daily living and basic care.
  ④ Senior citizen centers provide recreational programs for seniors.

66. Application, implementation, coordinated care (c)
  ❸ The patient's restless behavior is cause for concern, and the nurse should assess the patient before any intervention is done.
  ① The patient needs assessment before this is done, if needed.
  ② The nursing assistant should not restrain the patient before an assessment is done.
  ④ This may be required after the assessment, but the patient should be assessed first.

67. Application, implementation, safety and infection control (b)
  ❹ This is priority emergency care; the patient must have an intact airway before any other assessment can begin.
  ① This may cause injury prior to assessment.
  ②, ③ This is done after the patient's airway is secured.

68. Application, planning, reduction of risk potential (c)
  ❸ Any restless and confused behavior necessitates a cardiac and respiratory assessment; the patient may be hypoxic.
  ① The patient is not complaining of pain; a thorough assessment must be made before any intervention can be done.
  ② The spouse may provide valuable information about her husband's former cognitive status; however, the nurse needs to perform an assessment.
  ④ This may be appropriate if an emergency problem is found with the patient, but the nurse should first assess the patient.

69. Comprehension, implementation, coordinated care (b)
    ❹ The patient appoints an individual to make medical decisions for the patient should the patient become incapacitated.
    ① The healthcare proxy makes medical decisions for the patient.
    ② The patient usually chooses the individual; if the state makes the decision, a family member may or may not be chosen.
    ③ This more accurately describes a living will.

70. Comprehension, assessment, coordinated care (b)
    ❶ The Patient Self-Determination Act stipulates that information concerning advance directives be given to patients upon their admission to the hospital.
    ② It would be too late to give patients information during this time.
    ③ The information should be given when the patient is admitted into an acute care facility.
    ④ This is not always a comfortable issue, and patients may postpone the issue.

71. Comprehension, planning, coordinated care (b)
    ❸ Advance directives include living wills and healthcare proxy (durable power of attorney).
    ① Guardianship is established by the courts.
    ② Organ donation is not included under advance directives.
    ④ Active euthanasia is currently illegal in the United States, and passive euthanasia includes "do not resuscitate" (DNR) orders.

72. Application, planning, coordinated care (b)
    ❹ This is a true statement.
    ① Medicare covers only some of the expenses, such as those that would necessitate highly skilled care.
    ② Medicare generally covers very skilled nursing services, some of which do not last 1 or 2 years.
    ③ Social security payments will assist in paying for long-term care, but medicaid pays for most of the care.

73. Knowledge, assessment, growth and development through the life span (b)
    ❷ Older adults spend the latter part of their life dealing with the issues of ego integrity and despair. If the elderly patient reflects on his life and is pleased with the events, ego remains intact. If the patient is not happy with his life, then he will despair because it can't be changed.
    ① This is the task stage for early adulthood.
    ③ Adults (middle age) manage the tasks of generativity and stagnation.
    ④ Adolescents deal with the tasks of identity and role confusion.

74. Comprehension, implementation, prevention and early detection of disease (b)
    ❸ Chinese Americans are most likely to access alternative or traditional therapies before contacting the modern medical establishment.
    ① African-Americans utilize community and family resources readily and are likely to access healthcare in a short period of time.
    ② Jewish Americans are likely to readily access modern healthcare.
    ④ Hispanic Americans tend to access healthcare after consulting community and family relations.

75. Knowledge, planning, growth and development through the life span (b)
    ❹ The Hispanic culture values assisting the elderly at home; families are expected to care for the ill or elderly.
    ① Caucasians have the highest rate of nursing home utilization.
    ② Asian Americans have a low rate of nursing home utilization.
    ③ Jewish Americans tend to readily utilize long-term care.

76. Knowledge, assessment, coordinated care (b)
    ❸ Social Security provides the majority of the retired older adult's income.
    ① Medicare is a program that provides health coverage for the elderly.
    ② Medicaid is a program that provides health coverage for low-income individuals.
    ④ Tax-sheltered annuities may provide some of the older adult's income.

77. Comprehension, implementation, safety and infection control (b)
    ❹ OBRA heavily regulated the use of restraints in long-term care and passed regulations to safeguard the care of nursing home residents.
    ① The Administration on Aging provides nutritional programs, senior citizen centers, and home care services for the elderly.
    ② Provides federal monies for social programs for the elderly.
    ③ This Act ensures patients have information regarding decision-making for end-of-life care.

78. Comprehension, assessment, prevention and early detection of disease (b)
    ❶ The free-radical theory of aging postulates that free molecules eventually damage cells. The intake of vitamins A, C, and E (antioxidants) can decrease the damage done to the cells.
    ② This theory states that the structure of the collagen fibers in the body causes aging to begin.
    ③ This states that the body does not recognize changed cells and attacks them as foreign particles, initiating the aging process.
    ④ Lipofuscin are age pigments that accumulate in the cell, which may initiate the aging process.

79. Comprehension, assessment, growth and development through the life span (b)
    ❹ Stress over the loss of work-related role may have contributed to the patient's current health problem.
    ① There is no indication from the family or patient that this is the problem because the patient is retired.
    ② The patient may be excited to retire; however, the family member states that the patient has been depressed.
    ③ It is unlikely that the patient has met new friends or been involved in activities since he has been depressed.

80. Knowledge, implementation, prevention and early detection of disease (b)
    ❹ The focus of care for the majority of the older adult population encompasses the management of the symptoms of chronic illness.

① Although prevention is important, older adults have many chronic illnesses that must be managed.

② Prevention is always important; however, the elderly have many chronic illnesses that need symptom management.

③ Health maintenance is not usually associated with acute illnesses.

81. Application, implementation, coordinated care (b)
❹ This response correctly summarizes the trend of managed care within the healthcare system.
① This does not answer the family member's question.
② A cholecystectomy may not be simple for an older adult, and this statement does not correctly define diagnostic-related groups.
③ Although home health care providers visit individuals after discharge (if needed), this is not the major reason for short hospital stays.

82. Application, assessment, safety and infection control (b)
❸ These assessment data most strongly indicates that elder abuse may be a problem. The confusion could be due to excessive stress, and individuals who have had repeated abuse may have wounds in various stages of healing.
① These assessment data indicate changes in the patient's gastrointestinal system and could signify weight loss.
② Chronic cough and shortness of breath are symptoms associated with aging changes in the respiratory system.
④ Fatigue could be due to a variety of factors; pain on movement and palpation of the ankle is to be expected with a fracture.

83. Application, planning, safety and infection control (c)
❷ This is the best response because it solves the patient's problem while preserving independence.
① This may not be necessary, since the overdose has already been determined to be accidental.
③ This may alleviate the patient's problem; however, it does cause dependency.
④ This is an unnecessary expense and promotes dependency.

84. Application, implementation, coping and adaptation (b)
❹ This response correctly explains the role that aging has on the metabolism of alcohol.
① This does not address the family member's question.
② This is judgmental and does not answer the question.
③ This response is judgmental and threatening to the patient and family member.

85. Application, assessment, coping and adaptation (b)
❸ This is the only question that does not ask for a yes/no answer. By asking how much alcohol the patient drank that day, the nurse is more likely to get an accurate response.
① This is judgmental and is a yes/no question.
② This is important to know, but it is a yes/no question.
④ This may be relevant, but it closes communication because it is a yes/no question.

86. Knowledge, planning, psychosocial adaptation (b)
❹ Individuals in the latter stages of dementia do not orient well to reality and would not benefit from such programs.

① Individuals in the early stages of dementia orient well to the environment.
② This is a reversible condition, and individuals normally orient well to the environment; however, reality orientation programs may not be available in a hospital setting.
③ Confused patients reorient well to reality.

87. Application, implementation, pharmacological therapies (b)
❷ Cognex is a drug given to patients in early Alzheimer's disease to slow the progression of the disease.
① There is no cure for Alzheimer's disease.
③ There may be no visible improvement.
④ There will not be a noticeable improvement; the progression of the disease slow.

88. Knowledge, evaluation, growth and development through the life span (b)
❸ Circulatory changes cause drug distribution in older adults to be altered, increasing the chances for adverse drug reactions.
① Older adults do not excrete drugs more effectively.
② This is not a true statement; some muscle wasting occurs.
④ Absorption is altered, but it is due to decreased gastric motility.

89. Application, implementation, reduction of risk potential (b)
❷ This allows the older adult, who may have dry mucous membranes, to better swallow the medications.
① The head of bed should be at 60-90 degrees.
③ Medications given in this manner may not be compatible and may be overwhelming.
④ Medications should never be mixed with the patient's food.

90. Knowledge, assessment, prevention and early detection of disease (b)
❷ Cataracts, which are easily removed, cause more blindness than any other disorder.
① Glaucoma can cause blindness if not treated.
③ Presbyopia is the result of the normal changes of aging.
④ Macular degeneration causes blindness; however, more individuals suffer from cataracts.

91. Application, implementation, safety and infection control (b)
❸ This limits the chance for the patient to fall trying to get to the bathroom.
① This promotes dependence and incontinence.
② If the patient does not request a sedative, it should not be given for this reason.
④ A patient should not be restrained; this is inappropriate and fosters dependence.

92. Comprehension, implementation, pharmacological therapies (b)
❸ This is the most correct statement. Viagra is used to treat erectile dysfunction.
① This may not be true; Viagra does not promote a more intimate experience.
② This is judgmental; the individual obviously wishes to resume sex with his wife.
④ This is not a true statement.

93. Application, implementation, growth and development through the life span (b)
- ❸ Older adults do not take risks and will not fill in answers to multiple choice tests if they think they will get them "wrong."
- ① The slight brain shrinkage that older adults experience does not result in loss of intelligence.
- ② The nurse cannot generalize all older adults do not care about nutrition.
- ④ This assumes that all older adults have a profound loss of vision.

94. Application, planning, pharmacological therapies (b)
- ❷ Because Haldol is metabolized by the liver, jaundice may develop. The antipsychotic nature may cause excessive lethargy.
- ① Haldol normally causes urinary retention as a side effect.
- ③ These are not normally considered as side effects.
- ④ These are not significant side effects for Haldol.

95. Application, implementation, psychosocial adaptation (b)
- ❷ This promotes acceptance of the person's need for companionship.
- ① This is inappropriate and demeaning to the patient.
- ③ This response blocks communication; the resident merely expressed her thoughts.
- ④ This does not address the resident's needs.

96. Comprehension, implementation, basic care and comfort (b)
- ❸ The hearing aid should be turned on only when it is in the ear canal to decrease unpleasant noise from the aid.
- ① This will result in squealing and pain as it is inserted.
- ② Air flow will cause a high-pitched squeal, which is annoying and painful to the patient.
- ④ The patient should be encouraged to turn the aid on when it is safely in the ear canal so that the nursing assistant can help adjust the volume.

97. Application, implementation, basic care and comfort (b)
- ❶ This is the simplest and easiest way to ascertain if the aid is functioning.
- ② This may be necessary if it is found that the aid is working and the patient is still unable to hear.
- ③ This is an inappropriate response; the nurse should investigate the family's concern.
- ④ This may be necessary after checking the aid out and contacting the physician.

98. Comprehension, evaluation, safety and infection control (b)
- ❷ Hardwood floors may pose a risk for slippage, especially if scatter rugs are used.
- ① An electric stove is safer than gas stoves.
- ③ Non-glare lighting assists the elderly in reading.
- ④ Elevated toilet seats may assist the elderly in transferring to and from the toilet.

99. Knowledge, planning, safety and infection control (b)
- ❷ A walker would provide a stable mobility aid while fostering as much independent movement as possible.
- ① A cane is not as stable as a walker.
- ③ Crutches are a very dangerous mobility aid for a patient with vertigo.
- ④ Although a wheelchair is very stable, this patient needs to have as much independent movement as possible.

100. Application, assessment, coordinated care (b)
- ❸ This agency would most likely have a respite care program.
- ① Nursing homes provide skilled nursing care.
- ② Personal care homes care for individuals who live in the facility.
- ④ This agency is concerned with providing monetary benefits to the elderly and others who qualify.

CHAPTER 10

Emergency Nursing

This chapter emphasizes the nursing assessments and interventions essential to preserving the lives of victims of acute illness or injury. Rapid clinical assessment emphasizing airway, breathing, and circulation, establishment of care priorities, and implementation of lifesaving measures should be instituted until emergency medical care is available. The most serious and life-threatening injuries should be treated first, and all first aid measures carried out before transporting the victim(s).

Concurrent with emergency management of physical needs is the practitioner's recognition and understanding of the victim's emotional state. The feelings of the victim's significant others should also be acknowledged and responded to as realistically, gently, and expeditiously as possible.

Nurses should be familiar with the extent of protection and legal limitations of practice under the Nurse Practice Act and Good Samaritan Act, which vary from state to state.

The high incidence of AIDS and hepatitis B necessitates that nurses should consider all patients to be potentially infected; to have access to equipment that minimizes the need for mouth-to-mouth, mouth-to-nose, and mouth-to-stoma resuscitation; and to implement universal infection control precautions.

Current cardiopulmonary resuscitation literature raises the issues of cardiac pump theory versus thoracic pump theory; the effectiveness of abdominal compressions; and whether synchronized or interposed abdominal and chest compressions are more effective than chest compressions. No new cardiopulmonary resuscitation guidelines specific to these issues have been released by the American Heart Association as of the printing of this text.

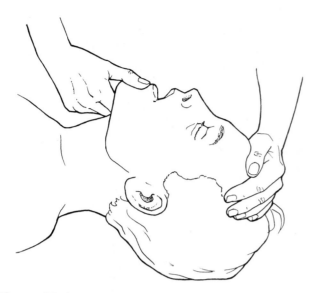

Figure 10-1   Head-tilt–jaw-thrust maneuver. Pull mandible forward using thumb and forefingers. (From Sheehy SB, Lenehan GP: *Manual of emergency nursing care,* ed 5, St Louis, 1999, Mosby.)

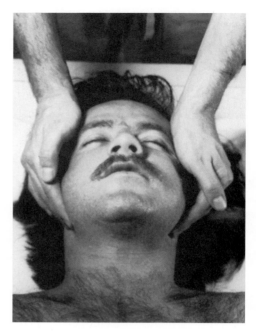

Figure 10-2   Jaw-thrust maneuver. (From Sheehy SB: *Emergency nursing: principles and practice,* ed 3, St Louis, 1992, Mosby. Photo by Richard Lazar.)

BASIC LIFE SUPPORT
Artificial Respiration

A. Simultaneously shake victim and shout to establish unconsciousness
B. Activate the EMS system (call 9-1-1) immediately when the victim is an adult; if an infant or child, call for help (even if you do not see anyone in the immediate vicinity), give 1 minute of CPR (20 cycles), check for pulse, and then activate EMS
C. Quickly place victim in supine position
D. Establish airway using the head-tilt–chin-lift maneuver or head-tilt–jaw-thrust maneuver (Fig. 10-1) if additional forward displacement of the jaw is required; for patients with possible neck or spine injuries, use only jaw-thrust maneuver (Fig. 10-2)
   1. Infant: maintain neck in neutral position
   2. Child: maintain neck slightly further back
E. Put your ear near victim's mouth and look, listen, and feel for breathing
F. Commence mouth-to-mouth, mouth-to-nose, or mouth-to-stoma resuscitation by delivering two breaths (1½ to 2 sec/breath) at the lowest possible pressure
G. Allow for victim's exhalation between breaths by removing your mouth; check the carotid pulse (brachial for infant) for 5 seconds
H. In the presence of a pulse, continue to deliver one breath every 5 seconds (12 breaths/min) for the adult and every 3 seconds (20 breaths/min) for the infant and for a child until breathing is restored (rescue breathing)

Cardiopulmonary Resuscitation

A. Follow steps A to G above; be sure victim is on a firm surface

B. In the absence of a pulse, place the heel of one hand on top of the other two finger-breadths above the victim's xiphoid process (Fig. 10-3)
   1. Child (1 to 8 years old): place heel of one hand two finger-breadths above the end of the sternum and deliver 100 compressions per minute
   2. Infant (less than 1 year old): place two fingers one finger-breadth below an imaginary line drawn between the nipples and deliver 100 compressions per minute
C. Compress the adult sternum 1½ to 2 inches for 15 compressions; then deliver two breaths
D. Compress the sternum of the child 1 to 1½ inches for 5 compressions; then deliver one breath
E. Compress the infant sternum ½ to 1 inch for 5 compressions; then deliver one breath
F. Continue the 15 compressions and two breaths sequence in the adult: 5 compressions and one breath sequence for infants and children
G. With two rescuers present for an adult deliver 5 compressions and one breath
H. Check the carotid pulse:
   1. After four cycles of 15:2 (1 minute) in the adult with one rescuer
   2. After 10 cycles of 5:1 (1 minute) in the adult with two rescuers
   3. After 20 cycles of 5:1 (1 minute) in the child
I. Check the brachial pulse after 20 cycles of 5:1 (1 minute) in the infant
J. If no pulse, resume CPR; if there is a pulse but no breathing, resume artificial respiration (rescue breathing)

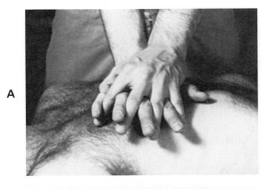

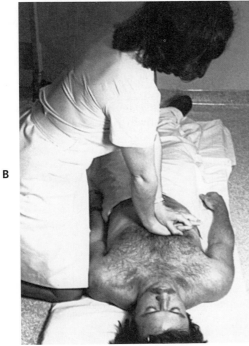

Figure 10-3 **A,** Hand position for chest compression: no weight on fingers. **B,** Body position for CPR. Rescuer should be kneeling, with knees slightly separated and elbows in straight, locked position. (From Sheehy SB: *Emergency nursing: principles and practice,* ed 3, St Louis, 1992, Mosby. Photos by Richard Lazar.)

Heimlich Maneuver

The Heimlich maneuver is used for management of foreign body airway obstruction (FBAO). Do not interfere if victim can cough, speak, or breathe
A. Conscious adult victim
1. Stand behind the victim, encircle his or her waist with your arms, place your fist above the umbilicus and below the xiphoid process with your thumb against victim's abdomen; grasp your fist with your other hand and apply pressure with an inward and quick upward motion (Fig. 10-4)
2. Repeat the thrusts until the obstruction is relieved, or switch to procedure for conscious victim who loses consciousness
B. Conscious adult victim who loses consciousness
1. Place victim in supine position, call for help, and activate Emergency Medical Service (EMS)

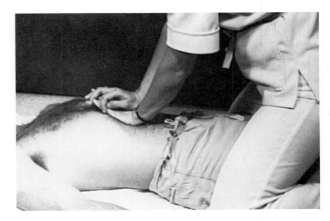

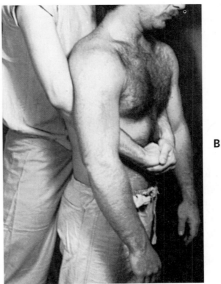

Figure 10-4 **A,** Heimlich maneuver, lying. **B,** Heimlich maneuver, standing. (From Sheehy SB: *Emergency nursing: principles and practice,* ed 3, St Louis, 1992, Mosby. Photos by Richard Lazar.)

2. Perform tongue-jaw lift and carefully sweep your curved finger in one direction along the back of the victim's throat to retrieve object
3. Establish airway using the head-tilt–chin-lift maneuver
4. Deliver two breaths
5. Kneel at level of victim's hips or straddle victim to deliver 5 abdominal thrusts by placing the heel of one hand above the umbilicus and below the xiphoid process; place your second hand on top of the first hand and apply pressure with an inward and upward motion
6. Perform the tongue-jaw lift and carefully sweep curved finger in one direction along the back of the victim's throat to retrieve object
7. Establish airway using the head-tilt–chin-lift maneuver
8. Attempt to ventilate by delivering one breath
9. Continue repeating abdominal thrusts, finger sweeps, and breathing attempts in rapid sequence

C. Unconscious adult victim
1. Simultaneously shake victim and shout to establish unconsciousness
2. Activate EMS
3. Quickly place victim in supine position
4. Establish airway using the head-tilt–chin-lift maneuver
5. Put your ear near victim's mouth and look, listen, and feel for breathing
6. Deliver two breaths
7. If unable to ventilate, reposition head and again attempt to deliver two breaths
8. Repeat steps 5 to 8 of conscious adult victim who loses consciousness until effective

D. Child
1. Same as adult, except:
2. Provide 1 minute of rescue support, then activate EMS
3. Do not perform finger sweeps; use tongue-jaw lift and remove object only if visualized

E. Obese victim and later stages of pregnancy
1. Conscious victim: deliver chest thrusts (place thumb side of fist on middle of breast bone) until foreign body is expelled or victim becomes unconscious
2. Unconscious victim
   a. Deliver chest thrusts with victim in supine position by placing heel of hand on lower half of sternum with other hand on top (CPR position)
   b. Follow Heimlich maneuver, finger sweep, ventilate sequence

F. Conscious infant
1. Supporting head and neck, position infant face down with head lower than trunk along rescuer's forearm
2. With heel of hand, administer 5 back blows between the shoulder blades
3. Continue to support head and turn infant over, keeping head lower than trunk
4. Compression location is directly below the point where the sternum is bisected by an imaginary line between the nipples
5. With the ring and middle fingers, administer 5 chest thrusts
6. Continue to administer back blows and chest thrusts until airway is cleared or infant becomes unconscious

G. Conscious infant who loses consciousness
1. Place in supine position, call for help, and activate EMS
2. Perform tongue-jaw lift and remove object only if you see it (DO NOT perform finger sweeps)
3. Establish airway using the head-tilt–chin-lift maneuver
4. Attempt to deliver two breaths; if unable to ventilate, reposition head and repeat
5. Administer 5 back blows
6. Administer 5 chest thrusts
7. Perform tongue-jaw lift and remove object only if you see it
8. Establish airway using head-tilt–chin-lift maneuver and deliver two breaths
9. Continue repeating back blows, chest thrusts, tongue-jaw lift, and breathing until effective

H. Unconscious infant
1. Simultaneously shake and tap victim to establish unconsciousness

2. Call for help even if you do not see anyone in the immediate vicinity
3. Quickly place infant in supine position while supporting the head and neck
4. Establish airway using head-tilt–chin-lift maneuver but do not tilt too far
5. Put your ear near victim's mouth and look, listen, and feel for breathing
6. Administer two breaths
7. If unable to ventilate, reposition head and again deliver two breaths
8. Activate EMS
9. Administer five back blows
10. Administer five chest thrusts
11. Perform tongue-jaw lift and remove object only if you see it
12. Attempt to ventilate
13. Repeat steps 9 through 12 until effective

HEMORRHAGE

A. Description: loss of a large amount of blood in a short period of time either externally or internally
B. Types
1. Venous: dark color; steady flow
2. Arterial: bright color; spurts
3. Capillary: red; oozes
C. Assessment for shock
1. Restlessness
2. Anxiety
3. Rapid, weak pulse
4. Cool, moist, pale skin
5. Rapid respirations
6. Thirst
7. Nausea/vomiting
8. Alteration in level of consciousness
9. Hypotension
10. If bleeding is internal (within a cavity or joint), pain will develop because the cavity is stretched by increasing blood volume
D. Intervention: external
1. Apply direct pressure with a clean cloth for at least 6 minutes (use gloves if available)
2. Elevate injured part above heart level
3. If arterial bleeding does not respond to direct pressure, attempt to control by applying direct pressure on supply artery (Fig. 10-5)
4. Tourniquets are not recommended unless an extremity is amputated or severely mutilated
   a. Leave tourniquet exposed (visible)
   b. Tag or label victim with location of tourniquet
   c. Apply proximal to wound
   d. Tourniquet should not be removed except by a physician
5. Cover victim to maintain body temperature; maintain supine position
6. Treat for shock and transport immediately
E. Intervention: internal
1. Cover victim to maintain body temperature
2. Keep in supine position
3. Monitor VS
4. Treat for shock and transport immediately

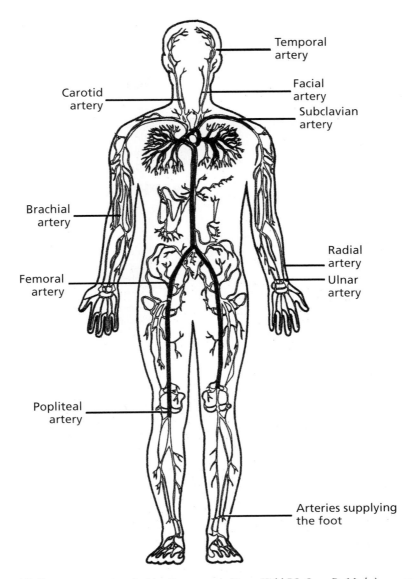

Figure 10-5 Pressure points for bleeding control. (From Kidd PS, Sturt P: *Mosby's emergency nursing reference,* St Louis, 1996, Mosby.)

F. Usual medical care:
 1. Replacement of fluids intravenously to expand blood volume
 2. Blood transfusions
 3. Locate source of and stop hemorrhage

Epistaxis (Nosebleed)

A. Description: bleeding from the nose caused by trauma, local irritation, violent sneezing, or chronic conditions such as hypertension
B. Assessment: obvious bleeding from one or both nares (most often unilateral)
C. Intervention
 1. Sit victim upright, head slightly forward to prevent swallowing blood
 2. Apply firm, continuous pressure (pinch nose) using thumb and forefinger
 3. Ice compress to nose
 4. Limit activity; avoid drinking hot or cold liquids
 5. Monitor vital signs
D. Usual medical care
 1. Nasal pack soaked in a topical vasoconstrictor
 2. Cauterization (silver nitrate or electrocautery)

SHOCK

A. Description: depressed state of vital body functions that, if untreated, could result in death
B. Types: (3 basic types) (Box 10-1)
 1. Hypovolemic: primarily a fluid problem caused by a loss of blood or fluid volume (for example: hemorrhage, severe burns, trauma, or dehydration)
 2. Cardiogenic: faulty pumping action resulting in reduced cardiac output (for example: myocardial infarction, cardiomyopathy, or diseases of the heart valves)

Box 10-1   Causes of Shock

Hypovolemic
External major bleeding
Hemothorax
Hemoperitoneum
Fractures
Gastrointestinal bleeding
Major vomiting
Major diarrhea
Major diaphoresis
Renal failure
Excessive diuretic use
Fluid loss from diabetes
Burns
Ascites

Cardiogenic
Myocardial infarction
Cardiomyopathy
Cardiac contusion
Dysrhythmia
Diseases of heart valve

Distributive
Sepsis
Anaphylaxis
Spinal cord injury
Overdose
Anoxia

Modified from Emergency Nurses Association: *Sheehy's emergency nursing: principles and practice,* ed 4, St Louis, 1998, Mosby.

3. Vasogenic or distributive: a vascular problem or disturbance in tissue perfusion caused by alteration in circulating blood volumes (vascular dilation); 3 types are as follows:
   a. Septic: massive bacterial infection resulting in release of endotoxin that causes vasodilation (e.g., gram-negative organisms)
   b. Neurogenic or spinal: disruption of arterioles and venules resulting in a decrease of circulating blood volume (e.g., spinal cord injury)
   c. Anaphylaxis: severe allergic reaction resulting in histamine release, increased capillary permeability with eventual dilation of arterioles and venules
C. Assessment: determination of the exact cause is vital to patient survival
   1. Shallow, rapid respirations
   2. Cool, pale, clammy skin
   3. Thirst
   4. Tachycardia
   5. Decreased blood pressure
   6. Weak, thready pulse
   7. Restlessness
   8. Decreased urine output
   9. Possible confusion or disorientation
D. Intervention: isolation of cause determines specific intervention strategies, which include:
   1. Ensure adequate airway and ventilation

2. Control bleeding if present
3. Place in supine position with legs elevated unless contraindicated (e.g., head injuries)
4. Insert urinary catheter
5. Monitor vital signs
6. Cover victim to conserve body heat
7. Remain with victim if possible
E. Usual medical care
   1. IV fluids
   2. Administer oxygen
   3. Medications depending on the type of shock

ANAPHYLACTIC REACTION
A. Description: a type of vasogenic or distributive shock (see Shock, above)
B. Assessment
   1. Pallor
   2. Diaphoresis
   3. Tachycardia or bradycardia
   4. Hypotension
   5. Wheezing, dyspnea
   6. Anxiety, restlessness
   7. Urticaria
   8. Edema
   9. Pruritus
   10. Rash
   11. Possible respiratory distress
   12. Diffuse erythema
C. Intervention
   1. Ensure adequate airway and ventilation
   2. Elevate feet slightly unless contraindicated (e.g., head injuries)
D. Usual medical care
   1. Administer oxygen
   2. Epinephrine
   3. Antihistamines
   4. Steroids
   5. IV fluids
   6. Drug therapy for cardiovascular support
E. Preventive measures
   1. Allergy history
   2. Medical identification tag for high-risk persons
   3. Insect (sting) emergency medical kits
   4. Skin testing when possible
   5. Question previous allergic reactions before administering medications

HEAD INJURIES
Traumatic damage to the head from blunt or penetrating trauma resulting in scalp, skull, and brain injuries

Scalp Injury

Type	Intervention
Abrasion	Wash with soap and water
Hematoma	Apply ice
Laceration	Stop bleeding by compression (only if no depression is present)
	Shave around laceration
	Cleanse wound
	Suture

Skull Fracture

A. Simple: linear crack in surface of skull with no displacement of bone
    1. Observation for alteration of respiration, vision, level of consciousness, pupils (dilated, fixed, pinpoint), motor strength, and speech
    2. X-ray examination
B. Depressed: skull fracture with depressed bone fragments resulting in a concave appearance
    1. Intervention
      a. Ensure adequate airway and ventilation
      b. Administer oxygen
      c. Control bleeding
      d. Treat for shock
      e. Observe for alteration of respiration, vision, level of consciousness, pupils (dilated, fixed, pinpoint), motor strength, and speech
      f. Maintain body temperature
      g. Protect cervical spine
      h. Monitor vital signs
    2. Usual medical care
      a. Surgical intervention
      b. Antibiotic therapy
      c. X-ray examination
C. Basilar: fracture located along base of skull
    1. Assessment
      a. Periorbital ecchymosis (black eyes)
      b. Cerebrospinal fluid (CSF) leak from nose or ear
      c. Ecchymosis behind ears (Battle's sign)
      d. Blood behind eardrum (hemotympanum)
    2. Intervention:
      a. Observe for alterations of respiration, vision, level of consciousness, pupils (dilated, fixed, pinpoint), motor strength, and speech; monitor vital signs
      b. If CSF leak noted, do not attempt to stop; apply a loose bulky dressing over area; protect cervical spine
    3. Usual medical care
      a. X-ray examination (although usually not visible)
      b. Antibiotic therapy if CSF leak is present

Brain Injury

A. Concussion: temporary alteration of neurologic functioning caused by a blow to the head, which results in jarring of the brain
    1. Assessment
      a. Nausea and vomiting
      b. Headache
      c. Possible brief period of unconsciousness and memory loss
      d. Possible skull fracture
      e. Confusion
    2. Intervention
      a. Observe for alteration of respiration, vision, level of consciousness, pupils (dilated, fixed, pinpoint), and motor strength
      b. Administer nonnarcotic analgesics as ordered
      c. Maintain hydration
      d. Protect cervical spine
B. Contusion: brain surface bruise resulting in structural alteration
    1. Assessment
      a. Nausea and vomiting

      b. Visual alterations (diplopia)
      c. Neurologic alterations (ataxia, confusion)
    2. Intervention
      a. Maintain adequate airway and ventilation
      b. Observe
      c. Protect cervical spine
      d. Monitor vital signs
    3. Usual medical care
      a. Hospitalization
      b. Antiemetics
C. Intracranial bleeding: hemorrhage or bleeding within the cranial vault
    1. Assessment
      a. Epidural (extradural) hematoma; bleeding between skull and dura mater; short period of unconsciousness followed by consciousness; severe headache, hemiparesis if conscious, bradycardia, and increased blood pressure
      b. Subdural hematoma; bleeding between dura mater and arachnoid membrane; can be acute or chronic; loss of consciousness, fixed dilated pupils, hemiparesis, and positive Babinski's sign
      c. Subarachnoid hematoma; bleeding between arachnoid membrane and the pia mater: severe headache, nausea and vomiting, delirium, syncope, or coma
    2. Intervention
      a. Maintain adequate airway and ventilation
      b. Administer oxygen
      c. Monitor vital signs
      d. Protect cervical spine
      e. Observe for alterations of respiration, vision, level of consciousness, pupils (dilated, fixed, pinpoint), and decreased motor strength (signs of increased ICP [intracranial pressure])
      f. Maintain body temperature
      g. Treat for shock
    3. Usual medical care
      a. Hospitalization
      b. CT scan
      c. Possible surgery

EYE INJURIES
Foreign Body in Eye

A. Evert eyelid (Fig. 10-6)
B. Touch particle gently with sterile swab moistened in sterile saline solution or water (do not remove if particle is on the cornea or if there is eyeball penetration)
C. Apply an eye patch after ensuring that the eye is closed

Foreign Body in Conjunctiva

A. Evert eyelid
B. Remove particle as described above
C. Irrigate with saline solution or water
D. Eye patch may be applied

Eyelid Contusion (Black Eye)

A. Cold compresses or ice pack intermittently for the first 24 hours
B. Warm compresses after 48 hours
C. Bilateral eye patches if intraocular hemorrhage is present

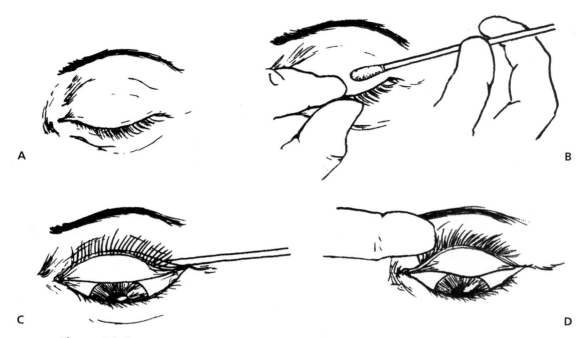

Figure 10-6   Steps in everting eyelid. **A,** Eyelid. **B,** Placement of cotton swab (eyelashes are pulled down and back over swab). **C,** Eyelid everted over swab. **D,** Examination of inside of eyelid and eye. (From Emergency Nurses Association: *Sheehy's emergency nursing: principles and practice,* ed 4, St Louis, 1998, Mosby.)

Corneal Abrasion

A. Assessment
  1. Pain
  2. Photosensitivity
  3. Spasms of the eyelid
  4. Excessive tear production
B. Intervention: apply eye patch to injured eye
C. Usual medical care: local ophthalmic antibiotics

Burns

A. Chemical
  1. If action of chemical is not enhanced by water, immediately flush area with copious amounts of normal saline solution or tap water for 15 minutes (damage increases with length of chemical contact)
  2. Usual medical care: topical application of antibiotics, administration of cycloplegic agents, or corticosteroids (alkali burns)
  3. The following solutions will neutralize the following types of burns
    a. Acid: sodium bicarbonate 2% solution
    b. Lime: ammonium tartrate 5% solution
    c. Alkali: boric or citric acid solution
B. Thermal (usually occurs with facial burns)
  1. Irrigate with normal saline solution or tap water
  2. Apply bilateral eye patches
  3. Usual medical care: analgesia, sedation, antibiotics, cycloplegics
C. Radiation
  1. Types
    a. Ultraviolet (sun)—severity depends on period of exposure
    b. Infrared (x-rays)—severity depends on wavelength and period of exposure (may cause loss of vision)

  2. Assessment
    a. Excessive blinking
    b. Excessive tear production
    c. Feeling that something is in the eye
    d. Pain
  3. Intervention
    a. Cold compresses
    b. Bilateral eye patches
  4. Usual medical care
    a. Topical antibiotics
    b. Cycloplegics
    c. Analgesics

Penetrating Eye Injuries

A. Place a protective shield, such as a paper cup, over the eye to prevent further damage by pressure
B. Apply eye patch to the uninjured eye
C. See an ophthalmologist immediately

SPINAL CORD INJURIES (Table 10-1)

A. Assessment
  1. Pain, tenderness
  2. Numbness, tingling, paralysis
  3. Weakness of extremities
  4. Alterations of sensation and motor function below level of injury
  5. Possible signs and symptoms of shock
B. Intervention
  1. Ensure adequate airway and ventilation; if helmet is on victim, leave it in place if airway is accessible; ***never attempt to remove helmet alone***
  2. Treat for shock
  3. Immobilization (movement may cause further damage)
  4. Maintain body temperature

TABLE 10-1 Cervical Spine and Spinal Cord Lesions and Resultant Physiological Function

Lesion	Resultant Function
C3, C4, or above	Respiratory arrest; flaccid paralysis; quadriplegia (tetraplegia)
C5, C6	Reduced respiratory effort; almost total dependence; flaccid paralysis; quadriplegia (tetraplegia)
C7	Reduced respiratory effort; almost total dependence; splints necessary for functioning of forearms; quadriplegia (tetraplegia)
T1	Reduced respiratory effort; partial dependence; paraplegia
T1, T2	Reduced respiratory effort; complete independence; paraplegia
T7	Complete independence; walking with long-leg braces; paraplegia
L4	Complete independence; walking with foot braces; paraplegia

From Sheehy SB, Lenehan GB: *Manual of emergency care,* ed 5, St Louis, 1999, Mosby.

    5. When help (EMS) arrives, place victim on board without flexing neck or back
    6. Transport immediately (EMS)

SOFT TISSUE NECK INJURIES
Fractured Larynx
A. Assessment
    1. Hoarse voice
    2. Cough with hemoptysis
    3. Difficulty breathing; respiratory distress
    4. Subcutaneous emphysema
B. Intervention
    1. Administer oxygen
    2. Observation
C. Usual medical care
    1. Emergency cricothyrotomy or tracheostomy
    2. Broad-spectrum antibiotics

Penetrating Neck Wounds
A. Assessment
    1. Noticeable penetrating wound
    2. Airway obstruction
    3. Signs and symptoms of hypovolemia, hemathorax, or shock
B. Intervention
    1. Ensure adequate airway and ventilation
    2. Control bleeding
    3. Surgery

CHEST INJURIES
Fractured Rib (Simple, Undisplaced)
A. Assessment
    1. Chest pain (increases on inspiration), tenderness
    2. Shortness of breath, shallow breathing
    3. Tachycardia
    4. Hypotension
    5. Ecchymosis
B. Intervention (individualized)
    1. Rest
    2. Intermittent ice for first 24 hours, then heat
    3. Observe for signs and symptoms of pneumothorax by monitoring breathing patterns and lung sounds
    4. Encourage deep breathing
    5. Administer analgesics sparingly

Flail Chest
A. Fracture of several ribs resulting in loss of chest wall stability; pulmonary or myocardial contusion may also be present because of force of injury; may be life threatening
B. Assessment
    1. Pain
    2. Difficulty breathing
    3. Shallow, rapid, noisy respirations
    4. Chest moves in opposite from normal direction: moves in on inspiration, out on expiration
    5. Tachycardia and cyanosis
    6. Possible bruising
C. Intervention
    1. Ensure adequate airway and ventilation
    2. Stabilization of chest wall
    3. Application of pressure dressing
    4. Position victim on affected side in semi-Fowler's position
    5. Monitor vital signs and lung sounds
D. Usual medical care
    1. Pain control
    2. Possible intubation and ventilation with severe flail
    3. Possible traction

Simple Pneumothorax
A. Description: air enters the pleural cavity; negative pressure is lost, resulting in partial or total lung collapse
B. Assessment
    1. Chest pain
    2. Shortness of breath (SOB) and tachypnea
    3. Decreased breath sounds
C. Intervention
    1. Ensure adequate airway and ventilation
    2. Place victim in semi-Fowler's position
    3. Administer oxygen
D. Usual medical care: possible chest tube placement

Tension Pneumothorax
A. Description: air enters the pleural cavity on inspiration and is trapped during exhalation, creating pressure that causes eventual collapse of the lung (same side) resulting in a life-threatening condition in which there is mediastinal shift that compresses the heart, great vessels, and the trachea as well as the opposite lung
B. Assessment
    1. Extreme shortness of breath
    2. Observed tracheal deviation
    3. Paradoxical movement of the chest
    4. Neck vein distention
    5. Hypotension
    6. Tachycardia
    7. Restlessness
    8. Cyanosis

9. Distant breath sounds
10. History of chest trauma
C. Intervention
   1. Ensure adequate airway, breathing, and circulation
   2. Administer oxygen
D. Usual medical care
   1. Needle thoracotomy
   2. Chest tube placement
   3. Intravenous fluids

Open Pneumothorax (Sucking Chest Wound)

A. Description: presence of air in the chest resulting from an open wound in the chest wall
   1. One-way flap: air enters pleural space but cannot escape (tension pneumothorax)
   2. Two-way flap: air enters and leaves pleural space
B. Assessment
   1. Audible sucking noise
   2. Shortness of breath
   3. Chest pain
   4. Cyanosis
   5. Shock
   6. Possible signs and symptoms of tension pneumothorax
C. Intervention
   1. Ensure adequate airway, breathing, and circulation
   2. Cover wound with air-tight dressing (depends on size of wound)
   3. Administer oxygen
   4. CPR may be necessary
D. Usual medical care
   1. Chest tube placement
   2. Antibiotic therapy
   3. Treat for shock

Spontaneous Pneumothorax

A. Description: presence of air in the intrapleural space resulting from rupture of lung tissue and visceral pleura with no evidence of trauma; can occur during periods of strenuous physical activity
B. Assessment
   1. Sudden, sharp chest pain
   2. Shortness of breath
   3. Diaphoresis
   4. Anxiety
   5. Hypotension
   6. Tachycardia
   7. Cessation of normal chest movement on affected side
C. Intervention
   1. Ensure adequate airway and ventilation
   2. Keep victim quiet
   3. Place in semi- or high-Fowler's position
D. Usual medical care
   1. Needle aspiration
   2. Chest tube
   3. IV fluids
   4. Oxygen

Hemothorax

A. Description: blood in the pleural space from traumatic injury (stabbing) or rupture of congenital blebs

B. Assessment
   1. Chest pain
   2. Shortness of breath
   3. Distant breath sounds
   4. Anxiety
   5. Shock
   6. Cyanosis
C. Intervention
   1. Ensure adequate airway and ventilation
   2. Treat for shock
D. Usual medical care: chest tube placement; thoracentesis

Pulmonary Embolism

A. Description: thrombus becomes detached and lodges in a branch of the pulmonary artery causing a partial or total occlusion resulting in a pulmonary infarct; commonly seen with trauma, surgery, or long-bone fractures
B. Assessment
   1. Sudden, sharp chest pain
   2. Shortness of breath
   3. Pallor, possible cyanosis
   4. Anxiety
   5. Tachycardia
   6. Rapid, shallow respirations (tachypnea)
   7. Possible hypotension, elevated temperature
   8. Possible cough, wheeze, hemoptysis
   9. Possible sudden death if large blood vessel is blocked
C. Intervention
   1. Ensure adequate airway, breathing, and circulation
   2. Treat for shock
   3. Administer oxygen
   4. Keep victim quiet
   5. Place patient in semi-Fowler's to high-Fowler's position if vital signs permit
D. Usual medical care
   1. Anticoagulant therapy
   2. IV fluids
   3. Surgical intervention in cases of profound shock or cardiovascular collapse

INTRAABDOMINAL INJURIES
Penetrating Wound

A. Description: wounds resulting from stabbings, shootings, impalement
B. Assessment
   1. Hypotension
   2. Shock
   3. Diminished bowel sounds
   4. Pain
   5. Tenderness
   6. Progressive abdominal distention
   7. Nausea or vomiting
C. Intervention
   1. Do not move victim
   2. Ensure adequate airway, breathing, circulation
   3. Control bleeding
      a. Look for entrance and exit wounds
      b. Apply compression for external bleeding
      c. Look for chest injuries
   4. Cover wounds with wet, sterile, or nonadhesive dressing(s) (e.g., saline or plastic wrap)
   5. Monitor vital signs

6. Treat for shock
7. Keep victim NPO
D. Usual medical care
   1. IVs
   2. Oxygen
   3. Tetanus prophylaxis
   4. Antibiotics
   5. Analgesics
   6. Indwelling catheter
   7. Nasogastric tube
   8. X-ray examination
   9. Possible surgery

Blunt Wound

A. Description: wounds resulting from a motor vehicle accident (MVA), contact sport injury, falls, or physical abuse (e.g., domestic violence)
B. Assessment
   1. Observable bruises and abrasions
   2. Abdominal pain, rigidity, palpable masses, or distention
   3. Signs and symptoms of shock
   4. Guarding
   5. Diminished bowel sounds
C. Intervention
   1. Do not move victim
   2. Ensure adequate airway, breathing, circulation
   3. Observe for hemorrhage
   4. Observe for chest injuries
   5. Monitor vital signs
   6. Treat for shock
D. Usual medical care
   1. Oxygen
   2. Nasogastric tube
   3. X-ray examination
   4. Peritoneal lavage
   5. Possible surgery

BURNS

A. Depth of Classification (Table 10-2)
B. Surface Area Classification
   1. The greater the body surface area (BSA) affected, the more serious the damage

TABLE 10-2 Burn Classification

Depth	Degree	Assessment
Superficial, partial thickness (involves only the epidermis)	First	Pain; red; minimal or no edema
Deep partial thickness (involves epidermis and part of the dermis)	Second	Pain; mottled color; blistering; wet appearance
Full thickness (involves epidermis and damage to subcutaneous layer, muscle, and bone)	Third	Gray, white, brown, leathery, or charred appearance; edema; minor or no pain

2. Use rule of nines (Fig. 10-7) to estimate percent of BSA affected

Major Burns

A. Burns are considered major or critical if they fulfill the following criteria:
   1. Deep partial-thickness burns: greater than 25% body surface area (BSA) in adults, or greater than 20% in children under 10 and adults older than 40 years of age
   2. Full-thickness burns: greater than 10% BSA in adults and children
   3. Electrical burns
   4. Burns involving face, eyes, ears, hands, feet, and perineum
   5. Burns in victims with preexisting chronic conditions (diabetes, cardiac conditions, renal failure)
B. Intervention
   1. Lay victim flat (standing forces him or her to breathe flames and smoke; running fans flames)
   2. Roll victim in carpet or blankets or use water to extinguish fire
   3. Remove any smoldering clothing that is nonadherent
   4. Ensure adequate airway and ventilation
   5. Administer oxygen
   6. Assess for inhalation burns
   7. Remove nonadherent, tight-fitting clothing
   8. Remove tight jewelry
   9. Apply cold soaks
   10. Cover burns with moist, sterile dressings or clean cloth
   11. Elevate affected parts if possible
   12. Cover victim
   13. Insert indwelling catheter
   14. Treat burned areas as ordered by physician
C. Usual medical care
   1. Tetanus prophylaxis
   2. Central venous pressure line

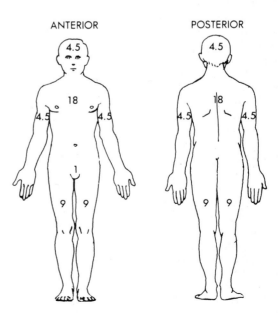

Figure 10-7   Rule of nines is used to estimate amount of skin surface burned. (From Phipps WJ, Sands JK, Marek JF: *Medical-surgical nursing: concepts and clinical practice*, ed 6, St Louis, 1999, Mosby.)

3. Pain management
4. Nasogastric tube
5. Standard Precautions
6. Intravenous therapy
7. Antibiotic therapy
D. Warnings
   1. Do not use salves, ointments, or oils
   2. Do not soak large burns unless you can maintain body warmth
   3. Do not use ice or ice water on deep partial-thickness or full-thickness burns; causes further injury and promotes hypothermia

Chemical Burns

A. Powdered chemicals: sweep off skin
B. Nonpowered chemicals: irrigate with copious amounts of water or saline solution
C. Cover loosely with a clean cloth
D. Usual medical care: treated as thermal burns (cleanse wound, open blisters and remove outer layer, apply topical antibacterial agent)

Electrical Burns

A. Assessment
   1. Discoloration
   2. Edema
   3. Cardiac irregularities
   4. Entrance and exit sites of current visible
   5. Confusion
   6. Unconsciousness
   7. Respiratory distress
B. Intervention
   1. Do not touch the victim
   2. Remove electrical source with a nonconductor and/or shut off current source
   3. If victim has no pulse and is not breathing, institute CPR
   4. Extremities should be handled minimally and with extreme caution
   5. Check victim for other injuries
   6. Monitor cardiac and renal function

Radiation Burns

A. Intervention
   1. Remove contaminated clothing
   2. Apply cool, moist compresses
B. Usual medical care: possibly antipyretics

Smoke Inhalation

A. Assessment
   1. History of exposure
   2. Singed hair in nares
   3. Mouth burns
   4. Brassy cough
   5. Respiratory distress
   6. Rales, rhonchi, or wheezes
   7. Restlessness
   8. Cyanosis
B. Intervention
   1. Ensure adequate airway and ventilation
   2. Administer oxygen
   3. Be prepared to initiate CPR

C. Usual medical care
   1. Hospitalization for 24 to 48 hours
   2. IV fluids
   3. Chest physical therapy
   4. Possible endotracheal intubation or tracheostomy
   5. Use of bronchodilators, steroids
   6. Nasogastric tube

WOUNDS

A. Open (break in skin integrity)
   1. Laceration: jagged cut through the skin and underlying tissue
   2. Abrasion: skin scrape or "brush burn"
   3. Avulsion: flap of skin and subcutaneous tissue torn loose
   4. Puncture: tissue penetration by a sharp object
   5. Abscess: localized pus formation
B. Closed (no break in skin integrity; e.g., contusion): injury to underlying tissue by blunt object
C. General management
   1. Stop bleeding
     a. Apply pressure dressing
     b. Elevate affected part
     c. Use digital pressure on supply artery
     d. Apply tourniquet only as a lifesaving measure and leave tourniquet visible
   2. Treat shock
   3. Control infection
     a. Wounds requiring medical care: it is generally recommended not to clean them until they are seen by a physician
     b. Cover open wounds with a clean, nonadhesive dressing
     c. Apply ice during the first 24 to 48 hours for closed wounds
     d. Minor wounds being treated at home: clean well with soap and water; thoroughly rinse; approximate wound edges with adhesive; cover with a clean dressing; seek medical care for signs of infection
   4. Puncture wounds
     a. Impaled object should be stabilized and left in place
     b. Medical attention should be sought
D. Special wounds
   1. Human bites
     a. May be self-inflicted or inflicted by another; evidenced by teeth marks and often by knuckle lacerations (occurs when fist hits another person's teeth during a fight)
     b. Intervention
       (1) Clean with soap and water
       (2) Rinse thoroughly
       (3) Apply clean dressing
       (4) Keep injured part elevated
     c. Usual medical care
       (1) Tetanus prophylaxis
       (2) Antibiotic therapy
       (3) Observe closely for systemic responses to bite: toxic shock syndrome, hepatitis, HIV, which can occur post-injury or during the healing process

2. Animal bites: potential for contracting rabies must be seriously considered with any animal bite
   a. Dog bites are most common, causing crushing injury to skin and underlying tissue or avulsion injuries should the victim attempt to pull away
   b. Cat bites are more likely to cause puncture wounds
   c. Intervention
      (1) Obtain history of bite
      (2) Clean minor wounds with soap and water
      (3) Rinse thoroughly
      (4) Flush with povidone-iodine (Betadine) or other cleansing solutions (hydrogen peroxide) if allergic to Betadine
      (5) Apply clean dressing
         NOTE: Major wounds (severe bleeding) require control of bleeding and medical attention
   d. Usual medical care
      (1) Antibiotic therapy for large, contaminated bites
      (2) Tetanus prophylaxis
      (3) Rabies prophylaxis if necessary
3. Snakebites
   a. Assessment
      (1) Teeth marks; possibly fang marks
      (2) Edema
      (3) Pain
      (4) Ecchymosis
      (5) Bleeding
      (6) Numbness of affected part
   b. Intervention
      (1) Have victim lie quietly in shaded area
      (2) Clean wound
      (3) Suction
         (a) Do not use mouth suction if you have open sores in your mouth
         (b) Suction wound using snakebite kit
         (c) Use mouth suction only if no other means is available
      (4) Apply clean dressing
      (5) Immobilize affected limb
      (6) Affected limb should be in dependent position
   c. Usual medical care
      (1) Analgesics
      (2) IV fluids
      (3) Tetanus prophylaxis
      (4) Antivenin therapy
4. Insect bites (bees, wasps, hornets)
   a. Assessment
      (1) Obtain detailed medical and activity history
      (2) Pruritus
      (3) Burning
      (4) Swelling
   b. Intervention
      (1) Remove the stinger by scraping; do not pull out because this releases more toxin; do not squeeze
      (2) Clean with soap and water
      (3) Apply ice (DO NOT apply heat)
      (4) Apply ammonia diluted with warm water or a paste of baking soda and water
   c. Usual medical care
      (1) Epinephrine
      (2) Antihistamines
      (3) Steroids
5. Tick
   a. Attaches to host with its teeth
   b. Releases a toxin that may cause tick paralysis or Lyme disease
   c. Squeezing tick releases more toxin
   d. If paralysis progresses to bulbar, respiratory failure and subsequent death may occur
   e. Paralysis will disappear after tick is removed
   f. Intervention
      (1) Grasp tick with tweezers and pull slowly and steadily
      (2) Wash area with soap and water
      (3) Seek medical treatment

FRACTURE

A. Description: a complete or incomplete break in bone continuity
   1. Fracture without displacement presents normal alignment despite the fracture
   2. Fracture with displacement presents a separation of bone fragments at fracture site
   3. Compound or open: bone protrusion through skin
   4. Simple or closed: no bone protrusion through the skin
   5. Incomplete: part of bone is broken
   6. Complete: breakage produces two fragments
B. Types of fractures (Box 10-2)
C. Assessment
   1. Five Ps (pain, pallor, pulses, paresthesia, and paralysis)
   2. Discoloration; ecchymosis
   3. Swelling
   4. Deformity, possible limb shortening and external rotation
   5. Crepitus (characteristic grating sound)
   6. Possible bone snap heard by victim
   7. External bleeding from associated wounds
   8. Tenderness (pain) relative to specific area of the body (sacrum, hip, symphysis pubis)
D. Intervention
   1. Control bleeding if necessary
   2. Treat for shock
   3. Immobilize affected part
   4. Splint above and below the fracture
   5. Apply ice
   6. Elevate affected part, if possible
   7. Observe for changes in sensation, temperature, and color (indicate nerve injury or circulation interference)
E. Usual medical care
   1. X-ray examination
   2. Possible cast application
   3. Possible surgery
   4. Analgesics
   5. Traction

DISLOCATION

A. Description: joint injury and bone displacement
B. Assessment
   1. Pain, tenderness
   2. Swelling
   3. Deformity

Box 10-2   Types of Fractures

Typical Complete Fractures

Closed (simple) fracture—Noncommunicating wound between bone and skin

Open (compound) fracture—Communicating wound between bone and skin

Comminuted fracture—Multiple bone fragments

Linear fracture—Fracture line parallel to long axis of bone

Oblique fracture—Fracture line at 45-degree angle to long axis of bone

Spiral fracture—Fracture line encircling bone

Transverse fracture—Fracture line perpendicular to long axis of bone

Impacted fracture—Fracture fragments are pushed into each other

Pathologic fracture—Fracture occurs at a point in the bone weakened by disease, for example, with tumors or osteoporosis

Avulsion—A fragment of bone connected to a ligament breaks off from the main bone

Extracapsular—Fracture is close to the joint but remains outside the joint capsule

Intracapsular—Fracture is within the joint capsule

Typical Incomplete Fractures

Greenstick fracture—Break on one cortex of bone with splintering of inner bone surface

Torus fracture—Buckling of cortex

Bowing fracture—Bending of bone

Stress fracture—Microfracture

Transchondral fracture—Separation of cartilaginous joint surface (articular cartilage) from main shaft of bone

From McCance KI, Huether SE: *Pathophysiology: the biological basis for disease in adults and children,* ed 3, St Louis, 1998, Mosby.

---

4. Alterations in function
5. Discoloration

C. Intervention
   1. Control hemorrhage if present (not usually seen with a simple dislocation)
   2. Immobilize the affected part
   3. Apply sterile dressing to any open wounds
   4. Splint above and below the site in the position found
   5. Apply ice
   6. Elevate affected part, if possible
   7. Check for fractures
   8. Monitor neurologic status (check pulses distal to the injury)

SPRAIN

A. Description: stretched or ruptured ligaments; sprain should be considered a fracture until proven otherwise by x-ray examination
B. Assessment
   1. Pain, tenderness
   2. Discoloration
   3. Swelling
   4. Alterations in function
C. Intervention
   1. Elevate affected part
   2. Apply ice intermittently for 72 hours
   3. Apply elastic (Ace) bandages
   4. Immobilize affected part

STRAIN

A. Description: muscle or tendon damage caused by excessive physical use
B. Assessment
   1. Pain
   2. Discoloration
C. Intervention
   1. Elevate affected part
   2. Apply ice intermittently for 72 hours
   3. Apply elastic (Ace) bandages
   4. Immobilize affected part
   5. Limited to no weight bearing

HYPERTHERMIA
Heat Stroke

A. Description: life-threatening emergency; body's mechanism for heat regulation breaks down, and excessive body heat is retained; occurs with overexposure to high environmental temperatures, especially those accompanied by high relative humidity and low wind
B. Assessment
   1. Hyperpyrexia to 106° or 107° F (41.1° to 41.6° C)
   2. Flushed, hot, dry skin or clammy and diaphoretic
   3. Dizziness
   4. Headache
   5. Confusion
   6. Nausea
   7. Tachycardia
   8. Hypotension
   9. Fixed and diluted pupils
   10. Seizures
   11. Possible altered level of consciousness
   12. Shallow, rapid breathing
   13. Delirium
C. Predisposing factors are:
   1. Age (elderly/infants)
   2. Obesity
   3. Alcoholism
   4. Preexisting illness (cardiovascular or neurological dysfunctions)
   5. Prescription medications that decrease perspiration (anticholinergics such as antihistamines and antispasmodics; diuretics and beta blockers such as propranolol)
   6. Excessive strenuous exercise
D. Intervention
   1. Ensure adequate airway, breathing, and circulation
   2. Move victim out of sun
   3. Loosen or remove clothing
   4. Provide rapid cooling, for example, immerse in cold water; apply towels soaked in cold water; air conditioning, fanning, and cool-water sponge

5. If conscious, provide cool water
6. Control shivering (this causes body temperature to increase)
7. Advise victim to avoid reexposure and warn of possible lowered tolerance to heat for a long time or indefinitely

E. Usual medical care
   1. Oxygen
   2. IV therapy

Heat Exhaustion

A. Description: ineffective circulating blood volume caused by excessive fluid loss and exposure to heat without sufficient fluid and electrolyte replenishment
B. Assessment
   1. Headache
   2. Dizziness, faintness
   3. Nausea and vomiting
   4. Marked diaphoresis
   5. Cool, pale, damp skin
   6. Muscle cramps
   7. Possible temperature elevation
   8. Orthostatic hypotension
   9. Tachycardia
   10. Dehydration
   11. Anxiety
   12. Anorexia, thirst
C. Especially at risk are:
   1. The elderly
   2. The very young
D. Intervention
   1. Move victim to cool, quiet area
   2. Loosen or remove constricting clothing
   3. Administer salted water if vomiting absent
   4. Provide rest
   5. Relieve muscle cramps (firm pressure against muscle with palm of hand)
   6. Advise victim of preventive measures: drink plenty of fluids and curtail activity on hot days

COLD INJURIES
Frostbite

A. Classification
   1. Superficial: superficial tissue below the skin freezes
   2. Deep: deep subcutaneous tissue freezes, and temperature of affected part is lowered
B. Most frequently affected areas: ears, nose, cheeks, fingers, and toes
C. Assessment
   1. Superficial
      a. Numbness, tingling, burning
      b. Gray-white appearance of affected parts
   2. Deep
      a. Hyperemic skin
      b. Edema
      c. Blister formation
      d. Discoloration
      e. Numbness
D. Intervention
   1. Superficial
      a. Remove wet, constricting clothing

      b. Give warm-water soaks
      c. Advise victim of preventive measures
   2. Deep
      a. Remove wet, constricting clothing
      b. Give warm-water soaks only if continuously available; otherwise keep area dry, place sterile gauze between affected fingers and toes, cover, and elevate frozen part
      c. If conscious, give warm liquids
      d. Do not allow use of frostbitten part
   3. Usual medical care
      a. Tetanus prophylaxis
      b. Analgesics
      c. Antibiotic therapy
E. Warnings
   1. Do not rub area with snow or ice
   2. Do not massage

Immersion Foot

A. Cause: wet foot in continuous contact with cold temperatures
B. Assessment
   1. Foot is cold and damp
   2. Foot appears shriveled
   3. Gangrene (if conditions were prolonged and repeated)
C. Intervention
   1. Dry footwear
   2. Warm-water soaks

Chilblain

A. Description: localized redness and swelling of the skin resulting from excessive exposure to cold
B. Commonly affected areas: fingers, toes, and earlobes
C. Assessment: burning, itching, blistering, and ulceration (similar to thermal burn) are possible
D. Intervention
   1. Protect part from cold and further injury
   2. Gentle warming
   3. Avoid use of tobacco products

Hypothermia

A. Description: exposure to cold resulting in heat loss and reduction in body temperature below the average normal range
B. Assessment (Table 10-3)
C. Intervention
   1. Ensure adequate airway and ventilation
   2. Administer oxygen
   3. Remove wet clothing and cover victim
   4. Give warm beverages high in sugar content
   5. Warm body gradually
      a. Passive rewarming: warm room, blankets, and draft prevention (mild hypothermia)
      b. Active external rewarming: heat packs, warming blankets, and overhead radiant warmers (mild to moderate hypothermia)
D. Usual medical care: (moderate to severe hypothermia) active internal warming)
   1. Warmed humidified oxygen

TABLE 10-3   Stages, Signs, and Symptoms of Hypothermia

Stage	Core Temperature	Symptoms
Mild	90°-95° F (32°-35° C)	Tachypnea, tachycardia, ataxia, shivering, lethargy, confusion, occasional atrial fibrillation
Moderate	86°-90° F (30°-32.2° C)	Rigidity, hypoventilation, decreased level of consciousness, increased myocardial irritability, hypovolemia, blood sludging with metabolic acidosis, Osborne or J wave (positive deflection in the RT segment)
Severe	<86° F (30° C)	Loss of reflexes, coma, hypotension, acidosis, apnea, cyanosis, ventricular fibrillation, asystole

From Kidd PS, Sturt P: *Mosby's emergency nursing reference,* St Louis, 1996, Mosby.

2. Warmed gastric and peritoneal lavage
3. Warmed intravenous fluids
E. Warning: Do not rub or massage the skin

POISONING
Food
A. Cause: pathogenic organisms transferred to victim from contaminated food; illness is caused by toxins produced by the organism
B. Botulism *(Clostridium botulinum)*
  1. Causes
    a. Improperly canned food
    b. Improperly cured food
  2. Assessment
    a. Headache
    b. Fatigue
    c. Nausea and vomiting
    d. Double vision (diplopia)
    e. Muscle incoordination
    f. Difficulty swallowing, talking, and breathing
  3. Intervention
    a. Ensure adequate airway and ventilation
    b. Be prepared to administer CPR
    c. Induce vomiting if consumption was recent, if victim has clinical and neurologic symptoms, no seizure activity, and no alterations in level of consciousness
    d. Usual medical care: antitoxin
C. *Staphylococcus aureus*
  1. Causes
    a. Secretions from respiratory tract and skin of food handlers
    b. Unrefrigerated cream-filled foods
    c. Fish
    d. Meat
  2. Assessment
    a. Nausea and vomiting
    b. Diarrhea
    c. Abdominal cramps
    d. Weakness
  3. Intervention
    a. Fluids
    b. Bed rest
  4. Usual medical care
    a. Possible IV therapy
    b. Antiemetics
    c. Antidiarrheals

D. *Salmonella*
  1. Causes: inadequately cooked meat, poultry, and eggs
  2. Assessment
    a. Nausea and vomiting
    b. Diarrhea
    c. Weakness
    d. Abdominal pain
    e. Elevated temperature
    f. Chills
  3. Intervention
    a. Bed rest
    b. Fluids
  4. Usual medical care
    a. Possible IV therapy
    b. Antiemetics
    c. Antidiarrheals

Accidental Poisoning
A. Description: ingestion, inhalation, or absorption of toxic substances or substances such as drugs, which, when taken in large amounts, are toxic to the body
B. Assessment: signs and symptoms will vary according to cause
  1. General
    a. Nausea and vomiting
    b. Abdominal pain
    c. Convulsions
    d. Change in level of consciousness
    e. Decreased pulse and respirations
  2. Drug poisoning: coma; flaccid muscles; hypotension (symptoms vary depending on drug)
  3. Chemical poisoning
    a. Burns around lips and mouth
    b. Excessive salivation
    c. Difficulty swallowing
    d. Breath odor (from cleaning or petroleum products)
  4. Inhalation poisoning
    a. Coughing and choking
    b. Headache; bright red skin (carbon monoxide—late indicator)
  5. Absorption poisoning: localized itching and burning (poison)
C. Intervention (Box 10-3)
D. Usual medical care
  1. IV fluids (severe cases)
  2. Hyperbaric oxygenation (carbon monoxide poisoning)

Box 10-3   Guidelines to Stop Absorption of Poisons

Inhaled Poison

Remove victim from source of toxic gas.

Assess cardiopulmonary status and give artificial ventilation if possible.

Give oxygen if available.

Contact Poison

Rinse skin with copious amounts of water.

Remove garments and rinse skin again.

Ingested Poison

If person is conscious:

A. Call physician or poison control center for assistance.

B. Substances other than caustics or hydrocarbons:
   1. Induce emesis by giving 15-30 ml syrup of ipecac; follow with full glass of warm water.
   2. Inactivate poison by giving activated charcoal (especially after drug ingestion).

C. Caustics or hydrocarbons (petroleum products):
   1. Give nothing by mouth.
   2. Seek immediate medical attention.
   3. Do not induce emesis.

If person is unconscious, transport without delay to medical facility.

From Phipps WJ, Sands JK, Marek JF: *Medical-surgical nursing: concepts and clinical practice*, ed 6, St Louis, 1999, Mosby.

DIABETES MELLITUS AND HYPOGLYCEMIA

A. Ketoacidosis: acute insulin deficiency (develops over a period of 2 to 3 days); hyperglycemia
   1. Assessment
      a. Polydipsia
      b. Weak, rapid pulse
      c. Hypotension
      d. Dry, warm, flushed skin
      e. Pallor
      f. Diaphoresis
      g. Acetone odor on breath
      h. Kussmaul's respirations
      i. Nausea and vomiting
      j. Alterations in consciousness
      k. Dehydration
      l. Weakness
      m. Headache
      n. Abdominal tenderness
   2. Intervention
      a. Ensure adequate airway and ventilation
      b. Monitor vital signs, fluid intake and output, and level of consciousness
      c. Provide fluids if conscious, for example, broth
   3. Usual medical care
      a. Regular insulin
      b. IV therapy: normal saline solution or 0.45% saline solution
      c. Monitor blood sugar and serum potassium levels

B. Hypoglycemia (low blood sugar; insulin reaction)
   1. Assessment
      a. Sudden onset of symptoms
      b. Weakness
      c. Pallor
      d. Hunger
      e. Nervousness; irritability
      f. Cool, moist skin
      g. Tachycardia
      h. Tremors
      i. Dizziness, syncope
      j. Headache
      k. Visual disturbances
      l. Drowsiness
      m. Confusion
   2. Intervention
      a. Ensure adequate airway and ventilation
      b. Administer quick-acting carbohydrate, for example, orange juice with sugar, honey, lump sugar, cola beverage, hard candy
   3. Usual medical care if unconscious
      a. IV therapy: 50% glucose
      b. Monitor blood sugar

DROWNING

A. Description: asphyxiation that results from aspiration of fluid into the lungs, which is inhaled as the individual panics or gasps for breath

B. Causes
   1. Accidental, for example, exhaustion, inability to swim, panic, injury, medical incident such as a seizure
   2. Intentional: suicide attempt

C. Intervention
   1. Remove victim from water
   2. If victim is not breathing, commence artificial respiration (may need to be instituted while victim is being removed from the water)
   3. If there is no carotid pulse, commence CPR
   4. Observe for pulmonary edema

D. Usual medical care
   1. IV fluids
   2. Oxygen under pressure

DRUG ABUSE

A. Description: Use of a substance in a manner or in amounts or in situations in which the drug use causes problems or greatly increases the chance of problems occurring

B. Assessment
   1. Needle marks on the body along the veins (many addicts wear long-sleeved shirts to conceal mainlining)
   2. Anorexia
   3. Abdominal cramping
   4. Constipation
   5. Nutritional deficiencies
   6. Watery, reddened eyes
   7. Runny nose
   8. Dilated or constricted pupils
   9. Central nervous system alterations (agitation, euphoria, seizures)
   10. Poor personal hygiene
   11. History of difficulty in school, on job, with interpersonal relationships

12. Accident-prone
13. History of personality change
14. Possibly hepatitis
C. Clinical manifestations and treatment (Table 10-4)
D. Intervention
    1. Ensure airway, breathing, and circulation
    2. Administer oxygen
    3. Insert indwelling catheter
    4. Monitor vital functions and neurologic status
    5. Take seizure precautions
E. Usual medical care
    1. Arterial blood gases
    2. Specific drug antagonist (e.g., naloxone hydrochloride [Narcan])
    3. IV therapy
    4. Central venous pressure line
    5. Possible dialysis
    6. High-protein, high-calorie diet
    7. Vitamin supplements
    8. Psychotherapy
    9. Withdrawal treatment: methadone hydrochloride (Dolophine); usually used for heroin addiction
       a. Legal synthetic drug addiction
       b. Supervised administration
   10. Rehabilitation

ACUTE ALCOHOLISM

A. Description: large alcohol intake in a short time
B. Assessment
    1. Alcohol on breath
    2. Slurring of speech
    3. Ataxia
    4. Agitation
    5. Belligerence
    6. Vomiting
    7. Drowsiness to stuporousness to unconsciousness
    8. Respiratory failure
    9. Death
C. Intervention
    1. Protect airway
    2. Observe for respiratory depression
    3. Monitor cardiac status
    4. Assess for head injury
D. Usual medical care
    1. Hydration
    2. Vitamin supplements
    3. High-protein diet
    4. Anticonvulsants to control or prevent seizures

Mild Alcohol Withdrawal

A. Assessment
    1. Nausea and vomiting
    2. Shaking
    3. Headache
    4. Ataxia
B. Intervention
    1. Rest
    2. Quiet environment
C. Usual medical care
    1. Analgesics
    2. Hydration

Delirium Tremens

A. Assessment
    1. Tachycardia
    2. Insomnia
    3. Hypertension
    4. Tremors
    5. Anxiety
    6. Hallucinations (auditory, visual, tactile, and [rarely] olfactory)
    7. Disorientation
    8. Amnesia
    9. Seizures
B. Intervention
    1. Ensure adequate airway and ventilation
    2. Treat for shock
    3. Hydration
    4. Monitor vital signs
    5. Crisis counseling
C. Usual medical care
    1. Treatment for seizures
    2. Anticonvulsant drugs
    3. IV therapy
    4. Sedation
    5. Vitamin therapy
    6. High-protein diet

Disulfiram (Antabuse) Reactions

A. Assessment
    1. Nausea and vomiting
    2. Diaphoresis
    3. Hypotension
    4. Consciousness alterations
    5. Tachycardia
    6. Headache
    7. Facial flushing
    8. Reddened conjunctiva
B. Intervention
    1. Ensure adequate airway, breathing, and circulation
    2. Administer oxygen
C. Usual medical care
    1. IV therapy
    2. Diphenhydramine hydrochloride (Benadryl)
    3. Chlorpheniramine maleate (Chlor-Trimeton)
    4. Ascorbic acid

SEXUAL ASSAULT

A. Victim should be examined and treated as quickly as possible
B. Notify police
C. Victim should not be left alone
D. Victim should be asked who they wish to have stay with them; offer to call family member, friend, or rape crisis center advocate
E. Provide immediate privacy
F. Kindness and support are crucial
G. Obtain history
H. Assess acuteness of physical and psychological needs
I. Assess victim's readiness for physical examination
J. Explain all procedures and encourage questions
K. Obtain necessary written permissions including consent to take photographs
L. Assist victim to undress

TABLE 10-4   Clinical Manifestations and Treatment of Acute Intoxication and Withdrawal of Mind-Altering Drugs

| Drug Group | Acute Intoxication | | Clinical Manifestations of Withdrawal |
	Clinical Manifestations	Treatment	
Narcotics	Respiratory depression, bradycardia, hypotension, cold clammy skin, decreased body temperature; deep sleep, stupor or coma, pinpoint pupils	Maintain ventilation; provide oxygen Give narcotic antagonist: naloxone (Narcan) 0.4 mg IV Monitor vital signs every 15-30 min until patient is conscious Treat for shock	(Not life-threatening) Early: restlessness, irritability, drug craving, yawning, lacrimation, diaphoresis, rhinorrhea, followed by "yen" sleep (intense desire to sleep; sleeps restlessly) Later: awakens with more severe symptoms, nausea, vomiting, anorexia, abdominal cramps, bone and muscle pain, tremors, piloerection (goose flesh)
Other CNS depressants	Same as narcotics (above)	Lavage if recent oral ingestion with possible activated charcoal treatment Maintain ventilation; provide oxygen Monitor vital signs every 15-30 min until patient is conscious Position patient side-lying or prone, not supine Treat for shock Hemodialysis for renal shutdown	(May be life-threatening) Insomnia, restlessness, tremors, anorexia, followed by convulsions, and symptoms similar to DTs (confusion, visual and auditory hallucinations), fever, dehydration
CNS stimulants	Labile cardiovascular symptoms (flushing or pallor, pulse and blood pressure changes, dysrhythmias), hyperpyrexia, mental disturbances (agitation, paranoia, hallucinations), convulsions, circulatory collapse	Give chlorpromazine, 25-50 mg IM Provide a quiet environment Orient patient to reality Monitor vital signs until stable	(Withdrawal is not severe) Somnolence, apathy, irritability, depression, fatigue
Hallucinogens	Physiological toxicity low at doses that produce strong psychological effects Acute panic reaction (bad trip) may lead to suicide "Flashback" episodes Prolonged psychotic disorders (paranoia, depression) Phencyclidine: CNS depression or stimulation may lead to death	Provide quiet, supportive environment and constant attention Give diazepam (Valium), 2-10 mg IM and/or major tranquilizers (Thorazine IM) for severe anxiety	No evidence of withdrawal symptoms
Cannabis	Adverse reactions infrequent Simple depression, paranoid ideation, confusion, disorientation, hallucinations	Provide support and reassurance Give tranquilizer for agitation	(Withdrawal symptoms rare) Insomnia, anorexia
Deliriants	Slowing of heart rate, brain activity, and breathing Slurred speech, blurred vision, inflamed mucous membranes, excessive tearing, and nasal secretions With high doses, loss of consciousness and seizures may occur Brain damage may occur (memory loss, depression, paranoia, hostility) Feeling of stimulation and energy Death may occur from suffocation or cardiac arrest	Maintain airway Maintain respirations Provide quiet environment and provide support Monitor vital signs Orient patient to reality	Chills, hallucinations, headaches, stomach pains, cramps, DTs

From Phipps WJ, Sands JK, Marek JF: *Medical-surgical nursing: concepts and clinical practice*, ed 6, St Louis, 1999, Mosby.

M. Observe for and ask about other possible injuries
N. Assist with physician's examination
1. A water-moistened speculum is used
2. History will indicate the body orifices from which specimens for semen analysis will be required
3. Pubic hair is combed for foreign hairs
4. Clothing is usually saved for analysis, and replacement clothing will be necessary; save in paper bags rather than plastic bags which retain moisture that could cause evidence to deteriorate
5. Follow protocol for collection of specimens that will be used as evidence
6. Testing done for sexually transmitted diseases (STDs), including HIV; follow-up testing done at appropriate intervals
7. STD prophylaxis
8. Pregnancy prophylaxis if contraception not in effect at time of attack: the "morning after" pill (norgestrel [Ovral]), a combination of estrogen and progesterone, given within 72 hours of sexual assault; treatment and side effects should be thoroughly explained
9. If possible and desired, offer accommodations for bathing and douching
10. Care for tissue trauma: immediate and follow-up
11. Care for psychological trauma: immediate and follow-up
12. If present, family and friends often require assistance and counseling

DISASTER

A. Definition: catastrophic event
1. Natural, for example, flood, earthquake, hurricane
2. Man-made, for example, riot, fire, train accident
B. May involve as few as 10 or more than 100 victims
C. Prevention
1. Community planning
2. Public education
D. Assessment
1. Civilian triage: care priority to those whose life is threatened
2. Military triage: care priority to those most likely to survive
E. Planning: the most capable person is designated to sort casualties
F. Intervention
1. First aid should be rendered before victims are transported
2. Care priorities
   a. Ensure airway, breathing, and circulation
   b. Control bleeding
   c. Treat for shock
      (1) Whole blood
      (2) IV fluids
      (3) Parenteral medications
      (4) Pain relief
      (5) Emergency wound care
   d. Preserve motor and sensory functioning
   e. Provide psychologic support
   f. Treat and transport

SUGGESTED READINGS

Anderson KN, Anderson LE, Glanze WD (editors): *Mosby's medical, nursing, and allied health dictionary,* ed 5, St Louis, 1998, Mosby.

American Red Cross: *First aid: responding to emergencies,* St Louis, 1991, Mosby.

Coleman E: Cardiac issues in CPR: what the future might hold, *Nursing 92* 22(4):54, 1992.

Emergency Nurses Association: *Sheehy's emergency nursing: principles & practice,* ed 4, St Louis, 1998, Mosby.

Kidd PS, Sturt P: *Mosby's emergency nursing reference,* St Louis, 1996, Mosby.

Phipps WJ, Sands JK, Marek, JF: *Medical-surgical nursing: concepts and clinical practice,* ed 6, St Louis, 1999, Mosby.

Sheehy SB, Lenehan GP: *Manual of emergency care,* ed 5, St Louis, 1999, Mosby.

Skidmore-Roth L: *Mosby's 2000 nursing drug reference,* St Louis, 2000, Mosby.

Spratto GR, Woods AL: *PDR nurse's drug handbook,* 2000 edition, Montvale, 2000, Medical Economics.

REVIEW QUESTIONS

1. Running to catch a bus, the nurse trips, falls, and sprains her wrist. Which of the following nursing interventions would be <u>most</u> appropriate?
   ① Application of dry heat
   ② Splinting above and below the wrist
   ③ Application of ice for 24 hours
   ④ Observation for sensation changes

2. In the presence of a pulse and a patent airway but the absence of respirations, which of the following actions would be most appropriate for an adult?
   ① Compress the sternum 1½ to 2 inches (3.75 to 5 cm)
   ② Turn the patient on her side
   ③ Sweep the back of the patient's throat
   ④ Continue to deliver breaths

3. A 52-year-old dockworker has come to the emergency room complaining of severe crushing sternal pain that radiates to his left arm. He is cool, pale, and diaphoretic. He believes he is having a heart attack. The first priority of nursing care for this patient is:
   ① Application of the cardiac monitor
   ② Administration of nitroglycerine sublingually
   ③ Prepare for administration of oxygen at 5 L/min
   ④ Insertion of a large-bore IV

4. A male, age 29, had been under stress from his job and has been having trouble sleeping. In an attempt to relax before bedtime, he drank 2 beers, then became confused, and accidentally overdosed himself with temazepam (Restoril) 45 mg. His wife became concerned and brought him to the emergency room. Which of the following assessments should the nurse complete <u>first</u>?
   ① Respiratory rate
   ② Temperature
   ③ Auscultation of lungs
   ④ Determination of pupil size

5. A conscious diabetic arrives at the emergency room with a blood glucose of 378 mg/dl. The treatment of choice is to:
   ① Administer regular insulin
   ② Administer 50% glucose intravenously
   ③ Initiate a dextrose intravenous infusion
   ④ Monitor the potassium level

6. A patient comes to the emergency room with signs and symptoms associated with food poisoning. The patient states he consumed hotdogs, potato salad, potato chips, and carbonated beverages during his picnic lunch. Which of the following foods is the most likely source of his food poisoning?
   ① Hotdogs
   ② Potato salad
   ③ Potato chips
   ④ Carbonated beverages

7. In caring for an unconscious victim of an airway obstruction, the nurse should take which of the following actions first?
   ① Immediately start cardiopulmonary resuscitation
   ② Open the airway using the head-tilt–chin-lift maneuver
   ③ Place victim in supine position on a firm, flat surface
   ④ Remove any foreign object obstructing the airway

8. A 32 year old is admitted to the hospital with an unstable fracture of the pelvis due to a serious motor vehicle accident. As part of the initial assessment of this patient, it is important the nurse identify which of the following?
   ① Nausea and vomiting
   ② External rotation
   ③ Pain on defecation
   ④ Symphysis pubis tenderness

9. The nurse's neighbor comes to the emergency room with a partial airway obstruction following ingestion of sirloin steak for dinner. Which of the following assessments would be consistent with a partial obstruction?
   ① Hacking cough and lethargy
   ② Absent respiratory effort
   ③ Flared nostrils and deep cough
   ④ Anxiety and labored use of accessory muscles

10. A 56-year-old male is brought to the emergency room with possible delirium tremens. Nursing actions would include:
    ① Applying restraints to both arms
    ② Placing him in Trendelenberg position
    ③ Putting a tracheostomy tray in his room
    ④ Initiating seizure precautions

11. When performing adult mouth-to-mouth resuscitation, the rescuer should deliver breaths that are:
    ① Full and quick
    ② Deep and forceful
    ③ Every 4 seconds
    ④ Every 5 seconds

12. A 19-year-old male arrived at the emergency room by a Life-Star helicopter. He had first-, second-, and third-degree burns over 70% of his body. He had been on a bass-fishing trip and was smoking a cigarette. Apparently, there was a small gasoline leak in the motor of the boat, and an explosion and fire occurred. The nurse knows that during initial management of a burn victim the first step to take is:
    ① Immediately begin intravenous fluids
    ② Establish and maintain an adequate airway
    ③ Assess if a cutdown for intravenous fluids is necessary
    ④ Give the burned areas initial care and cover with sterile dressings

13. A child has a bleeding occipital laceration, pain, discoloration, and swelling of the right ulna, and right-sided chest pain that increases on inspiration. Which of the following nursing actions will have the <u>highest</u> priority?
    ① Immobilizing the right arm
    ② Elevating the right arm and head
    ③ Applying ice to the right side of the chest
    ④ Stopping the bleeding and treating for shock

14. When one rescuer is performing cardiac compressions, the hands should be placed:
    ① Directly over the xiphoid process
    ② Two inches below the xiphoid process
    ③ Two finger breadths above the xiphoid process
    ④ Two finger breadths to the left of the xiphoid process

15. An acquaintance known to be taking lithium and under psychiatric care has taken cocaine. She telephones the hospital with abdominal cramps and extreme anxiety and asks what to do. The nurse's best response would be to:
    ① Refer her to the local emergency room
    ② Refer her to her psychiatrist
    ③ Refer her to the cocaine hotline number
    ④ Tell her the nurse cannot get involved right now

16. The nurse is caring for a rape trauma survivor. The initial assessment indicates that the patient appears calm and very much in control. Which characteristic psychologic reaction best describes the patient's behavior?
    ① Denial
    ② Humiliation
    ③ Hyperalertness
    ④ Reorganization

17. A new employee was opening cartons with a razor-sharp box-opener when he slashed a 6-inch gash across his abdomen. A loop of his intestines is protruding through the wound. Which of the following interventions should the nurse do first for this patient while waiting for the doctor?
    ① Cover the wound with a sterile dressing
    ② Apply sterile towels moistened with sterile saline
    ③ Establish a large-bore IV
    ④ Tuck the loop of bowel back into the body

18. To stop the bleeding from an occipital laceration, the best nursing action would be to:
    ① Apply pressure to the site
    ② Apply ice to the site
    ③ Elevate the head
    ④ Elevate the extremities

19. A 21-year-old construction worker was brought to the emergency room when he was found unconscious but breathing in a roadside ditch. He smells strongly of beer. His vital signs are stable. Initial treatment of this patient should include:
    ① Stabilization of the cervical spine
    ② Insertion of an endotracheal tube
    ③ Use of painful stimuli to rouse the patient
    ④ Insertion of a large-bore IV

20. For the rape survivor treated in the emergency room, an appropriate short-term expected outcome (goal) would be for the patient to:
    ① Initiate social interaction
    ② Express feelings about the attack
    ③ Return to her pretrauma level of functioning
    ④ Verbalize two methods of stress management

21. A 23-year-old insulin-dependent diabetic comes to the emergency room with hypoglycemia. Which one of the following signs and symptoms would the nurse expect to observe?
    ① Acetone odor on breath
    ② Complaint of hunger
    ③ Dry, warm skin
    ④ Kussmaul respirations

22. While watching children playing, the nurse notices one child fall and hit his face. His nose is bleeding. The nurse would place the child:
    ① Lying supine with his head elevated
    ② Right side lying, keeping his neck straight
    ③ Sitting upright with his head tilted forward
    ④ Semi-sitting with his head tilted back

23. A 32-year-old insulin-dependent diabetic comes to the emergency department in diabetic ketoacidosis. Which of the following signs and symptoms should the expect to observe?
    ① Sweating and tremors
    ② Increased hunger and thirst
    ③ Dry skin and mucous membranes
    ④ Anxiety and nervousness

24. The ER physician orders epinephrine (Adrenaline) for a patient whom he suspects is going into anaphylactic shock. The nurse is to avoid IM administration of this parenteral suspension into the buttocks because:
    ① Gas gangrene may occur
    ② Necrosis or pain may occur
    ③ It is to be given subcutaneous only
    ④ This site can cause more adverse reactions

25. While a neighbor was working in her garden, she was stung on the arm by a bee. The nurse's first action would be:
    ① Apply a dry sterile dressing
    ② Apply heat to her arm
    ③ Elevate her arm above her heart
    ④ Remove the stinger by scraping

26. The nurse arrives at the scene of a motor vehicle accident. Priority care should be given to the:
    ① Driver with a hoarse voice and coughing blood
    ② Passenger with a head laceration and complaining of knee pain
    ③ Passenger with a bleeding nose and complaining of headache
    ④ Passenger with an arm laceration and crying hysterically

27. While making midmorning rounds, the nurse finds a 60-year-old diabetic patient unconscious on the floor next to his bed. The nurse's immediate action should be to:
    ① Call the physician and prepare IV glucose
    ② Establish an airway
    ③ Administer regular insulin
    ④ Commence mouth-to-mouth resuscitation

28. The nurse's neighbor fell from a ladder and is complaining of pain in his right arm. The nurse notes deformity between the wrist and elbow; the first action would be:
    ① Check for a patent airway
    ② Observe for bleeding at the site
    ③ Apply a splint from the wrist to the elbow
    ④ Have him lie flat with his right arm elevated

29. During a major snowstorm, a 51-year-old male suffers from frostbite of both hands. Since continuous warm water soaks are not available, the nurse would:
    ① Rub the hands with snow
    ② Massage the hands vigorously
    ③ Do aggressive range of motion to both hands
    ④ Apply a dry dressing with gauze between the fingers

30. The nurse comes across a multiple trauma scene. Priority care should be given to the victim:
    ① With cyanosis of the earlobes and nailbeds
    ② Who is hemorrhaging
    ③ Who appears to be in a daze
    ④ With a suspected fracture of the femur

31. A patient dialed 911 after collapsing with a headache, dizziness, and nausea. The ambulance personnel found him unconscious but breathing. The suspect the victim was overcome by carbon monoxide as the result of a faulty furnace. Initial treatment for this patient should include the administration of oxygen at:
    ① 2 liters/minute via nasal cannula
    ② 5 liters/minute via nasal cannula
    ③ 40% per mask
    ④ 100% per mask

32. While sitting in the park in the midafternoon, the nurse hears cries for help from a young mother. The infant is not breathing and has no pulse. To commence CPR, the nurse places two fingers:
    ① At the nipple level
    ② The top half of the sternum
    ③ One finger width below the nipple level
    ④ Two finger widths above the xiphoid process

33. When two rescuers are performing cardiopulmonary resuscitation, the ratio of compressions to respirations is:
    ① 15 : 2
    ② 5 : 2
    ③ 15 : 1
    ④ 5 : 1

34. A friend falls down a set of stairs and dislocates her right shoulder. Which one of the following actions would the nurse perform first?
    ① Apply heat
    ② Check her airway
    ③ Monitor her vital signs
    ④ Apply a splint in the position found

35. Two teenagers are playing Frisbee in the park. Suddenly one of them sustains a blow to the nose from the Frisbee, resulting in rapid epistaxis. To prevent aspiration of blood, the victim should be placed in which of the following positions?
    ① Side-lying
    ② Supine
    ③ Upright with head tilted backward
    ④ Upright with head tilted forward

36. A nurse sees a motorcycle accident happen and stops at the scene. Her assessments include: the motorcyclist is alert, complains of an inability to move his legs, and still wears his helmet. The nurse's next action would be to:
    ① Drive for help
    ② Elevate his legs
    ③ Remove his helmet
    ④ Stay with him

37. A patient comes to the emergency room with a thermal burn to the left hand. The burned skin is red in color, does not blanch, is not painful, and is leathery in nature. The nurse would classify this burn as:
    ① Partial thickness
    ② Second degree
    ③ Full thickness
    ④ Fourth degree

38. While mowing his lawn, the nurse's neighbor steps on a nail. Her first action would be:
    ① Take him to the emergency room
    ② Ask when he had his last tetanus shot

③ Remove the nail and apply a dry sterile dressing
④ Stabilize the wound leaving the nail in place

39. A 40-year-old female is admitted to the ER bleeding profusely from an injury on the lower portion of her right arm. Emergency management of hemorrhage requires the nurse to implement which of the following actions first?
    ① Apply pressure to the bleeding area
    ② Apply a pressure dressing to the bleeding area
    ③ Elevate the injured area
    ④ Immobilize the injured area

40. A nurse witnesses a motorcycle accident in which the victim is thrown forcefully from the vehicle to the pavement. Upon initial assessment of the patient, the nurse notes a crack in the helmet. When administering care to this accident victim, which of the following should receive priority?
    ① Maintain an open airway
    ② Maintain normal body temperature
    ③ Minimize movement of the head
    ④ Monitor respirations

41. A 30-year-old male sustains a crush injury to his left lower arm in a tractor accident. Unable to palpate a radial pulse, the nurse should take which of the following actions?
    ① Check for a pulse in another major artery
    ② Commence cardiopulmonary resuscitation
    ③ Prepare to commence rescue breathing
    ④ Run to the phone and call 9-1-1

42. A resident of a nursing home has been found in cardiac arrest. The nurse arrives with another nurse, and two-rescuer CPR is begun. The nurse administering ventilations must give a breath:
    ① Whenever possible
    ② Immediately before the 5th compression
    ③ During the pause after the 5th compression
    ④ During the compression phase of every 5th compression

43. At the nurse's 12-year-old son's baseball game, she sees the center fielder slump to the ground. The nurse runs to him and determines that he is not breathing and has no pulse. She places her hand in position to deliver chest compressions. The correct depth of compression would be:
    ① ½ to 1 inch
    ② 1 to 1½ inches
    ③ 1½ to 2 inches
    ④ 2 to 2½ inches

44. Assessment protocol for a fracture of the right ulna should include which of the following nursing actions?
    ① Ascertaining range-of-motion (ROM) limitations
    ② Observing for changes in sensation, temperature, and color
    ③ Determining the presence of crepitus
    ④ Preventing limb shortening

45. A 36-year-old male is brought to the emergency room with an overdose of morphine. The first medication to administer is:
    ① Disulfiram (Antabuse)
    ② Epinephrine (Adrenalin)
    ③ Methylprednisone (Solu-Medrol)
    ④ Naloxone hydrochloride (Narcan)

46. A 23-year-old female arrives at the hospital in an agitated state, an elevated blood pressure, a temperature of 100.1° F, and reports having hallucinations. The nurse should suspect that the patient has consumed:
① Inhalants
② Stimulants
③ Depressants
④ Hallucinogens

47. While the nurse's 14-year-old neighbor boy is mowing her lawn, he is stung by a bee. He starts wheezing and complaining of difficulty breathing. The nurse takes him to the emergency room where he is diagnosed as having:
① Anaphylaxis
② Asthma
③ Hay fever
④ Pneumonia

48. While assessing a motor vehicle accident victim, the nurse notes fluid leaking from the right ear. The nurse suspects he has suffered a:
① Concussion
② Contusion
③ Basilar skull fracture
④ Intracranial bleeding

49. A 40-year-old female arrives in the emergency room with a fractured left wrist. Which assessment should be reported immediately?
① Complaints of pain in left wrist
② Complaints of fingers being swollen
③ Complaints of wrist being bruised
④ Complaints of numbness in fingers

50. While a nurse and a friend are hiking in the woods, the friend is bitten on the left ankle by a snake. The nurse's first action would be:
① Elevate the ankle
② Try to catch the snake
③ Immobilize the extremity
④ Help the friend walk back to the car

51. Which of the following would be a priority nursing concern for a victim with severe burns?
① Administering cardiopulmonary resuscitation
② Relieving pain
③ Stopping the burning process
④ Tetanus prophylaxis

52. The nurse is alone, caring for a neighbor's infant. When the nurse checks the napping baby, she sees that he is limp and has a bluish tint. The nurse commences CPR. After 20 cycles of compressions and ventilations, the nurse should:
① Activate EMS
② Check for breathing
③ Check for return of carotid pulse
④ Check for return of brachial pulse

53. A 20-year-old accident victim arrives at the emergency room after a bad car accident. He has lost so much blood that he is going into shock. The nurse knows that this type of shock is known as:
① Septic shock
② Neurogenic shock
③ Cardiogenic shock
④ Hypovolemic shock

54. The nurse is the first to arrive on the scene of a motorcycle accident. She notes that the bone is sticking out through the skin of the victim's leg. The nurse's first action would be to:
① Apply a splint to the victim's leg
② Only apply antibiotic ointment to the skin
③ Cover the area with a dressing
④ Push the bone back through the skin

55. While dressing for the prom, the nurse's 16-year-old daughter is complaining about wearing a medical identification tag. The nurse's best response would be:
① "You have to wear it so people will know you are diabetic."
② "If you promise to follow your diet, you can leave it at home."
③ "Your friends know you are diabetic, so you do not have to wear it."
④ "You can wear it around your ankle."

56. An 18 year old was on a rock-climbing expedition with his class when he fell 8 feet onto gravel. He is complaining of pain in his left elbow. It is obviously deformed when he presents to the emergency room. Which of the following should be included in the assessment of this patient's condition?
① Level of consciousness
② Presence of a radial pulse
③ Ability to adduct the elbow
④ Presence of ecchymosis on the upper arm

57. A 10 year old is stabbed in the abdomen on the school playground. The nurse responds to the other children's cries for help. By the time the nurse reaches the child, he has a rapid pulse, his lips are cyanotic, and he is pale and diaphoretic. The priority nursing action would be to:
① Elevate his feet to promote venous return
② Ensure a patent airway and maintain breathing
③ Administer fluids rapidly to restore blood volume
④ Cover him with a jacket to maintain body temperature

58. A mother reports that her 5-year-old son was found drinking from a bottle of wine. On the way to the hospital, he fell asleep. The nurse's first priority is to:
① Protect the airway
② Monitor cardiac status
③ Take seizure precautions
④ Document observations

59. A 3-year-old boy is brought to the emergency room from the day care center. He was bitten by another child. His parents should be instructed to:
① Contact a lawyer
② Wake the child every 2 hours
③ Obtain the name of the other child
④ Administer all the prescribed antibiotic

60. A 26-year-old female has come to the emergency room with lower right quadrant abdominal pain. She complains of feeling thirsty and is requesting a drink of water. To appease her thirst, the nurse should:
① Provide ice chips
② Provide a glass of water
③ Provide orange juice
④ Withhold fluids until tests are complete

61. A 58-year-old executive is admitted to the ER with a myocardial infarction. The nurse, assessing the patient for signs of shock, notes a stable blood pressure. Which of the following should the nurse also include in the assessment of shock?
    ① For tachycardia and skin temperature
    ② Pupils every 30 minutes
    ③ For elevated temperature
    ④ For mental confusion and slurred speech

62. When one rescuer is performing cardiopulmonary resuscitation on an adult, the rate of cardiac compressions is:
    ① 80 times per minute
    ② 5 times per minute
    ③ 60 times per minute
    ④ 15 times per minute

63. The treatment of choice for an <u>unconscious</u> diabetic diagnosed with hypoglycemia is to administer:
    ① 10 units regular insulin subcutaneously
    ② 50 cc 0.9% sodium chloride solution intravenously
    ③ 50% dextrose intravenously
    ④ 100 cc orange juice orally

64. The medication given to prevent pregnancy in a sexual assault survivor is:
    ① Cefixime (Suprax)
    ② Doxycycline (Vibramycin)
    ③ Estrogen-Progesterone (Oval)
    ④ Spectinomycin (Trobicin)

65. The police deliver to the ER a panicky man experiencing tremors, chills and sweating, intestinal cramps, and nausea. His eyes are watery and his nose is running. The nurse should suspect:
    ① Stimulant withdrawal
    ② Narcotics withdrawal
    ③ An overdose of narcotics
    ④ An overdose of hallucinogens

66. Paper bags are used to hold the clothing of a sexual assault survivor because:
    ① Paper bags are less expensive and can be reused
    ② Paper bags hide the evidence from view of any witnesses
    ③ Plastic bags hold air and would be more difficult to stack for the chain of custody
    ④ Plastic bags would hold moisture, which could cause deterioration of evidence

67. A hunter comes to the emergency room with feet that are cold, damp, and appear shriveled. He is most likely suffering from:
    ① Chilblain
    ② Frostbite
    ③ Hypothermia
    ④ Immersion foot

68. The nurse's neighbor shouts to come quickly, that her child has been stung by a bee. Which of the following skin manifestations would indicate that a general systemic reaction is developing?
    ① Body itching
    ② Facial pallor
    ③ Localized redness
    ④ Localized swelling

69. A high school student has chemicals splashed into his eyes during an experiment in chemistry lab. The school nurse's <u>first</u> action would be to:
    ① Call an ophthalmologist
    ② Flush his eyes with water
    ③ Notify his parents
    ④ Take him to the emergency room

70. The sleeve of a robe of a 45-year-old diabetic catches fire while she is cooking breakfast. She suffered superficial burns over 5% of her arm. Her burns would be classified as:
    ① Minor
    ② Moderate
    ③ Major
    ④ Simple

71. Which of the following patients would be most at risk for mortality following burn injury?
    ① A 7-year-old male
    ② A 38-year-old female
    ③ A 12-year-old female
    ④ A 78-year-old male

72. When a patient in diabetic ketoacidosis comes to the emergency room, blood electrolyte levels should be monitored. The nurse is aware that the <u>most important</u> electrolyte to monitor in this patient is:
    ① Calcium
    ② Chloride
    ③ Potassium
    ④ Sodium

73. Anticoagulant therapy is commonly used in which one of the following chest conditions?
    ① Flail chest
    ② Hemothorax
    ③ Pulmonary embolism
    ④ Sucking chest wound

74. A 79-year-old female comes to the emergency clinic appearing very anxious and complaining of nausea, headache, and muscle cramping. Suspecting heat exhaustion from the history given by the patient, the nurse's <u>first</u> action would be to:
    ① Call the physician immediately
    ② Monitor the patient's temperature
    ③ Administer an oral balanced salt solution
    ④ Move the patient to a cool, quiet room

75. A 47-year-old female comes to the emergency room with a gram-negative infection that is being treated by several antibiotics. She is complaining of "feeling funny, being thirsty, and being restless." The nurse's assessment findings include skin flushed and moist, temperature 103.8° F, pulse 124, respirations 30, and blood pressure 90/54. The nurse suspects that she is developing:
    ① Anaphylactic shock
    ② Hypovolemic shock
    ③ Neurogenic shock
    ④ Septic shock

76. A drug that can be used for treating the person with chronic alcoholism is:
    ① Disulfiram (Antabuse)
    ② Epinephrine (Adrenalin)
    ③ Methylprednisone (Solu-Medrol)
    ④ Naloxone (Narcan)

77. When assessing a trauma victim, the nurse observes that the chest moves inward when he breathes in and moves outward when he breathes out. This is a symptom of:
    ① Flail chest
    ② Pulmonary embolism
    ③ Simple rib fracture
    ④ Tension pneumothorax

78. Which individual is at greatest risk to suffer from heat stroke?
    ① 9-month-old infant girl
    ② 23-year-old male
    ③ 37-year-old female
    ④ 51-year-old male

79. The nurse knows that oils or ointments should not be applied to severe burns. Which is the chief reason for this principle?
    ① Burn areas should be left open to the air
    ② These products impede ice application to burn areas
    ③ These products prevent blisters from being broken
    ④ These products seal in heat

80. A young mother accidentally stepped on a nail as she ran to see why her children were crying. The nail is still embedded in her foot when she comes to the emergency room. When assessing the nature of the injury, the nurse should first:
    ① Remove the nail and cleanse the wound with hydrogen peroxide
    ② Secure the nail with tape until the physician sees the patient
    ③ Administer tetanus toxoid 0.5 cc IM
    ④ Copiously irrigate the foot with normal saline

81. The nurse knows that teaching is successful when a patient with chilblains states:
    ① "I should not use tobacco products."
    ② "I know I do not need to be careful when I go out in the cold."
    ③ "I know that I need to warm my fingers and toes rapidly."
    ④ "I should rub or massage my fingers and toes vigorously."

82. A 21-year-old unconscious male is brought to the ER by a friend. His breath smells of alcohol and the friend reports that they were at a fraternity party where there was heavy drinking. The nurse should:
    ① Treat for shock
    ② Ensure adequate airway and ventilation
    ③ Recommend rest in a quiet environment
    ④ Administer disulfiram (Antabuse) immediately

83. The new CPR recommendations for calling for help suggest "Phone first" for an adult and "Phone fast" for a child. The best explanation for this rule is:
    ① Children can go longer without oxygen
    ② An arrest in a child is usually caused by an obstructed airway
    ③ An arrest in an adult is usually caused by cardiac arrhythmias
    ④ It is usually too late by the time the first responder finds an adult

84. A laboratory employee has sustained chemical burns to his left forearm, thigh, and foot. Which of the following nursing actions should be taken initially?
    ① Apply ice to the burns immediately
    ② Cover the burns with wet, sterile dressings
    ③ Flush burns with cool, running water
    ④ Treat the victim for shock and tend to the burns later

85. During an intake interview in the ER, the nurse asks the patient if he is on any medication. He reports that he is on Methadone. The nurse knows that this patient is being treated for withdrawal from:
    ① Alcohol
    ② Heroin
    ③ Barbiturates
    ④ Benzodiazepines

86. While playing basketball, a 17-year-old male was hit in the right eye, resulting in a "black eye." Immediate first aid would be to apply:
    ① Antibiotic ointment
    ② Bilateral eye patches
    ③ A cold compress
    ④ A warm compress

87. A male, age 7, is brought to the emergency room on July 4th. A firecracker was thrown at him, and it exploded as it hit his bare left arm in the deltoid area. The nurse noted that the epidermis, dermis, and subcutaneous tissues were burned about 2.5 centimeters in diameter. There were also reddened areas all around the deltoid area. The child states that it doesn't hurt very much. This burn would be characterized as:
    ① First-degree burn
    ② Second-degree burn
    ③ Third-degree burn
    ④ Fourth-degree burn

88. An abdominal stab wound victim is brought to the emergency room. An assessment reveals a loop of the small intestine escaping the wound. The nurse's first action would be:
    ① Administer oxygen
    ② Administer tetanus toxoid
    ③ Take vital signs
    ④ Apply a wet dressing to the abdomen

89. A 42-year-old insurance broker sustained severe full-thickness burns to his pelvis and legs when he was trapped in a burning car. He was admitted to the ER and has been urinating red urine for several hours. The presence of red urine indicates this patient has possibly sustained:
    ① Kidney damage
    ② Liver damage
    ③ Muscle damage
    ④ Integumentary damage

90. Antibiotic therapy is commonly used in which one of the following chest conditions?
    ① Flail chest
    ② Hemothorax
    ③ Pulmonary embolism
    ④ Sucking chest wound

91. One morning a young mother was making chocolate chip cookies. She used one package mix that called for adding 3 eggs. She mixed the dough and was interrupted by a phone call. Her children, age 7 and 9, helped themselves to the cookie dough. That night both children were complaining of severe stomach cramps, vomiting, headaches, and fever. The nurse, in checking what the children ate that day, recognizes this could be:
    ① Botulism
    ② Salmonella
    ③ Trichinois
    ④ Anaerobic myositis

92. A 35-year-old male comes to the emergency room with electrical burns to one hand. These burns would be classified as:
    ① Minor
    ② Moderate
    ③ Major
    ④ Superficial

93. A young man has been diagnosed with a strain of the left ankle. He would be instructed to:
    ① Sit quietly with his foot on the floor
    ② Soak his ankle in warm water
    ③ Use crutches with no weight bearing
    ④ Wear white cotton socks

94. The nurse is driving in a rural area on an isolated country road and sees a child, approximately 12 to 15 years of age, lying in the middle of the road with an overturned bicycle not far away. Which of the following nursing actions should she take immediately?
    ① Keep driving to the nearest gas station and telephone for an ambulance
    ② Turn around and go back to the nearest main highway and hail a police car
    ③ Proceed with a rapid clinical assessment with emphasis on ABCs
    ④ Check with local authorities for specifics on the state's Good Samaritan law

95. The mother of a 3-year-old tells the nurse that her daughter has swallowed bleach, which was stored under the kitchen sink. A rapid assessment reveals no evidence of acute airway swelling. Which of the following interventions should the nurse take?
    ① Absorb the poison with activated charcoal
    ② Give nothing by mouth
    ③ Give water or milk
    ④ Induce vomiting with syrup of ipecac

96. A competitive racer had a near drowning accident when the canoe she was paddling tipped over and struck her on the head. Her lips and nails are cyanotic. Immediate emergency care for this patient's hypoxia includes:
    ① Insertion of chest tubes to drain the water
    ② Cricothyroid puncture to ensure a patent airway
    ③ Placing her in Trendelenburg position to facilitate fluid drainage
    ④ Bag-valve-mask resuscitation

97. After an earthquake, which of the following victims would be triaged with the highest priority?
    ① 4-year-old boy crying with a bleeding head laceration
    ② 26-year-old female dazed with a broken right arm
    ③ 48-year-old male unresponsive with contusions of the head
    ④ 70-year-old female alert diabetic with burns of both arms

98. The presence of human immunodeficiency virus infection is increasing. Which of the following measures is essential for the nurse to incorporate into care?
    ① Ask the patient his or her HIV status
    ② Have an HIV-positive health care worker attend to the patient
    ③ Adhere strictly to "standard precautions."
    ④ Observe standard precautions only if exposure to blood or body fluids is obvious

99. A known alcohol and substance user comes to the emergency room with a hand laceration. He has not consumed any alcohol or taken any drugs for 3 days. He starts having hallucinations. This is most likely caused by withdrawal from:
    ① Alcohol
    ② Hallucinogens
    ③ Narcotics
    ④ Stimulants

100. While exercising with a friend, an individual with diabetes complains of feeling weak and hungry. The friend's first action should be to:
    ① Have her lie down
    ② Give her some hard candy
    ③ Start cardiopulmonary resuscitation
    ④ Give her an injection of regular insulin

ANSWERS AND RATIONALES

1. Knowledge, implementation, basic care and comfort (a)
   ❸ This prevents edema, facilitates vasoconstriction, increases blood viscosity, and acts as a local anesthetic.
   ① Dry heat is appropriate for treating a strain.
   ②, ④ These two nursing interventions are appropriate for treatment of a fracture.

2. Application, implementation, psychosocial adaptation (a)
   ❹ Always continue breathing until help arrives or victim spontaneously resumes breathing.
   ① The sternum should not be compressed in the presence of a pulse.
   ② The victim must be in a supine position.
   ③ This measure is performed in the presence of an upper airway obstruction only.

3. Comprehension, implementation, physiological adaptation (b)
   ❸ Immediate oxygen may prevent pain and tissue damage.
   ① It is more important to try to save tissue.
   ② Further assessment needs to be done before any medication can be given.
   ④ An IV line should be inserted after assessment is completed.

4. Comprehension, assessment, reduction of risk potential (b)
   ❶ Sedatives combined with alcohol cause respiratory depression.
   ② Temperature is not affected by these drugs.
   ③ Lung sounds should be included in the baseline assessment.
   ④ Pupil size and reactivity are included in a neurologic assessment.

5. Comprehension, implementation, pharmacological therapies (b)
   ❶ Regular insulin is administered either intravenously or subcutaneously to treat the elevated blood glucose.
   ② This is the recommended treatment for hypoglycemia.
   ③ An intravenous infusion should be initiated with a normal saline solution not a dextrose solution.
   ④ Blood potassium levels should be monitored, but this is not a treatment.

6. Comprehension, assessment, physiological adaptation (b)
   ❷ Potato salad is made with salad dressing on mayonnaise, which are egg products. *Salmonella* poisoning is the most frequent cause of food-borne illness and is caused by contaminated eggs or egg spoilage.
   ① Hotdogs are highly processed/preserved meat products that are normally not associated with food-borne illness.
   ③, ④ These products are normally not associated with food-borne illness.

7. Application, implementation, physiological adaptation (c)
   ❸ With an unconscious victim, the priority is airway. To open the airway, the victim first has to be properly positioned.
   ①, ②, ④ These actions, while appropriate, are not done first as indicated in the rationale for #3.

8. Comprehension, assessment, physiological adaptation (a)
   ❹ This person will likely complain of pubic tenderness due to hemorrhage, a serious life-threatening complication; the physician should be notified immediately.
   ①, ③ This is not an important assessment at this time.
   ② This is indicative of a fractured hip.

9. Comprehension, assessment, physiological adaptation (b)
   ❹ Accessory chest muscles will aid in bringing oxygen to the lungs. Anxiety is common with air hunger.
   ① Lethargy is inconsistent with partial obstruction.
   ② Absence of spontaneous respirations indicates total airway occlusion.
   ③ A deep cough requires deep inspiration.

10. Application, implementation, safety and infection control (c)
    ❹ An individual with delirium tremens could have seizures.
    ①, ②, ③ These actions are not indicated at this time.

11. Knowledge, planning, physiological adaptation (b)
    ❹ This is standard rescue breathing procedure.
    ① Breaths should be full but at 1½ to 2 seconds per breath, allowing the lungs to deflate between breaths.
    ② Breaths should be given at the lowest possible pressure to avoid gastric distention.
    ③ This is not standard rescue breathing procedure.

12. Application, implementation, physiological adaptation (b)
    ❷ An open airway always takes first priority in any situation.
    ① Beginning intravenous fluids is the next step, after establishing airway and circulation maintenance.
    ③ Assessing for a cutdown for IV fluids can be done after determining the need for IV fluids.
    ④ Covering the burned areas with sterile dressings and gauze is done after airway maintenance and fluid maintenance are established.

13. Application, implementation, physiological adaptation (c)
    ❹ Priority is always airway, breathing, and circulation.
    ①, ②, ③ These are appropriate, but not the highest priority.

14. Knowledge, implementation, safety and infection control (b)
    ❸ This distance prevents damage to ribs and internal structures while providing adequate cardiac output.
    ① This may cause lower rib damage and low cardiac output.
    ② This may cause internal organ damage and no cardiac output.
    ④ This may cause left lower rib damage.

15. Application, implementation, safety and infection control (b)
    ❶ This victim requires immediate medical care.
    ② This is appropriate, but not the first priority.
    ③ This is inappropriate; the victim needs immediate medical care.
    ④ Referring a victim to a physician does not put the nurse at legal risk; not referring a victim to a physician could result in legal action being initiated against the nurse.

16. Comprehension, assessment, psychosocial adaptation (b)
    ❷ The acute stage, disorganization, immediately follows sexual assault and is either verbally expressed or hidden. Regardless of the manner of expression, the survivor experiences feelings of shock, restlessness, anger, guilt, confusion, and fear.
    ①, ③ These usually follow acute disorganization and precede reorganization.
    ④ Reorganization indicates that the survivor has put the event in perspective and moves toward some degree of recovery.

17. Comprehension, implementation, reduction of risk potential (c)
    ❷ Sterile towels moistened with saline will prevent the mucous membranes from drying out.
    ① A dry dressing may adhere to the bowel and cause more damage.
    ③ Preventing further damage to the bowel is the primary concern.
    ④ Only a physician should return body parts to their proper position.

18. Knowledge, implementation, physiological adaptation (b)
    ❶ The first step in treating hemorrhage is to apply pressure for at least 6 minutes.
    ② Application of ice is not an emergency measure.
    ③ Elevating the affected part aids in controlling the bleeding, but would not stop the bleeding.
    ④ This action would have no effect on occipital bleeding.

19. Comprehension, implementation, basic care and comfort (b)
    ❶ Because the nature of the injury is unknown, protection of the cervical spine is imperative.
    ② An endotracheal tube is not recommended; he is breathing on his own and his vital signs are stable.
    ③ Determining level of consciousness is secondary to preserving function.
    ④ Because his vitals are stable, insertion of an IV is not a priority.

20. Comprehension, planning, coping and adaptation (c)
    ❷ This is the only appropriately written short-term goal; it is patient centered, realistic, reachable, and time oriented; identifying and expressing feelings are essential to develop coping skills
    ①, ③, ④ These are long-term goals.

21. Knowledge, assessment, physiological adaptation (a)
    ❷ This is a symptom of hypoglycemia.
    ①, ③, ④ These are signs and symptoms of diabetic ketoacidosis.

22. Application, implementation, basic care and comfort (b)
    ❸ This position prevents blood from flowing down the back of the throat.
    ①, ②, ④ These positions are not appropriate because sitting upright prevents swallowing or aspiration of blood.

23. Comprehension, assessment, physiological adaptation (b)
    ❸ These are signs characteristically seen in diabetic ketoacidosis.
    ① Dryness is seen.

② These are signs of diabetes.
④ Lethargy is more common.

24. Knowledge, implementation, pharmacological therapies (c)
    ❶ Gas gangrene may occur because epinephrine reduces oxygen tension of the tissues, encouraging the growth of contaminating organisms.
    ② Necrosis caused by vasoconstriction usually occurs from repeated local injections.
    ③ Epinephrine can be given SQ or IM; if administered IM, site should be massaged to counteract possible vasoconstriction; the nurse should avoid IM administration of the parenteral suspension into the buttocks.
    ④ This site does not necessarily affect the adverse reactions to a drug that an individual may have. If an adverse reaction occurs, the physician will adjust the dosage or discontinue the drug.

25. Knowledge, implementation, basic care and comfort (a)
    ❹ Stingers should be removed by scraping. Pulling the stinger could release more venom.
    ① A dressing is not necessary.
    ② Ice would be applied rather than heat.
    ③ Elevating the arm is not necessary.

26. Application, evaluation, physiological adaptation (c)
    ❶ The driver could have a fractured larynx and may develop respiratory distress.
    ②, ③, ④ Pressure should be applied to all bleeding sites, but the passengers do not appear to have any potentially life-threatening injuries.

27. Application, implementation, physiological adaptation (a)
    ❷ With an unconscious victim, the priority is always airway, breathing, and circulation.
    ① This assumes that the patient is in insulin shock.
    ③ This assumes that the patient is in diabetic coma.
    ④ Mouth-to-mouth resuscitation cannot be given until a patent airway has been established.

28. Comprehension, implementation, basic care and comfort (a)
    ❸ The splint should be applied above and below the fracture.
    ①, ② Although this is important, there are no indications of these problems.
    ④ Although the fracture should be elevated, there is no need for him to lie flat.

29. Comprehension, implementation, reduction of risk potential (c)
    ❹ This action will prevent further injury to the fingers.
    ①, ② These actions are contraindicated.
    ③ The frostbitten parts should not be used.

30. Application, planning, physiological adaptation (a)
    ❶ Oxygenation is compromised in this situation, and airway is always the priority.
    ② Oxygenation will be compromised if the hemorrhaging is not controlled or stopped.
    ③ There is no immediate problem with airway, breathing, or circulation.
    ④ Fractures are suspected at multiple trauma scenes; the priorities are always airway, breathing, and circulation, in that order.

31. Comprehension, planning, basic care and comfort (b)
❹ Saturating the blood with oxygen may allow the body's tissues to remain oxygenated.
① This rate of flow would allow the carboxyhemoglobin to remain in place.
② This rate of flow would not provide adequate tissue oxygenation.
③ This rate of flow would not break the affinity of carbon monoxide for hemoglobin.

32. Knowledge, implementation, physiological adaptation (a)
❸ Sternal compression is performed approximately the width of one finger below the nipple level.
①, ② These positions are too high.
④ This is the position for children and adults.

33. Knowledge, planning, physiological adaptation (a)
❹ In two-rescuer CPR the standard ratio of compressions to breaths is 5:1.
① 15:2 is correct for one-rescuer CPR.
② This would be overventilation.
③ This is too many compressions for two-rescuer CPR.

34. Knowledge, implementation, reduction of risk potential (a)
❹ The dislocation should be splinted in the position found rather than risk further injury.
① Cold applications would be used rather than heat applications.
②, ③ Although these are good actions, they are not appropriate at this time.

35. Application, implementation, basic care and comfort (b)
❹ This is the only position that will prevent the victim from swallowing blood and being at risk for aspiration.
①, ②, ③ The victim is at risk for aspiration in any of these positions.

36. Application, planning, reduction of risk potential (b)
❹ The nurse should stay with him and continue to assess him until help arrives.
① The nurse should not leave him alone.
② The nurse should not move his legs; this could cause further damage.
③ Since the airway is adequate, the helmet must not be removed.

37. Application, assessment, physiological adaptation (c)
❸ This is also called a third-degree burn; the painless nature of this burn in conjunction with a lack of capillary refill and red, leathery skin are characteristics of a full-thickness burn.
① A first-degree (partial thickness) burn is normally painful and will blanch when the skin is compressed.
② A second-degree burn is normally painful in nature, with blistered skin, is wet and weepy, and blanches.
④ A fourth-degree burn, similar in appearance to a third-degree burn, has charring in the very deepest areas, and requires autografting for healing; if an extremity is involved, amputation is likely.

38. Comprehension, planning, reduction of risk potential (b)
❹ Removal of the nail could cause more damage. The wound must be assessed by a physician.
① Medical evaluation is needed, but the nail should be stabilized and left in place first.
② Although he will probably need a tetanus shot, it is not appropriate now.
③ Removal of the nail may cause further injury.

39. Comprehension, implementation, reduction of risk potential (a)
❶ All are correct interventions for hemorrhage, but the priority is to stop or control the bleeding.
② This is appropriate intervention after bleeding is under control.
③ After applying the pressure dressing, the affected body part should be elevated to further aid in control of hemorrhage.
④ Movement stimulates circulation; immobilization will also aid in controlling hemorrhage.

40. Application, implementation, physiological adaptation (c)
❶ The priority is always ABC: airway, breathing, and circulation.
② Although important, this is not the priority.
③ This is necessary and important, but not the priority.
④ A person cannot breathe unless the airway is patent.

41. Application, implementation, physiological adaptation (a)
❶ The radial artery can be sufficiently damaged in a crush injury so that it will not be palpable. Whenever a pulse cannot be palpated, move on to the next major artery to check circulation.
②, ③ There is no indication of need in this situation.
④ Take care of airway, breathing, and circulation first; send another person to activate EMS if possible.

42. Comprehension, implementation, physiological adaptation (a)
❸ The compression-to-ventilation ratio is 5:1 with a pause for ventilation of 1½ to 2 seconds consisting primarily of inspiration.
② With the correct ratio being 5:1, the fifth compression must occur before the respiration.
①, ④ Ventilation (inspiration) must occur during a pause; exhalation occurs during chest compression.

43. Knowledge, implementation, physiological adaptation (a)
❷ Standard CPR guidelines state that the child's chest should be compressed 1 to 1½ inches, or ⅓ to ½ of chest's total height.
① This is the appropriate depth for infants.
③ This is the appropriate depth for adults.
④ This is too deep for CPR compressions.

44. Knowledge, implementation, reduction of risk potential (b)
❷ These are appropriate assessments of circulation.
①, ③ This may cause further damage to the ulna.
④ Prevention is not part of assessment.

45. Knowledge, implementation, pharmacological therapies (a)
❹ Naloxone hydrochloride (Narcan) is the narcotic antagonist.
①, ②, ③ These drugs are not narcotic antagonists.

46. Comprehension, assessment, physiological adaptation (b)
❷ Effects of stimulant overdose include agitation, increased body temperature and blood pressure, hallucinations, convulsions, and possible death.
① Inhalant overdose will cause anxiety, but respirations will be depressed.

③ Depressants will not cause any of these symptoms.
④ Hallucinogens will cause hallucinations and elevated blood pressure, but not agitation.

47. Application, assessment, physiological adaptation (b)
❶ Wheezing and respiratory distress are symptoms of an anaphylatic reaction to the bee sting.
②, ③, ④ Although wheezing and respiratory distress are common with these disorders, the precipitating event was the bee sting.

48. Comprehension, assessment, physiological adaptation (a)
❸ This is a symptom of a basilar skull fracture.
①, ②, ④ This symptom is not seen in these conditions.

49. Application, assessment, reduction of risk potential (c)
❹ This could indicate nerve injury.
①, ②, ③ These are typical assessments for a fracture.

50. Application, implementation, physiological adaptation (c)
❸ Immobilize the extremity at or below the level of the heart to decrease spread of the venom.
① The ankle should be kept in a dependent position.
② This is not a priority.
④ The friend should be kept still to decrease the spread of the venom.

51. Application, implementation, physiological adaptation (a)
❸ The hemodynamic instability following burn injury must be stopped to proceed with airway, breathing, and circulation and to prevent further trauma to the victim.
① The situation does not indicate that CPR is necessary.
②, ④ This is appropriate, but not the priority.

52. Knowledge, implementation, basic care and comfort (a)
❶ Standard infant CPR procedure requires 1 minute of CPR, then activation of EMS.
②, ④ After activation of EMS, the rescuer should resume CPR by checking for return of breathing and brachial pulse.
③ Carotid pulse is not used in infant CPR.

53. Knowledge, assessment, physiological adaptation (b)
❹ Hypovolemic shock is a state of physical collapse and prostration caused by massive blood loss, circulatory dysfunction, and inadequate tissue perfusion.
① Septic shock results from complications of septicemia, a condition in which infectious agents release toxins into the blood.
② Neurogenic shock results from widespread dilation of blood vessels, caused by an imbalance in autonomic stimulation of smooth muscles in vessel walls.
③ Cardiogenic shock results from any type of heart failure.

54. Application, implementation, reduction of risk potential (c)
❸ The area should be covered with a dressing to reduce risk of infection until it can be evaluated.
① A splint could put pressure on the fracture site causing further injury.
② Although this is not totally inappropriate, the victim could be allergic to the ointment; the best action is to just apply a dressing.
④ Attempting to return the bone could cause further injury.

55. Application, implementation, prevention and early detection of disease (b)
❹ It is important that she take the medical identification tag with her in case of an emergency.
① Although she must wear the tag, it does not have to be conspicuous.
② Despite following her diet, she could be in an accident and would have no tag.
③ Despite her friends' awareness, she could be in an accident and have no tag.

56. Application, assessment, physiological adaptation (c)
❷ Determining the presence of the pulse is an indication of vascular intactness.
① If he is complaining of pain, he is alert.
③ The elbow is only capable of extension and flexion.
④ Bruising on the upper arm is likely as a result of the fall.

57. Application, implementation, physiological adaptation (a)
❷ The victim is displaying signs of shock; airway and breathing are the priorities.
①, ③, ④ These are interventions for shock that follow establishment of airway, breathing, and circulation.

58. Application, implementation, reduction of risk potential
❶ The risk is that the child will vomit and aspirate.
②, ③, ④ These are appropriate actions but not a first priority.

59. Application, planning, pharmacological therapies (b)
❹ Antibiotics are prescribed to prevent infection and the *full dose* should be administered.
① Although there is no need to contact a lawyer, this is clearly not within the realm of nursing practice.
② This is appropriate for a child with a head injury.
③ The name of the other child is probably a matter of record.

60. Comprehension, assessment, safety and infection control (b)
❹ The patient should be kept NPO because she may require immediate surgery.
① Because of the situation, an order for oral fluids would be necessary.
② Ingestion of water could delay surgery.
③ Clear liquids would be offered first, providing there was an order for liquids.

61. Application, implementation, physiological adaptation (c)
❶ Blood pressure does not always drop immediately. Increased heart rate and cold, clammy skin are signs of shock.
② Pupils will not indicate shock until the very late stages, after brain damage has occurred.
③ Elevated temperature will be a sign of cardiac damage, but not in the first 24 to 48 hours. It is not an indication of shock.
④ Mental confusion is a late sign of shock.

62. Knowledge, planning, physiological adaptation (a)
❶ Standard CPR procedure calls for a 15:2 count for 60 seconds providing 80 compressions in one-rescuer CPR.
②, ③, ④ These are inadequate compressions when administering CPR on an adult.

63. Application, implementation, pharmacological therapies (b)
  ❸ This is the treatment of choice for the unconscious diabetic; the intravenous route is the most appropriate and fastest manner in which to administer glucose.
  ①, ② These are not appropriate.
  ④ This would be appropriate treatment for the conscious diabetic.

64. Knowledge, planning, pharmacological therapies (a)
  ❸ This medication is used to prevent pregnancy.
  ①, ②, ④ These medications are used to treat sexually transmitted diseases.

65. Comprehension, assessment, physiological adaptation (b)
  ❷ Watery eyes and runny nose are telltale signs of narcotic withdrawal and are not associated with any other drug classification.
  ①, ④ These two situations would not cause the watery eyes and runny nose.
  ③ With a narcotic overdose, there would not be chills, sweating, or intestinal cramps; and the patient would be near coma.

66. Comprehension, implementation, basic care and comfort (c)
  ❹ Paper bags do not hold moisture, which could cause deterioration of evidence.
  ①, ②, ③ These are not appropriate responses.

67. Knowledge, evaluation, physiological adaptation (a)
  ❹ These are symptoms of immersion foot.
  ① Chilblain is evidenced by redness and swelling of the skin caused by excessive exposure to cold.
  ② Frostbite is the traumatic effect of extreme cold on skin and subcutaneous tissues evidenced by distinct pallor of exposed skin surfaces.
  ③ Hypothermia is an abnormal and dangerous condition in which the temperature of the body is below 95° F, usually caused by prolonged exposure to cold and/or damp conditions.

68. Comprehension, assessment, physiological adaptation (a)
  ❶ Body itching is the only systemic sign listed.
  ②, ③, ④ These are identified as localized signs.

69. Application, implementation, reduction of risk potential (a)
  ❷ Flushing of the eyes must occur immediately, before going to the emergency room.
  ① An ophthalmologist would be contacted to evaluate the damage
  ③ His parents should be notified as soon as possible after emergency intervention.
  ④ He will be taken to the emergency room, but flushing of the eyes should be done first.

70. Comprehension, assessment, physiological adaptation (a)
  ❸ Although the burns were superficial and about 5% of the arm, she is over 40 years of age and has a chronic condition (diabetes mellitus).
  ①, ②, ④ These not appropriate by definition.

71. Application, assessment, growth and development through the life span (b)
  ❹ The very young and the elderly are at greatest risk.
  ①, ②, ③ These are neither very young nor elderly.

72. Application, evaluation, physiological adaptation (c)
  ❸ Potassium is needed to allow the body to use insulin to metabolize glucose.

①, ②, ④ These electrolytes do not work with metabolism of glucose and insulin.

73. Knowledge, planning, pharmacological therapies (a)
  ❸ Anticoagulant therapy such as a heparin drip is used to prevent further clot formation.
  ①, ②, ④ Anticoagulant therapy is not appropriate for these conditions.

74. Application, implementation, reduction of risk potential (b)
  ❹ Heat exhaustion occurs when a prolonged fluid loss is caused by perspiration, diarrhea, or diuretics, and exposure to warm to hot temperatures without adequate fluid replacement. The fastest action is to remove one of the causes (the hot environment), then proceed to call the physician, monitor vital signs, and replace fluids as ordered.
  ①, ②, ③ These are appropriate, but not the first action that the nurse can implement that will eliminate one of the causes.

75. Application, assessment, physiological adaptation (c)
  ❹ Signs of septic shock include an elevated temperature, increased respirations, and tachycardia.
  ①, ②, ③ In these types of shock, the skin is cool, pale, and clammy.

76. Knowledge, implementation, pharmacological therapies (a)
  ❶ Disulfiram (Antabuse) is used for treatment of chronic alcoholism.
  ②, ③, ④ These drugs are not used for treatment of chronic alcoholism.

77. Knowledge, assessment, physiological adaptation (a)
  ❶ Flail chest is noted in a thorax in which multiple rib fractures cause instability in part of the chest wall and paradoxical breathing, with the lung underlying the injured area contracting on inspiration and bulging on expiration.
  ② Pulmonary embolism is a blockage of the pulmonary artery by foreign matter and is characterized by dyspnea, sudden chest pain, shock, and cyanosis.
  ③ Symptoms usually exhibited with simple rib fracture are pain on inspiration and rapid, shallow breathing.
  ④ Tension pneumothorax is air in the intrapleural space of the thorax caused by a rupture through the chest wall or lung parenchyma; air passes through the valve during coughing but can't escape during exhalation.

78. Knowledge, evaluation, growth and development (a)
  ❶ Heat stroke is more likely in the very young and the very old.
  ②, ③, ④ These age groups are not as likely to develop heat stroke.

79. Comprehension, implementation, pharmacological therapies (a)
  ❹ These products seal in the heat, causing further trauma to the victim.
  ① Burns left open place the victim at further risk for infection.
  ② Ice should not be applied because it causes body heat loss, thereby placing the victim at further risk.
  ③ Blisters should not be broken; intact skin prevents infection.

80. Comprehension, assessment, physiological adaptation (b)
    ❷ The nail may be tamponading a major blood vessel and should not be removed until the physician sees the patient.
    ① Impaled objects should not be removed until a doctor sees the patient
    ③ This will be necessary, but only after checking to see how recently her last tetanus shot was administered.
    ④ Once the nail is removed, irrigation will be necessary.

81. Application, evaluation, reduction of risk potential (c)
    ❶ A person with chilblains should not use tobacco products because they cause vasoconstriction.
    ② Affected parts should be protected from exposure to cold.
    ③ Warming should be done gently.
    ④ Rubbing or massage can cause further injury.

82. Knowledge, implementation, physiological adaptation (a)
    ❷ Vomiting from acute alcoholism can cause aspiration, and the depressed central nervous system can lead to respiratory arrest.
    ① Shock is associated with delirium tremens, not acute alcoholism.
    ③ This is appropriate for mild alcohol withdrawal; acute alcoholism requires observation.
    ④ Disulfiram (Antabuse) may be recommended as part of an aftercare program for the alcoholic who has already undergone withdrawal.

83. Knowledge, implementation, physiological adaptation (b)
    ❸ An arrest in an adult is usually caused by a cardiac arrhythmia such as ventricular fibrillation. Early defibrillation is necessary to revive the patient.
    ① Prolonged lack of oxygen in either the child or the adult will cause brain damage; this is not the correct explanation.
    ② Children need to be ventilated as quickly as possible, because an arrest in a child usually results from choking or suffocation. The child may revive quickly after CPR is begun.
    ④ Adults can be resuscitated many times, especially if defibrillation is done early. The rescuer must always try, unless the patient has obviously been without oxygen for a long time.

84. Application, implementation, reduction of risk potential (a)
    ❸ The chemical will continue to burn the victim as long as it remains on the skin.
    ① Ice or ice water should not be used in the treatment of burns because the burn has decreased the body's ability to retain heat. Overcooling will further increase metabolic demands.
    ② This is appropriate, but not the priority.
    ④ Treatment is to stop the burning first; then proceed with airway, breathing, and circulation.

85. Knowledge, assessment, pharmacological therapies (a)
    ❷ Methadone is used only for heroin withdrawal.
    ① Alcohol withdrawal is sometimes facilitated by administration of Valium, not Methadone.
    ③ Phenobarbitol is used for barbiturate withdrawal.
    ④ Withdrawal from benzodiazepines (Valium, Lithium) is done by administering progressively smaller doses of the drugs, not by substitution of another drug.

86. Knowledge, implementation, basic care and comfort (a)
    ❸ Cold compresses are used for the first 24 hours.
    ①, ② These actions are not indicated.
    ④ Warm compresses are applied after 48 hours.

87. Knowledge, assessment, physiological adaptation (b)
    ❸ When the epidermis, dermis, and subcutaneous tissues are involved, the burn is classified as a third-degree burn. Colors may vary in this type of burn, and there is little or no pain because nerves have been destroyed.
    ① A first-degree burn involves the epidermis with a red and pink color.
    ② A second-degree burn involves the epidermis and dermis. The color ranges from mottled pink to red, and there is usually some blistering.
    ④ The top three layers of skin are involved in a fourth-degree burn, and it may include fat, muscle, and bone.

88. Application, implementation, reduction of risk potential (c)
    ❹ It is imperative to keep the intestine moist to prevent tissue death.
    ①, ②, ③ These actions may also be performed, but it is important to prevent tissue death.

89. Comprehension, assessment, physiological adaptation (c)
    ❸ The presence of myoglobin in the urine indicates muscle damage.
    ① Renal damage is not indicated by the color of the urine.
    ② Hepatic damage is uncommon with these types of injuries.
    ④ Red urine is not associated with skin damage.

90. Knowledge, planning, pharmacological therapies (a)
    ❹ Since this is an open wound, there is a possibility of infection. Prophylactic antibiotics would be given.
    ①, ②, ③ Antibiotics would not be appropriate for these conditions.

91. Application, assessment, physiological adaptation (b)
    ❷ Salmonellosis is caused by eating raw eggs contaminated with the *Salmonella* bacteria; this organism can cause the symptoms of stomach cramps, vomiting, headaches, and fever.
    ① Botulism is caused by toxins produced by *Clostridium botulinum* bacteria and is characterized by double vision and respiratory difficulties.
    ③ Trichinosis is caused by a parasite, *Trichinella spiralis,* which is found in undercooked pork; the symptoms include vomiting, fever, chills, and muscle pain.
    ④ Anaerobic myositis or gas gangrene is caused by *Clostridium perfringens* bacteria, an anaerobic, gram-positive bacterium found in soil and in the intestinal tracts of humans and animals; it causes pain, swelling, and tenderness of wound area.

92. Comprehension, assessment, physiological adaptation (a)
    ❸ All electrical burns are considered to be major burns.
    ①, ②, ④ These are not appropriate by definition.

93. Comprehension, planning, basic care and comfort (b)
    ❸ Treatment for a strain includes limited to no weight bearing.
    ① His ankle should be elevated.
    ② Ice should be applied for 72 hours.
    ④ This is not applicable to the situation described.

94. Comprehension, assessment, physiological adaptation (b)
❸ Emergency nursing calls for a rapid clinical assessment with emphasis on airway, breathing, circulation, establishing priorities, and then the institution of life-saving measures.
① Although calling for help is important, it is not the priority.
② This is not a priority action.
④ The Good Samaritan law provisions should be known before traveling out of the home state.

95. Application, implementation, reduction of risk potential (a)
❸ Bleach is a corrosive substance that should be diluted only if the victim is conscious.
①, ② Nothing should be done besides calling the poison control center if the nurse is not absolutely sure of the antidote.
④ Vomiting should not be induced; this could cause burning of the esophagus, throat, and mouth.

96. Comprehension, implementation, physiological adaptation (b)
❹ Bag-valve-mask ventilation or AMBU ventilation provides oxygen to correct the hypoxia.
① Chest tubes drain only the pleural space.
② Cricothyroid puncture would be indicated if there were upper airway injury.

③ Trendelenburg position may assist with fluid drainage but will not help correct hypoxia. It may also cause dyspnea.

97. Application, evaluation, physiological adaptation (c)
❸ Unconscious victims need to be monitored for airway management.
①, ②, ④ These victims need care, but airway management is the first priority.

98. Application, planning, safety and infection control (b)
❸ CDC recommends using "standard precautions" at all times.
① In emergency situations, patients are often not able to provide accurate information.
② This is highly impractical and inappropriate.
④ It is inappropriate to rely on only the obvious.

99. Application, assessment, pharmacological therapies (c)
❶ Hallucinations are a symptom of alcohol withdrawal.
②, ③, ④ Hallucinations are not symptoms of withdrawal from these drugs.

100. Application, implementation, physiological adaptation (b)
❷ A conscious diabetic experiencing hypoglycemia should be given a quick-acting carbohydrate.
①, ③, ④ These are not appropriate actions for the situation at hand.

APPENDIXES

Appendix A | NANDA-Approved Nursing Diagnoses and Definitions

Activity Intolerance
The state in which an individual has insufficient physiological or psychological energy to endure or complete required or desired daily activities.

Activity Intolerance, Risk For
The state in which an individual is at risk of experiencing insufficient physiological or psychological energy to endure or complete required or desired daily activities.

Adaptive Capacity, Decreased: Intracranial
A clinical state in which intracranial fluid dynamic mechanisms that normally compensate for increases in intracranial volumes are compromised, resulting in repeated disproportionate increases in intracranial pressure in response to a variety of noxious and nonnoxious stimuli.

Adjustment, Impaired
Inability to modify lifestyle/behavior in a manner consistent with a change in health status.

Airway Clearance, Ineffective
Inability to clear secretions or obstructions from the respiratory tract to maintain a clear airway.

Anxiety
A vague uneasy feeling of discomfort or dread accompanied by an autonomic response; the source is often nonspecific or unknown to the individual; a feeling of apprehension caused by anticipation of danger. It is an altering signal that warns of impending danger and enables the individual to take measures to deal with threat.

*Anxiety, Death
The apprehension, worry, or fear related to death or dying

Aspiration, Risk For
The state in which an individual is at risk for entry of gastrointestinal secretions, oropharyngeal secretions, or solids or fluids into tracheobronchial passages.

Body Image Disturbance
Confusion in mental picture of one's physical self.

Body Temperature, Altered, Risk For
The state in which an individual is at risk for failure to maintain body temperature within normal range.

Bowel Incontinence
A change in normal bowel habits characterized by involuntary passage of stool.

Breastfeeding, Effective
The state in which a mother-infant dyad/family exhibits adequate proficiency and satisfaction with the breastfeeding process.

Breastfeeding, Ineffective
The state in which a mother, infant, or child experiences dissatisfaction or difficulty with the breastfeeding process.

Breastfeeding, Interrupted
A break in the continuity of the breastfeeding process as a result of inability or inadvisability to put the baby to the breast for feeding.

Breathing Pattern, Ineffective
Inspiration and/or expiration that does not provide adequate ventilation.

Cardiac Output, Decreased
A state in which the blood pumped by the heart is inadequate to meet the metabolic needs of the body.

Caregiver Role Strain
A caregiver's felt or exhibited difficulty in performing the family caregiver role.

Caregiver Role Strain, Risk For
A caregiver is vulnerable for felt difficulty in performing the family caregiver role.

Communication, Impaired Verbal
The state in which an individual experiences a decreased, delayed, or absent ability to receive, process, transmit, and use a system of symbols; anything that has meaning, i.e., transmits meaning.

Confusion, Acute
The abrupt onset of a cluster of global, transient changes and disturbances in attention, cognition, psychomotor activity, level of consciousness, and/or sleep/wake cycle.

Confusion, Chronic
An irreversible, long-standing, and/or progressive deterioration of intellect and personality characterized by decreased ability to interpret environmental stimuli, decreased capacity for intellectual thought processes and manifested by disturbances of memory, orientation, and behavior.

Constipation
A decrease in a person's normal frequency of defecation accompanied by difficult or incomplete passage of stool and/or passage of excessively hard, dry stool.

Constipation, Perceived
The state in which an individual makes a self-diagnosis of constipation and ensures a daily bowel movement through abuse of laxatives, enemas, and suppositories.

*Constipation, Risk of
At risk for a decrease in a person's normal frequency of defecation accompanied by difficult or incomplete passage of stool and/or passage of excessively hard, dry stool.

Coping, Community: Potential For Enhanced
A pattern of community activities for adaptation and problem solving that is satisfactory for meeting the demands or needs of the community, but can be improved for management of current and future problems/stressors.

Coping, Defensive
The state in which an individual repeatedly projects falsely positive self-evaluation based on a self-protective pattern that defends against underlying perceived threats to positive self-regard.

---

*New diagnosis approved at the thirteenth NANDA conference, 1998.

Coping, Family: Potential For Growth
Effective managing of adaptive tasks by family member involved with the patient's health challenge, who now is exhibiting desire and readiness for enhanced health and growth in regard to self and in relation to the patient.

Coping, Ineffective Community
A pattern of community activities for adaptation and problem solving that is unsatisfactory for meeting the demands or needs of the community.

Coping, Ineffective Family: Compromised
A usually supportive primary person (family member or close friend) is providing insufficient, ineffective or compromised support, comfort assistance or encouragement that may be needed by the patient to manage or master adaptive tasks related to his/her health challenge.

Coping, Ineffective Family: Disabling
Behavior of significant person (family member or other primary person) that disables his/her own capacities and the patient's capacities to effectively address tasks essential to either person's adaptation to the health challenge.

Coping, Ineffective Individual
Inability to form a valid appraisal of the stressors, inadequate choices of practiced responses, and/or inability to use available resources.

Decisional Conflict (Specify)
A state of uncertainty about the course of action to be taken when choice among competing actions involves risk, loss, or challenge to personal life values.

Denial, Ineffective
A conscious or unconscious attempt to disavow the knowledge or meaning of an event to reduce anxiety/fear to the detriment of health.

*Dentition, Altered
Disruption in tooth development/eruption patterns or structural integrity of individual teeth.

*Development, Risk For Altered
At risk for delay of 25% or more in one or more of the areas of social or self-regulatory behavior, or cognitive, language, gross or fine motor skills.

Diarrhea
Passage of loose, unformed stools.

Disuse Syndrome, Risk For
A state in which an individual is at risk for deterioration of body systems as the result of prescribed or unavoidable musculoskeletal inactivity; complications from immobility can include pressure ulcer, constipation, stasis of pulmonary secretions, thrombosis, urinary tract infection/retention, decreased strength/endurance, orthostatic hypotension, body image disturbance, and powerlessness.

Diversional Activity Deficit
The state in which an individual experiences a decreased stimulation from or interest or engagement in recreational or leisure activities.

Dysreflexia
The state in which an individual with a spinal cord injury at T7 or above experiences a life-threatening, uninhibited sympathetic response of the nervous system to a noxious stimulus.

*Dysreflexia, Risk For Autonomic
A lifelong threatening, uninhibited response of the sympathetic nervous system for an individual with a spinal cord injury or lesion at T8 or above, and having recovered from spinal shock.

Energy Field Disturbance
A disruption of the flow of energy surrounding a person's being that results in a disharmony of the body, mind, and/or spirit.

Environmental Interpretation Syndrome, Impaired
Consistent lack of orientation to person, place, time, or circumstances over more than 3 to 6 months, necessitating a protective environment.

*Failure to Thrive, Adult
A progressive functional deterioration of a physical and cognitive nature; the individual's ability to live with multisystem diseases, cope with ensuing problems, and manage his/her care are remarkably diminished.

Family Processes, Altered
A change in family relationships and/or functioning.

Family Processes, Altered: Alcoholism
The state in which the psychosocial, spiritual, and physiological functions of the family unit are chronically disorganized, leading to conflict, denial of problems, resistance to change, ineffective problem-solving, and a series of self-perpetuating crises.

Fatigue
An overwhelming sustained sense of exhaustion and decreased capacity for physical and mental work at usual level.

Fear
Fear is anxiety caused by consciously recognized and realistic danger. It is a perceived threat, real or imagined. Operationally, fear is the presence of an immediate feeling of apprehension and fright; the source is known and specific; subjective responses act as energizers but cannot be observed; and objective signs are the result of the transformation of energy into relief behaviors and responses.

Fluid Volume Deficit
The state in which an individual experiences decreased intravascular, interstitial, and/or intracellular fluid. This refers to dehydration—water loss alone without change in sodium.

Fluid Volume Deficit, Risk For
The state in which an individual is at risk of experiencing vascular, cellular, or intracellular dehydration.

Fluid Volume Excess
The state in which an individual experiences increased isotonic fluid retention.

*Fluid Volume Imbalance, Risk For
A risk of a decrease, increase, or rapid shift from one to the other of intravascular, interstitial, and/or intracellular fluid. This refers to the loss or excess of intravascular, interstitial, and/or intracellular fluid. This refers to the loss or excess or both of body fluids or replacement fluids.

Gas Exchange, Impaired
Excess or deficit in oxygenation and/or carbon dioxide elimination at the alveolar-capillary membrane.

Grieving, Anticipatory
Intellectual and emotional responses and behaviors by which individuals, families, communities work through the process of modifying self-concept based on the perception of potential loss.

Grieving, Dysfunctional
Extended, unsuccessful use of intellectual and emotional responses by which individuals, families, communities attempt to work through the process of modifying self-concept based on the perception of loss.

*Growth, Risk For Altered**
At risk for growth above the 97th percentile or below the 3rd percentile for age, crossing two percentile channels; disproportionate growth.

Growth And Development, Altered
The state in which an individual demonstrates deviations in norms from his/her age group.

Health Maintenance, Altered
Inability to identify, manage, and/or seek out help to maintain health.

Health-Seeking Behaviors (Specify)
A state in which an individual in stable health is actively seeking ways to alter personal health habits, and/or the environment in order to move toward a higher level of health.

Home Maintenance Management, Impaired
Inability to independently maintain a safe growth-promoting immediate environment.

Hopelessness
The subjective state in which an individual sees limited or no alternatives or personal choices available and is unable to mobilize energy on own behalf.

Hyperthermia
The state in which an individual's body temperature is elevated above normal range.

Hypothermia
The state in which an individual's body temperature is reduced below normal range.

Incontinence
See Bowel incontinence, Urinary incontinence.

Infant Behavior, Disorganized
Disintegrated physiological and neurobehavioral responses to the environment.

Infant Behavior, Disorganized, Risk For
Risk for alteration in integration and modulation of the physiological and behavioral systems of functioning (i.e., autonomic, motor, state, organizational, self-regulatory, and attentional-interactional systems).

Infant Behavior, Organized: Potential For Enhanced
A pattern of modulation of the physiological and behavioral systems of functioning of an infant (i.e., autonomic, motor, state, organizational, self-regulatory, and attentional-interactional systems) that is satisfactory but that can be improved resulting in higher levels of integration in response to environmental stimuli.

Infant Feeding Pattern, Ineffective
A state in which an infant demonstrates an impaired ability to suck or coordinate the suck-swallow response.

Infection, Risk For
The state in which an individual is at increased risk for being invaded by pathogenic organisms.

Injury, Risk For
The state in which an individual is at risk of injury as a result of environmental conditions interacting with the individual's adaptive and defensive resources.

Knowledge Deficit (Specify)
Absence or deficiency of cognitive information related to specific topic.

*Latex Allergy Response**
An allergic response to natural latex rubber products.

*Latex Allergy Response, Risk For**
At risk for allergic response to natural latex rubber products.

Loneliness, Risk For
A subjective state in which an individual is at risk of experiencing vague dysphoria.

Management of Therapeutic Regimen (Community), Ineffective
A pattern of regulating and integrating into community processes programs for treatment of illness and the sequelae of illness that are unsatisfactory for meeting health-related goals.

Management of Therapeutic Regimen (Families), Ineffective
A pattern of regulating and integrating into family processes a program for treatment of illness and the sequelae of illness that are unsatisfactory for meeting health-related goals.

Management of Therapeutic Regimen (Individual), Effective
A pattern of regulating and integrating into daily living a program for treatment of illness and its sequelae that is satisfactory for meeting specific health goals.

Management of Therapeutic Regimen (Individual), Ineffective
A pattern of regulating and integrating into daily living a program for treatment of illness and the sequelae of illness that is unsatisfactory for meeting specific health goals.

Memory, Impaired
The state in which an individual experiences the inability to remember or recall bits of information or behavioral skills. Impaired memory may be attributed to pathophysiological or situational causes that are either temporary or permanent.

*Mobility, Impaired Bed**
Limitation of independent movement from one bed position to another.

Mobility, Impaired Physical
A limitation in independent, purposeful physical movement of the body or of one or more extremities.

*Mobility, Impaired Wheelchair**
Limitation of independent operation of wheelchair within environment.

*Nausea**
An unpleasant, wave-like sensation in the back of the throat, epigastrium, or throughout the abdomen that may or may not lead to vomiting.

Noncompliance (Specify)
The extent to which a person's and/or caregiver's behavior coincides or fails to coincide with a health-promoting or therapeutic plan agreed upon by the person (and/or family, and/or community) and health care professional. In the presence of an agreed-upon, health-promoting or therapeutic plan, person's or caregiver's behavior may be fully or partially adherent or nonadherent and may lead to clinically effective, partially effective, or ineffective outcomes.

Nutrition, Altered: Less Than Body Requirements
The state in which an individual experiences an intake of nutrients insufficient to meet metabolic needs.

Nutrition, Altered: More Than Body Requirements
The state in which an individual experiences an intake of nutrients that exceeds metabolic needs.

Nutrition, Altered: Risk For More Than Body Requirements
The state in which an individual is at risk of experiencing an intake of nutrients that exceeds metabolic needs.

Oral Mucous Membrane, Altered
Disruptions of the lips and soft tissue of the oral cavity.

Pain

An unpleasant sensory and emotional experience arising from actual or potential tissue damage or described in terms of such damage; sudden or slow onset of any intensity from mild to severe with an anticipated or predictable end and a duration of less than 6 months.

Pain, Chronic

An unpleasant sensory and emotional experience arising from actual or potential tissue damage or described in terms of such damage; sudden or slow onset of any intensity from mild to severe with an anticipated or predictable end and a duration of greater than 6 months.

Parent/Infant/Child Attachment, Altered, Risk For

Disruption of the interactive process between parent/significant other and infant that fosters the development of a protective and nurturing reciprocal relationship.

Parental Role Conflict

The state in which a parent experiences role confusion and conflict in response to a crisis.

Parenting, Altered

Inability of the primary caretaker to create an environment that promotes the optimum growth and development of the child.

Parenting, Altered, Risk For

Risk for inability of the primary caretaker to create, maintain, or regain an environment that promotes the optimum growth and development of the child.

Perioperative Positioning Injury, Risk For

A state in which the patient is at risk for injury as a result of the environmental conditions found in the perioperative setting.

Peripheral Neurovascular Dysfunction, Risk For

A state in which an individual is at risk for experiencing a disruption in circulation, sensation, or motion of an extremity.

Personal Identity Disturbance

Inability to distinguish between self and nonself.

Poisoning, Risk For

Accentuated risk of accidental exposure to or ingestion of drugs or dangerous products in doses sufficient to cause poisoning.

Post-Trauma Syndrome

A sustained maladaptive response to a traumatic, overwhelming event.

*Post-Trauma Syndrome, Risk For

Risk for a sustained maladaptive response to a traumatic, overwhelming event.

Powerlessness

Perception that one's own action will not significantly affect an outcome; a perceived lack of control over a current situation or immediate happening.

Protection, Altered

The state in which an individual experiences a decrease in the ability to guard the self from internal or external threats, such as illness or injury.

Rape-Trauma Syndrome

A sustained maladaptive response to a forced, violent sexual penetration against the victim's will and consent.

Rape-Trauma Syndrome: Compound Reaction or Silent Reaction

The trauma syndrome that develops from actual or attempted forced violent sexual penetration against the victim's will and consent includes an acute phase of disorganization of the victim's lifestyle and a long-term process of reorganization of lifestyle.

Relocation Stress Syndrome

Physiological and/or psychosocial disturbances as a result of a transfer from one environment to another.

Role Performance, Altered

The patterns of behavior and self-expression do not match the environmental context, norms, and expectations.

Self-Care Deficit, Bathing/Hygiene

An impaired ability to perform or complete bathing/hygiene activities for oneself.

Self-Care Deficit, Dressing/Grooming

An impaired ability to perform or complete dressing and grooming activities for oneself.

Self-Care Deficit, Feeding

An impaired ability to perform or complete feeding activities for oneself.

Self-Care Deficit, Toileting

An impaired ability to perform or complete own toileting activities.

Self-Esteem, Chronic Low

Long-standing negative self-evaluation/feelings about self or self-capabilities.

Self-Esteem Disturbance

Negative self-evaluation/feelings about self or self-capabilities, which may be directly or indirectly expressed.

Self-Esteem, Situational Low

Negative self-evaluation/feelings about self that develop in response to a loss or change in an individual who previously had a positive self-evaluation.

Self-Mutilation, Risk For

The state in which an individual is at high risk to perform an act on the self to injure, not kill, that produces tissue damage and tension relief.

Sensory/Perceptual Alterations (Specify: Visual, Auditory, Kinesthetic, Gustatory, Tactile, Olfactory)

The state in which an individual experiences a change in the amount or patterning of incoming stimuli accompanied by a diminished, exaggerated, distorted, or impaired response to such stimuli.

Sexual Dysfunction

The state in which an individual experiences a change in sexual function that is viewed as unsatisfying, unrewarding, or inadequate.

Sexuality Patterns, Altered

The state in which an individual expresses concern regarding his/her sexuality.

Skin Integrity, Impaired

The state in which an individual has altered epidermis and/or dermis.

Skin Integrity, Impaired, Risk For

The state in which an individual's skin is at risk of being adversely altered.

*Sleep Deprivation

Prolonged periods of time without sustained natural, periodic suspension of relative unconsciousness.

Sleep Pattern Disturbance

Time-limited disruption of sleep (natural, periodic suspension of consciousness) amount and quality.

Social Interaction, Impaired

The state in which an individual participates in an insufficient or excessive quantity or ineffective quality of social exchange.

Social Isolation
Aloneness experienced by an individual and perceived as imposed by others and as a negative or threatened state.

*Sorrow, Chronic
A cyclical, recurring, and potentially progressive pattern of pervasive sadness that is experienced (by a patient [parent or caregiver, or individual with chronic illness or disability]) in response to continual loss, throughout the trajectory of an illness or disability.

Spiritual Distress (Distress of the Human Spirit)
Disruption in the life principle that pervades a person's entire being and that integrates and transcends one's biological and psychosocial nature.

*Spiritual Distress, Risk For
At risk for an altered sense of harmonious connectedness with all of life and the universe in which dimensions that transcend and empower the self may be disrupted.

Spiritual Well-Being, Potential For Enhanced
Spiritual well-being is the process of an individual's developing/unfolding of mystery through harmonious interconnectedness that springs from inner strengths.

Suffocation, Risk For
Accentuated risk of accidental suffocation (inadequate air available for inhalation).

*Surgical Recovery, Delayed
An extension of the number of postoperative days required for individuals to initiate and perform on their own behalf activities that maintain life, health, and well-being.

Swallowing, Impaired
Abnormal functioning of the swallowing mechanism associated with deficits in oral, pharyngeal, or esophageal structure or function.

Thermoregulation, Ineffective
The state in which an individual's temperature fluctuates between hypothermia and hyperthermia.

Thought Processes, Altered
The state in which an individual experiences a disruption in cognitive operations and activities.

Tissue Integrity, Impaired
The state in which an individual experiences damage to mucus membrane, or corneal, integumentary, or subcutaneous tissues. It is a state in which an individual has altered body tissue.

Tissue Perfusion, Altered (Specify Type: Renal, Cerebral, Cardiopulmonary, Gastrointestinal, Peripheral)
A decrease in oxygen resulting in the failure to nourish the tissues at the capillary level.

*Transfer Ability, Impaired
Limitation of independent movement between two nearby surfaces.

Trauma, Risk For
Accentuated risk of accidental tissue injury (e.g., wound, burn, fracture).

Unilateral Neglect
The state in which an individual is perceptually unaware of and inattentive to one side of the body.

Urinary Elimination, Altered
The state in which an individual experiences a disturbance in urine elimination.

Urinary Incontinence, Functional
Inability of usually continent person to reach toilet in time to avoid unintentional loss of urine.

Urinary Incontinence, Reflex
An involuntary loss of urine at somewhat predictable intervals when a specific bladder volume is reached.

Urinary Incontinence, Stress
The state in which an individual experiences a loss of urine of less than 50 ml occurring with increased abdominal pressure.

Urinary Incontinence, Total
The state in which an individual experiences a continuous and unpredictable loss of urine.

Urinary Incontinence, Urge
The state in which an individual experiences involuntary passage of urine occurring soon after a strong sense of urgency to void.

*Urinary Incontinence, Urge, Risk For
Risk for involuntary loss of urine associated with a sudden, strong sensation or urinary urgency.

Urinary Retention
The state in which an individual experiences incomplete emptying of the bladder.

Ventilation, Inability to Sustain Spontaneous
A state in which the response pattern of decreased energy reserves results in an individual's inability to maintain breathing adequate to support life.

Ventilatory Weaning Process, Dysfunctional
A state in which an individual cannot adjust to lowered levels of mechanical ventilator support, which interrupts and prolongs the weaning process.

Violence, Risk For: Directed at Others
Behaviors in which an individual demonstrates that he/she can be physically, emotionally, and/or sexually harmful to others.

Violence, Risk For: Self-Directed
Behaviors in which an individual demonstrates that he/she can be physically, emotionally, and/or sexually harmful to self.

*Walking, Impaired
Limitation of independent movement within the environment on foot.

From North American Nursing Diagnosis Association: *Nursing diagnoses: definitions and classification 1999-2000,* Philadelphia, 1999, The Association.

Appendix B — Classification of NANDA-Approved Nursing Diagnoses by Human Response Pattern (NANDA Taxonomy I–Revised)

1. **Exchanging**
   Altered nutrition: more than body requirements
   Altered nutrition: less than body requirements
   Altered nutrition: risk for more than body requirements
   Risk for infection
   Risk for altered body temperature
   Hypothermia
   Hyperthermia
   Ineffective thermoregulation
   Dysreflexia
   Risk for autonomic dysreflexia
   Constipation
   Perceived constipation
   Diarrhea
   Bowel incontinence
   Risk for constipation
   Altered urinary elimination
   Stress incontinence
   Reflex urinary incontinence
   Urge incontinence
   Functional urinary incontinence
   Total incontinence
   Risk for urinary urge incontinence
   Urinary retention
   Altered tissue perfusion (specify type)
   Risk for fluid volume imbalance
   Fluid volume excess
   Fluid volume deficit
   Risk for fluid volume deficit
   Decreased cardiac output
   Impaired gas exchange
   Ineffective airway clearance
   Ineffective breathing pattern
   Inability to sustain spontaneous ventilation
   Dysfunctional ventilatory weaning response
   Risk for injury
   Risk for suffocation
   Risk for poisoning
   Risk for trauma
   Risk for aspiration
   Risk for disuse syndrome
   Latex allergy response
   Risk for latex allergy response
   Altered protection
   Impaired tissue integrity
   Altered oral mucous membrane
   Impaired skin integrity
   Risk for impaired skin integrity
   Altered dentition
   Decreased adaptive capacity: intracranial
   Energy field disturbance

2. **Communicating**
   Impaired verbal communication

3. **Relating**
   Impaired social interaction
   Social isolation
   Risk for loneliness
   Altered role performance
   Altered parenting
   Risk for altered parenting
   Risk for altered parent/infant/child attachment
   Sexual dysfunction
   Altered family processes
   Caregiver role strain
   Risk for caregiver role strain
   Altered family processes: alcoholism
   Parental role conflict
   Altered sexuality patterns

4. **Valuing**
   Spiritual distress (distress of the human spirit)
   Risk for spiritual distress
   Potential for enhanced spiritual well-being

5. **Choosing**
   Ineffective individual coping
   Impaired adjustment
   Defensive coping
   Ineffective denial
   Ineffective family coping: disabling
   Ineffective family coping: compromised
   Family coping: potential for growth
   Potential for enhanced community coping
   Ineffective community coping
   Ineffective management of therapeutic regimen: individuals
   Noncompliance (specify)
   Ineffective management of therapeutic regimen: families
   Ineffective management of therapeutic regimen: community
   Effective management of therapeutic regimen: individual
   Decisional conflict (specify)
   Health-seeking behaviors (specify)

6. **Moving**
   Impaired physical mobility
   Risk for peripheral neurovascular dysfunction
   Risk for perioperative positioning injury
   Impaired walking
   Impaired wheelchair mobility
   Impaired transfer ability
   Impaired bed mobility
   Activity intolerance
   Fatigue
   Risk for activity intolerance
   Sleep pattern disturbance
   Sleep deprivation
   Diversional activity deficit
   Impaired home maintenance management
   Altered health maintenance
   Delayed surgical recovery

From North American Nursing Diagnosis Association: *Nursing diagnoses: definitions and classification 1999-2000,* Philadelphia, 1999, The Association.

Adult failure to thrive
Feeding self-care deficit
Impaired swallowing
Ineffective breastfeeding
Interrupted breastfeeding
Effective breastfeeding
Ineffective infant feeding pattern
Bathing/hygiene self-care deficit
Dressing/grooming self-care deficit
Toileting self-care deficit
Altered growth and development
Risk for altered development
Risk for altered growth
Relocation stress syndrome
Risk for disorganized infant behavior
Disorganized infant behavior
Potential for enhanced organized infant behavior

7. **Perceiving**
Body image disturbance
Self-esteem disturbance
Chronic low self-esteem
Situational low self-esteem
Personal identity disturbance
Sensory/perceptual alterations (specify)
Unilateral neglect
Hopelessness
Powerlessness

8. **Knowing**
Knowledge deficit (specify)
Impaired environmental interpretation syndrome
Acute confusion
Chronic confusion
Altered thought processes
Impaired memory

9. **Feeling**
Pain
Chronic pain
Nausea
Dysfunctional grieving
Anticipatory grieving
Chronic sorrow
Risk for violence: directed at others
Risk for self-mutilation
Risk for violence: self-directed
Post-trauma syndrome
Rape-trauma syndrome
Rape-trauma syndrome: compound reaction
Rape-trauma syndrome: silent reaction
Risk for post-trauma syndrome
Anxiety
Death anxiety
Fear

Appendix C	**Classification of Nursing Diagnoses by Gordon's Functional Health Patterns**

Health Perception–Health Management Pattern
Health-seeking behaviors (specify)
Altered health maintenance
Ineffective management of therapeutic regimen
Risk for ineffective management of therapeutic regimen
Effective management of therapeutic regimen
Ineffective family management of therapeutic regimen
Ineffective community management of therapeutic regimen
Noncompliance (specify)
Risk for infection
Risk for injury (trauma)
Risk for perioperative positioning injury
Risk for poisoning
Altered protection
Energy field disturbance

Nutritional-Metabolic Pattern
Altered nutrition: more than body requirements
Altered nutrition: risk for more than body requirements
Altered nutrition: less than body requirements
Adult failure to thrive
Ineffective breastfeeding
Interrupted breastfeeding
Effective breastfeeding
Ineffective infant feeding pattern
Impaired swallowing
Nausea
Risk for aspiration
Altered oral mucous membrane
Altered dentition
Fluid volume deficit
Risk for fluid volume deficit
Fluid volume excess
Risk for fluid volume imbalance
Impaired skin integrity
Risk for impaired skin integrity
Impaired tissue integrity
Latex allergy response
Risk for latex allergy response
Ineffective thermoregulation
Hyperthermia
Hypothermia
Risk for altered body temperature

Elimination Pattern
Constipation
Perceived constipation
Risk for constipation
Diarrhea
Bowel incontinence
Altered urinary elimination pattern
Functional urinary incontinence

Reflex urinary incontinence
Stress incontinence
Urge incontinence
Risk for urinary urge incontinence
Total incontinence
Urinary retention

Activity-Exercise Pattern
Activity intolerance
Risk for activity intolerance
Fatigue
Impaired physical mobility
Impaired bed mobility
Impaired transfer ability
Impaired wheelchair mobility
Impaired walking
Risk for disuse syndrome
Total self-care deficit
Self-care deficit, bathing/hygiene
Self-care deficit, dressing/grooming
Self-care deficit, feeding
Self-care deficit, toileting
Delayed surgical recovery
Altered growth and development
Risk for altered development
Risk for altered growth
Diversional activity deficit
Impaired home maintenance management
Dysfunctional ventilatory weaning response
Inability to sustain spontaneous ventilation
Ineffective airway clearance
Ineffective breathing pattern
Impaired gas exchange
Decreased cardiac output
Altered tissue perfusion (specify type)
Dysreflexia
Risk for autonomic dysreflexia
Disorganized infant behavior
Risk for disorganized infant behavior
Potential for enhanced organized infant behavior
Risk for peripheral neurovascular dysfunction
Decreased intracranial adaptive capacity

Sleep-Rest Pattern
Sleep pattern disturbance
Sleep deprivation

Cognitive-Perceptual Pattern
Pain
Chronic pain
Sensory/perceptual alterations (specify)
Unilateral neglect
Knowledge deficit (specify)
Altered thought processes
Acute confusion

From Gordon M: *Manual of nursing diagnosis,* ed 9, St. Louis, 2000, Mosby.

Chronic confusion
Impaired environmental interpretation syndrome
Impaired memory
Decisional conflict (specify)

Self-Perception–Self-Concept Pattern
Fear
Anxiety
Death anxiety
Risk for loneliness
Hopelessness
Powerlessness
Low self-esteem
Chronic low self-esteem
Situational low self-esteem
Body image disturbance
Risk for self-mutilation
Personal identity disturbance

Role-Relationship Pattern
Anticipatory grieving
Dysfunctional grieving
Chronic sorrow
Altered role performance
Social isolation
Impaired social interaction
Risk for violence: self-directed
Risk for violence: directed at others
Relocation stress syndrome
Altered family processes
Altered family process: alcoholism

Altered parenting
Risk for altered parenting
Parental role conflict
Risk for altered parent/infant/child attachment
Caregiver role strain
Impaired verbal communication

Sexuality-Reproductive Pattern
Altered sexuality patterns
Sexual dysfunction
Rape-trauma syndrome
Rape-trauma syndrome: compound reaction
Rape-trauma syndrome: silent reaction

Coping–Stress-Tolerance Pattern
Ineffective individual coping
Defensive coping
Ineffective denial
Compromised family coping
Disabling family coping
Ineffective community coping
Family coping: potential for growth
Potential for enhanced community coping
Impaired adjustment
Post-trauma syndrome
Risk for post-trauma syndrome

Value-Belief Pattern
Spiritual distress (distress of the human spirit)
Potential for enhanced spiritual well-being
Risk for spiritual distress

Appendix D | Guide to Common Drug Interactions*

Drug	Interacting Drug	Effect
Over-the-Counter Drugs and Substances		
Antacids		
Alumina and magnesia		Effects of dicumarol may be faster and/or increased with
Dihydroxaluminum sodium	Dicumarol	magnesium salts
carbonate	Digoxin	Effects of digoxin may be reduced with aluminum and
Magnesia	Tetracyclines	magnesium salts
	Doxycycline	Effects of tetracyclines may be reduced
	Tetracycline	Should be taken 1-3 hours apart
	Iron products	Effects of iron products may be reduced
Histamine H₂ Antagonists		
Cimetidine	Antidiabetic agents	
Ranitidine	Glipizide	Risk of low blood sugar
	Glyburide	Increased effect of warfarin
	Warfarin	Possible increased risk of bleeds
	Theophylline	Increased effect of theophylline
		Toxic effects may occur
Painkillers		
Acetaminophen	Alcoholic beverages	May cause liver damage with excessive use
Buffered acetaminophen		
	Blood-thinning drugs	High doses of acetaminophen may increase blood-thinning
	Warfarin sodium	effects of these drugs
	Tetracycline	Buffered form may cancel the effects of tetracycline
		Should be taken 1 hour apart
Ibuprofen	Alcoholic beverages	May cause internal bleeding or ulcers
	Blood-thinning drugs	May cause internal bleeding or ulcers
	Heparin	
	Warfarin sodium	
	Salicylates	May cause stomach upset without relieving symptoms; in
	Aspirin	combination may increase risk of internal bleeding or
	Aspirin and caffeine	ulcers
	Buffered aspirin	
Salicylates	Alcoholic beverages	May cause stomach ulcers or internal bleeding
Aspirin		
Aspirin and caffeine		
Buffered aspirin	Antidiabetics	May cause blood sugar level to drop too low
	Glipizide	
	Glyburide	
	Tolazamide	
	Blood-thinning drugs	Increases risk of internal bleeding
	Heparin	
	Warfarin sodium	
	Ibuprofen	May cause stomach upset without relieving symptoms; in
		combination may increase risk of internal bleeding or
		ulcers
	Tetracycline	Effects of tetracycline are reduced

From *Mosby's medical, nursing, and allied health dictionary,* ed 5, St Louis, 1998, Mosby.
*This table includes only common over-the-counter and prescription drugs. Some of these drugs may also interact with less common drugs and substances not described. When using any drug, always consult your doctor or pharmacist about possible interactions with other drugs, substances, or foods.

Continued

Drug	Interacting Drug	Effect
Over-the-Counter Drugs and Substances—cont'd		
Other Substances		
Alcoholic beverages	Acetaminophen Buffered acetaminophen	May cause liver damage; risk greater with high alcohol intake and high doses of acetaminophen
	Antidiabetics Glipizide Glyburide Tolazamide	Stomach upset, vomiting, cramps, headaches, low blood sugar
	Antiseizure drugs Carbamazepine Phenobarbital Primidine Valproic acid Diazepam Phenytoin	May cause extreme drowsiness
	Barbiturates Pentobarbital Phenobarbital Secobarbital Secobarbital and amobarbital	May cause drowsiness, increase effects of either drug, cause breathing to fail, or cause blood pressure to drop too low
	Ibuprofen	May cause internal bleeding or ulcers
	Narcotic analgesics Acetaminophen and codeine Meperidine Morphine Propoxyphene	May depress nervous system and breathing or cause blood pressure to drop too low
	Reserpine	May increase effects of alcohol and reserpine
	Salicylates Aspirin Aspirin and caffeine Buffered aspirin	May cause stomach ulcers or internal bleeding
	Tricyclic antidepressants Amitriptyline Amoxapine Doxepin	May cause extreme drowsiness
Sodium chloride (salt)	Lithium	Low-salt diet causes lithium to build up in body and is not advised
Tobacco (smoking)	Birth control pills Norethindrone with ethinyl estradiol	May increase chances of blood clot or heart attack
Tyramine-containing foods Avocados, bananas, beer, caffeine, cheese, chicken liver, chocolate, fava beans, fermented sausages (salami, pepperoni, bologna, etc.), canned figs, pickled herring, pineapple, raisins, red wine, sauerkraut, soy sauce, yeast extract, yogurt	MAO inhibitors Isocarboxazid Phenelzine Tranylcypromine	May cause severe and sometimes fatal high blood pressure Headache, vomiting, fever, and high blood pressure are warrning signals

From *Mosby's medical, nursing, and allied health dictionary,* ed 5, St Louis, 1998, Mosby.

Drug	Interacting Drug	Effect
Prescription Drugs		
Antibiotics		
Erythromycins Erythromycin Erythromycin lactobionate	Penicillins Amoxicillin Ampicillin	Could interfere with the effects of penicillins
Penicillins Amoxicillin Ampicillin	Birth control pills Norethindrone with ethinyl estradiol	May interfere with and result in unplanned pregnancy or menstrual problems
	Blood-thinning drugs Warfarin sodium	May increase blood thinning effects of these drugs
	Erythromycins Erythromycin Erythromycin lactobionate	May interfere with effects of penicillins
	Tetracyclines Doxycycline Tetracycline	May interfere with effects of penicillins
Tetracyclines Doxycycline Tetracycline	Acetaminophen Buffered acetaminophen	
	Antacids Alumina and magnesia Dihydroxaluminum sodium carbonate Magnesia	May decrease effects of tetracyclines and should be taken 1 to 3 hours apart
	Barbiturates Pentobarbital Phenobarbital Secobarbital Secobarbital and amobarbital	May decrease effects of doxycycline; other tetracyclines can be used
	Penicillins Amoxicillin Ampicillin	May interfere with effects of penicillins
	Salicylates Aspirin Aspirin and caffeine Buffered aspirin	Effects of tetracyclines are reduced
Antidepressants		
Lithium	Sodium chloride (salt)	Low-salt diet causes lithium to build up in body and is not advised
	Thiazide diuretics Furosemide Methyclothiazide	May cause lithium to have toxic effect
Tricyclic antidepressants Amitriptyline Amoxapine Doxepin Nortripthyline Imipramine Desipramine	Alcoholic beverages	May cause extreme drowsiness
	Antiseizure drugs Carbamazepine Chlordiazepoxide Diazepam Phenytoin	Effects of antiseizure drug may be decreased Dosage should be adjusted

Continued

Drug	Interacting Drug	Effect
Prescription Drugs—cont'd *Antidepressants*		
	Blood-thinning drugs Warfarin sodium	May increase effect of warfarin, thereby increasing the risk of internal bleeding
	MAO inhibitors Isocarboxazid	Severe seizure and death could result
	Phenelzine Tranylcypromine	Should be taken 14 days apart

	Narcotic analgesics
	  Acetaminophen and codeine
	  Meperidine
	  Propoxyphene
		May depress nervous system and breathing and cause blood pressure to drop too low

Selective Serotonin Reuptake Inhibitors (SSRIs)		

Paroxetine
Fluoxetine
Sertraline
	Tricyclic antidepressants
	  Amitriptyline
	  Imipramine
		Pharmacologic and toxic effects may occur

	Warfarin	Increased or decreased effect of warfarin Possible increased risk bleeds

	Antiseizure drugs
	  Carbamazepine
	  Phenytoin
		Increased toxic effects of seizure medication

	MAO inhibitors Phenelzine	Increased toxic effects Avoid use, especially with fluoxetine
Antidiabetics		
Glipizide Glyburide Tolazamide	Alcoholic beverages	May cause stomach upset, vomiting, cramps, headaches, low blood sugar

	Beta-adrenergic blockers
	  Metoprolol
	  Propranolol
		May increase risk of either high or low blood sugar levels
		May mask symptoms of low blood sugar

	Blood-thinning drugs Warfarin sodium	Blood-thinning effect will be increased at first, later it will be decreased May also cause low blood sugar and become toxic

	MAO inhibitors
	  Isocarboxazid
	  Phenelzine
	  Tranylcypromine
		Can cause extreme low blood sugar level

	Salicylates
	  Aspirin
	  Aspirin and caffeine
	  Buffered aspirin
		May cause blood sugar level to drop too low

Isophane insulin suspension	Beta-adrenergic blockers
	  Metoprolol
	  Propranolol
		These may mask symptoms of low blood sugar

	Birth control pills Norethindrone with ethinyl estradiol	May increase risk of high blood sugar levels Dosages should be adjusted

	MAO inhibitors
	  Isocarboxazid
	  Phenelzine
	  Tranylcypromine
		May cause extreme low blood sugar level

From *Mosby's medical, nursing, and allied health dictionary,* ed 5, St Louis, 1998, Mosby.

Drug	Interacting Drug	Effect
Prescription Drugs—cont'd		
Antiseizure drugs		
Carbamazepine Clonazepam Diazepam Phenytoin Phenobarbital Primidone Valproic acid	Alcoholic beverages	May cause extreme drowsiness

	Beta-adrenergic blockers
	  Metoprolol
	  Propranolol
		Could decrease the effect of beta-blockers

	Birth control pills
	  Norethindrone with
	    ethinyl estradiol
		Phenytoin and carbamazepine may interfere and increase risk of unplanned pregnancy
		May increase effect of diazepam

	Tricyclic antidepressants
	  Amitriptyline
	  Amoxapine
	  Doxepin
		Effects of antiseizure drug may be decreased (phenytoin)
		Dosage may need to be adjusted
		Central nervous system effects potentiated
		Complex interactions related to protein binding displacement may go either way

Barbiturates		
Pentobarbital Phenobarbital Secobarbital Secobarbital and amobarbital	Alcoholic beverages	May cause drowsiness, increase effects of either drug, cause breathing to fail, or cause blood pressure to drop too low

	Birth control pills
	  Norethindrone with
	    ethinyl estradiol
		Barbiturates may interfere with and result in unplanned pregnancy

	Blood-thinning drugs Warfarin sodium	May decrease blood-thinning effects of these drugs
	Doxycycline	May decrease effects of doxycycline; other tetracyclines can be used
Birth Control Pills		

Norethindrone with ethinyl estradiol	Antiseizure drugs
	  Carbamazepine
	  Diazepam
	  Phenytoin
		Will decrease effectiveness of birth control pills, resulting in unplanned pregnancy
		May decrease the effects of other antiseizure drugs

	Barbiturates
	  Pentobarbital
	  Phenobarbital
	  Secobarbital
	  Secobarbital and
	    amobarbital
		Barbiturates may interfere with birth control pills and result in unplanned pregnancy

	Isophane insulin suspension	May increase risk of high blood sugar levels; dosages should be adjusted

	Penicillins
	  Amoxillin
	  Ampicillin
		May interfere with birth control pills and result in unplanned pregnancy

	Tobacco (smoking)	May increase chances of blood clot or heart attack
Blood Pressure Drugs		

Thiazide diuretics
  Hydrochlorothiazide
  Methyclothiazide
	Beta-adrenergic blockers
	  Metoprolol
	  Propranolol
		Can cause extremely low blood pressure

Continued

Drug	Interacting Drug	Effect
Prescription Drugs—cont'd		
Blood Pressure Drugs—cont'd		
Loop diuretics	Digitalis glycosides	Can cause irregular heartbeat, which can be fatal
Furosemide	Digoxin	Can cause extremely low blood pressure
Bumetanide		
	Lithium	May cause lithium to have toxic effect
	Reserpine	Can cause extremely low blood pressure
Rauwolfia alkaloids	Alcoholic beverages	May increase effects of alcohol
Reserpine		May increase effects of rauwolfia alkaloids
	Beta-adrenergic blockers	May cause extremely slow heartbeat and low blood pressure
	Metoprolol	
	Propranolol	
	Digitalis glycosides	May cause irregular heartbeat
	Digoxin	
	MAO inhibitors	May cause slight to sudden and severe high blood pressure
	Isocarboxazid	May cause extreme high fever
	Phenelzine	Either effect could be life-threatening
	Tranylcypromine	
	Thiazide diuretics	Can cause extreme low blood pressure
	Hydrochlorothiazide	
	Methyclothiazide	
	Loop diuretics	
	Furosemide	
	Bumetanide	
Calcium channel blockers	Beta blockers	Potentiate effect on decreased heart contractility in some cases
Diltiazem	Propranolol	
Verapamil	Atenolol	
Nifedipine	Metoprolol	
Amlodipine		
	Digoxin	Levels of digoxin may be increased; risk of toxicity increases
	Other blood pressure	Increased effect on blood pressure lowering
	lowering drugs	
	Diuretics	
	Alpha-blockers	
	Prazosin	
Blood-Thinning Drugs		
Warfarin sodium	Acetaminophen	High doses of acetaminophen may increase blood-thinning
	Buffered acetaminophen	effects of these drugs
	Antacids	Effects of dicumarol may be faster and may also be increased
	Alumina and magnesia	
	Dihydroxyaluminum	
	sodium carbonate	
	Magnesia	
	Antidiabetics	Blood-thinning effect will be increased at first, later it will be
	Glipizide	decreased
	Glyburide	May also cause low blood sugar and become toxic
	Tolazamide	
	Barbiturates	Decreases blood-thinning effect
	Pentobarbital	
	Phenobarbital	
	Secobarbital	
	Secobarbital and	
	amobarbital	
	Heparin	May cause increased risk of internal bleeding
	Ibuprofen	May cause internal bleeding or ulcers
	Penicillins	May increase blood-thinning effects of these drugs
	Amoxicillin	
	Ampicillin	

From *Mosby's medical, nursing, and allied health dictionary,* ed 5, St Louis, 1998, Mosby.

Drug	Interacting Drug	Effect
Prescription Drugs—cont'd		
Blood-Thinning Drugs—cont'd		
	Salicylates	Blood-thinning effects will be increased
	Aspirin	May cause ulcers or internal bleeding
	Aspirin and caffeine	
	Buffered aspirin	
	Tricyclic antidepressants	May cause internal bleeding
	Amitriptyline	
	Amoxapine	
	Doxepin	
Heparin	Blood-thinning drugs	May cause increased risk of internal bleeding
	Warfarin sodium	
	Salicylates	Blood-thinning effects will be increased
	Aspirin	May cause ulcers or internal bleeding
	Aspirin and caffeine	
	Buffered aspirin	
Heart Drugs		
Beta-adrenergic blockers	Antidiabetics	May increase risk of either high or low blood sugar levels
Metoprolol	Chlorpropamide	May mask symptoms
Propranolol	Tolazamide	
	Antiseizure drugs	Could decrease the effect of beta blockers
	Carbamazepine	
	Diazepam	
	Phenytoin	
	Digitalis glycosides	May cause extremely slow heartbeat with a chance of heart block
	Digoxin	
	Isophane insulin	Beta blockers may mask symptoms of low blood sugar
	suspension	May also cause low blood sugar
	Reserpine	May cause extremely slow heartbeat and low blood pressure
	Thiazide diuretics	Can cause extremely low blood pressure
	Hydrochlorothiazide	
	Methyclothiazide	
	Loop diuretics	
	Furosemide	
	Bumetanide	
Digitalis glycosides	Antacids	Effects of digoxin may be reduced
Digoxin	Alumina and magnesia	
	Dihydroxaluminum	
	sodium carbonate	
	Magnesia	
	Beta-adrenergic blockers	May cause extremely slow heartbeat with a chance of heart block
	Metoprolol	
	Propranolol	
	Reserpine	May cause irregular heartbeat
	Thiazide diuretics	May cause extreme low blood pressure; may cause digitalis to become toxic
	Hydrochlorothiazide	
	Methyclothiazide	
	Loop diuretics	
	Furosemide	
	Bumetanide	
Angiotensin converting enzyme inhibitors (ACE inhibitors)	Potassium preparations	Increased potassium levels
Captopril	Potassium-sparing diuretics	Increased potassium levels
Enalapril		
Fosinopril	Digoxin	Increased digoxin levels
Lisinopril		
Others	Lithium	Increased lithium levels (risk toxicity)

Continued

Drug	Interacting Drug	Effect
Prescription Drugs—cont'd		
Heart Drugs—cont'd		
Antihyperlipidemic agents		
Lovastatin	Cyclosporine	Toxic effects on muscle may occur
Atorvastatin	Erythromycin	Monitor carefully
Simvastatin	Warfarin	Increased effect of warfarin possible
Monoamine Oxide Inhibitors (MAO Inhibitors)		
Isocarboxazid	Antidiabetics	Can cause extreme low blood sugar level
Phenelzine	Glipizide	
Tranylcypromine	Glyburide	
	Isophane insulin suspension	
	Tolazamide	
	Narcotic analgesics	May cause severe and sometimes fatal reactions
	Acetaminophen and codeine	
	Meperidine	
	Propoxyphene	
	Reserpine	May cause slight to sudden and severe high blood pressure
		May cause extreme high fever
		Either effect could be life-threatening
	Tricyclic antidepressants	Severe seizure and death could result
	Amitriptyline	Should be taken 14 days apart
	Amoxapine	
	Doxepin	
	Tyramine-containing foods	May cause severe and sometimes fatal high blood pressure
	Avocados, bananas, beer, caffeine, cheese, chicken liver, chocolate, fava beans, fermented sausages (salami, pepperoni, bologna, etc.) canned figs, pickled herring, pineapple, raisins, red wine, sauerkraut, soy sauce, yeast extract, yogurt	Headache, vomiting, fever, and high blood pressure are warning signals
Painkillers		
Narcotic analgesics	Alcoholic beverages	May depress nervous system and breathing
Acetaminophen and codeine		May cause blood pressure to drop too low
Meperidine		
Propoxyphene		
	MAO inhibitors	May cause many severe and sometimes fatal reactions
	Isocarboxazid	
	Phenelzine	
	Tranylcypromine	
	Tricyclic antidepressants	May depress nervous system and breathing
	Amitriptyline	May cause blood pressure to drop too low
	Amoxapine	
	Doxepin	
	Benzodiazepines	May cause increased drowsiness/confusion
	Diazepam	
	Alprazolam	
	Clonazepam	
	Chlordiazepoxide	
	Others	

From *Mosby's medical, nursing, and allied health dictionary*, ed 5, St Louis, 1998, Mosby.

Appendix E | Top 200 Best-Selling Drugs, Alphabetical Listing by Generic Name

Drug	FDA Drug Class(es)
Acetaminophen; codeine phosphate	Analgesics, general; analgesics-narcotic; analgesics-nonnarcotic; antitussives/expectorants/mucolytics
Acetaminophen; hydrocodone bitartrate	Analgesics, general; analgesics-narcotic; analgesics-nonnarcotic; antihistamines; antitussives/expectorants/mucolytics
Acetaminophen; oxycodone hydrochloride	Analgesics, general; analgesics-narcotic; analgesics-nonnarcotic
Acetaminophen; propoxyphene napsylate	Analgesics, general; analgesics-narcotic; antiarthritics
Acyclovir	Antifungals; antivirals; dermatologics
Albuterol	Antiasthmatics/bronchodilators; antihypertensives
Alendronate sodium	Calcium metabolism
Alprazolam	Antianxiety
Amitriptyline hydrochloride	Anorexiants/CNS stimulants; antidepressants
Amlodipine besylate	Antianginals; antihypertensives
Amoxicillin	Antihistamines; lincosamides/macrolides; penicillins
Amoxicillin; clavulanate potassium	Penicillins
Atenolol	Antianginals; antihypertensives; beta blockers
Atorvastatin calcium	Hyperlipidemia
Azithromycin dihydrate	Lincosamides/macrolides
Beclomethasone dipropionate	Adrenal corticosteroids; antiasthmatics/bronchodilators; antihistamines; nasal decongestants
Benazepril hydrochloride	ACE inhibitors; antihypertensives
Betamethasone dipropionate; clotrimazole	Analgesics, general; antifungals; dermatologics; topical steroids
Bisoprolol fumarate; hydrochlorothiazide	Antihypertensives
Buspirone hydrochloride	Antianxiety
Carisoprodol	Skeletal muscle hyperactivity
Cefaclor	Cephalosporins
Cefixime	Cephalosporins
Cefprozil	Cephalosporins
Cefuroxime axetil	Cephalosporins
Cephalexin	Cephalosporins; ocular antiinfective/antiinflammatory; penicillins
Cetirizine hydrochloride	Antihistamines
Cimetidine	Antacids; acid/peptic disorders
Ciprofloxacin hydrochloride	Antibacterials, miscellaneous; ocular antiinfective/antiinflammatory; quinolones/derivatives
Cisapride monohydrate	Acid/peptic disorders
Clarithromycin	Lincosamides/macrolides
Clonazepam	Antianxiety; anticonvulsants
Clonidine hydrochloride	Alpha agonists/alpha blockers; analgesics, general; antihypertensives
Codeine phosphate; promethazine hydrochloride	Antitussives/expectorants/mucolytics; cold remedies
Cyclobenzaprine hydrochloride	Skeletal muscle hyperactivity
Desogestrel; ethinyl estradiol	Contraceptives; estrogens/progestins
Dexamethasone; tobramycin	Aminoglycosides; ocular antiinfective/antiinflammatory
Diazepam	Anesthesia, adjuncts to/analeptics; antianxiety; anticonvulsants; skeletal muscle hyperactivity
Dicyclomine hydrochloride	Antispasmodics/anticholinergics; gastrointestinal, miscellaneous
Digoxin	Antiarrhythmics; cardiac glycosides
Diltiazem hydrochloride	Antianginals; antiarrhythmics; antihypertensives; calcium channel blockers; coronary vasodilators
Divalproex sodium	Anticonvulsants
Dorzolamide hydrochloride	Glaucoma
Doxazosin mesylate	Alpha agonists/alpha blockers; antihypertensives

From *Mosby's GenRx: the complete reference for generic and brand drugs,* ed 9, St Louis, 1999, Mosby.

Continued

Drug	FDA Drug Class(es)
Doxycycline	Antiasthmatics/bronchodilators; tetracyclines
Enalapril maleate	ACE inhibitors; antihypertensives
Erythromycin	Acne products; antihistamines; antineoplastics; cephalosporins; dermatologics; estrogens/progestins; lincosamides/macrolides; ocular antiinfective/antiinflammatory; topical antiinfectives
Estradiol	Dermatologics; estrogens/progestins
Estrogens, conjugated	Adrenal corticosteroids; antineoplastics; estrogens/progestins
Estrogens, conjugated; medroxyprogesterone acetate	Estrogens/progestins
Ethinyl estradiol; ethynodiol diacetate	Antineoplastics; contraceptives; estrogens/progestins
Ethinyl estradiol; ferrous fumarate; norethindrone acetate	Contraceptives; estrogens/progestins
Ethinyl estradiol; levonorgestrel	Contraceptives
Ethinyl estradiol; norethindrone	Contraceptives; estrogens/progestins
Ethinyl estradiol; norgestimate	Contraceptives; estrogens/progestins
Ethinyl estradiol; norgestrel	Contraceptives; estrogens/progestins
Etodolac	Analgesics, general; antiarthritics; NSAID
Famotidine	Acid/peptic disorders
Fexofenadine hydrochloride	Antihistamines
Fluconazole	Antifungals
Fluoxetine hydrochloride	Antidepressants
Fluticasone propionate	Corticosteroids-inhalation/nasal; dermatologics
Fluvastatin sodium	Hyperlipidemia
Fosinopril sodium	ACE inhibitors; antihypertensives
Furosemide	Antihypertensives; diuretics
Gabapentin	Anticonvulsants
Gemfibrozil	Hyperlipidemia; cerebral/peripheral vascular disorders
Glipizide	Blood glucose regulators
Glyburide	Blood glucose regulators
Guaifenesin; phenylpropanolamine hydrochloride	Antitussives/expectorants/mucolytics; cold remedies; nasal decongestants
Hydrochlorothiazide	Antihypertensives; diuretics
Hydrochlorothiazide; lisinopril	ACE inhibitors; antihypertensives; diuretics
Hydrochlorothiazide; triamterene	Antihypertensives; diuretics
Hydrocortisone; neomycin sulfate; polymyxin B sulfate	Deficiency anemias; ocular antiinfective/antiinflammatory; topical otics; vitamins/minerals
Ibuprofen	Analgesics, general; analgesics-nonnarcotic; antiarthritics; antigout; antimigraine/other headaches; antipyretics; NSAID
Insulin (human recombinant)	Blood glucose regulators
Ipratropium bromide	Antiasthmatics/bronchodilators
Isosorbide mononitrate	Antianginals; coronary vasodilators
Lansoprazole	Acid/peptic disorders
Latanoprost	Glaucoma
Levothyroxine sodium	Thyroid/antithyroid
Lisinopril	ACE inhibitors; antihypertensives
Loracarbef	Antibacterials, miscellaneous; cephalosporins
Loratadine	Antihistamines
Lorazepam	Anesthesia, adjuncts to/analeptics; antianxiety; sedatives/hypnotics
Losartan potassium	Antihypertensives
Lovastatin	Hyperlipidemia
Medroxyprogesterone acetate	Antineoplastics; contraceptives; estrogens/progestins
Metformin hydrochloride	Blood glucose regulators
Methylphenidate hydrochloride	Anorexiants/CNS stimulants; central nervous system; CNS, miscellaneous
Methylprednisolone	Adrenal corticosteroids; antiarthritics
Metoprolol succinate	Antihypertensives; beta blockers
Metoprolol tartrate	Antianginals; antihypertensives; beta blockers

From *Mosby's GenRx: the complete reference for generic and brand drugs,* ed 9, St Louis, 1999, Mosby.

Drug	FDA Drug Class(es)
Mometasone furoate	Adrenal corticosteroids; dermatologics; topical steroids
Mupirocin	Dermatologics; topical antiinfectives
Nabumetone	Antiarthritics
Naproxen sodium	Analgesics, general; antiarthritics; antigout; NSAID
Nefazodone hydrochloride	Antidepressants
Nifedipine	Antianginals; antihypertensives; calcium channel blockers
Nitrofurantoin; nitrofurantoin, macrocrystalline	Urinary tract antiseptics
Nitroglycerin	Antianginals; antihypertensives; coronary vasodilators; homeopathic products
Nizatidine	Acid/peptic disorders
Ofloxacin	Antibacterials, miscellaneous; ocular antiinfective/antiinflammatory; quinolones/derivatives
Omeprazole	Acid/peptic disorders; gastrointestinal, miscellaneous
Oxaprozin	Analgesics-nonnarcotic; antiarthritics
Paroxetine hydrochloride	Antidepressants
Penicillin V potassium	Penicillins
Phentermine hydrochloride	Anorexiants/CNS stimulants; thyroid/antithyroid
Phenytoin sodium	Anticonvulsants; central pain syndromes
Potassium chloride	Replacement/regulation of electrolytes/water balance; vitamins/minerals
Pravastatin sodium	Hyperlipidemia
Prednisone	Adrenal corticosteroids; antiarthritics; antineoplastics; ocular antiinfective/antiinflammatory
Promethazine hydrochloride	Anesthesia, adjuncts to/analeptics; antiemetics; antihistamines; antitussives/expectorants/mucolytics; sedatives/hypnotics; vertigo/motion sickness/vomiting
Quinapril hydrochloride	ACE inhibitors; antihypertensives
Ramipril	ACE inhibitors; antihypertensives
Ranitidine hydrochloride	Antihistamines; antivirals; acid/peptic disorders
Risperidone	Antipsychotics/antimanics
Salmeterol xinafoate	Antiasthmatics/bronchodilators
Sertraline hydrochloride	Antidepressants
Simvastatin	Hyperlipidemia
Sulfamethoxazole; trimethoprim	Antiarrhythmics; antibacterials, miscellaneous; urinary tract antiseptics; sulfonamides/related compounds; tetracyclines
Sumatriptan succinate	Antimigraine/other headaches; pharmaceutical aids
Tamoxifen citrate	Antineoplastics; hormonal/biological response modifiers
Temazepam	Sedatives/hypnotics
Terazosin hydrochloride	Alpha agonists/alpha blockers; antihypertensives; diuretics
Timolol	Glaucoma
Tramadol hydrochloride	Analgesics-nonnarcotic
Trazodone hydrochloride	Analgesics, general; antianxiety; antiarthritics; antidepressants
Tretinoin	Acne products; antineoplastics; dermatologics
Triamcinolone acetonide	Adrenal corticosteroids; antiasthmatics/bronchodilators; corticosteroids-inhalant/nasal; dental preparations; dermatologics; ocular antiinfective/antiinflammatory; sulfonamides/related compounds; topical steroids
Triamterene	Antihypertensives; diuretics
Venlafaxine hydrochloride	Antidepressants
Verapamil hydrochloride	Antianginals; antiarrhythmics; antiarthritics; antihypertensives; calcium channel blockers
Warfarin sodium	Anticoagulants/thrombolytics
Zolpidem tartrate	Sedatives/hypnotics

Appendix F   Tables of Weights and Measures

Metric System

Length	Weight	Volume
meter (m) basic unit	gram (g or gm) basic unit	liter (L) basic unit
1 micrometer (μm) = 0.000001 meter	1 microgram (mgc or μg) = 0.000001 gram	1 milliliter (ml)* = 0.001 liter
1 millimeter (mm) = 0.001 meter	1 milligram (mg) = 0.001 gram	1 centiliter (cl) = 0.01 liter
1 centimeter (cm) = 0.01 meter	1 centigram (cg) = 0.01 gram	1 deciliter (dl) = 0.1 liter
1 decimeter (dm) = 0.1 meter	1 decigram (dg) = 0.1 gram	1 dekaliter (Dl) = 10 liters
1 dekameter (Dm) = 10 meters	1 dekagram (Dg) = 10 grams	1 hektoliter (Hl) = 100 liters
1 hectometer (Hm) = 100 meters	1 hektogram (Hg) = 100 grams	1 kiloliter (kl) = 1000 liters
1 kilometer (km) = 1000 meters	1 kilogram (kg) = 1000 grams	

Apothecary System

Weight	Volume
20 grains (gr) = 1 scruple (Ꝫ)	60 minims (℔) = 1 fluidram (f℥ or ℥)
3 scruples (Ꝫ) = 1 dram (℥)	8 fluidrams (f℥) = 1 fluidounce (f℥ or ℥)
8 drams (℥) = 1 ounce (℥)	16 fluidounces (f℥) = 1 pint (O or pt)
12 ounces (℥) = 1 pound (lb)	2 pints (O) = 1 quart (qt)
	4 quarts (qt) = 1 gallon (C, Cong, or gal)

Household Equivalents

Volume

1 teaspoonful (tsp)	= 5 milliliters (ml)
1 dessertspoonful	= 10 milliliters (ml)
1 tablespoonful (tbsp)	= 15 milliliters (ml) or ½ ounce (℥)
1 teacupful	= 120 milliliters (ml) or 4 ounces (℥)
1 cupful	= 240 milliliters (ml) or 8 ounces (℥)

Other Commonly Used Equivalents (Approximate)

Weight	Volume
1 grain (gr) = 60 to 65 milligrams (mg)	1 minim (℔) = 0.06 milliliter (ml)
15 grains (gr) = 1 gram (g)	16 minims (℔) = 1 milliliter (ml)
kilogram (kg) = 2.2 pounds (lb)	1 fluidram (f℥) = 1 teaspoonful (tsp)†
	1 fluidounce (f℥) = 30 milliliters (ml)
	1 pint (pt) = 500 milliliters

*1 ml is considered equivalent to 1 cubic centimeter (cc).
†In medication orders, ℥i is commonly used to designate 1 tsp (5 ml).

Appendix G | Common Communicable Diseases

To prevents the spread of infection, any person with symptoms suggestive of a communicable disease should be kept away from others. Measures for control of communicable diseases are established either by law or by regulation in various states and communities. Because these may vary, practical nurses should keep in touch with local health authorities and cooperate with them in preventing the spread of disease.

Contagious Diseases

Disease and Synopsis of Symptoms	Incubation Period	Mode of Transmission	Period of Communicability
Actinomycosis Chronic disease most frequently localized in jaw, thorax, or abdomen; septicemic spread with generalized disease may occur. Lesions are firmly indurated areas of purulence and fibrosis.	Irregular; probably years after colonization in oral tissues, plus days or months after precipitating trauma and actual penetration of tissues.	Contact from person to person as part of normal oral flora.	Time and manner in which *A. israelii* becomes part of normal flora is unknown.
Amebiasis Infection with a protozoan parasite that exists in two forms: the hardy, infective cyst and the more fragile, potentially invasive trophozoite. Parasite may act as a commensal or invade tissues, giving rise to intestinal or extraintestinal disease.	Variation: from a few days to several months or years. Commonly 2 to 4 weeks.	Contaminated water or food containing cysts from feces of infected persons, often as complication of another infection such as shigellosis.	During period of cyst passing, which may continue for years.
Ascariasis (Roundworm Infection) Helminthic infection of small intestine. Symptoms are variable, often vague or absent, or ordinarily mild; live worms, passed in stools or regurgitated, are frequently first recognized sign of infection.	Worms reach maturity about 2 months after ingestion of embryonated eggs.	By ingestion of infective eggs from soil contaminated with human feces containing eggs, but not directly from person to person.	As long as mature female worms live in intestine. Maximum lifespan of adult worms is under 18 months; however, female produces up to 200,000 eggs a day that can remain viable in soil for months or years.
Balantidiasis Disease of colon characteristically producing diarrhea or dysentery accompanied by abdominal colic, tenesmus, nausea, and vomiting.	Unknown; may be only a few days.	By ingestion of cysts from feces of infected hosts; in epidemics, mainly by fecally contaminated water.	As long as infection persists.
Candidiasis (Monilliasis, Thrush, Candidosis) Mycosis usually confined to superficial layers of skin or mucous membranes with patients who have oral thrush, intertrigo, vulvovaginitis, paronychia, or onychomycosis.	Variable, 2 to 5 days in thrush of infants.	Through contact with excretions of mouth, skin, vagina, and especially feces from patients or carriers; from mother to infant during childbirth; and by endogenous spread.	Presumably for duration of lesions.

Modified from *Mosby's medical nursing and allied health dictionary*, ed 5, St Louis, 1998, Mosby.

Continued

Contagious Diseases—cont'd

Disease and Synopsis of Symptoms	Incubation Period	Mode of Transmission	Period of Communicability
Carditis, Coxsackie (Viral Carditis, Enteroviral Carditis)			
Acute or subacute myocarditis or pericarditis, which occurs as the only manifestation, or may occasionally be associated with other manifestations.	Usually 3 to 5 days.	Fecal-oral or respiratory droplet contact with infected person.	Apparently during acute stage of disease.
Chickenpox, Herpes Zoster (Varicella Shingles)			
Acute generalized viral disease with sudden onset of slight fever, mild constitutional symptoms, and a skin eruption that is maculopapular for a few hours, vesicular for 3 to 4 days, and leaves a granular scab.	From 2 to 3 weeks; commonly 13 to 17 days.	From person to person by direct contact, droplet, or air-borne spread of secretion of respiratory tract of chickenpox cases or of vesicle fluid of patients with herpes zoster.	As long as 5 days but usually 1 to 2 days before onset of rash, and not more than 6 days after appearance of first crop of vesicles.
Cholera			
Acute intestinal disease with sudden onset, profuse watery stools, occasional vomiting, rapid dehydration, acidosis, and circulatory collapse. Death may occur within a few hours.	From a few hours to 5 days, usually 2 to 3 days.	Through ingestion of food or water contaminated with feces or vomitus of infected persons or with feces of carriers.	Thought to be for duration of stool-positive stage, usually only a few days after recovery. Carrier stage may last for several months.
Conjunctivitis, Acute Bacterial			
Clinical syndrome beginning with lacrimation, irritation, and hyperemia of the palpebral and bulbar conjunctivae of one or both eyes, followed by edema of lids, photophobia, and mucopurulent discharge.	Usually 24 to 72 hours.	Contact with discharges from conjunctivae or upper respiratory tract of infected persons through contaminated fingers, clothing, or other articles.	During course of active infection.
Conjunctivitis, Epidemic Hemorrhagic (Apollo 11 Disease)			
Virus infection with sudden onset of pain or sensation of a foreign body in eye. Disease rapidly progresses (1 to 2 days) to full case of swollen eyelids, hyperemia of the conjunctivae, often with a circumcorneal distribution, seromucous disease, and frequent subconjunctival hemorrhages.	1 to 2 days or even shorter.	Through direct or indirect contact with discharge from infected eyes and possibly by droplet infection from those with virus in throat.	Unknown, but assumed to be for period of active disease, usually 1 to 2 weeks.
Dermatophytosis			
A. Ringworm of scalp and beard (tinea capitis, tinea kerion, favus).	10 to 14 days.	Direct or indirect contact with articles infected with hair from humans or infected animals.	As long as lesions are present and viable fungus persists on contaminated materials.

Modified from *Mosby's medical nursing and allied health dictionary,* ed 5, St Louis, 1998, Mosby.

Contagious Diseases—cont'd

Disease and Synopsis of Symptoms	Incubation Period	Mode of Transmission	Period of Communicability
Dermatophytosis—cont'd Begins as small papule and spreads peripherally, leaving scaly patches of temporary baldness. Infected hairs become brittle and break off easily. Kerions sometimes develop.			
B. Ringworm of nails (tinea unguium, onychomycosis). Chronic infectious disease involving one or more nails of hands or feet. Nail thickens, becoming discolored and brittle with an accumulation of caseous-appearing material beneath nail.	Unknown.	Presumably by direct extension from skin or nail lesions of infected persons. Low rate of transmission.	Possibly as long as infected lesion is present.
C. Ringworm of groin and perianal region (dhobie itch, tinea cruris).	4 to 10 days.	Direct or indirect contact with skin and scalp lesions of infected persons or animals.	As long as lesions are present and viable fungus persists on contaminated materials.
D. Ringworm of the body (tinea corporis). Characteristically appears as flat, spreading, ring-shaped lesions. Periphery is usually reddish, vesicular, or pustular and may be dry and scaly or moist and crusted.			
E. Ringworm of the foot (tinea pedis, athlete's foot). Scaling or cracking of skin, especially between toes, or blisters containing watery fluid are characteristic. In severe cases vesicular lesions appear on various parts of body.	Unknown.	Direct or indirect contact with skin lesions of infected persons or contaminated floors or shower stalls.	As long as lesions are present and viable spores persist on contaminated materials.
Diphtheria Characteristic lesion marked by patch or patches of grayish membrane with surrounding dull red inflammatory zone. Throat is moderately sore in faucial diphtheria, with cervical lymph nodes enlarged and tender; occasionally swelling and edema of neck.	2 to 5 days, sometimes longer.	Contact with patient or carrier; more rarely with articles soiled with discharges from lesions of infected persons. Raw milk has been a vehicle.	Variable, until virulent bacilli have disappeared from discharge and lesions. Usual period is 2 to 4 weeks but chronic carriers may shed organisms for 6 months or more.

Continued

Contagious Diseases—cont'd

Disease and Synopsis of Symptoms	Incubation Period	Mode of Transmission	Period of Communicability
Gastroenteritis, Viral			
A. Epidemic viral gastroenteritis. Usually self-limited mild disease that often occurs in outbreaks with clinical symptoms of nausea, vomiting, diarrhea, abdominal pain, myalgia, headache, malaise, low-grade fever, or a combination thereof.	24 to 48 hours; in volunteer studies with Norwalk agent, range was 10 to 51 hours.	Unknown; probably by fecal-oral route. Several recent outbreaks strongly suggest food-borne and water-borne transmission.	During acute stage of disease and shortly thereafter.
B. Rotavirus gastroenteritis (sporadic viral gastroenteritis of infants and children). Sporadic severe gastroenteritis of infants and young children characterized by diarrhea and vomiting, often with severe dehydration and occasional deaths.	Approximately 48 hours.	Probably fecal-oral and possibly respiratory routes.	During acute stage of disease and later while virus shedding continues. Virus is not usually detectable after eighth day of illness.
Giardiasis (Giardia Enteritis, Lambliasis)			
Protozoan infection principally of upper small bowel; often asymptomatic, it may also be associated with a variety of intestinal symptoms such as chronic diarrhea; steatorrhea; abdominal cramps; bloating; frequent loose, pale, greasy, malodorous stools; fatigue; and weight loss.	In a water-borne epidemic in United States, clinical illnesses occurred 1 to 4 weeks after exposure; average 2 weeks.	Localized outbreaks occur from contaminated water supplies. By ingestion of cysts in fecally contaminated water and occasionally by fecally contaminated food.	Entire period of infection.
Hepatitis, Viral			
A. Viral hepatitis A (infectious hepatitis, epidemic hepatitis, epidemic jaundice, catarrhal jaundice, Type A hepatitis). Onset is usually abrupt with fever, malaise, anorexia, nausea, and abdominal discomfort, followed within a few days by jaundice.	From 15 to 50 days, depending on dose; average 28 to 30 days.	Person to person by fecal-oral route. Common-vehicle outbreaks have been related to contaminated water and food.	Studies indicate maximum infectivity during latter half of incubation period, continuing for a few days, after onset of jaundice.

Modified from *Mosby's medical nursing and allied health dictionary,* ed 5, St Louis, 1998, Mosby.

Contagious Diseases—cont'd

Disease and Synopsis of Symptoms	Incubation Period	Mode of Transmission	Period of Communicability
Hepatitis, Viral B. Viral hepatitis B (type B hepatitis, serum hepatitis). Onset is usually insidious with anorexia, vague abdominal discomfort, and nausea and vomiting, sometimes arthralgias and rash, often progressing to jaundice. Fever may be absent or mild.	Usually 45 to 160 days, average 60 to 90 days. Variation is related in part to amount of virus in inoculum, mode of transmission, and host factors.	HB$_s$Ag, the infectious agent, has been found in virtually all body secretions, but only blood, saliva, and semen have been shown to be infectious. Transmission usually by percutaneous inoculation of infected blood and blood products; contaminated needles, syringes, and IV equipment.	From several weeks before onset of symptoms through clinical course of disease; carrier stage can last for years.
C. Hepatitis, non-A, non-B (non-B transfusion–associated hepatitis, hepatitis C). Chronic infection may be symptomatic or asymptomatic. Differential diagnosis depends on exclusion of hepatitis types A and B.	2 weeks to 6 months, model 6 to 8 weeks.	Most common posttransfusion hepatitis in United States and is more common when paid donors are used. Percutaneous transmission documented and other modes similar to those of hepatitis B virus are suspected.	Degree of immunity following infection is not known.
Herpangina, Hand-Foot-and-Mouth Disease, Acute Lymphonodular Pharyngitis			
Herpangina—grayish papulovesicular pharyngeal lesions on an erythematous base. *Hand-foot-and-mouth disease*—more diffuse oral lesions on buccal surfaces of cheeks, gums, and tongue. *Acute lymphonodular pharyngitis*—lesions are firm, raised, discrete, whitish to yellowish nodules.	3 to 5 days for herpangina and hand-foot-and-mouth disease. 5 days for acute lymphonodular pharyngitis.	Direct contact with nose and throat discharges and feces of infected (possibly asymptomatic) persons and by droplet spread.	During acute stage of illness and longer because virus persists in stools for as long as several weeks.
Herpes Simplex Viral infection characterized by localized primary lesion, latency, and a tendency to localized recurrence. In perhaps 10% of primary infections overt disease may appear as illness of varying severity marked by fever and malaise lasting 1 week or more.	2 to 12 days.	HSV type 1: Direct contact with virus in saliva of carriers. HSV type 2: Sexual contact.	Secretion of virus in saliva has been reported for as long as 7 weeks after recovery from stomatitis. Patients with primary lesions are infective for about 7 to 12 days, with recurrent disease for 4 days to 1 week.

Continued

Contagious Diseases—cont'd

Disease and Synopsis of Symptoms	Incubation Period	Mode of Transmission	Period of Communicability
Influenza Acute viral disease of respiratory tract characterized by fever, chilliness, headache, myalgia, prostration, coryza, and mild sore throat. Cough is often severe and protracted.	Usually 24 to 72 hours.	By direct contact through droplet infection; probably airborne among crowded populations in enclosed spaces.	Probably limited to 3 days from clinical onset.
Measles (Rubeola, Hard Measles, Red Measles, Morbilli) Acute, highly communicable viral disease with pro-dromal fever, conjunc-tivitis, coryza, bronchitis, and Koplik's spots on the buccal mucosa. A char-acteristic red blotchy rash appears on third to seventh day, beginning on face, becoming gener-alized, lasting 4 to 7 days and sometimes ending in branny desquamation. Leukopenia is common.	About 10 days varying from 8 to 13 days from exposure to onset of fever; about 14 days until rash appears; uncommonly longer or shorter human normal immune globulin (IG), given later than third day of incubation period for passive protection, may extend the incubation period to 21 days instead of preventing disease.	By droplet spread or direct contact with nasal or throat secretions of infected persons. Measles is one of most readily transmitted communicable diseases.	From slightly before beginning of prodromal period to 4 days after appearance of rash; com-municability is minimal after second day of rash.
Meningitis, Meningococcal (Cerebrospinal Fever, Meningococcemia) Characterized by sudden onset of fever, intense headache, nausea and often vomiting, stiff neck, and frequently a petechial rash with pink macules or, very rarely, vesicles. Delirium and coma often appear; occasional fulminating cases exhibit sudden prostration.	Varies from 2 to 10 days, commonly 3 to 4 days.	By direct contact, including droplets and discharges from nose and throat of infected persons, more often carriers than cases.	Until meningococci are no longer present in dis-charges from nose and throat. If organisms are sensitive to sulfonamides, meningococci usually disappear from naso-pharynx within 24 hours after institution of treat-ment. They are not fully eradicated from oronaso-pharynx by penicillin.
Meningitis, Haemophilus (Meningitis Caused by Haemophilus influenzae) Most common bacterial meningitis in children 2 months to 3 years old in U.S. Otitis media or sinusitis may be precursor. Almost always associated with bacteremia. Onset is sudden with symptoms of fever, vomiting, lethargy, and meningeal irritation.	Probably short—within 2 to 4 days.	By droplet infection and discharges from nose and throat during infectious period. May be purulent rhinitis. Portal of entry is most commonly nasopharyngeal.	As long as organisms are present, which may be for prolonged period even without nasal discharge.

Modified from *Mosby's medical nursing and allied health dictionary*, ed 5, St Louis, 1998, Mosby.

Contagious diseases—cont'd

Disease and Synopsis of Symptoms	Incubation Period	Mode of Transmission	Period of Communicability
Mononucleosis, Infectious (Glandular Fever, EBV Mononucleosis) Characterized by fever, sore throat (often with exudative pharyngo-tonsillitis), and lympha-denopathy (especially posterior cervical). Jaundice occurs in about 4% of infected young adults and splenomegaly in 50%. Duration is from 1 to several weeks.	From 4 to 6 weeks.	Person-to-person spread by oropharyngeal route via saliva. Spread may also occur via blood transfusion to susceptible recipients.	Prolonged; pharyngeal excretion may persist for 1 year after infection; 15% to 20% of healthy adults are oropharyngeal carriers.
Mumps (Infectious Parotitis) Acute viral disease charact-erized by fever, swelling, and tenderness of one or more salivary glands, usually parotid and sometimes sublingual or submaxillary glands.	About 2 to 3 weeks, commonly 18 days.	By droplet spread and by direct contact with saliva of an infected person.	Virus has been isolated from saliva from 6 days before salivary gland involvement to as long as 9 days there-after; but height of infec-tiousness occurs about 48 hours before swelling begins. Urine may be positive for as long as 14 days after onset of illness.
Paratyphoid Fever Frequently generalized bacterial enteric infection, often with abrupt onset, continued fever, enlarge-ment of spleen, sometimes rose spots on trunk, usually diarrhea, and involvement of lymphoid tissues of mesentery and intestines.	1 to 3 weeks for enteric fever; 1 to 10 days for gastroenteritis.	Direct or indirect contact with feces or urine of patient or carrier. Spread by food, especially milk, milk products, and shellfish. Files may be vectors.	As long as infectious agent persists in excreta, which is from appearance of prodromal symptoms, throughout illness, and for periods up to several weeks or months. Com-monly 1 to 2 weeks after recovery.
Pediculosis (Louse Infestation) Infestation of head, hairy parts of body, or clothing with adult lice, larvae, or nits (eggs), which results in severe itching and excoriation of scalp or scratch marks on body.	Under optimum conditions, eggs of lice hatch in 1 week and reach sexual maturity in approximately 2 weeks.	Direct contact with infected person and indirectly by contact with personal belongings, especially clothing and headgear. Crab lice are usually transmitted through sexual contact.	Communicable as long as lice remain alive on infested person or in clothing, and until eggs in hair and clothing have been destroyed.
The Pneumonias A. Pneumococcal pneumonia. Acute bacterial infection characterized by sudden onset with single shaking chill, fever, pleural pain, dyspnea, cough productive of "rusty" sputum and leukocytosis.	Not well determined; believed to be 1 to 3 days.	By droplet spread; by direct oral contact or indirectly, through articles freshly soiled with respiratory organisms is common.	Presumably until discharges of mouth and nose no longer contain virulent pneumococci in signifi-cant numbers. Penicillin will render patient nonin-fectious within 24 to 48 hours.

Continued

Contagious Diseases—cont'd

Disease and Synopsis of Symptoms	Incubation Period	Mode of Transmission	Period of Communicability
The Pneumonias—cont'd			
B. Mycoplasmal pneumonia (primary atypical pneumonia). Predominantly afebrile lower respiratory infection. Onset is gradual with headache, malaise, cough often paroxysmal, and usually substernal pain (not pleuritic). Sputum, scant at first, may increase later.	14 to 21 days.	Probably by droplet inhalation, direct contact with infected person or with articles freshly soiled with discharges of nose and throat from acutely ill and coughing patient.	Probably less than 10 days; occasionally longer with persisting febrile illness or persistence of the organisms in convalescence (as long as 13 weeks is known).
C. Pneumocystis pneumonia (interstitial plasma cell pneumonia). Acute pulmonary disease occurring early in life, especially in malnourished, chronically ill, or premature infants. Characterized by progressive dyspnea, tachypnea, and cyanosis; fever may not be present.	Analysis of data from institutional outbreaks among infants indicates 1 to 2 months.	Unknown.	Unknown.
D. Chlamydial pneumonia (pertussoid eosinophilic pneumonia). Subacute pulmonary disease occurring in early infancy, primarily in infants of mothers with infection of uterine cervix with causative organism.	Not known, but pneumonia may occur in infants from 1 to 18 weeks of age (more commonly between 4 and 12 weeks).	Presumed to be vertically transmitted from infected cervix to infant during birth, with resultant nasopharyngeal infection.	Unknown, but length of nasopharyngeal excretion can be at least 2 months.
Poliomyelitis (infantile paralysis)			
Acute viral infection whose symptoms include fever, malaise, headache, nausea, vomiting, and stiffness of neck and back with or without paralysis.	Commonly 7 to 14 days for paralytic cases, with a range from 3 to possibly 35 days.	Direct contact through close association. In rare instances milk, foodstuffs, and other fecally contaminated materials have been incriminated as vehicles. Fecal-oral is major route when sanitation is poor, but during epidemics and when sanitation is good, pharyngeal spread becomes relatively more important.	Not accurately known. Cases are probably most infectious during first few days after onset of symptoms.

Modified from *Mosby's medical nursing and allied health dictionary,* ed 5, St Louis, 1998, Mosby.

Contagious Diseases—cont'd

Disease and Synopsis of Symptoms	Incubation Period	Mode of Transmission	Period of Communicability
Respiratory Disease (Excluding Influenza) A. Acute febrile respiratory disease. Viral diseases of respiratory tract are characterized by fever and one or more constitutional reactions such as chills or chilliness, headache, general aching, malaise, and anorexia; in infants by occasional gastrointestinal disturbances.	From a few days to 1 week or more.	Directly by oral contact or may droplet spread, indirectly by hands or other materials soiled by respiratory discharges of infected person.	For duration of active disease; little is known about subclinical or latent infections.
B. Common cold (acute coryza). Acute catarrhal infections of upper respiratory tract characterized by coryza, sneezing, lacrimation, irritated nasopharynx, chilliness, and malaise lasting 2 to 7 days. Fever is uncommon in children and rare in adults.		Presumably by direct oral contact or by droplet spread; indirectly by hands and articles freshly soiled by discharges of nose and throat of infected person.	
Rubella (German Measles) A. Congenital rubella. Mild febrile infectious disease with diffuse punctate and macular rash. Sometimes resembling that of measles, scarlet fever, or both. May be few or no constitutional symptoms in children but adults may experience 1- to 5-day prodrome characterized by low-grade fever, headache, malaise, mild coryza, and conjunctivitis. As many as 20% to 50% of infections may occur without evidence rash; overall 50% are not recognized. B. Erythema infectiosum (fifth disease). Mild nonfebrile erythematous eruption occurring as epidemics among children. Characterized by striking erythema of cheeks, redding of skin, and lacelike serpiginous rash of body.	From 16 to 18 days with a range of 14 to 21 days.	Contact with nasopharyngeal secretions of infected person. Infection is by droplet spread or direct contact with patients and indirect contact.	For about 1 week before and at least 4 days after onset of rash. Highly communicable. Infants with congenital rubella syndrome may shed virus for months after birth.

Continued

Contagious Diseases—cont'd

Disease and Synopsis of Symptoms	Incubation Period	Mode of Transmission	Period of Communicability
Rubella (German Measles)—cont'd C. Exanthema subitum (roseola infantum). Acute illness of probable viral cause characterized by high fever that suddenly appears and lasts 3 to 5 days. A maculopapular rash on trunk and later on rest of body ordinarily follows lysis of fever.			
Shigellosis (Bacillary Dysentery) Acute bacterial disease primarily involving large intestine, characterized by diarrhea, accompanied by fever, nausea, sometimes vomiting, cramps, and tenesmus. In severe cases stools contain blood, mucus, and pus.	1 to 7 days, usually 1 to 3 days.	By direct or indirect fecal-oral transmission from patient or carrier. Infection may occur after ingestion of very few organisms.	During acute infection and until infectious agent is no longer present in feces, usually within 4 weeks of illness.
Staphylococcal Disease A. Staphylococcal disease in community, boils, carbuncles, furuncles, impetigo, cellulitis, abscesses, staphylococcal septicemia, staphylococcal pneumonia, osteomyelitis, endocarditis. Staphylococci produce variety of syndromes with clinical manifestations that range from single pustule to impetigo to septicemia to death. Lesion or lesions containing pus are primary clinical finding, abscess formation is typical.	Variable and indefinite. Commonly 4 to 10 days.	Major site of colonization is anterior nares. Auto-infection is responsible for at least one third of infections. Person with draining lesion or any purulent lesion or who is asymptomatic (usually nasal) carrier of pathogenic strain. Air-borne spread is rare.	As long as purulent lesions continue to drain or carrier state persists.
B. Staphylococcal disease in hospital nurseries, impetigo, abscess of breast. Characteristic lesions develop secondary to colonization of nose or umbilicus, conjunction, circumcision site, or rectum of infants with pathogenic strain.	Commonly 4 to 10 days but may occur several months after colonization.	Spread by hands of hospital personnel is primary mode of transmission within hospitals; to a lesser extent, air-borne.	Same.

Modified from *Mosby's medical nursing and allied health dictionary*, ed 5, St Louis, 1998, Mosby.

Contagious Diseases—cont'd

Disease and Synopsis of Symptoms	Incubation Period	Mode of Transmission	Period of Communicability
Staphylococcal Disease—cont'd C. Staphylococcal disease in medical and surgical wards of hospitals. Lesions may from simple furuncles or stitch abscesses to extensively infected bedsores or surgical wounds, septic phlebitis, chronic osteomyelitis, fulminating pneumonia, endocarditis, or septicemia.	Variable and indefinite. Commonly 4 to 10 days.	Major site of colonization is anterior nares. Autoinfection is responsible for at least one third of infections. Person with a draining lesion or any purulent lesion or who is an asymptomatic (usually nasal) carrier of a pathogenic strain. Air-borne spread is rare.	As long as purulent lesions continue to drain or carrier state persists.
Streptococcal Sore Throat Fever, sore throat, exudative tonsillitis or pharyngitis, and tender anterior cervical lymph nodes.	Short, usually 1 to 3 days, rarely longer.	Transmission results from direct or intimate contact with patient or carrier, rarely by indirect contact through objects or hands. Nasal carriers are particularly likely to transmit diseases.	In untreated uncomplicated cases 10 to 21 days; in untreated conditions with purulent discharges, weeks or months.
Syphilis, Nonvenereal Endemic Acute disease of limited geographical distribution, characterized clinically by eruption of skin and mucous membranes, usually without evident primary sore.	2 weeks to 3 months.	Direct or indirect contact with infectious early lesions of skin and mucous membranes. Congenital transmission does not occur.	Until moist eruptions of skin and mucous patches disappear—sometimes several weeks or months.
Trachoma Communicable keratoconjunctivitis characterized by conjunctival inflammation with papillary hyperplasia, associated with vascular invasion of cornea, and in later stages by conjunctival scarring that may eventually lead to blindness.	5 to 12 days (based on volunteer studies).	By direct contact with ocular discharges and possibly mucoid or purulent discharges of nasal mucous membranes of infected persons or materials. Flies *(Musca sorbens)* may contribute to spread of disease.	As long as active lesions are present in the conjunctivae and adnexal mucous membranes.

Continued

Contagious Diseases—cont'd

Disease and Synopsis of Symptoms	Incubation Period	Mode of Transmission	Period of Communicability
Tuberculosis Mycobacterial disease. Initial infection usually goes unnoticed; tuberculin sensitivity appears within a few weeks; lesions commonly heal, leaving no residual changes except pulmonary or tracheobronchial lymph node calcification. May progress to pulmonary tuberculosis or, by lymphohematogenous dissemination of bacilli, to produce miliary, meningeal, or other extrapulmonary involvement.	From infection to demonstrable primary lesion, about 4 to 12 weeks. Whereas subsequent risk of progressive pulmonary or extrapulmonary tuberculosis is greatest within 1 or 2 years after infection, it may persist for a lifetime as latent infection.	Exposure to bacilli in air-borne droplet nuclei from sputum of persons with infectious tuberculosis. Bovine tuberculosis results from exposure to tubercular cattle and ingestion of unpasteurized dairy products.	As long as infectious tubercle bacilli are being discharged.
Typhoid Fever (Enteric Fever, Typhus Abdominalis) Systemic infectious disease characterized by sustained fever, headache, malaise, anorexia, relative bradycardia, enlargement of spleen, rose spots on trunk, nonproductive cough, constipation more common than diarrhea, and involvement of lymphoid tissues.	Depends on size of infecting dose; usual range 1 to 3 weeks.	By food or water contaminated by feces or urine of patient or carrier.	As long as typhoid bacilli appear in excreta; usually first week throughout convalescence; variable thereafter. About 10% of untreated patients will discharge bacilli for 3 months after onset of symptoms; 2% to 5% become permanent carriers.
Whooping Cough (Pertussis) Acute bacterial disease involving tracheobronchial tree. Initial catarrhal stage has insidious onset with irritating cough that gradually becomes paroxysmal, usually within 1 to 2 weeks, and lasts for 1 to 2 months.	Commonly 7 days; almost uniformly within 10 days, and not exceeding 21 days.	Primarily by direct contact with discharges from respiratory mucous membranes of infected persons by air-borne route, probably by droplets. Frequently brought into home by older sibling.	Highly communicable in early catarrhal stage before paroxysmal cough stage. For control purposes, communicable stage extends from 7 days after exposure to 3 weeks after onset of typical paroxysms in patients not treated with antibiotics; in patients treated with erythromycin, period of infectiousness extends only 5 to 7 days after onset of therapy.

Modified from *Mosby's medical nursing and allied health dictionary,* ed 5, St Louis, 1998, Mosby.

Contagious Diseases—cont'd

Disease and Synopsis of Symptoms	Incubation Period	Mode of Transmission	Period of Communicability
Sexually Transmitted Diseases			
Acquired Immunodeficiency Syndrome (AIDS)			
Acute viral infection characterized by breakdown and failure of immune system, opening body to often lethal infections and disorders such as Kaposi's sarcoma, pneumonia, and meningitis. Symptoms begins with fever, weight loss, fatigue, shortness of breath, diarrhea, and neurologic disorders.	Variable.	By direct sexual contact and transmission of semen, saliva, blood, or other body fluids. Also by blood transfusion or contaminated syringes.	For duration of infection.
Chancroid (Ulcus Molle, Soft Chancre)			
Acute, localized, genital infection characterized by single or multiple painful necrotizing ulcers at site of inoculation, frequently accompanied by painful inflammatory swelling and suppuration of regional lymph nodes. Extragenital lesions have been reported.	From 3 to 5 days, up to 14 days.	By direct contact with discharges from open lesions and pus from buboes; suggestive evidence of asymptomatic infections in women. Multiple sexual partners and uncleanliness favor transmission.	As long as infectious agent persists in original lesion or discharging regional lymph nodes; usually until healed—a matter of weeks.
Conjunctivitis, Inclusion (Swimming Pool Conjunctivitis, Paratrachoma)			
In the newborn, acute papillary conjunctivitis with abundant mucopurulent discharge. In children and adults, acute follicular conjunctivitis with preauricular lymphadenopathy, often with superficial corneal involvement.	5 to 12 days.	During sexual intercourse; genital discharges of infected persons are infectious.	While genital infection persists; can be longer than 1 year in female.
Cytomegalovirus Infections, Congenital Cytomegalovirus Infection, Cytomegalic Inclusion Disease			
Most severe form of disease occurs in perinatal period, following congenital infection, with signs and symptoms of severe generalized infection especially involving central nervous system and liver.	Information inexact. 3 to 8 weeks following transfusion with infected blood. 3 to 12 weeks after birth.	Intimate exposure to infectious secretions or excretions. Virus is excreted in urine, saliva, cervical secretions, breast milk, and semen.	Virus is excreted in urine or saliva for months and may persist for several years following primary infection.

Continued

Contagious Diseases—cont'd

Disease and Synopsis of Symptoms	Incubation Period	Mode of Transmission	Period of Communicability
Sexually Transmitted Diseases—cont'd			
Gonococcal Infections			
A. Gonococcal infection of genitourinary tract (gonorrhea, gonococcal urethritis). *Males*—purulent discharge from anterior urethra with dysuria appears 2 to 7 days after infecting exposure. *Females*—few days after exposure initial urethritis or cervicitis occurs, frequently so mild as to pass unnoticed. About 20% of patients have uterine invasion at the first, second, or later menstrual period with symptoms of endometritis, salpingitis, or pelvic peritonitis.	Usually 2 to 7 days, sometimes longer.	By contact with exudates from mucous membranes of infected persons, almost always result of sexual activity.	May extend for months if untreated, especially in females who frequently are asymptomatic. Specific therapy usually ends communicability within hours except with penicillin-resistant strains.
B. Gonococcal conjunctivitis neonatorum (gonorrheal ophthalmia neonatorum). Acute redness and swelling of conjunctiva of one or both eyes, with mucopurulent or purulent discharge in which gonococci are identifiable by microscopic and cultural methods.	Usually 1 to 5 days.	Contact with infected birth canal during childbirth.	While discharge persists if untreated; for 24 hours following initiation of specific treatment.
Granuloma Inguinale (Donovanosis)			
Mildly communicable, nonfatal, chronic and progressive, autoinoculable bacterial disease of skin and mucous membranes of external genitalia, inguinal, and anal region. Small nodule, vesicle, or papule is present.	Unknown; probably 8 to 80 days.	Presumably by direct contact with lesions during sexual activity.	Unknown and probably for duration of open lesions on skin or mucous membranes.
Herpes Simplex			
Viral infection characterized by localized primary lesion, latency, and a tendency to localized recurrence. In perhaps 10% of primary infections overt disease may appear as illness of varying severity marked by fever and malaise lasting 1 week or more.	2 to 12 days.	HSV type 1: Direct contact with virus in saliva of carriers. HSV type 2: sexual contact.	Secretion of virus in saliva has been reported for as long as 7 weeks after recovery from stomatitis. Patients with primary lesions are infective for about 7 to 12 days, with recurrent disease for 4 days to 1 week.

Modified from *Mosby's medical nursing and allied health dictionary,* ed 5, St Louis, 1998, Mosby.

Contagious Diseases—cont'd

Disease and Synopsis of Symptoms	Incubation Period	Mode of Transmission	Period of Communicability
Sexually Transmitted Diseases—cont'd			
Lymphogranuloma Venereum (Lymphogranuloma Inguinale, Esthiomene, Climatic Bubo, Tropical Bubo)			
Venereally acquired infection, beginning with painless evanescent erosion, papule, nodule, or herpetiform lesion on penis or vulva, frequently unnoticed. Regional lymph nodes undergo suppuration followed by extension of inflammatory process to adjacent tissues.	Usually 7 to 12 days, with a range of 4 to 21 days to primary lesion. If bubo is first manifestation, 10 to 30 days, sometimes several months.	Direct contact with open lesions of infected persons usually during sexual intercourse.	Variable, from weeks to years, during presence of active lesions.
Syphilis, Venereal (Lues)			
Acute and chronic treponematosis characterized clinically by primary lesion, secondary eruption involving skin and mucous membranes, long periods of latency, and late lesions of skin, bone, viscerae, and central nervous and cardiovascular systems. Papule appears 3 weeks after exposure at site of initial invasion; after erosion, most common form is indurated chancre.	10 days to 10 weeks, usually 3 weeks.	By direct contact with infectious exudates from obvious or concealed moist early lesions of skin and mucous membrane, body fluids, and secretions of infected persons during sexual contact.	Variable and indefinite during primary and secondary stages and also in mucocutaneous recurrences; some cases may be intermittently communicable for 2 to 4 years.
Trichomoniasis			
Common disease of genitourinary tract, characterized in women by vaginitis, with small petechial or sometimes punctate hemorrhagic lesions and profuse, thin, foamy, yellowish discharge with foul odor; frequently asymptomatic. In men, infectious agent invades and persists in prostate, urethra, or seminal vesicles, but rarely produces symptoms or demonstrable lesions.	4 to 20 days, average 7 days.	By contact with vaginal and urethral discharges of infected persons during sexual intercourse and possibly by contact with contaminated articles.	For duration of infection.

Continued

Contagious Diseases—cont'd			

Disease and Synopsis of Symptoms	Incubation Period	Mode of Transmission	Period of Communicability
Sexually Transmitted Diseases—cont'd			
Urethritis, Chlamydial Urethritis, Nongonorrheal and Nonspecific			
Sexually transmitted urethritis of males caused by chlamydial agent. Clinical manifestations are usually indistinguishable from gonorrhea but are often milder and include opaque discharge of moderate or scanty quantity, urethral itching, and burning on urination. Infection of women results in cervicitis and salpingitis.	5 to 7 days or longer.	Sexual contact.	Unknown.

Modified from *Mosby's medical nursing and allied health dictionary,* ed 5, St Louis, 1998, Mosby.

Appendix H Nursing Guidelines for Advance Directives

The Patient Self-Determination Act (PSDA), which became effective December 1991, essentially mandates that health care facilities are responsible for ensuring that individuals enrolled in their facilities are informed of their right to formulate advance directives and their right to consent to or refuse treatment. This federal legislation affects virtually all health care facilities participating in Medicare and Medicaid programs: hospitals, nursing homes, home health agencies, hospices, and health maintenance organizations.

These agencies are required to:
- Provide education to the staff regarding these sensitive issues
- Maintain written policies and procedures for adherence to these requirements
- Ensure that the medical record reflects the patient's status regarding advance directives
- Not discriminate against any patient on the basis of individual decision making regarding advance directives

To ensure that the legislation addresses the problem as it was intended, nurses need to see that patients and their surrogates are aware of their right to formulate choices for the withholding or withdrawal of treatment under prespecified conditions.

Nurses need to:
- Formulate advance directives themselves
- Assist in the process of determining a patient's competency when there is reason to doubt it
- Ensure that the patient and family have sufficient information about the state statutes and the PSDA itself to make any desired decisions
- Recognize that not all individuals are ready to make decisions

- Be prepared to act on the patient's behalf if necessary
- Recognize the emotional state of the patient's family and help them to come to terms with the patient's advance directives formulated as a result of PSDA
- Ensure that agency administration has provided detailed policies and procedures, as well as thorough and comprehensive education of the individuals responsible for enforcing this statute (e.g., admission clerks, emergency room personnel)
- Facilitate discussions so that the involved individuals recognize that they are involved in a decision-making process, not a death-producing process
- Ensure that formative, summative, and ongoing evaluation mechanisms are in place in terms of implementation methodologies for enforcing the PSDA
- Serve and be active on ethics committees or, if necessary, establish one
- Ensure that no patient is discriminated against regarding type or quality of health care for any reason
- Ensure that whatever the patient's decision, it was not coerced—decisions must be strictly voluntary, and reflect the individual's values, desires, and wishes

To help in determining the competency of a patient, the following five questions should be considered:
1. Can the patient receive (hear or read) information?
2. Can the patient process and comprehend information?
3. Can the patient appropriately assess the relevant information?
4. Can the patient use relevant information to make a decision?
5. Can the patient make a decision and give a reason for it?

From Weber G: Tips on implementing the patient self-determination act, *Nursing and Health Care* 14(2), 1993. Excerpted with permission from National League for Nursing, New York.

Appendix I   State and Territorial Boards of Practical/Vocational Nursing—United States

ALABAMA
Board of Nursing
RSA Plaza, Suite 250
770 Washington Avenue
Montgomery, Alabama 36130-3900
Phone: (334) 242-4060
FAX: (334) 242-4360
http://www.abn.state.al.us

ALASKA
Board of Nursing
Department of Commerce & Economic Development
Division of Occupational Licensing
3601 C. Street, Suite 722
Anchorage, Alaska 99811-0806
Phone: (907) 269-8161
FAX: (907) 269-8196
http://www.dced.state.ak.us/occ/pnur.htm

AMERICAN SAMOA HEALTH SERVICES
Regulatory Board
LBJ Tropical Medical Center
Pago Pago, AS 96799
Phone: (684) 633-1222
FAX: (684) 633-1869

ARIZONA
State Board of Nursing
1651 East Morten, Suite 150
Phoenix, Arizona 85020
Phone: (602) 331-8111
FAX: (602) 906-9365
http://www.azboardofnursing.org

ARKANSAS
State Board of Nursing
University Tower Building
1123 S. University, Suite 8000
Little Rock, Arkansas 72204
Phone: (501) 686-2700
FAX: (501) 686-2714
http://www.state.ar.us/nurse

CALIFORNIA
Board of Vocational Nurse and Psychiatric Technician
  Examiners
2535 Capitol Oaks Drive, Suite 205
Sacramento, California 95833
Phone: (916) 263-7800
FAX: (916) 263-7859
http://www.bvnpt.ca.gov

COLORADO
Board of Nursing
1560 Broadway, Suite 880
Denver, Colorado 80202
Phone: (303) 894-2430
FAX: (303) 894-2821
http://www.dora.state.co.us/nursing

CONNECTICUT
Board of Examiners for Nursing
Division of Health Systems Regulation
410 Capitol Avenue, MS# 12HSR
P.O. Box 340308
Hartford, Connecticut 06134-0328
Phone: (860) 509-7624
FAX: (860) 509-7553
http://ww.state.ct.us/dph

DELAWARE
Board of Nursing
861 Silver Lake Blvd.
Cannon Building, Suite 203
Dover, Delaware 19904
Phone: (302) 739-4522
FAX: (302) 739-2711

DISTRICT OF COLUMBIA
Board of Nursing
Department of Health
825 N. Capitol Street, N.E.
2nd Floor, Room 2224
Washington, D.C. 20002
Phone: (202) 442-4778
FAX: (202) 442-9431

FLORIDA
Board of Nursing
4080 Woodcock Drive, Suite 202
Jacksonville, Florida 32207
Phone: (904) 858-6940
FAX: (904) 858-6964
http://www.doh.state.fl.us/mqa/nursing

GEORGIA
State Board of Licensed Practical Nurses
237 Coliseum Drive
Macon, Georgia 31217-1640
Phone: (912) 207-1300
FAX: (912) 207-1363
http://www.sos.state.ga.us/ebd-lpn

GUAM
Board of Nurse Examiners
P.O. Box 2816
1304 East Sunset Blvd.
Barrgada, Guam 96913
Phone: (671) 475-0251
FAX: (671) 477-4733

HAWAII
Board of Nursing
Professional & Vocational Licensing Division
Box 3469
Honolulu, Hawaii 96801
Phone: (808) 586-3000
FAX: (808) 586-2689

IDAHO
Board of Nursing
2800 N. 8th Street, Suite 210
P.O. Box 83720
Boise, Idaho 83720
Phone: (208) 334-3110
FAX: (208) 334-3262
http://www.state.id.us/ibn/ibnhome.htm

ILLINOIS
Department of Professional Regulation
James R. Thompson Center
100 W. Randolph, Suite 9-300
Chicago, Illinois 60601
Phone: (312) 814-2715
FAX: (312) 814-3145
http://www.state.il.us/dpr

INDIANA
State Board of Nursing
Health Professions Bureau
402 W. Washington St., Room W041
Indianapolis, Indiana 46204
Phone: (317) 232-2960
FAX: (317) 233-4236
http://www.ai.org/hpb

IOWA
Board of Nursing
RiverPoint Business Park
400 S.W. 8th Street, Suite B
Des Moines, Iowa 50309-4685
Phone: (515) 281-3255
FAX: (515) 281-4825
http://www.state.ia.us/government/nursing

KANSAS
State Board of Nursing
Landon State Office Building
900 SW Jackson, Suite 551-S
Topeka, Kansas 66612
Phone: (785) 296-4929
FAX: (785) 296-3929
http://www.ink.org/public/ksbn

KENTUCKY
Board of Nursing
312 Whittington Parkway, Suite 300
Louisville, Kentucky 40222
Phone: (502) 329-7000
FAX: (502) 329-7011
http://www.kbn.state.ky.us

LOUISANA
State Board of Practical Nurse Examiners
3421 N. Causeway Blvd., Suite 203
Metairie, Louisiana 70002
Phone: (504) 838-5791
FAX: (504) 838-5279

MAINE
State Board of Nursing
158 State House Station
Augusta, Maine 04333
Phone: (207) 287-1133
FAX: (207) 287-1149
http://www.state.me.us/pfr/auxboards/nurhome.htm

MARYLAND
Board of Nursing
4140 Patterson Avenue
Baltimore, Maryland 21215
Phone: (410) 585-1900
FAX: (410) 358-3530
http://dhmh1d.dhmh.state.md.us/mbn

MASSACHUSETTS
Board of Registration in Nursing
Commonwealth of Massachusetts
239 Causeway Street
Boston, Massachusetts 02114
Phone: (617) 727-9961
FAX: (617) 727-1630
http://www.state.ma.us/reg/boards

MICHIGAN
CIS/Office of Health Services
Ottawa Towers North
611 W. Ottawa, 4th Floor
Lansing, Michigan 48933
Phone: (517) 373-9102
FAX: (517) 373-2179
http://www.cis.state.mi.us/bhser/genover.htm

MINNESOTA
Board of Nursing
2829 University Avenue SE, Suite 500
St. Paul, Minnesota 55414
Phone: (612) 617-2270
FAX: (612) 617-2190
http://www.nursingboard.state.mn.us

MISSISSIPPI
Board of Nursing
1935 Lakeland Drive, Suite B
Jackson, Mississippi 39216
Phone: (601) 987-4188
FAX: (601) 364-2352

MISSOURI
State Board of Nursing
3605 Missouri Blvd.
Jefferson City, Missouri 65102-0656
Phone: (573) 751-0681
FAX: (573) 751-0075
http://www.ecodev.state.mo.us/pr/nursing

MONTANA
State Board of Nursing
Arcade Building, Suite 4C
111 N. Jackson
Helena, Montana 59620-0513
Phone: (406) 444-2071
FAX: (406) 444-7759
http://www.com.state.mt.us/License/POL/index.htm

NEBRASKA
Health and Human Services System
Department of Regulation and Licensure
Nursing Section
301 Centennial Mall South
P.O. Box 94986
Lincoln, Nebraska 68509-4986
Phone: (402) 471-4376
FAX: (402) 471-3577
http://www.hhs.state.ne.us/crl/nns.htm

NEVADA
State Board of Nursing
1755 East Plumb Lane, Suite 260
Reno, Nevada 89502
Phone: (775) 688-2620
FAX: (775) 688-2628
http://www.state.nv.us/boards/nsbn

NEW HAMPSHIRE
Board of Nursing
78 Regional Drive, Bldg. B
P.O. Box 3898
Concord, New Hampshire 03302
Phone: (603) 271-2323
FAX: (603) 271-6605
http://www.state.nh.us/nursing

NEW JERSEY
Board of Nursing
124 Halsey Street, 6th Fl.
P.O. Box 45010
Newark, New Jersey 07101
Phone: (973) 504-6586
FAX: (973) 648-3481
http://www.state.nj.us/lps/ca/medical.htm

NEW MEXICO
Board of Nursing
4206 Louisiana Boulevard NE, Suite A
Albuquerque, New Mexico 87109
Phone: (505) 841-8340
FAX: (404) 841-8347
http://www.state.nm.us/clients/nursing

NEW YORK
Board of Nursing
State Education Department
Cultural Education Center, Room 3023
Albany, New York 12230
Phone: (518) 474-3845
FAX: (518) 474-3706
http://www.nysed.gov/prof/nurse.htm

NORTH CAROLINA
Board of Nursing
3724 National Drive
Raleigh, North Carolina 27602
Phone: (919) 782-3211
FAX: (919) 781-9461
http://www.ncbon.com

NORTH DAKOTA
Board of Nursing
919 S. 7th Street, Suite 504
Bismarck, North Dakota 58504
Phone: (701) 328-9777
FAX: (701) 328-9785
http://www.ndbon.org

COMMONWEALTH OF THE NORTHERN MARIANA ISLANDS
Commonwealth Board of Nurse Examiners
Public Health Center
P.O. Box 1458
Saipan, MP 96950
Phone: (670) 234-8950
FAX: (670) 234-8930

OHIO
Board of Nursing
77 S. High Street, Suite 400
Columbus, Ohio 43215-3413
Phone: (614) 466-3947
FAX: (614) 466-0388
http://www.state.oh.us/nur

OKLAHOMA
Board of Nursing
2915 N. Classen Blvd., Suite 524
Oklahoma City, OK 73106
Phone: (405) 962-1800
FAX: (405) 962-1821

OREGON
State Board of Nursing
800 NE Oregon St., Box 25
Suite 465
Portland, OR 97232
Phone: (503) 731-4745
FAX: (503) 731-4755
http://www.osbn.state.or.us

PENNSYLVANIA
State Board of Nursing
124 Pine Street
P.O. Box 2649
Harrisburg, Pennsylvania 17101
Phone: (717) 783-7142
FAX: (717) 783-0822
http://www.dos.state.pa.us/bpoa/nurbd.htm

COMMONWEALTH OF PUERTO RICO
Board of Nurse Examiners
800 Roberto H. Todd Avenue
Room 202, Stop 18
Santurce, Puerto Rico 00908
FAX: (787) 725-7903

RHODE ISLAND
Board of Nurse Registration and Nursing Education
Three Capitol Hill
Cannon Health Building, Room 104
Providence, Rhode Island 02908
Phone: (401) 222-3855
FAX: (401) 222-2158

SOUTH CAROLINA
State Board of Nursing
110 Centerview Drive, Suite 202
Columbia, South Carolina 29210
Phone: (803) 896-4550
FAX: (803) 896-4525
http://www.llr.state.sc.us/bon.htm

SOUTH DAKOTA
Board of Nursing
4300 South Louis Ave., Suite C-1
Sioux Falls, South Dakota 57106-3124
Phone: (605) 362-2760
FAX: (605) 362-2768
http://www.state.sd.us/dcr/nursing

TENNESSEE
State Board of Nursing
426 5th Avenue North
1st Floor–Cordell Hull Building
Nashville, Tennessee 37247
Phone: (615) 532-5166
FAX: (615) 741-7899
http://170.142.76.180/bmf-bin/BMFproflist.pl

TEXAS
Board of Vocational Nurse Examiners
333 Guadalupe Street, Suite 3-400
William P. Hobby Bldg., Tower 3
Austin, Texas 78701
Phone: (512) 305-8100
FAX: (512) 305-8101
http://link.tsl.state.tx.us/tx/bvne

UTAH
Board of Nursing
160 East 300 South
Heber M. Wells Bldg., 4th Floor
Salt Lake City, Utah 84111
Phone: (801) 530-6628
FAX: (801) 530-6511

VERMONT
State Board of Nursing
109 State Street
Montpelier, Vermont 05609-1106
Phone: (802) 828-2396
FAX: (802) 828-2484
http://vtprofessionals.org/nurses

VIRGIN ISLANDS
Board of Nurse Licensure
Veterans Drive Station
St. Thomas, Virgin Islands 00803
Phone: (340) 776-7397
FAX: (340) 777-4003

VIRGINIA
Board of Nursing
6606 West Broad Street, 4th Floor
Richmond, Virginia 23230
Phone: (804) 662-9909
FAX: (804) 662-9512
http://www.dhp.state.va.us

WASHINGTON
State Nursing Care Quality Assurance Commission
Department of Health
1300 Quince Street SE
Olympia, Washington 98504-7864
Phone: (360) 236-4740
FAX: (360) 236-4738
http://www.doh.wa.gov/hsqa/hpqad/Nursing

WEST VIRGINIA
State Board of Examiners for Licensed Practical Nurses
101 Dee Drive
Charleston, West Virginia 25311
Phone: (304) 558-3572
FAX: (304) 558-4367

WISCONSIN
Department of Regulation and Licensing
1400 E. Washington Avenue
P.O. Box 8935
Madison, Wisconsin 53708
Phone: (608) 266-2112
FAX: (608) 267-0644
http://www.state.wi.us

WYOMING
State Board of Nursing
2020 Carey Avenue, Suite 110
Cheyenne, Wyoming 82002
Phone: (307) 777-7601
FAX: (307) 777-3519
http://commerce.state.wy.us/b%26c/nb

Appendix J | Registering or Licensing Authorities–Canada

ALBERTA
Alberta Association of Registered Nurses
11620 168th Street
Edmonton, Alberta
T5M 4A6
Phone: (780) 451-0043
FAX: (780) 452-3276
http://www.nurses.ab.ca

BRITISH COLUMBIA
Registered Nurses Association of British Columbia
2855 Arbutus Street
Vancouver, British Columbia
V6J 3Y8
Phone: (604) 736-7331
FAX: (604) 738-2272
http://www.rnabc.bc.ca

MANITOBA
Manitoba Association of Registered Nurses
647 Broadway Avenue
Winnipeg, Manitoba
R3C 0X2
Phone: (204) 774-3477
FAX: (204) 775-6052
http://www.marn.mb.ca

NEW BRUNSWICK
Nurses Association of New Brunswick
165 Regent Street
Fredericton, New Brunswick
E3B 3W5
Phone: (506) 458-8731
FAX: (506) 459-2838
http://www.nanb.nb.ca

NEWFOUNDLAND
Association of Registered Nurses of Newfoundland
55 Military Road, Box 6116
St. John's, Newfoundland
A1C 5X8
Phone: (709) 753-6040
FAX: (709) 753-4940
http://arnn.nf.ca

NORTHWEST TERRITORIES
Northwest Territories Registered Nurses Association
Box 2757
Yellowknife, Northwest Territories
X1A 2R1
Phone: (867) 873-2745
FAX: (867) 873-2336

NOVA SCOTIA
Registered Nurses' Association of Nova Scotia
1894 Barrington Street, Scotia Square
Barrington Tower, Suite 600
Halifax, Nova Scotia
B3J 2A8
Phone: (902) 491-9744
FAX: (902) 491-9510
http://www.rnans.ns.ca

ONTARIO
College of Nurses of Ontario
101 Davenport Road
Toronto, Ontario
M5R 3PI
Phone: (416) 928-0900
FAX: (416) 928-5607
http://www.cno.org

PRINCE EDWARD ISLAND
Association of Registered Nurses of Prince Edward Island
17 Pownal Street
Charlottetown, Prince Edward Island
C1A 3V7
Phone: (902) 368-3764
FAX: (902) 628-1430

QUEBEC
Ordre des infirmières et infirmiers du Québec
4200, boul. Dorchester Ouest
Montréal, Quebec
H3Z, 1V4
Phone: (514) 935-2501
FAX: (514) 935-1799
http://www.oiiq.org

SASKATCHEWAN
Saskatchewan Registered Nurses' Association
2066 Retellack Street
Regina, Saskatchewan
S4T 7X5
Phone: (306) 359-4200
FAX: (306) 525-0849
http://www.srna.org

YUKON
Yukon Registered Nurses Association
1114-1 Avenue, Suite 14
Whitehorse, Yukon
Y1A 1A3
Phone: (867) 667-4062
FAX: (867) 668-5123

COMPREHENSIVE EXAMS

COMPREHENSIVE EXAMINATION 1: PART 1

This examination contains individual questions, the majority of which relate to clinical situations. Read all questions carefully. There is only *one best answer* for each question.
Test time allotment (Part 1): approximately 2 hours
Answers and rationales begin on p. 652.

1. The primary role of the State Board of Nursing is to:
   ① Represent nurses in state government
   ② Protect the nursing profession
   ③ Protect the public
   ④ Issue nursing licenses

2. A patient is scheduled to begin a 24-hour urine collection for creatinine clearance at 8:00 AM. The nurse asks the patient to void at 8:00 AM. What should the nurse do with this urine?
   ① Send it to the lab for a urinalysis
   ② Pour it into the 24-hour collection container
   ③ Discard it
   ④ Test it for glucose and ketones

3. When auscultating a patient's blood pressure, the nurse should inflate the cuff until the sphygmomanometer reads:
   ① 200 mm Hg
   ② 10 mm Hg above the last recorded diastolic pressure
   ③ 30 mm Hg above the palpatory systolic pressure
   ④ The level at which the nurse last heard a beat

4. When feeding a patient with dysphagia, the nurse knows it is best to:
   ① Provide the patient with thin liquids
   ② Combine different food textures in one bite
   ③ Instruct the patient to swallow twice with each bite of food
   ④ Offer foods that the patient can pick up easily

5. A 56-year-old male has been admitted to have a biopsy of the bladder for suspected malignancy. He appears anxious during admission and tells the nurse "I probably will not leave here alive." The nurse's <u>best</u> response is:
   ① "You will get better."
   ② "That's ridiculous; don't even think that way."
   ③ "What does your family think and feel about all of this?"
   ④ "You may feel that way now, but much has been done in the treatment of this condition."

6. Oxygen therapy for the newborn must be administered with caution to prevent:
   ① Ophthalmia neonatorum
   ② ABO incompatability
   ③ Respiratory distress syndrome
   ④ Retrolental fibroplasia

7. A new patient needs instructions about the proper administration of Synthroid. Patient teaching should include which one of the following?
   ① Withholding medication and calling the physician if pulse rate is below 60 beats/minute
   ② Taking the medication at bedtime
   ③ Discontinuing drug therapy when all symptoms have subsided
   ④ Withholding medication and calling the physician if the pulse rate is over 100 beats/minute

8. A patient who has a diagnosis of hypothyroidism is placed on a thyroid replacement drug called Synthroid and is to return to the clinic in 2 weeks for follow-up lab studies. Which of the following are classic symptoms of hypothyroidism?
   ① Hirsutism, buffalo hump between the shoulder blades, hypertension
   ② Thirst, dry skin, urinary frequency
   ③ Fatigue, hypotension, urinary frequency
   ④ Muscle cramping, weakness, slow response time

9. The nutritional status of the elderly resident in long-term care requires regular monitoring. It is important for the nurse to know that in monitoring the status of an 86-year-old patient, the:
   ① Caloric requirements are greater than when the patient was younger
   ② Caloric requirements are less than when the patient was younger
   ③ Caloric requirements are the same as when the patient was younger
   ④ Nutritional requirements are greater now as the patient advances in age

10. A patient is admitted for surgery and the physician orders insertion of an indwelling Foley catheter. The nurse needs to take which of the following precautions while performing this procedure?
    ① Reverse isolation
    ② Medical asepsis
    ③ Surgical asepsis
    ④ Proper handwashing

11. A patient who has been having irregular heart rhythms has orders written for the nurses to take apical-radial pulses. Which of the following statements best describes this procedure?
    ① The nurse counts the apical pulse for one minute, then counts the radial pulse for one minute
    ② One nurse counts the apical pulse for one minute while a second nurse counts the radial pulse for one minute, both using the same watch
    ③ One nurse counts the apical pulse for one minute while another nurse counts the radial pulse for one minute, each using their own watch
    ④ A nurse counts the apical and radial pulses simultaneously for one minute

12. Treatment for a toddler with nephrotic syndrome will include:
    ① High-Fowler's position
    ② Regular diet
    ③ Diuretics as ordered
    ④ Sodium and potassium supplements

13. A patient is receiving oxygen therapy at 8 liters per minute continuously per a simple face mask. Which of the following symptoms would alert the nurse as being an early sign of oxygen toxicity?
    ① Fever
    ② Excessive mucus production
    ③ Dry cough
    ④ Moist breath sounds

14. A 32-year-old woman has been admitted for induction of labor. During the early stages of labor, the patient complains of feeling faint, particularly in the supine position. The nurse would:
① Take the patient's blood pressure
② Place the patient in Trendelenburg's position
③ Turn the patient on her left side
④ Begin preparation for an operative delivery

15. When caring for an AIDS patient on AZT (zidovudine), the nurse needs to monitor the patient for toxic effects of the medication. These toxic effects would include:
① Stomatitis and fevers
② Painful peripheral nerves
③ Headache and fatigue
④ Painful peripheral nerves and anemia

16. When performing wound irrigations, the nurse is best protected by:
① Raising the bed to a workable height
② Explaining the procedure to the patient
③ Handwashing before and after the procedure
④ Using personal protective apparel

17. A 73-year-old female patient complains that she can't hear as well as she used to. The nurse knows that hearing loss from nerve impairment is common in the elderly and that this is a condition known as:
① Tinnitus
② Presbycusis
③ Otosclerosis
④ Ménière's disease

18. When caring for an individual with AIDS, the nurse must follow standard precautions, which include:
① Sterile gloves and gown
② Gloves when in contact with blood or any body fluids
③ Mask and gloves at all times when caring for any HIV-positive client
④ Gloves at all times when in contact with any patient in the hospital

19. When contributing to the plan of care for a patient with high risk for injury due to debilitating illness, the nurse is aware that:
① This patient has a potential problem
② This is not a recognized nursing diagnosis
③ The statement is based on subjective data
④ The care plan addresses an actual problem

20. When evaluating a patient for possible pulse deficit, the nurse will need:
① The assistance of a second nurse
② An understanding of systolic murmur
③ The cooperative assistance of the patient
④ The availability of an electrocardiograph machine

21. The main reason the nurse explains procedure steps and purpose to the patient prior to performing a treatment is:
① It diminishes the likelihood of malpractice suits
② Patient anxiety is decreased with understanding
③ It allows the patient the opportunity to refuse the treatment
④ It provides the nurse with an opportunity to mentally review the procedure

22. When teaching a patient the procedure for collecting stools for occult blood, the nurse should include:
① Diarrhea stools are unacceptable sources for this examination

② The specimen should be kept warm until delivery to the laboratory
③ Small samples should be taken from two separate areas of the stool
④ The specimen should only be obtained from stool areas containing blood

23. The physician has ordered a urine sugar and acetone level. The best approach for obtaining this specimen would be to:
① Have the patient collect a midstream specimen
② Instruct the patient in the procedure for a clean-catch specimen
③ Discard the first voiding of the day and collect all following urines for 24 hours
④ Discard the first voided urine and collect the specimen as soon as the patient can void again

24. A 97-year-old patient is hospitalized for treatment of a fractured hip. On admission she is noted to have poor skin turgor and her son states she has not been drinking much prior to her fall. Of the following nursing diagnoses, which should receive the highest priority by the nurse providing care to the patient?
① Altered family processes related to stress of hospitalization evidenced by ineffective communication between family members.
② Risk for impaired gas exchange due to recent surgery and limited mobility.
③ Risk for skin breakdown related to limited mobility.
④ Fluid volume deficit related to limited oral intake evidenced by poor skin turgor and concentrated urine.

25. A mother has a 2-month-old daughter and a 5-year-old son. She brings the 5 year old to the clinic because he has started wetting the bed and having temper tantrums over the last month. A history and physical examination reveal no physical causes for this change in behavior. The nurse recognizes that the child is most likely showing signs of:
① Repression
② Displacement
③ Regression
④ Compensation

26. The physician orders meperidine (Demerol) 20 mg with atropine 0.08 mg IM as a preoperative medication. The meperidine is supplied at 50 mg/ml, the atropine at 0.2 mg/ml. The nurse should draw up a total volume of:
① 0.4 ml
② 0.8 ml
③ 1.0 ml
④ 1.2 ml

27. The patient, age 3, has to have blood drawn for a CBC. When she asks if it will hurt to have the blood drawn, the nurse's best response would be:
① "No, of course it won't hurt!"
② "It might hurt for a minute, but I will be here with you, and you can hold my hand if you want to."
③ "If you are a big girl, the blood test won't hurt you."
④ "It might hurt, but you have to have it done, so try not to cry."

28. Heparin sodium is ordered for a patient because of the potential for developing a blood clot due to immobility. To correctly administer heparin, the nurse would:
① Administer the heparin deep IM

② Aspirate before administering the heparin to ensure the injection is not in a blood vessel

③ Administer the heparin in the same site each time

④ Refrain from massaging the area after the injection

29. A patient has been receiving theophylline (Aminophylline) 80 mg per hour intravenously for exacerbation of acute asthma. He states he is feeling "jittery." His pulse is 120 beats per minute, respirations are 22 breaths per minute, and his lungs are clear to auscultation. The physician has ordered a theophylline level to be drawn. Which of the following titers are within therapeutic range?
   ① 4 mg/dl
   ② 14 mg/dl
   ③ 26 mg/dl
   ④ 34 mg/dl

30. A 24-year-old patient is to receive discharge information concerning home management following an appendectomy. In order for the patient to care for her wound, the nurse will instruct her to:
   ① Inspect her incision every 4 hours for signs of infection
   ② Gently wash the incision with soap and water daily and dry
   ③ Resume normal household activities upon her return home
   ④ Replace Steri-Strips with pieces of paper tape as needed

31. While the nurse is weighing and taking her vital signs, a patient expresses concern regarding weight gain related to her pregnancy. The *most appropriate* response by the nurse would be to explain that during pregnancy:
   ① Weight gain should not exceed 22 pounds
   ② Proper nutrition is more important than the actual number of pounds gained
   ③ Caloric intake is not to be restricted because metabolic needs increase
   ④ Only individuals who are greatly overweight need to be concerned about excessive weight gain

32. The order is to give heparin sodium 25,000 units in 1,000 cc of IV fluid at a rate of 40 cc per hour. How many units of heparin sodium per hour will the patient be receiving?
   ① 1,000 units per hour
   ② 10,000 units per hour
   ③ 100 units per hour
   ④ 40 units per hour

33. Warfarin sodium (Coumadin) therapy is regulated by which of the following laboratory tests?
   ① Partial fibrinogen time (PFT)
   ② Prothrombin time (PT)
   ③ Partial thromboplastin time (PTT)
   ④ Bleeding time

34. Which type of diuretic can the nurse expect the physician to order for treatment of hypovolemic shock during hemodialysis?
   ① Potassium-sparing diuretics
   ② Loop diuretics
   ③ Osmotic diuretics
   ④ Sodium-sparing diuretics

35. The nurse finds a patient lying on the floor in the hallway. What step should the nurse take *first*?
   ① Gently touch the patient and call his name

② Position the patient on his back and open his airway

③ Assist the patient back to bed and examine him for injuries

④ Call for help and begin chest compressions

36. Which of the following drugs should not be administered through a nasogastric tube?
   ① Digoxin (Lanoxin) tablets
   ② Potassium chloride (Klor) elixir
   ③ Acetaminophen (Tylenol) tablets
   ④ Theophylline anhydrase (Theo-Dur) tablets

37. Nursing interventions related to postoperative care of the patient who has just had a thyroidectomy performed include:
   ① Immediately report a moderate drop in body temperature less than 98.6° F, heart rate less than 80 beats per minute, and lethargy
   ② Place in Fowler's position, support head with sand bags, obtain vital signs every 2 to 4 hours
   ③ Report any signs of redness or discomfort to the physician
   ④ Assess for hypercalcemia, return of voice, and restlessness

38. The coronary arteries supply the heart muscle with oxygen. In coronary artery disease the arteries fail to supply the heart muscle with adequate oxygen. The nurse knows that the result is:
   ① General hypoxia of the tissues
   ② The heart gives out and beats at a slower rate
   ③ Decreased blood pressure
   ④ Cerebral hypoxia only

39. A newly admitted patient has a history of convulsions. The nurse is in the patient's room when suddenly he states: "I smell roses." The nurse understands the patient may be experiencing a(n):
   ① Aura
   ② Olfactory hallucination
   ③ Petit mal seizure
   ④ Pleasant aroma from his flowers

40. The nursing diagnosis for a 65-year-old patient who is 3 days postop hip replacement is potential for infection related to surgical incision. Identify the data that best reflects an evaluation statement:
   ① Temperature 100.9° F; white blood cell count 12,000; incision with small amount of redness, moderate swelling
   ② Temperature 99.0° F; white blood cell count 13,000; incision red with small amount of drainage
   ③ Temperature 99.0° F; white blood cell count 9,800; incision with redness and swelling with small amount of serosanguineous drainage
   ④ Temperature 98.6° F; white blood cell count 10,000; incision red; large amount of swelling with purulent drainage

41. An 18-year-old patient had a full body cast applied 3 days ago. He is complaining he feels "full," and his cast is too tight. The patient is also complaining of nausea and abdominal discomfort. The nurse recognizes that the patient is most likely experiencing:
   ① Pneumonia
   ② A claustrophobic reaction
   ③ An anxiety reaction
   ④ Decreased intestinal motility

42. A patient at the clinic tells the nurse that she is having trouble sleeping at night. What is the *first* action that the nurse should take?
    ① Instruct the patient to take an over-the-counter sleep aid about an hour before bedtime
    ② Ask the patient to describe her bedtime activities
    ③ Tell the patient to discuss the problem with the physician
    ④ Describe relaxation techniques that the patient might try when she has trouble falling asleep

43. The nurse is planning to teach a patient how to administer his insulin injections. Which goal would indicate that the nurse expects the patient to exhibit learning at the psychomotor domain?
    ① The patient will correctly explain how to administer his insulin injection by next Tuesday.
    ② The patient will correctly state the importance of taking his insulin at the same time every day by next Tuesday.
    ③ The patient will correctly demonstrate administration of his insulin by next Tuesday.
    ④ The patient will correctly identify the sites for insulin administration by next Tuesday.

44. Which of the following statements about central hyperalimentation (total parenteral nutrition) administration is most appropriate?
    ① It can be given via the antecubital vein
    ② It should be given very slowly
    ③ It can cause rebound hypoglycemia
    ④ It can be given via a central venous access catheter

45. A 4-year-old patient needs an antibiotic IM given that was ordered by the physician for a major inner ear infection. The best thing for the nurse to say to the patient before giving the injection is:
    ① "I have to give you an injection."
    ② "I have to give you a little shot."
    ③ "I need to put some medicine under your skin."
    ④ "I have to give you a shot that may sting a little bit."

46. One complication that is more common in cesarean section deliveries is ileus with abdominal distention. To reduce the likelihood of this, the nursing care plan for a patient who has had a cesarean section should include:
    ① A well-balanced diet with adequate bulk
    ② Splinting of the abdomen when deep breathing and coughing
    ③ Early ambulation
    ④ Kegel exercises

47. A patient has a diagnosis of primary dysfunction of the adrenal cortex. The physician has ordered replacement therapy. Which of the following is an important point to stress in patient teaching?
    ① The hormones will have to be taken for the rest of her life
    ② The hormones must be taken until the body's stores have been replenished
    ③ The hormones will only need to be taken during periods of stress
    ④ Daily visits to the physician will be necessary as the dose will be adjusted daily

48. Aerosol treatment, chest physiotherapy, and postural drainage are ordered for children with cystic fibrosis to:
    ① Decrease respiratory effort and mucus production
    ② Dilate the bronchioles and clear secretions
    ③ Increase efficiency of the diaphragm and gas exchange
    ④ Stimulate coughing and arterial oxygen consumption

49. When assessing a patient's chest pain, the nurse should note which of the following characteristics?
    ① Elevation of temperature
    ② Respiratory rate
    ③ Presence of incontinence
    ④ Radiation of pain to the jaw or arm

50. One of the major physical characteristics of the child with Down's syndrome is:
    ① Hypertonic musculature
    ② A single transverse crease on palms
    ③ Inflexibility of the joints
    ④ Janeway spots on the palms and soles

51. A patient is to have surgery. What is the responsibility of the nurse with regard to the surgical consent form.
    ① The nurse should obtain the patient's signature on the form.
    ② The nurse should witness the patient's signature on the form.
    ③ The nurse should check that the signed consent form is on the patient's chart before surgery.
    ④ The nurse should be sure that the patient understands what he is signing.

52. An Asian-American patient relates to her Anglo-American nurse that she has asked her family to bring a special herbal preparation to the hospital to help her to get well. Which statement is it most appropriate for the nurse to make?
    ① "That is fine. I should inform your physician before you use it."
    ② "It is not a good idea to try to treat illnesses with herbs. They are not as effective as the medications that your physician prescribed."
    ③ "Yes, it is fine if you want to use your herbal preparation. You may keep it in your drawer."
    ④ "Your physician knows what is best for you. You should just follow that treatment plan."

53. A hospitalized patient was recently diagnosed with lung cancer. While the nurse is providing care, the patient states, "If someone had only warned me that I would get lung cancer, I would have stopped smoking years ago." The nurse recognizes that this statement reflects which coping mechanism?
    ① Compensation
    ② Rationalization
    ③ Sublimation
    ④ Repression

54. A patient who is now clinically stable following a myocardial infarction is admitted on Monday to an extended care facility. The registered nurse identifies the following nursing diagnosis: activity intolerance related to low oxygen saturation evidenced by dyspnea after ambulating 10 feet. What is an acceptable goal for this nursing diagnosis?
    ① The patient will exhibit an oxygen saturation level of 95% by Saturday.
    ② The patient will use oxygen by nasal cannula before and after ambulating.
    ③ The patient will ambulate 12 feet without dyspnea by Saturday.
    ④ The patient will exhibit pink skin and mucous membranes by Wednesday.

55. The nurse is preparing to administer a dose from the following order: Demerol (meperidine) 75 mg IM every 4 hours as needed. What is it most important for the nurse to check before preparing the dose?
    ① The date and time that the order was written
    ② The time when the last dose of the medication was given
    ③ The amount of the medication that is left on hand
    ④ The effect of the last dose of the medication

56. A patient is taking Atrovent (ipratropium), an anticholinergic agent, for a respiratory condition. The nurse might expect the patient to exhibit which of the following adverse effects?
    ① Bradycardia
    ② Diarrhea
    ③ Dry mouth
    ④ Pupil constriction

57. A patient was seen 2 days ago at a clinic and diagnosed with arthritis in his knees and hips. He tells the nurse that the Motrin (ibuprofen) that the physician prescribed has not helped his pain. What should the nurse tell this patient?
    ① That he may need an opiate to relieve the pain.
    ② That Motrin (ibuprofen) is used to treat inflammation rather than pain.
    ③ That he should stop the medication until the nurse can discuss the problem with the physician.
    ④ That he has not been taking the medication long enough to have a therapeutic effect.

58. A patient was recently diagnosed with diabetes. While the nurse is teaching the patient about his condition, the patient states, "I am so afraid that I will lose my legs or my eyesight from this disease." Which response by the nurse is most appropriate?
    ① "Why are you so afraid of diabetes?"
    ② "If you follow your diabetic teaching carefully, that will not happen."
    ③ "Would you like to tell me more about your concerns?"
    ④ "Those things hardly ever happen anymore."

59. The nurse is assessing for signs of active tuberculosis (TB) in the patient who is in respiratory isolation. Which of the following best describes signs and symptoms of active TB?
    ① Night sweats, dyspnea, weakness
    ② Wheezing, insomnia, productive cough
    ③ Dyspepsia, being cold, fatigue
    ④ Loss of appetite, bloody stools

60. The nurse is assigned to a patient who was burned on her right upper extremity in an apartment fire 2 days ago. Eschar has developed over the burned areas. An escharotomy is planned to:
    ① Decrease caloric needs.
    ② Prevent infection of the underlying tissues.
    ③ Facilitate use of the extremity.
    ④ Prevent serous drainage.

61. A patient with second- and third-degree burns over 40% of his body is being treated by the open method. Which of the following interventions is most appropriate in his care?
    ① Wearing sterile gloves to apply the topical antimicrobial agents.

② Keeping the room temperature between 65° and 70° for patient comfort.
③ Providing a high-protein, high-fat diet to meet increased nutritional demands.
④ Elevating his arms on two pillows to prevent contractures.

62. A patient seen in the clinic has been diagnosed with seizures and is made aware that certain conditions may increase the potential for seizures. Which of the following conditions could lower the seizure threshold?
    ① Hyperglycemia
    ② Routine sleep habits
    ③ Fatigue
    ④ Antiseizure medications

63. The nurse just received lab results on her patient who is in acute renal failure. Which of the following statements accurately describes the lab findings common to patients in acute renal failure?
    ① Increased BUN and decreased creatinine levels
    ② Increased BUN and creatinine levels
    ③ Increased calcium levels and decreased BUN
    ④ Decreased BUN and potassium levels

64. Drugs can affect the urinary tract in several ways, even to the point of being nephrotoxic. Assessment of a patient's current and past use of medications, including over-the-counter drugs and herbs, is important. During a patient assessment the nurse would expect possible kidney problems if the patient gave a history of taking:
    ① Imipramine (Tofranil)
    ② Nitrofurantoin (Macrodantin)
    ③ Nifedipine (Adalat)
    ④ Ibuprofen (Advil, Motrin)

65. An indication that cord prolapse has occurred following rupture of an expectant mother's membranes would be related to which observation?
    ① Decreased fetal heart rate
    ② Increased fetal heart rate
    ③ Continuous leakage of fluid
    ④ Protrusion of the cord by 10 inches

66. The husband of a patient with hyperemesis gravidarum who was admitted that day, requests to stay overnight in his wife's private room. The nurse replies:
    ① "You may only stay tonight."
    ② "You may stay whenever you wish."
    ③ "She needs to rest, so you must leave."
    ④ "She needs to get used to staying alone."

67. After learning she has hydramnios, a pregnant woman asks the nurse what that means. The correct explanation is:
    ① "Dysfunctional labor will occur."
    ② "Postpartum hemorrhage will occur."
    ③ "There is a small amount of amniotic fluid present."
    ④ "There is a large amount of amniotic fluid present."

68. A patient was admitted 2 days ago in acute renal failure secondary to a severe infection. The infection has improved but the patient continues to have an output below 30 ml/hr. The nurse should instruct him that his diet will be:
    ① High carbohydrate, low protein, and low potassium
    ② High carbohydrate, high protein, and supplementary potassium
    ③ Low carbohydrate, low protein, and high potassium
    ④ Low carbohydrate, high protein, and low potassium

69. A patient experienced a pulmonary embolus and was immediately started on IV heparin. The goal is to maintain the partial thromboplastin time (PTT) at:
① 0.5 to 1 times normal
② 1.5 to 2 times normal
③ 2 to 3 times normal
④ 3 to 4 times normal

70. A patient with diabetes mellitus is currently in the hospital due to gangrene of the right lower extremity. Because she does not speak English the doctor explained to her in Spanish the need for a below-the-knee amputation and that her prognosis is good. The patient is crying and obviously grieving. The doctor notified her family. It is important that the nurse:
① Call in someone who speaks Spanish to listen to her and offer empathy
② Turn on the TV to a Spanish station
③ Give her an ordered prn mild sedative
④ Ask her if there is a clergy member she would like to visit with

71. A patient who had a right below-the-knee amputation is 3 days postop. She has no signs of infection and is doing well; however, she states that the pain she felt preoperatively continues to be present. She also states that at times it feels like her right lower leg is floating in mid air. The nurse should obtain an order for:
① A narcotic analgesic for pain prn
② Massage therapy to the residual limb
③ The application of cold to the residual limb
④ A TENS unit

72. The *first* thing a nurse should do for the patient who is experiencing phantom limb pain is:
① Apply a tourniquet above the amputation site
② Allow the patient to ventilate
③ Call the doctor
④ Explain that the sensations are normal and ask that he report them

73. A patient who has diabetes mellitus recently underwent a below-the-knee amputation. The nurse should instruct the patient:
① On the importance of foot care for the remaining foot
② To cut his toenails every week with a good nipper
③ To wear sandals to allow air to ventilate his foot
④ To soak his foot daily for 30 minutes prior to bathing

74. A 75 year old with hypertension has a history of passing out upon arising in the morning. The nurse should:
① Have her sit on the side of the bed for a few minutes before standing
② Advise her to take a multivitamin daily
③ Call the doctor
④ Increase her fluid intake

75. An 80-year-old resident in a local long-term care facility has Alzheimer's disease of 5 years duration. He paces the floor and wanders into other resident's rooms. One day he is found wandering outside the facility. What is the best thing the nurse should do to protect herself from being sued?
① Keep the family informed of his behavior
② Ask the aids to watch him more closely
③ Request a family member sit with him
④ Place him in a semiprivate room for company

76. A patient is 2 days postop from extensive abdominal surgery and is using the incentive spirometer as directed. The nurse notices crackles in the posterior right lower lobe. The nurse has him cough and deep breathe and should:
① Assess his lung sounds before and after deep breathing and coughing exercises
② Notify respiratory therapy to check his SAT level
③ Measure his vital signs prior to the deep breathing and coughing exercises
④ Position him in a semi-Fowler's position for the exercises

77. A patient is to have an IV started for blood administration. The nurse will:
① Insert a 22-gauge needle
② Ask if the patient is allergic to iodine
③ Take the patient's vital signs
④ Massage the insertion site first

78. The most serious complication of a ruptured appendix is:
① Peritonitis
② Hemorrhage
③ Intestinal obstruction
④ Ulceration of the duodenum

79. A patient with chronic obstructive pulmonary disease (COPD) is admitted to the hospital for an acute episode of respiratory distress. Which type of oxygen mask is the most appropriate for the nurse to administer oxygen to this patient?
① Venturi mask
② Non-rebreather mask
③ Partial rebreather mask
④ Simple mask

80. A woman who is postmenopausal and not taking estrogen should have a calcium intake of:
① 1200 mg per day
② 1000 mg per day
③ 1500 mg per day
④ 2000 mg per day

81. Patient/family education for ventilator care in the home addresses all of the following *except:*
① Patient care
② The weaning procedure
③ Ventilator care
④ Ventilator maintenance

82. Intravenous central hyperalimentation (total parenteral nutrition) is discontinued gradually to prevent:
① Rebound hypoglycemia
② Disequilibrium syndrome
③ Septicemia
④ Rebound hyperglycemia

83. The proper way to interpret a Mantoux skin test is to measure the amount of:
① Erythema in mm
② Induration and erythema in mm
③ Induration in mm
④ Lipohypertrophy in mm

84. The patient with Parkinson's disease experiences posture and gait changes. Which of the following describes how the gait is affected in this disease?
① Sways to the dominant side when ambulating
② Swings one leg across the other instead of straight forward

③ Takes short, accelerating steps

④ Slaps the feet to the floor with each step

85. The nurse is planning care for a patient who has been admitted for observation with a possible skull fracture. It is essential that the nurse observe for the possibility of changing levels of consciousness due to a venous bleed. Which type of hematoma is being described?
   ① Intracerebral
   ② Epidural
   ③ Subarachnoid
   ④ Subdural

86. The physician prescribes phenelzine (Nardil), a monoamine oxidase inhibitor (MAOI) for a patient with a diagnosis of depression. What should the nurse teach the patient about this medication?
   ① To limit foods that are high in potassium content
   ② To avoid foods that are high in tyramine content
   ③ To avoid exposure to direct sunlight
   ④ To expect to notice a therapeutic response within 3 days

87. The nurse administers meperidine hydrochloride (Demerol) 100 mg IM for pain. The nurse should plan to monitor the patient for which condition?
   ① Diarrhea
   ② Hypertension
   ③ Respiratory depression
   ④ Hypoglycemia

88. A patient has suffered a right-sided CVA and his safety is a nursing concern. The nurse would assess for:
   ① Intellectual impairment
   ② Impulsive behavior
   ③ Cautious behavior
   ④ Right-sided weakness

89. A nurse is measuring a patient's blood pressure using a mercury sphygmomanometer. Which of the following steps is performed correctly?
   ① The bell of the stethoscope is placed under the cuff in the antecubital space
   ② The arm is held at the level of the heart
   ③ The cuff is inflated until the sphygmomanometer reads 200 mm Hg
   ④ The air is released from the cuff at a rate of 1 mm Hg every 2 seconds

90. An employee who works in a lab splashed a chemical into her eyes. Her coworkers irrigated her eyes with plain water and then brought her to the emergency clinic. The patient is complaining of "burning" in the eyes. Both eyes and the surrounding tissue are reddened. The doctor orders that each eye be irrigated with 1000 ml of normal saline. The patient is placed in a reclining position in preparation for the irrigation. The nurse should direct the flow of fluid:
   ① From the outer canthus to the inner canthus
   ② From the inner canthus to the outer canthus
   ③ Directly on the center of the eyeball
   ④ Indirectly and slowly from the lower lid

91. When preparing to give an injection of NPH and regular insulin, the nurse knows to mix the two insulins in the same syringe to:
   ① Potentiate the action of the NPH insulin
   ② Potentiate the action of the regular insulin
   ③ Avoid two injections
   ④ Prolong the effects of both insulins

92. A patient receiving hemodialysis has been connected for 20 minutes and complains to the nurse that he is having some chest pain. The nurse observes that the patient is anxious, has a cough, and has respirations of 28. The nurse should:
   ① Check the needle insertion site and continue the procedure
   ② Clamp the venous line and stop the pump
   ③ Position the patient on his right side for 10 minutes
   ④ Stand the patient up and take his blood pressure

93. A neighbor's 16-year-old daughter has fallen and broken her right wrist. She is complaining of pain at the site and the wrist is swollen, contorted, and bluish in color. The nurse should:
   ① Apply heat to decrease swelling
   ② Advise not to move fingers of her right hand
   ③ Remove all jewelry from the right extremity
   ④ Place the extremity on her lap to decrease pain

94. When preparing a patient for an MRI, the nurse should instruct the patient:
   ① Not to eat 4 hours prior to the procedure
   ② About possible allergies to iodine
   ③ To remove dental bridges and jewelry
   ④ That he may feel a flushing sensation

95. A patient who recently underwent coronary bypass surgery has been recommended that he get 8 to 10 hours a night of sleep. The rationale for this recommendation is:
   ① Sleep allows the body to restore and heal itself
   ② His body lacks the oxygen necessary to stay awake for longer periods
   ③ His risk for infection is increased with less sleep
   ④ His muscles have weakened with his illness and need to rebuild

96. A patient has a serum K^+ level of 7.2 mEq/L. Which of the following substances will most likely be ordered?
   ① Potassium chloride (Kay Ciel)
   ② Sodium polystyrene sulfonate (Kayexalate)
   ③ Bananas
   ④ Strawberries

97. A patient with a history of an extremely stressful lifestyle underwent coronary bypass surgery a week ago. The multidisciplinary team decided that he needs to learn stress-management strategies. The principle behind this recommendation is that:
   ① A reduction in stress will decrease cardiac workload
   ② Stress reduction exercises are good for those who have had major surgery
   ③ Relaxation enhances the flow of blood to the periphery
   ④ Exercise increases the blood flow to the heart

98. The nurse should assess for signs of potassium imbalance when the patient has been:
   ① Febrile for 48 hours
   ② Without a bowel movement for 24 hours
   ③ Menstruating for 48 hours
   ④ Vomiting for 3 days

99. When irrigating a colostomy, the nurse should hold the irrigation bag:
   ① So that the bottom of the bag is even with the top of the patient's shoulder
   ② No higher than 15 inches
   ③ So that the bottom of the bag is even with the top of the patient's head
   ④ So that the water flows very slowly

100. When assessing a dying cancer patient for pain relief, the nurse should first focus her assessment on:
① Medication for the pain
② Quality of the pain
③ Source of the pain
④ Duration of the pain

101. The most common method of treatment for an infant weighing more than 30 lb with a simple fractured femur is:
① Surgery and placement of a pin to set the fracture
② Putting the child in skeletal traction
③ Immediate setting and casting of the fractured leg
④ Putting the child in Bryant's traction

102. The physician orders ampicillin 300 mg IVPB. Ampicillin is supplied as 500 mg/2 ml. What volume of ampicillin would the nurse draw up from the vial?
① 0.6 ml
② 0.8 ml
③ 1.2 ml
④ 1.4 ml

103. The patient reports to the nurse that the medication she is taking for her urinary tract infection (UTI) has stopped the frequency and urgency she had been experiencing. Which of the following medications works in this manner?
① TMP/SMZ, trimethoprim/sulfamethoxazole (Bactrim)
② Hyoscyamine (Anaspaz)
③ Ciprofloxacin (Cipro)
④ Amoxicillin (Amoxil)

104. A patient is admitted with hyperemesis gravidarum. Initially her diet should consist of:
① Dry toast and tea
② Low-fat foods three times a day
③ High protein foods six times a day
④ IV fluids of glucose, electrolytes, and vitamins

105. Which of the following statements is appropriate when giving medications to a 5-year-old patient?
① "Hi! It's time for your medicine. I know you don't like the flavor of the medicine, so I mixed it in your juice."
② "Are you finished with breakfast? I have some candy pills for you to take. They taste just like peppermint."
③ "I have a shot to give to you. I know shots hurt, but you need to have the medicine in the shot to make you better. Would you like me to give it to you now, or in 5 minutes?"
④ "Hi! It's time for your medicine. Your mom has to leave."

106. A patient, age 17 months, is admitted to the hospital with a diagnosis of meningitis. Which of the following findings would be noted relative to the patient's cerebrospinal fluid (CSF)?
① Reduced protein level
② Elevated glucose level
③ Reduced pressure
④ Cloudy

107. The physician has ordered an IV of D5.2NS to be infused at 100 ml/hr. If the IV tubing delivers 10 gtt/ml, at what rate would the nurse infuse the IV fluid?
① 10 gtt/min
② 12 gtt/min

③ 16 gtt/min
④ 18 gtt/min

108. Prior to emergency surgery for an epidural bleed, the patient was hyperventilated. The reason for this is that hyperventilation:
① Can cause constriction of cerebral vessels, which helps to keep ICP from increasing
② Prevents hypoxia, thereby decreasing ICP
③ Prevents hypercapnia
④ Prevents venous return from the brain

109. A patient has diabetes insipidus, and his doctor has ordered vasopressin. The nurse should expect to see:
① A decrease in blood pressure
② An increase in abdominal distention
③ A decrease in urinary output
④ An elevation in temperature

110. A 42-year-old woman was recently diagnosed with cancer. The doctor has informed the staff that the tumor has invaded the epidural space and the patient is beginning to show symptoms of spinal cord compression. The nurse caring for this patient is likely to document that the patient exhibits neck or back pain that:
① Is relieved with movement
② Is relieved by lying down
③ Is relieved by sitting
④ Has a sudden onset

111. Patient education is an important nursing action, especially when the patient is discharged with antimicrobial medications for a urinary tract infection (UTI). The nurse needs to make sure the patient understands the importance of:
① Taking warm tub baths
② Wiping from front to back after using the toilet
③ Taking the medications with grapefruit juice
④ Taking the entire course of the medication

112. A patient who has angina complained of chest pain to his wife, who then called 911. The patient has sublingual nitroglycerin ordered PRN. The EMT, a nurse, has administered 3 tablets at 5-minute intervals over a 15-minute period. The most appropriate action by the nurse will be to:
① Monitor the patient's blood pressure
② Hold the nitroglycerine until she hears from the doctor
③ Increase the dose to two tablets every 5 minutes while waiting for the doctor
④ Wait 5 minutes and administer the fourth tablet while waiting for the doctor

113. A patient is receiving oral anticoagulants. The nurse should instruct him to:
① Limit the amount of turnip greens, broccoli, and kale in his diet
② Use a disposable razor when shaving, to avoid the chance of infection
③ Take an extra aspirin daily to potentiate the effects of the anticoagulant
④ Use a hard-bristled toothbrush to massage and toughen the gums

114. When using an inhaler that contains albuterol (Proventil), the patient should be instructed to:
① Open his mouth and hold the inhaler 1 to 2 inches away

② Use the inhaler when he is extremely short of breath

③ Wash the inhaler after every use in warm, soapy water

④ Use mouthwash after each use

115. Which of the following should the nurse recognize as an early sign of retinal detachment?

① Purulent drainage

② Pain

③ Bloodshot eyes

④ Floaters

116. When performing a procedure on an uncooperative small child, which of the following actions would be the best for the nurse to try first?

① Sedate the child

② Use wrist and ankle restraints

③ Allow a parent to assist

④ Bring in another nurse to assist

117. When starting an infant on new foods, it is best to instruct the parents to:

① Mix the new food with one that the infant already likes

② Mix the new food with breast milk or formula

③ Feed the infant one new food at a time, to observe for possible allergic reactions

④ Try a new food at each feeding

118. The infant with diagnosed celiac disease should be given which cereal?

① Rice

② Wheat

③ Oat

④ Barley

119. The most serious complication of rheumatic fever is:

① Endocarditis

② Pneumonia

③ Arthritis

④ Meningitis

120. The morning after a vaginal birth, the patient's hemoglobin is 10.9 g/dL. The nurse expects the mother to experience:

① Dizzy spells

② Unstable vital signs

③ Difficulty performing small tasks

④ Managing basic care of herself and her infant

121. At her first prenatal visit, a patient is informed that her fundal height will be measured:

① At each visit

② At her last visit

③ Every 2 months

④ At the end of her first and second trimesters

122. A patient with trigeminal neuralgia (tic douloureux) has had surgical division of the trigeminal nerve. Which is most important to consider when a care plan is being developed?

① Facial pain

② Eating problems

③ Malocclusion of the teeth

④ Degenerative arthritis of the mandibular joint

123. A Denis Browne splint is a common method of treatment for:

① Scoliosis

② Congenital clubfoot

③ Developmental dysplasia of the hip (DDH)

④ Fractured femur

124. Papilledema is present in a patient with increased intracranial pressure (IICP). The nurse concludes there is:

① A brain abscess

② Swelling of the optic nerve

③ An increase of cerebrospinal fluid

④ The need for an electrophysiological test

125. During a myasthenia crisis a patient may experience several problems. Which is likely to necessitate an immediate response?

① Respiratory distress

② Slower speech rate

③ Difficulty chewing food

④ Weakness of arms and legs

COMPREHENSIVE EXAMINATION 1: PART 2

This examination contains individual questions, the majority of which relate to clinical situations. Read all questions carefully. There is only *one best answer* for each question.
Test time allotment (Part 2): approximately 2 hours
Answers and rationales begin on p. 663.

1. Preparation of a child for surgery should include all of the following *except:*
   ① Explaining all procedures and treatments before they occur
   ② Telling the child not to cry but to "be brave" if something hurts
   ③ Explaining anesthesia as a "special sleep"
   ④ Explaining where the incision or dressings will be after surgery

2. Nursing intervention for the child in sickle cell crisis is directed primarily toward:
   ① Maintaining active range of motion
   ② Oxygen therapy
   ③ Administration of blood
   ④ Maintaining adequate hydration

3. During a grand mal seizure, which of the following nursing actions is most appropriate?
   ① Protect head from injury
   ② Insert a padded tongue blade
   ③ Restrain extremities
   ④ Raise head of the bed

4. Which bandage turn should the nurse use when wrapping a joint, such as the elbow?
   ① Figure-of-eight
   ② Recurrent
   ③ Spiral
   ④ Circular

5. A patient is in respiratory alkalosis. Which of the following would assist this patient to increase his $PaCO_2$?
   ① Suctioning
   ② Postural drainage with cupping and clapping
   ③ Administering oxygen via nasal cannula
   ④ Using a rebreathing mask

6. A patient with diagnoses of diabetes mellitus and hypertension is being treated with Lasix (furosemide), 20 mg every morning. He tells the nurse that he has been waking up at night with leg cramps. What initial diagnostic test would the nurse expect the physician to order?
   ① Electromyelogram
   ② Arteriogram of the legs
   ③ Complete blood cell count
   ④ Potassium level

7. When entering the room of a patient who does not speak English, it is especially important for the nurse to:
   ① Greet the patient in his native tongue
   ② Always have an interpreter
   ③ Have a pen and paper with her
   ④ Offer a handshake

8. A patient was recently admitted to the hospital for treatment of congestive heart failure. Her admitting BP was 188/96. She has been taking Monopril 30 mg per day for 3 days. It is now time for her to take her dose of Monopril. The nurse finds her diaphoretic, pale, and weak. Her pulse is 96 and her blood pressure is 96/56. She is alert and talking. The nurse should first:
   ① Position her in a supine position with her legs elevated
   ② Call the doctor
   ③ Administer the Monopril
   ④ Place her in a high-Fowler's position

9. A patient has been diagnosed with Guillian-Barre syndrome. He is unable to turn his head, and his shoulders are drooping. The nurse informs the physician that she suspects involvement of the following cranial nerve:
   ① VII
   ② V
   ③ XI
   ④ IX

10. A baby with gastroesophageal reflux and failure to thrive (FTT) is classified as:
    ① Organic FTT
    ② Nonorganic FTT
    ③ Idiopathic FTT
    ④ Unstable FTT

11. A patient has end-stage cancer secondary to cancer of the colon. He is having difficulty with pain control. The nurse should:
    ① Administer narcotics indiscriminately
    ② Assess the effect of each pain intervention with a 1-10 scale
    ③ Instruct him on the use of guided imagery
    ④ Increase his fluid allowance

12. Techniques that minimize painful injections include:
    ① Injecting medications at room temperature
    ② Injecting prior to the alcohol drying
    ③ Having the client tighten the muscle
    ④ Inserting the needle slowly into the skin

13. A patient has a history of tonic-clonic seizures. Which of the following would best describe an aura that she may experience immediately before a seizure?
    ① Extreme anxiety
    ② Brief loss of consciousness
    ③ Automatic repetitive movements
    ④ Sensation of weakness or numbness

14. During which of the following assessment examinations should the nurse wear gloves?
    ① Assessing for drainage in the back of the throat
    ② Listening for lung sounds
    ③ Assessing bowel sounds
    ④ Checking skin turgor and texture

15. The incidence of hepatitis A in the community can be reduced by:
    ① A program of nutritional instruction
    ② A campaign against alcohol use
    ③ Early childhood immunizations
    ④ Effective sewage disposal

16. When a patient is stressed and the sympathetic nervous system is activated, the heart responds by:
    ① Slowing the conduction cycle
    ② Decreasing cardiac output

③ Increasing cardiac output

④ Stopping the beats

17. Which of the following is an expected outcome after giving a diuretic to decrease excess fluid volume?
① Weight gain
② Weight loss
③ Tachypnea
④ Oliguria

18. A patient is admitted to the hospital with gross hematuria and a history of a 20-pound weight loss during the last 3 months. The physician suspects bladder cancer. In obtaining a health history from the patient, the nurse recognizes which of the following as a significant risk factor for bladder cancer?
① Use of artificial sweeteners
② High caffeine intake
③ Excessive alcohol use
④ Cigarette smoking

19. When contributing to the nursing care plan, the nurse knows that an example of a short-term goal is:
① Assist patient in range-of-motion exercises
② Patient will transfer from bed to chair this week
③ Patient will return to previous level of functioning
④ Physical activity will improve muscle tone and function

20. A pregnant patient delivers quickly and without complications. The patient's husband arrives and is taken to the recovery room to see his wife. After visiting with her for a while, he asks to see the baby. It would be *best* for the nurse to suggest that:
① He go to the nursery to see the baby and let his wife sleep
② He visit with his wife for a while, then go home and see both his wife and the baby the next morning
③ The baby can be brought to the parents so they can begin the attachment process
④ Both parents go to the nursery to see the baby

21. A mother states that her 3-week-old infant has not been taking his formula well and is listless and unresponsive when she holds and cuddles him. He has lost 5 oz since birth. He is otherwise healthy and has no congenital defects. The pediatrician diagnoses the infant's condition as:
① Celiac disease
② Failure to thrive
③ Hirschsprung's disease
④ Pyloric stenosis

22. A young female patient comes to the clinic stating that she has missed a menstrual period. During her visit she tells the nurse that her last menstrual cycle was normal with a moderate amount of flow. It began on February 5th and ended February 11th. Using Nägele's rule, the nurse is able to calculate that her EDC (estimated date of confinement) would be:
① November 18th
② November 12th
③ November 4th
④ October 29th

23. A patient returns to her room from the ICU where she was nursed for 24 hours postoperatively. She is allowed to eat but must have a high protein intake. Which of these foods is highest in protein content?
① Dried beans and peas

② Eggs and cheese
③ Fresh vegetables
④ Cooked cereals

24. A popular 14-year-old female has just been diagnosed as having an extensive case of acne vulgaris and is concerned about her appearance. She asks the nurse why this happened. The nurse's *most appropriate* response should be:
① "It is caused primarily by overactivity of the sebaceous glands."
② "It is caused by overactivity of the sex glands during the adolescent period."
③ "It is caused by overactivity of the apocrine glands."
④ "It is caused by overactivity of bacterial growth on the skin."

25. A 6-week-old infant is admitted for surgical repair of a cleft lip. Vital signs are temperature, 100.8° F (38.2° C); pulse rate, 90 beats/min; respirations, 36/min; BP, 70/35. Which vital sign is abnormal and what should the nurse do about it?
① Respirations: call anesthesia
② Pulse rate: notify anesthesia
③ Temperature: notify admitting physician
④ Blood pressure: notify admitting physician

26. When placing a patient on a fracture pan, the nurse should place:
① The wide end toward the client's back
② The narrow end toward the client's back
③ Either end to the client's back
④ 8 ozs. of water in the pan first

27. An order is on the chart for a normal newborn to receive a hepatitis B injection. What should the nurse do first?
① Gather supplies
② Check vital signs
③ Obtain a signed permit from the parent/guardian
④ Check to see where the vitamin K injection was given

28. A female patient with Alzheimer's who has been looking through the window at the garden outside, suddenly becomes agitated when another patient approaches. Which of the following actions is most beneficial?
① Offering a high-protein drink
② Sending the patient to her room
③ Turning the day room television on
④ Taking the patient for a walk outside

29. When irrigating a colostomy, the object that is inserted into the ostomy is in the shape of a:
① Cone
② Cylinder
③ Long tube
④ Finger

30. Along with close monitoring, which nursing action is most essential to a patient scheduled for induction of labor?
① Hydrating with oral fluids
② Providing emotional support
③ Placing a "no visitors" sign on the door
④ Keeping the room temperature at a low setting

31. To promote a safe environment for a blind client, which of the following nursing measures is most appropriate?
① Leaving the door ajar
② Providing privacy at mealtime
③ Explaining the location of the call light
④ Rearranging the furnishings in the room

32. A 37-year-old male patient has been diagnosed with multiple sclerosis. In order to relieve fear and anxiety, which nursing action should be implemented *first?*
① Establishing a routine schedule
② Explaining the disease in detail
③ Initiating measures to prevent falls
④ Involving the family in the care plan

33. When utilizing a heat lamp, the nurse should:
① Keep the skin damp during treatment
② Cover the lamp with a pillow case after positioning it
③ Position the lamp 18 to 24 inches from the area being treated
④ Assess the patient every half hour

34. When administering the Tensilon test, the nurse should assess:
① Pupillary dilation
② Muscle strength
③ Irritability
④ Heart rate

35. A 90-year-old patient is admitted to the surgical unit following debridement of a decubitus ulcer. She is emaciated, has contractures of her extremities, and is in the end stages of Alzheimer's disease. The priority nursing goal is to promote/prevent:
① Nutrition
② Infection
③ Body alignment
④ A quiet environment

36. Following a physician's order, which one of the medications listed below would a nurse most likely administer to terminate status epilepticus in a patient?
① Diazepam (Valium)
② Doxazosin (Cardura)
③ Phenytoin (Dilantin)
④ Buprenorphine (Buprenex)

37. In order to promote tissue building in a patient who has had a right above-the-knee amputation, it is important that the patient's diet be:
① High in fats
② Low in carbohydrates
③ High in proteins
④ Low in calories

38. A patient with a new colostomy should be instructed on methods to prevent skin breakdown including which of the following?
① Shaving the area clean with a regular razor prior to applying the pouch
② Using tincture of benzoin as a skin barrier
③ Performing a patch test for allergies to new skin products
④ Washing the stoma area several times a day with soap and water

39. A patient is admitted for a colon resection. During the admitting assessment, the patient explains that she has a history of malignant hyperthermia. The nurse would:
① Administer dantrolene (Dantrium) prior to the surgery
② Notify the anesthesiologist
③ Serve only cold foods and water preoperatively
④ Take her temperature and record

40. A 68-year-old male is admitted to the telemetry unit following a routine visit to the doctor's office for his annual physical. Atypical changes were noted in his EKG. As part of the admission procedure, it is *most* important for the nurse to:
① Assess the occurrence of chest pain
② Question when and what he last ate
③ Start an IV of NS at 150 cc/hr
④ Question whether fatigue has increased

41. When applying antiembolism stockings, the nurse would apply the stockings:
① Before the patient arises
② 2 hours after the patient arises
③ Following the patient's bath
④ While the patient is sitting in a chair

42. A patient has recently been diagnosed with acute sinusitis. Her primary symptom is:
① Loss of appetite
② Nausea
③ Fever
④ Pain

43. A patient who is receiving an intensive course of chemotherapy for acute leukemia has developed leukopenia. His oral temperature is 100.1° F and his skin is warm and flushed. Which of the following nursing actions is *most* important?
① Direct a fan toward his bed
② Observe for undue bleeding
③ Force fluids to 3000 ml per day
④ Assess for the source of the infection

44. A patient underwent a cardiac catheterization this morning. Which of the following nursing interventions is most important during the first 4 to 6 hours after the procedure?
① Immobilize the involved leg
② Maintain the extremity used for the procedure in a flexed position
③ Keep the extremity elevated on at least two pillows
④ Limit the intake of fluids

45. When repositioning a patient from his back to his side, the nurse should:
① Position his feet perpendicular to his legs with a footboard
② Place his arms at his sides
③ Place a small pillow under his shoulder
④ Place a pillow between his legs

46. The patient being seen in the clinic for chlamydia is given a prescription for tetracycline; the patient should be instructed to:
① Avoid prolonged exposure to sunlight
② Empty the bladder every 2 to 3 hours
③ Drink a glass of milk when he takes the capsule
④ Take the medication with food

47. A 19 year old has had a nephrectomy. The doctor recommends that he withdraw from being an active member of the college football team. The reason for this recommendation is that:
① It will take at least a year to recover from surgery
② Major back, abdominal, and flank muscles have been compromised
③ He might injure the remaining kidney during play

④ The remaining kidney will not be able to meet the demands of his body

48. The three primary factors that influence the management of diabetes are:
① Diet, medication, and rest
② Diet, rest, and exercise
③ Diet, medication, and exercise
④ Rest, exercise, and medication

49. A 65 year old with osteoporosis has been recommended an exercise program by her physician. The primary reason for this recommendation is to:
① Build bone mass
② Increase circulation to the joints
③ Prevent constipation
④ Increase muscle strength

50. A patient who had a mastectomy for breast cancer is receiving prednisone as part of her therapy. The nurse will instruct her to observe for which of the following side effects?
① Hypotension
② Weight gain
③ Dehydration
④ Increase in muscle mass

51. The nurse is assigned to ambulate a patient who is non–weight bearing on the right. Physical therapy taught her how to use a three-point crutch gait. Which of the following indicates that the patient is performing the gait correctly?
① The patient advances the crutches, then advances both legs.
② The patient advances the crutches and the right leg, then advances the left leg.
③ The patient advances the right crutch with the left foot, then advances the left crutch with the right foot.
④ The patient advances the left crutch followed by the right foot, then the right crutch followed by the left foot.

52. While the nurse is preparing to apply antiembolism stockings, the patient states, "Boy, the back of my calf really hurts." What should the nurse do?
① Assess the patient for Homans' sign
② Apply the stocking as assigned
③ Tell the patient that the stockings will help the pain
④ Check the patient's Babinski reflex.

53. Which of the following dressing materials is most appropriate for an infected, draining stage III pressure ulcer?
① A hydrocolloidal dressing
② A transparent dressing
③ A dry sterile dressing
④ Gauze moistened with sterile normal saline solution

54. The nurse is teaching an individual with asthma the proper use of his Asmacort inhaler. He is to take 2 puffs twice a day and remember to:
① Rinse the mouthpiece at least twice a week
② Exhale quickly prior to inhaling the medication
③ Not shake the container prior to inhalation
④ Wait 30 seconds to 2 minutes between puffs

55. A patient exhibits a dry cough, in the absence of any other respiratory symptoms or fever. Following a thorough examination, the nurse would expect the physician to order which of the following medications?
① Robitussin (guaifenesin) syrup
② Phenergan (promethazine) with codeine elixir
③ Sudafed (pseudoephedrine) tablets
④ Benadryl (diphenhydramine) tablets

56. A patient is taking Synthroid (levothyroxine) for adult onset hypothyroidism. Which of the following observations might cause the nurse to suspect that the dose of the medication is insufficient?
① Lethargy
② Weight loss
③ Irritability
④ Tachycardia

57. A patient has a wound infection. The physician prescribes Aminopenicillin (ampicillin) 250 mg PO bid and Benemid (probenecid) 250 mg PO bid. What is the purpose of the probenecid?
① To reduce the risk of an anaphylactic reaction
② To promote metabolism of the ampicillin
③ To prevent an increase in the uric acid level
④ To increase the effect of the ampicillin

58. A patient is having postoperative urinary retention. Which cholinergic medication would the nurse expect the physician to order as treatment for this condition?
① Physostigmine (Antilirium)
② Tacrine (Cognex)
③ Bethanechol (Urecholine)
④ Pyridostigmine (Mestinon)

59. The physician orders Aldactone (spironolactone) 50 mg every morning to treat a patient with congestive heart failure. What patient teaching should be provided?
① Use a salt substitute to decrease sodium intake
② Increase foods such as bananas and oranges in her diet
③ Change positions slowly when moving from lying to standing
④ Maintain a record of monthly weights

60. A pregnant patient develops deep vein thrombosis. After the clots resolve, the physician prescribes heparin 5000 units subcutaneously every 12 hours for prophylaxis. While the nurse is teaching the patient how to administer her injections the patient asks, "Why can't I just take this as a pill?" How should the nurse respond?
① "Let me ask the physician if he will change the order to Coumadin (warfarin), which comes in a tablet form."
② "I will call the pharmacy and see if they stock heparin tablets."
③ "The physician wants you to take the injection because it is more effective."
④ "Heparin is the drug of choice for preventing blood clots during pregnancy and it is only given by injection."

61. The physician orders Sumycin (tetracycline) 500 mg qd to treat a patient's acne. Patient teaching for this individual should include instructions to:
① Take the medication with yogurt to prevent diarrhea
② Wear sunscreen to prevent a photosensitivity reaction
③ Take the medication in the morning with her vitamin and mineral supplement
④ Continue taking the medication for 2 days after the acne lesions subside

62. The nurse is providing discharge teaching for a patient following hospitalization for a myocardial infarction. One of his discharge prescriptions reads "Nitrostat (nitroglycerine) 0.4 mg SL up to 3 doses q 5 min prn for angina." How should the nurse explain this prescription to the patient?
① "You should place one, two, or three of these tablets under your tongue when you have chest pain. How many you used depends on the severity of the pain."
② "When you have chest pain, you can place one tablet under your tongue every 5 minutes until the pain is relieved, up to a maximum of three tablets."
③ "You should take one of these tablets every 5 minutes when you have chest pain and before activities that precipitate chest pain, but no more than three tablets."
④ "You can take up to three of these tablets with a full glass of water when you have chest pain."

63. A patient has a fractured nose and has clear fluid draining from each naris. Which of the following would be the best way to determine if the drainage is cerebrospinal fluid (CSF)?
① Do a spinal tap and evaluate the results
② Use a Dextrostick to identify the presence of sugar
③ Examine the drainage for the presence of bacteria
④ Perform a blood sugar test

64. An 18-year-old college student has a positive PPD. Her chest x-ray for tuberculosis is negative, as is her gastric analysis. She has been placed on isoniazid and vitamin B₆ and is to take the drugs for 6 to 9 months. The nurse should instruct her that the purpose of the B₆ is to:
① Decrease the chances of side effects from the isoniazid
② Potentiate the action of the isoniazid
③ Enhance her appetite
④ Enhance the side effects of the isoniazid

65. The physician prescribed the miscellaneous antidepressant agent Prozac (fluoxetine) for a patient with endogenous depression. Which of the following statements should be included when teaching this patient about his medication?
① "You should not eat any aged meats or cheeses when taking this drug."
② "You only need to take this medication when you feel depressed."
③ "You may take Benadryl (diphenhydramine) for your allergy symptoms."
④ "It may take a few weeks before you feel less depressed."

66. A 44-year-old patient with advanced multiple sclerosis is weak and dysphagic. To prevent respiratory complications, the nurse should:
① Administer supplemental oxygen when the patient attempts to cough and clear her lungs
② Provide the patient with an opportunity to talk about her anxiety to ease breathing
③ Inform the patient of the benefits of vitamin therapy to improve respiratory function
④ Sit the patient upright with head flexed forward toward the sternum while eating

67. The most appropriate nursing intervention for a patient scheduled for an echocardiogram would be to:
① Explain the procedure to the patient
② Inform the patient that he is to be NPO 4 hours prior to the procedure
③ Administer a sedative as ordered
④ Collect a clean-catch specimen

68. A relative of a newborn male infant is observed carrying the infant around in the hallway of the maternity unit. Which of the following statements by the nurse is most appropriate?
① "Stop; do you know what you are doing?"
② "Let me take the baby back to the nursery; it's time to take his vital signs."
③ "You need to place the infant back in his crib now and stay in the room with him."
④ "Hospital policy requires all newborns be transported in their cribs. We would appreciate your cooperation."

69. A primigravida is admitted to the maternity unit. After several hours it is well established she is in false labor. The patient expresses embarrassment to the nurse, whose best response is:
① "Don't worry; it happens to the best of us."
② "Forget about everything and enjoy a big meal."
③ "It's better to be safe than sorry; the next time you'll be here to have your baby."
④ "It's good you came to the hospital so the status of your contractions could be evaluated."

70. In addition to taking folic acid tablets, the expectant mother's dietary intake of this nutrient could best be met by eating:
① Melons
② Cucumbers
③ Fortified margarine
④ Green, leafy vegetables

71. After birth a preterm infant is placed in the high-risk nursery. Parents of the infant should be:
① Encouraged to touch their infant
② Allowed to see but not touch the infant
③ Informed that total care of the infant will be provided by the nurse
④ Instructed to learn all they can since nursing assistance will not be available after the infant goes home.

72. A patient is admitted with a left fractured tibia and fibula. The nurse assesses capillary filling to the left toes in order to determine adequate:
① Arterial peripheral circulation
② Venous peripheral circulation
③ Neurological functioning
④ Cardiac output

73. Individuals with glaucoma or benign prostatic hyperplasia (BPH) should be cautioned relative to taking which of the following drugs?
① Etodolac (Lodine)
② Furosemide (Lasix)
③ Dopamine hydrochloride (Intropin)
④ Atropine sulfate

74. Of the following medications, which reverses the effects of morphine sulfate?
① Hydromorphone hydrochloride (Dilaudid)
② Acetylcysteine sodium (Mucomyst)
③ Naloxone hydrochloride (Narcan)
④ Epinephrine hydrochloride

75. A 50 year old is admitted to the hospital in severe septicemia. Several days after admission he is diagnosed with disseminated intravascular coagulopathy (DIC). Which of the following drugs would the nurse expect the physician to use to treat this patient's condition?
① Protamine sulfate
② AquaMEPHYTON (vitamin K)
③ Heparin sodium
④ Warfarin sodium (Coumadin)

76. A patient with a new gastrostomy is silent and withdrawn as the nurse cares for the insertion site. Which of the following statements by the nurse is best for encouraging the patient to express his feelings?
① "Are you feeling angry?"
② "It must be tough for you."
③ "This will get better soon."
④ "You seem quiet today."

77. The nurse knows that _____ reverses the effect of heparin sodium therapy?
① Warfarin sodium (Coumadin)
② Naloxone hydrochloride (Narcan)
③ AquaMEPHYTON (Vitamin K)
④ Protamine sulfate

78. A patient with Ménière's disease is experiencing severe vertigo. Which of the following instructions can the nurse give to help the patient manage the vertigo?
① Wear dark glasses
② Listen to soft music
③ Avoid sudden movements
④ Rest on the involved side

79. While caring for a patient who had a total laryngectomy yesterday, the nurse would:
① Instruct the patient on tracheostomy care
② Assure the patient that his speech will not be impaired permanently
③ Have suction at the bedside
④ Report blood-tinged sputum

80. A 69-year-old patient is being admitted to the medical-surgical unit with pneumonia. As part of the assessment of the patient's respiratory system, the nurse will *first*:
① Auscultate the lung sounds
② Observe the rise and fall of the patient's chest
③ Measure the rate of respiration
④ Apply the pulse oximeter

81. A patient has an IV infusing at a rate of 1,000 cc every 8 hours. How many cc's will have infused in 7.5 hours?
① 800
② 838
③ 928
④ 938

82. A 30-year-old patient had a urinary tract infection 2 weeks ago. He calls the doctor's office and explains that he has not been able to void except for small amounts for 8 hours and is complaining of pain over the kidney. The nurse suspects that he may have:
① Ureteral obstruction
② Urinary tract infection
③ Prostate problems
④ Cancer of the bladder

83. A patient who had a renal transplant 3 weeks ago is suspected of rejecting his new kidney. The nurse recognizes which of the following as a symptom of rejection:
① Increased urine output
② Decreased serum creatinine
③ Loss of weight
④ Edema

84. The doctor has informed his patient that he has an infected finger secondary to a dog bite. The nurse knows that signs of infection include which of the following?
① Increased blood pressure
② Decrease in body temperature
③ Increase in white blood cells
④ Herpes simplex

85. A patient has a cast on his left leg. The nurse will assess him for neurovascular compromise. When monitoring an individual for neurovascular integrity, capillary refill should be less than:
① 1 second
② 2 seconds
③ 3 seconds
④ 4 seconds

86. Signs of compromised neurovascular integrity include which of the following?
① Increase in red blood cells
② Warmness of the involved extremity
③ Tingling and numbness in the involved extremity
④ Confusion

87. A patient recently had a total shoulder arthroplasty. Postoperatively, the nurse should monitor for injury to the:
① 8th cranial nerve
② Finger digits
③ Spinal cord
④ Brachial nerve plexus

88. A 77-year-old patient is 2 weeks postop from a total knee replacement. Which of the following should the home health nurse report to the physician?
① Reappearance of drainage
② Use of a walker to ambulate in the house
③ Mild discomfort with ambulation
④ Increase in appetite

89. The nurse is concerned that a patient who had an appendectomy 3 days ago is developing a paralytic ileus. The nurse should observe for:
① Increased bowel sounds
② Sudden relief of pain
③ Abdominal distention
④ Severe headache

90. A 50-year-old female had a left total hip replacement. The nurse should position her:
① On her left side with hips adducted with pillows
② On her right side with hips adducted with pillows
③ In Fowler's position for comfort
④ On either side with hips abducted with pillows

91. After using oral inhaled steroids, the patient should be encouraged to:
① Cough and deep breathe
② Blow his nose
③ Tilt his head posteriorly
④ Rinse his mouth with water

92. A 77-year-old patient is admitted with a diagnosis of status asthmaticus. The following should be considered when identifying her dietary needs:
    ① Muscle and lean tissue increase with aging and adipose tissue decreases
    ② Basal metabolic rate and physical activity decrease with aging, which slows the rate at which calories are burned
    ③ A daily intake of 1000 calories is the lowest recommended daily allowance to meet nutritional needs
    ④ When determining adequate caloric intake, disease processes are not considered

93. A 90-year-old has a stage III sacral decubiti. In order to promote tissue healing, the nurse should recommend the following diet option:
    ① Chicken, green peas, and rice
    ② Steak, deviled eggs, and macaroni and cheese
    ③ Hamburger, french fries, and a milkshake
    ④ Chicken soup and crackers

94. An 85-year-old patient presents to the primary care center with a complaint of recent weight loss. Assessment data reveals a weight loss of 15 pounds over the past 3 weeks. Factors to consider relevant to meeting the nutritional needs in the elderly population are:
    ① Economic, social, and physiologic factors
    ② Personal food preferences
    ③ Mealtimes
    ④ The ability to get to a grocery store

95. Identify the most appropriate measures to implement when caring for dementia patients to promote self-feeding:
    ① Place food in front of patient, instruct patient to eat within a specified time frame, and encourage staff members to check on the patient frequently
    ② Reduce interruptions, use placements, use finger foods, maintain consistency, and encourage with gentle prompting
    ③ Ask family members to be present at every mealtime
    ④ Insist the patient open all containers and eat everything on the tray

96. A patient is experiencing problems related to dysphagia. A teaching session is scheduled to discuss ways to promote adequate swallowing without choking. The best technique to utilize is to instruct the patient to:
    ① Tuck his chin and swallow
    ② Lie down immediately after eating
    ③ Drink plenty of water with his meals
    ④ Hyperextend his head and swallow

97. The institutionalized elderly are at increased risk of dehydration due to:
    ① Increased thirst perception and physical deficits
    ② Decreased thirst perception and urinary retention
    ③ Increased thirst perception and decreased physical deficits
    ④ Decreased thirst perception and physical, cognitive, mobility, and visual impairments

98. The important thing a nurse can do in the prevention and treatment of cerebrovascular accident (CVA) is to:
    ① Make the public aware of the signs and symptoms and what to do when they occur
    ② Make health care providers more aware of the need to treat within the first 60 minutes
    ③ Encourage patients to contact their physician as soon as they suspect they are having a stroke
    ④ Refer the patient immediately to a neurosurgeon

99. A 68-year-old patient is brought to the emergency department after being involved in a motor vehicle accident. She has been diagnosed with a fracture of the pelvis. In rendering care, the nurse knows that older adults:
    ① Often report pain very differently from younger patients
    ② Have an increased response to painful stimuli
    ③ Have a more rapid excretion of analgesic drugs
    ④ Will react much more vocally than their younger counterparts

100. An 82-year-old long-term care resident asks the nurse about the importance of regular exercise. She states, "I'm afraid if I exercise, I might get hurt or break a bone because my bones aren't so strong anymore." The most appropriate response by the nurse would be:
    ① "You're right; you get enough exercise walking around the facility."
    ② "Regular exercise is important because bone and muscle strength increase with exercise."
    ③ "Exercise when you feel like it; a little bit of exercise is better than none."
    ④ "I think it's important; you need to stay as active as possible for as long as possible."

101. The nurse is caring for a patient who was burned 72 hours ago. He has partial-thickness burns to 24% of his body surface and begins to excrete large amounts of urine. The nurse should monitor for signs and symptoms of:
    ① Infection
    ② Electrolyte disturbances
    ③ Respiratory obstruction
    ④ Shock

102. When assessing burns of the body, the nurse uses the rule of nines as a:
    ① Number of layers to classify the burn
    ② Formula for determining fluid volume replacement
    ③ Formula for determining amount of skin area burned
    ④ Comparison of body surface area burned to the patient's age

103. On the fourth postoperative day following a colectomy with subsequent colostomy, the patient is crying and tells the nurse she feels ugly. She is worried that her husband will not love her anymore. The nurse bases her interventions on the diagnosis of:
    ① Knowledge impairment related to inadequate education
    ② Noncompliance related to disinterest in self-care
    ③ Impaired social interaction related to depression
    ④ Body image disturbance related to creation of a colostomy

104. When assessing a patient at the onset of severe anaphylaxis, the breath sounds that indicate occlusion of the upper airways are:
    ① Wheezes
    ② Crackles
    ③ Rhonchi
    ④ Friction rubs

105. Which of the following nursing actions will minimize venous stasis?
    ① Ambulation

② Leg massage

③ Sitting with knees crossed

④ Placing pillows under the knee in a position of comfort

106. Which of the following nursing interventions would be most appropriate following an abdominal wound evisceration?

① Apply an abdominal binder

② Apply moist sterile dressings

③ Apply dry sterile cotton fluffy pads

④ Place the patient in a high Fowler's position

107. The nurse is helping a 2-day postoperative patient to ambulate. To evaluate the patient's tolerance for this activity, the nurse should:

① Auscultate lung sounds

② Auscultate heart sounds

③ Periodically assess the pulse rate

④ Ask the client if he is enjoying his walk

108. A patient has a history of renal calculi and is admitted to the hospital with gross hematuria and severe colicky left flank pain. In planning care for this patient, the nurse gives the highest priority to which of the following nursing diagnoses?

① Pain related to inflammation and urinary blockage

② Altered skin integrity related to immobility

③ Hypertension related to fluid overload

④ Altered health maintenance related to lack of information about kidney stones

109. If an anaphylactic blood transfusion reaction is suspected, the first nursing intervention is:

① Stop the transfusion

② Notify the charge nurse

③ Ambulate the patient

④ Administer epinephrine

110. A medical-surgical unit has reported many fall incidents in the last weeks. The nurse using critical thinking would:

① Get restraint orders for every patient

② Make sure all patients have their call lights within reach

③ Mandate that family members stay with patients

④ Analyze the causes in order to design the appropriate intervention

111. If the tuberculosis (TB) bacteria are walled off by capsules within the lung, the patient should still understand that it is possible to:

① React negatively to the TB skin test

② Be highly contagious

③ Continue to have active symptoms of TB

④ Have the bacteria break out and return to an active infection state

112. The nurse would suspect circulatory overload in a patient receiving IV therapy if which of the following were observed?

① Fever and chills

② Confusion and headache

③ Bounding pulse, dyspnea, and cough

④ Pain, edema, and erythema at the infusion site

113. A patient experiencing severe pain from cancer states that the pain medication is not working. The nurse has given the patient all the medications possible. The next nursing action should be to:

① Suggest the client try deep-breathing exercises

② Suggest the client try relaxation exercises

③ Contact the charge nurse and intervene on the client's behalf to have the dose changed

④ Emotionally support the patient and inform her that you will give her medication just as soon as time allows

114. The most important factor in the curing of cancer is:

① Chemotherapy

② Radiation therapy

③ Alternative therapy

④ Early diagnosis

115. A patient is 8 hours postop following an abdominal aortic aneurysm repair. Which of the following findings should the nurse report immediately?

① BP 130/80

② Diminished bowel sounds

③ Total urine output of 100 cc

④ Warm feet with equal strong pulses

116. Which of the following places the patient at high risk for AIDS?

① She is an IV drug user

② She breeds and sells poodles

③ She went to France for her vacation

④ She had surgery 6 months ago

117. One of the first things a patient with tuberculosis is taught to help decrease the spread of the disease is:

① Always wear a gown and gloves

② Avoid contact with all people

③ Wear a standard mask

④ Cover the nose and mouth when coughing and sneezing

118. A patient is admitted with diabetes mellitus. While doing routine checks at midnight, the nurse finds her lethargic, trembling, perspiring, and complaining of a headache. The nurse notifies the charge nurse and performs which of the following actions?

① Perform an EKG

② Administer 5 units of regular insulin IV

③ Give orange juice

④ Perform a blood glucose monitoring test

119. Which of the following acid-base disturbances would be the most characteristic of a patient with acute asthma?

① Respiratory acidosis

② Metabolic acidosis

③ Respiratory alkalosis

④ Metabolic alkalosis

120. A 16 year old has taken a spill on his bicycle and has sustained a head injury. He is groggy, confused, and does not remember what happened. A priority nursing assessment is:

① Degree of pain

② Number and location of bruises

③ Pattern of respirations and level of consciousness

④ Auscultation of lung, heart, and breath sounds

121. Which of the following is an appropriate short-term goal for the nursing diagnosis of pain?

① To be pain free by discharge

② To be free of constipation by discharge

③ To have a pain rating scale of less than 3 after analgesics are administered

④ To have a pain rating scale of greater than 5 after analgesics are administered

122. A patient with a left below-the-knee amputation is complaining of pain in the left foot. The nurse should:
① Encourage the client to grieve
② Administer an analgesic
③ Teach the client relaxation exercises
④ Discuss phantom limb pain

123. Which of the following suggest that a patient in a hip spica cast may be developing "cast syndrome"?
① The patient becomes nauseated and vomits
② The patient becomes feverish and delirious
③ The patient becomes tachycardic and hypotensive
④ The patient becomes confused and disoriented

124. After surgery to remove a brain tumor, a patient is conscious but lethargic. The nurse asks the patient to move her extremities to check for paralysis as well as to check for the patient's:
① Ability to hear
② Desire to do well
③ Willingness to cooperate
④ Ability to respond to and follow commands

125. Measures that are used to help prevent hepatic coma (hepatic encephalopathy) are:
① Give soap-suds enemas
② Reduce protein in the diet
③ Perform iced saline lavages
④ Reduce carbohydrates in the diet

COMPREHENSIVE EXAMINATION 2: PART 1

This examination contains individual questions, the majority of which relate to clinical situations. Read all questions carefully. There is only *one best answer* for each question.
Test time allotment (Part 1): approximately 2 hours
Answers and rationales begin on p. 674.

1. The nurse has taught the elderly patient with type 2 DM the importance of maintaining good glucose control. The nurse knows learning has occurred when the patient states:
   ① "My fasting blood sugar should be 100-140 mg/dL and between 120-180 mg/dL after eating."
   ② "My fasting blood sugar should be 180-240 mg/dL and between 250-300 mg/dL after eating."
   ③ "My fasting blood sugar should be between 75-100 mg/dL and 150-275 mg/dL after eating."
   ④ "My fasting blood sugar should be between 225-275 mg/dL and 276-375 mg/dL after eating."

2. A resident in a long-term care facility is unable to get out of bed and requires total assistance with positioning. When providing care it is important for the nurse to assess for the presence of pressure ulcers. The best way to prevent pressure ulcer formation is to:
   ① Ask the physician to order a pressure-reducing mattress
   ② Administer prophylactic antibiotics
   ③ Implement measures to decrease the duration/intensity of pressure to high-risk areas
   ④ Reposition the patient every 4 hours

3. A nursing home resident wears incontinence briefs due to urinary incontinence. Frequent inspection of the perineum is essential in preventing skin breakdown. The rationale for this intervention is:
   ① Skin that is waterlogged from constant wetness is more easily eroded by friction and more readily colonized by microorganisms than skin that is not overly wet
   ② To please the patient's family members
   ③ To prevent urinary retention
   ④ To prevent a urinary tract infection

4. Digoxin, a water-soluble drug, should be administered cautiously in the older adult for which of the following reasons?
   ① Digoxin is distributed in larger compartments in older adults
   ② Digoxin is less likely to accumulate to toxic levels
   ③ Digoxin dosing is the same in the older adult as it is in the younger adult
   ④ Digoxin is distributed in smaller compartments in older adults

5. A 75-year-old patient is recovering from a left-hemisphere stroke. The nurse knows that he will most likely have difficulty with:
   ① Ambulation
   ② Language function
   ③ Impulsive behavior
   ④ Impaired judgment

6. Six days after a partial gastrectomy, the patient, while eating a regular meal, suddenly becomes nauseated, flushed, diaphoretic, and dizzy. His blood pressure drops from 120/80 to 90/50. After controlling the episode, the nurse should instruct the patient that these episodes can be prevented by:
   ① Eating small amounts of food more frequently
   ② Remaining in an upright position after eating
   ③ Drinking lots of fluids with every meal
   ④ Taking an antacid after each meal

7. The nurse assesses the patient for wound hemorrhage after a thyroidectomy by:
   ① Inspecting the dressing and the back of the neck for blood
   ② Removing the dressing and checking the incision site
   ③ Monitoring hemoglobin and hematocrit levels
   ④ Inspecting the dressing for blood

8. When performing external cardiac compression, the victim must be positioned on a firm surface because:
   ① This position enables the rescuer to deliver more compressions
   ② The heart is compressed between sternum and spine
   ③ There is less risk of breaking the xyphoid process
   ④ Palpation of landmarks is easier

9. A 37-year-old patient is admitted with a diagnosis of multiple sclerosis. During the initial assessment she states "I'm too old to have this. I thought only children got this disease." Which of the following is the most appropriate reply by the nurse?
   ① "Multiple sclerosis is so rare that no one knows what age group is susceptible."
   ② "Symptoms usually occur between the ages of 20 and 40."
   ③ "You are correct. This is usually a disease of children."
   ④ "Symptoms usually occur after age 60."

10. A patient with a history of allergic reactions to bee stings should be taught which of the following to avoid an anaphylactic reaction?
    ① Take extra precautions when outdoors
    ② Carry epinephrine with him
    ③ Wear a Medic-Alert tag indicating an allergy to bees
    ④ Wear white clothing while outdoors

11. A patient develops a low-grade fever 24 hours postoperatively and has diminished breath sounds. Which of the following nursing actions is most appropriate to help reduce the fever and prevent complications?
    ① Administer Tylenol (acetaminophen)
    ② Administer antibiotics
    ③ Increase fluid intake
    ④ Encourage coughing and deep breathing

12. A 75-year-old patient is recovering from a right total hip replacement. The nurse has identified a diagnosis of impaired physical mobility related to decreased muscle strength and should plan to:
    ① Keep the right leg in extension and abduction
    ② Provide passive ROM to the right ankle
    ③ Provide active ROM to the right ankle
    ④ Encourage quadriceps-setting exercises

13. A patient with a transurethral resection of the prostate (TURP) and a 3-way Foley catheter is complaining of bladder spasms. The initial nursing action should be to:
    ① Reposition the patient in Trendelenberg position
    ② Check for obstructions in the catheter
    ③ Administer an antispasmodic
    ④ Administer a narcotic pain reliever

14. The nurse established a nursing diagnosis of fluid volume excess related to decreased glomerular filtration due to acute glomerulonephritis. Clinical data that support this nursing diagnosis include which of the following?
    ① Fever
    ② Thirst
    ③ Polyuria
    ④ Periorbital edema

15. A patient who has been admitted to the hospital with dehydration and electrolyte imbalance is confused and incontinent of urine. What nursing intervention does the nurse include in developing a care plan for the patient?
    ① Place incontinent pads on the bed
    ② Insert an indwelling catheter
    ③ Assist the patient to the bathroom q 2 hours
    ④ Restrict fluids

16. When caring for a patient with Alzheimer's disease, the nurse should:
    ① Provide for increased environmental stimulation
    ② Encourage frequent changes of environment
    ③ Provide external signs of orientation
    ④ Encourage group therapy

17. A patient is admitted with severe right flank pain, general weakness, and fever. He has a history of recurrent urinary tract infections and renal calculi. On the second hospital day, the patient's urine output drops to 300 cc in 24 hours and he complains of increased distention and pain in the suprapubic area. The nurse would evaluate which of the following to be the most likely cause for this change in status?
    ① Dehydration
    ② Urinary tract obstruction
    ③ Development of renal failure
    ④ Development of glomerulonephritis

18. The nurse performs a urinary catheterization immediately after a patient voids and obtains 30 cc of residual urine. The next step would be to:
    ① Immediately notify the physician of the results
    ② Continue intermittent catheterization after each voiding
    ③ Document the procedure
    ④ Restrict fluid intake

19. The best criteria for evaluating the care given based on the nursing diagnosis of altered nutrition: less than body requirements related to anorexia, nausea, and vomiting, include which of the following?
    ① Moist mucous membranes
    ② Absence of diarrhea
    ③ Stable body weight
    ④ Normal body temperature

20. When the nurse checks the lab results on a patient who has been receiving antineoplastic drugs for cancer treatment, the platelet count is below normal. Which of the following symptoms would be indicative of a low platelet count?
    ① Oliguria, weight gain, increased blood pressure
    ② Petechiae, hematuria, epistaxis
    ③ Fever, cough, chills
    ④ Dizziness, tremors, seizures

21. A patient who suffered a traumatic brain injury approximately 2 hours ago is placed on alteplase (Activase). The nurse would expect this drug to:
    ① Lower blood pressure
    ② Increase urinary output
    ③ Prevent development of clots
    ④ Dissolve existing clots

22. A patient is experiencing a generalized seizure. The nurse should:
    ① Leave the room, seeking assistance for the patient
    ② Insert a padded tongue blade into the patient's mouth
    ③ Note the type and location of body movements
    ④ Place the patient on his left side after the movements stop

23. The physician has determined that a patient has increased intracranial pressure. The nurse will position her in which of the following positions?
    ① Elevation of the head of the bed to 20 degrees
    ② Elevation of the head of the bed to 30 degrees
    ③ Elevation of the head of the bed to 60 degrees
    ④ Elevation of the head of the bed to 90 degrees

24. A patient has end-stage carcinoma secondary to multiple myeloma. The nurse will especially observe for which of the following electrolyte imbalances?
    ① Hyperkalemia
    ② Hypercalcemia
    ③ Hypokalemia
    ④ Hypocalemia

25. A recently admitted patient had a positive ELISA screening for AIDS, followed by a positive Western blot test. The nurse should instruct the patient that:
    ① HIV antibodies are present in his blood
    ② He has AIDS
    ③ He cannot transfer the virus to others
    ④ He will probably die within 10 years

26. According to the history of maternity care in the United States, the single greatest deterrent to maternal complications, particularly pregnancy-induced hypertension (PIH), has been:
    ① Discovery and use of antihypertensive drugs
    ② Good prenatal care
    ③ The advocation of salt-free diet
    ④ The age of the mother

27. The nurse is gathering data related to the growth and development of a 3-week-old infant. The nurse should expect to observe which of the following behaviors in the infant?
    ① Moro "startle" reflex
    ② Cooing and babbling
    ③ Recognizing a familiar face
    ④ Holding head erect

28. Which of the following activities *increases the risk* for development of urinary tract infection (UTI) in the *normal* female pediatric patient?
    ① Restricting fluids after supper to prevent bedwetting
    ② Taking daily tub baths
    ③ Using a front-to-back motion when wiping for toileting
    ④ Wearing tight panties or diapers

29. A 5 year old was bitten by a raccoon suspected of having rabies. He was taken to the pediatric clinic and received an intramuscular injection of HRIG (human rabies immune globulin) and HDCV (human diploid cell rabies vaccine). The nurse is reinforcing information about discharge instructions. Which of the following discharge instructions is *most* important?
    ① Cleanse wound b.i.d. with betadine solution
    ② Return to the clinic for suture removal in 7 days
    ③ Administer antipyretics for temperature elevation
    ④ Return to clinic *on exact scheduled dates* for HDCV injections

30. A mother must suction her 5-year-old son's tracheostomy. Which of the following statements by the mother indicates she has correct understanding of suction technique?
    ① Instill small amounts of hydrogen peroxide into the tube if the tube has caked secretions
    ② Set suction machine at 160 mm Hg pressure when suctioning
    ③ Insert the catheter no more than 0.5 cm beyond the tip of the tube
    ④ During each pass of the catheter, the catheter should remain in the tube no longer than 15 seconds

31. Which of the following activities may *precipitate* an asthma attack in a *pediatric* patient?
    ① Cleaning with an ammonia-based cleaner
    ② Learning a pet mouse died
    ③ Swimming laps at a pool
    ④ Using a fine cool mist humidifier in the house

32. Which of the following is the most appropriate nursing action when caring for a patient with meningitis?
    ① Strict isolation precautions
    ② Judicious handwashing
    ③ Wound precautions
    ④ Respiratory precautions

33. A 19 year old enrolled in a childbirth class asks the nurse when the preembryonic stage is over. The nurse replies:
    ① At birth
    ② At 9 weeks
    ③ About 3 weeks
    ④ Between the fourth and eighth week

34. A patient, pregnant for the fifth time, asks the nurse to refresh her memory and explain how waste products and nutrients are transmitted between the mother and the fetus. The nurse explains that the placenta is the organ primarily responsible for the exchange and that the connecting link is the umbilical cord which is composed of:
    ① Two arteries and one vein
    ② One artery and one vein
    ③ Two veins and one artery
    ④ Two veins only

35. When discussing nutrition with a 3-month pregnant gravida 1, para 0, the nurse explains that the most important consideration in her prenatal diet is to provide:
    ① An adequate diet to ensure optimum nutrition for mother and fetus
    ② A low-calorie diet to maintain the mother's weight
    ③ Limited fluid intake to prevent edema in the body tissues of both the mother and the fetus
    ④ A diet high in protein for nourishment of the fetus

36. The recommended total daily water intake for the older adult is:
    ① 2000-3000 ml of fluid each day
    ② 500-1000 ml of fluid each day
    ③ 2500-3500 ml of fluid each day
    ④ 1500-2000 ml of fluid each day

37. When assisting a patient receiving a lumbar puncture, the nurse helps the patient assume the knee-chest position in order to:
    ① Keep the patient from vomiting
    ② Keep the patient's vital signs stable
    ③ Keep the spinal cord as straight as possible
    ④ Allow the physician to more easily locate the correct site

38. A patient who drinks alcohol while taking chloropramide (Diabenese) can expect what specific type of reaction?
    ① Disulfiram (Antabuse)-type reaction
    ② Anaphylactic reaction
    ③ Reverse reaction
    ④ Antigen-antibody reaction

39. A nurse's 75-year-old mother is apparently in good health and lives independently in her own apartment. One morning, she tells her daughter that she would like to see an attorney to make arrangements for a will, a living will, and a durable power of attorney. The most appropriate response by her daughter, the nurse, would be:
    ① "We really don't need to discuss that right now."
    ② "Which attorney were you thinking of?"
    ③ "I know what you would want done."
    ④ "Mother, you are such a worrier."

40. The nurse in a local nursing home assigns a nursing assistant to an 87-year-old resident. The nurse will instruct the NA to help the resident with his total bath:
    ① Three times a week and to bathe with tepid water
    ② Once a week and to bathe with hot water
    ③ Every other week and to bathe with tepid water
    ④ Every other day and to bathe with cold water

41. The physician prescribes oral acyclovir (Zovirax) for a patient with genital herpes lesions. The nurse should include which of the following statements when teaching the patient about this medication?
    ① "Once the lesions disappear, you will be cured of genital herpes."
    ② "You may stop taking this drug once the pain and itching subside."
    ③ "You should drink at least three quarts of water every day while you are taking this medication."
    ④ "As long as you are taking the medication, your sexual partner will be protected from contracting the virus."

42. The physician prescribes propranolol (Inderal), a nonselective beta-adrenergic blocking agent, to treat a patient's hypertension. The nurse should monitor the patient for which side effect?
① Nervousness
② Photophobia
③ Tachycardia
④ Dyspnea

43. The patient care assistant asks whether it is permissible to apply a restraint to a patient who, in the opinion of the patient care assistant, is at risk for falling. What should the nurse do first?
① Direct the patient care assistant to apply a vest restraint
② Request a restraint order from the physician
③ Direct the patient care assistant to keep the patient in a visible area
④ Identify the factors underlying the patient's risk for falls

44. A patient who had an abdominal hysterectomy 3 days ago is to be discharged this morning. The nurse makes the following assessments: temperature, 101.2° F; pulse, 72; respirations, 16; BP 114/78; abdominal incision dry with staples intact; patient denies incisional pain. What action should the nurse take next with regard to the patient's temperature?
① Report the temperature and other data to the physician
② Administer Tylenol (acetaminophen) 650 mg PO as ordered
③ Reassess the patient's temperature
④ Record the temperature and other data in the patient's record

45. A patient with terminal cancer has been taking morphine sulfate, 10 mg, intramuscular every six hours for pain. Since the patient will be discharged to his home, the physician changes the order from the injectable to the oral form of the drug. The nurse would expect the physician to write which of the following orders?
① Morphine sulfate 5 mg by mouth every 6 hours
② Morphine sulfate 10 mg by mouth every 6 hours
③ Morphine sulfate 60 mg by mouth every 6 hours
④ Morphine sulfate 100 mg by mouth every 6 hours

46. To *best* assist a patient who has been on bed rest to prepare for ambulation, the nurse should:
① Dangle the patient's legs and swing them back and forth daily
② Have him push his popliteal space against the bed to the count of 5, several times daily
③ Perform passive range of motion exercises three times daily
④ Have him perform push-ups and use the bed trapeze bar as much as possible

47. To prevent constipation in CVA patients, the nurse should encourage them to:
① Take daily enemas
② Use a daily laxative
③ Increase fruits and fluids in their diet
④ Plan a bowel movement for early morning

48. In caring for a patient who has undergone a midthigh amputation, the nurse should *not* elevate the residual limb after the first 24 hours. This precaution is to prevent:
① Phantom limb pain
② Circulatory embarrassment
③ A hip flexion contracture
④ Damage to the peroneal nerve

49. A patient has had an above-the-knee amputation (AKA) because of complications stemming from long-standing, uncontrolled diabetes mellitus. Following an amputation, the *immediate,* most serious postoperative complication is:
① Infection
② Hemorrhage
③ Contractures
④ Pneumonia

50. A 36-year-old female has had a total hip replacement. The postoperative orders include aspirin, 5 grains (325 mg), PO, daily. The nurse is aware that the rationale for this treatment is to:
① Prevent joint inflammation
② Produce a mild anticoagulant effect
③ Provide better pain control
④ Maintain normal body temperature

51. Which set of laboratory values is it most important to monitor for the patient taking lithium carbonate (Eskalith) for a bipolar disorder?
① Complete blood cell count, platelet count, and serum albumin levels
② Blood urea nitrogen, creatinine clearance, and sodium levels
③ SGOT, SGPT, and serum bilirubin levels
④ Serum potassium, white blood cell differential, and platelet count

52. Before transferring a patient from the bed to the wheelchair, the nurse should:
① Leave the wheels of the chair unlocked so that the chair can be moved, if necessary, during the transfer
② Explain to the patient how the transfer will proceed to gain the patient's cooperation
③ Obtain the mechanical lift device to prevent injury to the nurse or patient
④ Raise the bed to a comfortable working height to reduce back strain for the nurse

53. When performing passive range of motion for a patient, the nurse should:
① Exercise the joint just past the point of stiffness to gradually increase joint motion
② Perform no more than five repetitions for each exercise to avoid tiring the client
③ Watch the patient's nonverbal communication to help evaluate the response to the exercise
④ Vary the order in which the exercises are performed so that the patient does not become bored

54. The nurse is inserting an indwelling catheter. As the nurse inflates the balloon, the patient complains of urethral pain. Which step should the nurse take next?
① Deflate the balloon and insert the catheter another inch
② Deflate the balloon and remove the catheter

③ Explain to the client that urethral pain is expected and continue to inflate the balloon

④ Encourage the patient to take a few deep breaths and continue to inflate the balloon

55. A patient is admitted for possible obstructive urinary retention due to an enlarged prostate gland. During the assessment the nurse would expect the patient to complain of:

① Hematuria

② Hesitancy in initiating voiding

③ Burning on urination

④ Nausea

56. A patient was recently discharged home with a diagnosis of cerebrovascular accident. He was discharged on warfarin 5 mg by mouth qd. When providing him with discharge instructions specific to warfarin, the nurse should instruct him to report which of the following symptoms?

① Nasal congestion

② Shortness of breath with hemoptysis

③ Constipation

④ Anxiety

57. When receiving physician's orders by telephone, the nurse must:

① Repeat the orders, then write the orders on the physician's order sheet

② Write the physician's name on the order sheet

③ Write the patient's name, next of kin, and date on the order sheet

④ Write the order as the physician gives the order, and repeat the order back to the physician for immediate verification

58. In caring for a patient with COPD, the nurse notes that the patient is more comfortable after:

① Being placed in the low-Fowler's position

② Having postural drainage

③ Fluids are restricted

④ He has provided all his own care

59. A patient with a diagnosis of sarcoidosis wants to know why the physician is planning to perform a biopsy of the lymph node. The nurse's most appropriate reply is:

① "He wants to see how far the sarcoidosis has spread."

② "Has the physician explained the procedure to you?"

③ "That is the way to definitely diagnose this disease."

④ "He can find out why your glands are swollen."

60. Frequent assessment of a patient with a fractured left leg would include maintaining proper alignment and:

① Checking sensation and circulation in the leg

② Increasing the weight of traction as necessary to maintain countertraction

③ Taking the apical pulse every 2 hours

④ Checking temperature and range of motion in his right leg

61. A nurse is assigned to administer medications to 20 patients. The gold standard for administering medications is to adhere to:

① The five rights of medication administration: right drug, dose, route, patient, time

② The five rights of medication administration: right drug, dose, route, patient, documentation

③ The five rights of medication administration: right drug, hospital policy, dose, patient, route

④ Computerized guidelines as defined by the pharmacist

62. Older persons may visit as many as two or three physicians in a relatively short period of time, with each writing the patient a different prescription. Identify the most serious potential problem related to multiple prescribed medications.

① Medications may be duplicated; therefore drug action and interaction may be affected leading to overdosage

② This will increase therapeutic effectiveness of the drugs previously prescribed

③ The patient may not be able to afford all of the medication prescribed

④ Potential problems are minimal for this patient

63. As the nurse places the medication in the patient's hand, the patient states, "This pill looks different than any pill I've ever taken." The most appropriate response by the nurse is:

① "These medications are correct; I pulled each pill out of your medication drawer."

② "The hospital changed medication vendors and so the pill looks different."

③ "I would never give you the wrong medication."

④ "I will return in just a moment, after I check to make sure this is the correct drug and dosage."

64. A 26-year-old woman with a fair complexion, blue eyes, and blond hair, arrives in the physician's office for an annual physical examination. She tells the nurse that she is going to the beach for vacation and asks for advice concerning sun exposure. Which of the following is the most appropriate response by the nurse?

① "Limit sun exposure between 10 AM and 3 PM."

② "Just use common sense."

③ "I hope you have a great time and come back very tanned."

④ "You know going to the beach means overexposure to the sun, so you shouldn't take the risk."

65. A patient has just arrived on the floor from the neurointensive care unit after intracranial surgery. Postoperative nursing care includes:

① Keep head and neck in flat position

② Maintain intravenous dextrose 5% in water

③ Maintain a patent airway

④ Maintain Trendelenburg position

66. A patient, age 10, has recently been diagnosed with epilepsy. The nurse knows that epilepsy is differentiated from convulsions based on the following criteria:

① Epilepsy is a permanent, recurrent seizure disorder; convulsion is one manifestation of a seizure

② Epilepsy is a one-time brief episode of abnormal electrical activity; convulsion is characterized by rigidity

③ Convulsion is a permanent, recurrent seizure disorder; epilepsy is one manifestation of a seizure

④ Epilepsy is an acute condition associated with brain injury; convulsion is a recurrent state of seizure activity

67. A patient is receiving intravenous heparin therapy. An important nursing intervention during heparin administration is to monitor:

① For signs of blood clotting

② For signs of hemorrhage and keep protamine sulfate available

③ For renal insufficiency and PT levels

④ Liver function studies

68. A 32-year-old patient is being admitted to the medical floor with a diagnosis of bronchiectasis. She has a chronic cough with expectoration of copious amounts of purulent sputum and hemoptysis. An appropriate *outcome criteria* is that:
    ① The patient will demonstrate improved ventilation and adequate oxygenation
    ② The nurse will encourage alternating rest and activity
    ③ The patient may have activity intolerance related to fatigue
    ④ The patient's arterial blood gases are improved

69. The *most* important aspect of nursing management specific to tracheostomy care is to:
    ① Elevate the head of the bed 30 to 45 degrees
    ② Discuss the importance of adequate intake in wound healing
    ③ Check the stoma and suctioned secretions for food particles that may indicate aspiration
    ④ Monitor for signs and symptoms of respiratory distress

70. Assessment of motor function in a patient who has had a stroke includes assessing:
    ① Cranial nerves VIII through XII
    ② Body position, level of consciousness, and mental status
    ③ Muscle movement, strength, and coordination
    ④ Intellectual function and speech pattern

71. A patient is admitted to the hospital with a diagnosis of hypergammaglobulinemia. She presents acutely ill with impaired ability to resist infection. An important measure for the nurse to implement is:
    ① Place the patient in contact isolation as soon as possible
    ② Implement protective isolation precautions and assess for signs of infection
    ③ Administer medications as ordered
    ④ Admit her to a semi-private room

72. A 60-year-old patient is being discharged after undergoing cardiac catheterization. Which of the following important instructions should the nurse include at the time of discharge?
    ① Do not change the bandage for 48 hours, and report site soreness to the physician
    ② Rest for 3 days and avoid heavy lifting/strenuous activity
    ③ Take a tub bath until the puncture site is healed
    ④ Drive a car that has an automatic transmission

73. A patient who was admitted to the medical floor with a diagnosis of thrombophlebitis of the right leg is receiving anticoagulant therapy and is placed on bed rest. Which of the following is an appropriate outcome criterion for this patient?
    ① Potential complication related to blood clot formation
    ② Both extremities are comparable in size, temperature, and color
    ③ To teach the patient how to prevent recurrences
    ④ Tissue will have adequate venous and arterial circulation

74. A 72-year-old patient is admitted to the cardiac floor with a diagnosis of acute myocardial infarction. The most reliable blood test to detect damage of heart muscle is:
    ① Complete blood cell count
    ② CK-MB (creatine kinase)
    ③ Fibrin split-products
    ④ Lactic dehydrogenase (LDH)

75. A patient's wife is very concerned about her family following her husband's recent heart attack. She tells the nurse, "I don't know what we'll do now that my husband can't work." An appropriate nursing diagnosis related to the patient's wife is:
    ① Anxiety related to concerns over lifestyle and family changes
    ② Risk for decreased cardiac output related to arrhythmias
    ③ Noncompliance related to denial of the circumstances
    ④ Ineffective individual coping related to worrying about the family's future

76. A 34-year-old patient is complaining of infertility, metrorrhagia, and dyspareunia. Examination reveals endometrial-like cells growing elsewhere in her pelvic cavity. The nurse knows this condition as:
    ① Endometriosis
    ② Endometritis
    ③ Pelvic inflammatory disease
    ④ Paraphimosis

77. To promote retraining of the affected side and a faster return to independence, CVA patients should be encouraged to:
    ① Comb their hair, wash their face, brush their teeth
    ② Participate actively in physical therapy
    ③ Perform daily push-ups
    ④ Use a pen with the affected hand

78. A 54-year-old patient underwent surgery for a suprapubic prostatectomy. Three days after surgery the cystotomy tube was removed. A specific nursing responsibility at this time is to:
    ① Force fluids
    ② Keep dressing dry
    ③ Encourage ambulation
    ④ Monitor fluid balance

79. A new mother asks the nurse at what age is it best to hang a new, colorful mobile for her newborn baby boy. The nurse can answer that newborns can follow bright and colorful objects at:
    ① 1 year of age
    ② First week of life
    ③ 9 to 10 months of life
    ④ 2 or 3 weeks of life

80. A 24-year-old mother of two comes to the clinic to obtain birth control information. The nurse tells her that the most reliable method of birth control is:
    ① Condom use
    ② Coitus interruptus
    ③ Oral contraceptives
    ④ Intrauterine device (IUD)

81. A patient receiving chlorpromazine (Thorazine) should be instructed to:
    ① Avoid certain foods containing tyramine
    ② Use a sunscreen when outdoors

③ Take medication with milk

④ Use prophylactic antacid

82. Which of the following statements regarding glycerin suppository insertion is the nurse expected to know to be true?

① Glycerin suppositories should be warmed to room temperature before insertion

② It is not necessary to lubricate glycerin suppositories before insertion

③ Glycerin suppositories should be inserted into a bolus of stool

④ Glycerin suppositories should be inserted before an attempt is made to toilet a patient in a bowel-retraining program

83. When preparing a patient for a bowel-retraining program, the nurse should understand that the most important factor for a successful retraining program is:

① Establishing regular day(s) and time to assist the patient to the toilet

② Making sure the patient understands the purpose of the program

③ Regular administration of a mild laxative

④ Skipping a day in the program if the patient has had more than one bowel movement the day before

84. An 84-year-old patient is a former WW II veteran who is experiencing extreme disorientation and agitation. A *priority* intervention for the nurse to implement is which of the following?

① Let the patient make his own care decisions

② Ask the physician for a temporary restraint order

③ Keep orienting the patient to time, place, and person

④ Limit the staff that is caring for and talking with the patient

85. A 52-year-old male is admitted for chronic alcoholism. His family tells the nurse that he now has had several episodes of short-term memory loss, is unable to learn new skills, and cannot hold a job because of these problems. The nurse recognizes this as:

① Addiction

② Habituation

③ Korasakoff's psychosis

④ Wernicke's encephalopathy

86. A patient on the mental health unit exhibits involuntary serpentine movements of the face, trunk, and extremities. This individual has been taking Thorazine for 6 years. Which of the following conditions is this individual exhibiting?

① Cowling's rule

② Chvostek's sign

③ Tardive dyskinesia

④ Sjögren's syndrome

87. A 26-year-old woman is admitted for AIDS-related *Pneumocystis carinii* pneumonia and dehydration. She states to the nurse that she feels depressed and is afraid of dying. The best therapeutic response for the nurse to make is:

① "You are afraid of dying?"

② "Does your family know how you feel?"

③ "Would you like me to call your pastor or priest?"

④ "Depression is sometimes repressed anger. Talking about it will help you feel better."

88. A nurse is working in the newborn nursery when a baby that one of his colleagues is feeding begins to choke on the formula. Immediately he assesses the situation and begins the procedure for obstructed airway on a *conscious infant*. To perform the procedure correctly, the nurse knows that he has to administer:

① Eight back blows and eight chest thrusts

② Six back blows and six chest thrusts

③ Five back blows and five chest thrusts

④ Four back blows and four chest thrusts

89. On arrival at the emergency room, a 3-year-old burn patient is semiconscious, whining, and calling for his mother. Once he has been transferred to the trauma room, the nurse begins to obtain baseline data—radial pulse rate, 160 beats/min; respirations, 32/min; and BP, 60/30. Based on the initial data, the nurse would report vital signs to the physician and assist as ordered in initiation of:

① Removal of clothing

② Central venous line

③ IV fluids

④ Antibiotics

90. Immediate physical observations of a burn patient would most importantly include:

① Physical development

② Head circumference

③ Height and weight

④ Quality of respirations

91. Normally preschoolers have little interest in eating and the anorexia associated with burns presents a problem of nutrition. A 3-year-old patient, whose parents have recently died, would most likely eat better if:

① Other children ate with him

② His grandmother ate with him

③ The nurse fed him

④ Tube feedings were given when he did not eat

92. To help a 4-year-old boy adjust to the newborn baby, the parents should be taught to:

① Make a plan to have him do simple chores around the house to increase his self-esteem and growing independence

② Buy him lots of presents too, since obviously the newborn will be getting presents

③ Make him cuddle and kiss the baby to teach him the concept of love

④ Include him in the care of the baby and plan to spend some time with him alone

93. A staff nurse on the psychiatric unit insists that her patient be up and bathed by 9 AM. The patient has difficulty complying, saying that she becomes flustered and nervous. This violates which of the following principles?

① Be aware of your own resources and limitations

② Respect the patient as a person; take time to listen to what is being said

③ Be honest

④ Help reduce anxiety by making few demands on the patient

94. A 62-year-old male was admitted 2 days ago with a diagnosis of CVA. His wife tells you, "Every time I go into the room he cries. I am afraid I have done something to upset him." The best response is:
① "He is trying to get your sympathy. You must ignore the crying and talk about other things."
② "He has no control over his crying. It is a symptom of his illness and does not mean that he is unhappy."
③ "He needs some time alone to sort out his feelings. You should consider staying away for a few days."
④ "He might benefit from a psychiatric consultation. Perhaps you could talk to your physician."

95. The primary purpose of instituting bed rest for a patient with hepatitis is to:
① Rest the liver by reducing the metabolic demands
② Control the spread of the disease
③ Reduce the risk of developing cardiac problems
④ Reduce the risk of hepatic coma

96. A 48-year-old man has just been diagnosed with glomerulonephritis. He states he has never heard of it before and asks the nurse what it is. The nurse's *best* initial reply would be which of the following statements?
① "It is an infectious disease that causes varying symptoms, primarily fatigue."
② "It is sometimes caused by a drug reaction and causes kidney damage."
③ "It is an inherited disease, and the cause is unknown; it can cause kidney damage."
④ "It is caused by your immune system's negative reaction to a previous infection."

97. A 70-year-old female has been hospitalized several times in the past year with complications from chemotherapy for metastatic breast cancer. She is placed on an antidepressant medication the day of her discharge. Discharge teaching for the patient should include which of the following:
① Fluids should be limited to three glasses a day while taking the antidepressant
② Call the physician immediately if dry mouth or orthostatic hypotension occurs
③ It may take 3 or more (even up to 12) weeks before symptoms improve
④ If this antidepressant fails to control depression, others won't be effective either

98. It is important that the nurse recognize which of the following as a recommendation made by the FDA and JCAHO about restraints?
① Restraints can be used indefinitely once the need for them has been documented
② Alternatives to restraints should be developed and implemented before using restraints
③ Restraints should be removed every 4 hours to allow for activities of daily living
④ Restraints should be tied with a square knot to the immovable part of the bed

99. One important complication to avoid following a cesarean section is a pelvic thrombosis. The nursing care plan would therefore include:
① Teaching good perineal care
② Encouraging early ambulation
③ Splinting the lower abdomen when coughing
④ Keeping the urinary and bowel tracts emptied by forcing fluids and offering stool softeners

100. If the amniotic sac is to be ruptured by the physician, what is the priority nursing responsibility?
① Time and check contractions afterward and report
② Note time and instrument used and check FHT after procedure
③ Note amount and characteristics of fluid, test with nitrazine, and report
④ Note time and amount and place pad on perineum

101. According to the theorist Erik Erikson, the first stage of development is focused on:
① Autonomy vs. shame and doubt
② Pleasure principle
③ Anal gratification
④ Trust vs. mistrust

102. A patient contracted AIDS from sharing contaminated needles with her husband. They have one 15-month-old child, whom her mother is caring for. She has just discovered that she is 5 months pregnant. To guide and help this patient and her husband, what is important for the nurse to know about AIDS?
① It is a highly contagious disease, so patients must be isolated
② It is likely that her unborn child will be infected with HIV and may have a shortened life expectancy
③ It is unlikely that her unborn child will be infected; the child may expect to enjoy a normal life
④ The nurse should read all she can about the etiology of the disease

103. While the nurse is teaching a group of single, pregnant teenage mothers about nutritional problems of pregnancy, one of the young mothers states that fat intake is only a problem if you eat a lot of meat. The nurse tells the group about other sources of fat that are "hidden" in such foods as:
① Tuna, banana, grapes, melons
② Apples, oranges, skim milk, rice
③ Creamed cottage cheese, ice cream, cashew nuts, chocolate
④ English muffins, water-packed tuna, uncreamed cottage cheese

104. A nurse observing a 2-day-old, full-term infant girl in the nursery notices that her hands and feet are cyanotic but that her body and cheeks are pink. She has passed greenish black stool and has lost several ounces since birth. This baby is:
① Premature
② Immature
③ Normal
④ Slightly abnormal

105. A 9 year old was admitted to the hospital in sickle-cell anemia crisis. Symptoms of sickle-cell crisis include all of the following *except:*
① Severe abdominal pain
② Elevated temperature
③ Joint pain
④ Elevated hemoglobin

106. When the nurse enters the patient's room, she finds a 22-year-old male with cystic fibrosis very short of breath. The first step the nurse should take is to:
    ① Take vital signs
    ② Call for help immediately
    ③ Raise the head of the bed
    ④ Obtain a brief health history

107. While the nurse is visiting a patient's home, the wife of the diabetic elderly man tells the nurse that he has been "crankier than usual" the last few days. He is also "moody and hungry as a horse." Which of the next following statements tells the nurse that she needs to check his blood sugar?
    ① He refuses to take a bath and stinks
    ② He has had a cough the last 3 or 4 days
    ③ He had diarrhea once last week in the middle of the night
    ④ He has been in the bathroom off and on all morning urinating

108. The nurse is teaching a 20-year-old male, who has been diagnosed with renal disease, about diet planning. The nurse knows that the patient with a chronic renal disease will possibly have potassium and phosphorus restricted, as well as sodium and:
    ① Fats
    ② Calcium
    ③ Protein
    ④ Carbohydrates

109. A patient is being admitted to the cardiac unit with ventricular arrhythmias. The nurse knows that the drug of choice for this condition is:
    ① Inderal
    ② Digoxin
    ③ Lidocaine
    ④ Morphine sulfate

110. A patient who is an alcoholic is to be started on Antabuse (disulfiram). The nurse knows that this drug, used to reinforce abstinence, can cause:
    ① Acne
    ② High-level energy
    ③ A sugar taste to foods
    ④ Insomnia and nightmares

111. An elderly patient who is going to have GI testing done has hematuria. The nurse needs to take a complete medication history because this condition can be caused by:
    ① Diuretics
    ② Pyridium
    ③ Macrodantin
    ④ Anticoagulants

112. Nurse Practice Acts are passed by state legislatures to:
    ① Accredit nursing programs
    ② Define legal standards of nursing
    ③ Ensure minimal safety performance of nurses
    ④ Set ethical standards for nurses

113. A 67-year-old male is admitted to the hospital with neurogenic atony of the bladder with urinary retention. The nurse knows that an effective acetylcholine derivative useful in managing nonobstructive urinary retention is known as:
    ① Mestinon
    ② Urecholine
    ③ Pilocarpine
    ④ Pro-Banthine

114. A retired schoolteacher whose husband is on a low-cholesterol diet following a heart attack says she is totally confused about cholesterol and its importance in the diet. Of the following statements about cholesterol, which should the nurse know to be true?
    ① It is best to be totally eliminated from the diet
    ② It is a normal component of blood and all body cells
    ③ It is not necessary for normal body functions
    ④ It is found in increased amounts in grain products

115. Assuming that the nurse's first action to control bleeding from a slashed wrist was correct but unsuccessful, the nurse should then:
    ① Apply a tourniquet
    ② Apply direct pressure for an additional 6 minutes
    ③ Apply pressure to the brachial artery
    ④ Apply pressure to the carotid artery

116. When caring for a patient who has just returned to the floor after having a cystoscopy, the nurse should instruct him to:
    ① Eat a soft diet for 2 days
    ② Decrease his fluid intake for 2 days
    ③ Take a warm sitz bath for discomfort
    ④ Decrease his fluid intake for 24 hours

117. A 14-year-old girl had a spina bifida repaired at birth. She has since developed a marked scoliosis and is now admitted to the hospital for spinal fusion and instrumentation. During her admission procedure the primary goal is to provide:
    ① Privacy
    ② Orientation to the ward
    ③ Her mother's presence
    ④ Introduction to her roommates

118. The primary reason that adverse drug reactions occur frequently in elderly patients is because the elderly have a:
    ① Higher percentage of body water
    ② Higher percentage of lean muscle
    ③ Lower percentage of body fat
    ④ Higher percentage of body fat

119. A patient with Alzheimer's disease is attempting to leave a long-term care facility. The most appropriate intervention for this patient would be to:
    ① Reorient the patient to time, place, and person and then escort the patient back to her room
    ② Validate the patient's feelings, but distract the patient with another activity
    ③ Call security and seek assistance to physically restrain the patient from leaving the facility
    ④ Allow the patient to leave the facility and bring the patient back to the facility when she becomes fatigued

120. A patient with diabetes who develops an infection should be taught to expect to:
    ① Need less insulin
    ② Need more insulin
    ③ Spill protein in the urine
    ④ Have severe hypoglycemic reactions

121. Three days after admission, a patient becomes confused. The nurse's care plan should recommend:
    ① Ambulation and maintaining mobility by ROM exercises
    ② Moving the patient to the psychiatric ward
    ③ Reviewing the medication regimen with the physician
    ④ Obtaining an order for medication to decrease confusion

122. While preparing to administer digitalis to a newly admitted patient, the nurse counted an apical pulse rate of 52 beats/min. The nurse would be correct to:
    ① Give the drug as usual
    ② Omit the drug and report it to the physician
    ③ Give the patient half the dosage
    ④ Give the drug but with twice as much water as usual

123. The nutritional requirements of a diabetic patient:
    ① Are the same as for a nondiabetic patient
    ② Will be lower in calories than for a nondiabetic patient
    ③ Will be lower in carbohydrates than for a nondiabetic patient
    ④ Will be higher in protein than for a nondiabetic patient

124. An 11-year-old female patient has an order for prochlorperazine (Compazine) 4 mg IM. On hand is Compazine 10 mg/ml. The nurse gives this patient:
    ① 0.2 ml
    ② 0.4 ml
    ③ 0.8 ml
    ④ 1.2 ml

125. Using Clark's rule, answer the following problem:
    Child's weight: 30 lb
    Average adult dose: 10 mg
    What is the child's dose?

    Clark's rule: $\dfrac{\text{Weight in pounds} \times \text{Adult dose}}{150}$

    ① 1 mg
    ② 2 mg
    ③ 2.5 mg
    ④ 3 mg

COMPREHENSIVE EXAMINATION 2: PART 2

This examination contains individual questions, the majority of which relate to clinical situations. Read all questions carefully. There is only *one best answer* for each question.
Test time allotment (Part 2): approximately 2 hours
Answers and rationales begin on p. 685.

1. Fluid and electrolytes are carefully monitored in patients with renal disease. A priority concern would be an increase in which of the following electrolytes?
   ① Calcium
   ② Chloride
   ③ Sodium
   ④ Potassium
2. When transferring a post–left lobectomy patient from the recovery room stretcher to the room bed, it is most important that the:
   ① Chest drainage tube be disconnected from the drainage bottle during transfer
   ② Physician be present in case massive hemorrhage occurs
   ③ Chest drainage tube be placed on a shelf above the patient's head
   ④ Chest drainage tube be kept below the level of the patient's chest
3. A patient admitted with a diagnosis of concussion and fractured left radius suddenly becomes agitated with the nurse and tries to climb out of bed. He starts talking incoherently and then becomes very lethargic. The nurse knows that these changes from his previous behavior are most likely due to:
   ① Mental illness
   ② Fat embolism
   ③ Compartment syndrome
   ④ Increased intracranial pressure
4. The nurse is preparing to ambulate a patient for the first time postoperatively. Which of the following actions should the nurse take to maintain patient safety?
   ① Use one person to assist
   ② Use two persons to assist
   ③ Give a narcotic 15 minutes before ambulation
   ④ Encourage the patient to dangle alone for 1 hour before ambulation
5. The reason for recommending that a patient stop smoking when he has peripheral vascular disease is:
   ① Smoke causes hypotension
   ② Nicotine constricts blood vessels
   ③ Smoke irritates the lungs
   ④ The tars in smoke decrease the RBC (red blood cell count)
6. When planning care, the nurse knows that due to thrombocytopenia, patients with leukemia are at great risk for:
   ① Anemia
   ② Anxiety
   ③ Infection
   ④ Bleeding
7. A patient has multiple soft-tissue injuries from a bicycle accident. Immediate medical management for these are:
   ① Aspiration of excessive fluid
   ② Rest and heat to control edema
   ③ Rest and cold to control edema
   ④ Immediate immobilization to halt pain
8. In caring for a patient with a penetrating foreign object in the cornea, the priority nursing intervention is:
   ① Pull out the object immediately with tweezers
   ② Cover both eyes and seek medical care
   ③ Cover the affected eye and seek medical care
   ④ Immediately irrigate with large amounts of tap water
9. A patient with a spinal cord injury at C6 is experiencing autonomic dysreflexia. What is the priority nursing intervention?
   ① Check for bowel impaction
   ② Give medication as ordered
   ③ Place the patient in an upright position
   ④ Place the patient in a supine position
10. A patient scheduled for colon surgery in the morning has the order "enemas 'til clear." Enemas are usually ordered before surgery to prevent:
    ① Impaction after surgery
    ② Paralytic ileus after surgery
    ③ Contamination of the surgical site
    ④ Injury of the colon during surgery
11. A patient is in a hip spica cast. For the nursing diagnosis risk of constipation due to decreased mobility, the appropriate goal for this patient is:
    ① Receive IV fluids at 50 cc/hr
    ② Drink 1000 cc/day
    ③ Drink 3000 cc/day
    ④ Receive an enema q.o.d.
12. A patient scheduled for an open reduction and internal fixation of the left hip due to a fracture should be taught that the immediate expected post-op outcome of this surgery relative to activity is:
    ① Bed rest only
    ② Pivoting into a chair
    ③ Ambulating with full weight bearing
    ④ Confinement in bed with skeletal traction
13. After a thyroidectomy a patient develops carpopedal spasms and tingling of the lips. Which of the following complications would the nurse consider as the most likely to be occurring?
    ① Hyperglycemia
    ② Hypocalcemia
    ③ Hyperkalemia
    ④ Thyroid storm
14. Which of the following nursing diagnoses would take priority when caring for a patient in anaphylactic shock?
    ① Altered comfort
    ② Risk for injury
    ③ Altered tissue perfusion
    ④ Altered bowel elimination
15. A patient is admitted to the hospital with burns to his upper chest and face. It would be most important for the nurse to assess him frequently for:
    ① Bradycardia
    ② Hypertension
    ③ Respiratory complications
    ④ Decreased level of consciousness

16. The nurse assesses a patient in an emergency situation in which of the following sequences?
    ① Breathing, airway, circulation
    ② Airway, breathing, circulation
    ③ Circulation, airway, breathing
    ④ Breathing, circulation, airway

17. A patient with bladder cancer is recovering from a cystectomy with an ileal conduit. An important nursing intervention is:
    ① Limiting acid-ash foods
    ② Prevention of tissue rejection
    ③ Maintenance of skin integrity
    ④ Maintenance of fluid and electrolyte balance

18. Other than taking baseline vital signs, an important nursing intervention to perform the morning of dialysis is to:
    ① Administer Benadryl
    ② Weigh the client
    ③ Do a urinalysis
    ④ Keep the patient NPO

19. Which of the following findings in the urine is significant in a patient with abdominal trauma?
    ① Pyuria
    ② Dysuria
    ③ Polyuria
    ④ Hematuria

20. When caring for a comatose patient, the nurse knows that it is not appropriate to discuss the patient's condition with the family at the patient's bedside because:
    ① It could confuse the patient
    ② It may upset the family
    ③ It may speed up the dying process
    ④ Hearing is one of the last senses lost

21. The nurse knows that family members assisting in the care of a dying loved one is beneficial because this:
    ① Prolongs the dying process
    ② Lessens the nurse's workload
    ③ Helps prevent the family from feeling helpless
    ④ Causes too much work for a grieving family

22. The nurse recognizes that the most frequent initial indication of coronary artery disease in women is:
    ① Mitral valve prolapse
    ② Endocarditis
    ③ Angina
    ④ Myocardial infarction

23. When caring for a patient with a tracheostomy, the nurse observes that the tube appears to be filling with dry mucus. Which of the following actions is appropriate for the nurse to implement at this time?
    ① Remove the inner cannula and clean with alcohol-soaked Q-Tips
    ② Remove the inner cannula and clean with hydrogen peroxide
    ③ Remove the outer cannula and clean with hot water
    ④ Remove the outer cannula and suction the trachea

24. A 45-year-old male was admitted a week ago with a diagnosis of cancer of the lungs. Since that time he has undergone a right lower lobectomy and is now being prepared for discharge. The nurse should instruct him to:
    ① Take his morphine sulfate as directed
    ② Practice breathing exercises daily
    ③ Keep smoking down to one to three cigarettes per day
    ④ Avoid lifting anything over 5 pounds until the incision is healed

25. A patient is being discharged following a suprapubic prostatic resection. He had an IV and a three-way Foley with continuous bladder irrigation, which was discontinued last evening. Which of the following is an appropriate discharge instruction for this patient?
    ① Use daily laxatives to avoid straining to have a bowel movement
    ② Limit fluid intake to what you had in the hospital to prevent stretching the bladder
    ③ If dribbling or incontinence occurs, use the Kegel exercises 10 to 20 times an hour
    ④ Don't worry if your urine turns a bright red because that is caused by passing clots

26. Administration of medication to a patient with aplastic anemia would be best achieved by which of the following routes?
    ① Intravenously, when possible
    ② Intradermally, when possible
    ③ Parenterally, when possible
    ④ Orally, when possible

27. The nurse is caring for a cognitively impaired older adult who is screaming and cursing as he enters the room. The most appropriate action for the nurse to take is:
    ① Remain calm while talking with a low, reassuring voice
    ② Speak loudly and ask him to be quiet
    ③ Shake him and instruct him not to shout or use profanity
    ④ Close the door and allow him to have his temper tandrum

28. A newly admitted clinic patient complains of extreme fatigue, weight loss, and anorexia. One of her nursing diagnoses is altered nutrition: less than body requirements. Which of the following is the most appropriate nursing intervention for this patient?
    ① Suggest use of hard candy, chewing gum, or artificial saliva to increase moisture in the mouth
    ② Discuss benefits of adequate moisture in the environment
    ③ Keep a dietary record of amount, type, and frequency of food intake
    ④ Plan low-calorie snacks into daily routine

29. When taking a nursing history from a patient with a diagnosis of cholelithiasis, which of the following questions is the most appropriate?
    ① Do you have gas?
    ② Do you get heartburn after a spicy meal?
    ③ Do you have an intolerance for fatty foods?
    ④ Are you more comfortable sleeping with your head up?

30. The major focus of care with a patient following a Whipple's procedure is:
    ① Monitoring renal function
    ② Maintaining chest tubes

③ Monitoring blood glucose levels
④ Monitoring hemoglobin and hematocrit (H&H)

31. After clamping the T-tube, the nurse notes the patient with the cholecystectomy begins to complain of abdominal pain and subsequently vomits. The most appropriate nursing intervention would be to:
① Administer an antiemetic
② Irrigate the NG tube
③ Unclamp the T-tube
④ Position the client upright

32. A patient has been placed in pelvic traction. Which of the following would indicate a problem with this traction?
① Weights are hanging free
② Head of bed is flat and two pillows are under knees
③ Belt is secured under the hips and skin is protected from irritation
④ Side straps are even and clear the bed for a straight line of pull

33. The nurse makes a diagnosis of altered sensory perceptions related to hemianopsia. Which of the following nursing interventions is appropriate?
① Cover the eyes with a blindfold
② Approach the patient on the right side
③ Teach the patient to scan the environment
④ Use artificial tears to prevent drying of the corneas

34. Which of the following nursing activities occurs during the assessment phase of the nursing process?
① Observing the patient's skin integrity
② Teaching the patient deep breathing exercises
③ Determining the priority patient care problem
④ Collaborating with the patient to determine a realistic diet plan

35. An MRI (magnetic resonance imaging) test is ordered for a patient. Before the MRI is performed, which nursing action is essential?
① Removal of the patient's dental bridge
② Administration of a pretest sedative
③ Insertion of a Foley catheter
④ Placing the patient on an EKG monitor

36. Which of the following would the nurse expect the drug of choice to be for treating a hypertensive crisis?
① Propanalol hydrochloride (Inderal)
② Enalapril maleate (Vasotec)
③ Nifedipine (Procardia)
④ Nitroprusside (Nipride)

37. The nurse should advise the patient with duodenal ulcer disease to seek immediate medical attention if he experiences:
① Heartburn
② Coffee-grounds emesis
③ Belching and flatulence
④ Pain when the stomach is empty

38. A patient is having an acute episode of GI hemorrhage. The physician orders are: IV of normal saline at 100 cc/hr, CBC, NG tube to low suction, NPO, oxygen 2 liters by nasal cannula. Which of these orders should the nurse consider a priority and do first?
① CBC
② IV with normal saline
③ Oxygen, 2 liters by nasal cannula
④ NG tube to low suction

39. The physician orders diazepam (Valium) 7.5 mg IV. Diazepam is supplied in a 10 mg/2 cc Bristoject container. How many cc should be administered?
① 0.5 cc
② 1.0 cc
③ 1.5 cc
④ 1.75 cc

40. Which of the following drugs would the nurse expect to be the drug of choice for treating left ventricular heart failure?
① Dopamine hydrochloride (Intropin)
② Furosemide (Lasix)
③ Nitroprusside sodium (Nipride)
④ Dobutamine hydrochloride (Dobutrex)

41. Which of the following would disqualify an individual as a blood donor?
① A body weight over 110 pounds
② History of a recent tattoo
③ Pregnancy 8 months ago
④ A hemaglobin greater than 12.5 gm/dl in a woman

42. A patient was recently diagnosed with myasthenia gravis. It is imperative that the nurse teach the patient the importance of:
① A high-protein diet
② Taking her medication 1 hour after meals
③ Going to a salon to tan for 30 minutes daily when possible
④ Energy conservation

43. A patient is admitted to the rehabilitation unit following a CVA. He has been experiencing dysphagia as a result of his brain infarct. In order to assist him, the nurse should put him in which of the following positions?
① Sitting in an upright position with head slightly forward
② Standing with legs abducted for 2 minutes then adducted for 1 minute
③ Sitting in a comfortable position to promote speaking
④ Turning him every 2 hours to a different position

44. When a patient is in status epilepticus, she is at risk for impaired respirations, which can cause systemic and cerebral hypoxia. IV administration of a rapid-acting anticonvulsant is indicated. Which of the following medications would the nurse expect to be the best choice?
① Valium
② Tegretol
③ Lithium
④ Magnesium sulfate

45. Following a seizure, the nurse knows to place the patient in which of the following positions?
① Side lying
② Prone
③ Supine
④ High Fowler's

46. A patient who had a cerebral vascular accident (CVA) yesterday was admitted to the unit. The nurse is to monitor her stools for blood. The rationale behind this is that:
① Hypersecretion of gastric juices occurs during stress
② Hyposecretion of gastric juices occurs during stress
③ Her medications are irritating to the bowel
④ Hemorrhoids frequently develop as a result of constipation

47. Besides a history of hypertension, diabetes, or high cholesterol levels, which of the following is a high risk factor for a CVA or TIA?
    ① Dehydration
    ② Epilepsy
    ③ Hyperthyroidism
    ④ Insomnia

48. The patient with Parkinson's disease experiences posture and gait changes. Which of the following statements best reflects how gait is affected in this disease?
    ① Patient displays muscle rigidity and brief, jerky motor movements
    ② Patient displays limp, fidgeting movement of legs when walking
    ③ Tremors cause the patient's ambulation to appear spastic
    ④ Patient is bedridden; ambulation is not possible.

49. A 34-year-old patient recently underwent a cystectomy. She is experiencing pain ranging between 2 and 3 on a scale from 1 to 10. The nurse is working with her on guided imagery. This type of pain control utilizes:
    ① The gate-control theory
    ② The specificity theory
    ③ Distraction theory
    ④ All-or-nothing theory

50. A 76-year-old woman is admitted to the surgical unit following hip replacement surgery. The nurse administers meperidine (Demerol) 20 mg IV, as ordered for pain. The patient sleeps for 3 hours and awakens confused, drowsy, and lethargic. The nurse should:
    ① Call the physician and report the patient's condition
    ② Not call the physician but chart the patient's response to the medication
    ③ Keep reminding the patient of where she is, the day, and the time
    ④ Observe the patient since the elderly metabolize drugs at a slower rate

51. A 25-year-old male patient had a tuberculin skin test (PPD). After measuring a 5 mm area of enduration, the nurse should:
    ① Gather more information
    ② Tell him he is negative
    ③ Retest in 3 months
    ④ Tell him he has active TB

52. A student questions the nurse about the common cold. Which of the following statements by the nurse is the most appropriate?
    ① Each infection is caused by a specific bacterium
    ② A person's susceptibility decreases with age
    ③ Symptoms appear in 7-10 days after exposure
    ④ The causative virus is constantly present in the upper respiratory tract

53. Health services at the college is open on Monday, Wednesday, and Thursday. A freshman student needs to have a tuberculin skin test (PPD). The nurse should schedule the student for her skin test on:
    ① Tuesday
    ② Wednesday
    ③ Monday
    ④ Thursday

54. A patient who is to have a fasting blood sugar in the morning, calls the nurse at 4 AM and asks what time she can expect breakfast. The nurse should instruct her that:
    ① She will be NPO until the lab worker arrives to draw her blood
    ② Breakfast will not be served until her blood is drawn
    ③ She is to save her first urine specimen in the morning
    ④ She may only have fluids this morning

55. A 30-year-old patient has been admitted to the neuro/surgical unit following surgery for a brain tumor. She reports to the nurse that she is seeing zig-zag lines in front of her face and hears voices singing. The nurse should *first*:
    ① Note her comments in the chart and refer them to her psychiatrist
    ② Have the patient lie down
    ③ Start an IV and administer IV Valium
    ④ Call the patient's physician

56. A patient with Parkinson's disease has been admitted to the hospital with a broken right foot. He had surgery yesterday and is doing well, and his family is visiting him at present. The nurse enters the room to serve him his lunch. The nurse should:
    ① Position him in a high Fowler's position
    ② See that he gets extra milk for lunch
    ③ Have the family feed him
    ④ Administer his L-dopa with his meal

57. A 19 year old who has type 1 diabetes is sexually active. The nurse is to teach her measures to prevent perineal irritation, vaginitis, and urinary tract infections. The nurse should instruct her to:
    ① Wear synthetic underwear
    ② Use petroletum products such as vasoline as a vaginal lubricant
    ③ Wear tight blue jeans if she wants
    ④ Drink 3000 ml a day of fluid

58. A patient who underwent a transurethral resection of the prostate has had his catheter removed and is placed on the four-bottle technique. He has just voided for the fifth time today. The nurse knows to discard the:
    ① Bottle contents on the left and place the bottle to the right
    ② Bottle contents on the right and place the bottle to the left
    ③ #2 bottle contents and place the bottle to the right
    ④ #3 bottle contents and place the bottle to the left

59. A patient is to have his stools tested for occult blood. When preparing him for this procedure the nurse will instruct him to:
    ① Eat no meat for 3 days prior to the procedure
    ② Collect the stool immediately prior to bedtime
    ③ Keep the specimen warm
    ④ Drink a quart of milk the day before the procedure

60. A 19-year-old patient who has type 1 diabetes mellitus is taking Ortho-Novum for birth control. She comes to the doctor's office complaining of an upper respiratory infection and is subsequently prescribed ampicillin to take for 1 week. The nurse should instruct her to:
    ① Use another means of birth control
    ② Perform a urine test to check her blood sugar
    ③ Take ampicillin until she feels better
    ④ Expect a rash from the ampicillin

61. A patient is post-op from a percutaneous transluminal coronary angioplasty. The left femoral vein was the site into which the catheter was inserted. When the nurse is instructing the patient on his care, she should instruct him:
    ① Not to drink fluids for 4 hours post-op
    ② That he may ambulate as soon as the sheath is out
    ③ To maintain his right leg in a flexed position
    ④ To keep his left leg straight and still for 3 hours

62. A patient has end-stage cancer of the liver. He has shortness of breath secondary to the ascites. The nurse can best monitor the progress of the ascites by:
    ① Weighing the patient every morning
    ② Monitoring his intake and output
    ③ Assessing his O_2 SAT level
    ④ Measuring his abdominal girth

63. The nurse assigned to a neurology floor is to assess a 21-year-old male patient admitted with facial trauma. The nurse then asks the patient to occlude each nostril separately and close his eyes while she presents sources of familiar odors. The nurse is assessing which of the following cranial nerves?
    ① I
    ② II
    ③ III
    ④ VII

64. The patient newly diagnosed with Guillain-Barré syndrome is closely monitored for:
    ① Skin breakdown
    ② Contractures
    ③ Respiratory distress
    ④ Dysphagia

65. A 16-year-old patient is admitted to the neurology floor after being involved in an automobile accident. His head hit the windshield and he is being admitted for observation. During the afternoon he begins to complain of a headache, has two episodes of vomiting, and is more difficult to arouse. The initial nursing intervention is to:
    ① Do nothing; he needs his rest
    ② Place him in a recumbent position, administer oxygen, and notify the physician immediately
    ③ Prepare him for emergency surgery
    ④ Assess his neurologic status, elevate the head of the bed slightly, and notify the physician immediately

66. A 45-year-old patient presents to the clinic with complaints of sudden, severe, and burning pain in the face area. She states, "It goes away as quickly as it began." She also complains of facial twitching with several episodes during a 24-hour period. The patient is diagnosed with trigeminal neuralgia. A priority nursing goal is:
    ① Pain related to nerve compression
    ② Patient's pain will be relieved or reduced to a tolerable level
    ③ Administer prescribed drugs
    ④ Encourage patient to chew on the opposite side

67. The nurse is assigned to provide care for a patient with temporomandibular joint (TMJ) syndrome. Appropriate nursing interventions would include which of the following?
    ① Teaching correct yawning technique
    ② Teaching correct chewing technique
    ③ Providing soft foods, nutritional liquid supplements, and pain-control management
    ④ Verbalizing decreases in jaw pain when joint is moved

68. A 35-year-old patient is status post-craniotomy. An expected outcome for him will be:
    ① Monitor for increased intracranial pressure
    ② Self-care deficit related to diminished level of consciousness
    ③ Intracranial pressure returns to normal
    ④ Turning in bed without help

69. An individual with a seizure disorder is being evaluated in the primary care center. Appropriate assessment data would include questioning the patient regarding:
    ① Events that occurred before or after the seizure
    ② Diet and exercise history
    ③ Social and educational levels
    ④ Work history

70. A priority teaching strategy for the nurse to include for the individual diagnosed with epilepsy is to:
    ① Control seizure activity and prevent injury
    ② Wear a Medic-Alert bracelet and avoid situations known to trigger seizures
    ③ Follow-up with the primary care physician on an annual basis
    ④ Refrain from going into crowded areas

71. Abrupt withdrawal of phenytoin may trigger:
    ① Hyperglycemia
    ② Tardive dyskinesia
    ③ Status epilepticus
    ④ Parkinsonism

72. A patient is taking Valium (diazepam) 20 mg by mouth four times a day. The nurse should monitor which of the following body systems closely?
    ① Gastrointestinal, relevant to decreased peristalsis
    ② Renal, relevant to increased urinary output
    ③ Respiratory, relevant to respiratory depression
    ④ Endocrine, relevant to decreased metabolism

73. A nurse is caring for a patient receiving total parenteral nutrition (TPN). Appropriate nursing interventions for this patient include:
    ① Weigh daily, monitor blood glucose levels, and wean from TPN gradually
    ② Assess for degree of hunger every shift
    ③ Monitor liver function, renal function, and cardiovascular function
    ④ Weigh every week, monitor for glycosuria, and discontinue TPN on the third day

74. A patient is receiving intravenous 5% dextrose in water (D5W). The physician writes an order to discontinue the IV. Appropriate documentation includes:
    ① The amount of total fluid infused and how the patient tolerated the procedure
    ② The time the IV was discontinued and the amount of remaining fluid
    ③ The time the IV was discontinued, the amount of fluid infused, and the appearance of the venipuncture site
    ④ How the patient tolerated the procedure, the time the IV was discontinued, and the appearance of the IV site

75. A 19-year-old patient presents to the emergency department with a gunshot wound to the chest. The nurse knows that he will require which of the following types of surgery?
① Urgent
② Elective
③ Required
④ Emergency

76. Most patients are allowed oral fluids within 4 to 24 hours after surgery. The nurse must *first:*
① Assess that the patient has recovered sufficiently from anesthesia to be able to swallow
② Check the physician's orders to make sure fluids are to be given
③ Introduce fluids slowly and in small amounts
④ Determine the patient's fluid preference

77. A 12-year-old patient presents to the emergency department with a dislocated shoulder following a playground accident. The physician orders Versed, 0.5 mg IV, prior to reducing the shoulder. Which of the following is an appropriate nursing diagnosis for this patient?
① Risk for ineffective breathing patterns
② Patient will have a normal respiratory pattern
③ Position head to allow for maximum ventilation
④ Stable respiratory pattern

78. Oral rehydration therapy is the treatment of choice for children with:
① Infectious gastroenteritis
② Hypertrophic pyloric stenosis
③ Viral meningitis
④ Celiac disease

79. One of the medications approved for use in children with AIDS that assists in slowing the progression of the disease is:
① IV gamma globulin (Gamamine N)
② Ceftazidime (Fortaz)
③ Vancomycin (Vancocin)
④ Azidothymidine (Retrovir)

80. The average 2- to 3-month-old infant:
① Babbles
② Has a crude pincer grasp
③ Has a closed posterior fontanel
④ Has one lower incisor

81. About 95% of all sudden infant death syndrome (SIDS) cases occur:
① In the first 10 weeks of life
② In the first 3 months of life
③ In the first 6 months of life
④ Between 6 and 12 months of age

82. The principal cause of mononucleosis is:
① Streptococcus
② The Epstein-Barr virus
③ Respiratory syncytial virus (RSV)
④ *H. influenzae*

83. A 72-year-old patient is taking diuretics for congestive heart failure. As part of his home care directions the nurse should instruct him to weigh himself:
① Each morning upon arising
② One hour after taking his medication
③ If he notices an increase in pedal edema
④ Whenever he develops shortness of breath

84. Which instruction is most appropriate for a COPD patient with copious bronchial secretions?
① Decrease fluid intake to solidify bronchial secretions
② Tracheal suctioning is the best method for removing heavy secretions
③ Try to drink several glasses of juice or water daily to loosen secretions
④ You'll find it easier to breathe if you sit up straight during postural drainage treatments

85. The nurse has been assigned to perform colostomy care for a 45-year-old recent hemicolectomy patient. She can best determine how the patient tolerated the procedure by:
① Noting all objective signs and symptoms during the procedure
② Asking the patient if anything is bothering him during the procedure
③ Questioning the patient regarding his well-being at the end of the treatment
④ Observing the patient's verbal and nonverbal actions throughout the procedure

86. A 67-year-old patient is admitted with excess fluid between the visceral and parietal pleural. The physician orders a thoracentesis to remove the accumulated fluid. Post-procedure the nurse would position the patient:
① On the affected side
② On the unaffected side
③ In a supine position
④ In high Fowler's position

87. Following a thoracentesis the patient is monitored closely for which of the following?
① Increased respiratory rate, chest tightness, and hypoxemia
② Decreased respiratory rate, low blood pressure, and decreased pulse rate
③ Bradycardia, dry hacky cough, hypotension
④ Normal sinus rhythm, normotension, and ventilation

88. A 75-year-old patient is being evaluated for a lower respiratory tract infection. Appropriate teaching strategies in the prevention of pneumonia are:
① Encourage deep breathing and coughing exercises every 2 hours
② Encourage bed rest every 2 hours
③ Administer a sedative to assist with sleep
④ Decrease fluid intake

89. A nurse happens on the scene of an accident and finds a man lying on the ground with his eyes closed. The nurse's first action should be to:
① Notify emergency personnel
② Open the airway with head-tilt, chin lift
③ Attempt to arouse the person
④ Start cardiopulmonary resuscitation

90. Tuberculosis is considered a communicable disease primarily affecting the lungs. Tuberculosis is commonly transmitted by:
① Indirect contact with a person who has the actual disease
② Direct contact with a person who has the active disease through the inhalation of droplets
③ Direct contact with a person who has the inactive disease

④ Indirect contact with a person who has the active disease for a brief period of time

91. A patient undergoes a cholecystectomy and duct exploration. She returns to the floor with an IV, nasogastric tube to low suction, and a T-tube in place. The purpose of the T-tube is to:
① Remove serous fluid from the abdominal cavity
② Provide an access to irrigate the operative area
③ Remove excessive bile from the intestines
④ Promote bile duct patency until edema subsides

92. In planning care for a patient with arteriosclerosis obliterans, the nurse would consider which of the following?
① Direct application of heat to improve circulation to the affected area
② Giving instructions in avoiding injury and maintaining circulation
③ Elevating the foot of the bed to increase arterial circulation
④ Massaging the extremities several times a day to improve circulation

93. A 32-year-old working mother was admitted for an evaluation of problems caused by severe anxiety. The nurse knows that anxiety is different than fear, in that anxiety:
① Is a response to an obvious threat
② Is a response to an unknown stimulus
③ Can usually result from an external threat
④ Occurs only in people who have mental health problems

94. A 14-year-old Boy Scout dove into a shallow pond while on a camping expedition. Friends rescued him from drowning when they saw he was in difficulty. When the emergency team arrived, they placed him on a stretcher, being especially careful *not* to:
① Move his extremities unnecessarily
② Flex his head
③ Put pressure on his diaphragm
④ Strap him to the stretcher too tightly

95. In providing health education to a patient with sarcoidosis, the nurse should most appropriately include:
① Ways to determine if the pulmonary system is getting more involved
② Agencies and methods to use to quit smoking
③ Methods to self-test for mediastinal node involvement
④ Symptoms of fibrosis of the advanced stage of disease

96. The patient is to receive ASA 600 mg. The label reads gr V. How many tablets should be given?
① 1.5
② 2
③ 2.5
④ 3

97. In reviewing the plan of care for a 24-year-old schizophrenic with regressive behavior, the nurse notes the following outcome (goal): patient will complete all ADLs and be neatly groomed within 2 days. The nurse may conclude:
① The goal is appropriate
② The goal is too broad
③ The goal is unrealistic
④ It is a long-term goal

98. According to Maslow's hierarchy, which basic needs must be met first?
① Esteem
② Love and belonging
③ Physiological
④ Safety and security

99. A male patient, age 53, slipped on icy steps and fractured his left tibia and fibula. He is in a long leg cast. Injury to the peroneal nerve as a result of pressure from the cast may cause:
① Numbness of the dorsal surface of the foot
② Volkmann's contracture
③ Dupuytren's contracture
④ Compartment syndrome

100. When caring for a patient with a blood sugar of 310, which one of the following is of highest priority for nursing care?
① Ensuring adequate rest
② Protecting patient safety
③ Checking nutritional intake
④ Bed rest because of potential dizziness

101. A female patient, age 42, calls the office for an appointment. She has noticed a red "butterfly" pattern over her cheeks and part of her nose. She also complains of soreness in walking and moving and is running an intermittent slight fever. All these symptoms and signs have occurred in the last 6 to 8 weeks. The nurse knows that one possible system disorder that can cause the above is:
① Scleroderma
② Raynaud's disease
③ Periarteritis nodosa
④ Systemic lupus erythematosus

102. A patient has a radioactive device implanted to treat carcinoma of the bladder. Of the following approaches, which would best address the safety of the nurse in performing daily care?
① Perform nursing measures as quickly and completely as possible
② Enter the patient's room frequently to assess the implanted device
③ Perform skills slowly to facilitate discussion of the patient's disease
④ Spend as much time with the patient as possible to decrease feelings of loneliness in the patient

103. While bathing a patient, the nurse notices a reddened area on the right hip. The appropriate nursing action is to:
① Massage the area every 2 hours and keep him off his right side
② Clean with alcohol and apply a sterile dressing
③ Apply warm, moist compresses intermittently
④ Apply lotion and powder before turning him on the right side

104. A postpartum patient complains that her left leg aches. The nurse notes that it is warm to the touch. What should the nurse do while awaiting the arrival of the physician?
① Apply ice bags to the leg
② Apply heat to the leg
③ Exercise the leg vigorously
④ Elevate the leg on pillows

105. A 23-year-old woman has discovered that she is about 3 months pregnant. She asks the nurse if it is safe for her to drink socially, about 3 to 4 drinks per week. The nurse's best response is:
① "Only 1 drink per week is advisable."
② "What you drink does not affect the baby."
③ "If you drink 5 or less drinks per week, it should be safe."
④ "The best thing you can do for your baby is to avoid any alcoholic beverages during the pregnancy."

106. Freud's understanding of human behavior is based on:
① Nine stages of ego development
② Sexuality and aggression
③ Cultural and environmental factors
④ Interpersonal conflict

107. A 28-year-old male stockbroker claims that he is the richest man in Michigan and a genius. He may be exhibiting:
① Tactile hallucinations
② Flight of ideas
③ Delusions of grandeur
④ Neurosis

108. A 42-year-old man has ingested 18 Valium (diazepam) tablets and 18 unidentified capsules. He is in the ER and is now alert after gastric lavage. He is calling his son to come and take him home. He is exhibiting which of the following defenses:
① Sublimation
② Projection
③ Denial
④ Regression

109. An 18-year-old woman, states, "It's such a beautiful day; will my new dog learn to sit up; give me some fruit." She is exhibiting:
① Confusion
② Flight of ideas
③ Delusions
④ Hallucinations

110. A patient who has been receiving antipsychotic drugs reports that he has a dry mouth, tight throat, and mouth movements. The nurse should consider that:
① These may be somatic delusions
② The patient is probably manipulating for more medication
③ These are transitory reactions that will disappear
④ These may be extrapyramidal reactions that require intervention

111. A 31-year-old patient is having a difficult pregnancy and is 4 weeks from her due date. The office physician asks the nurse to instruct the patient on doing a "kick" count at home daily. The nurse needs to advise the patient to call immediately if her kick count is:
① Under 3
② Seven or more
③ In the 4 to 6 range
④ In the 6 to 7 range

112. How would the nurse explain natural childbirth education to parents?
① "It is a method free from the use of drugs during labor and delivery."
② "Basically, it is preparation for labor and delivery by teaching relaxation exercises and breathing exercises to be used during pregnancy, labor, delivery, and postpartum."
③ "It prepares young couples to be good parents by teaching about newborns, nutrition, exercises, labor and delivery, and child care."
④ "It is preparing to have your baby in as natural a setting as you can, free from noise, in a quiet environment with soft music."

113. A patient with Alzheimer's is unable to recognize a cup as a receptacle to hold fluids. The nurse knows this is:
① Agnosia
② Projection
③ Displacement
④ Confabulation

114. Normal nutritional requirements of a preschooler include food from the Food Guide Pyramid. As a result of severe burns, a 3-year-old patient would need a diet:
① High in proteins, carbohydrates, and calories
② High in proteins, iron, and calcium
③ Low in sodium and cholesterol
④ Low in calcium and high in carbohydrates

115. When changing the burn dressing, the nurse would help a young patient control his feelings of fear and pain by:
① Having another nurse restrain the patient until the treatment is over
② Explaining firmly what is to be done and how he can help
③ Allowing the patient to cry until he is tired and less combative
④ Repeating administration of the prescribed pain medication

116. An 18-month-old infant is to have a long-acting antibiotic given IM. The nurse selects the best muscle or site to use, which is:
① Deltoid
② Gluteus maximus
③ Vastus lateralis
④ Ventrogluteal area

117. A 7-year-old girl is admitted with a tentative diagnosis of encephalitis. She recently had chickenpox. The nurse needs to focus care on monitoring:
① For jaundice
② Blood sugar
③ Blood pressure
④ Neurological status

118. A 4-year-old boy is admitted to a pediatric unit for initial IV treatment of osteomyelitis. The nurse knows that the peak incidence in children occurs between the ages of 3 and 15. It affects boys twice as often as girls. The nurse also knows that the bones most commonly affected are:
① Tibia, fibula, femur
② Fibula, tibia, patella
③ Patella, radius, ulna
④ Femur, tibia, humerus

119. A patient has sustained burns on the front and back of both her legs and her right arm. What percent of her body would the nurse estimate has been involved?
① 45%
② 54%
③ 72%
④ 18%

120. A neighbor runs into the nurse's yard screaming hysterically and the nurse sees that her bathrobe is on fire. The *immediate* nursing action is to:
① Instruct the neighbor to remove her bathrobe
② Call the fire department
③ Roll her in a blanket
④ Tell her to lie down

121. The nurse should know that the purpose of Good Samaritan laws is to:
① Mandate nurses and physicians to stop and render care at accident sites
② Encourage emergency aid at accident sites
③ Prevent any liability arising from care rendered at accident sites
④ Have universal laws mandating emergency aid at accident sites

122. Within the first few hours after treating a severe burn patient, the nurse should observe for which of the following?
① Laryngeal and tracheal edema
② Eschar formation
③ Absence of pain
④ Leathery appearance to skin

123. A small southern town has been devastated by a hurricane that has blown out to sea. The nurse is part of a volunteer rescue team searching for local missing persons. The team splits up; the nurse is alone and finds a man lying on his back moaning. Rapid assessment reveals a questionable back injury. Which of the following nursing actions should have the highest priority?
① Keeping the victim in supine position
② Positioning the victim in a side-lying position
③ Permitting the victim to assume the most comfortable position
④ Sitting the victim up to properly assess his pulmonary status

124. A patient complains of tenderness at her IV puncture site. On assessment the nurse notes redness and swelling. The nurse should first:
① Stop the flow of the IV fluids, and report this to the head nurse
② Notify the physician, and fill out an incident report
③ Elevate the arm, and apply warm compresses to the puncture site
④ Change the dressing over the puncture site using sterile technique

125. A patient with cystic fibrosis is intubated, on a ventilator, and must be suctioned every 2 to 3 hours for secretion control. Which of the following would be the most important goal for this patient at this time?
① Patient will be free of infection
② Patient will not experience arrhythmias
③ Patient will maintain a patient airway
④ Patient will have an equal intake and output

ANSWERS AND RATIONALES FOR COMPREHENSIVE EXAMINATIONS

COMPREHENSIVE EXAMINATION 1: PART 1

1. Knowledge, planning, safety and infection control (a)
   - ❸ Although the State Board of Nursing has many duties, its primary role is to protect the public health, safety, and welfare.
   - ① This is the role of the elected state officials; this is also assisted by professional nursing associations.
   - ② The protection of the nursing profession is the duty of nurses and nursing associations in conjunction with state government agencies making public laws and policies.
   - ④ Although this is a duty of the State Board of Nursing, it is not the Board's primary role. See rationale for #3.

2. Knowledge, implementation, reduction of risk potential (a)
   - ❸ The specimen is discarded to ensure that all of the urine in the container was collected during a 24-hour period. The voiding at 8:00 AM contained urine that was collected since the last voiding and would make the collection period longer than 24 hours.
   - ① The nurse would not send the specimen for urinalysis unless there was a physician's order to do so.
   - ② Adding the urine to the collection container would include urine outside of the 24-hour collection period.
   - ④ Although creatinine clearance reflects kidney function and the fact that renal impairment is a complication of diabetes mellitus, the information given does not indicate that the patient is a diabetic. Additionally, there is no mention of an order to test the urine for glucose and ketones.

3. Knowledge, assessment, prevention and early detection of disease (a)
   - ❸ The palpatory systolic pressure provides an estimate of the systolic blood pressure. This ensures inflating the cuff to an adequate level without applying undue pressure to the patient's arm.
   - ① If the nurse inflates the cuff to a set pressure for every patient, there is a risk of overinflating or underinflating the cuff. Overinflating causes undue pressure and congestion of the arm, while underinflation causes the nurse to miss the beats of a systolic pressure.
   - ② Inflating the cuff 10 mm Hg above the last diastolic would result in underinflation of the cuff.
   - ④ The nurse does not listen to Korotkoff's sounds while inflating the cuff.

4. Application, implementation, basic care and comfort (a)
   - ❸ Instructing the patient to swallow twice for each bite of food helps to ensure that food was swallowed and reduces the risk of choking.
   - ① Thickened liquids are generally tolerated better than thin liquids by individuals with dysphagia.
   - ② Combining more than one texture in a bite predisposes the patient to choking.

   - ④ Offering finger foods does not address swallowing problems associated with dysphagia; this type of food is more likely to cause choking than softer foods fed from the tip of a spoon.

5. Application, assessment, coping and adaptation (b)
   - ❹ The nurse needs to respond to the patient's feelings and thoughts as well as giving hope. The prognosis for bladder cancer can be good depending on the stage of the tumor.
   - ① This is false reassurance, and the nurse does not know what the outcome may be.
   - ② This is a put-down and belittles the patient; it also makes light of the patient's fears.
   - ③ Changing the subject by referring to his family is not appropriate at this point; the patient's feelings and thoughts need to be addressed first.

6. Knowledge, planning, prevention and early detection of disease (b)
   - ❹ Oxygen therapy for the newborn must be administered with great caution to prevent retrolental fibroplasia. This condition is caused by high levels of oxygen concentration and may result in blindness.
   - ① Ophthalmia neonatorum is a purulent conjunctivitis and keratitis of the newborn resulting from exposure of the eyes to chemical, chlamydial, bacterial, or viral agents.
   - ② ABO incompatibility is a hereditary condition that causes blood destruction in the fetus or the newborn; it is classified as a hemolytic disease of the newborn.
   - ③ Respiratory distress syndrome is an acute lung disease of the newborn caused by a deficiency of pulmonary surfactant.

7. Comprehension, implementation, safety and infection control (b)
   - ❹ Such a high pulse rate may indicate that too much thyroid hormone is in the system.
   - ① This is not a standard aspect of teaching for thyroid medication.
   - ②, ③ These are not part of the teaching protocol for this type of medication.

8. Knowledge, assessment, physiological adaptation (b)
   - ❹ These are classic symptoms of hypothyroidism.
   - ① These are symptom's of Cushing's disease.
   - ② These are seen in diabetes mellitus.
   - ③ Frequency is not a classic symptom.

9. Knowledge, assessment, physiological adaptation (b)
   - ❷ The elderly have a decreased need for calories.
   - ①, ③ Caloric needs decrease, not increase, as an individual advances in age.
   - ④ Nutritional needs are the same as those for other adults.

10. Knowledge, implementation, safety and infection control (a)
    - ❸ In a hospital setting, insertion of a Foley catheter must always be done using sterile technique.
    - ① Reverse isolation is not appropriate in this situation.
    - ② Medical aseptic technique can be used by patients in their home setting.
    - ④ Good handwashing is always a priority, but insertion of a Foley catheter must be done with sterile technique.

11. Comprehension, assessment, prevention and early detection of disease (a)
    ❷ Two nurses count simultaneously to compare the number of beats produced by the heart and the number of beats that are perfused to peripheral circulation; using the same watch ensures accuracy.
    ① By not counting the beats simultaneously, the nurse is unable to compare the number of beats produced with the number of beats perfused.
    ③ Two nurses count simultaneously to compare the number of beats produced and the number of beats perfused; using different watches may affect accuracy.
    ④ One nurse cannot accurately count the apical and radial beats simultaneously if there is a pulse deficit.

12. Application, implementation, pharmacological therapies (b)
    ❸ Use of diuretics is necessary because of the patient's edema.
    ① Semi-Fowler's is the most comfortable position to facilitate respiration.
    ② The normal diet for a child with nephrotic syndrome is a high-protein diet.
    ④ Sodium and potassium supplements are not usually given; sodium is limited.

13. Knowledge, evaluation, prevention and early detection of disease (a)
    ❸ Dry cough is an early sign of oxygen toxicity.
    ① Fever might indicate presence of infection associated with the effects of oxygen toxicity on the mucosal lining, but is not an early sign of the condition.
    ② Excessive mucus production may result from the on-going effects of oxygen toxicity, but it is a later sign of the condition.
    ④ Moist breath sounds may result from the ongoing effects of oxygen toxicity, but this is a later sign of the condition.

14. Application, implementation, reduction of risk potential (b)
    ❸ Failure of venous return of blood from the legs and pelvis may be caused by compression of the inferior vena cava by the uterus while the patient is in a supine position during labor. Turning the patient on her left side relieves the pressure on the inferior vena cava and is the best and simplest nursing measure for comfort and relief.
    ①, ②, ④ These are inappropriate nursing actions that are unnecessary and would not correct the situation.

15. Knowledge, evaluation, pharmacological therapies (c)
    ❸ These symptoms, along with malaise and fever, are the symptoms of toxicity that a patient on AZT (zidovudine) may experience.
    ① These are toxic effects of ddC (dideoxycytidine).
    ② Painful peripheral nerves are caused by the drug ddI (dideoxyinosine).
    ④ These symptoms are caused by d4T (dideoxythymidine).

16. Comprehension, implementation, safety and infection control (a)
    ❹ Wound irrigation presents the danger of splashing or spraying. Goggles, gown, and mask should be worn.

① The bed should be at a workable height for all nursing procedures; bed height does not offer protection from fluid splash or spray.
② Explaining the procedure encourages patient cooperation; it does not protect the nurse from fluid splash or spray.
③ While handwashing is indicated before and after all patient contact, it does not offer protection from fluid splash or spray.

17. Knowledge, planning, reduction of risk potential (b)
    ❷ Presbycusis is progressive hearing loss and is associated with aging.
    ① Tinnitus is a ringing in the ear that has various causes.
    ③ Otosclerosis is an inherited bone disorder impairing conduction by causing structural irregularities in the stapes.
    ④ Ménière's disease is the term for the episodic symptoms created by fluctuations in the production or reabsorption of fluid within the inner ear lobe.

18. Application, implementation, safety and infection control (a)
    ❷ Standard precautions advise that gloves are to be worn whenever the nurse comes into contact with blood or any body fluid.
    ① It is not necessary to wear sterile gloves; they cannot be kept sterile anyway. A gown is not necessary unless the patient is also in wound/drainage isolation.
    ③ A mask is not necessary unless the AIDS patient has active tuberculosis or an MRSA infection.
    ④ Gloves are not necessary unless the nurse will come into actual contact with any body secretion.

19. Comprehension, planning, prevention and early detection of disease (c)
    ❶ High-risk nursing care plans address the needs of patients more vulnerable to developing a health problem.
    ② High-risk nursing problems are NANDA-approved nursing diagnoses.
    ③ There is no indication of how this statement was formulated. Subjective data include information supplied by the patient, which cannot be easily measured.
    ④ Actual problems represent conditions that presently exist. This statement describes a condition that might occur.

20. Comprehension, planning, coordinated care (b)
    ❶ The pulse deficit examination requires one nurse to take the radial pulse while the second nurse takes the apical pulse at the same time.
    ② Pulse deficit does not determine systolic murmur.
    ③ The assistance of a second nurse is more necessary than patient cooperation.
    ④ The electrocardiograph is a diagnostic tool that measures electrical currents in the heart; it is not needed to measure pulse deficit.

21. Comprehension, planning, coordinated care (a)
    ❷ Knowledge of the procedure diminishes patient fear, which improves patient cooperation and promotes the expected outcome of the procedure.
    ① Competent nursing practice reduces the likelihood of malpractice suits.
    ③ Procedures are not explained to avoid them, although this may be a secondary aspect of patient teaching.
    ④ The nurse must review the procedure before explaining it to the patient to provide complete information.

22. Knowledge, implementation, coordinated care (a)
   ❸ This procedure increases the likelihood of detecting occult blood in the stool.
   ① Diarrhea stools are acceptable sources provided they are not contaminated with urine.
   ② Stools for ova and parasites must be kept warm and delivered to the laboratory immediately.
   ④ Occult blood is hidden or unseen blood.

23. Knowledge, planning, coordinated care (a)
   ❹ The second voiding is the best measure of how much glucose the kidneys are clearing at that time.
   ① A midstream voiding reduces the number of tissue and skin bacterial contaminants in the urine specimen.
   ② A clean-catch specimen reduces the number of tissue and skin bacteria contaminants in the urine specimen.
   ③ Urine sugar and acetone is not a 24-hour specimen.

24. Application, planning, coordinated care (b)
   ❹ The need for nutrition and hydration falls under the physiological needs, which are the most basic of needs and therefore receive the highest priority when planning care.
   ① Altered family processes falls under love and belonging needs, which are two levels up from the basic needs according to Maslow's hierarchy of needs.
   ② Although the need for oxygenation is also a basic physiological need, an actual problem is given a higher priority than a potential problem.
   ③ Skin integrity is part of the safety and protection needs, which is one level above the basic physiologic needs. In addition, an actual problem is given a higher priority than a potential problem.

25. Comprehension, assessment, coping and adaptation (b)
   ❸ The child is most likely demonstrating regressive behavior, following the birth of his sister, due to feeling that she is receiving some of the attention to which he is accustomed to receiving. This new sibling poses a threat to his security.
   ① Repression involves excluding unacceptable thoughts and feelings from the unconscious mind.
   ② Displacement means that the person directs pent-up frustrations toward another object or person.
   ④ Compensation is a defense mechanism whereby the person makes up for an area that is lacking by taking advantage of a strength.

26. Application, implementation, coordinated care (b)
   ❷ Meperedine: DD = 20 mg
   $$DH = 50\ mg$$
   $$V = 1\ ml$$
   $$\frac{DD}{DH} = \frac{20\ mg}{50\ mg} \times 1\ ml = 0.4\ ml$$
   Atropine: DD = 0.08 mg
   $$DH = 0.2\ mg$$
   $$V = 1\ ml$$
   $$\frac{DD}{DH} = \frac{0.08\ mg}{0.2\ mg} \times 1\ ml = 0.4\ ml$$
   $$0.4\ ml + 0.4\ ml = 0.8\ ml$$
   ①, ③, ④ This is not the correct amount.

27. Application, implementation, coping and adaptation (b)
   ❷ This is the most honest, helpful answer the nurse can give.
   ① This is a lie.
   ③ At 3 years of age, she is not a "big girl"; she is a child and should be allowed to act like one.
   ④ She should be allowed to cry if the procedure hurts. Telling her not to cry only gives her something else to worry about.

28. Application, implementation, safety and infection control (b)
   ❹ Massaging after administering the heparin can cause bleeding in the tissue.
   ① Heparin is usually given subcutaneously.
   ② Aspirating can cause bleeding in the tissue.
   ③ All injection sites should be rotated.

29. Knowledge, assessment, pharmacological therapies (c)
   ❷ The therapeutic range for theophylline is 10 to 20 mg/dl.
   ① This is subtherapeutic.
   ③ This level is above the therapeutic range.
   ④ This level is toxic.

30. Application, planning, safety and infection control (b)
   ❷ Cleansing removes resident bacteria and decreases the risk of infection.
   ① Checking the incision daily is often enough.
   ③ Heavy lifting should be avoided. Normal activities should be resumed over a 2- to 3-week period.
   ④ Once the Steri-Strips fall off, there is no need to replace them.

31. Comprehension, implementation, physiological adaptation (b)
   ❷ Proper nutrition during pregnancy is critical. The exact number of pounds gained may depend on many other variables.
   ① This is the approximate average weight gain resulting from pregnancy; individuals vary significantly.
   ③ If there is no control of intake, many individuals will gain excessively.
   ④ Even nonpregnant individuals may find it difficult to lose excessive weight gained.

32. Application, implementation, pharmacological therapies (b)
   ❶ 1,000 units per hour is correct. 25,000 units ÷ 1,000 cc = 25 units per cc; 25 units per cc × 40 cc per hour = 1,000 units per hour.
   ② 10,000 units per hour is 10 times greater than the prescribed dosage.
   ③ 100 units per hour is 10 times less than the prescribed dosage.
   ④ The concentration is not 1 unit per 1 cc.

33. Knowledge, planning, physiological adaptation (a)
   ❷ This test measures the extrinsic pathway of the clotting process and is used to regulate warfarin sodium (Coumadin) therapy.
   ① There is no such test.
   ③ This test helps regulate heparin sodium therapy.
   ④ This test is used for assisting in the diagnosis of bleeding disorders, not in regulating therapy of anticoagulants.

34. Comprehension, planning, pharmacological therapies (c)
   ❸ Osmotic diuretics such as mannitol are effective because they increase the plasma osmolality, which increases the intravascular volume.
   ① Potassium-sparing diuretics affect the distal tubule of the nephron and therefore will not be of benefit.
   ② Loop diuretics affect the loop of Henle and therefore will not be of benefit.
   ④ There is no classification of diuretics called sodium sparing.

35. Knowledge, assessment, physiological adaptation (a)
   ❶ Touching the patient and calling his name establishes level of responsiveness, which should be done prior to beginning any resuscitative measures or examining the client for injuries.
   ② Repositioning the patient and opening the airway are done after checking for responsiveness.
   ③ The patient should be assessed for injuries after assessing for unresponsiveness and any necessary resuscitative measures. The patient should not be moved until after he is assessed for injuries.
   ④ Chest compressions are indicated only after determining unresponsiveness, opening the airway, administering rescue breaths, and determining that the patient has no carotid pulse.

36. Comprehension, planning, pharmacological therapies (b)
   ❹ Theophylline anhydrase (Theo-Dur) should not be given via a nasogastric tube because it is an extended-release medication.
   ① Other than checking the apical heart rate prior to administering, this route is acceptable.
   ② Other than giving with 3-4 ounces of juice, this route is acceptable.
   ③ Although Tylenol elixir would be easier than tablets, this route is acceptable.

37. Application, implementation, coordinated care (c)
   ❷ Fowler's position facilitates breathing and decreases swelling of the operative site; sandbags relieve tension on suture lines; frequent monitoring of vital signs allows for early intervention should complications arise.
   ① A complication of a thyroidectomy is a thyroid crisis, which causes a sudden increase in thyroxine. Signs of thyroid crisis are body temperatures as high as 106° or higher, an increased heart rate of 200 beats per minute or greater, increased respiratory rate, apprehension, and restlessness. If the crisis is not arrested, death may occur.
   ③ Redness, some swelling, and discomfort at the operative site are expected.
   ④ Tetany secondary to hypocalcemia is a possible complication of the surgery secondary to accidental removal of the parathyroid glands.

38. Comprehension, assessment, physiological adaptation (c)
   ❶ General hypoxia of the tissues causes fatigue and dyspnea especially on exertion, which results in increased oxygen demands.
   ② The compensatory mechanism of the heart to meet oxygen demands is to increase heart rate.
   ③ The blood pressure is usually increased because of the decreased lumen size of coronary arteries, secondary to the disease process.

   ④ Coronary artery disease causes general hypoxia, not limited to a single system.

39. Comprehension, assessment, safety and infection control (a)
   ❶ Many patients experience an aura or unusual sensory perception before having a seizure.
   ② Hallucinations are auditory or visual and are mental stimuli not based in reality.
   ③ Petit mal seizures are usually confined to children without an associated aura. Petit mal is classified as a brief loss of consciousness.
   ④ This has nothing to do with seizure activity.

40. Knowledge, evaluation, reduction of risk potential (b)
   ❸ The data support absence of infection with normal physiological responses expected after surgery.
   ① The data suggest the patient has developed an infection.
   ② The data suggest the patient has developed an infection, especially with a white blood cell count of 13,000.
   ④ A reddened incision site with purulent drainage indicates the presence of an infection.

41. Comprehension, assessment, basic care and comfort (b)
   ❹ Compression of the mesenteric blood supply can cause constipation.
   ① Pneumonia usually presents with fever and coughing.
   ② Body casts may cause a claustrophobic reaction, but this patient's symptoms are more consistent with constipation.
   ③ Anxiety reactions usually produce sweating, tachycardia, and a general feeling of unease.

42. Application, assessment, coping and adaptation (b)
   ❷ The nurse should assess the patient's complaint before suggesting other actions.
   ① The nurse should suggest non-drug approaches to help the patient sleep, rather than initially suggesting medications, and only after assessing the problem.
   ③ This action suggests that the nurse is not interested in her problem.
   ④ Although relaxation techniques may help, the nurse should assess the problem before describing possible interventions.

43. Application, planning, coordinated care (b)
   ❸ The psychomotor domain of learning involves physically performing a task or skill.
   ① Stating or explaining information that has been provided indicates learning at the cognitive domain.
   ② Stating the importance of doing something is cognitive learning. Applying that knowledge in life situations indicates learning in the affective domain.
   ④ Identification indicates learning at the cognitive domain.

44. Comprehension, planning, physiological integrity (c)
  ❹ Because the glucose concentration of central hyperalimentation is greater than 10%, it should be administered via a central venous access catheter to prevent vein irritation and possible extravasation into the surrounding tissue.
  ① Because the glucose concentration of central hyperalimentation is greater than 10%, it should be administered via a central venous access catheter to prevent vein irritation and possible extravasation into the surrounding tissue.
  ② These solutions can infuse at rates of 75-100 cc/hour.
  ③ These solutions can cause hyperglycemia at least initially. Rebound hypoglycemia can occur if the infusion is abruptly discontinued.

45. Knowledge, implementation, basic care and comfort (b)
  ❸ This is the least threatening thing the nurse can say to a 4 year old.
  ① A 4 year old does not have the vocabulary to understand the term *injection*.
  ② There is no such thing as a "little shot" to a 4 year old.
  ④ This is not quite truthful; most antibiotics sting considerably.

46. Comprehension, planning, reduction of risk potential (b)
  ❸ Early ambulation helps promote the return of intestinal peristalsis, thereby decreasing the likelihood of ileus.
  ① Until bowel sounds are present, the patient should not receive solid food.
  ② Splinting of the abdomen will do nothing to promote normal bowel function.
  ④ Kegel exercises promote urinary control and do not affect the intestines.

47. Application, planning, coordinated care (a)
  ❶ In primary hypofunction (not the result of a pituitary disturbance), the therapy is lifelong.
  ②, ③, ④ Hormonal therapy is not classically adjusted on a day-to-day basis, nor is hormonal therapy, in this case, temporary or intermittent.

48. Knowledge, assessment, reduction of risk potential (a)
  ❷ The main function of aerosolized bronchodilators and chest physiotherapy is to dilate the bronchioles and loosen and move secretions out of the lungs.
  ① Nothing has been shown to be effective in decreasing mucus production.
  ③ Efficiency of the diaphragm is not a problem in cystic fibrosis.
  ④ Although chest physiotherapy may stimulate coughing to some degree, it is not done to increase oxygen consumption.

49. Comprehension, assessment, coordinated care (b)
  ❹ Chest pain that radiates is a significant finding.
  ①, ③ These are not associated with chest pain.
  ② Increase in respiration caused by anxiety is common.

50. Knowledge, assessment, coordinated care (a)
  ❷ This is a classic sign seen in children diagnosed with Down's syndrome.
  ① These children are hypotonic.
  ③ These children have hyperflexibility of the joints.
  ④ This is a symptom seen in bacterial endocarditis.

51. Knowledge, assessment, coordinated care (a)
  ❸ The nurse, as part of the preoperative routine, ascertains that the signed consent form is on the chart.
  ① The physician and anesthesiologist should obtain the patient's signature after explaining the procedure to the client.
  ② The nurse sometimes witnesses the consent form, but it is not a responsibility of the nurse.
  ④ The surgeon and anesthesiologist are responsible for ascertaining that the patient understands what he is signing.

52. Application, implementation, coping and adaptation (b)
  ❶ This shows that the nurse accepts the cultural difference, but also recognizes that the herbal preparation may interact with other parts of the treatment plan, especially medications.
  ② This response disregards the patient's cultural practices and imposes the opinions of Western medicine.
  ③ This shows cultural acceptance but does not consider the potential interactions with other areas of the treatment plan.
  ④ This response disregards the patient's cultural practices and also gives the patient advice based on the nurse's opinion rather than allowing the patient to make informed choices.

53. Knowledge, assessment, coping and adaptation (b)
  ❷ The patient is relieving himself of his responsibility to quit smoking by placing the blame on those who should have warned him about the consequences.
  ① Compensation is striving for excellence in one area to make up for a weakness in another area.
  ③ Sublimation involves replacing an unacceptable or unrealistic action with an acceptable alternative.
  ④ Repression means that the person forgets about the situation that is causing stress.

54. Application, planning, physiological adaptation (b)
  ❸ This goal is realistic, contains an observable behavior, includes a target date, and addresses the manifestation of the nursing diagnosis.
  ① This goal addresses the etiology rather than the manifestation of the nursing diagnosis.
  ② This statement is a dependent nursing intervention rather than a goal statement.
  ④ Although this statement describes a desired outcome for a patient with dyspnea, it does not address the manifestation of the nursing diagnosis.

55. Application, assessment, pharmacological therapies (a)
  ❷ The nurse should check to be sure that the medication has not been given in the last 4 hours.
  ① Narcotic orders may, by institutional policy, have automatic stop dates; the discontinuation date should be determined and noted when the order is transcribed.
  ③ Since, by law, schedule II drugs must be accounted for, the amount left on hand should be checked. This is done with change-of-shift narcotic counts, and when the medication is signed out after preparing and administering the dose.
  ④ The effect of the last dose should be checked when the dose peaks, rather than just before the next dose.

56. Comprehension, evaluation, pharmacological therapies (b)
❸ Anticholinergic agents reduce secretions, resulting in dry mouth.
① Anticholinergic agents tend to increase heart rate.
② Anticholinergic agents reduce gastrointestinal motility, resulting in constipation.
④ Anticholinergic agents cause pupil dilation

57. Comprehension, implementation, pharmacological therapies (b)
❹ It may take 3 to 4 weeks of routinely taking an antiinflammatory medication before the patient experiences pain relief.
① Although opiates provide a greater degree of analgesia, antiinflammatory medications are more appropriate for the treatment of inflammatory conditions such as arthritis.
② Motrin (ibuprofen) has both analgesic and antiinflammatory properties, as well as antipyretic effects.
③ The patient needs to continue taking the medication routinely in order to achieve a sufficient serum drug level to produce a therapeutic response (pain relief).

58. Application, implementation, coping and adaptation (b)
❸ This response demonstrates interest and concern on the part of the nurse; it provides a broad opening that allows the patient to choose whether he wants to discuss his fears with the nurse and how much information he wants to disclose.
① A "why" question demands that the patient defend his statement
② This leads the patient to believe that these consequences can be avoided by following a rigid regimen.
④ This statement is not necessarily true, in addition to belittling the patient's fears.

59. Comprehension, assessment, basic care and comfort (b)
❶ Symptoms of active TB include a cough lasting longer than 2 weeks, fever, night sweats, malaise, irritability, weakness, fatigue, and dyspnea.
② These symptoms may be present in asthma or chronic bronchitis.
③ Feeling cold, tired, and having stomach upset may reflect a gastrointestinal problem, anemia, or anxiety.
④ Bloody stools may reflect a gastrointestinal problem.

60. Comprehension, planning, physiological adaptation (b)
❸ The eschar can constrict tissues causing ischemia and possibly necrosis.
① Caloric needs are based on the hypermetabolic state required for healing and a positive nitrogen balance.
② Infection is always a possibility when the first line of defense, the skin, is damaged.
④ An escharotomy may allow for drainage.

61. Application, implementation, basic care and comfort (b)
❶ Sterile technique is necessary due to the loss of the body's first line of defense, intact skin.
② The room temperature should be closer to 80° to 85°.
③ A diet high in protein and carbohydrates is appropriate for any burned patient.
④ When positioning extremities the nurse must consider the possibility of flexion contracture.

62. Comprehension, implementation, reduction of risk potential (b)
❸ Fatigue is a stress on the body. Anything that increases stress may decrease the seizure threshold and potentially increase seizure activity.
① Hypoglycemia lowers the seizure threshold.
② Sleep is not considered to be a stress on the body; insomnia is.
④ Antiseizure medications increase the seizure threshold.

63. Comprehension, assessment, reduction of risk potential (b)
❷ In acute renal failure, potassium, BUN, and creatinine increase due to the kidneys' inability to filtrate resulting in an accumulation of nitrogenous wastes in the blood.
①, ③, ④ See rationale for #2. The BUN increases, the creatinine increases, potassium is increased, and calcium is decreased.

64. Application, assessment, reduction of risk potential (b)
❹ These are NSAIDS, which may be nephrotoxic.
① This is an tricyclic antidepressant that may be prescribed for urinary incontinence.
② This drug is a urinary antiseptic that may change the urine's color.
③ Calcium channel blockers may affect the ability of the bladder or sphincter to contract or relax normally.

65. Comprehension, assessment, reduction of risk potential (b)
❶ Fetal distress is present and is a sign of cord prolapse following rupture of the membranes.
② The opposite is true, as the fetal heart rate decreases.
③ Amniotic fluid may continue to leak and is not an indication of cord prolapse.
④ There is not a certain length of cord protrusion to make this answer correct; the cord may be hidden inside with the presenting part against it.

66. Comprehension, implementation, coping and adaptation (a)
❷ She is in a private room, and the couple's needs are being met.
① This deprives the patient of the emotional support of her husband.
③ This is an insensitive response and does not help the patient to cope.
④ The patient may have a short or longer stay and does not need to be lonely.

67. Knowledge, implementation, coping and adaptation (a)
❹ This explanation correctly defines the term.
①, ② There is a risk for these, but they are not the definition.
③ This is an incorrect response that is opposite of what actually is present.

68. Comprehension, planning, reduction of risk potential (c)
❶ The diet is high in carbohydrates, usually 2500 to 3000 calories per day, to prevent the breakdown of fats that would produce ketosis. It is low in protein to reduce the BUN. Potassium is restricted because patients in renal failure retain potassium and are at risk for hyperkalemia.
②, ③, ④ These diets are inappropriate for this patient and would further compromise the patient's condition. See rationale for #1.

69. Knowledge, planning, pharmacological therapies (c)
    ❷ 1.5 to 2 times the amount of the control is considered thin enough to prevent further clot formation with minimal risk for undue bleeding.
    ① This would present a risk for clot formation
    ③, ④ These would present a high risk of hemorrhage

70. Application, implementation, coping and adaptation (c)
    ❸ This would calm her down so that she could face her problems more easily in order for her to ventilate her concerns to someone. The medication would have time to take effect before the interpreter arrived.
    ① It is important that the patient be allowed to grieve. She needs to be able to ventilate her concerns. Someone who speaks her language would be able to communicate with her and help her to view her situation realistically, although the medication should be given first.
    ② The patient is extremely emotionally upset. The TV would not provide her the opportunity to talk to someone about her problem.
    ④ She would not understand what the nurse was asking her.

71. Application, implementation, physiological adaptation (c)
    ❹ Stimulation of a different site may override the phantom sensation.
    ① Narcotics are not effective for phantom limb pain.
    ② Massage therapy might be ordered after 2 weeks.
    ③ Cold would increase phantom limb pain.

72. Application, implementation, physiological adaptation (a)
    ❹ The patient may feel he is abnormal and be hesitant to complain.
    ① This would cut off circulation.
    ② This would not help the pain.
    ③ This is not an immediate priority.

73. Application, implementation, reduction of risk potential (b)
    ❶ Daily care is important to prevent injury to the remaining foot secondary to the diabetes. Care includes:
    • Daily foot bath
    • Thorough drying
    • Daily inspection for signs of infection, calluses, infection, etc.
    • Professional nail cutting
    • Clean socks at all times
    • Sturdy shoes
    ② Nails should only be cut by a podiatrist.
    ③ Shoes should be sturdy and supportive to prevent injury.
    ④ Foot bathing is important but daily soaking could increase the chance of injury.

74. Application, implementation, physiological adaptation (a)
    ❶ The patient is experiencing orthostatic hypotension, which results in her blood pressure dropping upon standing. Having her sit up prior to standing will allow her circulation to stabilize to her brain.
    ② This will have no effect on her orthostatic hypotension.
    ③ This is not necessary at this point. Her blood pressure needs to be evaluated lying, sitting, and standing before calling. She may need a lower dose.

④ This would not help her orthostatic hypertension but may increase her hypertension, which could prove harmful.

75. Comprehension, planning, reduction of risk potential (b)
    ❶ Family members expect, and it is their right, to be kept informed of their loved one's care.
    ② The nurse should record anything she does; asking without documentation means nothing. Simply asking them to keep a close eye on him is a weak attempt at controlling the situation.
    ③ He is in the home because the family couldn't manage him. It is the responsibility of the facility to care for him.
    ④ Generally, another resident would not want a person with Alzheimer's in their room. It is not the responsibility of the other residents to take care of him.

76. Application, evaluation, reduction of risk potential (b)
    ❶ This helps the nurse to evaluate the effectiveness of the deep breathing and coughing exercises.
    ② Nurses usually have a pulse oximeter on the unit for spot checks of a client's blood O_2 levels.
    ③ This is not necessary.
    ④ He should be positioned in the highest position possible so as to not interfere with gas exchange.

77. Comprehension, assessment, reduction of risk potential (b)
    ❷ The skin will be prepared with betadine. If the client is allergic, only alcohol would be used.
    ① The gauge is generally 18 or 20 in order for the blood to flow freely.
    ③ The vital signs would be taken prior to beginning the blood infusion but not prior to the start of an IV.
    ④ Massage is not necessary.

78. Knowledge, assessment, reduction of risk potential (a)
    ❶ Peritonitis is the most serious complication of a ruptured appendix.
    ② Although some hemorrhage may occur, the development of peritonitis is more problematic.
    ③ Although a paralytic ileus or intestinal obstruction may occur, peritonitis is more problematic.
    ④ Ulceration of the duodenum is not a complication from a ruptured appendix.

79. Application, planning, coordinated care (b)
    ❶ The Venturi mask is correct. It can provide precise concentrations of oxygen through a noninvasive route and avoids risk of suppressing the patient's hypoxic drive to breathe.
    ②, ③, ④ This mask is not able to provide precise oxygen concentrations, which could suppress the patient's hypoxic drive to breathe.

80. Knowledge, planning, physiological adaptation (b)
    ❸ Older women need an increased intake to compensate for decreased absorption, thereby decreasing the symptoms of osteoporosis.
    ① Individuals up to the age of 24 should receive 1200 mg per day as bone mass is forming.
    ② Adults should receive 1000 mg per day to maintain bone mass and to prepare for postmenopausal losses.
    ④ This level is not recommended for any age group by the National Osteoporosis Association.

81. Comprehension, planning, coordinated care (c)
  ❷ The weaning procedure is not part of the patient/family education process. If the patient could be weaned from the ventilator it would have occurred prior to discharge to the home environment.
  ① Patient care is always applicable to discharge or ongoing education efforts.
  ③, ④ Since the ventilator is going home with the patient, someone in the home needs to know the basic procedures involved in care of the ventilator.

82. Comprehension, planning, reduction of risk potential (c)
  ❶ Rebound hypoglycemia may occur due to a sudden withdrawal of glucose in the presence of large levels of endogenous insulin that develop because of the high glucose concentration in the central hyperalimentation.
  ② This syndrome may occur during hemodialysis.
  ③ Blood infections may result from a contaminated container of central hyperalimentation but not from its discontinuance.
  ④ Hyperglycemia may occur at the onset or during treatment with central hyperalimentation, but not as a result of its discontinuance.

83. Analysis, evaluation, physiological adaptation (b)
  ❸ The amount of induration (hardness and or elevation) in mm at the greatest diameter is the proper method. 0-4 mm is nonsignificant; 5-10 mm may be significant; greater than 10 mm is considered significant.
  ① The amount of erythema (redness) is not helpful in interpretation.
  ② Only the amount of induration is used for interpretation.
  ④ The Mantoux test is intradermal. Lipohypertrophy occurs in the subcutaneous layer of the skin and is usually related to multiple subcutaneous injections.

84. Application, assessment, physiological adaptation (b)
  ❸ This is also known as a festinating gait. The alteration in equilibrium causes the client to assume this type of gait in an attempt to maintain an upright position while walking.
  ① This may be seen in patients who have had a CVA, have a space-occupying lesion, or a balance problem. It is a wide-based gait with lateral veering; may be called an ataxic or cerebellar gait.
  ② This is a scissor gait, with a criss-cross motion in walking; may be present in bilateral hemiglegia.
  ④ This is a severe gait ataxia seen in tabetic neurosyphilis. Patients walk with feet wide apart and depend on visual clues to maintain balance.

85. Comprehension, planning, physiological adaptation (b)
  ❹ Subdural hematomas usually are caused by venous bleeding; 50% are associated with skull fractures.
  ① With intracerebral hematomas, blood occurs in the parenchymal tissue; may be caused by head trauma or secondary to hypertensive bleeding.
  ② Epidural hematomas generally result from arterial bleeding.
  ③ Subarachnoid hematomas usually result secondary to rupture of intracranial aneurysms, AV malformation, or hypertensive bleed.

86. Comprehension, planning, reduction of risk potential (b)
  ❷ Tyramine stimulates the production of norepinephrine (a monamine), which elevates blood pressure. Since this drug inhibits the action of monamine oxidase, and therefore blocks the destruction of norepinephrine, the patient's blood pressure could rise to critical levels.
  ① Potassium levels do not affect the action or effects of monoamine oxidase inhibitors.
  ③ Monoamine oxidase inhibitors do not increase the patient's risk of sunburn.
  ④ It takes at least 1 to 4 weeks for the therapeutic effects of a monoamine oxidase inhibitor to be evident.

87. Comprehension, planning, pharmacological therapies (a)
  ❸ Meperidine hydrochloride and other narcotic analgesics tend to depress the respiratory center located in the medulla oblongata.
  ① Narcotic analgesics commonly lead to slowing of peristalsis, predisposing the client to constipation rather than diarrhea.
  ② Narcotic analgesics usually lower blood pressure.
  ④ Narcotic analgesics have no effect on blood sugar.

88. Application, assessment, reduction of risk potential (b)
  ❷ Patients with right-sided CVAs tend to demonstrate a lack of judgment and more impulsive behavior. They tend to make inaccurate assessments of their abilities and are prone to falls.
  ① Intellectual impairment is not consistently prevalent in patients with a right-sided CVA.
  ③ Cautious behavior is seen more in patients who have suffered a left-sided CVA.
  ④ Usually the contralateral side of the body is affected in individuals who suffer a CVA; that is, right-sided CVA affects the left side of the body, and left-sided CVA affects the right side of the body.

89. Knowledge, implementation, reduction of risk potential (a)
  ❷ Holding the arm level with the heart promotes an accurate measurement of the blood pressure.
  ① Placing the bell (or diaphragm) of the stethoscope under the cuff alters the fit of the cuff and may affect the accuracy of the measurement.
  ③ The nurse should first obtain the palpatory systolic pressure, then inflate the cuff 30 mm Hg higher than that reading. Automatically pumping to 200 mm Hg may cause the nurse to inflate the cuff with excessive pressure, or to miss a high systolic pressure.
  ④ The air should be released from the cuff at a rate of 2 to 3 mm Hg per second. Releasing the air too slowly may congest the vessels and alter the reading.

90. Application, implementation, safety and infection control (b)
    - ❷ Eyes are irrigated from the inner to the outer canthus because the inner canthus could absorb the chemical into the patient's system. It is also easier to catch the overflow from the outer canthus rather than from the side of the face. The chemical could also be breathed into the nose if draining toward the inner canthus.
    - ① This is an inappropriate direction of irrigating fluid; see rationale for #2.
    - ③ Irrigating directly onto the eyeball would be painful, and the fluid would drain into the inner canthus.
    - ④ While the fluid should be directed along the lower conjunctiva, it is more important it be directed from the inner to the outer canthus.

91. Application, implementation, pharmacological therapies (a)
    - ❸ Giving two injections increases risks for lipodystrophy (hypertrophy of subcutaneous tissue) or lipoatrophy (atrophy of subcutaneous tissue).
    - ①, ②, ④ NPH and regular insulin mix well; mixing will have no effect on their respective actions.

92. Comprehension, assessment, reduction of risk potential (c)
    - ❷ The patient is exhibiting signs and symptoms of air embolism. As little as 10 ml of air can be significant. Clamping the line and stopping the pump can stop the infusion of air.
    - ① Monitoring the insertion site is necessary throughout the dialysis procedure but not a priority here.
    - ③ When air embolism is suspected, the patient is positioned on the left side with the feet elevated for 30 minutes. This prevents air from going to the head. Rather, the air is trapped in the right atrium and the right ventricle where it is kept away from the pulmonary circulation.
    - ④ This is an inappropriate action; see the rationale for #3.

93. Application, implementation, basic care and comfort (b)
    - ❸ As the extremity swells, the jewelry will have a tourniquet effect and decrease circulation. This will promote swelling and pain. All jewelry must be removed.
    - ① Cold should be applied for the first 24 hours to decrease swelling.
    - ② The patient should be instructed to move her fingers to enhance circulation.
    - ④ This would increase pain since the blood would flow to the area. The extremity should be elevated to direct the flow of blood away from the wrist to decrease swelling and relieve pain.

94. Application, planning, reduction of risk potential (b)
    - ❸ The MRI (magnetic resonance imaging) uses high-intensity magnetic fields; they are powerful enough to harm the client if metal is left in place.
    - ①, ②, ④ These are all actions for a CT scan. A contrast medium is not used with an MRI.

95. Comprehension, planning, physiological adaptation (c)
    - ❶ The body heals itself at a faster rate when we sleep.
    - ② O$_2$ levels are not dependent on sleep.
    - ③ This may be true but is not the primary reason for the recommendation; the heart and the body need to heal so that infection does not occur.
    - ④ Muscle strength is not restored with sleep but with exercise.

96. Comprehension, planning, pharmacological therapies (b)
    - ❷ Sodium polystyrene sulfonate (Kayexalate) will most likely be ordered to decrease the serum K$^+$ level. The normal serum K$^+$ level range is 3.8-5.5 mEq/L.
    - ① This is a K$^+$ supplement and would increase the serum K$^+$ level.
    - ③ Bananas are a source of K$^+$ and should not be encouraged at this time.
    - ④ Strawberries are a source of K$^+$ and should not be encouraged at this time.

97. Comprehension, planning, reduction of risk potential (c)
    - ❶ Stress causes the release of epinephrine, which in turn speeds the heart up while constricting blood vessels and raising blood pressure. This increases the demands on the heart and can lead to failure.
    - ② Stress reduction exercises are good for anyone, not just those who have had surgery. This answer is too general.
    - ③ Relaxation will direct the flow of blood away from the periphery.
    - ④ Exercise would be a part of the treatment for managing stress but is not the principle behind the recommendation.

98. Comprehension, assessment, reduction of risk potential (b)
    - ❹ The most common causes of hypokalemia are abnormal losses, either via the kidneys or GI tract. GI tract losses from diarrhea, vomiting, fistulas, NG suction, and ileostomy drainage can cause hypokalemia. Renal losses include diuretics, elevated aldosterone levels causing sodium retention in the kidneys and potassium loss in the urine, and magnesium deficiency leading to increased urinary excretion of potassium. Other causes are skin losses through diaphoresis and dialysis.
    - ① There is an inverse relationship between sodium and potassium reabsorption in the kidneys.
    - ② The normal frequency of bowel movements varies per individual from 1 to 3 days.
    - ③ There is no direct correlation between potassium and blood loss through menstruation.

99. Application, implementation, basic care and comfort (b)
    - ❶ At a lower height, the water may not flow easily.
    - ② The water would not flow easily.
    - ③ At this height, the water would flow with too much force causing cramping.
    - ④ The water should flow easily, not slowly.

100. Application, implementation, basic care and comfort, (b)
    - ❸ Pain is not always due to tissue destruction. Pain from different sources requires different interventions.
    - ① This might be a consideration but not the first consideration.
    - ②, ④ These are considerations but not the first focus of the initial assessment.

101. Comprehension, assessment, coordinated care (b)
    - ❹ Bryant's traction is the usual method of treatment for an infant with a fractured femur as it immobilizes both extremities.
    - ① This is more extensive treatment than is usually needed.

② Skeletal traction is not usually used for infants with fractured femurs; often used in older children.

③ Traction is usually necessary before casting can be done if the fracture is to heal properly.

102. Application, implementation, safety and infection control (b)
❸ DD = 300 mg
DH = 500 mg
V = 2 ml
$$\frac{DD}{DH} = \frac{300 \text{ mg}}{500 \text{ mg}} \times 2 \text{ ml} = 1.2 \text{ ml}$$
①, ②, ④ This is not the correct amount.

103. Analysis, evaluation, pharmacological therapies (c)
❷ This is an example of an antispasmodic that may be given in UTI to decrease frequency and urgency.
①, ③, ④ These are all antimicrobials that may be used to treat UTIs; they may have this effect indirectly.

104. Comprehension, planning, basic care and comfort (a)
❹ This form of intake would be the choice until oral food and fluids are tolerated.
① This diet is not recommended until nausea and/or vomiting subsides.
② The patient is not able to tolerate this diet upon admission.
③ Frequent feedings are not advised due to the patient's intolerance of food.

105. Application, implementation, coping and adaptation (a)
❸ It is important not to lie to children when a shot or procedure is going to hurt. Allowing them to decide whether to get the shot "now, or in 5 minutes" gives them some control in the situation.
① Medicine should not be mixed in juice.
② The nurse should always be honest with the child when giving medicine; medicine should never be called candy.
④ The parent is the child's support system.

106. Knowledge, assessment, physiological adaptation (b)
❹ The CSF of a child with meningitis is cloudy because of the increased WBC count.
① Meningitis causes an increased protein level.
② Meningitis causes a decreased glucose level.
③ There is an increase in the CSF pressure in meningitis.

107. Knowledge, implementation, coordinated care (b)
❸ This is the correct rate of infusion.
①, ② This rate is too slow.
④ This rate is too fast.

108. Knowledge, planning, reduction of risk potential (c)
❶ Hyperventilation (blowing off CO_2) aims to maintain the $PaCO_2$ of 30 mm Hg, which causes constriction of cerebral vessels.
②, ③ Preventing hypoxia and hypercapnia is better accomplished by the administration of a high percentage of oxygen. CO_2 is a potent vasodilating agent. More blood is delivered to the brain, causing ICP to rise.
④ The goal in this patient situation is to keep the ICP from rising; venous return from the brain is therapeutic.

109. Comprehension, assessment, pharmacological therapies (b)
❸ Diabetes insipidus is caused by a deficiency of antidiuretic hormone (ADH). Vasopressin acts as replacement therapy for ADH. ADH acts in the renal tubules to increase the reabsorption of water back into the blood. Therefore, the amount of urine formed is decreased.
① This would be a side effect and not an expected outcome.
② Abdominal distention would decrease.
④ This should not effect temperature.

110. Comprehension, implementation, basic care and comfort (c)
❸ Pain resulting from spinal cord compression will be relieved when the patient sits because this decreases the pressure caused by the tumor.
① Movement increases the pressure on the nerves.
② Lying down stretches the spine and promotes the pain caused by spinal cord compression.
④ The pain of spinal cord compression has a gradual onset as the tumor increases in size.

111. Comprehension, implementation, pharmacological therapies (a)
❹ As with any antimicrobial therapy, the full ordered course must be taken to ensure recovery and decrease the possibility of a drug-resistant strain of organism developing.
① Showers should be taken.
② This is the proper way for females to wipe after voiding or defecation, and although this is a correct statement, the focus is on medications.
③ Grapefruit juice and citrus juices may irritate the bladder and may make some medications ineffective.

112. Application, implementation, physiological adaptation (b)
❶ Nitroglycerine increases blood pressure, so BP should be monitored while administering nitroglycerine.
②, ③, ④ Recommendations are to begin transport to the nearest emergency room after three tablets.

113. Application, implementation, reduction of risk potential (b)
❶ These foods have high amounts of vitamin K, which will decrease the effect of the anticoagulant. These foods should be eaten in small amounts.
② An electric razor should be used to avoid nicking the skin and bleeding.
③ Aspirin will increase the effects of the anticoagulant and should not be taken without the doctor ordering it.
④ A soft-bristled toothbrush should be used to avoid damage and subsequent bleeding of the gums.

114. Knowledge, implementation, pharmacological therapies (b)
❶ This is the proper method for using an inhaler.
② The inhaler should be used as ordered and before the individual becomes this short of breath.
③ This is unnecessary with inhalers; if a spacer is used cleaning is recommended.
④ Some individuals may find this comforting, but it is not required for the therapeutic effect.

115. Comprehension, assessment, reduction of risk potential (a)
   ❹ Floaters and/or flashing light sensation are early complaints in retinal detachment.
   ①, ②, ③ These symptoms are not seen in retinal detachments. Purulent drainage reflects an infection. Pain may be present with glaucoma, trauma, or infection. Bloodshot eyes may be present in a variety of conditions from overuse, irritation, infection, etc.

116. Application, planning, coping and adaptation (b)
   ❸ Having a parent assist in procedures often helps to calm the child, making it much easier to perform the procedure.
   ① Sedation is used only as a last resort when absolutely necessary.
   ② Restraints may be needed if assistance by a parent or by another nurse has not been effective.
   ④ Bringing in another nurse may frighten a small child; strange faces may upset the child instead of help calm him.

117. Application, implementation, prevention and early detection of disease (b)
   ❸ Introducing new foods one at a time helps to determine the infant's likes, dislikes, and possible allergies to certain foods.
   ① Mixing the food with formula does not allow the infant to taste the new food.
   ② Mixing the food with other foods does not allow the infant to taste the new food.
   ④ New foods should be introduced one at a time for 2 to 3 days to determine possible allergies the infant might have.

118. Comprehension, planning, safety and infection control (a)
   ❶ Rice cereal is digested properly in the infant with celiac disease.
   ②, ③, ④ Because of the defect in metabolism in the child with celiac disease, ingestion of wheat, oats, or barley leads to impaired fat absorption.

119. Comprehension, assessment, safety and infection control (c)
   ❶ This is the most common, serious complication of rheumatic fever; the endocardium and valves become inflamed and often are permanently damaged.
   ② This is not a common complication of rheumatic fever.
   ③ Arthritis is a symptom of rheumatic fever but not the most serious complication.
   ④ This is not a complication of rheumatic fever.

120. Comprehension, evaluation, physiological adaptation (b)
   ❹ A slight drop in hemoglobin is normal, and the mother is able to care for herself and her infant.
   ① Usually this is not associated with a slight drop in hemoglobin.
   ② Unless other problems are identified, vital signs are generally normal.
   ③ Performing basic tasks is usually within her realm and not a problem.

121. Knowledge, planning, growth and development through the life span (a)
   ❶ This is routinely done on each visit to ensure proper growth is occurring.
   ② There would be a long interval when possible problems would not be observed.
   ③ This is not the correct time sequence.
   ④ These are not "landmark" times for the mother to be checked.

122. Comprehension, planning, basic care and comfort (b)
   ❷ Some permanent loss of sensation can occur when the mandibular nerve branch is severed.
   ① Surgical division of the nerve has provided pain relief.
   ③ This is often associated with temporomandibular joint problems.
   ④ This may occur when there is a problem with the temporomandibular joint.

123. Comprehension, assessment, coordinated care (b)
   ❷ The Denis Browne splint is often used for the treatment of congenital clubfoot.
   ①, ③, ④ This type of splint is not used to treat scoliosis, DDH, or a fractured femur.

124. Comprehension, assessment, physiological adaptation (b)
   ❷ There is interference with venous drainage from the eyeball, which may be seen upon examination with an ophthalmoscope.
   ① This is not specifically associated with papilledema.
   ③ Papilledema does not cause an increase in cerebrospinal fluid.
   ④ This test is not associated with papilledema; it is performed to show any slowing in the conduction of nerve impulses.

125. Comprehension, assessment, reduction of risk potential (b)
   ❶ Respiratory distress would need immediate attention.
   ② This is associated with the disease but is not a priority need.
   ③ This problem needs to be met but doesn't take precedence.
   ④ The needs resulting from this problem could be met later.

COMPREHENSIVE EXAMINATION 1: PART 2

1. Application, planning, coping and adaptation (b)
   ❷ The child should not be told to be brave; children should be allowed to cry if something hurts.
   ①, ③, ④ Should be covered during preoperative preparation of the child.

2. Comprehension, implementation, reduction of risk potential (b)
   ❷ Oxygen therapy to prevent tissue deoxygenation is of primary importance in sickle cell crisis.
   ① This is part of the treatment for children with chronic sickle cell disease.
   ③ This may be part of the treatment in chronic sickle cell disease.
   ④ Hydration is important in treating sickle cell crisis; however, oxygen therapy ranks first in order of importance.

3. Application, implementation, reduction of risk potential (b)
   ❶ Protecting the head prevents a possible concussion from the seizure activity.
   ② Padded tongue blades are dangerous because they can obstruct the airway or injure the mouth.
   ③ Restraint of any part of the body is discouraged because such action could result in sprains and/or fractures.
   ④ The patient should be lowered to the floor and away from all objects to prevent injury.

4. Knowledge, implementation, basic care and comfort (a)
   ❶ The figure-of-eight turn allows the bandage to lay smoothly and provides support for the joint.
   ② The recurrent turn is used to cover distal areas such as the head, a digit, or a stump.
   ③ The spiral turn is used on cylindrical parts such as the forearm.
   ④ The circular turn is used to anchor the beginning and end of the bandage.

5. Comprehension, implementation, reduction of risk potential (c)
   ❹ This is the purpose of a rebreathing mask.
   ①, ②, ③ These are appropriate interventions for a client in respiratory acidosis.

6. Comprehension, assessment, pharmacological therapies (b)
   ❹ The leg cramps are most likely due to hypokalemia, a common side effect of loop diuretics such as Lasix.
   ① An electromyelogram tests for the presence of electrical impulses in a muscle when the muscle is active and at rest.
   ② The arteriogram assesses arterial circulation. Limited arterial circulation is common in diabetic clients; however, the associated leg cramps (claudication) are usually evident during activity rather than during rest.
   ③ Anemia can cause muscle cramps due to a lack of hemoglobin to carry oxygen to cells, but these cramps would be more likely to occur during activity rather than at rest.

7. Comprehension, implementation, coping and adaptation, (b)
   ❶ Greeting the client in his language shows that the nurse cared enough to go out of her way to learn this. It helps to build trust, which is very important to someone from another culture.
   ② The nurse will need an interpreter for important instructions, but not for routine care. The body language of an individual generally communicates enough information.
   ③ A pen and paper may be handy for communicating with pictures or if family wants to leave notes but is not a priority here.
   ④ This would be a nice gesture, but #1 is better.

8. Comprehension, assessment, reduction of risk potential, (c)
   ❶ The patient is exhibiting excessive hypotension and going into shock. It is important to get the blood to her head in order to maintain consciousness. Her blood pressure has undergone a marked change since admission. A patient receiving antihypertensives should have blood pressure monitored regularly and compared with the admitting baseline.
   ②, ③ The nurse will call the doctor after the patient is immediately seen to. She will hold the Monopril, since this is the source of the problem. The dosage may need to be adjusted.
   ④ This position would take blood away from the brain and place the patient at risk for loss of consciousness.

9. Knowledge, assessment, physiological adaptation (c)
   ❸ The accessory nerve (spinal accessory) has two branches and is a motor nerve. One branch controls the trapezius and the sternocleidomastoid. The trapezius functions to raise and pull back the shoulder and extend the head. The sternocleidomastoid flexes the neck and rotates the head.
   ① Involvement of the facial nerve will decrease the ability of the patient to wrinkle the forehead or close the eyes.
   ② Involvement of the trigeminal nerve will cause the patient to have loss of facial sensation, forehead, and temples. He will also have problems chewing.
   ④ The glossopharyngeal nerve (cranial nerve IX) controls taste, secretions of the parotid gland, and swallowing.

10. Knowledge, assessment, coordinated care (b)
    ❶ Gastroesophageal reflux is an organic (physical) cause of FTT.
    ② Nonorganic FTT is usually caused by psychosocial factors.
    ③ Idiopathic FTT has no explainable cause.
    ④ There is no classification with this name.

11. Comprehension, evaluation, basic care and comfort (c)
    ❷ Assessing the effects of each intervention will serve as a guideline for subsequent interventions to all involved in his care.
    ① Medications, including narcotics, are never used indiscriminately.
    ③ Guided imagery could be useful for mild pain, but not for moderate or severe pain.
    ④ Increasing his fluid intake would have no effect on pain control.

12. Application, implementation, basic care and comfort (b)
    ❶ Giving medications that are refrigerated hurt more because of the temperature difference. Room temperature is closer to body temperature and therefore more compatible.
    ② Injecting prior to the alcohol drying may cause some of the alcohol to be tracked into the deeper layers of the skin, which will cause pain.
    ③ Tightening of the muscles increases the resistance for the flow of the medication into the tissue, thereby increasing pain.
    ④ Inserting a needle slowly into the skin gives the brain longer to comprehend the pain. It also stimulates more pain receptors. A swift dart-like motion is always less painful.

13. Knowledge, assessment, safety and infection control (a)
    ❹ This is a typical example of an aura.
    ① This may likely be seen in the preictal phase, prior to the aura.
    ② This occurs after the aura and during the seizure.
    ③ These may be seen with partial seizures and are termed *automatisms*.

14. Knowledge, planning, safety and infection control (a)
    ❶ Oral assessments may involve contact with body fluids.
    ②, ③, ④ It would not be necessary to wear gloves unless skin breakdown or drainage were present.

15. Comprehension, planning, prevention and early detection of disease (b)
    ❹ Hepatitis A is spread by direct contact through the fecal-oral route; therefore sanitation methods will reduce the incidence.
    ① Hepatitis A is not a nutritional disorder.
    ② Hepatitis A is not a consequence of excessive alcohol use.
    ③ There is no effective vaccine for hepatitis A.

16. Knowledge, assessment, physiological adaptation, (b)
    ❸ The sympathetic nervous system increases heart rate thereby increasing cardiac output (heart rate times stroke volume)
    ① The sympathetic nervous system speeds up heart rate rather than slowing it down.
    ② The sympathetic nervous system increases heart rate and cardiac output.
    ④ The sympathetic nervous system does not cause cardiac arrest.

17. Comprehension, evaluation, pharmacological therapies (a)
    ❷ Diuretics act to remove fluids from the body therefore decreasing water weight.
    ① Losing fluids will result in weight loss, not gain.
    ③ A rapid respiratory rate is not an expected outcome of diuretic therapy.
    ④ Loss of fluids will result in high, not low, urine output.

18. Comprehension, assessment, physiological adaptation (b)
    ❹ Cigarette smoking has been correlated with increased risks of lung, bladder, mouth, pharynx, larynx, and pancreas cancers.
    ① Use of artificial sweeteners has not been shown to increase cancer risk.
    ② Caffeine intake has not been shown to increase cancer risk.
    ③ Excessive alcohol use has been correlated with increased risks of oral, larynx, esophageal, and liver cancers but not bladder cancer.

19. Application, planning, coordinated care (b)
    ❷ This is an expected outcome of the nursing action that should occur within a short period of time.
    ① This is a nursing intervention. It outlines the actual nursing activity.
    ③ This is a long-term goal, outlining the overall purpose of the nursing actions.
    ④ This is the rationale; it explains why the action is being implemented.

20. Comprehension, implementation, psychosocial adaptation (b)
    ❸ It is important to promote attachment of the family to the infant. This is best done by providing an environment in which the family is able to touch the infant and to interact as a unit.
    ①, ②, ④ These do not promote family interaction and sharing.

21. Comprehension, assessment, physiological adaptation (b)
    ❷ These are classic signs and symptoms of the condition known as failure to thrive.
    ① These are not symptoms of celiac disease.
    ③ These are not symptoms of Hirschsprung's disease.
    ④ These are not symptoms of pyloric stenosis.

22. Application, assessment, growth and development through the life span (b)
    ❷ Using Nägele's rule, add 7 days to the first day of the last menstrual period, then subtract 3 months.
    ① This calculation incorrectly started using the last day of the menstrual cycle.
    ③ This calculation incorrectly subtracted 7 days instead of adding 7 days.
    ④ This date has no relation to the application of Nägele's rule.

23. Comprehension, planning, physiological adaptation (a)
    ❷ These are high in protein as well as calcium.
    ① This provides protein but little else.
    ③, ④ These do not provide any protein.

24. Knowledge, implementation, growth and development through the life span (a)
    ❶ Disturbance of androgen-estrogen balance affects the activity of the sebaceous glands.
    ② Sex glands do not have a direct relationship; it is the androgen-estrogen balance.
    ③ Secretory cells are not the direct cause of the condition.
    ④ The bacteria are not the direct cause; the condition of the androgen-estrogen balance causes this to occur.

25. Comprehension, implementation, safety and infection control (c)
    ❸ If a patient scheduled for OR has an elevated temperature, the admitting physician should be notified.
    ① Respirations are within normal limits; the physician should be notified of abnormal vital signs, not anesthesia.
    ② Pulse is within normal limits; the physician should be notified of abnormal vital signs, not anesthesia.
    ④ Blood pressure is within normal limits.

26. Application, implementation, basic care and comfort (a)
    ❷ The narrow end is made to promote comfort for the client.
    ① The wide end has a narrow rim and would cut into the client's buttocks.
    ③ The narrow end is made to slide easily under the client's buttocks.
    ④ The water could be easily spilled and would take up space in the pan.
27. Knowledge, planning, reduction of risk potential (b)
    ❸ The parent/guardian must provide a written consent before the medication is given.
    ① This would be done after the permit has been signed.
    ② This is not imperative unless a problem is anticipated.
    ④ It is important to check so the hepatitis B is given in the opposite thigh; this is done after the permit is signed.
28. Comprehension, implementation, coping and adaptation (b)
    ❹ A form of distraction may provide relief from the current situation.
    ① This is not a remedy for this situation.
    ② The patient may get lost on the way to her room and does not need to be isolated.
    ③ Excess stimulation may add to her agitation.
29. Knowledge, implementation, basic care and comfort (b)
    ❶ A cone is inserted into the ostomy to direct the irrigating solution into the stoma.
    ②, ③, ④ Long tubes or cylinders are inappropriate and would not obtain maximum results when irrigating a colostomy.
30. Application, implementation, coping and adaptation (a)
    ❷ It is important to maintain a caring attitude.
    ① It would depend on how well she is progressing and if orders were received.
    ③ This is not routinely done unless requested.
    ④ The temperature should be kept at a level comfortable for the patient; it is not the top priority.
31. Knowledge, planning, safety and infection control (a)
    ❸ The patient will be able to call the nurse when the need arises. It will help relieve anxiety and may prevent an accident.
    ① It is dangerous to leave the door ajar. It should be left all the way open or be closed.
    ② It is not essential for the patient to eat alone unless this is a personal request.
    ④ Accidents may be avoided if the patient is informed of any rearrangement of furnishings.
32. Application, implementation, coping and adaptation (b)
    ❹ It is important to talk with the family first so they can be involved first-hand with care issues.
    ① While this is important, it is not the first thing to be done.
    ② This may be done later based on the needs of the patient and family.
    ③ After the care plan has been developed, this may be a priority.
33. Knowledge, implementation, safety and infection control (a)
    ❸ This delivers adequate heat and will not damage skin from this distance.
    ① Skin should be kept dry during treatment.
    ② Lamp should be left uncovered.
    ④ The patient is assessed every 10 minutes while the heat lamp is in use.
34. Application, evaluation, pharmacological therapies (c)
    ❷ Muscle strength (grip) is assessed at 1 minute, 2 minutes, 5 minutes, and 10 minutes after the administration of Tensilon.
    ①, ③, ④ These are not a routine part of the test.
35. Comprehension, planning, basic care and comfort (b)
    ❶ Without good nutrition, healing will not occur and infection will ensue.
    ② While a priority, aseptic techniques would be used with all patients.
    ③ This is good care but not vital.
    ④ This is good care since patients with Alzheimer's become agitated with stimuli, but this is not the priority here.
36. Application, implementation, pharmacological therapies (b)
    ❶ This is the medication used to terminate status epilepticus.
    ② This is used to treat hypertension.
    ③ This medication is used for control and maintenance of seizures but is not the drug of choice for status epilepticus.
    ④ This is an opioid analgesic for management of moderate to severe pain.
37. Comprehension, planning, physiological adaptation (a)
    ❸ Protein is necessary for tissue building and healing.
    ① This is not healthy and causes increased heart risk.
    ② Low carbohydrates may not meet calorie demands.
    ④ To give low calories, one would have to assume the patient was overweight; that is not a known factor here.
38. Application, implementation, reduction of risk potential (b)
    ❸ The patient with a colostomy is at increased risk for peristomal skin breakdown. All skin care products should be evaluated for allergic reaction. A patch test should be performed on an area of the abdomen away from the stoma.
    ① If shaving is necessary, an electric razor should be used. A blade increases the risk of irritation or cuts.
    ② Tincture of benzoin is drying to the skin and is not an effective barrier.
    ④ Soaps should be avoided except when showering.
39. Comprehension, implementation, reduction of risk potential (c)
    ❷ Malignant hyperthermia is caused by an idiosyntric reaction to drugs and anesthetics administered during surgery.
    ① Dantrium is given after malignant hyperthermia occurs.
    ③ This would have no effect on the occurrence.
    ④ Routine admitting vital signs are taken, not just the temperature. This action would have no effect on the potential problem.

40. Application, assessment, physiological adaptation, (c)
    ❹ Fatigue is a common symptom of heart failure.
    ① The elderly frequently have no chest pain. Shortness of breath is more common than pain.
    ② This is not pertinent information unless surgery is scheduled.
    ③ A line is always established on a telemetry unit. Normal saline would not be the solution of choice unless labs indicated it, and not at 150 cc an hour. This rate could put a client with possible heart failure into circulatory overload.

41. Application, implementation, reduction of risk potential (a)
    ❶ They are applied before feet and legs have a chance to swell.
    ② The patient's legs will be collecting fluid through gravity and decrease in venous return after they arise.
    ③ The stockings may be removed for the bath and reapplied immediately.
    ④ The legs would be in a dependent position and venous return would be decreased; better if lying down.

42. Knowledge, assessment, physiological adaptation (b)
    ❹ Pain occurs in sites related to the sinus involved. For example, if the pain is in the maxillary sinus, the pain will be intense over the cheeks and may radiate down to the teeth. If the infection is in the frontal sinus, the pain will be in and above the eyes.
    ①, ②, ③ Nausea, fever, and anorexia may be present in acute sinusitis but are not the primary symptom.

43. Application, implementation, physiological adaptation (c)
    ❹ The source of the infection must be found in order to eliminate it.
    ① This would help to control the temperature but not eliminate the cause of the fever.
    ② Observing for bleeding is an ongoing assessment in clients with leukemia.
    ③ Forcing fluids will help hydrate the patient but does not eliminate the cause of the infection.

44. Application, implementation, reduction of risk potential (c)
    ❶ Immobilization promotes clot formation around the catheter insertion site.
    ②, ③ The extremity is maintained in an extended position to promote circulation to the area and to enhance clot formation at the insertion site.
    ④ Clients may have fluids postprocedure.

45. Knowledge, implementation, basic care and comfort (a)
    ❹ A pillow place between the patient's legs helps to promote proper alignment of the hips and prevents skin to skin contact, helping to prevent skin breakdown.
    ① A footboard is generally not used in the lateral position.
    ② In the lateral position, the arms should be positioned comfortably in front of the client, with the upper arm supported on a pillow.
    ③ A small pillow should be placed under the head rather than the shoulder.

46. Application, implementation, pharmacological therapies (b)
    ❶ Persons taking tetracycline should be cautioned to avoid sunlight and ultraviolet light due to photosensitivity.
    ② There is no need to give this instruction related to tetracycline.
    ③, ④ This medication should be taken on an empty stomach.

47. Comprehension, planning, reduction of risk potential (b)
    ❸ Trauma to the remaining kidney would place the patient's renal function at risk. He should not be allowed to play contact sports ever again.
    ①, ② It will take about a year for the major back, abdominal, and flank muscles to heal, but this is not the reason for withdrawal from the football team. However, heavy lifting should be avoided for that year.
    ④ It takes only one kidney to meet the body's demand for kidney function.

48. Knowledge, planning, physiological adaptation (b)
    ❸ A balance of these three factors is necessary for the control of diabetes. The blood glucose level in diabetes mellitus is naturally elevated. It is important to eat a diet low in simple carbohydrates. Since the body does not make enough insulin, a supplement has to be given. Or in the case of type II, a stimulant is given in the form of a medication to enhance the production of more insulin to meet the body's needs. If a patient exercises excessively or becomes inactive without adjustments being made in the other two factors (diet, medication) then the body will be either hyperglycemic or hypoglycemic. Exercise uses glucose. Diet adds glucose to the system. Insulin uses glucose. The three have to be in balance.
    ①, ②, ④ Rest is important to everyone. It is critical, however, that an individual with diabetes maintain proper balance of the three factors indicated in #3 in order to maintain control of this condition. Refer to the rationale for #3.

49. Comprehension, planning, physiological adaptation (b)
    ❶ Regular exercise enhances bone formation and decreases bone loss. It also provides increased agility and decreases the chance of falling.
    ②, ③, ④ All are true but not the primary reason. Since the client has osteoporosis, building and preservation of bone strength take priority.

50. Comprehension, evaluation, pharmacological therapies (b)
    ❷ Weight gain frequently occurs due to the increase in appetite and fluid retention.
    ① Hypertension is more apt to occur related to fluid retention.
    ③ Fluid retention is more apt to occur, not dehydration.
    ④ Muscle mass will atrophy with extended use of cortisones and the client's strength will weaken.

51. Knowledge, evaluation, basic care and comfort (a)
    ❷ This describes the three-point crutch gait.
    ① This technique is the swing-through crutch gait.
    ③ This statement describes the two-point crutch gait.
    ④ This technique describes the four-point crutch gait.

52. Application, assessment, reduction of risk potential (b)
    ❶ The patient's pain may be related to a blood clot (deep vein thrombosis); a positive Homans' sign is indicative of a blood clot.
    ② The nurse should ensure that the possibility of a blood clot has been ruled out. The action of applying the stockings may dislodge the clot into general circulation.
    ③ If the pain is related to a blood clot, the stockings will not help the pain and may contribute to a pulmonary embolism.
    ④ Babinski's reflex is part of the neurologic assessment and has nothing to do with calf pain.

53. Comprehension, planning, physiological adaptation (b)
    ❹ Gauze moistened with normal saline will absorb drainage from the wound and allow for second intention wound healing.
    ① Occlusive dressings, such as hydrocolloidal dressings, are contraindicated with infected wounds, because they trap the microorganisms within the wound.
    ② A transparent dressing will not accommodate the drainage from an infected wound.
    ③ A dry sterile dressing will absorb drainage, but will not promote second intention wound healing.

54. Application, planning, pharmacological therapies (b)
    ❹ Waiting 30 seconds to 2 minutes between puffs gives the medication time to disperse.
    ① Rinsing the mouthpiece daily minimizes the presence of bacteria.
    ② The patient should exhale slowly so that the airway is completely empty when the medication enters.
    ③ The container should be shook for 3 to 5 seconds to allow thorough mixing of the medication.

55. Application, planning, pharmacological therapies (b)
    ❷ Codeine exerts antitussive properties by direct action on the cough center in the medulla oblongata.
    ① Guaifenesin is an expectorant that is indicated for congested coughs, to help thin mucus and promote expectoration.
    ③ Pseudoephedrine is an adrenergic agent that elicits a decongestant effect by causing vasoconstriction of nasal vessels.
    ④ Diphenhydramine is an antihistamine used to treat allergic reactions.

56. Comprehension, evaluation, pharmacological therapies (b)
    ❶ An insufficient dose of levothyroxine would lead to signs of hypothyroidism such as lethargy.
    ② An insufficient dose of levothyroxine would cause weight gain rather than weight loss.
    ③ Irritability is a sign of an excessive dose of levothyroxine.
    ④ An insufficient dose of levothyroxine would cause bradycardia rather than tachycardia.

57. Comprehension, planning, pharmacological therapies (b)
    ❹ Probenecid, an antigout agent, decreases the excretion of penicillin antibiotics thereby prolonging the action and increasing the effect of the ampicillin.
    ① Probenecid will not reduce the risk of anaphylaxis.
    ② Probenecid reduces the excretion of penicillin antibiotics and does not affect the metabolism.

③ This is the action of probenecid when it is used to treat gout, but in this case, it is used to prolong the action of the ampicillin.

58. Comprehension, planning, pharmacological therapies (b)
    ❸ Bethanechol is the drug of choice to treat postoperative urinary retention.
    ① Physostigmine is used as an antidote to tricyclic antidepressant overdose.
    ② Tacrine (Cognex) is used in the treatment of Alzheimer's disease.
    ④ Pyridostigmine (Mestinon) is used in the treatment of myasthenia gravis.

59. Application, implementation, pharmacological therapies (b)
    ❸ Postural hypotension is a common side effect of diuretics that causes a transient but symptomatic drop in blood pressure.
    ① Most salt substitutes contain potassium chloride and should be avoided when a client is taking a potassium-sparing diuretic such as spironolactone.
    ② These foods are high in potassium, which could lead to hyperkalemia.
    ④ The patient should be taught to maintain a record of daily rather than monthly weights. Daily fluctuations provide a reflection of fluid status.

60. Comprehension, implementation, pharmacological therapies (b)
    ❹ This response explains the physician's decision and directly answers the patient's question.
    ① Warfarin, although useful in treating blood clots, crosses the placental barrier and is contraindicated during pregnancy and lactation.
    ② Heparin is not available in oral form.
    ③ It is true that the physician ordered the injection, but that is the only way heparin is available. This response may lead the patient to believe that there is an oral form available.

61. Knowledge, planning, pharmacological therapies (b)
    ❷ Photosensitivity (increased sensitivity to ultraviolet radiation), a frequent adverse reaction to tetracycline, causes the patient to develop sunburn more readily than usual. In addition to sunscreen, the nurse might teach the patient to wear protective clothing and avoid tanning beds.
    ① Yogurt helps to replace some of the normal flora that are often destroyed by antibiotic therapy; however, the calcium in yogurt binds with the tetracycline, forming an insoluble complex that will not absorb into circulation.
    ③ The iron and other minerals in the supplement bind with the tetracycline, forming an insoluble complex that will not absorb into circulation.
    ④ The patient should continue to take the medication until it is discontinued by the physician.

62. Application, implementation, pharmacological therapies (b)
    ❷ This explanation clearly describes when and how the client is to take the medication.
    ① This explanation does not clearly describe how the client is to take the medication.
    ③ This explanation describes how to carry out the prescription but does not inform the client to stop taking the tablets if the pain subsides. In addition, Nitrostat is indicated for treatment of acute angina, not prophylaxis of anginal attacks.
    ④ Aside from being an incomplete explanation of the order, this explanation describes taking the medication by the wrong route.

63. Comprehension, implementation, prevention and early detection of disease (b)
    ❷ Sugar is present in spinal fluid but not nasal mucosal discharge. Therefore, the presence of sugar would confirm the finding of a CSF leak.
    ① A spinal tap would be contraindicated and is a function of medicine and not nursing.
    ③ Bacteria could grow from any body fluid and therefore would be non-specific.
    ④ This is an unrelated test and would not help the physician with the differential diagnosis.

64. Application, implementation, pharmacological therapies (b)
    ❶ The isoniazid depletes the body's stores of vitamin B_6; therefore a supplement is necessary since peripheral nerve damage could occur.
    ②, ④ Has no effect on the actions of isoniazid.
    ③ Has no effect on the patient's appetite.

65. Application, implementation, pharmacological therapies (b)
    ❹ Miscellaneous antidepressants may take from 1 to 4 weeks to produce the desired effect.
    ① These foods are high in tyramine, a substance that is contraindicated with monoamine oxidase inhibitors (MAOI) but not with miscellaneous antidepressant medication.
    ② Antidepressants need to be taken routinely in order to maintain a consistent blood level of the medication.
    ③ Miscellaneous antidepressants tend to produce sedation, as does Benadryl (diphenhydramine). Combining these two medications can lead to additive sedation.

66. Comprehension, implementation, reduction of risk potential (c)
    ❹ An upright position with head flexed toward sternum improves swallowing thereby reducing the risk of aspiration—the key respiratory complication in patients with dysphagia.
    ① Supplemental oxygen may improve blood oxygen level but does not prevent the respiratory complication of aspiration.
    ② There is no indication in this question of an abnormal breathing pattern.
    ③ Vitamin therapy may help with healing and tissue function but will not prevent aspiration.

67. Application, implementation, basic care and comfort (b)
    ❶ The procedure is always explained and opportunity is given for the patient to ask questions; no additional preparation is required for this procedure.
    ② A fasting state is not routinely required for this procedure unless it is and transesophageal echocardiogram and then the client is NPO 8 hours prior to the procedure.
    ③ A sedative is not required.
    ④ Collection of a urine specimen is totally unrelated to this procedure.

68. Application, implementation, safety and infection control (a)
    ❹ The nurse politely informs the relative of hospital policy and expects cooperation.
    ① This implies the relative is behaving in a wrongful manner.
    ② This is an excuse and does not teach hospital policy.
    ③ This is a punitive statement, and no explanation is given.

69. Application, implementation, coping and adaptation (b)
    ❹ A positive attitude and promotion of self-esteem is provided, and emotional support is given by the nurse.
    ① This is a cliché and lacks sensitivity.
    ② This is not an appropriate response.
    ③ The nurse does not know for sure if the patient will deliver on her next admission.

70. Knowledge, planning, growth and development through the life span (a)
    ❹ This is an appropriate source of folic acid.
    ①, ② These are sources of vitamin C.
    ③ Vitamins A and D are in this type of food.

71. Comprehension, planning, psychosocial adaptation (b)
    ❶ Touching will promote bonding with their infant.
    ② This may have been true previously, but most parents are now encouraged to touch and talk to their infant.
    ③ Parents are taught care of the infant by observing and assisting the nurse.
    ④ Home visits, phone calls by nursing staff, and other resources are usually available.

72. Comprehension, assessment, reduction of risk potential (a)
    ❶ A check of capillary filling, also known as the blanching test, is done to determine adequate arterial blood flow. Slow or no capillary filling would be indicative of compartment syndrome.
    ② An obstruction of venous peripheral circulation would be manifested by edema.
    ③ Impaired neurological function such as seen in compartment syndrome would be manifested by paralysis and sensory loss.
    ④ Although capillary filling is affected by cardiac output, that is not what the nurse is assessing in this case. The nurse is looking for signs and symptoms of compartment syndrome.

73. Comprehension, planning, pharmacological therapies (b)
    ❹ Atropine sulfate can increase intraoccular pressure and precipitate urinary retention.
    ① Etodolac (Lodine) is a nonsteroidal antiinflammatory drug (NSAID) and not usually contraindicated for persons with these disorders.

② Furosemide (Lasix) is a diuretic and not usually contraindicated for persons with these disorders.

③ Dopamine hydrochloride (Intropin) is an alpha- and beta-adrenergic and not usually contraindicated for persons with these disorders.

74. Knowledge, planning, pharmacological therapies (a)
❸ Naloxone hydrochloride (Narcan) is the narcotic antagonist used to reverse morphine sulfate.
① Hydromorphone hydrochloride (Dilaudid) is an opoid analgesic.
② Acetylcysteine sodium (Mucomyst) is a mucolytic that is used as an acetaminophen antidote.
④ Epinephrine hydrochloride is a sympathamometic drug.

75. Comprehension, planning, pharmacological therapies (c)
❸ Heparin sodium may retard the clotting process so the clotting reserves can be restored, thus allowing the DIC to reverse.
① This is used to reverse heparin sodium but has no effect on DIC.
② This reverses the effects of warfarin sodium (Coumadin) but has no effect on DIC.
④ This is not therapeutic in DIC.

76. Comprehension, implementation, coping and adaptation (b)
❹ Stating observations can clarify verbal and nonverbal clues and encourage expression of feelings.
① This is a closed-ended question that does not encourage the patient to elaborate further.
② This is a presumption of the patient's feelings, which often closes all conversation.
③ This is a false promise that can undermine the trust needed for communication.

77. Knowledge, planning, pharmacological therapies (b)
❹ Protamine sulfate reverses the effect of heparin sodium.
① Warfarin sodium (Coumadin) is an anticoagulant.
② Naloxone hydrochloride (Narcan) is a narcotic antagonist.
③ AquaMEPHYTON (Vitamin K) reverses the effects of warfarin sodium (Coumadin).

78. Comprehension, implementation, physiological adaptation (b)
❸ Lying immobile and keeping the head in one position will minimize the vertigo.
① Dark glasses may prevent migraines or light halos but not vertigo.
② Soft music is soothing but will not diminish vertigo.
④ Resting will help vertigo, but which side the patient rests on does not matter.

79. Application, implementation, reduction of risk potential (b)
❸ The nurse will have to be prepared to suction the patient frequently the first few days.
① This is too soon for instructions to begin.
② His speech will be permanently impaired.
④ Blood-tinged secretions are expected the first day or two; continued bleeding should be reported.

80. Application, assessment, reduction of risk potential (c)
❷ Visual inspection is the first step in assessment of the lungs, followed by the processes of palpation, percussion, and auscultation.

① Examination of the body is an orderly process. Auscultation of the lungs is done last.
③ Measuring of vital signs including the respirations would be done after the visual inspection.
④ This is not a routine measurement but may be done without an order in most hospitals since it is noninvasive. If the nurse wanted the information as part of the assessment, it could be done either before or after the examination.

81. Application, evaluation, pharmacological therapies (b)
❹ 1,000 cc/8 hours = 125 cc/hour; 125 cc/hour × 7.5 hours = 937.5 cc or 938 cc.
①, ②, ③ These choices are incorrect.

82. Comprehension, assessment, physiological adaptation (c)
❶ Primary symptoms of ureteral obstruction include decrease in urine output and pain over the kidney area.
② Urinary infection would be more apt to have painful urination, fever, and hematuria.
③ Blockage of the prostate could include these symptoms, but he is young and therefore it is not apt to be the prostate.
④ The most obvious symptom of cancer of the bladder would be painless hematuria.

83. Comprehension, assessment, physiological adaptation (c)
❹ Edema would be present as the kidneys became unable to handle the proteinuria.
① The urine output would decrease.
② The serum creatinine would increase.
③ Weight would increase as fluid was retained.

84. Knowledge, assessment, physiological adaptation (b)
❸ The white blood cells will increase as the body prepares to defend itself against the infection.
① Blood pressure has no bearing on the presence of infection.
② The body temperature will increase.
④ Herpes simplex may appear as a result of a weakened immune response, which may occur when an infection is present but is not considered a sign of infection.

85. Knowledge, assessment, physiological adaptation (b)
❸ Prolonged capillary refill time indicates diminished capillary perfusion, so it should not take longer than 3 seconds.
①, ② Capillary refill in 1 or 2 seconds is acceptable; it should not take longer than 3 seconds.
④ Refer to #3

86. Knowledge, assessment, physiological adaptation (b)
❸ The decrease in circulation to the involved extremity causes tingling and numbness.
①, ④ These are not factors in compromised neurovascular integrity.
② The extremity would feel cool.

87. Knowledge, assessment, reduction of risk potential (b)
❹ The brachial nerve plexus is close to the surgical field.
①, ②, ③ These are not involved in the surgery.

88. Comprehension, assessment, reduction of risk potential (a)
❶ Drainage that reappears after it has stopped is an indication of infection.
② Use of an ambulatory aid is expected for a few weeks. Full function should not be expected for 6 months.
③ Mild discomfort is expected until the knee is fully healed and functional.
④ This is not related to the surgery.

89. Comprehension, assessment, reduction of risk potential (b)
    ❸ Due to manipulation of the gut, the patient may experience a reflex paralysis of the ileus. When peristalsis is stopped, the gut continues to produce gas. The gut also is not moving the contents along its pathway. This results in abdominal distention. Paralytic ileus typically occurs 3 to 5 days postoperatively.
    ① The patient with a paralytic ileus will have decreased or absent bowel sounds.
    ② The pain may be localized, sharp, and intermittent.
    ④ Headache is not a result of paralytic ileus.

90. Comprehension, planning, reduction of risk potential (b)
    ❹ The patient may be turned to either side unless the physician orders otherwise. Always maintain abduction with pillows when turning.
    ①, ② Adduction of the hip places the patient at a high risk of dislocation of the hip.
    ③ Fowler's position should be avoided since it can dislocate the prosthesis.

91. Knowledge, implementation, reduction of risk potential (b)
    ❹ Rinsing with water will help decrease the incidence of oral fungal infection.
    ① Other than helping prevent atelectasis, this does not affect the medication or its usage.
    ② This is not relevant, as the medication was inhaled via the mouth, not the nose.
    ③ This applies to nasally administered medications; inhaled steroids are administered orally.

92. Application, assessment, growth and development through the life span (b)
    ❷ Basal metabolic rate decreases with aging in response to a decrease in muscle and lean tissue and an increase in adipose tissue. Decreased physical activity is a normal finding with aging and contributes to burning calories at a slower rate.
    ① Muscle and lean tissue mass decrease and adipose tissue increases with age.
    ③ A daily intake of 1200 calories is the lowest recommended to adequately meet nutritional needs.
    ④ When determining an adequate caloric intake, disease processes must be considered. Diseases may either decrease caloric intake (diseases that restrict mobility) or increase caloric intake (infection or injury).

93. Comprehension, planning, physiological adaptation (b)
    ❶ Chicken, green peas, and rice are good sources of complete proteins needed for tissue repair without large amounts of fat.
    ② Steak, deviled eggs, and macaroni and cheese are good sources of protein; however, these food sources are high in fat content.
    ③ Hamburger, french fries, and a milkshake contain proteins and are high in fat.
    ④ Chicken soup is an appropriate source of protein, but this selection is low in calories, which could lead to poor tissue healing.

94. Comprehension, assessment, basic care and comfort (b)
    ❶ Financial resources determine the quality, quantity, and access to nutritious foods. Eating is part of social interactions; therefore, older adults eat better when eating with someone else than if eating alone. Physical impairments or deficits may interfere with food intake.
    ② Personal preferences should be one consideration among many.
    ③ Food intake may be influenced by the time of day the meal is served; however, this factor is not considered in isolation.
    ④ Transportation is important in terms of obtaining food; however, this is not the most complete answer. Other factors must also be considered.

95. Application, implementation, basic care and comfort (c)
    ❷ In cognitively impaired patients, overstimulation may lead to dependence as opposed to independence.
    ① Cognitively impaired patients have difficulty with memory retention; therefore, instructions with reminders or prompting are quickly forgotten.
    ③ This is not a realistic intervention for all dementia patients.
    ④ This is inappropriate and reflects disrespect and lack of knowledge relevant to the care of patients with dementia.

96. Application, implementation, reduction of risk potential (b)
    ❶ This technique allows for smoother passage of food into the stomach because the trachea is partially closed, therefore, food is less likely to be aspirated into the lungs.
    ② This is inappropriate and may cause aspiration of food into the lungs.
    ③ Liquids should be thickened to assist with swallowing difficulties.
    ④ Hyperextension of the neck is uncomfortable and may increase the possibility of aspiration.

97. Knowledge, assessment, reduction of risk potential (a)
    ❹ Decreased thirst perception and physical, cognitive, mobility, and visual impairments in the institutionalized older adult predispose patients to dehydration. The greater the impairments, the greater the dependence on someone else to meet basic needs.
    ① Older adults have decreased thirst perception.
    ② Urinary frequency is a common reason older adults give for not drinking adequate amounts of fluid. Urinary retention is a complication of the urinary system, not a problem directly associated with dehydration.
    ③ The older adult has a decreased thirst perception and many have an increase in physical and cognitive deficits.

98. Application, planning, prevention and early detection of disease (c)
    ❶ Increased public awareness regarding signs and symptoms and what to do in the event of a CVA will relay the importance of seeking prompt medical attention; "time is brain" in patients having a stroke.
    ② Health care providers understand the need to treat promptly to facilitate recovery. To best decrease delays in seeking treatment, the general public needs to be more knowledgeable because ignorance prevents patients from seeking treatment.
    ③, ④ When a stroke is suspected, the first course of action is to call 911.

99. Comprehension, assessment, basic care and comfort (b)
    ❶ Older adults often report pain differently from younger patients as a result of physiological, psychological, and cultural differences associated with aging.

② Older adults usually have a decreased response to painful stimuli.

③ Older adults have a slower excretion rate of drugs due to age-related renal changes.

④ Many older adults are very stoic regarding pain. Nurses must also rely on nonverbal behaviors when assessing pain, especially in the older adult.

100. Application, implementation, physiological adaptation (b)
❷ A regular program of exercise increases bone and muscle strength; it will increase mobility and decrease immobility problems.
① This response is not appropriate or accurate information.
③ A regular program of exercise will provide optimal effectiveness in terms of maintaining muscle size and strength.
④ This is a non–knowledge-based answer to an important question.

101. Comprehension, assessment, reduction of risk potential (c)
❷ Polyuria 72 hours after a burn indicates the diuretic phase of burn recovery. The nurse should monitor for electrolyte disturbances (sodium, potassium), which often accompany massive diuresis.
① Signs and symptoms of skin infection are fever, redness, and swelling.
③ Signs and symptoms of respiratory obstruction are shortness of breath, dyspnea, and wheezing.
④ Signs and symptoms of shock are hypotension, tachycardia, and oliguria.

102. Knowledge, assessment, reduction of risk potential (a)
❸ The rule of nines is used to determine the total body surface area (BSA) of burns.
① The number of layers burned defines first-, second-, and third-degree burns
② The fluid replacement is based on the BSA (total body surface area) burned.
④ There are comparison charts to alter the rule of nines to fit with the patient's age.

103. Comprehension, planning, coping and adaptation (a)
❹ Body image disturbance is a known consequence of any body-altering procedure.
①, ② This diagnosis does not match with this scenario.
③ Depression may be occurring, but there are no data to support impaired social interaction.

104. Knowledge, assessment, physiological adaptation (a)
❶ Wheezes are produced by airflow through narrow airways as would be seen in the bronchospasms of anaphylaxis.
② Crackles are produced by fluid in the bronchioles and alveoli, usually due to pulmonary edema.
③ Rhonchi are produced when fluid or mucus blocks the larger airways such as seen with infection.
④ Friction rubs are due to pleural inflammation.

105. Knowledge, planning, reduction of risk potential (a)
❶ Ambulation is the most effective way of keeping blood circulating and preventing pooling of blood in the extremities.
② Leg massage is contraindicated because it may loosen an already formed clot and create an embolus.
③ Sitting with knees crossed cuts off venous return and contributes to venous stasis.

④ Pillows under the knees cut off venous return and contributes to venous stasis.

106. Knowledge, implementation, reduction of risk potential (a)
❷ Moist sterile dressings will maintain the viability of the tissue until surgery can be performed to repair the damage.
① An abdominal binder will cut off circulation to the affected bowel.
③ Dry sterile cotton fluffy pads will stick to the tissue and dry it up.
④ Placing the client in a high Fowler's position will worsen the evisceration by placing more strain on the surgical incision.

107. Application, evaluation, physiological adaptation (b)
❸ Pulse rates are an objective indicator of heart workload and therefore are utilized to measure tolerance to physical activity.
① Lung sound changes do not correlate with physical activity but with the disease process itself.
② Heart sound changes do not correlate with physical activity but with the disease process itself.
④ This is a subjective assessment of well-being, not necessarily tolerance to physical activity.

108. Comprehension, planning, basic care and comfort (b)
❶ The top priority in this client's care is pain management.
② Altered skin integrity may not occur since there is no indication the client is immobile.
③ There is no indication in this scenario that hypertension is occurring.
④ The priority problem during the acute phase is pain relief. Discharge teaching, if necessary, will be a priority at the end of the acute episode.

109. Comprehension, implementation, reduction of risk potential (b)
❶ Stopping the transfusion immediately will remove any more trigger for the anaphylactic reaction.
② The second step would be notifying the charge nurse.
③ Ambulating the patient would further tax the cardiovascular system.
④ The third step would be administering medication.

110. Application, planning, safety and infection control (c)
❹ Critical thinking involves the problem-solving method, which includes an analysis of the causes before solutions are utilized.
① This may be a solution but is inappropriate.
② This may be a solution but does not demonstrate critical thinking.
③ This may be a solution but it is not realistic.

111. Comprehension, planning, safety and infection control (b)
❹ A compromised immune system or other stress can cause the capsule to open and release active TB bacteria.
① The TB skin test would be positive since antibodies have been formed against the TB bacteria.
② To be contagious, there must be active disease.
③ Walling off the TB bacteria eliminate the active symptoms.

112. Comprehension, assessment, reduction of risk potential (b)
    ❸ An increase in blood volume can result in hypertension, bounding pulses, and pulmonary edema (dyspnea, cough).
    ① This indicates possible systemic infection.
    ② These indicate CNS involvement or hypoxia.
    ④ This indicates local infection.

113. Application, planning, pharmacological therapies (b)
    ❸ Pain needs to be relieved since the consequences of pain (hypertension, tachycardia, immobility) can severely compromise a patient's physical functioning. Being a patient advocate means intervening in order to relieve pain.
    ① Deep-breathing exercises are not effective against severe cancer pain.
    ② Relaxation exercises are not effective against severe cancer pain.
    ④ This is not intervening to help the patient.

114. Knowledge, assessment, prevention and early detection of disease (a)
    ❹ Early diagnosis and the type of cancer are the primary factors that increase survival (cure) rates.
    ①, ②, ③ Cancer treatments are utilized because the cancer has spread beyond the boundaries of what could be immediately surgically removed and cured.

115. Comprehension, assessment, reduction of risk potential (b)
    ❸ Any urine output of less than 30 cc/hr (240 cc for a 8 hour period) is immediately reported because it may indicate impending renal failure.
    ① This is normal.
    ② This is normal postsurgically.
    ④ This is normal and expected.

116. Knowledge, assessment, prevention and early detection of disease (a)
    ❶ IV drug use is a known high-risk behavior since it involves sharing needles and blood exchange.
    ② Dog breeding is not a high-risk behavior.
    ③ Travel to western European countries is not a high-risk factor.
    ④ Surgery itself is not a high-risk factor, and blood transfusions associated with surgery are a low-risk activity.

117. Knowledge, planning, safety and infection control (b)
    ❹ The simplest and most effective technique for preventing spread is to cover the nose and mouth when coughing and sneezing.
    ① TB is spread by droplets, so a gown and gloves don't help.
    ② TB patients are not longer isolated and can resume normal lives.
    ③ A standard mask allows the TB particles to pass through.

118. Comprehension, implementation, reduction of risk potential (b)
    ❹ These signs and symptoms along with the admitting diagnosis are the most characteristic of hypoglycemia. To confirm this assessment, the nurse would perform a blood glucose monitoring test.

① The first suspicion should be hypoglycemia, not a heart problem.
② Giving insulin could worsen the hypoglycemia.
③ Giving orange juice is the second priority after the glucose test to confirm the problem.

119. Comprehension, assessment, physiological adaptation (c)
    ❶ The narrowing of the airways traps carbon dioxide. This buildup of carbon dioxide produces carbonic acid and the net result is respiratory acidosis.
    ② The metabolic system is not involved in this acute respiratory problem.
    ③ High carbon dioxide levels result in acidosis, not alkalosis.
    ④ The metabolic system is not involved in this acute respiratory problem.

120. Comprehension, assessment, reduction of risk potential (b)
    ❸ The chief danger in head injury is the possibility of increased intracranial pressure, which would be manifested by a decreased level of consciousness and altered patterns of respiration.
    ① Assessing pain is important but not a priority.
    ② The number and location of bruises is part of the overall assessment but is not a priority.
    ④ Auscultation of lung, heart, and breath sounds may provide a clue to other complications but not the main concern, which is increased intracranial pressure.

121. Comprehension, planning, basic care and comfort (b)
    ❸ This goal is measurable and attainable over a short period of time.
    ① This goal is unrealistic and long term.
    ② This goal has nothing to do with the diagnosis.
    ④ A pain rating scale of greater than 5 is not an acceptable goal.

122. Comprehension, implementation, basic care and comfort (b)
    ❷ Phantom limb pain is due to continued irritation of the nerve tracts. It is real and should be treated with pain relievers.
    ① The grieving process is necessary to accept the loss of a limb but won't relieve the acute phantom limb pain.
    ③ Relaxation will not relieve acute phantom limb pain.
    ④ Phantom limb pain will diminish with time, but until then it needs to be treated.

123. Comprehension, assessment, reduction of risk potential (b)
    ❶ Cast syndrome is due to acute obstruction of the duodenum and results in nausea and vomiting
    ② These are signs and symptoms of infection
    ③ These are signs and symptoms of shock
    ④ These are signs and symptoms of fat embolism

124. Comprehension, assessment, reduction of risk potential (a)
    ❹ The ability to respond and follow commands assesses the return of normal cerebral cortex function after brain surgery.
    ① Hearing is an assessment of the eighth cranial nerve and not overall brain function.
    ②, ③ These relate to the patient's attitude, not physiological function.

125. Comprehension, planning, prevention and early detection of disease (c)

❷ Hepatic coma is due to an inability to metabolize ammonia and other substances. Proteins are avoided because one of their breakdown products is ammonia.

① Soaps-suds enemas will not help prevent hepatic coma.

③ Iced saline lavages are used for GI hemorrhaging, not hepatic coma.

④ Carbohydrates are necessary in the diet to provide energy for healing.

ANSWERS AND RATIONALES FOR COMPREHENSIVE EXAMINATIONS

COMPREHENSIVE EXAMINATION 2: PART 1

1. Analysis, evaluation, reduction of risk potential (c)
   ❶ Health care professionals generally agree that elderly people with diabetes are best managed by maintaining a fasting blood glucose in the 100-140 mg/dL range and postprandial glucose in the 120-180 mg/dL range.
   ②, ③, ④ This is incorrect information; therefore learning has not occurred.

2. Application, planning, reduction of risk potential (b)
   ❸ Individuals should be positioned so they are not sitting or lying on reddened areas of the body, which promote skin breakdown. The degree of skin breakdown directly depends on the duration and intensity of pressure to pressure points.
   ① Pressure-reducing mattresses reduce the intensity of pressure, not the duration. These special mattresses do not take the place of frequent positioning. Deterioration may occur if position changes do not take place every 2 hours.
   ② Antibiotic therapy is useful in treating a bacterial infection but is ineffective in preventing pressure ulcers.
   ④ Immobile patients should be repositioned every 2 hours.

3. Comprehension, planning, reduction of risk potential (b)
   ❶ Waterlogged skin is more likely to develop broken areas leading to microorganism colonization, ulceration, and dermatitis.
   ② Although this intervention may be pleasing to the family, appropriate delivery of competent nursing care is based on knowledge, theory, and established nursing practice standards.
   ③ Frequent inspection of the skin in the perineal area will not prevent urinary retention.
   ④ A urinary tract infection may occur after desquamation has occurred; the focus is on prevention of skin breakdown.

4. Comprehension, planning, pharmacological therapies (c)
   ❹ Normal changes of aging include reduction in total body water and muscle mass, which results in a greater risk of adverse drug reactions. Digoxin is a water-soluble drug and is distributed in smaller compartments, placing the older adult at risk for drug toxicity.
   ① In the older adult a water-soluble drug is distributed into smaller compartments, causing an increased risk of drug toxicity.
   ② In the older adult digoxin is more likely to accumulate to toxic levels in association with physiological changes.
   ③ Digoxin dosing in the older adult is usually smaller than the dose prescribed for the younger adult because of a decrease in total body water and muscle mass, and an increase in total body fat.

5. Comprehension, assessment, physiological adaptation (c)
   ❷ Patients with a left-hemisphere stroke will have difficulty understanding speech or written language and/or have difficulty expressing themselves.
   ① Patients with right-hemisphere strokes cause motor and sensory deficits.
   ③ Patients with right-hemisphere strokes often demonstrate impulsive behavior.
   ④ Patients with right-hemisphere strokes often demonstrate impaired judgment.

6. Application, implementation, reduction of risk potential (c)
   ❶ The combination of the type of surgery and symptomology are characteristic of dumping syndrome. This is due to a bolus of hypertonic food inducing rapid gastric emptying. To control this syndrome it is recommended to eat six small meals daily.
   ② An upright position would worsen the dumping syndrome; a reclining position is recommended.
   ③ Excessive fluids worsen dumping syndrome.
   ④ Antacids decrease stomach acidity and have no effect on dumping syndrome.

7. Application, assessment, reduction of risk potential (b)
   ❶ Bleeding from the incision may flow to the back of the neck and shoulders due to gravity.
   ② Dressings are not routinely removed because they act as pressure bandages to decrease wound bleeding.
   ③ Hemoglobin and hematocrit levels do not decrease immediately and can be affected by other factors such as fluid levels.
   ④ Blood may flow to the back of the neck and shoulders due to gravity.

8. Comprehension, planning, physiological adaptation (b)
   ❷ A firm surface provides support so that the heart is adequately compressed between the sternum and spine.
   ① The speed of compressions is not affected by the surface composition.
   ③ The risk of breaking the xyphoid process is dependent on the hand position on the chest wall.
   ④ Palpation of landmarks is not affected by the surface composition.

9. Comprehension, assessment, coping and adaptation (a)
   ❷ The onset of symptoms is usually between 20 and 40 years of age.
   ① MS is a common degenerative neurological disease.
   ③ MS is not common in children.
   ④ The onset of MS symptoms is not common in older adults.

10. Comprehension, planning, reduction of risk potential (b)
    ❶ To prevent an anaphylactic response to an antigen the patient needs to avoid exposure to the antigen, in this case, bees.
    ② Epinephrine is the drug of choice for treating anaphylaxis but does not prevent it.
    ③ A Medic-Alert tag enables other persons to recognize a possible anaphylactic reaction should anything happen.
    ④ White clothing has not been shown to repel bees or prevent bee stings.

11. Application, implementation, reduction of risk potential (b)
    ❹ Atelectasis (collapse of lung tissue) is a common postoperative complication due to shallow breathing and manifested by dyspnea, tachypnea, and fever. The appropriate intervention is to encourage coughing and deep breathing to reopen the lung tissue.
    ① Tylenol should reduce the fever but will not prevent the complications of atalectasis such as pneumonia.
    ② Antibiotics should counteract any bacterial infection present but cannot reopen lung tissue.
    ③ Increasing fluid intake will loosen secretions helping to clear the airways but cannot reopen the lung tissue.

12. Comprehension, planning, reduction of risk potential (b)
    ❹ Quadriceps muscles must be strengthened to allow for ambulation.
    ① Extension and abduction should prevent possible dislocation of the prosthesis but does not strengthen muscles.
    ② Passive ROM to the ankle will prevent joint freezing but does not strengthen muscles.
    ③ Active ROM to the ankle will prevent joint freezing but does not strengthen muscles.

13. Application, implementation, basic care and comfort (b)
    ❷ Obstruction of the catheter with blood clots is the primary cause of bladder spasms; relief of that obstruction will reduce the spasms.
    ① Trendelenberg position is contraindicated, as urine would flow backward into the bladder.
    ③ Antispasmodics are used to relieve bladder spasms but are not the first choice of action.
    ④ Narcotics are effective for pain but not for bladder spasms.

14. Comprehension, assessment, physiological adaptation (a)
    ❹ In acute glomerulonephritis an immune response occurs, which damages the kidney and reduces glomerular filtration. This results in fluid volume excess, which is characterized by periorbital edema, lung crackles, distension of neck veins, and weight gain.
    ① Typically fever is characteristic of inflammation, infection, or injury. A client with glomerulonephritis can manifest a fever, but this is not due to the decreased glomerular filtration rate.
    ② Thirst is characteristic of fluid volume deficit, not excess.
    ③ Polyuria is urination of large volumes, which does not occur with decreased glomerular filtration rates.

15. Knowledge, planning, basic care and comfort (a)
    ❸ The least-invasive intervention would be to make certain the patient has access to bathroom facilities.
    ① Placing incontinent pads on the bed will only absorb the urine and not assist with the incontinence problem.
    ② An indwelling catheter will temporarily eliminate the incontinence problem but is invasive and carries with it a significant risk of infection.
    ④ Restricting fluids is contraindicated in a patient with dehydration.

16. Application, implementation, psychosocial adaptation (b)
    ❸ Alzheimer's disease is characterized by lack of orientation to time, place, and person, so external signs of orientation such as clocks and calendars help reorient the patient.
    ① In an atmosphere of increased environmental stimulation, Alzheimer's patients become more confused because they cannot handle the stimuli.
    ② Frequent changes of environment also confuse these patients.
    ④ Group therapy provides too much stimulation and confuses the patient.

17. Comprehension, assessment, physiological adaptation (c)
    ❷ The history of the patient (previous renal calculi) and the symptoms of oliguria and pain (renal colic) are all characteristic of a urinary tract obstruction due to renal calculi.
    ① Dehydration is typically characterized by dry mucous membranes, poor skin turgor, and oliguria; pain is not a typical finding.
    ③ Renal failure is typically characterized by oliguria along with fluid volume excess, anorexia, nausea, and vomiting; pain is not a typical finding.
    ④ Glomerulonephritis is typically characterized by a history of previous infection and periorbital edema, lung crackles, distension of neck veins, and other typical manifestations of fluid excess; pain is not a typical finding.

18. Knowledge, implementation, basic care and comfort (a)
    ❸ Less than 50 cc of residual urine is a normal finding and does not require further intervention. All procedures should be documented immediately after performance.
    ① A physician is not usually immediately notified of a normal finding.
    ② Unless specifically ordered by the physician there is no reason to continue catheterization for a normal bladder.
    ④ There is no indication of the need to restrict fluids which would decrease urine output.

19. Comprehension, evaluation, physiological adaptation (b)
    ❸ The outcome of care related to less-than-normal nutrition would be stable body weight indicating a maintenance of nutritional status.
    ① Moist mucous membranes would be an appropriate outcome of care for dehydration.
    ② Absence of diarrhea would be an appropriate outcome of care for altered GI status: diarrhea.
    ④ Normal body temperature would be an appropriate outcome of care for altered body temperature: higher than normal.

20. Comprehension, assessment, reduction of risk potential (a)
    ❷ A low platelet count (thrombocytopenia) can result in an inability of blood to clot normally. Clinical signs and symptoms would include petechiae, hematuria, epistaxis, and gingival bleeding.
    ① Blood clotting abnormalities are not associated with oliguria, weight gain, and increased blood pressure; these may be characteristic of CHF or renal failure.
    ③ Fever, cough, and chills are typical signs and symptoms of infection which could be due to low WBC count, not platelets.
    ④ Dizziness, tremors, and seizures are indicative of neurological impairment. A brain hemorrhage could occur due to low platelets, but the signs and symptoms would be different (lowered level of consciousness, pupil dilation, and posturing).

21. Comprehension, planning, pharmacological therapies (b)
    ❹ This drug is a clot buster and should be given within 3 hours of the accident.
    ① Alteplase has no effect on blood pressure.
    ② This drug does not increase urinary output.
    ③ Alteplase is not given to prevent clot formation.

22. Application, implementation, safety and infection control (a)
    ❸ In order to assist with identifying the type of seizure, as well as the effects of medications the patient may be taking, the nurse would note the movements.
    ① The nurse should remain with the patient for the patient's safety.
    ② Once the seizure has started, it is too late. The nurse or the patient could get hurt.
    ④ The patient is placed on either side to promote drainage of secretions after and during the seizure if possible.

23. Application, implementation, reduction of risk potential (b)
    ❷ This degree allows for the best circulation and drainage of CNS fluid.
    ① This is not enough elevation.
    ③ This is too much elevation.
    ④ This would be uncomfortable and could promote flexion of the neck, which would increase pressure.

24. Knowledge, assessment, physiological adaptation (c)
    ❷ Hypercalcemia (serum calcium >11 mg/dL) is a common complication of end-stage cancer. It occurs most often in multiple myeloma, breast cancer, and metastatic bone cancer, owing to disturbed calcium reabsorption.
    ①, ③, ④ This is not usually a consequence of end-stage cancer.

25. Comprehension, implementation, prevention and early detection of disease (c)
    ❶ If both the ELISA and the Western blot are positive, then the client is positive for HIV. This means that HIV antibodies are present in the blood.
    ② By CDC definition (1993), the diagnosis of AIDS means that at least one AIDS-defining condition is present. Examples include:
    • CD4 cell count below 200/mm^3
    • Kaposi's sarcoma
    • Candidiasis of bronchi, trachea, or lungs.
    ③ He is contagious and is capable of passing the virus onto others.
    ④ People with HIV are living longer, more productive lives due to rigid retroviral treatment regimens.

26. Knowledge, planning, prevention and early detection of disease (a)
    ❷ Absence of prenatal care precludes early detection so that the condition can be watched and controlled.
    ① Hypertensive drugs were discovered and used for primary hypertension and were adopted for use by obstetricians; poor answer.
    ③ Controversial; recent studies reveal may have no effect.
    ④ PIH may occur at any age; number of pregnancies is of more concern, that is, whether first baby; although PIH is more likely in teenagers or older women, this is not the best possible answer.

27. Knowledge, assessment, growth and development through the life span (b)
    ❶ The primitive Moro reflex is still present at 3 weeks of age.
    ②, ④ Vocalizations and holding head erect are behaviors which can be observed in the 2-month-old infant. This infant does not have the neuromuscular development to perform these behaviors.
    ③ Recognizing familiar faces occurs at approximately 3 months. Before this time, younger infants may start to recognize familiar voices.

28. Comprehension, assessment, safety and infection control (c)
    ❹ Tight undergarments may result in perineal inflammation, which may inhibit the flow of urine during micturition. If the bladder is unable to empty fully, urine stasis results. Urine stasis is a major risk factor for UTI.
    ① Restriction of fluids at night only will not increase the risk of UTI as long as adequate fluids have been consumed during the day.
    ② Daily tub baths in plain water are not harmful. Tub baths may facilitate keeping the perineal area clean, which reduces the risk for UTI. Adding bubble bath to the water in contrast may increase the risk.
    ③ Because of the short female urethra and the close proximity to the rectum, it is recommended that females use a front to back motion when wiping to decrease the likelihood of *E. coli* contamination from the rectum.

29. Comprehension, planning, prevention and early detection of disease (c)
    ❹ To stimulate the immune system to produce antibodies against the rabies virus, the entire series of HDCV injections must be completed on the exact recommended dosing schedule. Failure to follow this schedule could result in development of rabies in the patient, which is usually fatal.
    ① Although some type of wound care may be ordered, it is not the priority in discharge instructions.
    ② Same as #1. Also in many cases these wounds are not sutured because of the danger of infection by other bacteria, because the wound is usually considered a dirty wound.
    ③ Temperature elevation is a potential side-effect of the injections but not the priority in discharge instructions.

30. Application, evaluation, safety and infection control (b)
    ❸ Insertion of the catheter no farther than 0.5 cm beyond the tip of the tube depth will prevent excessive damage to the tracheal mucosa.
    ① Hydrogen peroxide should never be instilled into the trach tube. It can, however, be used to remove crusts externally around the stoma or to clean the inner cannula when removed during tracheostomy care.
    ② The suction gauge should be set at no more than 120 mm Hg pressure; greater pressures will result in damage to the tracheal mucosa and possible excess depletion of oxygen, causing hypoxemia.
    ④ Leaving the suction catheter in the tube longer than 5 to 10 seconds may result in depletion of oxygen, resulting in hypoxemia.

31. Comprehension, assessment, safety and infection control (c)
    ❶ Inhalation of noxious fumes as produced by ammonia may precipitate an asthma attack caused by irritation of respiratory passages.
    ② Emotional upset will not precipitate an asthma attack in children. It may, however, exacerbate an attack already in progress.
    ③, ④ Cool humidification of respiratory passages as could occur while swimming or when using a humidifier does not usually precipitate an attack. Respiratory passages may be soothed.

32. Application, implementation, safety and infection control (b)
    ❷ *Streptococcus pneumoniae* is the most common cause of meningitis and a common cause of upper respiratory infections. It may result in meningitis due to extension of the infection into the CNS. Only good handwashing is needed.
    ① Strict isolation is not required for the strep organism but is for meningococcal meningitis to prevent transmission of the organism.
    ③ Meningitis transmission usually does not occur through wounds.
    ④ Respiratory precautions are necessary only as a part of strict isolation for meningococcal meningitis.

33. Knowledge, assessment, physiological adaptation (b)
    ❸ The zygote is implanted in the uterine wall at about 3 weeks and thus ends the preembryonic stage.
    ① At birth, the fetus becomes a neonate.
    ② The fetal stage is from 9 weeks to birth.
    ④ The embryonic stage occurs from the fourth to eighth week, and consists of rapid growth and differentiation.

34. Application, implementation, physiological adaptation (b)
    ❶ The umbilical cord has two arteries, which return waste from the system, and one vein, through which nutrients pass from the mother to the fetus.
    ②, ③, ④ This is incorrect. There are two arteries and one vein in the umbilical cord.

35. Comprehension, planning, growth and development through the life span (b)
    ❶ A balance of all nutrients provides a favorable environment for the developing fetus.
    ② An adequate amount of calories is needed for protein utilization and fat metabolism.
    ③ Fluid intake facilitates the clearance of creatinine, urea, and other waste products of fetal and maternal metabolism.
    ④ A well-balanced diet is recommended for adequate metabolism.

36. Knowledge, planning, reduction of risk potential (b)
    ❹ 1500-2000 ml of fluid per day is recommended in the older adult to maintain adequate fluid balance, renal function, and hydration.
    ① 2000-3000 ml of fluid each day exceeds the recommended intake in the older adult. Older adults have a total water decrease of approximately 8%, with a greater decrease of fluid in the intracellular and interstitial spaces than younger adults.

    ② 500-1000 ml of fluid each day is not sufficient to meet metabolic, hydration, or fluid balance needs.
    ③ 2500-3000 ml of fluid each day exceeds total daily water intake in the older adult.

37. Knowledge, planning, physiological adaptation (a)
    ❹ A bent spinal position enables the physician to more easily locate the correct site for puncture.
    ① This position does not decrease the potential for vomiting.
    ② This position does not help to stabilize vital signs.
    ③ This position does not keep the spine straight.

38. Knowledge, planning, coordinated care (c)
    ❶ A disulfiram (Antabuse)-type reaction can occur, causing severe nausea and vomiting.
    ②, ④ There are no significant literature reports of this occurring.
    ③ Since the two substances should not be taken together, this answer is not correct.

39. Comprehension, implementation, growth and development through the life span (b)
    ❷ Preparation for death is one of the normal developmental tasks of aging.
    ① This response blocks further conversation.
    ③ This response indicates assumption.
    ④ This response is definitely inappropriate and a put down.

40. Comprehension, planning, basic care and comfort (a)
    ❶ As a result of the decreased glandular function of the skin in the elderly, they have dryer, thinner, and extremely fragile skin. The elderly also tolerate extreme heat and extreme cold poorly.
    ② Hot water could damage the skin, causing scalds.
    ③ This is not frequent enough.
    ④ Cold water would cause chilling and discomfort.

41. Comprehension, implementation, reduction of risk potential (c)
    ❸ Fluid intake of at least 2400 ml should be encouraged to prevent crystalluria; the nurse should use terms the patient will understand (3 quarts rather than 3 liters or 3000 ml).
    ① Acyclovir (Zovirax) helps to reduce the duration of the lesions but does not eradicate the virus.
    ② The patient should be encouraged to complete the full prescribed course of the medication.
    ④ The medication will not protect a sexual partner from contracting the virus. The patient should be instructed to use condoms for or abstain from sexual intercourse.

42. Comprehension, planning, pharmacological therapies (b)
    ❹ Non-selective beta-adrenergic blocking agents may affect the $beta_1$ receptors leading to bronchoconstriction or bronchospasm producing dyspnea.
    ① Stimulation, rather than blocking, of the adrenergic receptors causes nervousness.
    ② Photophobia is a result of pupil dilation as occurs with adrenergic stimulation, not blocking.
    ③ An increase in heart rate is caused by the simulation, rather than the blocking, of adrenergic receptors.

43. Application, assessment, safety and infection control (b)
❹ The nurse should identify the potential cause of the behavior and try appropriate alternatives before deciding to apply a restraint.
① Prior to applying a restraint, alternatives should be tried. If a restraint becomes the most appropriate option, then the nurse should obtain a physician's order for the least-restrictive restraint.
② The nurse should try alternatives to address the potential risk factors before asking the physician for a restraint order.
③ This may be an acceptable alternative to restraints, but the nurse must first identify the risk factors before determining interventions.

44. Analysis, evaluation, physiological adaptation (a)
❸ The temperature is higher than the nurse might expect given the rest of the assessment data, so the nurse should take the temperature again to ensure its accuracy.
① Since the temperature is inconsistent with the other assessment data, the temperature should be reassessed before the data are reported to the physician.
② Since the temperature is inconsistent with the other assessment data, the temperature should be reassessed before an antipyretic medication is administered.
④ Since the temperature is inconsistent with the other assessment data, the temperature should be reassessed before the temperature is recorded in the chart.

45. Comprehension, planning, coordinated care (c)
❸ Morphine sulfate has a high first-pass metabolism rate, which means that a large percentage of the drug molecules are distributed to the liver via portal circulation, and metabolized before reaching the site of action; 60 mg of oral morphine sulfate provides the equianalgesic dose of 10 mg given intramuscular.
①, ② A higher oral dose is required due to the effect of first-pass metabolism.
④ Although a higher dose in necessary when giving morphine sulfate by the oral rather than parenteral route, 100 mg given orally exceeds the equianalgesic dose for 10 mg given parenterally; the client would likely experience life-threatening side effects such as respiratory depression and sedation.

46. Comprehension, planning, basic care and comfort (b)
❷ Quadriceps setting exercises improve the strength of muscles needed for walking.
①, ③, ④ These actions will not strengthen muscles as indicated in #2.

47. Knowledge, planning, basic care and comfort (a)
❸ An increase in fruits in the diet will increase bulk in the intestines. Increasing bulk and fluids in the intestines will promote normal elimination.
①, ② These are not appropriate means of encouragement as a routine to follow.
④ This may not be possible.

48. Comprehension, implementation, reduction of risk potential (b)
❸ Hip and knee contractures can occur after surgery.
①, ②, ④ These are not generally the prime consideration for the identified nursing measure.

49. Comprehension, assessment, reduction of risk potential (a)
❷ The *foremost* complication is hemorrhage.
① This is possible during the postoperative period.
③ These are possible if an exercise regimen is not adhered to.
④ This is possible after any surgery.

50. Comprehension, planning, pharmacological therapies (a)
❷ Thromboembolic problems are a postoperative complication of hip surgery. Low-dose aspirin reduces the risks of this complication.
① This dose is too low for an antiinflammatory effect.
③, ④ These are not the primary purpose behind such an order.

51. Comprehension, assessment, reduction of risk potential (c)
❷ Lithium is excreted intact by the kidneys, so it is most important to monitor the values that reflect renal function; hyponatremia predisposes to lithium toxicity.
① Complete blood cell count and platelet count reflect the composition of the blood and bone marrow function, neither of which are related to lithium therapy; serum albumin may reflect the number of protein binding sites for distribution of the drug.
③ SGOT, SGPT, and serum bilirubin levels reflect the function of the liver rather than the kidneys; since lithium is not metabolized by the liver and is excreted by the kidneys, it is more important to monitor renal function.
④ Serum potassium, white blood cell differential, and the platelet count are not significantly affected by lithium.

52. Comprehension, planning, basic care and comfort (a)
❷ Explaining the procedure helps to reduce the patient's anxiety and promotes cooperation.
① The wheels of the bed and the wheelchair should be locked to prevent rolling, which could contribute to injuries for both the patient and the nurse.
③ The nurse should determine whether the mechanical lift device is needed before obtaining it; not all patients require the mechanical lift device.
④ Raising the bed for a transfer increases the risk of injury for both the patient and the nurse, since the patient will not be able to place his feet on the floor.

53. Comprehension, planning, basic care and comfort (a)
❸ The patient's nonverbal responses may indicate pain or discomfort associated with the exercise.
① The joint should not be exercised past the point of pain or stiffness to prevent joint injury.
② Each exercise should be repeated at least two to five times; the number of repetitions varies among patients.
④ The exercises should be performed in a consistent order to prevent overlooking a joint.

54. Application, implementation, safety and infection control (b)
❷ The balloon may be in the urethra; deflating the balloon prevents further urethral injury, and removing the catheter reduces the risk of infection.

① Deflating the balloon prevents further urethral injury; the catheter was contaminated when the nurse grasped it with her fingers to inflate the balloon, so inserting the catheter further may introduce more microorganisms into the urethra.

③ Urethral pain is not expected and may indicate that the balloon is being inflated in the urethra; continuing to inflate the balloon increases the risk of urethral damage.

④ Deep breaths may help the patient to relax, but continuing to inflate the balloon increases the risk of urethral damage.

55. Comprehension, assessment, physiological adaptation (b)
❷ This is a frequent symptom with prostate enlargement.
① This is more common with bladder carcinoma or upper UTI.
③ This is more common with an UTI.
④ This symptom is vague; nausea may occur with various disease states.

56. Comprehension, implementation, reduction of risk potential (b)
❷ Shortness of breath with pink-tinged sputum may indicate bleeding at the capillary bed due to an increased bleeding time. Warfarin is an anticoagulant and prolongs bleeding time.
① Nasal congestion is not an expected side effect in association with the administration of warfarin.
③, ④ These are not common side effects in association with the administration of warfarin.

57. Application, implementation, safety and infection control (a)
❹ Nurses always write the orders as the physician gives orders and then repeat the orders for verification.
① Orders are written as given, then repeated for verification.
② Telephone orders are signed by the nurse receiving the order with the physician counter-signing the order within a specified time period.
③ The steps are to write the orders as the physician is giving the order, verify the orders, then make sure the patient's name appears on the order sheet. The next of kin is not information found on the order sheet.

58. Application, evaluation, basic care and comfort (b)
❷ Postural drainage helps drain sections of the lung, aids in coughing and removing secretions, and improves breathing.
① High-Fowler's position (45- to 90-degree elevation) is most effective in relieving dyspnea.
③ Fluids should be forced to liquefy secretions.
④ Patient should have rest and conserve energy.

59. Comprehension, implementation, prevention and early detection of disease (a)
❸ Lymph node biopsy is the most definitive diagnostic procedure for sarcoidosis.
① This would give the patient a false sense of spreading disease.
② The question was not understood properly.
④ Swollen glands are symptomatic of sarcoidosis.

60. Comprehension, assessment, reduction of risk potential (a)
❶ Circulation and sensation are periodically assessed to determine the presence of pressure areas that may obstruct circulation and nerve pathways.
②, ③, ④ These are inappropriate actions.

61. Knowledge, planning, safety and infection control (a)
❶ The gold standard for administering medications is the five rights: the right drug, dose, patient, route, and time.
② Four rights are presented in this response. Documentation has been considered by many as the sixth right.
③ Hospital policy should be followed but is not considered one of the components in the standard.
④ This is an inaccurate response.

62. Comprehension, assessment, safety and infection control (b)
❶ The patient may end up with several medications that duplicate drug actions or cause a drug-drug interaction or overdosage.
② One drug may potentiate the action of another; however, several drugs administered together may also cause toxicity. More than one physician prescribing medications may lead to potential toxic conditions.
③ The cost of medications may be a factor, but there is a greater degree of concern because different physicians have prescribed different medications to the same patient leading to potential problems.
④ The degree of risk is directly proportional to the number of medications ingested by individuals.

63. Application, implementation, safety and infection control (a)
❹ When a patient indicates that a drug is different in any way, the nurse's responsibility is to verify that the drug is correct based on the physician's order. The drug is not given until validation of the physician's order takes place.
① Just because medications are placed in a specific patient's drawer does not mean that the medications are correct for that patient. The nurse must follow the five rights of medication administration.
② This response invalidates the patient's concern.
③ Everyone is capable of making an error relevant to passing medications.

64. Application, implementation, prevention and early detection of disease (b)
❶ Limiting sun exposure is most important, along with use of sunscreens with an SPF rating of at least 15, wearing of wide-brimmed hats, and avoidance of purposeful tanning.
② This response is vague and lacks professional advice.
③ This response is inaccurate and does not address the patient's concern.
④ This response is judgmental and lacks patient respect.

65. Comprehension, planning, reduction of risk potential (b)
   ❸ A priority intervention for the patient having intracranial surgery is to assess for increased intracranial pressure and maintain airway patency.
   ① The head and neck are positioned midline.
   ② Dextrose 5% in water is not administered in the patient who has undergone brain surgery. After the dextrose is metabolized out, the solution becomes hypotonic, placing the patient at increased risk of intracerebral edema.
   ④ The head of the bed is elevated per physician's order to decrease intracranial pressure.

66. Comprehension, assessment, physiological adaptation (c)
   ❶ Epilepsy is defined as a chronic recurrent pattern of seizures. Convulsion is defined as one manifestation of a seizure, characterized by spasmodic contractions of a muscle.
   ②, ③ These are incorrect responses based on the criteria given. Refer to #1.
   ④ Epilepsy may occur as a complication after brain injury, but this is not relevant to the differential criteria between epilepsy and convulsion. The second part of the sentence is inaccurate.

67. Comprehension, planning, reduction of risk potential (a)
   ❷ The most common adverse effect of heparin is hemorrhage. Protamine sulfate is kept available if it becomes necessary to counteract the effects of heparin.
   ① Prevention of blood clotting is the reason heparin is being administered.
   ③ Renal insufficiency is not considered an adverse effect of heparin therapy. The lab test to monitor therapeutic effectiveness for heparin therapy is the partial thromboplastin time (PTT).
   ④ This is not a requirement with the administration of heparin.

68. Comprehension, planning, physiological adaptation (c)
   ❶ This is an outcome criteria statement.
   ② This is a nursing intervention.
   ③ This is an appropriate nursing diagnosis.
   ④ This is an appropriate evaluation statement.

69. Comprehension, planning, reduction of risk potential (a)
   ❹ Priority nursing management of the patient with a tracheostomy is airway, breathing, and circulation.
   ① The head of the bed should be elevated 30 to 45 degrees to facilitate expectoration of secretions, second to maintaining a patent airway.
   ② Nutritional intake is important to wound healing, after airway, breathing, and circulation status is managed.
   ③ Checking the stoma and secretions suctioned are appropriate nursing actions after monitoring respiratory status.

70. Application, planning, physiological adaptation (c)
   ❸ Assessment of motor function includes muscle movement, size, tone, strength, and coordination of muscle groups.
   ① Cranial nerve VIII is responsible for hearing; CN IX and X are responsible for the gag reflex and ability to speak. Cranial nerve XI allows the person to raise the shoulders, and CN XII allows movement of the tongue.

② Body positioning is evaluated during the inspection portion of the assessment; mental status and level of consciousness are assessed throughout the examination and are not specific to motor function.
   ④ Intellectual functions and speech patterns are components of a neurological examination but are not included in the motor function assessment.

71. Application, planning, safety and infection control (c)
   ❷ Hypergammaglobulinemia occurs when excessive amounts of gamma globulins are produced, causing an impaired immune response. Patients with this disorder are at risk for developing infections; therefore, the nurse should place the patient in protective isolation and assess for signs of infection.
   ① Contact isolation is not indicated.
   ③ Medication administration per physician's order is an appropriate nursing action, but the patient's primary health risk is an overwhelming infection.
   ④ This is inappropriate for a patient with a depressed immune response.

72. Comprehension, implementation, reduction of risk potential (b)
   ❷ Rest and avoidance of heaving lifting or strenuous activity promotes healing and decreases intraabdominal pressures to the puncture site. Heavy lifting or strenuous exercise may precipitate a bleeding episode. Large volumes of blood can be lost should bleeding occur; therefore prompt medical attention is required.
   ① The bandage can be changed in 24 hours; the puncture is expected to be sore for several days, however progressive.
   ③ Tub baths are contraindicated until the puncture site is healed due to placing undue stress at the puncture site.
   ④ Driving and climbing stairs are contraindicated for 24 hours following catheterization due to an increased risk of bleeding.

73. Comprehension, planning, physiological adaptation (c)
   ❹ Adequate tissue perfusion is an appropriate outcome criteria statement for thrombophlebitis.
   ① This is a nursing diagnosis.
   ② This is an evaluation statement.
   ③ This is a nursing intervention.

74. Knowledge, assessment, physiological adaptation (b)
   ❷ Creatine kinase (CK-MB) is found mainly in cardiac muscle and rises 4-12 hours after infarction, peaks in 24 hours, and returns to normal in 3-4 days.
   ① The white blood cell count may be elevated by the third day due to the inflammatory response. This test is not specific, however, to myocardial infarction.
   ③ This is a test used primarily to screen for disseminated intravascular coagulation (DIC).
   ④ This is a test useful in the diagnosis of several disorders: anemia, cardiomyopathy, congestive heart failure, delirium tremens, hypothyroidism, inflammation, leukemia, muscle injury, myxedema, pulmonary infarction, and renal infarction. LDH will be elevated 24-48 hours after infarction, peaks in 3-6 days, and returns to normal in 7-14 days.

75. Comprehension, assessment, coping and adaptation (b)
   ❶ Anxiety is defined as a state in which an individual experiences feelings of uneasiness or apprehension.

② This nursing diagnosis is applicable to the patient but not to the family member.

③ The data do not suggest noncompliance. Noncompliance is defined as the state in which an individual or group desires to comply with health-related advice given by health professionals.

④ Ineffective individual coping is defined by destructive behavior in response to an inability to manage internal or external stressors.

76. Knowledge, assessment, physiological adaptation (b)
   ❶ This is the correct response.
   ②, ③, ④ Incorrect responses; these are inflammatory conditions; #2 and #3 are related to the female, and #4 to the male.

77. Application, planning, physiological adaptation (a)
   ❶ These activities will put the arm through range of motion (ROM) as the patient assumes some responsibility for personal care.
   ② This is part of daily routine in rehabilitation.
   ③ This is an inappropriate activity.
   ④ This is too fine a movement and one that does not allow full range of motion.

78. Comprehension, planning, safety and infection control (b)
   ❷ A wet dressing must be changed as soon as possible because it will be a source of infection and is irritating.
   ①, ④ These are not specifically related to the question.
   ③ The patient should be ambulatory before removal of the tube.

79. Knowledge, implementation, growth and development through the life span (a)
   ❹ At this age, the baby should be able to follow bright lights and objects.
   ① Vision is 20/100 at 1 year of age. Because it is not yet normal, this is the age at which babies keep bumping into things.
   ② Visual acuity is about 20/300, and babies can see only at a very close range.
   ③ By 9 to 10 months of age, depth perception is developing.

80. Knowledge, implementation, reduction of risk potential (c)
   ❸ Oral contraceptives are considered the most effective method of birth control if taken correctly. They also have few side-effects.
   ① Condoms are sheaths that prevent sperm from entering the cervix and have been known to tear or leak. Some find putting them on correctly a problem. Condoms are recommended to prevent spread of AIDS. They are not 100% effective for birth control.
   ② Coitus interruptus is difficult to control, and sperm can escape.
   ④ Intrauterine devices are controversial. There is some danger that the device can dislodge and remain in the vagina so a woman may think she is fully protected. There is also literature addressing infections and other problems caused by IUDs.

81. Knowledge, implementation, safety and infection control (a)
   ❷ Chlorpromazine makes skin sensitive to sunlight.
   ① This is related to monoamine oxidase (MAO) inhibitor.
   ③, ④ Not related.

82. Knowledge, assessment, basic care and comfort (b)
   ❶ The nurse should never use a suppository directly from refrigerator, because cold causes constriction.
   ② Lubrication ensures easy, painless insertion.
   ③ The suppository is ineffective when inserted into a bolus of stool.
   ④ Glycerin suppositories are inserted after 20 minutes if the patient has not had a bowel movement.

83. Comprehension, planning, physiological adaptation (a)
   ❶ Pattern is essential with retraining.
   ② It is not necessary for the patient to understand the program for the program to be successful.
   ③ Laxatives are never used with bowel retraining.
   ④ Regular days and times must be strictly followed to establish a pattern.

84. Application, implementation, coping and adaptation (c)
   ❹ The best thing a nurse can do for a patient with disorientation and anxiety is limit the staff and people who have contact with him.
   ① When a patient is agitated and disoriented, he is not capable of making his own care decisions.
   ② Asking the physician for a restraint order or medications should be done only as a last resort.
   ③ Orienting the patient to time, place, and person can add to his agitation.

85. Knowledge, assessment, psychosocial adaptation (c)
   ❸ Korsakoff's psychosis is a form of amnesia seen in advanced alcoholism; the person is unable to learn new skills and suffers from short-term memory loss.
   ① Addiction is defined as compulsive, uncontrollable dependence on a substance or habit.
   ② Habituation is defined as a psychological and emotional dependence on a drug, tobacco, or alcohol substance without the need to increase the dosage.
   ④ In Wernicke's encephalopathy, there are lesions in several areas of the brain that cause the brain to deteriorate.

86. Comprehension, assessment, pharmacological therapies (b)
   ❸ Tardive dyskinesia is an irreversible syndrome of involuntary movements of the face, trunk, and extremities associated with antipsychotic medications.
   ① Cowling's rule is a method of calculating pediatric drug dosages.
   ② Chvostek's sign is a spasm of facial muscles when the cheek is stroked; it is seen in tetany.
   ④ Sjögren's syndrome is a group of symptoms including rheumatoid arthritis and xerostomia seen in postmenopausal women.

87. Application, implementation, coping and adaptation (b)
   ❶ Using open-ended questions by picking a key word used by the patient (dying) is a good way to lead to more sharing.
   ② The patient said this to the nurse, not the family. The nurse needs to pursue fears here and now. Many AIDS patients are abandoned by their families, and the nurse does not know the situation in this case.
   ③ This would be a cop-out by the nurse and is not an appropriate response at this time.
   ④ This is not true. Depression may be repressed anger. Talking may or may not help one feel better when dealing with death.

88. Application, implementation, safety and infection control (b)
    ❸ This is correct per the 1993 changes instituted by the American Heart Association.
    ① Incorrect; eight back blows and eight chest thrusts were never a recommended sequence for obstructed airway in an infant.
    ② Incorrect; six back blows and six chest thrusts were never a recommended sequence for obstructed airway in an infant.
    ④ Incorrect; four back blows and four chest thrusts were the recommended sequence for obstructed airway in an infant *before the changes instituted early in 1993.*

89. Application, implementation, pharmacological therapies (b)
    ❸ In assisting the physician, the nurse would prepare an IV fluid administration set and fluids (as ordered) for the immediate replacement of fluids lost from the burn site(s).
    ①, ②, ④ These are correct but not vital at this time.

90. Comprehension, assessment, reduction of risk potential (a)
    ❹ An immediate physical observation of a person burned in the area of the face is assessment of respiration (difficulty, rate, sound).
    ①, ②, ③ These are not immediate physical observations during an emergency.

91. Comprehension, assessment, coping and adaptation (a)
    ❷ A preschooler enjoys the close family relationship of mealtimes. Parents are usually the significant persons during the preschool years. Since his parents are dead, his grandmother will become the significant person in his life now.
    ① Not for his age group.
    ③, ④ These would be inappropriate before attempting #2.

92. Knowledge, planning, psychosocial adaptation (a)
    ❹ This lets him share, yet gives him his own special time.
    ① The parents should not separate him from the major activity (newborn) at this time; poor timing of such a plan.
    ② Presents will not substitute for presumed neglect or inattention.
    ③ They should never force a child to cuddle and kiss someone he feels is threatening.

93. Comprehension, assessment, coordinated care (b)
    ❹ The demands of the nurse lead to increased anxiety rather than a reduction of it.
    ① The patient may not be aware of her limitations.
    ② This is not specifically related to the situation.
    ③ This is not related to situation.

94. Comprehension, evaluation, coping and adaptation (a)
    ❷ Depression is a natural response to catastrophic illness. Other psychological problems manifested by cerebral damage include emotional lability, hostility, frustration, and noncooperation.
    ①, ③, ④ These are inappropriate nursing responses showing clearly that the nurse lacks understanding of the disease process.

95. Comprehension, planning, physiological adaptation (a)
    ❶ Bed rest promotes liver regeneration and increased blood filtration through the liver.

② Enteric precautions and proper hygiene prevent the spread of the virus.
③ Cardiac effort is reduced, but the primary aim is to rest the liver.
④ This will not reduce the risk of hepatic coma.

96. Comprehension, implementation, coordinated care (b)
    ❹ Glomerulonephritis usually results from an immune reaction to a streptococcal infection.
    ① Glomerulonephritis is not an infectious disease.
    ② Glomerulonephritis is not caused by a drug reaction.
    ③ Glomerulonephritis is not an inherited disease.

97. Comprehension, implementation, pharmacological therapies (b)
    ❸ It may take as long as 12 weeks for antidepressants to achieve their full therapeutic effect.
    ① There is no reason to limit fluids while taking antidepressants.
    ② Dry mouth and orthostatic hypotension are common bothersome side-effects of antidepressants.
    ④ If the first antidepressant fails to control depression, other effective medications are available.

98. Knowledge, planning, safety and infection control (c)
    ❷ Alternatives to restraints should be tried before resorting to restraints.
    ① Restraints are to be used only for a specific period of time.
    ③ Restraints should be removed at least every 2 hours to allow for activities of daily living.
    ④ Restraints should be tied with knots that can be quickly released and secured to parts of the bed that move with the patient.

99. Comprehension, planning, reduction of risk potential (b)
    ❷ Ambulation stimulates circulation and prevents the formation of thrombi, besides aiding in breaking up clots.
    ① This is to relieve pain, promote healing, and prevent infection.
    ③ Splinting helps to diminish pain and discomfort.
    ④ Keeping urinary functions at a maximum aids in promoting involution, and offering stool softeners relieves initial pain and discomfort during the postpartum period.

100. Knowledge, implementation, basic care and comfort (a)
    ❷ This is the first priority.
    ① This is not first priority.
    ③ Physician knows; it is not necessary to do test unless the nurse is asked.
    ④ Pads are not used during labor and delivery.

101. Knowledge, assessment, psychosocial adaptation (b)
    ❹ Trust vs. mistrust is Erikson's first stage.
    ① This is appropriate for a later stage.
    ② This is Sullivan's theory, not Erikson's.
    ③ This is Freudian theory.

102. Knowledge, comprehension, safety and infection control (b)
    ❷ This is a true statement.
    ① Though highly contagious, there must be direct bloodstream contact with the virus.
    ③ The fetus of an HIV-infected pregnant mother is likely to become infected.
    ④ It is important that all nursing personnel familiarize themselves with all aspects of AIDS.

103. Knowledge, implementation, growth and development through the life span (a)
❸ These foods, including favorites of teenagers, are very high in fat. The fat is known as invisible or hidden fat because one cannot see it.
① These foods are very low sources of fat.
② These foods have only a trace of fat.
④ These foods have 1 gram total fat per serving.

104. Comprehension, assessment, physiological adaptation (a)
❸ These signs are normal for a 2-day-old newborn.
① This is a full-term infant, so she cannot be premature.
② There is no indication in the situation that the infant is immature.
④ Nothing abnormal is reported in the situation.

105. Knowledge, assessment, physiological adaptation (b)
❹ The hemoglobin is decreased, not increased, in sickle cell crisis.
①, ②, ③ These are common symptoms of sickle cell crisis.

106. Application, assessment, basic care and comfort (b)
❸ The nurse should raise the head of the bed first, because many times this will bring a patient back in control of his respirations. It will make breathing easier.
① The nurse should take vital signs after raising the head of the bed, or the shortness of breath will continue.
② It is not necessary to call for help unless he does not respond to raising the head of the bed.
④ His health history should already be documented and on the chart. To determine if he has been short of breath before is not necessary, as this goes along with the disease process of cystic fibrosis.

107. Application, assessment, reduction of risk potential (b)
❹ Excessive urination is one of the classic signs and symptoms that blood sugar levels may be off.
① Refusing to bathe is no indication that diabetes is out of control.
② A cough does not indicate that diabetes needs to be checked.
③ One diarrhea stool last week does not need further assessment.

108. Comprehension, planning, basic care and comfort (b)
❸ Protein is limited to help reduce the amount of excretory work demanded of the kidneys.
① Fats are not restricted. They are necessary to fulfill energy requirements and should be polyunsaturated.
② Calcium supplements may be prescribed to prevent osteomalacia. Calcium is not restricted.
④ Carbohydrates are not restricted and are used to fulfill energy requirements. If energy requirements are not met by fats and carbohydrates, ingested protein or body tissue will be metabolized for energy.

109. Comprehension, planning, pharmacological therapies (b)
❸ Lidocaine is the drug of choice for ventricular arrhythmias; it depresses ventricular irritability.
① Inderal is a beta-adrenergic blocking agent that depresses cardiac function; it is contraindicated in ventricular arrhythmias.
② Digoxin is a drug used to strengthen ventricular contractions.
④ Morphine sulfate will not prevent or help arrhythmias.

110. Knowledge, assessment, pharmacological therapies (c)
❶ Antabuse has been known to cause acne. This is a common side effect that will usually disappear as the body adjusts to the drug.
② Antabuse usually causes fatigue and energy loss.
③ Antabuse gives foods a metallic aftertaste.
④ Antabuse causes drowsiness and is not known to cause nightmares or sleep disturbances.

111. Comprehension, assessment, reduction of risk potential (b)
❹ Anticoagulants can cause blood to show up in urine.
① Diuretics alter the urine quantity output.
② Pyridium will alter the urine color to a red or orange color but will not test positive for blood.
③ Macrodantin alters the color of urine to a harmless brown.

112. Knowledge, assessment, safety and infection control (b)
❷ Legal standards of nursing are developed by legislative actions.
① State boards of nursing and other agencies accredit nursing programs.
③ Licensure ensures minimal safety performance of nurses.
④ Professional organizations set ethical standards for nurses.

113. Knowledge, planning, pharmacological therapies (c)
❷ Urecholine (bethanecol chloride) is a cholinergic that has side usage for urinary bladder retention, as long as the cause is not an obstruction.
① Mestinon is a cholinergic drug used in myasthenia gravis.
③ Pilocarpine is a cholinergic used in the treatment of glaucoma.
④ Pro-Banthine is used in adjunctive therapy to treat peptic ulcer.

114. Knowledge, assessment, basic care and comfort (a)
❷ Cholesterol is found in blood and body cells, especially brain and nervous tissue.
① It should not nor can it be eliminated totally from the diet.
③ It is necessary for normal body functioning.
④ It is mainly through animal sources—meat, eggs, and saturated fats.

115. Comprehension, planning, reduction of risk potential (c)
❸ Brachial artery is the supplying artery; this is done when application of direct pressure does not control bleeding.
① Tourniquets are not recommended unless an extremity is amputated or severely mutilated.
② Direct pressure has already been applied unsuccessfully.
④ This is not the immediate supplying artery.

116. Application, implementation, basic care and comfort (b)
❸ A warm sitz bath is recommended to help with pain and comfort after a cystoscopy.
① There are no diet restrictions after having had a cystoscopy.
② One is to increase fluid intake after a cystoscopy.
④ One is to increase fluid intake after a cystoscopy, not decrease the fluid intake.

117. Comprehension, planning, psychosocial adaptation (c)
❶ Modesty and sensitivity are of prime importance to this age group.
②, ④ This is part of the normal admission procedure for any age group.
③ Not so for this age group.

118. Comprehension, assessment, reduction of risk potential (c)
❹ The elderly have a higher percentage of body fat, which affects the metabolism and storage of medications.
① The elderly have a lower percentage of body water.
② The elderly have a decrease in lean muscle mass.
③ The elderly have a higher percentage of body fat.

119. Application, planning, safety and infection control (c)
❷ Validating the feelings that are being manifested by the wandering behavior allows the client to feel understood. Distraction allows the client to expend energy in something other than wandering.
① Reality orientation is not effective in demented clients.
③ Attempting to restrain the client may lead to a catastrophic event.
④ Safety needs of the individual cannot be met in an open, free environment.

120. Comprehension, planning, physiological adaptation (b)
❷ The presence of an infection triggers the sympathetic nervous system, which converts glycogen into glucose. The blood glucose levels will rise, thus requiring more insulin.
① Less insulin will only worsen the hyperglycemia.
③ Protein is spilled into the urine when severe kidney damage has occurred.
④ Hyperglycemia occurs, not hypoglycemia.

121. Comprehension, planning, reduction of risk potential (c)
❸ Abrupt onset of confusion relates to side-effects of antihistamine, benzodiazepine, beta blocker, and cardiac glycoside combination.

① This would not resolve the situation.
② This would not resolve the situation and is not necessary.
④ This is not necessary.

122. Application, assessment, safety and infection control (a)
❷ Pulse rate is below 60 beats/min.
①, ③, ④ These could lead to adverse reactions.

123. Knowledge, assessment, physiological adaptation (a)
❶ Dietary requirements for a diabetic patient are calculated on the basis of age, sex, body build, weight, and activity. They should be the same as those of a nondiabetic patient.
② The diet will be lower in calories only if the diabetic patient is overweight.
③ The diabetic diet contains approximately 50% to 60% carbohydrates, equal to a well-balanced diet of a nondiabetic patient.
④ The diet should be equal in protein to that of a nondiabetic patient.

124. Application, implementation, pharmacological therapies (a)
❷ DD = 4 mg
DH = 10 mg
V = 1 ml
$$\frac{DD}{DH} = \frac{4\ mg}{10\ mg \times 1\ ml} = 0.4\ ml.$$
①, ③, ④ This is not the correct amount.

125. Application, implementation, safety and infection control (a)
❷ $$\frac{Weight\ in\ pounds\ (30) \times Adult\ dose\ (10\ mg)}{150} =$$
$$\frac{300}{150} = 2\ mg.$$
①, ③, ④ This is not the correct answer.

COMPREHENSIVE EXAMINATION 2: PART 2

1. Comprehension, assessment, reduction of risk potential (b)
   ❹ An increase in potassium can result in cardiac irregularities.
   ① An increase in calcium has side effects, but they are not as serious as potassium.
   ② An increase in chloride does not have significant side effects.
   ③ An increase in sodium has side effects, but they are not as serious as potassium.

2. Knowledge, planning, reduction of risk potential (a)
   ❹ Drainage should always be kept below chest level to prevent backflow.
   ① The tube should never be disconnected; air will rush into the thoracic cavity and collapse the lung.
   ② Physicians do not need to be present during a routine transfer.
   ③ Placing the drainage above chest level will result in backflow.

3. Analysis, evaluation, reduction of risk potential (c)
   ❹ Altered levels of consciousness are the first warning signs of increased intracranial pressure.
   ① He may have a mental illness, but the first priority is to rule out a physical cause for his changes in behavior.
   ② The signs and symptoms of fat embolism are tachypnea, dyspnea, and petechiae.
   ③ The signs and symptoms of compartment syndrome are absent pulse, cool temperature, and parasthesia.

4. Knowledge, implementation, safety and infection control (a)
   ❷ Two persons to assist will maintain safety and provide assistance should the patient become dizzy.
   ① One person cannot provide adequate assistance in the case of a fall.
   ③ Giving a narcotic will relieve any pain but may contribute to potential falls.
   ④ The patient should never dangle alone for the first time postoperatively; this is extremely unsafe.

5. Knowledge, planning, prevention and early detection of disease (a)
   ❷ Nicotine is a potent vasoconstrictor, and the further narrowing of the arterial walls will worsen peripheral vascular disease.
   ① Smoke causes hypertension, not hypotension.
   ③ Smoke does irritate the lungs, but this is not the mechanism by which it worsens peripheral vascular disease.
   ④ Smoke does not decrease RBC.

6. Knowledge, planning, reduction of risk potential (a)
   ❹ Thrombocytopenia is a decreased number of platelets, which could cause bleeding problems.
   ① Anemia is caused by decreased numbers of RBCs.
   ② Leukemia does not physiologically cause anxiety.
   ③ Infection could be due to a decreased number of WBCs.

7. Knowledge, implementation, basic care and comfort (a)
   ❸ Cold is vasoconstricting and will reduce swelling and therefore pain.
   ① Aspiration of edema in the soft tissues cannot be done.
   ② Heat is vasodilating and will increase swelling immediately after the injuries.
   ④ Soft-tissues injuries often cannot be immobilized.

8. Knowledge, implementation, reduction of risk potential (b)
   ❷ Penetrating eye injuries are treated by covering both eyes (to prevent eye movement) and seeking a physician to remove the object.
   ① The nurse should never remove the object herself; this can cause further injury.
   ③ Covering only one eye will still allow movement in the affected eye, which could cause further injury and pain.
   ④ Irrigation is used to remove non-penetrating foreign bodies in the eye.

9. Comprehension, implementation, reduction of risk potential (b)
   ❸ Emergency care for a patient with autonomic dysreflexia involves placing the patient in an upright position immediately to help decrease the hypertension.
   ① The second priority is to check for any trigger to the autonomic dysreflexia.
   ② The third priority is to administer medication to reduce blood pressure. This is not the first priority because medications can cause side effects so the nurse should attempt non-pharmacological measures first.
   ④ Placing the patient in a supine position will worsen the hypertension.

10. Knowledge, planning, safety and infection control (a)
    ❸ Enemas 'til clear are ordered to flush out the bowel and remove fecal bacteria that could contaminate the surgical site.
    ① Enemas will loosen an impaction, but that is not why they are ordered preoperatively.
    ② Paralytic ileus is due to the nature of the surgery and anesthetic effects; enemas given preoperatively will not prevent this.
    ④ Enemas given preoperatively will not prevent possible injury to the colon.

11. Comprehension, planning, reduction of risk potential (b)
    ❸ Increasing the oral intake to 3000 cc/day will help prevent constipation and possible impaction.
    ① IV fluids of 50 cc/hr (1200 cc/day) are not sufficient to prevent constipation.
    ② Drinking 1000 cc/day is not sufficient to prevent constipation.
    ④ Enemas are intrusive, potentially dangerous, and treat rather than prevent the constipation.

12. Comprehension, knowledge, safety and infection control (a)
    ❷ The client will be able to get out of bed and pivot into a chair with no weight bearing on the affected leg.
    ① Bed rest is not needed and increases the risk of deep-vein thrombosis.
    ③ Full weight bearing is not appropriate immediately postoperative.
    ④ No skeletal traction is utilized for this type of procedure.

13. Comprehension, assessment, reduction of risk potential (b)
    ❷ Hypocalcemia can occur after a thyroidectomy due to inadvertent removal of parathyroid tissue. The signs and symptoms of this complication are numbness and tingling of fingertips, toes, and lips, carpopedal spasms, tachycardia, tachypnea, and hypertension.
    ① Hyperglycemia is not a usual consequence of thyroid surgery, and the signs and symptoms are polydipsia, polyuria, and polyphagia.
    ③ Hyperkalemia is not a usual consequence of thyroid surgery, and the signs and symptoms would include cardiac rhythm disturbances.
    ④ Thyroid storm can occur postsurgically, but it is characterized by severe tachycardia, severe hypertension, and hyperthermia.

14. Comprehension, planning, reduction of risk potential (b)
    ❸ Altered tissue perfusion is a consequence of the hypotension and subsequent cardiovascular collapse seen in anaphylactic shock; this is a life-threatening process and therefore takes priority.
    ①, ④ These are not a priority focus.
    ② Falls or other injuries could occur as the patient collapses, but this is not the priority concern; the nurse needs to focus on preventing the collapse.

15. Comprehension, assessment, reduction of risk potential (b)
    ❸ Facial burns are associated with smoke and fire inhalation, which could produce life-threatening respiratory complications.
    ① Bradycardia is not associated with burns.
    ② Hypertension could occur due to IV fluid resuscitation but is not the most important assessment.
    ④ This could be a sign of hypoxia, but that would also indicate respiratory problems.

16. Application, assessment, reduction of risk potential (a)
    ❷ The standard assessment model for any emergency situation is always ABC—airway, breathing, circulation. The patient must have an open airway to have effective breathing, and effective breathing must be present to have effective circulation.
    ①, ③, ④ This is not the correct sequence.

17. Comprehension, planning, reduction of risk potential (b)
    ❸ An ileal conduit plants ureters onto a loop of the ileum, which is then brought to the surface of the abdominal wall. Because of urine drainage, skin integrity can be compromised.
    ① Limited acid-ash food diets are used to minimize the development of urinary stones.
    ② No foreign tissue has been transplanted in this procedure.
    ④ Fluid and electrolyte balance is not usually affected by ileal conduit surgery.

18. Comprehension, assessment, physiological adaptation (a)
    ❷ Fluid balance and removal of excess fluids is one of the primary goals of dialysis. Comparing predialysis and postdialysis weights will measure the effectiveness of therapy.
    ① Benadryl is not routinely given for dialysis.
    ③ Urinalysis is not necessary since blood tests are used to measure kidney function.
    ④ Patients do not need to be NPO.

19. Comprehension, assessment, reduction of risk potential (a)
    ❹ The chief danger in abdominal trauma is hemorrhage. Blood in the urine can indicate bladder trauma.
    ① Pus in the urine is usually due to infection.
    ② Difficulty voiding and pain on urination is usually a problem with the prostate or a urinary tract infection.
    ③ Excessive urine is usually due to fluid overload or the administration of a diuretic.

20. Comprehension, planning, basic care and comfort (a)
    ❹ Comatose patients can still hear what is being said and may react to that physiologically.
    ①, ③ There are no data to support this.
    ② The family may be upset by bad news, but that is not the reason to avoid bedside conversation.

21. Knowledge, planning, psychosocial adaptation (a)
    ❸ It aids in family grieving and allows the family to feel useful.
    ① There is no evidence to support the prolongation of the dying process.
    ② Actually, it increases the workload, because the nurse must assist the family and their psychosocial needs.
    ④ Family members often want to help and don't view it as work.

22. Knowledge, assessment, reduction of risk potential (b)
    ❸ Angina is the most frequent presenting symptom of coronary artery disease in women.
    ① Mitral valve prolapse occurs more frequently in women, but it is not a sign of coronary artery disease.
    ② Endocarditis usually has fever, chest pain, and shortness of breath as symptoms.
    ④ Myocardial infarction is the most common indicator in men of coronary artery disease.

23. Knowledge, implementation, basic care and comfort (a)
    ❷ The inner cannula is removed and hydrogen peroxide used to break up the dried mucus.
    ① Q-Tips are never used because they can leave behind tiny cotton fibers, which could be inhaled.
    ③, ④ The outer cannula is never removed.

24. Knowledge, planning, reduction of risk potential (a)
    ❹ Heavy lifting (over 5 pounds) is to be avoided because healing will be hindered.
    ① Non-pharmacologic measures and OTC analgesics would be recommended for pain control.
    ② Breathing exercises are performed three to four times per day.
    ③ Smoking is an irritant to lung tissue and is prohibited.

25. Comprehension, planning, reduction of risk potential (b)
    ❸ This is an appropriate discharge instruction; Kegel exercises help strengthen the perineal floor muscles.
    ① This is an unsafe instruction that may cause further bleeding.
    ② This is an unsafe instruction; fluids should be encouraged to 10 to 12 glasses a day.
    ④ This is an unsafe instruction; any increased redness of the urine should be reported as it may indicate hemorrhage.

26. Comprehension, implementation, reduction of risk potential (b)
    ❹ The client with aplastic anemia is extremely susceptible to infection and to bleeding. Administering medications orally does not traumatize tissue.
    ①, ②, ③ These routes invite the risk of bleeding or infection.

27. Comprehension, implementation, coping and adaptation (b)
    ❶ Progressive dementia is associated with deteriorating language and communication skills. Reframing vocal outbursts is essential to effective assessment and care. Loud, busy environments may precipitate vocal outbursts. The nurse must probe for underlying meanings; the best way to accomplish this is to remain calm and in control.
    ② This may exacerbate the vocalizations as loud environments frequently intensify vocal outbursts in the cognitively impaired.
    ③ This would be overstimulation, and demands by the nurse will only intensify the vocalizations; demanding environments may intensify vocal outbursts.
    ④ To ignore the vocalizations is to ignore the patient; every effort should be made to probe the meaning underlying the disruptive communication.

28. Application, implementation, basic care and comfort (b)
    ❸ A dietary record will assist the nurse in determining problem areas.
    ① This intervention will promote salivation but does not affect food/caloric intake.
    ② This intervention will promote elasticity of the skin but does not affect food/caloric intake.
    ④ This is an appropriate intervention for the diagnosis altered nutrition: more than body requirements.

29. Comprehension, assessment, basic care and comfort (a)
    ❸ Indigestion after eating food high in fat is a characteristic sign of cholecystitis and cholelithiasis. This is because the decreased amount of bile decreases fat absorption.
    ① Gas is a normal characteristic.
    ② Heartburn is characteristic of GERD (gastroesophageal reflux disease).
    ④ This is also characteristic of GERD.

30. Comprehension, evaluation, reduction of risk potential (c)
    ❸ A Whipple procedure, also known as a pancreatoduodenectomy, involves the removal of part of the pancreas. Since insulin is produced by the pancreas, blood glucose levels may be affected.
    ① Monitoring renal function is done for all surgeries.
    ② Chest tubes are not normally found with a Whipple procedure.
    ④ Monitoring H&H is done for all surgeries.

31. Comprehension, implementation, reduction of risk potential (b)
    ❸ T-tubes allow for drainage of bile until the common bile duct edema is resolved. If the common bile duct is not open, clamping the T-tube traps bile and results in nausea and vomiting. Unclamping the T-tube will resolve this problem.

① This will help the symptoms but not resolve the cause of the problem.
②, ④ This has no effect on bile drainage.

32. Knowledge, assessment, basic care and comfort (a)
    ❷ In pelvic traction the knees are never supported by pillows. This interferes with the correct line of pull necessary to align and stabilize the fracture.
    ①, ③, ④ This is normal and expected.

33. Comprehension, implementation, physiological adaptation (b)
    ❸ Hemianopsia is blindness of half of the visual field. In order for the patient to maximize eyesight, it is necessary to scan the environment.
    ① This will further blind the patient.
    ② Both eyes have lost half the vision.
    ④ The problem is not dry corneas.

34. Knowledge, assessment, basic care and comfort (a)
    ❶ In the assessment phase, the nurse observes the physiological, psychosocial, health, and safety needs of clients.
    ② Teaching is part of nursing intervention.
    ③ Prioritizing problems is part of the planning phase.
    ④ Collaborating to determine a plan of care if part of the planning phase.

35. Knowledge, implementation, safety and infection control (a)
    ❶ No metal objects can be subjected to an MRI field.
    ②, ③, ④ Not necessary for an MRI.

36. Knowledge, planning, pharmacological therapies (c)
    ❹ Nitroprusside (Nipride) is preferred because of its quick vasoactivity and short half-life.
    ① Propanalol hydrochloride (Inderal) is a maintenance drug for hypertension.
    ② Enalapril maleate (Vasotec) is primarily used for maintenance therapy of hypertension.
    ③ Nifedipine (Procardia) is used as a maintenance drug for hypertension.

37. Comprehension, implementation, reduction of risk potential (a)
    ❷ Coffee-grounds emesis is a sign of GI hemorrhage, a potential life-threatening emergency.
    ① Heartburn is a sign of gastroesophageal reflux disease (GERD) and is not life threatening.
    ③ Belching and flatulence are generally signs of food intolerance.
    ④ Pain when the stomach is empty is a sign of a duodenal ulcer.

38. Comprehension, planning, physiological adaptation (b)
    ❸ The nurse should first raise the oxygen level and prevent potential brain damage from hypoxia.
    ① CBC will help the diagnosis but is not necessary to do first.
    ② IV fluids will replace lost blood volume, but that blood needs to be oxygenated.
    ④ NG tube will remove the excess blood from the GI tract but is not necessary to do first.

39. Application, implementation, pharmacological therapies (b)
    ❸ This is correct; 7.5 mg/x × 2 cc/10 mg = 1.5 cc.
    ①, ②, ③ These are incorrect.

40. Comprehension, planning, pharmacological therapies (c)
❹ Dobutrex increases cardiac contractility. Decreased contractility is the basic mechanism of heart failure.
① Intropin at doses greater than 5 mcg/kg/min cause vasoconstriction and increases arterial blood pressure. This would increase afterload, making the already weak heart work harder. Doses less than 5 mcg/kg/min would increase renal artery perfusion. Neither dosage would directly improve myocardial contractility.
② Lasix would increase the urinary output and decrease preload, but it would not directly increase myocardial contractility.
③ Nipride causes vasodilation and is used to treat hypertensive crisis.

41. Knowledge, assessment, safety and infection control (a)
❷ Because needles are utilized, the risk of hepatitis would exclude the individual.
① A weight less than 110 pounds would exclude donation.
③ Pregnancy within the last 6 months would exclude donation.
④ A hemaglobin level less than 12.5 gm/dl in a woman would exclude donation.

42. Comprehension, planning, physiological adaptation (b)
❹ Rest periods should be scheduled when her medication levels are low. She should learn to space her tasks in conjunction with her medication.
① Diet is not a consideration in myasthenia gravis; the patient may eat what she wishes.
② Medications should be administered 1 hour before meals in order to provide energy for chewing.
③ Ultraviolet light has been known to trigger myasthenic crisis.

43. Comprehension, implementation, physiological adaptation (c)
❶ Since the patient is having difficulty swallowing, this position will create a gravity force for downward motion of food.
② This position would put him in danger of injury if he should fall.
③ This position would not help his dysphagia.
④ This position would not help.

44. Comprehension, planning, pharmacological therapies (b)
❶ IV valium is the drug of choice for status epilepticus. It is a strong anticonvulsant probably due to potentiating gamma-aminobutyric acid (GABA), which inhibits neurotransmitters.
② Tegretol is given by mouth; it is useful in the prevention of seizures.
③ Lithium is given for bipolar disorder; not used for treatment of seizures.
④ Magnesium sulfate is useful in eclamptic seizures.

45. Application, implementation, reduction of risk potential (a)
❶ Lying the patient on the side lessens the danger of aspiration of secretions.
②, ③, ④ These are not practical and could cause injury to the patient in a postictal state.

46. Comprehension, planning, physiological adaptation (c)
❶ When the body is undergoing increased stress such as with a stroke, myocardial infarction, or any other severe illness, the stomach secretes more gastric juices, which are irritating to the gastric mucosa and may result in an ulcer.
② Hyposecretion would not cause gastric irritation or bleeding.
③ No information was given about medications. Aspirin, which is frequently given as a blood thinner, can cause gastric irritation but not usually bowel irritation.
④ Hemorrhoids can develop as a result of constipation, but information was not given that the client was constipated.

47. Comprehension, assessment, prevention and early detection of disease (b)
❶ Dehydration may lead to stasis and/or a hypercoagulability state. Other risk factors include sickle cell disease, coagulation disorders, hypothyroidism, and oral contraceptive use.
②, ④ There is not a common link between these states and CVA or TIA.
③ There has been a link with hypothyroidism and CVA/TIA but not with hyperthyroidism.

48. Analysis, evaluation, physiological adaptation (b)
❶ The muscle rigidity caused by the involuntary contraction of striated muscles may inhibit fluid voluntary movement. This results in the "cogwheel" jerking motor contractions that are a characteristic manifestation of this disease.
② Movement may appear weak, especially when the client is fatigued.
③ The tremors associated with Parkinson's usually lessen with voluntary movement.
④ The goal is to get the client as physically active as long as possible.

49. Comprehension, implementation, basic care and comfort (c)
❸ Distraction theory involves anything that distracts the patient from the pain. It is only useful for mild pain and should not be attempted in moderate to severe pain. It includes relaxation techniques and slow, rhythmic breathing as well as guided imagery.
① The gate-control theory states that all pain goes through a gate that can be cut off by sensory stimulation of fibers other than the source. Use of the TENS unit or the application of Ben-Gay ointment are examples.
② The specificity theory is obsolete; it does not explain the differences in individuals' interpretation of pain.
④ This theory is applicable to the contraction of a muscle and has nothing to do with pain relief.

50. Analysis, evaluation, pharmacological therapies (b)
❶ There has been an unexpected change in the patient's condition, especially with the confusion, so the physician has to be notified.
② This would be negligent.
③ Reality orientation is in order but is not a priority.

④ The elderly do not absorb drugs the same as younger adults do. However, simply observing would be negligent since the physician has to be kept current; the medication may not be causing the confusion.

51. Application, evaluation, prevention and early detection of disease (b)
    ❶ A 5-mm area of enduration is positive for people who are in close contact with an individual who has active TB and it is positive for those who have HIV infection. It is considered negative in all others. Therefore, the nurse would need to gather more information.
    ② The nurse is unaware of the patient's recent contacts and should assess further; see rationale for #1.
    ③ A repeat is not necessary for most people. A two-step testing procedure is sometimes done on the elderly. The test is repeated routinely due to the elderly's slower immune response. It is seldom done on an individual under 65. A chest x-ray would be ordered instead.
    ④ This may or may not be true; see rationale for #1.

52. Knowledge, implementation, prevention and early detection of disease (a)
    ❹ Coryza (common cold) is caused by one of several viruses that are in the upper respiratory tract at all times.
    ① Each infection is caused by a specific virus, not by a bacterium.
    ② Susceptibility increases with aging.
    ③ Symptoms appear in 24-48 hours after exposure.

53. Knowledge, planning, prevention and early detection of disease (a)
    ❸ The test has to be read in 48 to 72 hours.
    ① Health services is not open on Tuesday.
    ② The test would have to be read on Friday, and health services is not open.
    ④ The test would have to be read on Saturday or Sunday; health services is not open on those days.

54. Knowledge, implementation, basic care and comfort (a)
    ❷ The patient is fasting for a blood sugar test, which means she gets no food. If she eats, the food will be converted to glucose and quickly enter her bloodstream. Her glucose level will rise rapidly, and the test would not be valid.
    ① The patient may not know what NPO means.
    ③ The urine has nothing to do with this particular test.
    ④ The client is to be fasting, with no food and no fluids.

55. Comprehension, assessment, reduction of risk potential (c)
    ❷ The patient is experiencing an aura, which can appear as any sensory sensation. An aura is a precursor to a seizure. The nurse will have her immediately lie down in order to protect her from injury should she fall.
    ① The nurse would note her comments later but needs to stay with her at this point; there is no need to contact a psychiatrist.
    ③ IV Valium would probably be given, but only with an order.
    ④ Her medical doctor would be called to inform him of the seizure, but this would be done later.

56. Comprehension, planning, basic care and comfort (b)
    ❶ Patients with Parkinson's disease are at risk of aspiration and impaired swallowing. This position enhances swallowing, as well as the propelling of food down the esophagus with gravity.
    ② The patient should be receiving a low-protein diet during the day and a little higher in the evening due to the fact that protein binds up the L-Dopa. Milk is high in protein.
    ③ The patient needs to be as independent as possible.
    ④ L-Dopa should be administered 45 minutes prior to eating.

57. Comprehension, planning, reduction of risk potential (b)
    ❹ Elevated blood sugar levels enhance bacterial growth in the vagina and urinary tract; increased fluid intake helps to wash away the bacteria in the urine.
    ① Cotton underwear should be worn since air can flow through its fibers.
    ② A water-soluble lubricant should be used such as KY jelly; an oil-based lubricant retains bacteria.
    ③ Tight jeans rub the perineal area and are irritating.

58. Analysis, evaluation, physiological adaptation (c)
    ❶ One of the purposes of the four-bottle technique is to observe the color changes in the urine to assess for blood over time. Normally, the urine lightens in color as bleeding decreases. Therefore the oldest specimen is discarded, which would be the one to the left.
    ②, ③, ④ These choices do not follow proper procedure for such a technique; refer to the rationale for #1.

59. Knowledge, planning, physiological adaptation (b)
    ❶ Eating meat could give a false-positive result.
    ② It does not matter when the specimen is collected.
    ③ This is not necessary; the temperature of the stool will not affect the results of the test.
    ④ This will have no effect on the outcome of the test.

60. Comprehension, implementation, pharmacological therapies (b)
    ❶ Many antibiotics, including ampicillin, decrease the effects of Ortho-Novum 1/50 and other oral contraceptives.
    ② Blood sugar should be checked; ampicillin can cause a false-positive urine sugar result.
    ③ The full course of antibiotics should be completed to decrease the chances of a superinfection.
    ④ A rash is indicative of an allergic reaction and is to be observed for but is not an expected effect of treatment.

61. Comprehension, implementation, reduction of risk potential (c)
    ❹ This promotes stasis of the heart and the artery and helps to avoid bleeding or an embolus.
    ① Fluids are encouraged immediately after the procedure to wash the dye out of the system.
    ② He may ambulate 6 hours after the sheath is removed.
    ③ He can move his right leg after the procedure to whatever position is comfortable.

62. Comprehension, planning, reduction of risk potential (b)
❹ Ascites is the accumulation of fluid in the peritoneal cavity and can be quantitatively monitored by measuring the abdominal girth on a daily basis.
① Weighing daily is the best method for monitoring overall body fluid retention but is not specific to the abdominal area.
② Measuring intake and output will serve as a guideline for what amount is being retained but does not present an exact picture.
③ A decrease in the SAT level will occur as the ascites increases and pressure is put on the diaphragm. Breathing is impaired, the lungs are not well ventilated, and subsequently the patient has lower O_2 levels.

63. Application, implementation, physiological adaptation (b)
❶ Cranial nerve I (olfactory) is assessed following the technique described. A normal finding occurs when the person correctly identifies odors presented.
② Cranial nerve II (optic) is the nerve that controls sight.
③ Cranial nerve III (otic) is the oculomotor nerve.
④ Cranial nerve VII (facial) is the facial nerve and provides symmentry of facial movement.

64. Comprehension, planning, reduction of risk potential (b)
❸ The primary area of concern is respiratory function. Progressive muscle weakness that begins often in the legs and moves upward. Muscle weakness is followed by paralysis. If the diaphragm is affected, then the individual's ability to oxygenate is compromised.
① Skin breakdown is a potential problem associated with immobility and should be monitored. Airway, breathing, and circulation are considered priority areas of assessment.
②, ④ Both are potential problems as the disease progresses; see response to #1.

65. Analysis, implementation, reduction of risk potential (c)
❹ A change in neurologic status may indicate increased intracranial pressure. A thorough neurological assessment is indicated. Placing the head of bed in a slightly elevated position will aid in decreasing the pressure rise. The physician should be notified immediately in case emergency interventions are required.
① This is an inappropriate and negligent action.
② In suspected increased intracranial pressure, the head of the bed is slightly elevated to decrease intracranial pressure.
③ Preparing the patient for emergency surgery may be indicated, but the nurse must begin with assessment of the patient's status and subsequent notification of the physician.

66. Comprehension, planning, physiological adaptation (b)
❷ This is a goal statement.
① This is a nursing diagnosis.
③, ④ These are nursing interventions.

67. Application, implementation, basic care and comfort (c)
❸ Signs and symptoms of TMJ are jaw pain, pronounced muscle spasm, and tenderness of the masseter and temporalis muscles. Nursing management includes diet modifications, implementing pain control measures, and encouraging the use of a bite guard during sleep.

① The pain or clicking may be worse during yawning, however, a correct yawning technique does not exist.
② Soft foods, nutritional liquid supplements, and abstaining from foods that are difficult to chew may decrease pain.
④ This is an outcome statement not nursing intervention.

68. Comprehension, planning, physiological adaptation (b)
❸ An appropriate outcome criteria statement is intracranial pressure returns to normal (1-15 mm Hg).
① This is a nursing intervention.
② This is a nursing diagnosis.
④ This activity increases intracranial pressure and should be avoided until intracranial pressure returns to normal.

69. Knowledge, assessment, basic care and comfort (a)
❶ Assessment data relevant to seizure disorder includes obtaining a complete history, medication history, and allergy history. Data collection should be specific to the seizure disorder, such as onset, duration, behavior before and after, type of body movements, loss of consciousness, incontinence, and awareness of seizure afterward.
② Diet and exercise history is not specific to the seizure disorder.
③ Social and educational levels are not relative to this disorder.
④ Work history is not relative to this disorder.

70. Comprehension, implementation, physiological adaptation (b)
❷ Patient teaching should include instructing the patient in the importance of wearing a Medic-Alert bracelet, tag, or other medical identification. The person is taught to avoid situations known to trigger seizures such as flashing or blinking lights, stress, or lack of sleep.
① This response is an expected outcome of the nursing and medical treatment plan.
③ Persons with a diagnosis of seizure disorders are frequently evaluated many times throughout the year and should be encouraged to keep follow-up medical appointments as well as appointments to have blood drawn for lab work.
④ This response supports social stigmas associated with epilepsy. Individuals in the community need education regarding seizure disorders. Individuals with a seizure disorder are encouraged to live normal lives.

71. Comprehension, planning, pharmacological therapies (c)
❸ Abrupt withdrawal of any anticonvulsant drug may trigger status epilepticus; the drug must be gradually withdrawn.
① Hyperglycemia is not a condition associated with the withdrawal of an anticonvulsant.
② Tardive dyskinesia is associated with the administration of psychotropic drugs and characterized by slow, rhythmical, automatic stereotyped movements.
④ Parkinsonism is associated with Parkinson's disease and characterized as a fine, slowly spreading tremor; muscular weakness and rigidity; and a peculiar gait.

72. Knowledge, assessment, pharmacological therapies (a)
❸ A primary side effect of benzodiazepines is respiratory depression. Close observation of respiratory function is a priority.
① The gastrointestinal system should be assessed for decreased peristalsis, but this has a lower priority than assessment of the respiratory system.
② Urinary output will probably be decreased as a result of slowing down of system functions associated with benzodiazepines.
④ Metabolism will not be affected.

73. Comprehension, implementation, physiological adaptation (b)
❶ Appropriate nursing actions in the administration of TPN is to weigh the patient daily, monitor blood glucose levels regularly to assess the patient's ability to metabolize concentrated glucose, and wean gradually to avoid a sudden drop in blood sugar.
② This response reflects a lack of knowledge relevant to the rationale for administering TPN. The patient may express hunger sensations but may be physiologically compromised, requiring TPN for nutritional support.
③ Monitoring liver, renal, and cardiovascular function is required of any patient receiving fluids but is not specific to the administration of TPN.
④ Incorrect response; refer to #1.

74. Knowledge, assessment, safety and infection control (b)
❸ Documentation required upon discontinuing an IV is the time the IV was discontinued, the amount of fluid infused, and the appearance of the venipuncture site, which could indicate a potential problem such as phlebitis.
① The amount of fluid infused is one component of appropriate documentation. There are at least two important components missing; how the patient tolerated the procedure is not a missing component.
② This response indicates missing components, which need to be documented; the amount of fluid remaining in the bottle is not important.
④ This response is an important consideration; however, not all aspects of discontinuing the IV are listed.

75. Knowledge, planning, reduction of risk potential (a)
❹ *Emergency* surgery is required when the patient's condition is life threatening.
① *Urgent* surgery is indicated when prompt attention, usually within 24-30 hours, is necessary.
② *Elective* surgery is indicated when the patient will not be harmed if surgery is not performed but will benefit if it is performed.
③ *Required* surgery is indicated when the patient needs to have surgery at some point, e.g., for cataracts.

76. Knowledge, assessment, coordinated care (b)
❷ The nurse must first check to make sure that the physician's orders allow fluids to be given.
① This response is accomplished only after the physician's orders have been checked.
③ While this may be true, physician orders must be checked and the patient recovered enough to accept fluids.
④ This too is appropriate, but only after physician orders have been checked.

77. Comprehension, planning, psychological adaptation (b)
❶ The effect of conscious sedation requires careful monitoring of the airway; therefore, the risk for ineffective breathing pattern is appropriate.
② This response is a goal statement.
③ This response is a nursing intervention.
④ This response is an evaluation statement.

78. Comprehension, intervention, coordinated care (a)
❶ This type of fluid replacement is favored for treatment of all ages of children with infectious gastroenteritis.
②, ③, ④ Incorrect treatment for this disease.

79. Knowledge, planning, pharmacological therapies (a)
❹ Azidothymidine (AZT) (Retrovir) is approved for children and assists in slowing the progression of AIDS.
① IV gamma globulin (Gamamine N) may be used in children with AIDS to compensate for B-lymphocyte deficiency.
② Ceftazidime (Fortaz) is an antibiotic and does not affect the progression of AIDS.
③ Vancomycin (Vancocin) is an antibiotic used for severe staphylococcal infections.

80. Knowledge, assessment, physiological adaptation (a)
❸ The posterior fontanel closes by this age.
① This develops at 6 to 7 months of age.
② This develops at 8 to 9 months of age.
④ This occurs at 7 to 8 months of age.

81. Knowledge, assessment, prevention and early detection of disease (a)
❸ Although some SIDS cases occur later, most occur by 6 months of age.
①, ②, ④ This is not true of SIDS.

82. Knowledge, assessment, safety and infection control (b)
❷ Mononucleosis is an acute infectious disease caused by this virus.
① Mononucleosis is a viral disease; *Streptococcus* is a bacteria.
③ RSV is not the cause of mononucleosis; it is responsible for 50% of the cases of bronchiolitis seen in infants.
④ *H. influenzae* is not the cause of mononucleosis.

83. Application, implementation, physiological adaptation (b)
❶ Weight should be measured at the same time each day, in the same clothing.
② There is not enough information to assume this. The patient may be taking medication several times a day or at irregular intervals.
③ Daily weights are a more accurate measurement of fluid retention.
④ Daily weights will indicate early fluid retention, avoiding symptoms of advancing congestive failure.

84. Application, implementation, prevention and early detection of disease (b)
❸ Increased fluid intake decreases the tenacity of respiratory secretions, making sputum removal easier.
① Low hydration makes respiratory secretions tenacious and difficult to expel.
② Tracheal suctioning is invasive and should be employed only if the patient is unable to expel secretions independently.
④ Postural drainage relies on gravity to assist with expulsion of secretions. Affected lung areas vary and must be vertical for this to occur.

85. Comprehension, evaluation, physiological adaptation (b)
    ❹ A full assessment includes both subjective and objective data.
    ① Objective signs do not address cues that the patient himself can provide when evaluating progress.
    ② Limiting data collection to subjective information ignores the observable, measurable symptoms not offered by the patient.
    ③ Data must be gathered throughout the procedure to fully determine their effect upon the patient.

86. Comprehension, implementation, physiological adaptation (b)
    ❷ When the procedure is completed, the patient is placed on bed rest and usually lies on the unaffected side for at least 1 hour to promote expansion of the lung on the affected side.
    ①, ③ Incorrect response; see #2.
    ④ While Fowler's position may be indicated to promote adequate ventilation, lying on the unaffected side for 1 hour promotes lung expansion and is the priority.

87. Comprehension, assessment, reduction of risk potential (b)
    ❶ Increased respiratory rate, chest tightness, and hypoxemia are signs of complications following a thoracentesis and should be reported to the physician immediately.
    ② Respiratory rate would be increased, as would the pulse; hypotension would be noted.
    ③ Bradycardia is not an early sign of respiratory distress. Low blood pressure may occur secondary to removing a volume of fluid and should be monitored. A dry, hacky cough is usually not indicative of respiratory distress.
    ④ A normal sinus rhythm indicates adequate cardiac function, normotension reflects blood pressure within normal limits, and ventilation is the act of moving air into and out of the lungs.

88. Comprehension, planning, reduction of risk potential (a)
    ❶ Deep breathing and coughing exercises every 2 hours will improve lung expansion and facilitate expectoration of secretions.
    ② Bed rest every 2 hours may promote secretion accumulation. Rest and activity should be well balanced.
    ③ Sedatives should be administered cautiously due to respiratory depression.
    ④ Oral fluids should be increased to thin and liquefy secretions.

89. Knowledge, assessment, physiological adaptation (a)
    ❸ Assessment begins with first determining unresponsiveness.
    ① Activation of the emergency medical system occurs after responsiveness is determined.
    ②, ④ These actions are initiated only following determination of responsiveness.

90. Knowledge, assessment, safety and infection control (b)
    ❷ Tuberculosis is most commonly transmitted by direct contact with a person who has the active disease through inhalation of droplets produced by coughing, sneezing, or spitting. Brief contact does not usually result in infection.
    ①, ③, ④ Incorrect response; see rationale for #2.

91. Comprehension, planning, physiological adaptation (a)
    ❹ When the bile duct is explored for stones, edema could ensue and block the duct, hindering bile flow. The T-tube maintains patency.
    ①, ③ The tube is not placed in the abdominal cavity nor in the intestines.
    ② This is not the primary purpose of the tube in this situation.

92. Comprehension, planning, prevention and early detection of disease (b)
    ❷ Injury could lead to infection. The tissues are already compromised of oxygen and nutrients; certain positions (legs crossed, knees flexed) hamper circulation.
    ①, ③, ④ Measure could lead to greater compromise in circulation and burns.

93. Knowledge, assessment, psychosocial adaptation (b)
    ❷ An unknown stimulus is known to cause anxiety. Stress reactions happen when there is a source believed to be threatening and when it is not obvious to the person involved.
    ① An obvious threat causes fear, not anxiety.
    ③ Fear usually results from external threats.
    ④ Everyone experiences anxiety at some point in their lives; this can be mild, moderate, or severe.

94. Knowledge, implementation, reduction of risk potential (a)
    ❷ Suspected spinal cord injuries should be handled with care to prevent further damage to the spinal cord.
    ① Spinal cord injury is the main concern; fractures of extremities are secondary.
    ③, ④ These are not relevant to the situation.

95. Application, implementation, prevention and early detection of disease (a)
    ❷ Smoking decreases pulmonary function; sarcoidosis compromises lung capacity.
    ① Treatment should focus on healing; the patient cannot assess pulmonary function.
    ③ Physician will monitor any increased involvement; this is too complicated for the patient.
    ④ Treatment should focus on positive aspects of healing because course of disease is to resolution.

96. Application, planning, pharmacological therapies (a)
    ❷ 60 mg = 1 gr
    60 × 5 = 300 mg/tablet: 2 tablets = 600 mg.
    ①, ③, ④ Incorrect dose.

97. Comprehension, evaluation, psychosocial adaptation (c)
    ❸ The goal is inappropriate and too difficult for this type of patient.
    ① See rationale for #3.
    ② The goal itself is not too broad, just unrealistic.
    ④ It is not long-term as stated (48 hours).

98. Knowledge, planning, physiological adaptation (a)
    ❸ This is the first level of the hierarchy.
    ①, ② High level of the hierarchy.
    ④ This is the second level of the hierarchy.

99. Application, assessment, physiological adaptation (b)
    ❶ Paresthesia may result from pressure on a nerve.
    ② Volkmann's contracture affects the arm.
    ③ Dupuytren's contracture affects the hand.
    ④ Compartment syndrome occurs when there is increased fluid in an encapsulated muscle.

100. Comprehension, assessment, safety and infection control (b)
- ❷ Protecting patient safety is the highest priority, and steps need to be taken immediately with a blood sugar this high. The nurse needs to call the physician stat.
- ① Ensuring adequate rest is not a high priority when a blood sugar is too high.
- ③ Checking nutritional intake can be done after notifying the physician of the patient's blood sugar and getting orders for insulin.
- ④ Bed rest does not take priority over taking steps to notify the physician.

101. Knowledge, assessment, prevention and early detection of disease (b)
- ④ Systemic lupus erythematosus causes a red "butterfly" pattern on the face, as well as a slight fever and soreness in joints. It is believed to be an autoimmune disorder and affects collagen.
- ① Scleroderma is a condition in which the skin becomes tight and smooth. Movement becomes difficult. It is thought to be an autoimmune disorder.
- ② Raynaud's disease is a cardiovascular problem characterized by periodic constriction of arteries, usually manifested in the fingers. It can occur in the toes, causing them to become red and eventually cyanotic.
- ③ Periarteritis nodosa is a disorder that causes nodules that appear along a course of arteries. The nodules cause muscle and joint pain.

102. Application, planning, safety and infection control (c)
- ❶ This allows the nurse to perform skills completely, yet decreases the amount of time that the nurse must spend in the radioactive environment.
- ② Entering the patient's room frequently exposes the nurse to the radioactive environment: the implant should not be visible for the nurse to assess.
- ③ This increases the amount of time the nurse spends in the radioactive environment.
- ④ Although it is important to decrease the loneliness of an isolated patient, this measure would increase the amount of time the nurse is in the radioactive environment.

103. Knowledge, implementation, reduction of risk potential (a)
- ❶ Massaging the area and avoiding repeated pressure will enhance circulation.
- ②, ③, ④ This is inappropriate nursing action for pressure areas.

104. Comprehension, implementation, reduction of risk potential (a)
- ④ This will encourage circulation and alleviate pain; symptoms may be indicative of a femoral vein thrombus.
- ① This treatment has not been ordered.
- ② This is an unauthorized treatment.
- ③ The nurse should be aware of possibility of thrombus in postpartum patient; should not move leg until the physician examines it.

105. Knowledge, implementation, prevention and early detection of disease (b)
- ④ This is the best advice to give any pregnant woman, because many birth anomalies have been associated with alcohol.

- ① No alcohol during pregnancy is best; fetal alcohol syndrome is always a potential problem with drinking during pregnancy.
- ② As stated in #4, no alcoholic beverages are recommended during pregnancy. Alcohol is a drug and CNS depressant.
- ③ No alcohol during pregnancy is best; statistics show a high incidence of birth defects with moderate drinking.

106. Knowledge, assessment, psychosocial adaptation (a)
- ❷ Freud believed the struggle between internal forces to be the basis of human behavior.
- ① Freud theorized that there are three stages of ego development.
- ③ Freud did not take environmental factors into consideration to any great extent.
- ④ Freud did not give much consideration to interpersonal conflict.

107. Comprehension, assessment, psychosocial adaptation (a)
- ❸ Exaggerated ideas of one's power or influence are usually delusions of grandeur.
- ① Tactile hallucination refers to the false sense that there is something on one's skin.
- ② Flight of ideas refers to scattered thoughts, which are manifested by illogical connections made during verbalization.
- ④ Neurosis is not usually characterized by delusion.

108. Comprehension, assessment, coping and adaptation (a)
- ❸ Denial is indicated by the patient's inability to recognize the seriousness of his act and his belief that he can go home.
- ① Sublimation is the process by which negative impulses are channeled into more acceptable outlets.
- ② Projection is the placing of unacceptable impulses onto another person.
- ④ Regression is the moving back to an earlier time or developmental level during periods of stress.

109. Comprehension, assessment, psychosocial adaptation (a)
- ❷ Flight of ideas refers to scattered thoughts, as evidenced by illogical connections made during verbalizations.
- ① Confusion is usually a matter of being disoriented as to time, place, or person.
- ③ Delusions are fixed false beliefs.
- ④ Hallucinations are the perceptions of sensory stimuli when no external objects are present.

110. Knowledge, assessment, reduction of risk potential (a)
- ④ This is a correct assessment.
- ① These are not likely to be delusions.
- ② This is unlikely.
- ③ This is incorrect; symptoms may worsen.

111. Knowledge, implementation, prevention and early detection of disease (b)
- ❶ If the fetal movements felt in 1 hour while resting and doing a kick count are 3 or under, the patient needs to phone immediately. This is serious, and hypoxia may be developing.
- ② Seven or more kicks are normal but unusual when the mother is resting.
- ③, ④ These are within normal range, although 10 kicks is not unusual within a 20-minute to 2-hour period.

112. Knowledge, implementation, growth and development through the life span (a)
   ❷ This is true; it includes all pertinent phases of childbearing.
   ① This is untrue; drugs may be requested or even given when necessary, such as with dystocia.
   ③ It is preparation for labor and delivery; not necessarily "young" parents; does not include child-rearing classes.
   ④ This is more a description of the Bradley method.

113. Knowledge, assessment, basic care and comfort (b)
   ❶ Agnosia is the inability to recognize commonly used objects of daily living.
   ② Projection is a defense mechanism manifested by blaming another for one's own faults.
   ③ Displacement is a defense mechanism characterized by the rationalization of one's own actions.
   ④ Confabulation is a technique used by demented patients to fabricate explanations for events that they may not remember.

114. Knowledge, planning, growth and development through the life span (b)
   ❶ This diet provides essential nutrients that encourage tissue repair and replacement, energy for increased metabolic demands, and carbohydrates to prevent utilization of protein for energy.
   ②, ③, ④ These are inappropriate diets for this situation.

115. Comprehension, implementation, psychosocial adaptation (a)
   ❷ Informing the patient of what is expected of him during the procedure will lessen his anxiety and increase his capability to control his feelings.
   ①, ③, ④ These are inappropriate responses indicating lack of understanding and concern.

116. Knowledge, implementation, basic care and comfort (b)
   ❸ The vastus lateralis is the recommended muscle and site to be used for a patient this age.
   ① The deltoid muscle is not developed enough to safely give an IM injection in a patient this age.
   ② The gluteus maximus should not be used because it is not developed enough, and also the sciatic nerve and artery are in this area.
   ④ The patient should be over age 2 years to use the ventrogluteal area.

117. Knowledge, implementation, reduction of risk potential (b)
   ❹ The nurse needs to monitor the neurological status of a patient suspected of having encephalitis; the patient may have a seizure or go into a coma.
   ① Jaundice is not a problem with encephalitis.
   ② Blood sugars are not a problem with encephalitis unless the patient is a diabetic.
   ③ Blood pressure, like *all* vital signs, needs to be monitored closely, but the neurological status takes priority.

118. Knowledge, planning, physiological adaptation (c)
   ❹ The femur, tibia, and humerus are the bones in which osteomyelitis occurs in children.
   ① This is not commonly found in the fibula.
   ② This is not commonly found in the fibula or patella.
   ③ This is not commonly found in the patella, radius, and ulna.

119. Knowledge, assessment, reduction of risk potential (b)
   ❶ Follow rule of nines.
      Left leg = 18%
      Right leg = 18%
      Right arm = 9%
      Total = 45%
   ②, ③, ④ Does not follow rule of nines.

120. Application, implementation, safety and infection control (b)
   ❸ Roll victim in carpet or blankets to extinguish fire or use water.
   ①, ④ Victim is screaming hysterically and should not be relied on to hear or follow instructions.
   ② Extinguish the fire and have someone call the fire department.

121. Comprehension, planning, safety and infection control (a)
   ❷ Many states have Good Samaritan laws to encourage medical aid at the scene of an accident by limiting the legal liability that might arise.
   ① It is not mandatory for nurses or physicians to render emergency aid.
   ③ It is expected that the person rendering aid will act as a reasonable, prudent person would act under similar circumstances. A higher standard of medical aid would be expected of a nurse, physician, and members of a first-aid squad than that of the average general public.
   ④ Laws vary in each state.

122. Comprehension, evaluation, reduction of risk potential (b)
   ❶ Victim should be observed for laryngeal and tracheal edema because the degree of inhalation burns is unknown.
   ②, ③, ④ Characteristic of second-degree burns; it was previously determined that the victim has second-degree burns.

123. Application, planning, reduction of risk potential (b)
   ❶ A victim suspected of having an injury to the spine is never moved because of the risk of causing paralysis.
   ②, ③ Any movement may cause further damage.
   ④ This is not the proper procedure for assessing pulmonary status.

124. Comprehension, implementation, reduction of risk potential (a)
   ❶ Stop the flow of the IV fluids to prevent further swelling and report to charge nurse.
   ②, ③, ④ Inappropriate responses that will not correct the stated situation.

125. Comprehension, planning, physiological adaptation (c)
   ❸ Because of the large amount of secretions, the maintenance of a patent airway is the most important goal for this patient.
   ① Although the frequent suctioning could lead to respiratory infections, this is not the most pressing need at this time.
   ② Although a problem associated with repeated suctioning, arrhythmias are not the most pressing need at this time.
   ④ An equal intake and output is important to maintain liquifaction of secretions; however, this is not the primary concern.

INDEX

Endocrine system disorders, diagnosis of, 252-253
  nursing assessment of, 249-252
  nursing care of, 253
Endometriosis, 278
Endometrium, 277-278
Endoscopy, 228
Enemas, 39
Engagement of fetus, 408
Engle, George, grieving defined by, 372
Enteral administration, 87
Enteric fever, 602
Enteric isolation, 25
Enteritis, regional, 233-234
Enteroviral carditis, 592
Enuresis, 262
Environmental factors, 44-45
  influencing health, 21-22
Environmental hazards, reduction of, 42
Enzymes, serum, 208
Epidemic hemorrhagic conjunctivitis, 592
Epidemic viral gastroenteritis, 594
Epidermis, 283
Epididymis, 268
Epidural administration, 88
Epidural hematoma, 541
Epidural space, 241
Epiglottis, 195-196
Epiglottitis, 463
Epilepsy, 468
Epiphyseal disk, 183
Epiphysis, 183
Episiotomy, 413, 414f
Epispadias, 459
Epistaxis, 200, 539
Epithelial membranes, 183
Epithelial tissue, 182
Equipment, hospital, care of, 42
Erb-Duchenne paralysis, 421
Erb's palsy, 421
Erepsin, 227
Erikson, developmental stages of, 361, 362t-365t, 500, 501f
Erythema, 284
Erythema infectiosum, 599
Erythema toxicum neonatorum, 417
Erythrocyte indexes, 219
Erythrocyte sedimentation rate (ESR), 188, 208, 219
Erythrocytes, 207
Erythromycin, 119
Esophageal atresia, 457, 458f
Esophageal varices, 230-231
Esophagitis, 230
Esophagus, 225
ESR; *see* Erythrocyte sedimentation rate
Esteem, 26
Esthiomene, 605
Estriol level study, 392, 397
Estrogens, 115
Ethical considerations in mental illness, 374
Ethics, code of, 13

Eversion of eye, 541, 542f
Examinations, 1, 4-5, 12-13, 18
Exanthema subitum, 600
Excoriation, 284
Excretion, 89, 262
Excretory urogram, 29
Exercise needs, nursing measures for, 40-41
Exocrine glands, 249
Expectorants, 108-109
Expiration, 198
Expressive aphasia, 242
Expulsion of fetus, 408
Extended-care facilities, 20
Extension of fetus, 408
External ear, 291
External fetal monitor (EFM), 409
External radiotherapy, 50
External rotation of fetus, 408
Extracts, 87
Extradural hematoma, 541
Extrasystole, 206
Exudate, 284
Eye, foreign bodies in, 541, 542f
  injuries of, 541-542, 542f
    penetrating, 542
Eye care professionals, 289
Eyelids, contusion of, 541
Eyes, disorders of, diagnosis of, 289
  hot compresses for, 47
  nursing assessment of, 288-289
  nursing care of, 47, 289
  in toddlers, 464
  elderly hygiene of, 509
  fixed, 244
  irrigation of, 47, 47f
  lazy, 464
  medications for, 116-117
  nursing assessment of, 242

F

Facial paralysis of newborn, 421
Failure to thrive (FTT), 452
Fallopian tubes, 272
False imprisonment, 13
Family, assessment of, 450
  communal, 21
  development of, 21
  single parent, 21
Family planning, 425-426
Farsightedness, 290
Fascial membranes, 183
Fastin, adverse reactions of, 105
Fatigue, 209, 220
Favus, 592-593
FBAO; *see* Foreign body airway obstruction
FDA; *see* Food and Drug Administration
Febrile seizures, 455
Fecal impaction, digital removal of, 39
Fecal incontinence, retraining for, 518

Federal Controlled Substances Act of 1970, 14, 88
Feeding of newborns, 419
Feedings, oral, 122-123
Feet hygiene for elderly, 509-510
Female pelvis, 383f, 393
Female reproductive system, anatomy and physiology of, 271-272, 271f
  disorders of, diagnosis of, 274-275
  nursing assessment of, 272-274
  nursing care of, 275
  drugs for, 115-116
Fenfluramine hydrochloride, adverse reactions of, 105
Fertility drugs, 115
Fertilization, 393-394
Fetal monitor, external, 409
Fetoscope, 409
Fetoscopy, 392
Fetus, 394, 407-408
  circulation of, 394, 396f
  death of, 390
  heart tone of, 390, 393
  monitoring of, 409
  movement of, 393
  physiology of, 394-395
Fever blisters, 285-286
Fibrocystic breast disease, 281
Fibrous membranes, 183
Fields of vision, 289
Fifth disease, 599
Finasteride, 270
Fire prevention, 42
Fissure, 284
Fixed eyes, 244
Flaccid, 242
Flail chest, 543
Flat bones, 183
Flexion of fetus, 408
Flora, normal, 22
Fluid and electrolyte balance, 23
Fluid extracts, 87
Fluid needs, nursing measures for, 36
Fluids, 122-123
Fluoroquinolones, 120
Foams, 87
Focus charting, 26
Foley catheters, care of, 37
  removal of, 38
Folic acid deficiency anemia, 221
Follicle-stimulating hormone (FSH), 274
Fontanels, 407
Food, Drug, and Cosmetic Act, 88
Food and Drug Administration (FDA), 89
Food-drug interactions, 89
Food exchange list, ADA, 256
Food poisoning, 550
Food stamps, 490
Foods, with high sodium content, 211
  with purine, 189
  tyramine-containing, interactions of, 580

Newborns, abnormal, 419-425
  congenital malformations of, 422-423
  of diabetic mothers, 424
  drug addiction in, 424
  ecchymosis of, 420
  facial paralysis of, 421
  feeding of, 419
  hemolytic disease of, 423-424
  infections of, 422
  normal, 417-419
  rash of, 417
  reflexes of, 418
  skeletal injuries of, 420-421
  skin of, 417
  subconjunctival hemorrhage of, 420
NF; see National Formulary
NFLPN; *see* National Federation of
        Licensed Practical Nurses
Nidation, 393
Nikethamide, adverse reactions of, 105
Nitrofurantoins, 120
NLN; *see* National League for Nursing
NLNAC; *see* National League for Nursing
        Accrediting Commission
Nocturia, 262
Nodule, 284
Non-A, non-B hepatitis, 595
Non-B transfusion-associated hepatitis,
        595
Nonopioid/antiinflammatory analgesics,
        97, 99t
Nonpathogens, 21
Nonsteroidal antiinflammatory drugs, 97
Nonstress test, 393
Nonstriated muscles, 183
Nonvenereal endemic syphilis, 601
Nonverbal communication, 26
North American Nursing Diagnosis
        Association, approved nursing
        diagnoses and definitions,
        570-574
    Gordon's functional health patterns
        classification of, 577-578
    human response pattern classification
        of, 575-576
Nose, 195
Nose hygiene for elderly, 509
Nosebleed, 200, 539
Nosocomial infections, 25
Nothing by mouth after midnight (NPO
        p-MN), 29
Nothing by mouth (NPO), 29
NPO; *see* Nothing by mouth
NPO p-MN; *see* Nothing by mouth after
        midnight
NSAIDs; *see* Nonsteroidal
        antiinflammatory drugs
NST; *see* Nonstress test
Nuchal rigidity, 242
Nurse-patient relationship in mental
        health nursing, 356
Nurse Practice Act, 12

Nurses, drug addiction among, 12
Nurses' notes, 26, 26f-27f
Nursing, maternity, 389-426
  medical-surgical, 181-294
  mental health; *see* Mental health
        nursing
  pediatric, 449-478
  practical; *see* Practical/vocational
        nursing
  primary, 13
  team, 13
  trends in, 10-18
  vocational; *see* Practical/vocational
        nursing
Nursing and Health Care, 16
Nursing assessment, 28-33
  data gathering methods for, 29
  data sources for, 28-29
  nursing interventions required, 33
  in pharmacology, 86
  subjective *vs.* objective data in, 29
Nursing boards, 12, 608-612
Nursing care, functional, 13
Nursing care planning in pharmacology,
        86-88
Nursing homes, 20
Nursing organizations, 15-17
  Canadian, 18
Nursing process, 26, 28-34
Nutrients, 122-123
Nutrition, 149-165
  for elderly, 508-509
Nutrition counseling during pregnancy,
        398
Nutritional needs nursing measures for,
        36-37
Nutritional problems, in older adult, risk
        factors for, 509
Nutritional requirements in pregnancy,
        399t
Nystagmus, 242

O

Obesity, 370
  Heimlich maneuver in, 538
OBRA; *see* Omnibus Budget
        Reconciliation Act of 1991
Observation of patients, 29
Obsessive compulsive disorder (OCD),
        368-369
Obstetrics, abbreviations in, 390
  historical development of, 390
  legislation affecting, 390
  operative, 413-414
  organizational resources for, 426
  terminology of, 390-391
  trends in, 391-392
Obstruction, 233
OCD; *see* Obsessive compulsive disorder
Oculists, 289
Odors, 44

Office of Human Development Services,
        19
Oil glands, 283
Oil-retention enemas, 39
Ointments, 87
Older adulthood; *see* Elderly
Older Americans Act, 499
Olecranon, 183
Olfactory sense of elderly, 508
Oliguria, 244
Omnibus Budget Reconciliation Act
        (OBRA) of 1991, 499
Omphalocele, 457
Ontario Association for Nursing
        Assistants, 17
Onychomycosis, 593
OOB; *see* Out of bed
Open pneumothorax, 544
Open wounds, 546
Operative obstetrics, 413-414
Ophthalmologists, 289
Ophthalmoscope, 289
Opiate abuse, 371
Opioid analgesics, 97, 98t
Opticians, 289
Optometrists, 289
Oral administration, 92, 93t
  in children, 96
Oral cholecystography, 228
Oral contraceptives, 425-426
Oral feedings, 122-123
Oral hygiene for elderly, 509
Oral hypoglycemic agents, 117-118
Oral temperature, measurement of, 31
Organic anxiety syndrome, 513
Organic brain syndrome, 371
Organic delusional syndrome, 513
Organic hallucinosis, 513
Organic mental syndromes, 513
  factors associated with, 514t
Organic mood syndrome, 513
Organic personality syndrome, 513
Organizations, alumni, 17
  nursing, 15-17
    Canadian, 18
Oropharynx, 195
Oroscopy, 292
Orthopnea, 31, 198
Oscillometry, 209
Osteitis deformans, 192
Osteoarthritis, 189
Osteogenic sarcoma, 191
Osteomalacia, 191-192
Osteomyelitis, 190-191
Osteoporosis, 191
Otitis media, acute, 454
Otosclerosis, 294
Out of bed (OOB), 40
Outcome criteria, 86
Ovarian cyst, 280
Ovarian tumors, 280
Ovaries, 249, 271-272, 271f

Over-the-counter drugs, interactions of, 579-580
Overeating, compulsive, 370
Overflow incontinence, 262
Ovum, 394
Oxazolidinediones, adverse reactions of, 102
Oxygen, administration of, 35
  masks for, 35
  need for, nursing measures for, 34-35
Oxytocic drugs, 116
Oxytocin, 114

P

Package inserts, 89
Paget's disease of bone, 192
Paget's disease of the breast, 282
Pain, 209, 229
  nursing measures for, 41-42
Painkillers, interactions of, 579, 586
Pancreas, 227
  cancer of, 238
Pancreas scans, 229
Pancreatitis, 238
Papanicolaou smear test, 274
Papilledema, 242
Papule, 284
Paraesophageal hernia, 231, 231f
Paralysis, 244-245
  Erb-Duchenne, 421
  facial, of newborn, 421
  Klumpke's, 421
Paranoid behavior in elderly, 516
Paranoid personality, 370
Paraplegia, 244
Parasympathetic blocking agents, 106
Parasympatholytic blocking agents, 106
Parathyroid glands, 249, 250f, 251t
  medications affecting, 11t
Paratrachoma, 604
Paratyphoid fever, 597
Pare, Ambroise, 390
Parent education classes, 398
Parenteral administration, 87, 92-93, 93t
Parenteral medications, 87
Paresthesia, 242
Parkinsonian syndrome, 514
Parkinson's disease, 248
Parotitis, infectious, 597
Paroxysmal, 198
Partial seizures, 245
Passive immunity, 23
Paste, 87
Pasteur, Louis, 390
Patent ductus arteriosus (PDA), 459
Pathogens, 21
Patient advocates, 14-15
  for elderly, 499
Patient care planning, 33-34
Patient discharge, nursing measures for, 50-51, 475
  early, impact on obstetrics, 391

Patient rights, 14-15
  for mentally ill, 374
Patient Self-Determination Act (PSDA), 499, 607
Patient teaching in pharmacology, 86, 92, 104
Patient transfer, to another service/floor/agency, 50-51
  from bed, 42
Patient's Bill of Rights, American Hospital Association, 14
Pavlik harness, 460f
PDA; see Patent ductus arteriosus
PDR; see Physicians' Desk Reference
Peck, development stages of, 501f
Pediatric; see Children
Pediatric nursing, 449-478
Pediculosis, 44, 469, 597
Pelvic examination, 274
Pelvic inflammatory disease (PID), 278-279
Pelvis, female, 383f, 393
Penetrating wounds, intraabdominal, 544-545
  of neck, 543
Penicillin substitutes, 119
Penicillins, 118-119
Pepsin, 225
Peptic ulcers, 232-233
Perception, 369
Percussion, 34
Percutaneous administration, 88
Perianal region, ringworm of, 593
Pericarditis, 214
Pericardium, 205
Perineal prostatectomy, 270
Periosteum, 183
Peripheral nervous system, 241
Peripheral vascular disorders, diagnosis of, 215
  nursing assessment of, 215
  nursing care of, 215-216
  vasodilator drugs for, 109
Peritoneal dialysis, 267, 267f
Peritonitis, 239
Pernicious anemia, 221
Personality, of elderly, 515
  elements of, 361
Personality development, 361
  stages of, comparison of, 362t-365t
Personality disorders, 370-371
Personality structures, 361
Pertussis, 602
Pertussoid eosinophilic pneumonia, 598
PET; see Positron emission tomography
Petechia, 284
Petit mal seizures, 245
Pharmacokinetics, 89-90
Pharmacology, 85-123
  evaluation in, 86-88
  nursing assessment in, 86
  nursing care plan implementation in, 86-88
  planning in, 86

Pharynx, 195, 225
Phendimetrazine tartrate, adverse reactions of, 105
Phenothiazines, 104
Phentermine hydrochloride, adverse reactions of, 105
Phenylpropanolamine hydrochloride, adverse reactions of, 105
Pheochromocytoma, 259
Phlebitis, 217-218
Phobias, 368
Phocomelia, 423
Phonotransducer, 409
PHS; see Public Health Service
Physical development, of adolescents, 471
  of children, 465, 467
  of infants, 450-452
  of toddlers, 462
Physical examination, 29
  positioning and draping for, 30f
Physical therapy, chest, 34-35
Physicians' Desk Reference (PDR), 89
Physiological needs, 26
Pia mater, 241
Piaget, developmental stages of, 362t-365t
PID; see Pelvic inflammatory disease
PIE; see Problem, Intervention, Evaluation
PIH; see Pregnancy-induced hypertension
Pineal glands, 249, 250f, 251t
Pinna, 291
Pinworms, 468
Pituitary glands, 249, 250f, 251t
Placebos, 42
Placenta, 394
Placenta previa, 402-403, 402f
Plantar flexion, 40
Plasma, 207
Plasters, 87
Platelet count, 220
Platelets, 207
Platypoid pelvis, 383f, 393
Pleurisy, 202
PN/NA; see Practical nursing/nursing assistant
Pneumococcal pneumonia, 597
Pneumocystis pneumonia, 598
Pneumonia, 201-202, 597-598
Pneumothorax, 202-203, 543-544
  open, 544
  simple, 543
  spontaneous, 544
  tension, 543-544
Point of service (POS), 20
Poisoning, 550-551
Poliomyelitis, 598
Polydactyly, 423
Polymyxins, 120
Polyps, colon, 234-235
  nasal, 201
Polyuria, 262
Pondimin, adverse reactions of, 105